TOXICOLOGY

MEMOIRS

TOXICOLOGY

by

WILLIAM D. McNALLY, A.B., M.D.

*Assistant Professor of Medicine, Lecturer in Toxicology,
Rush Medical College, University of Chicago; At-
tending Toxicologist, Presbyterian Hospital;
Attending Staff, St. Joseph's Hospital,
Chicago; Formerly Toxicologist
to the Coroner of Cook
County, Chicago,
Illinois*

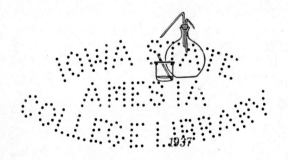

INDUSTRIAL MEDICINE

CHICAGO

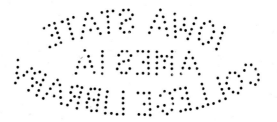

FOREWORD

SOCRATES, were he permitted to return to life today, might be amazed to learn that his "juice of the hemlock" was not "a poison" but a galaxy of poisons. With endless fecundity the many "hemlocks" of an ancient day have yielded a profusion of toxic entities serving and harming mankind in proportion to the propriety of their application. In some measure it may be maintained that the number of toxic agents surrounding a people constitutes an index of its cultural development. Inescapably intelligent man in his desire to make the best use of materials about him will uncover and produce limitless combinations of elemental substances, some of which will prove to possess dangerous properties. No guilt may be attached to that chemist who, because of a laudable curiosity to learn of what a lump of coal consists, first produced benzene. This plentiful substance, like a myriad of others, is at the same time one of man's helpful servants and one of his treacherous enemies.

While the number of "poisons" knowingly or fortuitously isolated by the technologists of a race may mark its milestones of racial advancement, the "poisonings" of human beings in proportion to their number serve as an index of a people's degradation. Whether by vicious design, accident, carelessness, unconcern, ignorance or superstition, poisonings among a people tangibly represent deficiencies in the plans for human living.

It may be conceived that, in a remote day, those human brains best equipped with information as to poisons were engaged in the preparation of better poisons—agents that acted with dispatch, leaving the fewest tell-tale marks and the least gore. Today, in a world still far removed from human perfection, toxicologists foremostly serve in just the opposite capacity. Theirs is the duty to detect the nature and mechanism of poisonings with such exactness that the guilty may be punished as a deterrent to others who might elect similar activities; to guide therapeutists as to the thresholds demarking safe and beneficent actions of man's natural and synthetic agents from those direful actions associated with use in larger amounts; to plan with industry and commerce for the controlled use of baneful substances and machines, lest the hu-

man elements of industry and commerce be damaged in the
performance of their obligations. Thus the toxicologist takes
a place alongside the lawmaker, the educator, the healer, the
minister, the engineer, as a unit in the orderly organization of
mankind—all participating in the conservation of the public
well being.

Since the mighty among the toxicologists may not with
their own voices and hands directly touch all the agencies requiring their services, they are obligated to record their experience, to appraise and compile the observations of others, and
to disseminate their learning to the end that knowledge may
not disappear from the earth; that remote man may enjoy the
benefits of learning gathered in centers of technical activity;
that succeeding generations of technologists may escape the
necessity of oft repeated elemental investigations and instead
may devote their capacities to needed new endeavors. In this
present book one widely experienced and highly skilled toxicologist meets, but does not necessarily finally discharge, his
obligations to those about him and to coming generations.

Medicine, in its slow growth toward complete control of
its problems, must always progress both as an art and a science. Toxicology is one of those branches of medicine which,
more than most others, holds the promise of becoming an almost exact science. In present day America, with its un-
precedented complexity of industrial and scientific pursuits,
numberless and intricate situations demand a full measure of
exactness in toxicologic guidance. In this country there are
outstanding   toxicologists,   many   meritorious   toxicologic
achievements, numerous praiseworthy isolated journal pub-
lications, but conversely all too few comprehensive toxicologic
books. The advent at this period of this book is no chance
happening. Inevitably its arrival hinges on the operation of
unvoiced, unseen and unmeasured scientific needs.

It is a refreshing characteristic of this new publication that
it treats the outmoded observations of bygone periods only on
their historical merits. This book is singularly liberated from
the ancient thralldom of the occult in toxicology, and its distinguished author, in breaking with the past save for historical
reference, may be marked as the man who replaced many of
toxicology's threadbare garments with a raiment suited to a
rapidly expanding science.

Time is the master appraiser of all books. Only on the basis of a claimed consortship with future time may any foreword writer seek to act as time's harbinger. Conceded this consortship, let it be said that time will be generous in its increasing recognition of the influence of this book on all the affairs to come to the world of toxicology.

The prime function of any foreword writer is not to praise any author or his writings nor to extoll the merits of any publisher or his printings. Instead, the great duty is to challenge the chance reader who stands hesitant between the title page and the author's introduction. To you who have reached this point, permit the foreword writer to serve you through saying "The world may be made richer if you plunge deeply into the contents of this good book."

CAREY P. McCORD, M.D.

Detroit, Michigan,
October 1, 1937.

PREFACE

THIS volume has been compiled so that the medical and legal professions may have a modern toxicological text that contains the results of recent research in the field of toxicology as well as the fundamental facts and basic principles.

The subject matter has been the basis of a course of lectures given students of the Rush Medical College of the University of Chicago, and is considered detailed in description. Sources for the compilation of the subject matter include standard textbooks, reference books, and original literature. Among the textbooks used in this work are: LEGAL MEDICINE AND TOXICOLOGY, Peterson, Haines, and Webster; NOXIOUS GASES, Henderson and Haggard; LEHRBUCK DER INTOXIKATIONEN, Dr. Rudolf Kobert; LEHRBUCK DER CHEMISCHEN TOXIKOLOGY UND ANLEITUNG ZUR AUSMITTELUNG DER GIFTE, J. Gadamer; the UNITED STATES PHARMACOPEIA, Eleventh Decennial Revision; DIE GEWERBLICHEN VERGIFTUNGEN UND IHRE BEKÄMFUNG, E. Brezina; CLINICAL TOXICOLOGY, Erich Leschke; and INDUSTRIAL TOXICOLOGY, Alice Hamilton. Credit is given to all authorities in instances where experiments are noted and definite results have been obtained.

The author has endeavored to produce a text that will be valuable both as a classroom adjunct and as a source for evidence in the courtroom, based upon the analysis of organs from many thousands of human bodies. Considerable space is devoted to carbon monoxide, lead, and arsenic, as these subjects are more frequently encountered in court and in industrial work.

WILLIAM D. MCNALLY, M.D.

Chicago, Illinois,
October 1, 1937.

CONTENTS

CONTENTS

CONTENTS vii

Corrosive Acids 59
Sulphuric Acid 60
Nitric Acid 66
Hydrochloric Acid 69
Oxalic Acid 74
Corrosive Alkalis 79
Ammonium Hydroxide 81

METALS AND NON-METALS

Phosphorus 84
Potassium Chlorate 88
Potassium Permanganate 89
Boric Acid and Borax 89
Fluorine 91
Iodine 108
Bromine 110
Chlorine 111
Tellurium 115
Thallium 116
Silver 124
Vanadium 125
Chromium 126
Cadmium 129
Nickel 132
Manganese 134
Barium 140
Lead 147
Chronic Lead Poisoning 154
Mercury 199
Corrosive Sublimate 202
Chronic Mercury Poisoning 211
Calomel 219
Arsenic 219
Arsenic Trioxide 227
Chronic Arsenical Poisoning 236
Organic Arsenicals 267
Carbarsone 269
Tryparsamide 269
Arsphenamin 270
Neo-Arsphenamin 275
Sodium Arsphenamin 277
Silver Arsphenamin 277
Sulpharsphenamin 278
Copper 280
Bismuth 284
Antimony 285
Antimony Chloride 286
Tartar Emetic 286
Tin 290

CONTENTS

VOLATILES, DISTILLATES AND SOLVENTS

DRUGS AND MISCELLANEOUS

ILLUSTRATIONS

TABLES

TOXICOLOGY

IN THE history of ancient medicine, records show that even before the development of systematic chemistry there was in the field of medicine a knowledge of the action of poisons and venoms upon the animal organism. Although the "medical profession" of the early ancients consisted much of superstitious beliefs and divinations, it was due to the very practice of divination that there developed a school of anatomical observation. This was the observation of the entrails of animals for the purpose of divination. The action of poison was, therefore, observed. Ancient literature, too, bears many allusions to the knowledge of poisons. Ovid, the poet, for example, between the years 43 B.C. and 17 A.D., wrote that the arrows of Hercules were charged with the venoms of the Lerneian serpent. It is from this method of poisoning that the word poison (Latin—**toxicum**-poisoning—originally Arrow-poisoning) is derived.

GENERAL CONSIDERATIONS

TOXICOLOGY (**toxic**-poison, and **ology**-science) is defined as the science treating of poisons, their origin, properties, physiological action, treatment of their noxious effects and their detection by chemical or other means. POISON is defined by Webster as **any agent** which, introduced into the animal organism, may produce a morbid noxious or deadly effect. Webster is wrong in defining poison as **any agent** which introduced into the animal organism may produce a morbid noxious or deadly effect, for fragments of glass, steel, or other hard or sharp substances may produce a morbid noxious or deadly effect due to mechanical action. Also nearly all medicines if administered in too large a dose may produce a morbid noxious or deadly effect. Foods which are in daily use may, under certain conditions of the body, produce a like effect. Not only these, but also many other agents, classified as producers of morbid noxious or deadly effects, known generally as poisons, may in certain forms and quantities and in certain conditions of the body act as therapeutic measures.

A definition which I have found to withstand the onslaught of the legal fraternity is the following: A poison is a substance which, when it has been introduced into or upon the body and is absorbed into the blood stream, and acting chemically, is capable of seriously affecting health or destroying life; and this is the usual effect upon the healthy body. According to the definition, it must be a substance which acts after the absorption into the blood. It would be difficult to include in this definition substances such as the corrosive acids and alkalis, whose chief effect is a local one. However, as a certain part of the corrosives does enter the circulation and produces harmful noxious effects, I shall include them in this text as poisons.

Not every substance which produces deleterious effects by an unusual action or by causing injury upon a diseased body can be classed as a poison. Some common articles of food occasionally cause distressing symptoms when taken by people who have an idiosyncrasy to them. Muskmelons and strawberries cannot be eaten by some people without causing an urticaria and other unpleasant effects. Allergens should not come within the definition of a poison, as the toxic results noted are not their usual effects. The particular amount, large or small, of a substance necessary to produce death, affords no basis for determining that certain substances are poisons as distinguished from others which are not poisons. Half an ounce of oxalic acid may prove as fatal as half a grain of strychnine. However, we usually look upon poisons as substances which in small amounts are capable of producing death.

Poisons Classified.—Poisons may be classified first, according to the effects produced upon the system, and secondly, as to the origin or nature of the substance.

From the physiological action a simple general division can be made into Corrosives, Irritants and Neurotics according to whether the chief effect is one of local corrosion, gastro-intestinal irritation, or action upon the nervous system.

Under Corrosives are included the strong acids and alkalis, whose chief action is a local destruction of tissues.

Under Irritants are included arsenic, antimony, mercury, phosphorus, bromine, iodine, a number of organic substances like cantharides, and croton oil, whose most conspicuous effects are usually a gastro-intestinal irritation shown chiefly by local pain, vomiting, and purging.

Under Neurotics are alcohol, strychnine, carbon monoxide, opium, and carbolic acid; the toxic action being exerted chiefly upon the nervous system, producing delirium, convulsions, and coma, with disordered circulation and respiration as the outstanding symptoms.

There is a great overlapping in this classification; a small dose of a corrosive might act as an irritant, and a large dose of an irritant may act as a corrosive; arsenic as an irritant poison might fail to show its characteristic gastro-intestinal symptoms and exhibit only the neurotic type.

From the standpoint of origin, the classification of Chapuis[1] is probably the most useful, and is the one I have used in my class work for many years. The division is as follows: (1) Inorganic poisons, (2) Gaseous poisons, (3) Alkaloidal poisons, (4) Non-Alkaloidal poisons, and (5) Food poisons.

From the analyst's view I use in the laboratory a classification based upon the method of isolation, namely: Volatile poisons, Metallic poisons, Alkaloidal and Non-Alkaloidal poisons. Either one of these classifications brings together poisons of a similar nature.

From a long experience in the Cook County (Illinois) Coroner's Office, I have classified deaths by poisons from the history of the case with reference to the circumstances surrounding their origin, for purposes of statistics into four groups: (1) Homicidal, (2) Suicidal, (3) Accidental, and (4) Undetermined.

Among the homicidal cases I include all cases which from the Coroner's records indicate a murder, even if the case was not brought before a grand jury. To the fourth class, "undetermined," belong all cases where the history and Coroner's record are hazy as to how the poison was obtained and why it was administered. Accidental poisonings are those that occur without intent to cause death. As in the case of children picking up a bottle of Hinkle laxative pills containing strychnine, eating fifteen to twenty of these tablets, and later dying of strychnine, the poisoning would be accidental. However, having such dangerous articles within the reach of a child shows ignorance, and even criminal negligence. Industrial poisonings due to the exposure of workmen to poisonous substances and gases are accidental, but nevertheless the managment is held liable under the Workmen's Compensation Act. Food poisonings are the result of eating articles of food which have been rendered toxic either by the unintentional or the fraudulent addition of mineral poisons, or by the generation of poisons in the body, elaborated by bacteria. Such cases are numerous in our large cities, where, for example, whole families may be

1. CHAPUIS: Precis de toxicologie, 3rd ed., 119, 1897.

attacked by eating a cream-filled cake that has stood in a warm place.

Accidental poisonings by a mistake of both pharmacist and physician are of too frequent occurrence. I have seen a case where a prescription calling for barium sulphate was filled with barium sulphide which when taken by the patient caused death. On the other hand a physician prescribed barium carbonate for barium sulphate with fatal results.

Poisonings may be classified as acute, subacute, or chronic. Acute cases follow the administration of large doses of poison which acts rapidly, with violent symptoms. Subacute are cases of short duration and extreme violence which may include some symptoms of chronic poisoning. Chronic poisonings usually result from a repeated and continuous absorption of small quantities of poison, are of a milder character than the acute, and may have certain added symptoms not seen in the acute type.

Absorption of Poisons.—Orfila was the first chemist to demonstrate the presence of arsenic in the blood and urine after the administration per mouth, first, in a series of experiments with animals in 1839,[2] and later in the human subject in the famous case of Scoufflard. Since that time chemists have shown the presence of a great number of poisons in the tissues of the body, and in the urine and stool, either in the original form in which it was administered or in its decomposed products. In embalmed bodies dead from hydrocyanic acid, the cyanide may be changed to an isonitrile for which we do not have a good method of detection.

The rate of absorption of poisons depends on several factors: first, diffusibility of the substance; second, its form, whether in solution or solid; third, conditions favoring or impeding solution or diffusion; fourth, the very same conditions that modify the action of drugs for systemic effects also modify the action of poisons.

Some poisons are more diffusible than others, depending upon variations in conditions influencing the solution, as it is necessary to have them in solution before we can have diffusion or absorption. Anything which intensifies the concentration of the poison in solution increases its rate of absorption, while any condition which retards the substance going into solution

2. *Mem. Acad. roy de med.*, 8:376, 1840.

retards absorption. For instance, phosphorus, if administered in butter or oils, is much more rapidly absorbed, while the opposite effect is noted with powdered white arsenic. Oils favor the solution of the phosphorus and retard the solution of the arsenic. Insoluble substances, such as barium sulphate, are non-poisonous, but if the barium is given in a soluble form, as barium chloride, it becomes a very active poison. All poisons are much more rapidly absorbed in solution. If given in solid form, time is necessary in order that the solid be acted upon by the hydrochloric acid of the stomach or by the fluid intake. The absorption of poisons is greatly impeded if taken upon a full stomach, but when taken upon an empty stomach the absorbent surfaces are large and the poisons become quickly absorbed, while by hypodermic injection the rapidity with which the poisons enter the absorbent surfaces is greatly increased.

The motives for poisoning are the same as for the commission of crime by other means. Four motives exist: first, financial gain, as in the collection of insurance of the victims; second, love and passion; third, hatred; and fourth, revenge. Usually the prosecution advances the motive, as the important element of proof as bearing upon the question of intent and premeditation.

The crime of secret poisoning is as old as the hills; it was known to the ancient Greeks, to the people of the far East, and even before them. A poison need not be tasteless; I have been consulted in many murder cases where strychnine was given per mouth. Sometimes the poison is given in divided doses, as with arsenic, or in one overwhelming dose, or, again, small doses may be used over a long period of time and then one large dose given to hasten the end, as in the Baker case. (See p. 229.) Many famous cases of poisoning have been planned by pharmacists and physicians who have selected this means because of easy access and familiarity with poisons.

Absorption by the Respiratory Tract.—An injection of cocaine into the nasal mucous membrane may cause death. The mouth, pharynx and epiglottis are easily reached by gargling, and the administration of a corrosive by this method could very likely do considerable damage in a short time. The absorption of vapors takes place rapidly when they are inhaled; the effect induced by inhalation does not depend upon the quantity given, but upon the concentration of the gas and the time during which the absorption takes place; the action is very rapid through the lungs because the rich capillary area of the alveoli is one of the best absorbent surfaces in the body. If fluids and dissolved substances are introduced through the trachea, absorption takes place quickly. If ferrocyanide in solution is injected into the trachea, it can be demonstrated in the carotid blood in two minutes. Absorption of fluid from the lungs surpasses our usual conception. Dogs and rabbits have received 30 to 200 cc. of fluid into the trachea without apparent damage.

Oral Administration.—This method of administration of poison is the most ancient, the most natural, and the most likely method to cause the least suspicion. Absorption of poisons by the mouth is of no great importance, as the poison rarely is retained in the buccal cavity long enough to permit of any extensive injury. Corrosives may remain long enough in the mouth to cause great pain, edema and even ulceration. Nicotine or hydrocyanic acid, when applied to the tongue may cause symptoms of poisoning in a few seconds to half a minute.

Alimentary Tract.—The absorbing power of the stomach is relatively low, the stomach acting more as an organ of preparation for the later absorption of foods by the small intestine. However, some substances are rapidly absorbed in the stomach. I have detected mercury in the blood of dogs two minutes after the administration of bichloride per mouth.[3] Drugs dissolved in alcohol are more quickly absorbed than in water solution.

Absorption rates in the stomach vary with different kinds of animals. Otto[4] found that strychnine is absorbed from the ligated stomach in cats and dogs, but not in rabbits or guinea pigs. Substances such as morphine, bichloride of mercury, and sodium fluoride are reabsorbed into the stomach.

The contents of the stomach pass into the small intestine, where more favorable conditions for absorption of poisons and medicines exist. The extensive surfaces, the folds and villi and the peristaltic movements with the long period of retention, make the small intestine the essential organ of absorption. The rectal administration of a solution of poison causes a rapid

3. Burmeister, W. H., and McNally, W. D.:   *J. Med. Research, Bost.,* 31:1, 1917. See also Mentin: *J. Med. Research, Bost.,* 43:315, 1922.

4. Otto: *Arch f. Verdauungskr.,* 8:427, 1902.

absorption. Instances of murder by this method are not frequent, but suicides and accidental deaths have occurred by this
method. A prisoner, desiring to conceal tobacco, inserted it in
the rectum, dying of nicotine poisoning.

The length of time in which a poison is absorbed from the
alimentary canal will depend upon the form in which the toxic
substance is taken, and to what extent the poison is rendered
inert by antidotes, and whether it is removed by vomiting or
by lavage.

The skin can absorb some poisons very rapidly. This is
very evident from the absorption of nitrobenzene from shoes
which have not had sufficient time to dry after the removal of
dye or blacking. Kalenberg has also shown that traces of boric
acid can be detected in the urine if the feet are immersed in a
saturated solution of boric acid for five minutes. I have killed
rabbits in eleven days by a daily application of 4 cc. of wood
alcohol to a shaved area on their backs. The skin is most important for use in the systemic therapy in mercurial inunction.
Absorption is greater where the epidermis is thin, as in the
axilla, loins, and inner surface of the arms and thighs. The
broken skin exposing the vascular subcutaneous tissue becomes
a more active absorbent surface.

The genito-urinary tract has been a frequent place of absorption of poisons. I have seen a number of cases of mercurial
poisoning from the use of bichloride of mercury solutions as
vaginal douches, and from the use of this drug in attempts at
committing abortion. Administration of arsenic by the vagina
has caused serious illness and death.

Diagnosis of Poisoning.—The diagnosis of poisoning before
death is many times easy, sometimes difficult, and, with the
present methods, occasionally impossible. When one considers
the large number of poisons available, how the same poison
varies in its action depending on the size of the dose, the form
in which it is given, and whether it is given on an empty or
full stomach, it is no wonder at all that a diagnosis is difficult.

Again, many of the same symptoms seen in poisoning can
also come from certain diseases. The one point, however, to
bear in mind is that the symptoms of poisoning come suddenly
upon a person who previously has been in good health, while
disease is usually preceded by a number of hours, days or even
weeks of local or general indisposition. The physician in a case

of poisoning must observe carefully all of the symptoms, take possession of any suspected medicine or food, and preserve the vomitus and urine for a chemical examination. The symptoms when related to the toxicologist may enable him to shorten the time of the analysis. The analysis should never be undertaken by one who has not had an extensive experience in this kind of work. This is a specialty that is out of the field of the practicing physician or the commercial chemist. The physician, in case of a judicial inquiry, is expected to have some knowledge of how poisons act and of the general treatment.

There are many diseases simulating poison; those causing greatest confusion with irritant poisons are acute indigestion, ulceration of the stomach or duodenum, gastro-enteritis, appendicitis, intestinal obstruction, and hepatic or renal colic. Symptoms of a neurotic poison may be caused by hysteria, inflammation of the brain and its coverings, cerebral hemorrhage and thrombosis, epilepsy, tetanus, and organic heart disease.

As an aid to the differential diagnosis, I have placed in Table I the common poisons and diseases causing the same symptoms.

With the aid of the foregoing table and a physical examination, the physician can usually arrive at a correct diagnosis. The odor of the breath should always be noted, as the odor of phenols, cyanides and alcohol will frequently aid the medical examiner in the detection, and in the treatment of the person. The odor of the vomitus and the color of the urine will be of further assistance. The luminosity of the stomach contents would indicate phosphorus; solid particles in the vomitus might be arsenic. It is well always to keep in mind that the symptoms usually appear after partaking of food, drink or medicine. If the symptoms appear in several people, after taking the same food or drink, the conclusion that a poison had been ingested is materially strengthened.

Diseases are generally much slower in their progress and are preceded by circumstances such as exposure, recognized symptoms, and general or local indisposition lasting for hours, days or weeks. In disease, remissions of the several symptoms frequently occur, while with poisoning (unless of the subacute, as with arsenic) such remissions do not occur.

When poisons are mixed with medicines and given to a person already suffering from a disease, the diagnosis is diffi-

TABLE I.*
Symptoms Caused by Poisons and Disease

Vomiting (frequently associated with purging and abdominal pain)
POISONS: Arsenic, antimony, aconite, corrosive acids and alkalis, barium, colchicum, cantharides, digitalis, copper, iodine, mercury, phosphorus, phenols, wood alcohol, veratrum, zinc, poisonous foods.
DISEASES: Gastritis, gastro-enteritis, gastric and duodenal ulcer, cholera, cholera morbus, cholera infantum, uremia, acidosis, onset of many acute infectious diseases, the early stages of pregnancy, brain tumor.

Convulsions
POISONS: Aspidium, brucine, camphor, cyanides, santonin, strychnine.
DISEASES: Uremia, puerperal eclampsia, tetanus, epilepsy, many acute cerebrospinal disturbances, especially meningitis.

Coma
POISONS: Opium and most of its derivatives, hydrated chloral, sulphonal, trional, veronal and other barbituric acid derivatives, paraldehyde, chloroform, cyanides, carbon monoxide, carbon dioxide, atropine, hyoscine, the various alcohols and phenols.
DISEASES: Uremia, puerperal eclampsia, acidosis, cerebral hemorrhage, cerebral thrombosis and embolism, brain injury, epilepsy and other brain diseases.

Dilatation of Pupil
POISONS: Belladonna, stramonium, hyoscyamus, scopola, and their derivatives, gelsemium, cocaine, nicotine.
DISEASES: Certain nervous diseases causing optic atrophy sympathetic irritation, or weakness of oculomotor nerve.

Contraction of Pupil
POISONS: Opium and its derivatives, physostigmine and its derivatives, pilocarpine, muscarine.
DISEASES: Certain nervous diseases, such as tabes.

General and Partial Paralysis
POISONS: Cyanides, carbon monoxide, carbon dioxide, botulism.
DISEASES: Apoplexy, brain tumor, meningitis.

Slow Respiration
POISONS: Opium and its derivatives, carbon monoxide.
DISEASES: Uremia, compression of brain as from hemorrhage.

Rapid Respiration
POISONS: Atropine group, cocaine, carbon dioxide.
DISEASES: Acute respiratory diseases, lesions of the medulla oblongata, hysteria.

Delirium
POISONS: Atropine group, cannabis indica, cocaine.
DISEASES: Epilepsy, insanity, delirium tremens, organic brain diseases, such as meningitis, visceral diseases, such as nephritis.

Dyspnea
POISONS: Strychnine (in the convulsions), cyanides, carbon monoxide.
DISEASES: Diseases of cardiac and respiratory system, lesions of medulla oblongata and of vagus nerves.

Cyanosis
POISONS: Nitrobenzene, anilin, acetanilid, opium.
DISEASES: Same as under dyspnea, prolonged convulsions from any cause producing cardiac dilatation.

* Peterson, Haines and Webster: Legal Medicine and Toxicology, 2:24, 1923.

cult. In the case of Mr. T., strychnine was put in the medicine, which happened to be alkaline, and the symptoms of poisoning did not appear until the last few teaspoonfuls were taken. The examination of the medicine showed sufficient strychnine to

---

TABLE II*
URINE CHANGES IN POISONING

1. Reaction very acid.	Mineral acids, acid, metallic salts.
2. Reaction strongly alkaline.	Corrosive alkali, sodium carbonate, salts of organic acids (except oxalic acid.)
3. Violet odor.	Turpentine and other ethereal oils.
4. Garlic odor.	Tellurium or bismuth preparations containing tellurium.
5. Odor of ammonia.	Catarrah of the bladder poisoning through strong bases.
6. Yellow to deep red.	Picrates, picric acid, serenium, pyridium, acriflavin.
7. Red in color after addition of sodium hydroxide (to be free of blood pigments.)	Phenolphthalein, senna leaves, cascara sagrada, hematoxylin, fuchsin, pyramidon, antipyrin.
8. Port wine color through hematoporphyrin.	Sulphonal, trional, chronic lead, tetronal.
9. Urine contains conjugated sulphates.	Phenol, creosol, lysol, resorcin, creosote, guaiacol, anilin, paramidophenol, acetanilid, phenacetin.
10. Urine contains leucin and tyrosin.	Phosphorus, acute yellow atrophy of liver, pellagra.
11. A small drop of urine in cat's eye causing dilatation of pupil.	Atropine, hyoscyamine, scopolamine, cocaine, tropocaine.
12. A small drop of urine causing tetanus in frog or small mouse.	Strychnine.
13. Garlic odor obtained by adding urine to culture of penicillium brevicaule.	All compounds of arsenic except triphenyarsines. Selenium, and tellurium compounds.

* (KOBERT: Kompendium der Toxikologie, 1912.)

---

have caused death if the administration of it had been continued. The only way to be certain of the diagnosis is to have a chemical examination made of the vomitus, medicine or food. For most of the poisons this would take considerable time, but in the case of heavy metals, such as mercury or arsenic, we have the quick and reliable Reinsch test.

Circumstantial Evidence.—The family physician can obtain considerable information to assist the authorities in the investigation of a criminal case of poisoning. He knows the environment, actions, and family history; and the words, looks, and behavior of the suspected person while he is in the home, may be of great assistance in solving the crime. The physician should make notes in every suspected case of poisoning to fortify his memory, if the case does come to trial.

In a case of poisoning, a third party seldom is a witness to the administration of a poison. However, in the case of Mrs. W., of Charleston, Illinois, an old woman was present when the husband administered poison to his wife. She heard the wife exclaim how bitter the medicine was and heard the husband tell her to wash it down with a dipper of water. This woman saved the spoon in which the medicine was given and, after Mrs. W. died of strychnine poisoning, gave it to the authorities. I found strychnine in the residue left on the spoon as well as in the organs of Mrs. W. The husband was given a life sentence.

The changes occurring in the urine will assist in the diagnosis (See Table II).

THE PROGNOSIS OF POISONING

THE prognosis depends upon the nature and the strength of the poison taken. The prognosis in general depends upon the size of the dose, its solubility and its concentration, whether it was taken upon an empty or a full stomach, the age of the patient, whether young or old, and, probably the most important, how soon medical attention was given and if the patient is in a coma from an acute intoxication.

GENERAL TREATMENT

SPECIFIC treatment will be taken up under each poison.

1. Wash out the stomach with plain water or one teaspoonful of baking soda to the pint unless an alkali has been taken. If a stomach pump is not handy give copper sulphate gr. V, or zinc sulphate gr. XV, or a hypo of 1/10 grain of apomorphine.

2. Removal of poisons by enema.

3. Immobilize the parts by tourniquet, as in bites of snakes or animals, to prevent absorption.

4. Schafer's method of resuscitation when respiration is failing, or, if in a hospital, give oxygen with 5% CO_2.

5. Intubation or tracheotomy where unable to swallow or breathe as in case of acids, alkalis, or bichloride of mercury.

6. Cold compresses to head and sponging of the body until temperature is normal.

7. Sweating tends to remove some poisons.

8. Passive massage of limbs to improve circulation.

9. Give gelatinous drinks in case of corrosive poisons.

10. Pieces of ice to hold in the mouth in alkali poisoning.

11. Catheterize urinary bladder, in case of morphine poisoning, to prevent reabsorption of the alkaloid and also for chemical examination.

12. For dilution of poison in the blood give hypodermoclysis, using Fischer's solution or normal saline.

In case the poison is known give the appropriate antidote in Table III, otherwise use a general antidote composed of magnesium oxide two parts, and one part each of activated charcoal, tannic acid, and Fuller's earth.

The mixture may be given in doses of a heaping teaspoonful stirred with water or milk, and can be repeated several times if necessary. The stomach should be washed out after each dose. The treatment of poisoning may be briefly summarized by stating that the first step should be the removal of the poison from the stomach. The contents and washings should be saved in a perfectly clean jar or bowl and inspected carefully to determine if any poison can be ascertained by its physical properties. The odor of cyanides, or the green or blue colored tablets of corrosive sublimate, are aids in prescribing the appropriate treatment. A portion of the vomitus or lavage should be saved, in case of judicial inquiry. Secondly, antidotes may act chemically or mechanically. Under the chemical antidotes we usually have another chemical either neutralizing the first poison or detoxifying it by rendering it insoluble. Thus in the case of a corrosive alkali we would neutralize the effect of the alkali by adding a weak acid, such as vinegar or lemon juice.

Caution should be used in the selection of an antidote, because if given in excess, it might cause as much harm as the substance to be neutralized. The weak acids mentioned would be preferable to using sulphuric acid. If a soluble barium salt had been taken we would render it insoluble by the adminis-

TABLE III
Poisons and Antidotes

(Consult the Section on the Specific Poison.)

Universal Antidote: When the poison is not known give a heaping teaspoonful of two parts of activated charcoal, one part of magnesium oxide, one part of Fuller's earth, and one part tannic acid in a glass of water. If the above mixture is not at hand wash out the stomach with a pint of water containing a teaspoonful of baking soda and induce vomiting. Give, by hypo 1/10 grain of apomorphine, or, by mouth, copper sulphate grs. V, or zinc sulphate grs. XV, in three ounces of water.

Acids, Mineral: Give an ounce of milk of magnesia or lime water. Repeat at frequent intervals. Give ice to relieve thirst and pain, and stimulants to combat collapse. Give demulcent drinks, such as linseed tea, starch water, and follow with a pint of milk containing whites of two eggs. An enema of strong coffee or three to five grains of caffein citrate is a valuable stimulant if administration by mouth is difficult.

Alcohol, Ethyl: Wash out the stomach with a pint of water containing a teaspoonful of baking soda. Keep the patient warm. Give hot, strong coffee, aromatic spirits of ammonia. Inhalation of 7% carbon dioxide with 93% oxygen. For collapse symptoms—digitalis, strychnine. If in coma, warm baths, followed by cold affusions.

Alcohol, Wood: Give an emetic, or wash stomach with a solution of sodium bicarbonate. As a purgative give magnesium sulphate or one to two drops of croton oil suspended in a little water. Give artificial respiration for pulmonary or cardiac failure. Stimulants per hypo and pilocarpine hydrochloride 1/10 to 1/6 grain to cause perspiration for elimination of poison. After treatment: One-half gm. of sodium bicarbonate every two to three hours; bowels must be kept open. Give strong coffee enemas, and inhalations of ammonia and fresh air.

Alkalis, Caustic: Patient should be given immediately copious draughts of water, alone, or acidulated with vinegar or lemon juice. Melted butter, olive oil, salad oil or fat should be given to change alkali to soap. In case of shock give atropine, strychnine or digitalin, by hypo. Control pain by opiates.

Aniline and Derivatives (Acetanilid): Give artificial respiration, pulmotor and administration of oxygen to overcome cyanosis. Use an emetic or stomach tube to empty stomach. Give strychnine, atropine, or digitalin by hypo, as stimulant.

Arsenic: Give emetics of mustard or zinc sulphate if vomiting is not present. Follow with intravenous injection of 1 gm. of sodium thiosulphate, repeat in four hours, and give one injection a day for several days. Give demulcents. Give one ounce of castor oil to clean out intestines. Give morphine to relieve pain and strychnine or digitalis if necessary.

Atropine: Give gastric lavage with tannic acid solution, strong coffee, or activated charcoal. Give injections of pilocarpine or physostigmine.

Barbital Group: Wash out the stomach. Give 1/30 grain of strychnine, repeat if necessary. Give strong coffee. Injections of coramine and cardiazole have the same effect. Artificial respiration with oxygen may be necessary.

Barium: Give one tablespoonful of epsom salts or other soluble sulphate in water. Wash out stomach. Give demulcents. Give aromatic spirits of ammonia and injections of strychnine.

Benzene: If inhaled, remove rapidly from exposure and give artificial respiration; blood transfusion; pentnucleotide. If by mouth—give bicarbonate of soda, stomach lavage, emetics, belladonna. Later, injections of liver extract.

Boric Acid: Give calcium chloride, 2 gm. to an ounce or wash out stomach with lime water. Give intravenous injection of calcium gluconate.

Bromine: Wash out the stomach with a pint of water containing a teaspoonful of sodium bicarbonate. Give demulcents. Apomorphine 1/10 grain by hypo; morphine by hypo for pain.

Carbolic Acid (Lysol, cresols): Wash out stomach with lime water. Epsom salts may be given to delay absorption. Apomorphine by hypo as emetic. Give demulcents. Morphine by hypo for pain. Stimulants.

Carbon Monoxide: Give inhalations of 7% carbon dioxide and 93% oxygen. Give artificial respiration in absence of apparatus for carbon dioxide inhalation.

Carbon Tetrachloride: Give calcium gluconate intravenously; glucose by mouth; digitalin and strychnine by hypo.

Chloroform and Chloral Hydrate (Knockout drops): Wash out stomach with warm water or milk; keep body flat and warm; treat persistent vomiting by hypodermoclysis of physiological salt and 5% glucose. Give respiratory stimulants, strychnine, caffeine, atropine; cardiac tonic —digitalis.

Cocaine: If by mouth, give gastric lavage with water containing activated charcoal. Artificial respiration; amyl nitrate, brandy. To relieve convulsions—barbituric hypnotics.

Corrosive Gases (Chlorine, bromine, ammonia fumes): Fresh air. Inhalation of dilute ammonia for chlorine and bromine. Inhalation of acetic acid vapor for ammonia fumes, then inhale alcohol or ether vapor for soothing. Salyrgan or atropine sulphate by hypo, to counteract edema of lungs; inhalations of oxygen; alkaline salt injection to counteract cyanosis.

Cyanides: Intravenous injections of methylene blue; 3% solution of hydrogen peroxide in large quantities or equal volume of freshly prepared 5% ferrous sulphate and sodium carbonate followed by immediate evacuation of stomach. Artificial respiration and pulmotor.

Digitalis: Give tannic acid, wash out stomach or give emetics. Give cautiously tincture of aconite.

Ergot: Wash out stomach, give purgatives (calomel or castor oil). In collapse, give warm baths with cold affusions, hot strong coffee or tea. Strychnine may be administered. Inject sodium tetrathionate.

Fluorides: Give soluble calcium salts by mouth and intravenously to render fluorides inert. Ten grains of calcium gluconate should be given intravenously.

Iodine: Wash out the stomach with water containing 2 gm. of sodium thiosulphate. Give patient thin starch water paste. Give demulcents. Give morphine to quiet pain.

Lead: Wash out stomach with a pint of water containing a teaspoonful of sodium magnesium sulphate. Give an intravenous injection of calcium gluconate. Eggs and milk may be given. Afterward, control pain by morphine.

Mercury: Give white of egg in a pint of milk. Wash out stomach with water containing 2 gm. of activated charcoal. Repeat until washings show no mercury by the Reinsch test. Give morphine to control pain. Give fifteen grains of sodium thiosulphate, intravenously.

Morphine: Give copious stomach lavage with 0.5% permanganate solution, also activated charcoal. One half teaspoonful to each pint of water used. Give strong black coffee. Artificial respiration with pure oxygen may be necessary. Give atropine sulphate, 1/20 grain hypo, and stimulants as strychnine and caffeine. Give high bowel enemas.

Mushrooms (Poisonous): Give emetics; glucose to protect the liver; atropine by hypo; cardiac and respiratory stimulants.

Nitrobenzene: Give emetic; large amounts of water and stomach tube; artificial respiration, pulmotor, with administration of oxygen. Give stimulants.

Nitric Oxides: Inhalation of oxygen; ampoule of salyrgan daily; 100 cc. of 50% glucose intravenously if lungs are edematous.

Oxalic Acids and Oxalates: Give milk of lime or lime water; emetics; demulcents; morphine. Give an intravenous injection of calcium gluconate or lactate.

Phosphorus: Wash out the stomach with a 1% solution of permanganate. As emetic, use one to five grains of copper sulphate in eight ounces of water, adding a teaspoonful of activated charcoal which aids in adsorption.

Phosgene: Same treatment as under nitric oxides.

Pyridine: Emetics. Two gm. of tannic acid in 50 cc. of water; artificial respiration and pulmotor. Stimulants by hypo.

Silver Salts and Organic Compounds: Wash out the stomach with a pint of water containing two teaspoonfuls of salt.

Snake Bites: Apply tourniquet above bite. Give anti-venom; injections of permanganate solution (1:3000) into the tissues around bite.

Strychnine (Nux-vomica): Wash out stomach immediately with water containing activated charcoal, tannic acid or tea. Give 1/10 to 1/5 grain doses of apomorphine, or give intravenously 1/10 grain of pentobarbital per pound of body weight. Keep patient very quiet. Give ether or chloroform to quiet patient; between spasms chloral hydrate can be given. Artificial respiration may be necessary.

Tear Gas: For the eyes apply a solution of 0.4 gm. sodium sulphite in 25 cc. of water and 75 cc. of glycerine. Wash off skin with 4% solution of sodium sulphite.

Thallium: No certain antidote. Give 2 gm. doses of sodium iodide and calcium lactate by mouth.

Trichlorethylene: Remove from exposure. Give inhalations of oxygen. If decomposition products are phosgene give injections of salyrgan and glucose.

Zinc Chloride: Wash out the stomach with water containing sodium bicarbonate, one teaspoonful to the pint. Give intravenous injection of 100 cc. of 50% glucose. Give opiates to stop pain and diarrhea.

tration of a soluble sulphate, as magnesium sulphate, to precipitate the harmless barium sulphate.

Under mechanical antidotes are those substances that reduce the absorption of the poison by enveloping it with a coating of oil or fat or the white of eggs. The stomach walls covered by the administration of any of these substances also prevent the absorption of the poison until it is removed. The effects of the poison can be altered by the use of "physiological antidotes," as in the treatment of strychnine poisoning by the use of chloral hydrate or chloroform.

The elimination of the poison can be aided by the use of diuretics, cathartics, enemas, and hot packs. Many poisons are eliminated through the kidneys, and large drafts of water should be administered after the removal of the poison from the stomach, and potassium acetate, caffein, digitalis, theobromine or other diuretics may be administered unless contraindicated. Hot packs over the abdomen and over the region of the kidneys will increase their activity when they are congested by the poison. If the patient is unable to void naturally, the bladder should be emptied by a catheter. As most cathartics are too slow in action, the bowel should be emptied by means of soapsuds enemas or plain water. In certain poisons it will be found of value to increase the activity of the skin by the use of a hypodermic injection of pilocarpine.

Diluting the poison in the blood and favoring the action of the organs, elimination can be accomplished by the hypodermic injection into the breast of normal salt solution (hypodermoclysis). Where it is not possible to set up an apparatus for hypodermoclysis, a saline solution can be administered as a retention enema in the lower bowel (enteroclysis).

Where there is considerable pain anodynes can be administered. In cardiac trouble, give strychnine, digitalis, camphorated oil, or caffeine with sodium benzoate. Chloral or chloroform can be given in controlling convulsions if the convulsions are not due to methyl chloride or other poisons of this series. Patients should be given the best nursing service possible, and visitors should be kept out of the room until all danger is past. Electric pads and hot water bottles may be applied to the body or the extremities in case of coldness or chills.

Detection of Poisons.—It is amusing to read how the experts prior to the eighteenth century determined whether or not a person had been poisoned. If a healthy person became ill suddenly, poison had been taken. If the body became livid, and the hair and nails fell out easily and the latter became dark after death, their suspicion became certain. The bodies of poisoned persons did not putrefy easily. Persistent vomiting was another indication to the expert at that time that poisons had been taken. The vomitus was fed to hens; if poisons were present the hens died. This last test was a very good one, but all poisons do not kill hens; for instance, strychnine in doses that would kill a human being can be given to hens without effect.

A study of Table I (page 9) will show that symptoms of acute poisoning can occur in instances of sudden death from ulceration and perforation of the stomach and bowels, from rupture of the heart, gall-bladder and Fallopian tubes, from unsuspected diabetes, Bright's disease, and other causes.

The development of methods in medicolegal recognition of poisoning, to the point which they have reached at the present time, and which we believe far short of what they will be in the future, has followed the advances made in those sciences upon which they mainly depend, chemistry and pathology.

The advances made in spectrum and violet-ray analysis may shorten some of the cumbersome methods now in use. The great value of a postmortem examination in a case of suspected poisoning lies in the determination of whether appearances such as are usually produced by poisoning are present both grossly and microscopically, and in the disclosure of the presence or absence of natural causes of death. For example, a gross appearance of the stomach may be that of corrosion, walls may be black and tarry in color, without any disclosure to the pathologist that this was due to mercury, or if the amount of mercury taken was small there may not be any change at all.

One of the greatest aids a toxicologist can have is the able assistance of a competent pathologist who can report upon the gross and microscopical examination of the heart, kidneys, liver, brain, and, if possible, the spinal cord. A bacteriological and microscopical examination of the blood and bowels may also give valuable information. However, with a good clinical history and with the discovery of a considerable quantity of poison in the organs, these extended examinations are rarely necessary.

Chemical Examination.—The expert to whom the organs are sent for analysis must be a chemist of experience. He should be a graduate of medicine and familiar with the methods used in pharmacological investigation. The analysis should be conducted by persons who have a reputation for honesty and who have made a special study of the subject of toxicology.

In a case of suspected poisoning the pathologist or physician making the autopsy should submit the stomach and content, part of the liver, both kidneys, and at least 500 gm. of bowel. Too often only the stomach is submitted for a chemical analysis because the popular opinion seems to be that the poison will always be found in the stomach. Although the stomach and its content are extremely important, a person may die from the effects of a poison and none be detected in the stomach, it having entirely disappeared by vomiting and absorption.

I have found cases of death by poison where none of the poison was found by analysis of the usual parts of the body submitted for a chemical examination. Aside from a scientific phase of demonstrating the distribution of various poisons in the body, the brain, spinal cord, heart, lungs, blood, and urine are of great value to the toxicologist.

It should be understood that the poison in the stomach usually is not the toxic material that has caused death. The poison has not entered the circulation, and any damage that may have been done is purely local; in other words, the poison, in the liver, kidneys, etc., is the portion that has caused the death of the person. In murder cases where a number of people have died under suspicious circumstances over a period of years the analyst should request that portions of the skeleton be submitted for chemical examination. During life in a suspected case of arsenic poisoning the hair and nails will give valuable information and assist in the treatment of cases of polyneuritis.

The chemist should report the amount of poison found per 100 gm. of tissue examined, so that persons working in this special field will be able to compare the amounts of that poison taken under similar conditions. The report should also give the amount of poison found in the total organ calculated from the aliquot part. The amount in the metric system may be transposed to the apothecary's system for the benefit of the Coroner, the State's Attorney, and the jury, as they are more familiar with the latter system.

The examination of the organs should be conducted in a room in which no other work is being done at the time. To demonstrate the importance of this, I wish to cite an instance in which a serious mistake would have been made if the work had not been checked by another chemist. A chemist, assigned to test for volatile poisons only, handled the copper foil used in testing for heavy metals. An examination of the subliming tube (see Reinsch test, page 26) revealed the presence of mercury in a case where quantitative examinations were under way for another poison. Investigation of the steps in the process indicated that the chemist testing for volatile poisons had been using the Millon's reagent. The washings of his hands showed clearly the presence of mercury. In large laboratories, doing routine toxicological work, one chemist should be assigned to the preparation of the samples, such as weighing of the organs submitted, the grinding and starting of the extraction of the alkaloids, the volatile distillate, and the tests for a metallic poison. A second chemist, in a separate room, should test for volatile and alkaloidal poisons, so there will not be any opportunity of contamination of the samples being tested.

The apparatus used need not be new for every analysis, but must be scrupulously clean; glassware and porcelain should be cleansed with chromic acid, then washed thoroughly with an abundance of warm water.

It is of the utmost importance to obtain a clinical history, as the symptoms and the postmortem appearances are valuable guides in suggesting what shall be sought for in the chemical examinations. This is all the more important in cases in which there is insufficient material or the authorities wish to keep down the expense, so that tests may be made for a specific poison or for a group of poisons suspected.

The toxicologist desires plenty of material, and if communicated with, before the autopsy is made, he can specify the amount needed. Then, without a clinical history, he can proceed with the analysis for the common poisons.

ROUTINE METHODS OF EXAMINATION

A NOTEBOOK should be maintained for a complete record and description of all material received for examination.

A method which I followed for many years while serving as Coroner's chemist and toxicologist was to receive personally all material and give it a number. Under this number were recorded the name of the deceased, address if known, suspected cause of death, the name of the Coroner's physician submitting the material, and, if the material was submitted by a police officer, his number, name, the station from which he worked, and the name of his commanding officer. In the case of clothing, guns, knives, and other weapons, each article was marked with my name, number, and date, and kept in a sealed locker in a room to which no other person had access. The jars of organs, after being properly marked, were turned over to one chemist who weighed and inspected each organ, removing a small section to be used later, if necessary for a microscopical examination. The contents of the stomach, vomited matter, and blood were always weighed.

The stomach walls and stomach contents should be examined with the unaided eye and with a small hand magnifying glass for the presence of undissolved poison, as arsenic trioxide, seeds, parts of tablets, and the character of the food. The reaction toward litmus paper and the odor should be noted. A fragment of the stomach content should be placed on a slide and examined under a microscope of medium power. In this way, if the digestion is not too far advanced, it will be possible to identify muscle fibers, starch granules and vegetable tissue. This examination frequently aids the prosecutor in determining whether or not a witness is telling the truth about the time the deceased had his last meal.

The second step after weighing is to bring the tissue to a finely comminuted state by means of a pair of scissors or a hashing machine. The material is thoroughly mixed, one portion, usually 100 gm., is used for the volatile distillate, another 100 gm. for alkaloidal poisons, and the remainder set aside until a further examination indicates the next step to be employed for the detection or quantitative examination for poisons. When the amount of material submitted amounts to only 100 gm. or less, one portion may be used for the volatile and mineral poison test and the second portion for organic poison, no portion being retained for reserve or check analysis. If the history points to the administration of an organic substance it may be necessary to use 200 gm. of each tissue submitted. On the other hand, if the Reinsch test shows the presence of arsenic or mercury in considerable quantities, a small sample of 25 gm. of each organ may be sufficient for analysis.

Whenever possible, it is advisable to retain a reserved portion, as unexpected tests or accidents may happen requiring additional tissue for examination. Where there is a shortage of material, the residue from the volatile distillate may be used for the detection of mineral poison, controlled tests being made upon the tartaric acid, phosphoric acid, or magnesium oxide used in the separation of the volatile poisons.

VOLATILE POISONS

THE tissue to be examined is prepared as above and placed in a 700-cc. Kjeldahl flask, 100 cc. of distilled water are added, the solution is acidulated with tartaric acid, and the flask is connected with a Liebig condenser and a copper steam

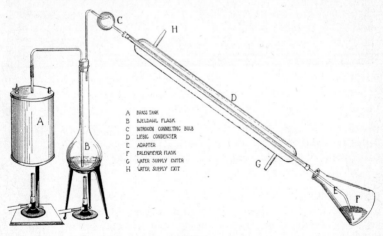

A   BRASS TANK
B   KJELDAHL FLASK
C   NITROGEN CONNECTING BULB
D   LIEBIG CONDENSER
E   ADAPTER
F   ERLENMEYER FLASK
G   WATER SUPPLY ENTER
H   WATER SUPPLY EXIT

FIG. 1.
Steam Distillation Apparatus for
Volatile Poisons (McNally)

generator as seen in Fig. 1. In the absence of a copper boiler a Kjeldahl or other flask may be used for the generation of steam. An adapter should be attached to the Liebig condenser, the end dipping into about 5 cc. of distilled water. One cc. of distillate should be distilled for each gram of material used. If phosphorus is suspected the distillation may be conducted in the apparatus shown in Fig. 3. This apparatus consists of an upright Liebig condenser which has been painted with an asphaltum paint, leaving an upright band three-eighths of an inch wide free of paint. This Liebig condenser is placed inside an asbestos box, dimensions 20 in. x 6 in. x 6 in., which

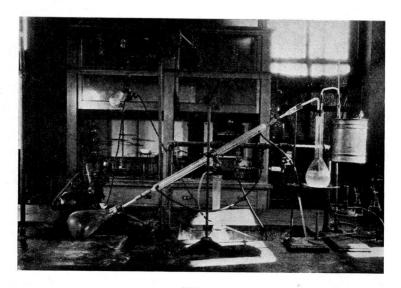

FIG. 2.
Operation of Apparatus Diagrammed
in Fig. 1

has one side covered by a split piece of asbestos board. The chemist places over his head and the box a dark cloth, similar to that used by photographers, which enables him to see the phosphorescence of phosphorus. After 100 cc. of distillate have been collected (except in the case of cyanide, where it may be necessary to distill several hundred cc.) the contents of the distilling flask are rendered alkaline by calcined magnesium oxide, and 100 cc. collected as before, (except where nicotine is present, when the distillation will have to be continued until the distillate fails to show the presence of nicotine).

In the beginning of the process a small flame should be placed under the flask holding the organs, otherwise considerable steam will condense. To prevent bumping, small pieces of glass tubing are placed in the flask before distillation begins. The distillation of urine or blood will be accompanied by considerable frothing, and small amounts should be used if the frothing is not stopped by the addition of a piece of paraffine wax.

The distillate obtained from the first part of the process may contain grain alcohol, methyl alcohol, phosphorus, formaldehyde, acetone, amyl nitrite, iodoform, hydrogen sulphide, ethers, chloroform, chloral hydrocarbons, camphors, essential oils, phenols, salicylic acid, benzoic acid, nitrobenzene, hydrocyanic acid, iodine, bromine, hydrochloric and other volatile acids; in the second part of the process, or in the alkaline distillate, may be found ammonia, amines, anilin, conine, nicotine, chloroform (from chloral hydrate), and other volatile bases.

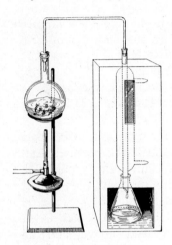

FIG. 3.
Apparatus for Phosphorus
Distillation (McNally)

Some of the volatile substances mentioned, such as benzoic acid, camphor, salicylic acid, anilin, and nicotine, may appear in the various extractions in the examinations for alkaloids and other organic poisons.

The residue, after the alkaline volatile distillate, should be saved and used for the detection of inorganic or mineral poisons if there has not been enough material submitted to examine directly for mineral poisons.

EXAMINATION FOR MINERAL POISONS

WITH the advancement of the methods for the chemical identification of poisons there have been devised a number of methods for the separation of mineral poisons. The poisons found in this group are the compounds of arsenic, antimony, barium, bismuth, chromium, copper, lead, mercury, silver, tin, zinc, thallium, tellurium, and cadmium. The finely ground and well mixed sample must be weighed for each analysis, as a quantitative examination should be a part of every toxicological examination.

In order to test for mineral poisons the organic matter of the food or tissues must be destroyed. The most rapid method is that of burning or ashing, but as some poisons like arsenic, lead, mercury, and zinc suffer a loss by volatization, it is not the method of choice. It may be used when looking for non-volatile metals, as barium. The material should be dried and heated in a porcelain crucible until a gray ash is obtained; after cooling it is extracted with dilute hydrochloric or nitric acid. The ashing can be hastened by the addition of nitric acid or ammonium nitrate. The undissolved ash is saved for future examination for insoluble compounds, such as barium sulphate and lead sulphate. This method is simple, and is the method of choice for testing urine for the presence of lead as in the Fairhall method.

When an extended examination for metals is to be made, the method of Fresenius and von Babo is the method that I have found best, and the method of Gautier[5] as modified by Chittenden and Donaldson for the non-volatile mineral poisons.[6]

Method of Fresenius and von Babo. — Take 100 to 150 gm. of the ground organs as prepared above and add sufficient water to make the mass fluid; add 25 cc. of hydrochloric acid and 2 gm. of sodium chlorate; the mixture is heated over a low flame with frequent additions of sodium chlorate being made from time to time until the content of the flask is yellow and fluid. If the fluid remains clear, except for fatty matter that comes to the top or is in suspension, after one-half hour of heating without the addition of chlorate, the process can be said to be completed. This usually takes from six to eighteen hours. If during the heating and with the addition of chlorate there is little or no evolution of chlorine, 10 cc. of hydrochloric acid may be added to each 100 gm. of tissue being digested.

The procedure is best conducted in a liter Kjeldahl flask, with a funnel placed in the neck of the flask, to prevent evaporation and also to add the sodium chlorate, which can be added from a saturated solution, drop by drop. Allow

5. *Ann. de chim. et phys., Par.,* 5th series, 8:384, 1876.
6. *Am Chem. J., Balt.,* 2:235, 1880, 1881.

the digestion to cool and filter off the fat, washing the filter paper several times with boiling hot water. The residue on the filter paper should be saved, as it may contain barium sulphate, lead sulphate, and particles of glass. The acid solution is partially neutralized by the addition of sodium carbonate which aids in the expelling of the excess of chlorine. The remainder of the chlorine is then removed by a rapid current of carbon dioxide through the warm solution. The filtrate now contains in solution any of the mineral poisons which may have been present in the original tissue with the exception of silver and lead, a portion of which may remain in the undissolved residue. If mercury is present in metallic form it is only very slowly dissolved by this method, and may remain as a metallic deposit if the digestion of the tissue has been completed rapidly.

Some authorities recommend the addition of sodium sulphite to reduce any arsenic present in the liquid to arsenous acid, in which state it is much more easily precipitated by hydrogen sulphide; however, I never use a sulphite for this purpose as arsenic is estimated much more accurately by other methods, and if it had been indicated by the preliminary Reinsch test the method of Fresenius and von Babo (F. and B. method) would not be indicated. Into the slightly acid liquid a washed stream of pure hydrogen sulphide is passed slowly through the liquid for one hour. The flask is well stoppered and set aside in a warm place for eighteen hours. The liquid is agitated several times during this period and then filtered, and the precipitate well washed with water containing a little hydrogen sulphide in solution. The precipitate upon the paper contains, in the form of sulphides, any arsenic, antimony, cadmium, bismuth, copper, gold, mercury, platinum, lead, and tin that may be present. In the filtrate are all of the other metals excepting silver and probably a part of the barium which may have been precipitated as the sulphate and left in the residue after the destruction of the organic matter by sodium chlorate. The precipitated sulphides and the filtrate may be examined by recognized methods of qualitative or quantitative analysis.

A chemist should assure himself that the reagents which he uses do not contain impurities in a quantity sufficient to interfere with his quantitative analysis or in any way to reflect upon the report that he submits to a jury. And every chemical he employs should be tested for its purity by control experiments, and should be kept under seal by the analyst for future use. Thus the hydrogen sulphide used to precipitate the above-mentioned metals should be prepared in a generator by the use of arsenic-free ferrous-sulphide and arsenic-free sulphuric acid. Certain manufacturers make a specialty of manufacturing zinc and sulphuric acid arsenic-free, but even with such reagents it is always advisable to have a blank control in which negative results should be controlled under similar conditions as actually carried out in the search for the specific poison.

There are several objections to this method. First, it does not readily detect the presence of arsenic in certain organic compounds which are used in medicine. Second, the destruction of organic matter is not complete, a portion of the mineral matter being retained by the fat upon the filter paper. Third, a small amount of mercury and also arsenic is lost by volatilization. Fourth, the large quantity of chlorate and hydrochloric acid used in the digestion may contain traces of arsenic. Fifth, if the volume of the resulting digestion is too large after neutralization, traces of metal may not be precipitated by hydrogen sulphide.

Process of Ogier.[7]—To overcome the objection that the arsenic may be volatilized as arsenic trichloride, Ogier modified the above method by passing a stream of hydrochloric acid gas (liberated from the aqueous acid by allowing sulphuric acid slowly to drop into it) into the organic material containing one part of chlorate to ten parts of the solids to be destroyed. As more accurate methods are available for the estimation of arsenic this modification is little used.

Many other methods have been suggested for the destruction of organic matters, such as the method of Grigorijew[8] in which sulphuric acid is added to the dried pulverized tissue and heated. After cooling, 10 cc. of fuming nitric acid are added and the digestion continued with the occasional addition of nitric acid until the digestion does not froth. The mixture is then transferred to a Kjeldahl flask and heat applied slowly until the mass begins to boil, adding 5 cc. of sulphuric acid

7. Le Lab de Toxicol., 44, 1891.
8. *Vrtljschr. f. gerichtl. Med., Berl.,* 29:74, 1905.

until brown fumes are no longer given off and the mass has become light yellow. The cool liquid is diluted with five volumes of water, heated upon the hot plate until the nitric vapors are expelled, then treated as above under the F. and B. method. The method of Pouchet[9] decomposes material with 20% of its weight of monopotassium sulphate, and its own weight of fuming nitric acid is added. The carbonized mass is extracted with water and hydrochloric acid. The method of Meillers[10] uses a mixture of sulphuric and nitric acids in place of nitric acid alone as in the method of Pouchet. The method of Gautier[11] is a combination and perfection of the method of Orfila, 1839, and a modification as later suggested by Filhol, 1848. This method has been modified by other authors, as Chittenden and Donaldson,[12] and by Chapuis.[13] McNally's modification of the Gautier process as used in the Cook County (Illinois) Coroner's laboratory is as follows: Twenty-five to 100 gm. of the ground material to be examined are placed in a large casserole and 25 gm. of nitric acid are added and allowed to stand for one hour. The casserole is then heated gently, and if the material begins to foam it is removed from the source of heat. This heating is continued until the mixture liquefies and assumes an orange to a dark yellow color. One cc. of arsenic free sulphuric acid is added and gentle heat applied. Continue to add 1 cc. of sulphuric acid until about 8 cc. have been added. The mixture now becomes thick and dark brown in color. It is now heated over a small flame with stirring until carbonization begins, and then removed from the source of heat and allowed to cool. About 15 cc. of nitric acid are poured around the edges of the black mass around the casserole, when it is again heated until white vapors of sulphur dioxide begin to come off. If any yellow appears on the edge of the casserole add 2 or 3 cc. of sulphuric acid. The stirring and heating are continued until the mass begins to pulverize. It is allowed to cool, and pulverization is completed by means of a glass pestle; 50 to 100 cc. of water are added, and the mixture is boiled for several minutes and filtered while hot. The water extraction

9. LEGRAND DU SAULLE BERRYER, and POUCHET: *"Med. Leg.,"* *Compt. rend. Acad. d. sc.,* Par. 1424, 1881.
10. *J. de pharm. et chim.,* Par., 15:97, 1902.
11. *Ann. de chim. et phys.,* Par., fifth series, 8:384, 1876.
12. *Am. Chem. J., Balt.,* 2:235, 1880, 1881.
13. CHAPUIS: Precis de toxicologie, 150, 1897.

of the carbonaceous material is repeated three times, the filtrate being made up to a definite volume. In the case of 25 gm. it is usually made up of 100 cc.

The Reinsch Test[14] is an exceedingly useful and simple method for the detection of arsenic, mercury and antimony. For clinical use the rapidity with which this test can be conducted makes it of great value to the physician. Although it is a qualitative test, using the tube with a capillary constriction as devised by the author, the relative quantity of the arsenic or mercury present can be readily determined by weighing the constricted portion with and without the deposited metal. The Reinsch test, however, is not quantitative. According to Cownley the following reaction takes place:

$$6 \; Cu_5As_2 = 5 \; Cu_6 \; As + 7As$$

from which can be seen that only seven-twelfths of the arsenic is deposited in elementary form whereas the remainder is combined with the copper.

The material prepared as above is put in a porcelain dish or casserole, mixed with a quarter of its bulk of arsenic-free hydrochloric acid, adding an equal quantity of water to bring it to a thin consistency to which a piece of pure copper foil three-quarters of an inch long and one-eighth of an inch wide is added. The mixture is boiled for five minutes, or until the substance under examination is thoroughly disintegrated. The copper foil should be polished by rubbing with fine emery paper and a control test made with the copper foil and the hydrochloric acid used. This strip of thin copper foil is removed from the casserole by decanting the mixture which has just been boiled. The foil is gently washed with water, alcohol and ether; it should not be allowed to come in contact with the hands, being handled all the while with a pair of tweezers previously heated in a flame.

The copper foil is placed in the long end of the McNally tube and over the constricted area is placed a strip of filter paper, about one inch wide, which has been dipped in cold water. This refrigerates the capillary tube and causes a deposition of extremely small quantities of metal. The index finger is pressed tightly to the end of the tube and heat is applied by means of a small Bunsen burner, just beneath the copper foil. The amount of air entering the tube can then be

14. *J. f. prakt. Chem., Leipz.*, 24:244, 1841.

regulated by the forefinger. In case of mercury very little heat should be applied, as there is danger of loss of the sublimate in the tube. If the foil has not been thoroughly washed there is danger of volatilizing fat adhering to the copper foil.

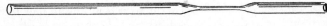

FIG. 4.
McNally Reinsch Tube

After the tube has cooled, the filter paper acting as a refrigerating agency is removed, and the capillary tube is carefully dried and examined under the low power microscope. Arsenic will be seen as octahedral crystals, the mercury will

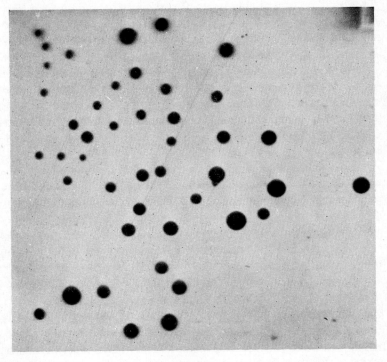

FIG. 5.
Globules of Mercury in Reinsch Tube as Seen
Under Low Magnification

be found to exist as an aggregation of shiny globules of mercury. (Figs. 4 and 5). The antimony deposit is closer to the point at which the heat was applied, and a portion of it may be in that part of the tube which is in the flame. The antimony deposit is generally amorphous and is very difficult to identify. Clark[15] has proposed dissolving off the black film by potash and hydrogen peroxide. The solution is boiled and any copper hydrate filtered off. The antimony will then exist as potassium antimonate. Any arsenic that might be present can be decomposed and reduced by ferrous chloride and hydrochloric acid. The arsenic is distilled as arsenic trichloride, and can be recognized by precipitation with hydrogen sulphide. Antimony, if present, will remain in the flask and can be precipitated as antimony sulphide.

A dark gray deposit may be of antimony or arsenic. The arsenic stain, according to Lippart,[16] is a true alloy consisting of one part arsenic to five parts of copper. If the deposit is of a silvery cast this would indicate the presence of considerable mercury. This deposit on the copper is not formed in the presence of powerful oxidizing agents, such as chlorates. With organic arsenical preparations, or with an arsenate, it is only slowly formed and in the usual time of heating it might be entirely missed. A stain upon the copper may appear in the case of decomposed organs from the sulphur compounds present or from selenium, gold, platinum, palladium, silver, bismuth, and antimony.

If the presence of arsenates be suspected, reduce to arsenites by sulphur dioxide, expelling the excess of the gas by boiling before applying the Reinsch test. With experience, 0.0065 mg. of arsenic and still smaller amounts of mercury can be detected.

If octahedral crystals resembling those of arsenic are found in the capillary tube they can be distinguished from the latter by the fact that they require a higher degree of heat, 700° C. to 800° C., while those of arsenic are sublimed at a much lower temperature. The globules of mercury found in the constricted area are so characteristic that it is not necessary to add iodine to the tube and allow it to stand for the conversion of the mercury present to the mercuric iodide. The glass tubing selected should be absolutely free from bubbles and should be cut in six-inch lengths, thoroughly washed with water, and allowed to stand covered with chromic acid ready for use.

15. Clark: *J. Chem. Soc. Lond.*, 1893.
16. *J. f. prakt. Chem., Leipz.*, 13:168.

The tubes are thoroughly washed with water and alcohol, and allowed to drain and draw out, so that the capillary will be about one inch long and the long arm of the tube at least two and one-half inches long. These tubes should not be permitted to stand open in the laboratory, as they collect small particles of dust which are confusing to the analyst while examining under the microscope. After arsenic or mercury has been found the ends of the tube can be sealed off and held for court evidence or for future reference. Where mercury has been found in small quantities the tubes must not be left unsealed over night, as the mercury will volatilize at the temperature of the laboratory room.

Volatile Poisons.—To 100 gm. of the material as prepared above, add sufficient water to make it the consistency of a thin gruel, add a small piece of tartaric acid, and place in a 1000-cc. Kjeldahl flask which is connected with a steam generator and a Liebig condenser and allowed to dip in 5 cc. of distilled water. The distillation is continued until there is 1 cc. for each gram of material placed in the flask. In the case of cyanide or nicotine a smaller quantity of material may be used and the distillation continued until there is no longer a test given by the distillate for these poisons. For a volatile substance like ether the collecting flask must be kept packed in salt and ice. If phosphorus is present use the special apparatus for distilling. (Fig. 3, page 21.)

The distillate as thus obtained, should be labelled "acid distillate," and may contain grain alcohol, wood alcohol, ether, carbolic acid and other phenols; formaldehyde, iodine, phosphorus, chloroform, chloral hydrate, turpentine, hydrogen, sulphide, amyl nitrite, camphor substances volatile with steam.

After the distillation from the acid mixture has been made, it is then rendered alkaline by the addition of magnesium oxide. The mixture is distilled until 100 cc. of distillate are obtained. The distillate from the alkaline mixture may contain aniline, conine, nicotine, chloroform if chloral hydrate has been present, ammonium and other volatile bases. Some of these same poisons, such as aniline, conine, nicotine, chloral hydrate and phenol, may appear in the extractions for alkaloidal poisons. The material after the two distillations have been completed should be saved, as it can be used for the examinations of inorganic or mineral poisons. However, if there is an abundance of material a fresh sample should be taken for this examination.

ALKALOIDAL POISONS

TO DETERMINE the presence of an alkaloid, a method of extraction must be used which will obtain the alkaloid free from salts, fatty matter, protein, and other extraneous material that would interfere with the melting point, color reactions and other tests used in the identification of the alkaloid. The. method usually employed is one of extraction by immiscible solvents modified after the method first used by Stas in the famous Bocarme's case. This method was founded upon the facts that tartrates of the alkaloids are readily soluble in water and alcohol, and that these alkaloids can be separated in aqueous solutions of their salts by ammonia and other powerful bases. The alkaloids thus liberated can be separated by ether, chloroform, and other liquids immiscible with water. The evaporation of these solvents leaves the alkaloids and other organic substances usually in an amorphous form. Further treatments with suitable solvents are necessary to obtain crystals.

The Author's Method.—An aliquot part of the material above prepared, usually 100 gm., is placed in a large Erlenmeyer flask and covered with 150 cc. of 50% alcohol acidified with tartaric acid, the flask being stoppered with a bark stopper, connected with a reflux tube about thirty inches in length. (Fig. 6). This flask is allowed to stand in a warm place over night, warmed on a hot plate the following morning until the alcohol begins to boil, and the material is then filtered through several layers of cheesecloth. This operation is repeated three times, allowing the material to boil on the hot plate with the reflux tube for two hours, and again filtered. The residue upon the cheesecloth with other residues from the purification is saved for future reference. The combined filtrates are now filtered through a filter paper. The filtrate is placed in a large Kjeldahl flask connected with a Liebig condenser which is connected with a vacuum pump. Under reduced pressure the alcohol and water are evaporated to about 20 cc. To this residue in the flask 80% alcohol is added. A fine curdy precipitate is formed, which can be readily filtered. If the alcohol used is too strong, a gummy mass may be obtained which will have

to be redissolved, and the precipitation will have to be repeated, as the gummy mass may retain some of the alkaloid.

The filtrate is again evaporated down, using a vacuum, and
the residue is purified with stronger alcohol each time, until
94% alcohol fails to produce a precipitate in the flask. The
Kjeldahl flask is always kept heated in a water-bath so as not
to get too high a temperature, as that might destroy the alkaloid
present. The residue in the flask is
taken up with 5 to 20 cc. of 0.5%
hydrochloric acid and filtered
through a small filter paper into a
Squibb's separatory funnel. The filtered liquid is now extracted with
20 cc. of petrolic ether in three separate portions. The combined petrolic ether extracts are washed
with 5 cc. of distilled water. The petrolic ether is separated, and filtered through a small piece of cotton into a small beaker. The petrolic
ether is allowed to evaporate at
room temperature or on the hot
water-bath.

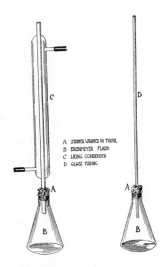

A STOPPER, WRAPPED IN TINFOIL
B ERLENMEYER FLASK
C LIEBIG CONDENSER
D GLASS TUBING

FIG. 6.
Condensers used in Alkaloidal
Extraction

The residue will contain fat, the
alkaloid-piperine, bitter principals,
absinthe, capsicin, and hop bitter;
acids: salicylic, benzoic, cinnamic,
and picric (very slightly), creosol, thymol, menthol, camphor,
terebene, copaiba, cubebin, sanatol, cumarin, vanillin, styrone,
acetanilid, phenacetin, antipyrine, subcutin, chloretone, brome-
tone, epicarin, chloral hydrate, neuronal, sulphonal, trional,
barbituric acid compounds (slightly), and dormiol. The characteristic odors will be noticed if camphor, menthol, copaiba,
styrone, thymol, terebene, sanalol, coumarin, and vanillin are
present. The aqueous solution in the separatory funnel is now
shaken out three times with ether. The solvents are separated,
washed with water, filtered into a small beaker, and evaporated
over the steam-bath. This removes certain substances not completely removed by the petrolic ether. The residue will contain emodin, elaterin, picrotoxin, colchicine, acetanilid, phena-
cetine, santonin, gelsemic acid, narcotine, cantharidine, digi-

taline, benzoic and salicylic acids, phenolphthalein, aspirin, phenol, pyrogallol, vanillin, resorcinol, sulphonal, trional, barbital, phenobarbital, and caffeine, which are a few of the common substances removed by this solvent.

Unless there is some organic substance that is more soluble in chloroform than in ether, I omit the chloroform extraction from the acid solution and proceed with the alkaline ether. To the acid solution in the separatory funnel add an equal amount of sulphuric ether and make alkaline with ammonia water. If a green color appears this would indicate apomorphine. If a red color appears after adding ammonia, physostigmine may be present. Shake out four times with ether, wash the combined solvents with 5 cc. of distilled water, separate the ether, filter into a beaker, and evaporate at room temperature or over a steam-bath. A large number of substances will be removed by this solvent. The most important are the following: aconitine, adrenalin, anesthesin, antipyrin, apomorphine, atropine, brucine, codeine, dionin, emetine, ephedrine, gelsemine, gelseminine, heroin, homatropine, hydrastine, hyoscyamine, novacaine, nupercaine, nicotine, veratrine, physostigmine, pilocarpine, quinine, quinidine, quiniline, sanguinarine, sparteine, strychnine, anilin and pyridin. The alkaline solution is now made acid with 0.5% hydrochloric acid, warm chloroform is added, and the solution is made alkaline with ammonia, and shaken. If an emulsion forms it may be run into a beaker, brought to a boil, and then separated as usual. Repeat the extraction three times more, making acid and then alkaline, wash combined solvents with water, filter through cotton into a beaker, and evaporate over the steam-bath. The air from an electric fan blowing over the beakers assists in the evaporation. Many of the substances found in the alkaline ether will also be found in this extraction, as aconitine, atropine, apomorphine, berberine, brucine, cephaeline, cinchonine, cinchonidine, codeine, emetine, heroin, hydrastine, hyoscyamine, methylene blue, morphine, papaverine, pelletierine, physostigmine, quinidine, sabadinine, sanguinarine, strychnine, and scopolamine.[17] Dragendorff devised a more elaborate process for the extraction of nearly all non-volatile organic compounds of toxicological interest by making all three extractions from the acid solution by means of petrolic ether, benzene, and chloroform;

17. DRAGENDORFF'S METHOD: Ermittelung der Gifte, 149, 1895.

also four extractions from the alkaline solution using petrolic ether, benzene, chloroform, and amyl alcohol. In my method I omit the amyl alcohol from the alkaline solution unless I am looking for morphine, and in this way save time and solvents in a routine examination involving thousands of extractions. I use the Squibb separatory funnel, which can be obtained from dealers in scientific apparatus.

The distilled water used in washing the various solvents is extracted with the same type of solvent that has just been used, as there is always danger of losing some of the organic substance in the wash water.

The wash water and the residue in the extraction flask should be saved in every instance until the case has been disposed of by the authorities. Quantitative determinations of the purified extracts are always less than the amount originally present in the tissue. Where methods are available for volumetric or colorimetric determination the gravimetric should always be checked. In many instances the substances can be tested by the use of experimental animals.

Kippenberger's method[18] is based upon the formation of soluble alkaloidal compounds and the insolubility of protein compounds in a mixture of tannic acid and glycerine. A weighed portion of 100 gm. of finely ground tissue is digested for two days at 40°C., in glycerol containing 1% of tartaric acid and 10% of tannic acid. The liquid is pressed out and the residue washed several times with water containing glycerol in a cloth bag, the washings being removed by means of a press. The combined extracts are heated to 50°C., cooled, and immediately filtered, with the addition of water if necessary. The filtrate is shaken with petrolic ether and then with chloroform. The liquid in the separatory funnel is then rendered faintly alkaline with sodium hydroxide and extracted with chloroform. Sodium bicarbonate is now added to the alkaline liquid to convert any excess of alkaline hydroxide into the carbonate, and the mixture extracted with chloroform containing about 10% of alcohol. The alkaline solution is saturated with sodium chloride and shaken out with chloroform containing about 15% of ether. (1) The petrolic ether extraction in the above method, contains traces of jervine, and veratridine with fat. (2) After the removal

18. *Ztschr. f. anal. Chem., Wiesb.,* 34:294, 1895.

of the petrolic ether in the acid liquid, chloroform removes from the acid solution colchicine, digitaline, picrotoxine, cantharadine, papaverine, aconitine, narcotine, jervine, geissospermine, traces of deliphin, brucine, veratrine, thebaine, narceine, and strychnine. (3) Chloroform removes from the alkaline solution sparteine, coniine, nicotine, atropine (hyoscyamine, scopolamine) codeine, pilocarpine, brucine, strychnine, emetine, delphinin, apomorphine, and substances not completely removed in No. 2. (4) After the addition of a concentrated solution of sodium carbonate and shaking with chloroform alcohol mixture, morphine and narceine are obtained. (5) After the saturation with sodium chloride the ether chloroform removes strophanthine.

Kippenberger[19] has suggested the use of acetone in conjunction with tannic acid. This avoids the great difficulty of pressing out the viscid fluid attending the use of glycerine described in the original method. To the solution thus obtained a small quantity of glycerine and a little hydrochloric acid are added, the acid is evaporated off, and the resulting acid aqueous solution is extracted by immiscible solvents.

SEPARATION OF PTOMAINES

IN THE foregoing methods for the extraction of organic substances, the residues in the beakers, from the extraction by the immiscible solvents, will contain products of putrefactive decomposition. Ptomaines are always present in cadavers, especially in those parts which are in advanced state of putrefaction. Like alkaloids they give precipitates with the general alkaloidal reagents, and certain ptomaines react with special reagents to resemble some alkaloids. This fact makes ptomaines greatly important in toxicological investigations since their presence may lead to mistakes in the identification of an alkaloid. Most of the ptomaines are strong reducing agents. They will immediately convert potassium cyanide into ferrocyanide, a reaction given by several alkaloids like morphine. It is fortunate that a resemblance of a ptomaine to a vegetable base is frequently confined to one reaction with the foregoing and never extends to several reactions characteristic for that particular alkaloid. Peterson, Haines and Webster[20] recommend that after the

19. Ztschr. f. anal. Chem., Wiesb., 39:627, 1900.
20. Legal Medicine and Toxicology, 62, 1923.

solvent has been evaporated in a flat-bottomed evaporating dish, the residue be heated on a water-bath and put aside in a warm place for two or three days, which causes ptomaines and other products of protein decomposition when exposed to the air to take up oxygen, resinify, and otherwise change so as to lose their identity. "The ether, chloroform, amyl alcohol, or other immiscible solvent used in extracting the alkaloid is allowed to evaporate in a capacious watch glass or flat-bottom evaporating dish so that the residue may present a large surface to the action of the air. After the solvent has evaporated, the residue is gently heated on a water-bath for an hour or two, and afterward put aside in a warm place for two or three days. The more or less resinified material is then extracted with very dilute sulphuric acid, the solution filtered, the acid filtrate shaken repeatedly with ether, alkalinized and shaken out with appropriate immiscible solvent. The latter is allowed to evaporate, and if the residue is still found to be impure, the treatment above described is repeated one or more times, sometimes many repetitions being necessary. Eventually, if care is taken with all the details of the process, the alkaloid is usually obtained in a practically pure condition."

Other methods for the separation of poisons have been included in textbooks, but have not been found practical or necessary in my experience covering many thousands of cases. Two of these methods will be briefly mentioned. The separation of alkaloidal poisons, or mineral poisons from organic mixtures by dialysis, is based upon the discovery of Graham that crystalline substances pass through animal membranes from their solution into pure water on the other side of the membrane, while protein and other non-crystalline substances do not. The Soxhlet extraction apparatus is ideal for material already dry, but for tissues that have to be dried, other methods are more rapid. Separation of alkaloids from fat during the purification of the alcoholic extracts can be accomplished by adding acidulated water with hydrochloric acid to the brown residue left in the flask after the evaporation of the first alcohol. The acidulated aqueous solution is filtered through paper which retains most of the fatty substances. The filtrates can then be treated with alcohol, and the protein material removed, as given under purification. The acid petrolic ether extract can be purified of fat and oily substances by extraction with warm acid water, filtering off the fat and re-extracting the filtrate with petrolic ether. In case the extracts obtained by the evaporation of the immiscible solvents contain impurities, the alkaloid can be precipitated from its acidulated solution by means of Wagner's reagent. The precipitate usually flocculent can be filtered off. By adding a solution of sodium thiosulphate to the alkaloidal precipitate the alkaloid is dissolved, the periodide being reduced to a hydriodide. The solution is made alkaline with ammonia and extracted with the appropriate immiscible solvent, the evaporation of which gives the alkaloid in a fairly pure condition. The process can be repeated, keeping in mind that with every purification there is a loss of the alkaloid.

Cremation of the body destroys all of the organic poisons and volatilizes practically all the mineral poisons, with the exception of copper and lead. From the medicolegal standpoint it should not be permitted for at least thirty days after death, unless there has been an autopsy and organs removed for chemical examination, as relatives in distant parts are not informed of the death immediately, especially in cases where there has been foul play. Several States have already passed laws to this effect.

The toxicological examination of an embalmed body should offer no difficulties, as the usual embalming fluid contains formaldehyde and other substances not usually taken as poison. Many States prohibit the sale of fluids containing arsenic, mercury and carbolic acid. (Such a law should be enforced in every State.) What is of greater importance at the present time is the presence of arsenic in "hardening compounds," that are used after a postmortem examination. To cite a specific instance, a man died in Princeton, Indiana, after an automobile accident. The coroner who had held only one or two postmortems, made an autopsy and reported "death due to a ruptured stomach." The body was prepared for burial by an undertaker. The following day several insurance companies, holding policies for $140,000, demanded a second autopsy. Material was removed for a chemical and microscopical examination. A report was given that "death was due to arsenical poisoning." The insurance companies refused to pay the policies. After the insurance companies had introduced testimony of the pathologist and chemist to the effect that they had found arsenic, and that death was due to arsenical poisoning, the lawyer for the family put on the undertaker as a witness who testified that he had used a certain embalming fluid and a certain hardening compound, samples of which he identified as having been submitted to me for examination. I was placed on the stand and testified that the embalming fluids did not contain arsenic but that the hardening compound contained over 50% of arsenic trioxide. The insurance companies paid the policies in full. In this case the erroneous reporting of an arsenical poisoning jeopardized the life and freedom of an innocent woman. I cannot lay too much stress upon the fact that it is criminal to use arsenic in any form for the embalming of a dead body. In every case a toxicologist should have a sample of the hardening compound and the embalming fluid. Hardening compounds sometimes contain zinc chloride.

Where a postmortem is to be made, it should be made before the body is embalmed, as formaldehyde may interfere with the detection of cyanides and certain other poisons, which will be taken up under the specific poisons.

FORENSIC QUESTIONS

IN NEARLY every case of poisoning certain questions of medicolegal importance appear during the investigation. The expert must be prepared to answer these questions, as they are frequently essential in the proper solving of the case. Some of these questions have already been formulated by Tardieu,[21] and other authors, such as Kobert.[22] And some have been discussed, in different places. They are summarized here for convenience. No attempt should be made to evade a question, and if the expert does not know, he should admit the fact, for, later on, incorrect answers may be a source of embarrassment to him. The expert should clothe his answers with as few technical terms as possible; the language should be simple, and said in a clear voice. The expert must bear in mind that the judge and jury do not have any medical training, and that they depend upon the witness for an opinion and expect the witness

21. Etude Medico-Legale et Clinique sur l'Empoisonnement, 2nd. ed., 113, 1875.
22. KOBERT: Lehrbuch der Intoxikationen, 119, 1902.

to assist the court by his special knowledge and experience. No attempt should be made to argue with the lawyers for the defense or the prosecution. The expert should impress the court by his gentlemanly manner, and his conduct, when under a severe cross-examination. If the question is not clear and the attorney asks for a direct "yes" or "no" answer, the witness should refuse unless he is allowed to explain.

The medical witness should never take any side in an action, but should assist in bringing forth the truth whether called upon in behalf of the defense or the prosecution. The highest compliment that can be paid an expert is to be called as a witness for both sides.

1. Was Death or Illness Caused by Poison?—This is the most important question, and the one to be answered by expert evidence. The expert must establish beyond a doubt the fact that a poisoning has or has not occurred. Before a definite answer can be given the expert must know: (1) the symptoms known to be caused by the poison were observed during life; (2) the postmortem examination shows the presence of such lesions as the poison is capable of producing, and the absence of other causes of death; and (3) the poisonous substance is demonstrated to be present in the cadaver or in the vomit or excretions of the person poisoned.

1. The symptoms shown by the victim would furnish the first indications of poison. As before stated, symptoms of poisoning make their sudden appearance while the individual is in good health, and almost always after the ingestion of food or drink. The rapidity of these symptoms is followed frequently by a fatal termination. Where more than one poison is found in the body it is difficult for the expert to say which one caused death. I have had cases where the individuals took potassium cyanide and then shot themselves; and other cases where phosphorus had been taken and then carbon monoxide. Questions like this have to be determined in each case by the jury, from the evidence offered by the expert. If the victim does not die, the symptoms may have been caused by a disease, which may give symptoms practically identical to those produced by poison. Where a chemical examination shows the presence of arsenic in the urine, the finger-nails and the hair, the expert can give an opinion based upon the symptoms and the chemical report. In September, 1931, the author was called

to Nogales, Arizona, to testify for a Mrs. M., who was accused
of murdering her husband, and also to give an opinion as to the
cause of her illness. Having found arsenic in the hair and urine
(a sample of which was submitted to me) in amounts such as
are found in people dying of arsenical poisoning, I gave an
opinion from the symptomatology and the chemical examination that Mrs. M. was poisoned by arsenic. Mrs. M. had been
poisoned on two different occasions. One of her physicians, a
former student of mine, consulted me regarding her illness. I
advised him by telegram to isolate the patient because of the
dangerous amount of arsenic found in the urine. When this
information was given to the lady she shot her husband, whom
she had for some time suspected of poisoning her.

2. When death follows a suspected poisoning, a postmortem examination furnishes important evidence as to the
cause of death. The pathologist is able to testify whether or
not the individual died from natural causes; and further, that
the changes found grossly and microscopically are compatible
with the theory of poisoning. Certain lesions may be found in
the body that could have been responsible for death, but if they
did not cause symptoms during life similar to those prevailing
after the ingestion of the specific poison discovered by the
toxicologist, then it can be assumed that the poison caused the
death.

3. One of the most important factors in determining death
by poisoning is the finding of a substance in the organs of the
victim capable of causing the death. It is possible that a poison
may have been administered and none detected. This is especially true of certain organic poisons and of the cyanides after
the body has been embalmed with formaldehyde.

II. What Poison Produced the Illness or Death?—In nearly
every murder trial where poison is alleged to have been the
cause of death, the defense invariably asks the expert what
was the nature of the poison found. In a case of poisoning by
arsenic trioxide the toxicologist is rarely able to isolate the
crystals of arsenic trioxide except in those cases in which it
may have been taken or given in large quantities and is found
to be adhering to the mucous membrane of the stomach or intestines. In numerous cases of poisoning by Paris green I have
been able to separate from mere traces, to as much as 31 gm.

The chemical examination of a suspected case of arsenical poisoning shows the presence of an arsenical mirror, as in the Marsh test, or by the coating of a copper, as in the Reinsch test, or by the color developed by the mercuric bromide paper, or by the precipitation of a sulphide of arsenic, or other tests. The same may be said of the alkaloids and other organic poisons. We separate the base and identify by color, or by precipitation tests which are very definite for that particular compound. In exceptional cases only is the analyst able to determine the acid radical that accompanies the alkaloid. Occasionally, the toxicologist may be unable to detect the presence of a poison in the organs of the victim. Then we must rely on other evidence than the findings of the poison in order to ask for an indictment. It is not always necessary to find a poison for the establishment of the fact that a poisoning has taken place, as in the well known Palmer-Cook case,[23] which occurred in England, in 1855. Palmer was tried, convicted and executed for killing Cook with strychnine. Although the chemical examination failed to reveal the poison in the body after death, the incriminating circumstances were so strong and the symptoms displayed by the deceased so characteristic, as to prove conclusively the guilt of the accused. The pathological changes in many cases of poisoning are so few that it is only when an irritant or a corrosive poison has been taken that the pathologist is able to assist in determining the character of the poison. Marsh tubes, Reinsch tubes, and other evidence of the substance isolated should be held for court exhibits by the toxicologist.

III. Could the Substance Administered Cause Illness or Death?—A substance may be administered with a desire to cause death, yet from the character or form of administration be incapable of causing death. In answering this question one must take into consideration the definition I have given of a poison. It must be something which when absorbed or acting chemically must be capable of seriously affecting health or causing death. Tardieu[24] cites the case of a woman who tried to poison her husband with pure copper filings. If the copper had been combined with some other chemical, as the chloride or the sulphate, it would then have been of importance. So it is essential for the expert to be able to answer whether the

23. TARDIEU: *Ann. d'hyg., Par.,* 6:371, 1856.
24. TARDIEU: Empoisonnement, 2nd. ed., 123.

substance is capable of causing death in the manner in which it was found.

IV. Was the Substance Found by the Chemist the Poison which Caused Death?—When a poison is present in large amounts in an exhumed body as in the Princeton, Indiana, case, already cited, postmortem introduction must be entertained. If the chemical examination on the other hand shows only a small amount of the poison, it may have entered the body in medicine, food, or drink. If the analyst is not an experienced individual in toxicological work, traces of arsenic from chemicals used might appear to him as the poison that caused the death of the individual. With the usual precautions advised earlier in the text this part of the question could not arise.

V. Is a Substance Given in a Minute Quantity, a Poison?— The expert will not be confronted with this question unless the quantity administered is known to be small. This does not apply to cases where the quantity of the dose is unknown and only minute amounts have been separated by analysis. When the poison has been given in such small amounts or extreme dilution that it is incapable of causing injury, it does not come within the definition of a poison. "Whether its administration in such an amount or form with criminal intent is punishable is a legal question and one which does not concern the toxicologist except in so far as he may be called upon to fix the limit of quantity or dilution below which the substance will be incapable of causing deleterious effects."[25]

VI. Was the Poisoning Suicidal or Accidental?—Circumstances attending the administration of the poison would answer this question. The Coroner's jury after hearing the evidence would be in a better position than the expert to answer the question.

The physical properties, or the amount which was found to be present, may raise a presumption in favor of suicide. For instance, in one case I separated 34.05% of Paris green from the stomach walls. A poison with such marked color as Paris green would not be swallowed by an adult in complete possession of his faculties. Accidental poisonings may be entirely cleared up by a chemical examination. In the case of Mrs. Waters the husband claimed that the medicine prescribed by

25. WITTHAUS and BECKER: Medical Jurisprudence, Forensic Medicine and Toxicology, IV: 211, 1911.

the doctor was responsible for his wife's death. The examination of the tablets given by the physician did not disclose strychnine. However, the residue on the tablespoon with which the medicine was given did contain strychnine. Whether the case is homicidal is again for the jury to decide, and not the expert. A person with a defective sense of taste would not be able to detect the presence of strychnine. For a number of years, while giving laboratory work in Materia Medica and Toxicology at Rush Medical College, I tried the effects of diluted solution of strychnine upon the students, and found four or five students every year who were unable to distinguish the bitterness of strychnine sulphate in a dilution of 1 to 20,000.

VII. Could the Substance Found have been Administered as a Medicine?—In general, this must be answered in the affirmative, as it may have been taken by the individual or may have been given upon the advice of a physician. Where the amount recovered by analysis far exceeds the average dose recognized by the U. S. Pharmacopeia, it is necessary for the District Attorney to have copies of the physician's prescription to show what drugs were prescribed. However, this would not be sufficient, as the pharmacist could have made the mistake in compounding the prescription, and a chemical examination of the capsule should be made. On the other hand, the prescription for strychnine could have been properly prescribed and compounded and still contain a poisonous dose of the strychnine. Someone, knowing that strychnine was in the prescription could add a lethal dose to several of the capsules for the purpose of murder.

Claims may be made that the poison found by the toxicologist was introduced as an impurity in a medicine legitimately administered, as arsenic and bismuth subnitrate. With the high degree of purity of drugs manufactured today, this contention seldom appears. If the drug should contain an impurity, such as arsenic, then the expert should show the absurdity of this contention by asking how many ounces, pounds, or quarts if it was liquid, would have to be taken to obtain the amount of poison found by analysis. For instance, in a celebrated cyanide poisoning case where the author found potassium in considerable amounts, a claim was made that sodium cyanide was given to commit murder. The late Dr. Ralph Webster, expert for the prosecution, was forced by the experts for the defense to admit that it would take several pounds of cyanide of the sample in question to produce the potash discovered, thus eliminating the sodium cyanide found on the farm of the defendant as the source of the poison.

From the quantitative distribution, in several organs of the body, of the poison and alleged drug carrying the poison, the expert could arrive at a conclusion whether it was present as an impurity. However, an analysis of a part of the original drug administered would be better evidence.

Where mere traces of arsenic have been found in cases in which there is a suspicion of poisoning, where evidence is offered to show it was previously administered to the deceased in medicine, the question naturally would arise whether the same poison found in the cadaver may not be a portion un-eliminated from the medicine. Against this we must revert to the circumstances, the quantity of poison found, and the time that has elapsed since the last dose of medicine was taken. The answer to this question would be greatly strengthened by the nature of the symptoms in the final attack and the report of the pathologist upon the gross and microscopical examination of the organs.

VIII. When and How was the Poison Taken?—It is frequently a great aid to the District Attorney to establish with certainty the exact time of the commission of the crime. With rapidly acting poisons, such as nicotine or the cyanides, the time can be very closely established. With poisons acting less rapidly, modified by the action of food in the stomach, and the form in which the poison was taken, the time of administration can be set down as within the hour of the time the first symptoms appeared.

Most poisons are administered by mouth. The symptoms would appear much quicker if the poison were of such a character that it could be given hypodermically, intravenously, or inhaled, than when given by mouth, therefore the answer must be formulated with these points in mind. The finding of the poison in the stomach in more than mere traces would indicate its administration by mouth, keeping in mind that some poisons such as morphine, mercury and sodium fluoride are reabsorbed by the stomach. However, I have failed to find poison in the stomach when it had been given or taken by mouth, as it was completely removed by vomiting or had been completely absorbed before death. This is especially true of organic poisons.

IX. May a Poisoning have Occurred and the Poison Either Be or have Become Undetectable?—Certain poisons which cause death may escape detection, because they are extremely volatile, such as some of the refrigerating gases. Good methods for the chemical and physiological detection may not be available or may be insufficiently studied for certain poisons. Poisons may be removed from the stomach and intestines by repeated vomiting, purging, and absorption, so that none will be found in these organs by a chemical examination. Repeated washing out of the stomach by the physician may also remove all traces of the poison. All of the absorbed poison may be eliminated from the body if life continues sufficiently long. If the body had been embalmed, hydrocyanic acid may escape detection. Inorganic poisons can be detected for a longer period than organic poisons. Either class of poisons, however, may have been eliminated from the organs before the examination was made.

X. Could the Poison have been Simulated?—Frequently samples of food or drink are submitted to the toxicologist for analysis by persons describing symptoms that may or may not come from poisoning. Most of the examinations give negative results for poisoning, but occasionally a specimen of food will contain poison.

As previously mentioned, the symptomatology of poisoning very frequently resembles that of some natural disease so that a differential diagnosis without a chemical examination is difficult or may be impossible. The great similarity occasionally gives rise to groundless suspicion of poisoning, which if the person dies may be disproved by the finding at the postmortem of some lesion adequate to cause the symptoms observed during life.

The introduction of a poison into a cadaver for the purpose of manufacturing evidence to bolster up a false accusation of criminal poisoning is possible, but has not occurred in my experience. However, in the famous Orpet case, at Waukegan, Illinois, in which Marion Lambert met her death by potassium cyanide, I believe such an attempt was made to strengthen the prosecution. Miss Lambert was found dead on February 9, 1915. The stomach and contents were submitted to the late Dr. Ralph Webster, who gave me half of the specimen for a quantitative examination. Several months later, in July, Mr. Carl Miner, a consulting chemist, requested me to testify in this case for the defense. The prosecution, when informed that the defense wanted me, submitted a coat said to have been worn by the young woman, who died of cyanide. On the outside of this coat three inches below the top button, were four white stains about an inch apart, having a distinct odor of cyanide. The stains looked suspicious, and I made tests which confirmed my suspicion that sodium cyanide in a fabric exposed to air for a period of four months, would not retain its shape or odor. After the acquittal of Orpet, an evening paper had the spots examined by Professor W. S. Haines and Mr. Carl Miner, who found the stains had been made with sodium cyanide, while the girl died of potassium cyanide. Here was clearly an incident where someone for the prosecution tried to bolster up a weak case which had circumstances looking like suicide and others that looked like murder. Motive paralleled motive; opportunity paralleled opportunity for the possession of the cyanide, and in connection with other circumstances in the case. The author was called by both the prosecution and the defense.

POSTMORTEM APPEARANCES

IRRITANT and corrosive poisons are the only ones giving characteristic postmortem appearances. Some other poisons such as carbon monoxide give well marked evidence of their effects. The corrosive acids and alkalis do not always leave evidence of their action, death occurring from shock before the tissues have time to become disorganized. The ulcerations from the corrosives are usually large and ragged, while ulcerations from disease are generally small with edges smooth. Table IV gives some of the outstanding appearances of some of the common poisons.

EVIDENCE OF POISONING FROM THE DEAD BODY

THE examination of the body is divided into four parts: First, the examination of the clothing, if the person is dressed, for containers of poison, and for letters indicating a reason, if it be suicide. Second, the autopsy, giving the appearance of the body and the appearance of the organs grossly, noting whether there is a natural cause for death, or whether

TABLE IV
EVIDENCE OF POISONING FROM POSTMORTEM APPEARANCES

POSTMORTEM APPEARANCES	LEAD US TO SUSPECT DEATH BY
Stains about the mouth, brownish or yellowish.	Strong mineral acids, oxalic acid, carbolic acid, lysol.
Corrosion and softening of tissues of mouth and throat.	Alkalis.
Bright red spots on skin.	Hydrocyanic acid, cyanide, carbon monoxide.
Tissues abnormally red.	Potassium (or sodium) nitrate, carbon monoxide.
Multiple hemorrhages in skin and surfaces of internal organs.	Phosphorus, poisonous mushrooms. (Heat stroke.)
Skin cyanotic.	Hydrocyanic acid, phenol, nitrobenzol, carbon dioxide, silver nitrate.
Pupils contracted.	Belladonna, stramonium, henbane, scopolamine, gelsemium.
Odors (more marked on opening the body).	Opium or some of its preparations. (Not always.)
Dark line on gums.	Lead, mercury, silver, bismuth.
Putrefaction markedly delayed.	Alcohol, arsenic, mercury.
Putrefaction rapid, absence of rigor mortis.	Poisonous mushrooms.
Protracted rigor mortis.	Strychnine.
Dry gangrene of extremities.	Ergot.
Blood much disorganized and chocolate colored.	Potassium chlorate.
Contents of stomach green or bluish green.	Paris green, copper salts.
Shining green particles.	Cantharides.
Contents of stomach yellow, or reddish yellow.	Picric acid, potassium bichromate, lead chromate, orpiment, acriflavin, selenium, pyridium.
Contents of stomach luminous.	Phosphorus.
Walls and contents of stomach turn black on exposure to ammonium sulphide.	Lead, mercury, copper, bismuth.
Villi of small intestine turn black spontaneously on exposure to light.	Silver.
Fatty degeneration of liver, and other internal organs.	Phosphorus, arsenic, mercury.
White deposit or granules on mucous lining of stomach, each granule the center of an inflamed spot.	Arsenic, antimony.

abnormal conditions are present. Third, the pathological examination, by which the presence or absence of changes in the tissues caused by the action of the poisons, or by disease, is determined by the microscopical examination of sections of the organs. Fourth, the toxicological examination to demonstrate the presence of poison in the organs.

Where a sudden death has occurred, the police in most large cities are requested by the Coroner, or the medical examiner, to leave the body where it was found until the Coroner's physician, arrives to take charge of the case. Notes can then be made of the body and its surroundings. Such observations frequently are of great assistance in determining whether the case is one of accident, murder, or suicide. These notes should include the following points: the date and place of the examination; second, who found the body; third, the names of the persons present; fourth, the position of the body— whether on the floor, in a chair, or in bed; fifth, whether fully or partially clothed and whether the condition of the clothing indicated a struggle; sixth, had the deceased vomited, and if so, the relation of the stains of vomit to the position of the cadaver; seventh, description of any cup, spoon, bottle, other vessel, paper, or weapon found near the body, and the position of the same relative to the body, with marks of identification, all of these to be held in the possession of a police officer or representative of the Coroner's office; eighth, had the stains of vomit or excretion been made while the body was in the position in which it was found, or had the body been moved subsequently before or after death; ninth, when an exhumation is made, note the position of the grave, getting the section and lot number, take a sample of the soil, note the condition of the casket, copy any inscription on the plate upon the casket. The condition of preservation of the body should be noted, as well as any evidence of the body having been covered by ground water; samples of the fabric in and outside of the coffin, artificial flowers, and any portion of the burial clothes and casket trimmings, should be taken. In case arsenic is found in the body the defense will claim that it was derived from this source. It is much easier to take these samples at the time of the original exhumation, than to have a second exhumation. A jury is always favorably impressed by thoroughness in these details.

THE AUTOPSY

THE postmortem examination should be made in a thorough manner by qualified persons, to determine the presence or absence of disease, and to disclose the remote effects of the poison. The postmortem examination should be conducted in a room with good light and running water; wherever possible the body should be removed to an undertaking establishment or a morgue provided by the county officials. The pathologist and toxicologist should be the only persons present at the postmortem examination. The toxicologist should provide chemically clean, wide-mouthed glass bottles with glass covers, for organs necessary for the chemical examination. If the organs are to be sent by a messenger, express, or parcel post, the bottles should be sealed with adhesive tape across the top of the cover of the jar, at right angles, and again around the neck of the bottle. Where the two tapes cross, sealing wax should be applied and an imprint of a seal made in the wax. Before the wax is applied, the initial of the autopsy surgeon and other officials present at the postmortem should be made at the intersections of the tape so that part of the initial will cover both pieces of tape. Metal of any kind should not come in contact with the organs. Zinc mason-jar tops, should be absolutely forbidden. The defense could claim that arsenic if found in the organs came from the metal tops. (See Fig. 7.) A complete history of the case should be available to the pathologist, so that the principal points may be given special atten-

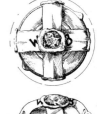
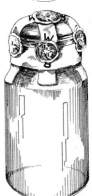

FIG. 7.
Manner of Sealing Glass Jars Containing Organs

tion. The body should be identified to the operator, either by relatives or friends. If the body is unknown, it is the duty of the physician to make note of the color of the hair, the color of the eyes, the condition of the teeth, describing any dental work that may have been done, any scars upon the body, any deformities. If possible a photograph should be taken of the body as it was found, and also of the face. In the Cook County morgue Chicago, I included in the plans of the new morgue a room where scraps of clothing could be retained in glass jars for assistance in identification. The tag attached to the jar contained the morgue number and a description of jewelry and all other articles found upon the body. The number of the watch and any marks of jewelers who have repaired it should be noted as further aids in the identification.

The data should include:

1. The apparent age.
2. The sex.
3. The height. (This has been of service on several occasions, in showing substitution, in insurance cases, where a sick individual's name has been put in a policy for which a healthy person of a different height was examined; for instance, the Bonifiglio case where the height of the deceased was two inches more than that of the person examined.)
4. The weight, exact if an examination is made in the county morgue; approximate if a scale is not at hand.
5. Race.
6. Development: thin, emaciated, muscular, obese, etc.
7. The condition of the hands, labor or office man.
8. The color and condition of the hair, eyes, eyebrows.
9. The color of the skin.
10. The condition of the teeth, describing any dental work, extractions or plates.
11. Describe scars, tattoo marks, evidence of disease, wounds, stains, and any external peculiarities.
12. External evidence as to disease or injury, time since death, conditions under which the body has been exposed since death, as in the water.
13. If the body is in a fit state, photographs, of both full face and profile should be taken. Pictures are to be kept in chronological order in a large book, giving morgue number and other data.

External Examination.—If the body is clothed, an examination should be made regarding tears, loss of buttons, dust or dirt upon the clothes, burns or blackening from the discharge of firearms, and blood stains. Stains on the clothing due to corrosives, alkalis, acids or vomit should be saved for a chemical examination. The clothes, when removed, should be taken off intact if possible, otherwise they should be split up at the seams. The anterior and posterior surfaces of the body should be examined from head to foot for evidence of external violence, old scars, rigidity, lividity, and putrefaction. If the body is that of an unknown person, the details given above under identification should be followed closely. Indications of diseases, such as edema of the legs, dropsy, skin diseases, and eruptions, marks of corrosives on the lips and mouth or the smell of alcohol, cyanide, or carbolic acid, should be noted. The external examination should include the natural orifices, also examination of the bony structures for fractures.

Internal Examination.—It does not take long for a person engaged in medicolegal work to learn that a complete examination of the viscera should be carried out in all cases, even when a condition is found which would be sufficient to give as a cause for death. If this is not done, the defense attorney may ask questions that will cause a great deal of embarrassment. Some pathologists will open the head first, others will begin with the chest and abdomen. A definite plan should be adopted so that there are no omissions in the examination of the organs. Accurate observations and thoroughness are necessary to obtain a correct diagnosis. The usual method is to make an incision from just above the sternum to the pubis, taking care that when the abdominal cavity is opened the intestines are not injured. The skin of the chest wall and the deeper tissues of the neck are reflected, paying particular attention to the skin and deeper tissues of the neck in cases of suspected strangulation. The sternum is removed by cutting the costal cartilages and sawing the clavicles if necessary. The conditions of the thoracic cavity should be observed before anything is disturbed, to ascertain if any blood is in the cavity. The same precautions should be taken in the examination of the abdominal cavity, having dictated notes to an assistant. The attachments of the tongue are separated by passing a knife around the inner side of the lower jaw, the tongue is pulled down into the opening, and with it are separated the hyoid bone, pharynx, larynx, trachea and esophagus from the posterior wall. In this way the operator is given a perfect view of the fauces and larynx, enabling him to note any pathological conditions. These structures are now cut into, and a complete examination is made. The hyoid bone is examined for fractures. An incision is made into the trachea, which is continued into the bronchi in order to detect the presence of foreign bodies, as blood and froth in the lungs. Note whether there are adhesions existing between the parietal and visceral pleura. These are separated with the fingers, or cut across with a knife. If desired, the lungs may be removed by cutting across the bronchi and the vessels at the root of each. It is better, however, to leave the lungs attached, removing the organs from the neck and chest as above described.

The Pericardium.—The pericardium is opened by making an incision in the center of the anterior surface, elevating the pericardium so that the heart will not be injured. The cut in the pericardium is extended downward to the left and right, and upward as far as its reflection upon the large vessels. The amount of fluid and the surface of the sac should be examined. The heart should be examined as to position, size, and shape, as well as the condition of the coronary vessels. The chambers of the heart are opened while the heart is still attached, in order to determine the condition of the blood.

The best description for the examination of the heart is that by Drs. L. Hektoen and E. R. LeCount[26]: "Place the left hand under the heart and draw it downward and to the left, make a vertical incision with blunt pointed scissors into the pulmonary conus, and extend this distally into the pulmonary artery. This part of the examination is to be carried out with as little handling of the heart as possible before it is greatly disturbed in any way so as to allow the contents of the pulmonary artery and its two branches to be examined, for emboli lodged in them may be loosened or have their location changed unless this examination is made early before the organs of the thorax in general have been much disturbed. This is especially necessary with sudden death, particularly in puerperal women. Then an incision is made into the right auricle, between the entrances of the superior and the inferior vena cava. Then open the right ventricle by an incision beginning below the circular furrow, and running downward to near the apex, along the right margin and in line with the cut made into the auricle; the contents of these cavities may now be examined.

"To incise the cavities of the left side, grasp the heart so that the fingers of the left hand lie upon the anterior surface and the thumb upon the posterior, the apex resting in the hollow

26. PETERSON, HAINES and WEBSTER: Legal Medicine and Toxicology, 102, 1923.

of the hand. Make an incision from the left superior pulmonary vein through the auricular wall nearly down to the transverse furrow, and then another into the cavity of the left ventricle, commencing below the transverse furrow and extending along the left margin down to the apex. The contents of these cavities are now removed and examined.

"Next, the heart is removed by lifting it directly upward and cutting successively the vessels that enter and leave it, as near to the pericardium as possible. (Fig. 8.) The competency of the semilunar valves is next tested with water; all coagula

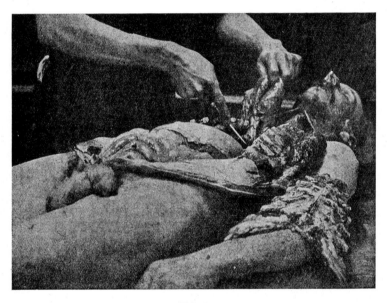

FIG. 8.
Illustrating Technique of
Removal of the Heart

are removed, the aorta and pulmonary artery are trimmed down, so that the behavior of the valves can be observed as the water is poured into the vessels, while the heart is suspended by the auricles, so that the plane of the orifices is horizontal. Competent valves meet exactly under the column of water, whereas the segments of incompetent valves fail to meet and allow the water to trickle away.

"The heart is now opened completely by passing the blunt end of an enterotome into the right ventricle, ventral to the attachment of the papillary muscle to the anterior wall, and cutting through the wall as much to the left as possible, continuing the incision out through the pulmonary artery. It will be found that when the scissors are held as far to the left as the septum between the ventricle permits, the division will pass between two valve segments without injury to either.

"The left ventricle is opened by passing the enterotome upward into the cavity from the incision already made, cutting along the interventricular septum (Fig. 9) and then between the pulmonary artery and the auricle, through the aorta; one of the aortic segments is unavoidably cut in two by this incision.

"The auricles may be opened still more by prolonging the incisions made out through the veins on each side, a good view being thus obtained of their interior and also of the auricular aspect of the mitral and tricuspid valves. Finally, the original incisions into the auricles and ventricles on each side may, if desirable, be united by cuts that divide the mitral and tricuspid rings; but these cuts may spoil the characteristic appearance of stenosis of the orifices, as well as other changes.

"When it is desired to obtain exact measurements of the size of the orifices of the heart, by means of graduated cones, the foregoing procedures are so modified that the cones are inserted into the orifices before the incisions described have divided the semilunar and auriculoventricular rings; naturally these cones are inserted with great gentleness, so as not to detach the inflammatory vegetations and thrombotic deposits. The diameter of the mitral and tricuspid orifices is often estimated by carefully inserting the fingers from the auricular aspect—in the adult the mitral normally admits three fingertips; the tricuspid, four. There is, however, a rigor mortis of the heart which may alter these dimensions.

"Having removed and opened the heart, the examiner is now ready to make a detailed examination of all its parts. The valvular and the mural endocardium are to be looked over, the foramen ovale and the membranous part of the ventricular septum are inspected, the size of the ventricles as to the depth and thickness of the wall may be measured, while the weight should always be determined, as it gives the most accurate indication of absolute increase or diminution in substance. The condition of the coronary orifices in the commencement of the aorta must be investigated; these orifices may be seriously involved in the sclerotic changes so often found immediately above the aortic valves. In all cases of sudden death from obscure causes, the coronary arteries must be searched for arteriosclerotic and other changes, and for this purpose they are cut open from their beginning in the aorta to the smallest

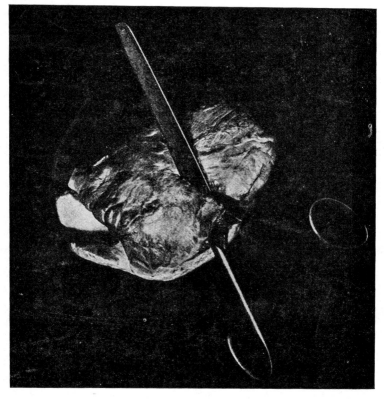

FIG. 9.
This figure shows the blunt point of the scissors projecting from the pulmonary artery when the right ventricle is opened by cutting along the interventricular septum (LeCount)

branches. In the event of doubtful coronary disease and secondary myocardial changes microscopic examination may show astonishingly extensive lesions. The myocardium, especially of the left ventricle, is finally exposed by a number of incisions, either parallel with, or vertical to, the surface of the heart.

"Having examined the lungs and the heart wholly or

partially in situ, the remaining thoracic organs and the organs of the neck are removed in toto. The left hand grasps the organs of the neck and pulls them downward, the right and left subclavian arteries and veins and other structures are cut across by a curved incision on the left side at the superior opening of the chest, and the cellular tissue between the esophagus and the thoracic aorta and the spinal column rapidly separated as far as the diaphragm, while the organs are drawn downward. Then the esophagus is ligated near the diaphragm and divided above the ligature, at which time the aorta, the inferior vena cava, and the parietal pericardium are also cut across. The organs are then placed upon a tray, the esophagus being uppermost. This latter is then divided along the posterior wall, in continuation of the incision already made into it. Turning the mass around, the arch of the aorta is laid open; then the trachea is opened by continuing the incision already made into it and this opening may be continued into the right bronchus; but in order to open the left bronchus the aorta must first be freed and taken out of the way.

"The peribronchial lymphatic glands are also to be incised, and their relation, if perchance tuberculous, to adjacent vessels determined. If necessary, the lungs may be detached and weighed. In the case of aneurysms of the aorta, tumors, and other swellings of the mediastinum caution must be used in removing the organs from the chest, so that instructive specimens are not marred by unskillful dissection, and the relations disturbed."

After the examination of the chest and its contents, each organ of the abdomen should be examined in turn, for the presence of disease or injury. The peritoneum should be examined before removal of the organs. The order of examination depends upon the individual operator. Sections of every organ should be saved, even if the material is not saved for chemical examination. The abdominal organs are of chief interest to the toxicologist. For, with the opening of the abdomen, the characteristic odors may be noted, as the peach blossom of hydrocyanic acid, or the characteristic odor of lysol and carbolic acid.

Stomach.—The external surface of the stomach and its degree of distention by food or gas are noted. The contents of the stomach are removed by making an incision with the scissors at the most dependent part of the stomach. The contents of the stomach are examined as to odor, reaction to litmus paper, and for the presence of particles of drugs. If the stomach is sent to the laboratory with both ends tied off, the stomach and content can be weighed, and after removal of the contents, as above, the weight of the stomach ascertained. The stomach should be placed in a separate wide-mouthed jar, so that the organs cannot be contaminated and given erroneous quantitative distribution of the poisons found. An alkaline reaction of the stomach contents may be due to sodium bicarbonate or magnesium oxide administered as antidotes. The alkaline reaction may also be due to caustic alkalis or alkaline cyanides. An acid reaction may be due to acid salts or to acids. The mucous surface of the stomach can be examined for solid particles adhering to the surface. Crystals of white arsenic accompanied by particles of carbon, indicate that the poison taken was such as "rough on rats." A green color adherent to the walls of the stomach may indicate poisoning by Paris green. Look for ulceration and erosion in the stomach wall from the effect of corrosives. If the death is from an acute irritant poison the stomach wall may show a marked redness or even hemorrhage. In some cases of bichloride of mercury or sulphuric acid poisoning, the stomach contents and wall of the stomach may be as black as tar. The stomach has a harsh feeling with sulphuric acid, and a soapy slippery feeling with the caustic alkalis. Similar changes may be seen in the esophagus, pharynx, and mouth.

The intestines are carefully examined and then removed completely from the body; they are washed after opening unless a portion is to be cut away for analysis. The small bowel is opened along its mesenteric attachment, so as not to mutilate the Peyer's patches, which may show changes of importance, especially when the defense intimates, in a poison case, that the prolonged illness was due to typhoid fever. The large bowel is opened and examined in the same manner, looking for evidence of irritant poisons. The upper part of the small intestine may be colored from Paris green, the large bowel may show the corrosive action of bichloride of mercury.

The liver, kidneys and heart may show fatty degeneration caused by arsenic, phosphorus, antimony, and chloroform. The gall-bladder is opened, the color and consistency of the bile

noted, and the appearance of the wall, whether thin or thickened. The size and weight of the liver should be recorded,
before exposing the interior. The kidneys are removed, the
adrenals are detached and incised in the longest diameter.
A careful examination of the adrenals for tuberculosis should
be made, as a sudden death in an undiagnosed, non-pigmented
Addison's disease can be explained on this basis. Each
kidney is measured, weighed, and divided into halves by
an incision from the convex margin to the pelvis. The capsule
of the kidney is removed; portions of the cortical substance may
be adherent as the result of chronic inflammation. The mucous
membrane of the pelvis is examined, and the ureters are
opened as far as the bladder.

If the urinary bladder contains urine it should be removed
and put in a clean bottle for chemical examination. The appearance of the wall of the bladder should be noted.

Cranial Cavity.—A postmortem examination is never complete unless the cranial cavity has been examined—as, even in
cases of poisoning, where only small amounts of poison have
been found, the defense attorney will ask: "How do you know
death was not due to cerebral hemorrhage?" The head should
be supported upon a paving block or on a couple of bricks to
elevate it from the table. The hair is parted along the con-
templated line of incision, from the mastoid process behind the
ear, over the vertex, to the mastoid of the opposite side. This
saves the hair so that the line of incision can be covered up after
the completion of the examination. Following the incision of
the soft parts down to the periosteum, the scalp is pulled over
the forehead. It may be necessary to loosen the scalp with a
scalpel. The other portion is pulled backward to the occiput.
The skull cap is now removed by means of a saw following a
line previously made by a knife in the greatest circumference
of the skull. Care should be exercised that the saw does not
enter the brain tissue. If the skull cap sticks, it may be removed
by gently applying pressure with a small chisel in the line of
the sawing. After the removal of the skull cap the exposed
surface of the dura is now examined. The degree of tension
should be tested by pinching up a fold near the apex of the
frontal lobes; the longitudinal sinus is incised, and its contents
examined. The next step consists in dividing the dura on each
side along the sawed edge of the skull, from the anterior to the

posterior extremity of the falx cerebri, with the point of a scalpel or small scissors, using great care not to puncture the pia. The dura over each half of the convexity is then folded in turn over upon the opposite half, so as to expose the under surface to full view; abnormal contents of the subdural space are now readily seen. The color, vascularity, etc., of the pia are now readily made out, and the brain is removed from its cavity in the following manner:

Place the block under the neck, so that the head hangs backward a little; pass the fingers of the left hand between the skull and the frontal lobes, and gently draw these backward. As the brain mass slowly leaves the cavity by its own weight, supported all the time by the left hand, everything that connects the brain with the base of the skull is divided, to wit: the olfactory nerves, the optic nerves, the carotid vessels, the peduncle of the hypophysis, and the third, fourth, and sixth nerves. When the tentorium cerebelli is reached, it is cut with the point of the knife along its attachment to the superior margin of the petrous portion of the temporal bone, great caution being used not to damage the cerebellum. Before cutting any blood vessels the cerebrospinal fluid can be collected with pipets, and as much as possible secured in case chemical examination for either wood or grain alcohol is desired, or tests for syphilis, cultures, etc. After cutting the fifth to the twelfth nerves, as well as the vertebral arteries, the spinal cord is the only remaining connection of the brain, and this should be divided as nearly at right angles as possible by means of the sharp myelotome. The division should always be made as far below the medulla as practicable. The base of the skull is now examined, the dural sinuses are incised and inspected, and the pachymeninx is loosened and removed so that the inner surface of the bones may be inspected for fractures and other lesions. The hypophysis may be removed from the sella turcica by carefully cutting away the dural diaphragm which covers this cavity. The brain may be sectioned at the time of the postmortem, or if it is possible, it may be hardened in Mueller's fluid, or solutions of formaldehyde, and sectioned at a later period. In cases of suspected poisoning such as arsenic, ether, chloroform, ethyl alcohol, or methyl chloride, the brain should be given to the chemist for examination, without sectioning, and without the addition of any preservative.

INORGANIC POISONING

THE mineral poisons are commonly classified into two groups, the corrosives and the irritants; both of which exert their action locally, the effect depending upon the concentration of the poison. Under the first group are classified the corrosive acids, oxalic and carbolic acids, and metallic irritants such as bichloride of mercury. All of these destroy the tissues by direct chemical action and are, therefore, corrosive. The acids convert the proteins into acid-proteinates which are soluble in concentrated and very weak acids, but are insoluble in moderately strong acids. The concentrated acids have an affinity for water and withdraw this from the cells. This is illustrated in the case of concentrated sulphuric acid, in which not only the formed water is withdrawn from the tissues, but also the elements hydrogen and oxygen are split off from the chemical combination leading to carbonization. The second group is composed of the corrosive alkalis, which produce swelling and clearing up of the mucous membranes, with a dark color due to the presence of altered hematin.

CORROSIVE ACIDS

POISONING by the mineral acids is chiefly suicidal and accidental. It would be difficult to administer these chemicals to a person, because of their intense action. They might, however, be given to an intoxicated or a sleeping person or to an infant. When the concentrated mineral acids come in contact with the skin there is an intense inflammation. When strong mineral acids are swallowed, there is an immediate burning sensation in the mouth and esophagus. When the acid reaches the stomach the pain is intense, and there may be vomiting of brown or black matter mixed with blood. The vomited material may contain portions of the mucous membrane of the stomach. Swallowing may be very painful and difficult because of the swollen condition or stricture of the esophagus. When the corrosive action has involved the larynx and trachea, there may be difficulty in speech and some coughing. There is a small and weak pulse. The skin may be clammy and cold. The mouth and lips are generally blistered; however, in cases of suicide where the poison has been gulped down, such signs may be absent. Breathing is difficult, and death may occur either from suffocation or from shock. Where the acids are dilute the above changes are not so pronounced and only stimulation and irritation may be pronounced. All of the acids cause intense pain, depending upon the concentration, with extensive scar formation.

SULPHURIC ACID (H_2SO_4)
(Molecular Weight 98.086. Synonym: Oil of Vitriol)

E NORMOUS quantities of sulphuric acid are produced each year. It is used for the preparation of other mineral acids, the refining of petroleum, the manufacture of fertilizers, dye stuffs, and explosives; the pickling of steel and iron, the charging of storage batteries, nitration of cellulose and benzol derivatives. In the United States in 1929, there were produced 2,166,898 short tons of sulphuric acid; in 1934, 1,519,504 tons were produced. Official statistics for German sulphuric acid production in 1933, gave 1,207 million tons (985,000 tons of sulphuric trioxide). In 1934 the production was increased to 1.4 to 1.5 million tons.

With this enormous production of sulphuric acid it is surprising how very few cases of poisoning are seen, since it enters into the manufacture of so many other acids and commodities.

Poisoning from this acid usually occurs by accident, as it is sometimes mistaken for such liquids as whiskey or medicine. In several of the cases I have had, the acid was in a flask which was labelled "Bourbon Whiskey," and had become colored from the action upon the cork stopper. The individuals drank the liquid straight, without diluting it with water. I have seen only a few cases of suicide by this poisoning. The acid is occasionally thrown in the face in revenge for some fancied wrong. It is popularly known as oil of vitriol. Witthaus[27] collected 388 cases from the journals, of which 256 were fatal, 120 recovered; fifty-three were homicidal, 189 suicidal, and

TABLE V
CASES OF SULPHURIC ACID POISONING

	Cases	Deaths	Recoveries	Homicides	Suicides	Accidents
Sulphuric acid	388	256	120	53	189	99
Hydrochloric acid	126	89	106	6	57	40
Nitric acid	89	70	15	17	43	14

27. WITTHAUS and BECKER: Medical Jurisprudence, Forensic Medicine and Toxicology, IV:228, 1911.

ninety-nine accidental. Since that time I have found only fifty-two cases of poisoning with eleven deaths reported, as with many other poisons—reports of deaths are seldom seen in medical journals.

Leymann's statistics show that the diseases of the respiratory tract are more frequent in sulphuric acid workers than among other chemical workers. Industrial injuries and burns to the eyes from sulphuric acid are not uncommon.

Properties: The chemical formula is H_2SO_4. The commercial acid is sometimes colorless, but it may be gray or black. The pure acid has a specific gravity of 1.85, the commercial acid is 1.545. When the acid is added to water, heat is given out, the temperature may rise to 212°F. Sulphuric acid absorbs water from the air, increasing in volume. When brought in contact with organic material it abstracts water, leaving frequently a carbonized mass. When the dilute acid is added to zinc, there is an evolution of hydrogen gas. When the concentrated acid is heated with metals, sulphur dioxide gas is liberated.

Two weaker forms are used for medicine: a dilute of 10%, and the aromatic of 20% sulphuric acid. It is applied externally as a powerful caustic in the shape of Ricord's paste, made with powdered charcoal, or Michael's paste made with powdered asbestos. Valade[28] reported a case of carcinoma of the scalp which he thought had developed from the treatment of an ulcer with sulphuric acid paste.

Symptoms: The severity of the intoxication from this group of poisons depends upon the concentration of the acid used. Concentrated acids cause severe corrosive effects in a short time. If they come in contact with the mucosa of the mouth, they produce a whitish discoloration. Nitric acid, however, produces a yellowish discoloration. The irritation of the pharynx is usually so intensive that cough and reflex irritations may be produced. As soon as the acid comes in contact with the mouth, there is an intense pain, which extends down the throat and stomach. If only a few cubic centimeters of concentrated acid are introduced into the stomach, grave symptoms are produced immediately. Vomiting occurs, the material being of a dark brown or black color mixed with blood, frequently containing fragments of the mucous membrane. The tongue swells, and may be coated white or a dark brown. There

28. *J.A.M.A.*, 100:37, 1933.

is an intense thirst with great difficulty in swallowing, obstinate constipation, diminution or suppression of urination, extreme tenderness of the abdomen, restlessness and collapse. The majority of the patients experience a sensation of anxiety and often fear, particularly if they become dyspneic. Other cases display motor symptoms, and the pulse usually becomes rapid shortly after the ingestion of the poison. The signs of absorption include spasms, dilatation of the pupil, fainting, and motor weakness. In some cases consciousness is maintained throughout. The pulse is small and rapid. The skin is cold and covered with perspiration. The voice is hoarse, and speech may be weak or impossible. With the retching, vomiting, and destruction of the tissue, the patient becomes weaker, and death may occur from shock.

Fatal Dose: One drachm (3.88 gm.) is the smallest dose reported to be fatal to an adult. One half that amount has been reported as the cause of death in a child one year old. With prompt and appropriate treatment recovery has taken place after four ounces had been taken. Bruce[29] reported a case of a plumber who, by mistake, drank three ounces of commercial sulphuric acid. Within twenty-five minutes his stomach was washed out, but he went home without any further instructions. The next day he vomited a blackish fluid, and at the end of a week he was unable to take food. On examination a complete obstruction of the pylorus was found. A jejunostomy was performed and the patient improved rapidly, making an uneventful recovery.

Lord Moyniham in an examination of several museum specimens found the worst injury is inflicted on the pylorus, and in several cases the whole mucous membrane may be affected. In these cases food is intolerable and vomiting is an early symptom.

Fatal Period: Death usually occurs within sixteen to twenty-four hours, from the local action, or the patient may recover partially only to die in a few days or weeks from weakness and exhaustion. Stricture of the esophagus may eventually result in complete closure, or injury of the stomach may result in impairment or destruction of the digestive juices and the patient die of starvation.

Treatment: In all acid poison cases you are dealing with a

29. BRUCE, H. A.: *Tr. Am. Surg. Ass., Phila.,* 48:123, 1930.

desperate condition, the patient is going to die unless the acid is removed. Unless there is a definite disorganization of the tissues, introduce a Rehfuss tube, and wash out the stomach with plain water, if alkaline substances are not at hand to put in the wash water. The first thought is neutralization of the acid: lime water, white wash, calcined magnesia, plaster from the wall, baking soda, or chalk. In the use of baking soda or other carbonates, caution should be exercised in not giving too much of the carbonate so as to cause a distention of an already weakened stomach wall. After the washings are free of the acid, give milk, whites of eggs, demulcent drinks, such as linseed tea and starch water. The pain is intense and should be controlled by the use of opiates. Retention enemas of 5% glucose, and 3% sodium bicarbonate will aid in neutralization and nutrition. Surgical interference may be necessary if edema of the glottis occurs or if a stricture of the esophagus results.

If the lesion is confined to the pylorus, jejunostomy followed by gastro-enterostomy are the operations of choice. Hoebeke and Brasseur[30] described a case in which the mouth was not burned. Burns of the skin should be washed with an abundance of water. If the acid has been thrown into the eyes, immerse the whole head in a pail of water. The eyes should be washed with water containing one teaspoonful of baking soda to the quart of water. In a treatment of chemical burns of the eye it is far better to use plain water than a neutralizing agent which causes an increase in the irritation. In industrial first aid kits, a 2% solution of sodium bicarbonate in water may be kept on hand for emergency purposes.[31]

Postmortem Appearances: Postmortem appearances will depend upon the strength of the acid used, and the length of time after the poison has been swallowed. The lips will be found corroded and brown in color. Spots on the skin will have a similar appearance. The cheeks may be soft, swollen and corroded. The esophagus may have the same appearance and be intensely red. The stomach may have a black tarry appearance, and, if the acid is not strong enough to cause corrosion, may be intensely red. The stomach walls have a harsh dry feeling, differing markedly from alkaline corrosion, which has

30. *Presse méd. belge, Brux.,* 48:105, 1896.
31. McNally, W. D.: *J.A.M.A.,* 98:45, 1932.

a soapy feeling. The pylorus is generally contracted. There may be a perforation of the stomach with an escape of the contents into the peritoneal cavity causing severe damage to neighboring organs. The duodenum may show corrosion. If the acid is not absorbed, its chief action is a local one where it comes in contact with the organs. If life is prolonged for several days, the appearances will differ according to the length of the survival of the patient, owing to the various changes caused by necrosis and repair.

TESTS FOR SULPHURIC ACID

THE mineral acids turn blue litmus paper red, decolorize red phenolphthalin, and turn cochineal yellow. Litmus paper will be turned red by acid salts and by the organic acids of digestion. Therefore it is not the proof of the presence of free mineral acids. Congo paper is turned a dark blue by mineral acids, while organic acids give a violet color.

If some of the acid that has been taken is available in a glass or bottle, the following tests may be applied:

The Barium Chloride Test: Take one or two drops of the solution, add distilled water and a few drops of hydrochloric acid (to prevent a precipitation by salts of carbonic, phosphoric and oxalic acid), and add a few drops of barium chloride, which will give a white precipitate of barium sulphate in the presence of sulphates. . If too much hydrochloric acid is added the barium chloride will be thrown out, and a precipitate will form, confusing the test.

The Veratrine Test: Add to a minute fragment of the alkaloid a drop of the free acid. A yellow color will be obtained, finally changing to crimson. If the acid is dilute, concentrate by evaporation. A crimson color will be obtained on the edge of the residue.

The Charring Test: Evaporate some of the acid in a porcelain dish with a small particle of sugar. A black carbonaceous residue will be produced by free sulphuric acid.

The Barium Rhodizonate Test depends upon the production of a red brown precipitate which is decolorized by sulphuric acid or sulphate. Upon a filter paper add one drop of barium chloride and one drop of freshly prepared sodium rhodizonate solution. A red brown precipitate will develop, which is decolorized when the test solution contains an acid or an alkaline sulphate.

Detection: If the strong acid has been dropped upon black clothing, a damp spot will develop which at first is red and later becomes dark brown, and the fabric easily disintegrates. If the cloth is colored with indigo there will be no red stain. White linen or cotton will turn black and disintegrate. Spots on clothing may be extracted with distilled water and the tests applied as given above.

Unless death occurs suddenly after the administration or the taking of sulphuric acid, the free acid will not be found by chemical examination. Extract the finely divided stomach with cold absolute alcohol. Allow the alcohol to remain upon the material until the albuminous residue has settled, then filter. The filtrate will contain sulphuric acid, but not the sulphates. Evaporate the alcohol, using a suction pump to hasten evaporation. Take up the residue with a few cc. of alcohol. Heat to the boiling point to saponify the ethyl sulphuric acid which was formed during the extraction. Apply the tests as given above. For the quantitative estimation of the acid either the gravimetric or the volumetric methods may be used. In the absence of soluble sulphates, precipitate as barium sulphate, or titrate with a normal alkaline solution using phenolphthalein as an indicator.

Sulphates are found in our foods and in many medicines, therefore the reporting of the presence of sulphates does not mean sulphuric acid. A mixed meal contains about 10 grains of sulphates. A water extraction can be made of a portion of the stomach and contents. The barium sulphate determination will give both free and acid soluble sulphates. The determination of the sulphuric acid in the alcohol extract will give the amount due to free sulphuric acid. One hundred parts of barium sulphate precipitate represent forty-two parts of absolute sulphuric acid.

Garnier* noted that the alcohol ether extract from the alimentary tract was strongly acid, yet sulphuric acid was absent. This acidity was ascribed to phosphoric acid liberated from the phosphates by sulphuric acid. If lesions are found in the viscera appearing as if caused by corrosives, the presence of phosphoric acid is a strong confirmation that sulphuric acid had been previously present, that is if the phosphoric acid had not been given in the form of medicine.

* *Ann. d'hyg.*, 17:148, 1887.

NITRIC ACID (HNO₃)

(Molecular Weight 63.05.   Synonym: Aqua Fortis, Engraver's Acid)

V ERY few cases of poisoning by this acid are seen by the physician. Schultz-Brauns[32] have reviewed the literature and reported in tabular form 150 cases which ended fatally. Most of these cases came from the inhalation of the oxides of nitrogen, in working with or in handling nitric acid. Fatal poisonings which have been produced by vapors, derived from nitric acid in contact with organic matter such as paper packing and wood filings, will be taken up under the subject of poisoning by gaseous oxides of nitrogen. Most of the cases are suicidal. Nitric acid would be difficult to administer to an adult unless he were made unconscious by drunkenness or in a deep sleep, because of the oxidizing action upon organic matter. Nitric acid is a very strong corrosive and is volatile. The symptoms produced are very similar to those of sulphuric acid. It turns the skin with which it comes in contact a yellow color, differing from strong sulphuric acid, which chars.

Properties: Pure nitric acid of the United States Pharmacopeia is a colorless, fuming, heavy liquid with a specific gravity of 1.403, containing 68% of nitric acid. It is a strong oxidizing agent, and in the presence of air and sunlight it decomposes into oxygen, water, and the oxides of nitrogen. The peroxide will contain lower oxides of nitrogen, imparting a yellow color to the acid. The commercial acid is weaker, having a specific gravity of 1.25, and is nearly always colored and fumes with an orange-colored vapor of the mixed lower oxide. It is used as an oxidizing agent, in the separation of gold and silver, and in etching and corrosion of metals. It is used in the manufacture of explosives, celluloid, photographic films, nitrobenzol, nitrophenol; in the production of dyes and drugs; in the bright dipping of copper and brass. It corrodes organic matter by oxidation, producing a deep yellow, the color of picric acid.

Symptoms: The effects of the administration of nitric acid are similar to those of sulphuric and hydrochloric acid. There is intense pain, vomiting, and thirst. The tissues are stained yellow, turning to deep orange upon the addition of ammonia. If seen several days after the nitric acid has come

32. SCHULTZ-BRAUNS: *Virchows Arch. f. path. Anat.*, 277:174, 1930.

in contact with the skin an eschar may conceal the yellow stain. The stain produced on the fingers by the acid remains for several days, gradually peeling off.

Fatal Dose: The fatal dose varies with the strength of the acid, and with the area with which the acid comes in contact. A small quantity entering the larynx would produce death from asphyxia. The fatal dose for adults is generally placed at three fluid drams.[33]

Fatal Period: Of fifty-four fatal cases in which the duration is reported, death occurred in less than three hours in five cases, or 9.2%; and during the first twenty-four hours in twenty-one cases, or 61.19%. Death may occur in a few minutes in an infant, while in an adult life may be prolonged for several years.

Treatment: The administration of chalk, milk of magnesia, and eggs as antidotes will assist in neutralizing the acid. In the absence of these use ordinary baking soda or bicarbonate of soda, a half teaspoonful to a glass of water. Have the patient rinse out his mouth thoroughly before swallowing the dilute alkali. Inasmuch as we are dealing with an acid which has great oxidizing powers it is imperative that haste be employed in using in dilute form whatever neutralizing agent is at hand. A physician seldom arrives promptly enough to retard the action of this acid by the administration of antidotes. The symptoms as they appear can be treated on general principles. Give morphine for pain, oils and mucilaginous drinks, gradually increasing the nourishment. Rectal feeding may have to be resorted to.

Postmortem Appearances: The changes are as extensive as with sulphuric acid. The stomach, esophagus, pharynx and tongue are usually yellow in color. The tissues are never as hardened as with sulphuric acid, nor do we see any charring, but the stomach, esophagus and bowel may show ulceration and sloughing, with shreds of mucous membrane. Perforation has been reported, but I have never seen such a condition.[34]

Tests: Nitric acid oxidizes all ordinary metals: it does not act upon chromium, gold, or platinum. Most of the tests for the identification of nitric acid are by deoxidation; disengaging a lower oxide, or by complete deoxidation, forming ammonia.

33: WITTHAUS and BECKER: Medical Jurisprudence, Forensic Medicine and Toxicology, IV: 297, 1911.

34. JACQUEMART: *Marseille-méd.*, 32:208, 1895.

The Brown Ring Test, for nitrates or nitric acid can be conducted in several ways. The one usually preferred is to pour into a test-tube about 2 cc. of ferrous sulphate solution, add two or three drops of the solution under examination, mix thoroughly, incline the tube, and add carefully an equal volume of concentrated sulphuric acid (best by means of a small pipet) so as to form two separate layers. Cool and let stand. At the junction of the two liquids a brown ring will form in the presence of a nitrate or nitric acid. Delicate to one part in 25,000.

The Ammonium Test: Treat the solution with KOH and aluminum wire; warm until gas is evolved. Pass the gas into water containing a few drops of Nessler's solution. A yellowish brown precipitate indicates the presence of nitric acid. Nothing interferes with this test, but the action is delayed by chlorine and many other oxidizing agents.

The Diphenylamine Test: Take 1 mg. of diphenylamine, add a few drops of water and make up to 100 cc. volume with concentrated sulphuric acid. On a porcelain dish or plate add a drop of the unknown to 0.5 cc. of the reagent; a blue color will be obtained in the presence of nitrates or nitric acid. Delicate to one part in 100,000.

The Brucine Test: To a drop of the unknown add a few mg. of brucine and 1 cc. of pure concentrated sulphuric acid. If a nitrate or nitric acid is present, a red color will develop. Upon standing, this color changes to a brown red. Delicate one to 800,000. The reagent is best prepared as 0.02 of 1% of brucine in sulphuric acid prepared just before making the test. Dilute the acid with water until it has a specific gravity of 1.4 and heat on the cover of a platinum crucible with the unknown solution, so that any nitrates will be changed to nitric acid.

Detection: Nitrates are found as constituents of a number of food materials such as bacon, ham, and corned beef, therefore the reporting of the presence of nitrates should be considered with caution. If the vomited material is acid and responds to the tests given above, one can be certain that free nitric acid is present. Stains left on clothing will be of a yellow color, intensified by ammonia water and the alkalis. If the yellow stain has been produced by tincture of iodine, the color will be discharged by potassium hydroxide or ammonia water; in a yellow stain made by acriflavine, the color is affected by ammonia water. Some of the color can be removed by soaking the fabric in water. The addition of an acid will make the solution fluorescent. The usual tests for mineral acids and the specific tests for nitric acid can be applied to the filtered solution of the stained fabric.

HYDROCHLORIC ACID (HCl)
(Synonym: Muriatic Acid, Spirits of Salt)

POISONING by hydrochloric acid is more common than by sulphuric or nitric acid (not including oxides of nitrogen). Tunik[35] reported that from 1922 to 1932 there had occurred 1,630 cases of poisoning by means of acids and alkalis in the Leningrad Hospital. Of these 250 died in the first few days; only thirteen gave a subsequent history of stenosis. Hydrochloric acid is not important from an industrial toxicological point of view. Cases of industrial poisoning observed in England, were four in 1917; ten in 1922; thirty-five in 1923; twenty-eight in 1924; thirty-five in 1925; five in 1927; three in 1929, and not any in 1930. Its irritating vapors are produced during the cleaning process of raw products. Lehmann[36] reports the maximum concentration allowable for prolonged exposures ten parts of hydrogen chloride per million parts of air. Lehmann, Kohn-Abrest,[37] and Leymann,[38] report that 1000 to 2000 parts of hydrogen chloride for even short exposure are dangerous. It has been found that hydrochloric acid causes suppurative wounds which can be prevented by immediately washing with water any part that has come in contact with the acid. Most of the cases that I have examined have been suicides, with an occasional accidental poisoning. I have never seen a case of an attempted homicide, the reason in all probability being that the strong irritative action of the acid warns the individual something is wrong. Witthaus[39] reported five alleged cases of homicides by this corrosive acid, two of the victims being adults. Accidental poisonings have occurred in children and in adults who had consumed the hydrochloric acid

35. Tunik: Anschutz W., and Seiffert, A.: *Zentralbl. f. Chir.*, 61:1504, 1934.

36: Lehmann, K.: *Arch. f. Hyg.*, 5:1, 1886.

37. Kohn-Abrest: *Ann. des Falsifications*, 8:215, 1915.

38. Leymann: *Concordia*, 13:120, 1906.

39. Witthaus and Becker: Medical Jurisprudence, Forensic Medicine and Toxicology, IV:278, 1911.

from bottles which had formerly contained "Bourbon." The severity of the intoxication depends upon the concentration of the acid.

Properties: The commercial acid is a yellow liquid containing about 32% of hydrochloric acid; and owes its color to the ferric chloride which it contains. It also frequently contains arsenic trichloride, traces of free chlorine, thallous chloride and selenium. The hydrochloric acid of the United States Pharmacopeia, contains not less than 31% and not more than 33% of hydrochloric acid, having a specific gravity of 1.155 at 25°C. It is usually prepared by the action of sulphuric acid upon sodium chloride as a by-product of soda ash. The dilute acid of the Pharmacopeia contains 10% by weight, of the anhydrous acid. The strong acid when exposed to air, forms white fumes, due to the condensation with aqueous vapor of the air. The fumes have a strong, pungent odor, and an acid taste, irrespirable, one-quarter heavier than air. If a rod is moistened with ammonia, then passed over hydrochloric acid, a dense white cloud of ammonium chloride is produced. The acid is used extensively in soldering flux, and in the pickling of iron. Hydrochloric acid reacts readily with iron and zinc in the formation of a soluble chloride, and in the evolution of hydrogen. Each bubble of hydrogen as it is evolved is coated with a film of acid which is carried into the air. The fumes from hydrochloric acid are occasionally encountered in large quantities by firemen in burning buildings containing carboys of these acids. The anhydrous gas is seldom encountered except in the course of its manufacture.

Symptoms: If only a few cc. of concentrated acid are introduced into an empty stomach, grave symptoms are produced immediately. An acute laryngeal inflammation may occur from the irritating fumes due to its volatility. The lips, tongue, and throat are at first white, later becoming a dark brown. Where the acid has been thrown back into the throat there may be no burning on the lips. The symptoms are practically the same as in the two preceding acids: instant pain in the mouth, throat, abdomen, difficult swallowing, vomiting, feeble pulse, and general weakness. The majority of the patients experience a great feeling of anxiety and fear. Dyspnea is present. The signs of absorption include nervous symptoms, such as spasms, dilatation of the pupil, fainting and motor weakness. In some cases consciousness is maintained throughout. The vomited material usually has a coffee-ground appearance. Surviving these acute symptoms the patient remains subject to bronchitis and dry pleurisy from inhalation of the fumes; or he may develop a stricture of the gullet or pylorus, with a loss of function of the stomach. Noetzel[40] reported a case of a twenty-one year old patient who had ingested a considerable quantity of hydrochloric acid. About six weeks later an x-ray showed a complete displacement of the pyloric outlet. A gastroenterostomy was performed. The patient made a complete recovery. He was seen seven years later, and was found to be in excellent condition. Anschutz and Seiffert[41] reported a case of a forty-six year old workman who drank by accident, from a beer bottle, a mouthful of 16% hydrochloric acid, four hours after a copious meal. He vomited immediately. A physician was consulted who instituted a gastric lavage and prescribed a diet. During the subsequent days, the patient experienced several attacks of hematemesis, and later his stools became bloody. About two weeks later he felt fatigued, and from then on he lost considerable weight. He vomited repeatedly, and finally was unable to ingest anything, not even liquid food. An x-ray of the stomach showed a marked constriction in the region below the cardia. This condition became much worse, and an operation was performed. It was found that the stomach had been converted into a sausage-like stricture. The stomach was opened anteriorly, and the muscularis was found to be edematous, hard and brittle. The gastric mucosa could be seen only in places. The surface was badly ulcerated and certain areas showed a brownish discoloration. A temporary duodenal fistula was made. The patient was given food through the fistula, also injections of glucose. The stenosed portions were gradually dilated by means of bougies and ten months later the fistula was closed, the patient being able to ingest food. This case is interesting because stenosis in acid poisoning is usually observed at the pylorus. Cases in which the stomach and esophagus are involved simultaneously, are not rare. Pienniz and Tunnik observed this in about 35% of their cases. Pop

40. NOETZEL, W.: *Arch. f. klin. Chir.*, 173:475, 1932: CLELAND, J. B.: *M. J. Australia*, 1:170, 1920.

41. ANSCHUTZ, W., and SEIFFERT, A.: *Zentralbl. f. Chir.*, 61:1504, 1934.

and Samondi[42] report pancreatic necrosis developing as the result of acute poisoning.

Death may occur if a few drops enter the larynx. Death may follow the rapid swallowing of a fluid dram. Stratford[43] reported a case of a young man recovering after the taking of three ounces of fuming hydrochloric acid, following a heavy meal.

Fatal Period: Death may occur in two hours or may be prolonged twenty-four hours. In two of the seventy-one cases which have been reported, death occurred in less than three hours. In the first twenty-four hours, thirty-three, or 46.5% died; during the first week 66.2%; and during the first month 80%.

Treatment: Institute the same therapy as was given for sulphuric acid (see page 62). The acid can be neutralized by magnesia, chalk, plaster, and the alkaline bicarbonates given with milk, water, or eggs. Bismuth subcarbonate with vegetable oil is very soothing to the patient after the acid has been neutralized. Treat symptomatically.

Postmortem Appearances: The pathological changes found after death are very much different from those in sulphuric or nitric acid. In many of the cases which I have seen, the stomachs were intensely red, with no darkening or hardening as reported by Noetzel. Hydrochloric acid does not stain or destroy tissues like sulphuric or nitric acid. Internally we may find in addition to the signs of intense inflammation, a shrivelled condition of the mucous membrane, which has a white or brownish color. If considerable acid had been taken, the esophageal mucous membrane and the stomach will be coated black, due to the destruction of tissue. The esophagus has been found dilated in two instances, and twice perforated.[44] The pathology that has been seen in the stomach and esophagus differs widely from that reported in most textbooks, probably owing to the fact that these people had early treatment, but died later from the effects of the poison. The stomach and bowel may be perforated, but these cases are again rare.

Tests: The free acid responds to the test given for free mineral acids. If the acid is poured upon zinc, hydrogen is

42. POP, A., and SAMONDI, G.: *Zentralbl. f. Chir.*, 58:2382, 1931.

43. STRATFORD, H.: *Brit. M. J.*, 2, 1920.

44. HEDDEN: *Tr. Path. Soc., Lond.*, 51, 84, 1889-90; GEHLE: *Berl klin. Wchnschr.*, 21:337, 1884.

evolved, and if heated with manganese dioxide, the greenish-yellow colored gas bleaches a piece of moist litmus paper suspended in the test-tube. White clouds of ammonium chloride are evolved when a glass rod wet with the acid is held near a bottle of ammonia water.

The Silver Nitrate Test: When silver nitrate test solution is added to a few drops of the suspected hydrochloric acid, a heavy, curdy, white precipitate of silver chloride will be obtained which is soluble in ammonium hydroxide, but is insoluble in nitric acid. This test is given by soluble chlorides.

The Chromium Chloride Test: Take a cubic centimeter of the distillate, neutralize with sodium hydroxide. Transfer the solid substance into a small test-tube of 2 cc. capacity. Add

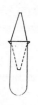

a small crystal of bichromate and two drops of sulphuric acid. Close the test-tube with a tube drawn out to a capillary as in Fig. 10. The capillary contains a liquid column of one mm. high of 1% alcoholic solution of diphenylcarbazid. Heat is applied for a few minutes. In the presence of chlorides, chromium chloride (CrO_2Cl_2) causes a violet discoloration of the reagent. This is delicate to one part in 33,000.

FIG. 10

$$K_2Cr_2O_7 + 6HCl = 2CrO_2Cl_2 + 2KCl + 3H_2O$$

If the vomited material is strongly acid, hydrochloric acid can be separated by distillation, distilling the material to nearly dryness, as hydrochloric acid does not begin to distill until the concentration is about 10%. In the absence of other acids, the distillate can be titrated with 0.1 N sodium hydroxide solution using phenolphthalein as an indicator, or it may be estimated gravimetrically. Precipitate with silver nitrate and weigh as silver chloride. Where it is desired to determine the free acid in the stomach and contents where the amount is insufficient to warrant distillation, we may then resort to a water extraction. An aliquot part of the stomach and contents is extracted three times with warm water, combining the extracts and making up to a definite volume, 250 cc. Take 100 cc. of the combined filtrates and evaporate to dryness in a porcelain dish. In a second porcelain dish place another 100 cc. making it alkaline with sodium hydroxide, and evaporate to dryness. Take up with distilled water the residue in the first dish (B) and titrate with N/10 silver nitrate, using Volhard's method. Titrate the solution of the residue from the second 100 cc. (A). The difference in the titration of A and the titration of B will give the number of cc. of N/10 silver nitrate due to the presence of free hydro-chloric acid.

Detection: As most of the cases coming to autopsy have been treated by the family physician or in the hospital, the toxicologist will rarely find the presence of free acid in the stomach. If vomited materials are submitted, care must be taken in reporting the presence of free hydrochloric acid, as the stomach normally contains 0.2% in the gastric juice.

OXALIC ACID ($C_2H_2O_4$)
(Molecular Weight 90.01. Synonym: Acid of Sugar— Salt of Sorrel)

OXALIC acid is prepared by the action of nitric acid upon sugar or starch, or by the action of an alkali hydroxide upon sawdust. It crystallizes in transparent prisms, which effloresce on exposure to air and lose water slowly, but com-pletely at 100°C. Oxalic acid and its salts are widely present in nature, being found in the dock, night shades, rhubarb (used in pies), sorrell (used for greens), and in tobacco.[45] It is used for its bleaching properties by workers in leather, marble and brass, and by makers of straw hats and bonnets. Before the sand air-blast, it was used, and is still used, for the cleaning of porcelain and brick work on buildings. Accidents occur in homes, where it remains unlabelled after some of it has been used to remove ink stains from linen, when it is taken for Epsom salts which it resembles very closely. It was commonly used for suicide, owing to the fact that it could be obtained cheaply from any pharmacist. It would be difficult to commit murder by this acid because of its taste and the rapidity of its effect. I know of no acute cases of industrial poisoning, but have been consulted in several chronic cases where it was used in cleaning marble and wood work. It is the most rapid in action of all the common poisons, and this effect is observed when the poison is given either in a dilute or a strong solution, entirely differing from the mineral acids already discussed. The effect of the poison is exerted on the central nervous system, and on the heart. Very few cases of chronic poisoning have been reported.

45. BEHRENS: *J. Landw. Verst. Sta.*, 43:271, 1894. RIDGWAY, C. S.: *J. Agric. Research, Wash.*, 7:269, 1916. SCHMUCK, A.: U. S. S. R. State Inst. Tobacco Investigations, Bull. 50 (in Russian), 1929.

Grolnick[46] reported a case of early gangrene in a painter who has used (at intervals, for two years) a solution of oxalic acid in cleaning floors. He never used rubber gloves. The gangrene began in his fingers; they became so stiff he could hardly bend them. The soft tissues of his hands and the tips of his fingers were tense. There was a sensation of numbness and the fingers felt cold to touch. His condition improved under hot Epsom salt baths, dry heat, and woolen wrappings around the hands. Howard[47] reported a second case of chronic poisoning by oxalic acid, in a man fifty-three years of age, who was employed in repair work involving the use of a strong solution of oxalic acid in cleaning automobile radiators. In this process he introduced the oxalic acid crystals through the radiator filler opening, and in doing so his fingers came in contact with the crystals of the acid. From the fingers the substance was conveyed to the mucous membranes of the nose and mouth. Vapors rising from the boiling fluid in the radiators caused him to inhale considerable amounts of oxalic acid. Initial symptoms were repeated spells of vomiting. There was rapid loss of weight. The patient coughed, raising small pieces of what appeared to be shreds of mucous membrane. He was extremely nervous and any little noise would upset him. He was unable to get out of bed, and seemed to be paralyzed from the waist down. He had a bronchial cough, and his skin was dry and pale. Potassium iodide and salicylates were given as routine treatment.

The poisonous action is due to the withdrawal of calcium from the blood, ultimately affecting the nervous system. There is usually a profound renal disturbance owing to the fact that the kidney tubules become obstructed by the insoluble calcium oxalate. Blyth has observed that the poison lasts for a long time and the kidney becomes less rich in blood. Microscopical examination shows the oxalates are increased in the kidney. Allen states that the oxalic acid in the heart, liver, kidney and urine is in combination. Taylor describes a chronic case, in which, during the first month, there was a numbness and loss of voice. He attributes that to a remote effect on the spinal nervous system. Chronic poisoning is rare; most of the cases recorded involved the swallowing of a solution of the drug.

46. GROLNICK: Industrial Toxicology, 184, 1929.
47. HOWARD, CHARLES D.: *J. Indust. Hyg.*, 14:283, 1932.

Properties: Crystals of oxalic acid are colorless, four-sided, prismatic, closely resembling the appearance of those of magnesium sulphate and zinc sulphate. Crystals are soluble in ten parts of cold water, and two and a half parts of cold alcohol; and very sparingly in ether. It can be distinguished from magnesium and zinc sulphate by heating on a platinum cover, as it sublimes without leaving any residue.

Symptoms: After ingestion of the poison there are violent stomach pains and dark masses are vomited. There is a burning in the mouth, stomach, and throat, and swallowing is difficult. The pulse becomes slow. Dyspnea and tremors occur, and the patient suffers from cramps and pains. Oxalic acid and oxalates are powerful kidney poisons, and violent pains in the kidneys are among the early symptoms. The urine contains albumin, along with casts, red cells and octahedral crystals. The secretion of urine decreases, and edema is produced. The anuria is due to a nervous disturbance affecting the excretory glomeruli, even with a good circulation.[48]

The smallest dose that has been fatal is given as one dram (3.88 gm.)[49] A dose of one-half to one ounce would be more certain to cause death than the one dram. Recovery has been reported after a dose of two ounces.[50]

Leschke,[51] reports recovery of a nineteen year old working girl who had taken twenty grains of salts of sorrel, whose stomach was washed out with lime water, and who was given copious amounts of lime water to drink. After a few days she was free from symptoms of poisoning. An unusual case of chronic poisoning was reported by Leschke in a twelve year old girl, who fell ill with head and stomach pains, had pain on passing of urine, vomited blackish-brown matter, had stiffness of the limbs and brown stains on her finger-nails. The mother had given her salts of sorrel instead of bicarbonate of soda, for several months. The internal organs were found to contain, besides oxalic acid, succinic acid, which had been formed probably as a result of disorders of the intermediate protein metabolism. If antidotes are given, recovery may be expected from much larger doses.

48. KOCH, F.: *Deutsches Arch. f. klin. Med.,* 161:100, 1931.
49. BARKER: *Lancet,* 2:1073, 1885.
50. TAPSON: *London Medical Gazette,* 1:491, 1842.
51. LESCHKE: *Clinical Toxicology,* 1934.

Fatal Period: Ogilvie[52] reported a death occurring in three minutes due to gastric hemorrhage. Witthaus[53] reports eighty-six cases, of which seventy-eight lasted less than twenty-four hours; twelve victims of this number were found dead; in eight death occurred "soon"; for seven in less than ten minutes; for nineteen in from ten to thirty minutes; for eleven in one-half to one hour; for three in two hours; for nine in from three to nine hours. Death may occur at a later period; one man lived for fourteen days after the accident.[54]

Treatment: After the diagnosis of oxalic acid poisoning is made, give intravenously one ampoule containing fifteen and one-half grains of calcium gluconate, in solution. Some soluble calcium salt should be given by mouth in order to precipitate the oxalate in an insoluble form, and the stomach should be washed out repeatedly with lime water.[55] Finely divided chalk, calcium, magnesium, and carbonate, suspended in a large quantity of water, may be given. After this the patient may be given calcium gluconate wafers, calcium lactate, or other calcium salts by mouth, to aid in the formation of the insoluble calcium oxalate.

Postmortem Appearances: There may be no stains upon the lips and face, but the tongue, throat and esophagus are white, and the mucous membrane is loose and eroded in patches. I have seen several cases where only a slight redness appeared in the mouth, and an intense redness in the stomach. Occasionally the stomach is dark red to black from extensive venous engorgement, and contains blood. The mucous membrane may be pale and smooth, or detached in shreds. Similar appearances are observed in the upper part of the small bowel. Microscopically, in the tubules of the kidney, may be found calcium oxalate crystals.

Tests: The contents of the stomach will be acid in reaction to litmus, unless alkaline therapy had been instituted. To separate the oxalic acid, make a water extract of the material, filter, and evaporate the water. Take up the residue with alcohol, making three extractions with 75, 80, and 94% alcohol. The alcohol is evaporated and the residue tested for the pres-

52. OGILVIE: *Lancet*, 2:205, 1845.
53. WITTHAUS and BECKER: Medical Jurisprudence, Forensic Medicine and Toxicology, IV:830, 1911.
54. FRASER: *Edinb. M. & S. J.*, 14:260, 1818.
55. Liquor Calcii Hydroxidi, U.S.P., XI.

ence of free oxalic acid. The material left undissolved by alcohol, in the preparation of the free oxalic acid, may contain oxalates which can be recovered by extracting with alcohol acidulated with hydrochloric acid. This alcoholic extract can be evaporated, taken up with a little water, and tested for oxalic acid, which may have been present in the form of soluble oxalates. The oxalic acid of the insoluble oxalates, in the residue from the foregoing extractions, can be obtained by boiling for two hours with a solution of potassium carbonate, evaporating the solution, and extracting the residue with alcohol, as before.

First Test: In neutral or alkaline solutions, soluble calcium salts with oxalic acid will produce a white precipitate, calcium oxalate, which redissolves in hydrochloric acid.

Second Test: Oxalic acid decolorizes a dilute solution of potassium permanganate acidified with sulphuric acid.

Third Test: Silver nitrate solution produces a white precipitate, silver oxalate, which dissolves in ammonium hydroxide solution, and also in nitric acid. The silver oxalate, collected and dried, when heated upon a platinum foil explodes with the production of a white smoke. The oxalates are all dissociated on ignition.

Fourth Test: Heated upon the cover of a platinum dish, the acid crystals slowly sublime at as low a temperature as 100° C., and disappear entirely at 150° C. By rapid heating, the acid is in part decomposed to carbon monoxide (which can also be used as a test), carbon dioxide, formic acid, and water.

Detection: The vomited matters should be searched for crystals, leaves of sorrel, or rhubarb. A person dying ten to twenty minutes after taking a crystalline salt which tasted strongly acid, having no stains upon the mouth and having symptoms of a corrosive poison would point strongly to oxalic acid. The extraction method given above would isolate the oxalic acid. For quantitative determination precipitate as calcium oxalate, determine gravimetrically or volumetrically.

Potassium binoxalate occurs in colorless monoclinic crystals soluble in forty parts of water at 15° C., slightly soluble in dilute alcohol. It is sold by druggists to remove rust and ink stains. The symptoms, treatment, and postmortem appearances are similar to oxalic acid. It gives the same tests with calcium salts and silver nitrate as oxalic acid.

CORROSIVE ALKALIS

POISONING by caustic alkalis is comparatively rare in the United States. Accidental cases were more common many years ago when it was customary in rural communities to extract lye from ashes. This crude lye was used for making soap at home and for cleaning; many children were accidentally poisoned, mistaking the lye for candy.

Those bent on self destruction have found, in the use of carbon monoxide gas from the service pipes of homes or the exhaust from an automobile, a much easier method than by way of the painful corrosive poisons. Aezul reports that in Budapest in the ten years from 1887 to 1897, out of 1,032 suicides, 415 were due to poisoning by caustic alkali. Jankovich[56] found that in Hungary between the years 1915 and 1925 there occurred nearly 3,000 cases of lye poisoning.

Properties: The common forms of potash are potassium hydroxide (KOH) in solid or solution, potassium carbonate (K_2CO_3), and pearl ash, an impure commercial product. Soda is found in commerce as sodium hydroxide (NaOH), sold in powder lumps or granules, as the carbonates (Na_2CO_3), washing soda, or as the bicarbonate ($NaHCO_3$). All of these substances are white to grayish-white in color, depending upon the purity of the product. The two hydroxides of sodium and potassium impart a soapy feeling when handled, have a soapy taste, and give a strong alkaline reaction to litmus. Both the hydroxides deliquesce rapidly in the moist state, freely taking up carbon dioxide from the air to form potassium carbonate. Potassium hydroxidum (U.S.P.) is very soluble in water, and fairly soluble in alcohol. It is used as a caustic to remove warts, and to soften epidermis in a 2% solution. Liquid potassium hydroxidum (U.S.P.), a 5% solution, is sometimes used internally as an alkali in doses of 1 cc. well diluted with water. Similar preparations of sodium hydroxide are found in the U.S.P. The hydroxides of sodium and potassium corrode the skin, while the carbonates produce inflammation and necrosis. Mild alkaline salts, such as the bicarbonates, merely soften the epithelium. The free alkalis combine with fats to form soaps, and form alkaline albuminates with tissue ele-

---

56. JANKOVICH: *Deutsche Ztschr. f. d. ges. gerichtl. Med.,* 16:352, 1930, 1931.

ments, withdrawing water from the cells, aiding in the necrosis of the tissues.

Symptoms: Large doses of the caustic soda or potash, or the carbonate, cause a soapy nauseous taste, and a burning pain in the mouth, throat and stomach. Violent vomiting may take place at once, and the vomited material may contain mucous shreds stained with blood. The mucous membranes of the mouth and adjacent tissues become white and swollen. The lips and tongue may become edematous and turn brown. Respiration is difficult, due to constriction of the pharynx. The face is extremely anxious, the pulse becomes feeble and rapid. The skin is cold and clammy. If death does not occur immediately, it may occur later from obstruction of the air passages or from starvation owing to the constriction of the esophagus, unless there is surgical intervention.

Fatal Dose: Ordinarily about one-half of an ounce (15.5 gm.) of the caustic hydroxide will cause death. Willmot reported recovery of 1.6 gm. of caustic soda from the vomited material of a woman who had taken about 60 gm. of solid soda dissolved in half a tumbler of water. Immediately after ingestion she vomited, complained of burning pain in the mouth, throat, and stomach, became exhausted, her pulse grew almost imperceptible, and twenty-nine and a half hours after the ingestion of the poison she died.

Fatal Period: Death may occur within three hours, and may be prolonged from secondary effects for weeks. Generally death occurs within twenty-four hours.

Postmortem Appearances: The lips, mouth and esophagus are very much softened, swollen and white. The mucous membranes of the stomach and intestines are dark red or black, and may be partially destroyed and disorganized in some areas. Ulcerations are quite characteristic. The stomachs all have a soapy feeling, not harsh as with the acids.

Treatment: The patient should be given immediately copious draughts of water, alone or acidulated with vinegar. Caution must be employed in the selection of an antidote so as not to use one which would increase the inflammation or chemical action already started. Diluted lemon or orange juice may be given in the absence of a weak acid such as vinegar. Milk. melted butter, salad oil, olive oil, or lard will assist in the neutralization of the alkalis, though the formation of a soap will not act as promptly as a weak acid. The pain can be controlled by the use of opiates. Stricture of the esophagus calls for surgical treatment. Threatened starvation can be treated by nutritive enemata.

Tests: Red litmus paper is turned blue by the alkalis. In the absence of ammonia, the potassium salts can be precipitates, as the chloroplatinate. Sodium salts impart an intense yellow color, which the spectroscope places at the bright D line. To a colorless flame potassium gives a violet hue, when viewed through a cobalt glass. When viewed by the spectroscope there is seen a characteristic combination of a dull-red band with a faint violet hue. Zinc uranyl acetate can be used as a microchemical reagent for sodium. A drop of the reagent is added to the unknown; a test solution gives characteristic crystals of $NaOAcZn(OAc)_2\text{-}3UO_2(OAc)_2.6H_2O$. This is a very sensitive test and can be applied in the presence of potassium, ammonia, or alkaline earth metals.[57]

Detection: The alkalinity of the gastric contents free from the odor of ammonia would point to the ingestion of one of the fixed alkalis. The alkali can be separated from the undissolved matter by dialysis, the clear liquid can be titrated with normal sulphuric acid and tested in another container for the presence of potassium by the platinic chloride test. Inasmuch as potassium is a normal constituent of food and medicine, a quantitative determination should be made. If the container of the undissolved substance can be obtained, the task of identifying the alkali is made much easier.

AMMONIUM HYDROXIDE (NH₄OH)
(Synonym: Ammonium Hydrate—Ammonia Water)

AMMONIA, being a volatile substance, differs from the preceding alkalis discussed. It is a common household article, being used in the laundry and in the softening of water. The U. S. Pharmacopeia, XI, recognizes aqua ammoniae containing about 10% by weight of NH_3; also aqua ammoniae fortior, or stronger ammonia water, containing between 27% and 29% by weight of NH_3. Both solutions lose ammonia rapidly. The latter is a colorless transparent fluid and has a very caustic and alkaline taste, having a specific

57. MALITZKII, V. P., and TUBAKAIEV, V. A.: *Mikrochemie*, 7:334, 1929. KOLTHOFF, J. M.: *Ztschr. f. anal. Chem. Wiesb.*, 70, 398, 1927.

gravity of 0.897 at 25° C. It should never be tasted or smelled unless greatly diluted. It is produced during the decomposition of nitrogenous substances. It finds extensive use in the dyes and refrigerating industries.

Symptoms: The symptoms are very much similar to those described for the fixed alkali, but not as destructive of the tissue. The respiratory passages are involved by the inhalation of the ammonia fumes. Ammonia will be taken up again under Refrigerants.

Fatal Dose: A fluid dram of the stronger ammonia water has proved to be fatal. Recovery has taken place from much larger doses, such as fifteen fluid drams.

Fatal Period: Death occurs in a few hours, or may not occur for many months, the individual finally dying of starvation due to stricture of the esophagus and the pylorus.

Treatment: Treatment consists of the administration of lemon juice, a weak solution of vinegar, vegetable oil, animal fats, or milk.

Postmortem Appearances: Postmortem appearances are never as severe as seen with the fixed caustic alkalis. There is an intense inflammation of the mouth, throat, esophagus, and stomach.

Tests: The odor is quite characteristic. Ammonia gas turns red litmus blue, and when brought in contact with hydrochloric acid causes a dense cloud of smoke. Platinum chloride yields a yellow precipitate. A dilute solution of copper sulphate is turned blue. Mercuric chloride, $HgCl_2$, forms in a solution of ammonium hydroxide or ammonium carbonate the "white precipitate" of nitrogen dihydrogen mercuric chloride NH_2HgCl.

Nessler's Test: A solution of potassium mercuric iodide, K_2HgI_4, containing also potassium hydroxide produces a brown precipitate of NHg_2I, dimercur-ammonium iodide soluble in excess of potassium iodide and HCl, not soluble in potassium bromide.

Para-Nitrodiazobenzol Test: Upon a porcelain crucible cover add a drop of the ammonia solution, and a drop of para-nitrobenzol solution in the presence of a small piece of calcium oxide. In the presence of ammonia salts a zone of red will be formed around the fragment of calcium oxide. The reagent can be prepared by dissolving 1 gm. of paranitranilin with the aid of heat in 20 cc. of water, and 2 cc. of hydrochloric acid. This is diluted to 160 cc. with shaking; after cooling, 20 cc. of a 2.5% of sodium nitrate solution are added. The reagent becomes cloudy and must be filtered each time before use.

METALS AND NON-METALS

PHOSPHORUS (P)
(Atomic Weight 31.0)

SINCE yellow phosphorus has been prohibited in the manufacture of matches, very few cases of acute or chronic poisoning occur. Occasionally, a person attempting suicide will use rat paste containing phosphorus. In one instance the phosphorus acted very slowly so the individual took illuminating gas containing 24% of carbon monoxide. Small children sometimes chew upon fireworks known as "sons of guns" and become poisoned by the phosphorus contained in them. A small boy stealing food from an icebox on a porch became an unfortunate victim of phosphorus poisoning. He picked up a piece of bologna which had been mixed with phosphorus and ate it. Death occurred within twenty-four hours. Stacy[58] reported the death of a child fifteen months old, which occurred on the fourth day following the eating of an unburned portion of certain fireworks, containing phosphorus.

Properties: There are two varieties of phosphorus, the red or amorphous which is non-poisonous, and the yellow or crystalline phosphorus which is poisonous. The yellow phosphorus must be kept under water where it becomes coated with a thin white crust, as it oxidizes readily in the air. It should be handled carefully with forceps, as painful burns can be sustained if it comes in contact with the skin. If such burns should occur, a lotion of chlorinated soda or a paste of chlorinated lime should be applied immediately. It is sparingly soluble in water, alcohol, and glycerine; ether dissolves 0.9%, while carbon disulphide dissolves ten to fifteen times its own weight. It has the odor and taste of garlic. It is never found in nature. It is found in the primitive rocks as calcium phosphate and occasionally as aluminum, iron or lead phosphates.

Ordinary phosphorus is prepared from bones. It ignites spontaneously in the air at 60° C., producing much heat. Red phosphorus is a dull carmine red and tasteless mass made by heating the ordinary form in a closed vessel without air for thirty-six hours. The red variety needs no special precaution for its preservation. The medicinal use of elementary

58. *J.A.M.A.*, 27:1514, 1921.

phosphorus has been practically dropped since the use of viosterol, and the extensive use of cod and halibut-liver oils.

Symptoms: The symptoms at first are those due chiefly to local irritants upon the stomach and intestinal tract, followed later by jaundice and profound blood changes. The patient complains of a garlic-like smell. There is pain in the throat, gullet and stomach, accompanied by vomiting and purging. If the room is dark, the breath is phosphorescent and the ejected materials will emit light when agitated in a dish. Death may occur from collapse, as in the child above referred to, but usually the irritation stops and jaundice sets in after two or three days and may continue for several weeks. If the jaundice continues the blood changes increase. The skin and the conjunctiva become yellow, and there is an increase in tenderness over the liver. Insomnia, headache and itching eruptions of the skin are common. The urine may be scanty, albuminous and bloody, containing tube casts and occasionally leucin and tyrosin, and is of a saffron yellow or olive green color. Extreme weakness may follow, resulting in heart failure due to the degeneration of the muscular tissues including the heart muscle. Delirium, convulsions, and syncope may end in death. A rare form of acute phosphorus poisoning is that in which the nervous phenomena are the most conspicuous. Many cases undoubtedly have been reported as acute yellow atrophy of the liver when the real cause was phosphorus poisoning.

Fatal Dose: A quantity as small as one-eighth of a grain has proved to be fatal; however, one and one-half grains may be considered as the fatal dose for an adult. A child is reported to have died after sucking the heads of matches containing about one-fiftieth of a grain of phosphorus. Three babies under two months of age were given five drops of oil containing phosphorus, twice in one day, dying within twenty-four hours. The analysis of the oil showed it to contain one one-hundredth of a grain of phosphorus per dose.

Fatal Period: Death may occur in less than one hour or be prolonged for many weeks. Seventy-five per cent of the cases die within one week. Formerly, phosphorus was used for suicide and as an abortifacient. Hammer[59] reports a case of a woman forty-six years of age who destroyed herself in

59. HAMMER: *Prag. Med. Wchnschr.,* 14:79, 1889.

nine hours time by swallowing about 3,000 match heads.

Treatment: The stomach may be washed out with a 1% solution of potassium permanganate, which renders the phosphorus inert by oxidation. A teaspoonful dose of animal charcoal can be administered at the same time. The stomach may also be washed out with a weak solution of copper sulphate. Three grains of copper sulphate may be used to eight ounces of wash water, adding a teaspoonful of activated charcoal to each eight ounces administered.

Postmortem Appearances: Upon opening the body the garlic smell can be noticed. The liver may be enlarged, undergoing various degrees of fatty degeneration. The kidney sections are hyperemic, and when the capsule is stripped, hemorrhagic areas are found. Microscopically, the epithelial cells and the walls of the blood vessels may be seen to be infiltrated with fat. The heart undergoes fatty degeneration. Extravasation may be seen in the tubules of the kidneys and in the endocardium.

Tests: Phosphorus may be detected easily by its phosphorescence in the dark, and in the formation of phosphine when boiled with potassium hydroxide, and by its oxidation to phosphoric acid, also in the precipitation of this acid as ammonium phosphomolybdate.

Detection: The vomited materials in the presence of much phosphorus will have a luminous appearance in the dark. The easiest way to detect it is by Mitscherlich's method. The stomach contents or portions of the organs are acidulated with sulphuric acid and put in an Erlenmeyer flask, containing portions of the vomited material, and connected to an upright Liebig condenser, three-quarters of the surface of this condenser having been painted with black asphalt paint. The Liebig condenser dips into a flask containing dilute nitric acid. The Liebig condenser is surrounded by an asbestos cabinet, the front of which has a removable window, so that when the contents begin to boil in flask A, the steam and the volatilized phosphorous will pass up B, and the condenser tube C, and be seen by the operator through the removable window in the front of the cabinet. (See Fig. 3, page 21.) If a dark room is not available a black cloth can be put over the operator's head which will make the cabinet darker and freer from shadows coming from lights in the room. There are a number of sub-

stances, such as iodine, calomel, mercury, turpentine, petroleum, creosote, ammonia, chlorine, hydrogen sulphide, and
most essential oils, which interfere with the phosphorescence.
I have been able to detect one part per million of phosphorus
in the presence of formaldehyde.

The Fresenius-Neubauer Method:[60] "Generate hydrogen
in flask A (Fig. 11) from pure phosphorus-free zinc and dilute
sulphuric acid. Fill U-tube C with pieces of pumice stone
saturated with concentrated potassium hydroxide solution to
absorb any hydrogen. Use hard glass for tube D and have

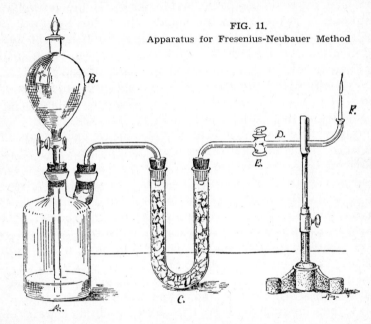

FIG. 11.
Apparatus for Fresenius-Neubauer Method

the tip F of platinum. The part marked E is a glass stop-cock
or screw tap. Reservoir B serves to hold liquid from A when
cock E is closed. A platinum tip is essential, otherwise the
flame instead of being colorless will always be yellow from
sodium in the glass. The place where the platinum tip is
fused into the glass should be cooled by wrapping cotton
around the glass and keeping it moist.

"Procedure: Open E and let hydrogen from A pass for
some time through the apparatus to expel air. Then close E

60. FRESENIUS, C. R.: Qualitative Chemische Analyse, 16th ed.,
521.

and liquid in A will rise into B. Now open E just enough to allow hydrogen to burn with a small flame which should be colorless in the dark. If there is no trace of green in the inner cone and a porcelain dish depressed upon the flame does not show an emerald green coloration, hydrogen is phosphorus-free. It is well to repeat this test. To test the silver precipitate for phosphorus, wash it with the paper into B with a little water.

"When the entire precipitate is in A, close E until all the liquid has risen from A into B. Then open E, light the hydrogen and examine the flame in the dark. If the precipitate contains a trace of silver phosphide, the inner cone will be green and a porcelain dish depressed upon the flame will show an emerald-green coloration. Have the hydrogen flame small so that its color may be observed for some time."[61]

Quantitative Estimation: The free phosphorus may be estimated in the acid distillate prepared and described in the distillate of the Mitscherlich method. Oxidizing the phosphorus with dilute nitric acid, the phosphoric acid is precipitated as the ammonium magnesium phosphate with magnesium mixture. The best method given is that of the Association of Official Agricultural Chemists,[62] in which an aliquot part of the distillate has been oxidized, and the phosphoric acid precipitated as ammonium phospho-molybdate. The precipitate, after washing with ammonium nitrate, is dissolved with ammonium hydroxide. Then neutralize with hydrochloric acid, add magnesia mixture and 10 cc. to 15 cc. of strong ammonia. Allow to stand two hours, filter, wash until chloride-free with dilute ammonium water, dry, burn at low heat then intensely to grayish-white, cool, and weigh as magnesium pyrophosphate ($Mg_2P_2O_7$). Calculate and report grains of phosphorus present.

POTASSIUM CHLORATE (KClO₃)

POTASSIUM chlorate occasionally causes poisoning. The drug acts as a gastro-intestinal irritant causing destruction of the red corpuscles and the formation of methemoglobin. There is acute pain in the abdomen, vomiting, diarrhea, and

---

61. AUTENRIETH, W.: The Detection of Poisons and Powerful Drugs (Trans. by W. H. Warren), 10, 1915.

62. Association of Official Agricultural Chemists, 20, 1935.

even collapse. This sort of poisoning is very rare in the United States.

POTASSIUM PERMANGANATE (KMnO₄)

IN THE solid state or in solution, if swallowed, it acts as a corrosive or a strong irritant, causing a gastro-enteritis. Adler[63] reported the suicide of a woman thirty-seven years of age who took 10 gm. of the solid.

BORIC ACID AND BORAX

THE potential danger of boric acid as a food preservative is such that its use has long been forbidden in the United States, France, Germany, Holland, Italy, and Spain. Great Britain has only recently prohibited its use, following a prolonged investigation of the various methods of preserving foods. Boricized milk has caused serious bowel disorders in infants. A mixture of three parts of boric acid and one part of borax has been found to be a very effective preservative for milk, butter, and meat products. Its common use in medicine, as a milk disinfectant, in washing the nose, throat, eyes, and cavities, coupled with its use in compresses, has helped very materially to create an impression of harmlessness. In 1928, I reported[64] the case of six babies, in a Chicago hospital, who died as a result of the administration, by accident, of a solution of boric acid. I had previously had for examination, the organs of a woman fifty-three years of age, who died after eating four pancakes made from flour containing 51.12% of sodium borate. Bazin[65] reported the case of a boy fifteen years of age who died after the first injection into the rectum of forty-eight teaspoonfuls of boric acid powder during a period of six days. Death occurred in seven days. Gonzales, Vance and Helperin[66] reported a patchy exfoliation of epidermis in a case of poisoning with boric acid in a baby accidentally administered by subcutaneous injection. Death after two days. Best[67] reported a fatal result from the packing of six ounces of boric acid powder into a wound after an operation. Maguire,[68] Brose,[69]

63. *Med. Klin.*, 33, 1914.
64. McNally, W. D.: *J.A.M.A.*, 90:382, 1928.
65. Bazin, A. T.: *Canad. M. A. J.*, 14:419, 1924.
66. Gonzales, Vance, and Helperin: Legal Medicine and Toxicology, 523, 1937.
67. Best, C. H.: *Tr. Chicago Path. Soc.*, 6:161, 1903.
68. Maguire, G. C.: *Practitioner*, 97:580, 1916.
69. Brose, L. D.: *Med. News*, 43:199, 1883.

Moldenow,[70] and Schurzer,[70] and Dopfer[71] report somewhat similar cases in which postmortem examinations were made. Potter[72] reported the death of an adult who took by mistake for a saline laxative, a mixture of pure boric acid. On July 29, 1937, a young man, aged twenty-three years, took a heaping teaspoonful of boric acid crystals for a laxative, vomited several times, made a complete recovery. Boric acid causes a gastro-enteritis. Schwyzer[73] reported the death from one-half ounce used as an abortifacient. A girl died in twenty-four hours having taken an unknown amount of boric acid.[74] Kahlenberg[74-A] found that boric acid when applied to the skin may be detected in the urine. Achner[75] says boric acid will appear in appreciable quantities in the urine within an hour after application to the skin. Boric acid or boracic acid (H_3BO_3) occurs as a white powder, soluble in eighteen parts of water. The average dose is eight grains (U.S.P.,XI). It is extensively used in solution as an eye lotion.

Symptoms: The symptoms of these substances are practically the same. Nausea, severe vomiting, diarrhea, signs of gastro-intestinal irritation with an irregular pulse and often raised temperature, muscular debility and collapse.[76] Wiley's experiments upon man prove that "both boric acid and borax when continuously administered in small doses for a long period or when given in large quantities for a short period create disturbances of appetite, of digestion, and of health." Before June 21, 1906, boric acid was used extensively by the packers in the preservation of chipped beef, corned beef, and other meat products.

Detection: The vomited material or portions of organs are ashed in the presence of an excess of sodium hydroxide solution in a Hoskins electric furnace at a low red heat in the usual manner. The material is extracted with hot water and the insoluble material is ashed a second time. Extract with hot water and combine the extracts. The boric acid can be assayed by titrating the free boric acid with sodium hydroxide

70. In TILLMAN: Textbook of Surgery, 7th Germ. ed., 1:162, 1901.
71. *München. med. Wchnschr.*, 52:764, 1905.
72. POTTER, CARYL: Borax Poisoning, *J.A.M.A.*, 76:378, 1921.
73. *J.A.M.A.*, 76:385, 1921.
74. *Brit. M. J.*, 1695, 1907.　74-A. *J. Biol. Chem.*, 62, 1924.
75. *J.A.M.A.*, January 20, 1917.
76. WILEY: Circ. No. 15, U. S. Dept. of Agriculture, Bureau of Chemistry, 27, 1908.

in the presence of glycerin, according to the method described in the Official and Tentative Methods of Analysis of the Association of Official Agricultural Chemists.[77] In this method hydrochloric acid is added to the extraction until the reaction is distinctly acid. Filter into a 100-cc. volumetric flask and wash with a little hot water; the volume of the filtrate should not exceed 50 to 60 cc. Return the filter containing any unburned carbon to the platinum dish, make alkaline by wetting thoroughly with lime water, dry on a steam-bath, and ignite to a white ash. Dissolve the ash in a few cc. of dilute hydrochloric acid (one to three) and add to the liquid in the 100-cc. flask, rinsing the dish with a few cc. of water. To the combined solutions, add 0.5 gm. of calcium chloride and a few drops of phenolphthalein indicator, then 10% sodium hydroxide solution until a permanent light pink color is produced, and finally dilute to the mark with lime water. Mix and filter through a dry filter. For a rough estimate of the amount of boric acid in foods and meat products, the combined extracts as prepared above can be made to a definite volume with 100 cc. hydrochloric acid and water. Five cc. can be placed in a beaker and a strip of turmeric paper allowed to dip into the beaker. Control tests can be made so that the liquid will be absorbed by the filter paper for comparison with a one-thousandth of a per cent, one-hundredth of a per cent, and one-tenth of a per cent of boric acid solution. The amount of red color developed on the turmeric paper by standing over night will, by comparison, give the approximate amount of boric acid in the unknown.

HALOGENS
FLUORINE (F)
(Atomic weight 19.05)

SODIUM fluoride (NaF) is a white powder crystallizing in colorless cubes, with a specific gravity of 2.766, which, on heating, melts at about 900° C. volatilizing slightly at a lower temperature; is of an acrid bitter taste; and is soluble one part in twenty-five parts of water. (One hundred parts saturated solution contains 4.3 gm. of NaF at 18° C.)[78] It is a general protoplasmic poison having a strong local irritant

77. Washington, D. C., 436, 1935.
78. MYLEIUS and FUNK: *Ber. d. deutsch. chem. Gesellsch., Berl.*, 30:1718, 1897.

action. It exerts an alkaloid-like action, in addition to the changes in the tissues wrought by the loss of calcium, similar to·that of oxalic acid poisoning. In the lower organisms not requiring lime, oxalic acid, in contrast with the fluorides, does not exert this alkaloid-like action.[79] One part of the salt in 200 parts of water, or one part in 500 of a fermentable liquid such as the sour mash of distilleries, stops the growth of bacteria. Tappeiner[80] believes the local and antiseptic action due to change of salts to hydrofluoric acid. It has an inhibiting action on lipase.

A small amount of fluoride is normally found in the bones and teeth.[81] The bones and teeth of dogs do not contain more than 0.3% of fluorine. The fluorine content was raised to 1.73% in bones and 1.29% in teeth, by feeding dogs sodium fluoride.[82] The diaphyses of fresh bone contain four times as much as the epiphyses.[83] Dry flat bones are poorer in fluoride than the diaphyses of long bones. Fluoride is a constant constituent of food,[84] the amount ranging from 0.059 to 13.87 mg. in 100 gm. of the dried material. Fluoride is most abundant in the leaves. The skins of the banana and apple contain more than ten times as much as the pulp. Traces of fluorides are found in potable waters.[85] Small quantities are found in the epidermis, hair, thymus, testis, blood, milk, and in all the organs.[86] Gautier[87] found from 0.57 to 8.0 mg. per 100 gm. of dried tissue, those of low vitality containing the most fluorine.

Fluorine exists in two chief forms: In the most important tissues it is combined with phosphorus in a nitrogenous organic substance, and in the epidermal tissues in an inorganic

79. Loew: *Allg. bot. Ztg.*, 94:330, 1905.

80. *Arch f. exper. Path. u. Pharmakol*, 26:108, 1890.

81. Gabried: *Ztschr. f. physiol. Chem.*, 18:261, 1894. Harms: *Ztschr. f. Biol.*, 38:487, 1899.

82. Sonntag, G.: *Arb. a. d. k. Gesellsch.*, 50:307, 1916; *Chem. Zentralbl.*, 50:1095, 1916.

83. Gautier and Clausman: *Compt. rend. Acad. d. sc.*, 156:1425, 1913.

84. Gautier and Clausman: *Compt. rend. Acad. d. sc.*, 162:105, 1916.

85. Charles: *Rev. chim. applicado*, 4:181, 1919. Gautier and Clausman: *Compt. rend. Acad. d. sc.*, 158:1389, 1631; 1914.

86. Kickton and Belinke: *Ztschr. f. nahr. Genuss*, 20:193, 1910.

87. Gautier, A.: *Compt. rend. Soc. de biol.*, 76:107, 1914; *Compt. rend. Acad. d. sc.*, 156:1425, 1913.

combination with phosphorus resembling apatite. Zdarek[88] determined fluorine gravimetrically as calcium fluoride in the ash of the organs of two healthy men accidentally killed, the kidney, liver and spleen containing the greatest amounts. The kidney contained 1.34 and 1.54 mg., the spleen 0.82 and 2.35 mg., and the liver 0.68 and 0.80 mg., respectively, per 100 gm. of dried tissue. The fresh blood of one patient contained 0.21 mg. in 100 gm. Sodium fluoride is used as a wood preservative;[89] with sulphuric acid it is used in the etching of glass; also as a food preservative,[90] and as an insecticide.[91] The amount of sodium fluoride varies from 16% to 63.6% in roach powders. It is in the latter connection that we are chiefly interested from a toxicological standpoint. Hydrofluoric acid has been responsible for several deaths and many serious cases of poisoning. In 1801 an Italian named Morchini found fluorine for the first time in the enamel of the teeth and the bones. In 1887 Tammann, Brandl, and then Tappeiner, found it in the organs of the human body. This was followed by the work of Jodlbauer,[92] who attempted to estimate fluorine, but the method he used was not reliable. The first reliable work along this line was done by Armand Gautier,[93] who discusses the sources from which fluorine was derived and introduced into the organism, its assimilation, and the formation.

Horsford[94] reported the presence of fluorine in the brain. Later Gay-Lussac and Berthollet[95] found fluorine in the enamel of normal teeth. Zdarek[96] studied the distribution of fluorine with reference to the human organs. Gautier and Clausman[97] in 1913 reported the fluorine content of these same materials, coming to the conclusion that fluorine substances are

88. ZDAREK, E.: Ztschr. f. phys. Chemie, 69:127, 1910.

89. TEESDALE, R. S.: Forest Prod. Wood Preserving, 3:80, 1916; 4:6, 1917.

90. BLOXAM: Chem. Ztg., 1244, 1893.

91. EFRONT: Compt. rend. Acad. d. sc., 18:1420, 1894.

92. JODLBAUER, A.: Arch. f. exper. Path. u. Pharmakol., 164:127, 1910.

93. GAUTIER, A.: Compt. rend. Acad. d. sc., 158:167, 1914.

94. HORSFORD, E. N.: Am. Chem. Pharm. Bd., CXLIX:S. 202, J. B. 815, 1869.

95. Ann. de chimie, IV (series 1): 258, 1805.

96. ZDAREK, E.: Ueber die Verteilung des Fluors in den einzelnen Organen des Menschen, Ztschr. f. phys. Chemie, 69:127, 1910.

97. Compt. rend. Acad. d. sc., 157:94, 1913.

in greater or lesser amounts in the diaphyses of bones and in the epidermis, hair, thymus gland, testis, and blood in the hemispheres of the brain. The author speaks of a definite P/F ratio for any given organ. Within one and the same organ the fluorine varies much with age. The gray matter of the brain contains about as much fluorine as the white matter, and the medulla oblongata seems to be richer in fluorine than the rest of the cerebral matter. The fluorine intake usually exceeds one milligram per day. According to Steinkoenig,[98]

TABLE VI
FLUORINE CONTENT OF ORGANS, EXCRETIONS, ETC.

Organ, Excretion, etc.,	Milligrams of fluorine per 100 grams organ (or excreta)	
	Fresh	Dried
Brain, adult	0.71	3.07
(newborn)	0.18	1.70
Thymus (newborn)	2.60	11.11
Thyroid gland	0.54	2.12
Testis	0.82	4.24
Lungs	0.44	2.44
Liver, adult	0.64	2.13
(newborn)	0.37	1.19
Kidney	0.26	0.95
Muscle	0.16	0.57
Heart (newborn)	0.19	0.45
Blood	0.46	2.30
Milk (aver. observed in four normal women)	0.048	0.38
Feces	0.42	1.48
Urine	0.018	0.41

fluorine in soil amounts to about 0.03%. Phosphate rock contains 2.62%. Carles[99] found mineral water to contain 0.0001 to 0.018%. Gautier and Clausman obtained values for bone, varying from 17.5 gm., and 123.0 mg. F per 100 gm. of ash. The table (Table VI) refers only to human organs and gives the amount of fluorine found per 100 gm. of organ.

The Panhandle, West-Texas, region constitutes the largest mottled enamel area in the United States.[100] Smith, Lantz and Smith[101] reported that the mottled teeth in humans in

98. STEINKOENIG, L. A.: J. Indust. & Eng. Chem., 11:463, 1919.
99. CARLES, P.: Compt. rend. Acad. d. sc., 144:37, 1907.
100. DEAN, H. T., DIXON, R. M., and COHEN, C.: Reprint No. 1678, Pub. Health Reports, No. 13, 50:424, 1935.
101. SMITH, M. C., LANTZ, E. M., and SMITH, H. V.: Arizona Agricultural Experiment Sta. Technical Bull., No. 32, June 10, 1931.

certain areas in Arizona were caused by an excess of fluorides in the water. They found that the water contained 3.8 to 7.15 mg. fluorine per liter. Gautier and Clausman[102] estimate a daily excretion of fluorine by man of 1 mg. per day. They found a loss of fluorine in the hair, nails and epidermis. I have advanced the theory that the presence of fluorides in the blood accounts for the formation of fibrous tissue from inhaled silica and strengthens the opinion previously rendered that silicosis is caused by a chemical action rather than by traumatic action. A government rule should be made to regulate the amount of fluorides in water, beer, fruits, and foods, as harmful amounts may be found in any of these products. The work of Clifford[103] indicates the effect of fluorides on the enzymatic decomposition of starch. It is known that fluorides do not prevent a decrease in glycogen of muscle pulp undergoing fermentive changes, but do prevent the formation of lactic acid.[104] Fluorides also inhibit alcoholic fermentation by yeast.[105] Dickens and Simer[106] have confirmed the essential facts brought out by Lipmann, and conclude in part that fluoride forms an inactive compound with some substance essential for glycolysis. Jacoby[107] first observed that fluorine inhibits the reaction of urease. Subsequent research[108] by this investigator has brought out the following facts regarding the urease effect: (1) Fluorine is most effective at optimum conditions for enzymic reactions; (2) it is most active against urease in acid solution; (3) the effect is more pronounced in buffered solutions on account of the reaction being influenced by the ammonia formed in the hydrolysis; (4) the fluorine effect cannot be duplicated with oxalic or citric acids; (5) iodine salts are also very active against urease. (For dichloro-difluoro methane see Refrigerants.)

Hydrofluoric acid has been therapeutically used for the treatment of pulmonary tuberculosis. Various observers report cases of healing, or at least improvement, and report these

102. *Compt. rend. Acad. d. sc.,* 157:94, 1913.
103. CLIFFORD, W. M.: *Biochem. J.,* 19:218, 1925.
104. LANG, H.: *Ztschr. f. physiol. Chem.,* 137:105, 1924. DAVENPORT, H. A., and CATONIO, M.: *J. Biol. Chem.,* 72:463, 1927. EULER, H., and CRAMER, H.: *Biochem. Ztschr.,* 60:25, 1914.
105. LIPMANN, F.: *Biochem. Ztschr.,* 196:3, 1928.
106. DICKENS, F., and SIMER, F.: *Biochem. J.,* 23:936, 1929.
107. JACOBY, M.: *Biochem. Ztschr.,* 74:107, 1916.
108. JACOBY, M.: *Biochem. Ztschr.,* 198:163, 1928; 214:368, 1929.

due to the germicidal action of the acid. Other authors have investigated this problem, but without any marked success. In 1897 Kobert[109] found that the addition of solutions of sodium fluoride to methemoglobin forms fluormethemoglobin, which is a little more red than methemoglobin, having a characteristic absorption spectrum in the orange, and a second one in the blue which is more difficult to see. Bloxam[110] in 1893 used sodium fluoride as a food preservative, and as an insecticide. Tammann[111] found in 102 gm. of fresh egg yolk 0.0023 gm. of potassium fluosilicate corresponding to 0.012 gm. of fluorine. According to Zaleski, bone contains 0.23% of fluorine. In 189 gm. of the fresh brain of a thirty day old calf, analysis showed the presence of 0.0027 gm. of potassium fluosilicate corresponding to 0.0014 gm. of fluorine. One liter of cow's milk was ashed with 5 gm. of potassium fluosilicate corresponding to 0.0004 gm. of fluorine; in another case it yielded 0.0006 gm. corresponding to 0.0003 gm. of fluorine. The salts of hydrofluoric and fluosilic acid are poisonous to plants. Hydrofluoric acid (HF) is a colorless, intensely corrosive gas, soluble in water, reddens litmus paper and corrodes glass, porcelain, and the metals, except platinum and gold.   Both the solution and its vapors act on the skin as an insidious and virulent caustic, causing painful wounds and obstinate ulcers. The anhydrous acid at 25° C. has a vapor density of 20, indicating that the molecule at that temperature is H_2F_2. In the production of acid phosphates for fertilizing, large amounts of this acid are produced and cause severe irritation of the air passages in men mixing the sulphuric acid with the phosphate rock. The fumes coming from the mixture of the sulphuric acid and the phosphate rock are carried for blocks in such a concentration that the windows of buildings are etched. Where the acid has come in contact with the skin it should be immediately washed with ammonia or lime water. Inhalation of ammonium vapors will assist in the mixing of the irritant when the acid fumes have been inhaled. The inhaled fumes have been responsible for four deaths.[112] Huppert re-

109. KOBERT: Kompendium der Toxocologie, 5th ed., 205, 1912.
110. *Chem. Ztg.*, 1244, 1893.
111. TAMMANN, G.:   Ueber das Vorkommen des Fluors in den Organismen, *Ztschr. f. phys. Chemie*, 12:322, 1888.
112. KING: *Tr. Path. Soc. Lond.*, 24:98, 1873. STIMSON: *Brit. M. J.*, 2:1145, 1899. WITTHAUS: Man. Toxic., 309, 1911.

ported a case of poisoning in a worker in a mineral water factory who drank etching liquid. He died within an hour.[113] Exposure to concentrations of hydrogen fluoride above 1.5 mg. per liter for any period of time is dangerous for rabbits and guinea pigs.[114]

Sodium fluorosilicate ($SiFNa_2$), when added in excess as a preservative of food causes nausea, eructation, vomiting, and a slow pulse. Sodium fluosilicate ($NaSiF_6$) is an easily crystallizable substance and has a remarkably high density; it dissolves in water at room temperature to the extent of 0.66%. The solutions have an acid reaction; one molecule of the salt is neutralized by four molecules of sodium hydroxide, using phenolphthalein as the indicator. Hence the following equilibrium is established in aqueous solution:

$$Na_2SiF_6 + 2H_2O \rightleftarrows 2NaF + SiO_2 + 4HF$$

Wieland and Kurtzahn[115] found that the lethal dose of sodium fluosilicate was between 0.074 and 0.149 gm. per kilo weight of the animal, corresponding to 0.045 and 0.09 gm. of F respectively per kilo weight. When the sodium fluosilicate comes in contact with hydrochloric acid of the stomach, undissociated hydrochloric acid is formed, penetrating the mucosa.

Symptoms: Schultz,[116] and Schwyzer,[117] found that there was a loss of chlorine and calcium in the bones following the intramuscular injection in animals of from 1 to 2 mg. of fluorine per kilogram of weight. Schultz found that subcutaneous injections of sodium fluoride acted on the central nervous system, and that a paralysis of the brain and of the spinal cord occurred. Rabbits dusted daily with a mixture of one-half ounce of sodium fluoride and five pounds of fine silica dust suffer loss of weight, a stiffness of the vertebral column and finally a spinal cord paralysis. One hundred mg. of calcium fluoride produce a marked trembling of the whole body in man after intravenous injection.*

The symptoms depend upon the size of the dose. In man

113. *Deutsches Ztschr. f. d. ges. gerichtl. Med.*, 8:424, 1926.
114. MACHLE, W., THAMANN, F., KITZMILLER, K., and CHOLAK, J.: *J. Indust. Hyg.*, 16:129, 1934.
115. WIELAND, H., and KURTZAHN, G.: Zur. Kenntnis der Fluorwirkung, *Arch. f. exper. Path. u. Pharmakol.*, 97:489, 1923.
116. *Arch. f. exper. Path. u. Pharmakol.*, 21:326, 1889.
117. SCHWYZER, F.: *Biochem. Ztschr.*, 60:32, 1914.
* SIMONIN and PIERRON: *Compt. rend Soc. de biol.*, 124:133, 1937.

there is vomiting, diarrhea, salivation, shallow, rapid and difficult respiration, convulsive seizures with tonic and clonic spasms, deep sleep and cyanosis; the pulse is small and rapid. The face is covered with a cold, clammy perspiration; the sweat may contain sufficient amounts of fluoride to cause a burning sensation on the face of a second person who has come in contact with it.[118] The disturbance of calcium metabolism causes a severe damage of the vasomotor and respiratory centers with subsequent death by respiratory failure.   In chronic poisoning the mottling of the teeth has been reported by Smith, Lantz, and Smith.[119]

Dean, Sebrell, Breaux, and Elvove[120] report that as little as twenty-five parts per million of sodium fluoride in the drinking water of white rats produces changes in the teeth which are manifested by minute, transverse, brown striations. When 150 parts per million are used, the striations lose their uniformity and become irregular brown patches. If 300 parts per million of sodium fluoride are used, the teeth become creamy in color, and no striations are seen. If 500 parts per million are used, some of the animals die and the teeth of the survivors become white, chalky, and very brittle.[121]

Fatal Dose: Jodlbauer[122] found that in fluoride intoxications the calcium content of the blood plasma diminishes. This decrease in blood calcium is greater in acute (but not fatal) intoxication and less in chronic (but fatal) intoxication; the calcium decrease in acute fluoride poisoning with fatal outcome amounted to 50%, in chronic fluoride poisoning to 13%. Christiani and Gautier[123] noted that in these cases which

118. McNally, W. D.: *J.A.M.A.*, 81:811, 1923.
119. Smith, M. C., Lantz, E. M., and Smith, H. V.:   Arizona Agricultural Experiment Sta. Technical Bull. No. 32, June 10, 1931.
120. Dean, H. T., Sebrell, W. H., Breaux, R. P., and Elvove, E.: Pub. Health Reports, 49:37, 1075, 1934.
121. Sebrell, H., Dean, H. T., Elvove, E., and Breaux, R. P.: Pub. Health Reports, 48:437, 1933. Bergara, Carlos: *Compt. rend. Soc. de biol.*, 97:600, 1927.
   Chaneles, Juan: Talleres Graficos Ferrari Hnos., Buenos Aires, 1930.
   McClure, F. J., and Mitchell, H. H.:   *J. Biol. Chem.*, 90:297, 1931.
   Pierle, C. A.:   *J. Am. Dent. A.*, 13:999, 1926.
   Smith, M. C., and Lantz, E. M.:   *J. Biol. Chem.*, 101:677, 1933.
   Eager: U. S. Pub. Health Reports, 16:25, 1901.
122. Jodlbauer, A.:   *Arch. f. exper. Path. u. Pharmakol.*, 164:464, 1932.
123. Christiani, H., and Gautier, R.:   *Compt. rend. Soc. de biol.*, 92:946, 1925.

were following a subacute course the general symptoms appeared more rapidly and were more severe, except the loss of weight, which was less pronounced. Meanwhile one could easily discover a cachectic state in those cases where death occurred during the third week; in these cases one could easily notice a few days before the death of the animal a peculiar posture referable to stiffness of the vertebral column and extremities, particularly the posterior ones. Death occurred following medullary and spinal symptoms, difficulty of respiration, muscular rigidity, tremors and convulsions. I found the same in rabbits which were being dusted with silicon dioxide and sodium fluoride. The fatal dose is about 0.5 grains per kilogram of body weight when taken by mouth, and about 0.015 grains per kilogram when injected intravenously in mammals. Using white rats I found the lethal dose to be 0.1 grains of the chemically pure sodium fluoride per kilogram weight when given by mouth, death being delayed from eight to twenty-six hours. Schultz[124] found that when subcutaneously injected, the lethal dose for rabbits was 0.2 to 0.4 gm.; for dogs, 0.3 gm; for frogs, 0.005 gm. Heidenhain[125] found from 0.05 to 0.10 gm. per kilogram of weight to be fatal to dogs when injected into the blood stream. Weinland[126] found that sodium fluoride in 2.10% strength killed the mucous membrane from the throat of a frog in one minute; sodium iodide, 7.5% in ten minutes; sodium bromide, in forty-five minutes; sodium chloride, 2.9% in sixty minutes. Grutzner,[127] using equimolecular proportions of the foregoing salts, found the same order of sensitiveness for nerves. Czrellitzer,[128] reviewing the work of others, concludes that sodium fluoride is an active poison for micro-organisms of all kinds, algae, nerves, and muscles of the higher organisms.

Elimination: The insoluble calcium fluoride formed by it is stored in the liver, skin and other tissues. Masses of these crystals accumulating in the bones impair their nutrition and make them whiter, harder, and more brittle. Gautier claims that 1 mg. is eliminated per day.

124. SCHULTZ: *Arch. f. exper. Path. u. Pharmakol.,* 25:236, 1889.
125. HEIDENHAIN: *Arch. f. d. ges. Physiol.,* 56:579, 1894.
126: WEINLAND: *Arch. f. d. ges. Physiol.,* 58:105, 1894.
127. GRUTZNER: *Arch. f. d. ges. Physiol.,* 53:83, 1892.
128. CZRELLITZER: Zur Kentniss des Fluornatrium, Inaug. Dies., Breslau, 1895.

Fatal Period: Hickey[129] records the death of a girl, aged ten years, who was given one teaspoonful of sodium fluoride by mistake for potassium and sodium tartrate, and died in one hour. In case No. 3 which I reported,[131] death occurred in three quarters of an hour. Death usually occurs within eight hours. Baldwin[130] has reported a number of cases of poisoning and death from accidental ingestion of sodium fluoride. In one case, a man ate three or four pancakes prepared by using a roach powder in mistake for baking powder. Death occurred within twelve hours. The fatal dose was estimated at 10 gm. In 1923 I reported four cases of fluoride poisoning, three accidental and one with suicidal intent.[131]

CASE No. 1. C.Y., a woman, aged fifty-nine, made an omelet on February 16, 1921, using an unknown amount of roach powder in place of starch. A few minutes later, at 6:30 P.M. she complained of a chilly feeling and weakness. There were no gastro-intestinal symptoms. She died at 10:00 P.M. Necropsy on the embalmed body gave no noteworthy alterations in the organs of the thorax and abdomen, except in the stomach and bowel. The stomach walls were edematous, with areas of congestion and small hemorrhages. The mucosa of the small bowel was congested and edematous. A chemical examination of the organs demonstrated the presence of sodium fluoride. The powder used for starch contained 63.64% of sodium fluoride.

CASE No. 2. M.C., a woman, aged forty-five, took from 4.5 to 5 gm. of a white powder for a laxative at 3:00 P.M. on February 5, 1923. In a few minutes she was found in the bathroom, complaining of nausea and cramps. There was an excessive thirst. She complained of muscular weakness, and was unable to walk. There was vomiting of bloody fluid, diarrhea, paralysis of the facial muscles, and loss of speech. A physician was not called until 5:00 o'clock. The patient died at 7:00, four hours after the poison was taken. The cause of death on the burial certificate was given as carcinoma. Six weeks later the body was exhumed, and no evidence of carcinoma was found. The gross pathologic changes were similar to those recorded in the preceding necropsy. A chemical examination of the organs re-

129. HICKEY: Bull. Massachusetts Board of Health, 341, 1911.
130. BALDWIN: J. Am. Chem. Soc., 21:517, 1899.
131. McNALLY, W. D.: J.A.M.A., 81:811, 1935.

vealed the presence of sodium fluoride as shown in Table VII.

CASE No. 3. A.C., a woman, aged thirty-six, sister of the preceding patient, took 17 gm. of the same laxative in a glass of water at 7:00 P.M., March 14, 1923. The taste was bitter and caused a severe burning, pain, and a feeling of nausea. Within five minutes severe vomiting occurred; in ten minutes, the patient was moaning, with great pain over the whole abdomen; she became very pale, and then purple spots appeared on the

TABLE VII

PRESENCE OF SODIUM FLUORIDE IN FOUR CASES

	Case 1	Case 2	Case 3	Case 4
Stomach	0.0329	0.2432	0.2096	0.1343
Liver	0.0056	0.0154	0.2524	----------
Kidney	Trace	R0.1306 L0.1234	0.0712	----------
Bowel	0.0218	0.2388	0.4864	----------
Bowel content	----------	0.0094	----------	----------
Spleen	----------	0.2354	----------	----------
Pancreas	----------	Negative	----------	----------
Blood	----------	0.1446	----------	----------
Lung	----------	0.1560	----------	----------
Heart	----------	0.1946	----------	----------

face. Ptyalism was noted. The lower extremities became paralyzed, with simultaneous loss of speech. Excessive cold perspiration was wiped off the face by a sister, who put the same handkerchief to her face and noted a burning sensation. The fluoride was probably excreted in the sweat. The vomitus was bloody. There was great thirst, the same as in Case No. 2. Death occurred in three-quarters of an hour. Gastric lavage, syrup of ipecac and 1/10 grain of apomorphine were used for treatment.

A postmortem showed that there were no external visible marks of violence on the body. The lungs presented an acute edema. The heart grossly was without changes of note. The liver, spleen, pancreas, suprarenals and urinary bladder presented no gross changes. The gastric mucosa was hemorrhagic, the wall edematous and the mucosa in part necrotic. The mucosa of the duodenum and the jejunum was edematous. The stomach contained about 100 cc. of turbid, sanguineous fluid of an alkaline reaction.

A chemical examination of the stomach, liver, kidneys, and bowel showed the presence of sodium fluoride. The white substance in a wrongly labelled bottle contained 90% of sodium fluoride.

CASE No. 4. A.S., a woman, aged nineteen, took two tea-spoonfuls of a rat poison with suicidal intent. A severe burning pain in the stomach, vomiting, diarrhea, with muscular para-lysis and loss of speech, occurred as in the previous cases. An examination of the principal organs of the thorax and abdomen gave evidence of congestion and marked hyperemia. The stomach walls were edematous, with a few small scattered hemorrhages. A chemical examination of the stomach gave tests for sodium fluoride.

Huppert[132] records a case of poisoning in a worker in a mineral water factory who drank etching liquid. He died in an hour without special clinical phenomena being noted. The mucous membrane of the pharynx, esophagus, stomach, duo-denum, and jejunum was of a grey color, and swollen. Luhrig,[133] reported two fatal cases of poisoning by silico-fluoride common-ly sold as insect powder. In one of these, half a teaspoonful of the salt was taken by mistake. Fluorine was found in various organs, including the kidneys and liver. Criminal poisonings by this agency are very rare. Sedlmeyer, however,[134] reported a case of criminal poisoning, when a wife gave rat poison to her husband, aged twenty-nine. He became ill with nausea, vomit-ing, and general exhaustion. Death occurred from paralysis of the respiratory muscles and cardiac insufficiency. For com-prehensive review see the monograph by Chaneles,[135] who quotes 215 papers with the review of fluorine and its physio-logical effects.[136] Flamm reports the death of a twenty-two year old man who took a mouthful of "Montanin" which had been kept in a beer bottle. He complained of cramp-like pains in the abdomen, of a burning sensation in the pharynx and esophagus; he also vomited and passed diarrheic stools, and showed vasomotor disturbances. The stomach was washed out and oxygen was administered. He was seized with tonic and clonic spasms and became cyanotic; the respiration was shallow

132. HUPPERT: *Deutsche Ztschr. f. d. ges. gerichtl. Med.*, 8:424, 1926.

133. LUHRIG: *Chem. Ztschr.*, 49:805, 1925.

134. SEDLMEYER: *Deutsche Ztschr. f. d. ges. gerichtl. Med.*, 15:369, 1930.

135. CHANELES, J.: Estudios sobre el Fluor, Buenos Aires, 1930.

136. CHANELES, J.: *Compt. rend. Soc. de biol.*, 102:860, 1929.

and rapid; the pulse was small and rapid, and he died four days after the accident.[137] Wirthlin reported a death occurring two and a half hours from drinking water containing a half-pound of sodium fluoride.

Treatment: In suspected cases of poisoning, the soluble sodium salt may be rendered inert by conversion to the insoluble calcium fluoride by copious and repeated gastric lavage with lime water or a weak solution of calcium chloride. Calcium gluconate should be given intravenously immediately after washing out the stomach. All insecticides containing fluoride powders should be covered with a 10% lampblack or other coloring matter and be distinctly labelled "Poison," giving the name and amount of the fluoride present. This would assist the doctor in diagnosis, and prevent accidental poisoning.

Postmortem Appearances: In Flamm's case[137] the palpebral conjunctiva showed a bluish discoloration, the vessels were highly injected, and there were pin-point petechiae. Case No. 3 (page 101), where postmortem findings are reported, is typical of this type of poisoning. The gastric mucosa was hemorrhagic and the mucosa of the duodenum and the jejunum was edematous. Microscopically, the kidney showed extensive and severe parenchymatous degeneration. The epithelium of the uriniferous tubules is not extensively necrotic, and blood cells may be found within the tubules. The histologic examination includes changes of the gastric mucosa but very rarely changes in the muscularis or in the serosa. The blood vessels are very much dilated, hemorrhages are numerous, particularly between the gastric glands, and in very severe cases the cells of these glands show marked changes. The results of experimental investigations show conclusively that there is a disturbance of calcium metabolism which causes a severe damage of the vasomotor and respiratory centers with subsequent death by respiratory failure.

Detection: Fluorine is a normal constituent of animal tissues, especially of the bones and teeth. Quantitative determination should always be made on this account. In the last few years there has been a great deal of work done on the quantitative determination of fluorine. Brunnig and Quast recommend the etching test for the detection of fluorine con-

137. FLAMM, M.: *Deutsche Ztschr. f. d. ges. gerichtl. Med.*, 22:21, 1935. And for WIRTHLIN: see *U. S. Nav. Med. Bull.*, 35:255, 1937.

ducted as follows:[138]   25 gm. of the finely divided material
are kneaded in a suitable nickel crucible with 10 cc. of lime
water (50 gm. CaO per liter of water); 10 cc. of a 10% solution of copper sulphate is added, and the mass is well stirred.
The mixture is then dried and ashed, a process which requires
about fifteen minutes, provided there is no large amount of fat
present. In order to insure a more rapid combustion, heat may
be also applied from above. The red-hot contents of the crucible
may also be blasted, inasmuch as the cupric oxide forms a solid
mass.   The residue is now transferred into a small platinum
crucible and is moistened with dilute sulphuric acid, about 1
cc. being sufficient.   After cooling, 5 cc. of concentrated sulphuric acid are added, cautiously and gradually, and after each
addition the crucible is immediately covered with a shellacked
(not paraffinized) watch glass. The shellac film on the watch
glass must be dry and must have been suitably prepared before
use.

The platinum crucible is now heated over a small flame.   In
one to one and one-half hours the test is usually completed.
The watch glass is freed from the shellac layer by washing it
in chloroform, and is then carefully examined.   In this connection it is well to bear in mind that small quantities of fluorine
yield an etching which it not always easily recognizable.   The
etched portion is best examined with a hand lens, and the watch
glass should be held against a light and dark background
(window frame, for example); with this method lines as fine as
hair may be detected. Willard and Winter[139] use the following
procedure for determining fluorine: Ash the organs in a
platinum dish, place the ash in a small distilling flask, and add
a few glass beads or pieces of porous plate, 5 cc. of 60% perchloric acid, and sufficient water to cause the solution to boil at
100°C. or less.   Place the flask on an asbestos mat with an opening large enough so that about one-third of the flask will be
exposed to the flame.   Close with a two-hole rubber stopper
through which pass a thermometer and a capillary tube, both
of which extend down into the liquid.   Connect a dropping
funnel with the capillary tube so that water may be added dur-

138. Brunnig, A., and Quast, H.:   Ztschr. f. ang. Chemie, Berl.,
44: 656, 1931.
139. Willard, H. H., and Winter, O. B.:   Volumetric Method for
Determination of Fluorine, Indust. & Eng. Chem., 5: 7, 1933.

ing the process of distillation, and fill this with water. Connect the flask with a water condenser. The distillate may be collected in an open container. Distill until the boiling point of the solution reaches 135°C. and hold at about that temperature by allowing water to run into the flask from a dropping funnel, until all of the fluorine has been volatilized. This is usually accomplished by distilling over 50 to 75 cc. Add six drops of the zirconium-alizarin mixture and dilute sodium hydroxide drop by drop until the color of the indicator appears. Add an equal volume of ethyl alcohol, and then dilute acid until the color of the indicator just about disappears (at this point it is advisable to cause the color to appear and disappear two or three times so as to be sure of having the solution only very slightly acid). Titrate with thorium nitrate as previously directed under the determination of soluble fluorides. The test described by these authors is carried out as follows: (a) determination in soluble fluorides with no interfering elements, i.e., any ion which forms a precipitate or non-dissociated salts with fluorine or with thorium such as calcium, barium, ferric, aluminum, and phosphate ions.

The reagents used for determining fluorine in solution when no interfering elements are present are as follows:

1. Zirconium nitrate: 1 gm. of Zr $(NO_3)_4.5H_2O$, in 250 cc. of water.

2. Alizarin red: 1 gm. of sodium alizarin sulphonate in 100 cc. of ethyl alcohol. Filter off the undissolved residue and add 150 cc. of ethyl alcohol to the filtrate. The two solutions are kept in stock and mixed, three parts of (1) and two parts of (2) as needed. The color should be violet-red when mixed.

3. Thorium nitrate solution, standardized against a known fluoride solution.

4. Standard fluoride solution, lithium fluoride, 0.02 N solution or a specially purified sodium fluoride of the desired concentration.

5. HCl, approximately one to fifty.

Dissolve a weighed amount of the fluoride in water and make up to a given volume. Transfer an aliquot of the solution to be analyzed to a small tall-form beaker, add water to make a volume of approximately 20 cc. and three drops of zirconium-alizarin mixture. If necessary, add just enough dilute HCl to destroy the color. Add an equal volume of neutral ethyl alcohol, and titrate over a white surface in good light with the standard thorium nitrate to a faint permanent reappearance of color. The reaction is slow near the end point. When titrating with 0.01 N thorium nitrate, make a correction for the fluorine which combines with the indicator. Determine this by titrating the number of drops of indicator used in the titration with 0.01 N fluoride solution to the disappearance of the color. The maximum error is approximately 4%.

Other methods have been described for the colorimetric estimation of fluorine based on the bleaching action exerted by fluorine. Quantities of 0.01 to 0.02 mg. of fluorine can be determined using Nessler tubes for the comparison. Mayrhofer, Schneider, and Wasitsky[140] describe an indirect method by colorimetric means in which silicomolybdic acid is formed and upon the addition of hydroquinone a blue color is obtained. The color intensity usually reaches its maximum after about one hour and remains unchanged for an additional hour.

De Boer[141] describes a colorimetric method for hydrofluoric acid using zirconium salt mixed with alizarin in which the red color of the reagent is turned yellow by the presence of hydrofluoric acid.[142]

Smith and Dutcher,[143] recommend the zirconium-quinalizarin reagent in which the fading of the color of the zirconium-quinalizarin is a function of time, temperature and acidity. After fifteen minutes at room temperature the change is very slow and the color remains sufficiently constant for comparisons. Kolthoff and Stansby[144] used the purpurin-zirconium test; a colorimetric method that can be used for quantities of fluorine between 0.01 and 0.05 mg. is also described which is accurate to 0.002 mg. of fluorine. The fluorine is separated by the "distillation method." The fluoride is distilled off as silicon tetrafluoride, which is collected in the pink purpurin-zirconium reagent. The distillation apparatus consists of a wide-mouth

140. MAYRHOFER, A., SCHNEIDER, C., and WASITSKY, A.: *Biochem. Ztschr.*, 251:70, 1932.

141. DEBOER, J. H.: *Chem. Weekbl., Amst.*, 404, 1924; *Chem. Zentralbl.*, 1:133, 1925.

142. See also *Chem. Analyst*, 20:14, 1931.

143. SMITH, O. M., and DUTCHER, H. A.: *Indust. & Eng. Chem., Analytical Ed.*, VI:1:61, 1934.

144. KOLTHOFF, I. M., and STANSBY, M. E.: *Indust. & Eng. Chem., Analytical Ed.*, VI:2:118, 1934.

Pyrex flask of about 150 cc. capacity. It is fitted with a ground-glass stopper containing an inlet tube extending to the bottom and a second tube ending below the neck of the flask, the other end of which is bent down and sealed in a small test-tube. (Fig. 12.)

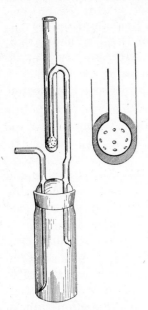

FIG. 12.
Apparatus for Fluorine
Determination

The dry sample is introduced into the flask with about 1 gm. of quartz or silica powder and 25 cc. of concentrated sulphuric acid. One cubic centimeter of the purpurin-zirconium reagent is put into the small test-tube. A stream of air, dried through concentrated sulphuric acid, is passed through the flask and the latter heated to 140°C. in an oil bath. It is essential that the entire apparatus be perfectly dry before the test is begun. The temperature should never exceed 160°C. A blank test run for one hour without any fluoride gave no change in the color of the reagent in the small test-tube. Longer heating resulted in a gradual change of color of the reagent to orange. The speed with which the reagent changes color depends on the amount of fluoride present as shown in Table VIII.

TABLE VIII

DETECTION OF FLUORINE BY DISTILLATION METHOD

Fluorine (Mg.)	Time (Min.)	Color of Reagent	Fluorine (Mg.)	Time (Min.)	Color of Reagent
1.0	0.33	Yellow	0.01	15	Orange
0.1	1	Yellow	0.01	20	Yellow
0.05	3	Yellow	0.005	30	Orange-yellow
0.03	3	Orange	0.005	40	Yellow
0.03	5	Yellow			

The test is sensitive to 0.005 mg. of fluorine with a time of heating of forty minutes. With 0.0025 mg. of fluorine and fifty minutes of heating the reagent had become orange-yellow.

Phosphates, bromides, chlorides, sulphates, sulphites, acetates, oxalates, and sulphides do not interfere. Boric acid in the absence of fluoride turns the reagent an orange color which is easily distinguished from the yellow color with fluorides. It is easy to detect as little as 0.01 mg. of fluorine in the presence of 500 mg. of boric acid. Nitrates and nitrites interfere and destroy the purpurin in the reagent, which turns cloudy yellow. Interference by nitrates and nitrites can be eliminated by dissolving some salicylic acid in the sulphuric acid used, thus transforming the acids into nitro and nitroso compounds. Petrey[145] describes the spectral determination of fluorine in water, where the fluorine is present from 0.05 to 1.5% in the mineral residue of water.

IODINE (I)
(Atomic Weight 126.85)

IODINE occurs as heavy, bluish-black, brittle rhombic plates having a distinctive odor. One gm. of iodine is soluble in 2950 cc. of water, 12.55 cc. of alcohol, 80 cc. of glycerin and in 4 cc. of carbon disulphide at 25° C. It is easily accessible to the public in the form of tincture of iodine containing 7% of iodine, and 5% of potassium iodide; also in Lugol's solution (liquor iodi compositus of the U.S.P.) which contains 5% iodine and 10% potassium iodide. Acute iodine poisoning happens occasionally in people who take these preparations with suicidal intent.

Symptoms: When applied in the form of tincture to the skin it causes a tingling sensation, resulting in a disagreeable burn unless promptly removed. When taken internally it acts as a powerful irritant upon the stomach and bowel. There is pain in the mouth, throat, and stomach, vomiting and purging, fainting attacks and collapse. I have seen a number of attempted suicides in women who took from one-half to one ounce of the tincture in water. Nausea and burning in the mouth and throat followed.

Fatal Dose: Recovery has followed a dose of one fluid ounce of the tincture. Death has been reported from one fluid dram of the tincture containing less than two grains of the element.

Fatal Period: Death may occur in a few hours or be delayed for several weeks. Culpepper[146] reports that a boy

145. PETRY, A. W.: *Indust. & Eng. Chem., Analytical Ed.,* VI: 5: 343, 1934.
146. CULPEPPER: *Therap. Gaz., 3S,* 4: 225, 1888.

eleven years of age was poisoned by the absorption of iodine upon the raw surface extending on both legs from the knees to the feet. He died on the sixth day, suffering from suppression of urine, hemorrhagic stools, vomiting, and purging.

Treatment: When informed that a patient has taken tincture of iodine, order the patient to be given starch water immediately and continue washing out the stomach with starch water until the vomited materials cease to have a blue color.

Postmortem Appearances: Postmortem appearances are such as are found following a gastro-intestinal irritation.

Detection: If the iodine is in a free state, a steam distillation as directed under volatile poisons will give iodine in the acid distillate, where it can be separated by carbon disulphide, giving a violet color to the solvent. If the iodine is in a combined form, a very small quantity of chlorine water can be used to liberate it. In water solution a yellow to black color is noted, a violet color when dissolved in carbon disulphide, a reddish in chloroform, and a blue with a starch solution. The presence of tannic acid interferes with the usual tests for iodine unless a drop or two of ferric chloride solution is added. Organs can be ashed in the presence of a small amount of NaOH, the ash digested in hot water, and the iodine obtained by distillation with manganese dioxide and sulphuric acid.

Iodism: Iodism manifests itself by rashes, coryza, headache, laryngitis, and conjunctivitis. Some people are more sensitive to the presence of iodides than others. There are persons who can take iodides for months without showing any ill effects, others will complain of a coryza within twenty-four hours. The skin breaks out in irregularly scattered pimples, chiefly on the face, shoulders and neck. In some individuals with nephritis, the iodides are more slowly excreted, with the production of acne, furuncles, erythema, purpura, urticaria, and vesication. The treatment is mainly the lowering of the dosage or discontinuing altogether. Magnesium citrate may be given and calcium gluconate wafers taken every two hours for a day or so, until the eruption stops. Iodides should not be given without the supervision of a physician, as over dosage of patients with extensive chronic hyperplasia may give symptoms of hyperthyroidism. These reactions are not pro-

voked until the patient has taken about seventy grains of
potassium iodide.[147]

BROMINE (Br)
(Atomic Weight 79.95. Synonym: Bromum)

BROMINE is a brown-red, intensely caustic liquid evolving
brown vapors, having a suffocating chlorine-like odor.
Indigo, litmus, and other organic substances are bleached by
it. A solution of starch is colored slightly yellow. It reacts
with potassium hydroxide similarly to chlorine, or by electrolysis of the mother liquor at a low temperature, and then
distills in a current of steam. It is obtained chiefly from the
mother liquor of the salt works, which is treated with
manganese dioxide and sulphuric acid. Bromine dissolves in
thirty parts of water at 15°C., forming an orange-yellow
solution. The water solution is permanent, but slowly
decomposes into hydrobromic acid and oxygen. It is soluble
in carbon disulphide, ether, and alcohol.

Symptoms: When the vapors of bromine are inhaled, they
cause violent catarrhal inflammation of the air passages, with
cough, constriction of the chest, and hemoptysis. It causes a
diminution of the number of blood cells and the hemoglobin
content of the blood.[148] Leukocytosis is produced at the same
time. When swallowed it acts as a caustic, producing pain in
the throat and stomach. It causes burns when coming in
contact with the tissues. When its vapors are inhaled, they
cause a bronchial irritation, very much like chlorine and
phosgene gas, which was used in the World War for hand
grenades. Bromides in large doses should be avoided in
mental and physical debility, old age and melancholia, because
of the depressant effects and the lowered resistance produced.

Fatal Dose and Period: Death by bromine is very rare.
A fatal case is reported of a child, ten years of age, taking two
grains of bromine.

Treatment: Wash out the stomach with a solution of
sodium bicarbonate, one teaspoonful to a half pint of water.
Give vegetable oils or animal fats or mucilaginous drinks

147. Oswald, A. D.:   Arch. klin. Med., 551, 1915. Kimball:
I.A.M.A., 85:1709, 1925.
148. Marino: Arch. di farmacol. sper., Roma, 29:48, 1920; Chem.
Abs., 15:1763, 1921.

after removal of the bromine by means of the stomach pump.

Postmortem Appearances: When bromine comes in contact with the skin it leaves a brown stain. The mucous membranes of the mouth, throat and stomach are inflamed, softened, loosened, and there may be hemorrhages of the stomach.

Detection: The bromine of bromides may be freed by adding a little chlorine water, and extracted with carbon d:sulphide which becomes a reddish-yellow color. If present in quantities the color is brown to brown-black. In this case add more of the carbon disulphide, when the reddish-yellow color of the bromine will be distinguished from the violet color of iodine. In starch solution it gives a yellow color with bromine, but the reaction is less delicate than with carbon disulphide.

Bromism.—The bromides are used as sedatives and many times are purchased by people without a doctor's prescription. Long continued use of bromides induces an acneiform eruption. By extinction these take on various forms, such as bullae and pustules. The distribution of these lesions is similar to those from acne vulgaris. In infants and children, and sometimes in adults, the lesions consist of round, nut-shaped, elevated hard nodules and flattened plaques. The bromide is transmitted through the milk to a child; the children exhibiting bromism without the mother manifesting any reactions. One case of bromine intoxication was reported simulating typhoid fever.[149] Long continued use of bromides leads to nutritional disturbances and psychic deterioration.

CHLORINE (Cl)
(Atomic Weight 35-45. Synonym: Chlorum)

CHLORINE is a greenish-yellow suffocating gas, not combustible in oxygen, burns in hydrogen, and in the sun light combines explosively, forming hydrochloric acid. It is readily liquefied, and its boiling point is negative 33.5°C. It is handled commercially in the form of a liquid in steel cylinders and tank cars. Chlorine is obtained during the electrolysis of sodium chloride in the manufacture of sodium hydroxide. It is used extensively to disinfect the water supply of large cities, and has lowered the incidence of typhoid fever to practically

149. Mayrhofer, H., and Fissler, A.: *Wien. klin. Wchnschr.*, 43: 1315, 1930.

nothing. It is used for purification of sewage, in the manufacture of bleaching powder, and as a whitening agent in the bleaching of papers and textiles. It is given off in the dye industry, especially in the manufacture of aniline chloride, benzl chloride, and nigrosin. It is used in the chlorination of a large number of organic compounds; it is also used as a disinfectant in sugar manufacturing. Shrubbery and trees are affected for long distances in the direction of the prevailing winds, as for instance at a midwestern town where chlorine fumes from a chemical manufacturing works caused destruction of vegetation for miles around. It is the active agent found in the household bleaching powder which is used as a disinfectant. The chlorinated lime, or calx chlorinata of the U. S. Pharmacopeia, should yield not less than 30% of available chlorine. Chlorine gas in the air, to the extent of one-thousandth of one per cent causes cough, dyspnea, bronchial catarrh and, if excessive quantities are breathed, great respiratory distress and rapid death. Chlorine is nearly twenty times as toxic as hydrochloric acid, which can be explained on the grounds of its low solubility and its great oxidizing power. It abstracts hydrogen from the water present in the tissues, with liberation of nascent oxygen and the formation of hydrochloric acid. Its use on April 22, 1915, during the World War, marked the beginning of gas warfare, although carbon monoxide and sulphur dioxide had been used many hundred years before in the wars of the Athenians and Spartans, 431-404 B. C., when the Spartans saturated wood with pitch and sulphur, burning it under the walls of Platea and Belium.

TABLE IX

PHYSIOLOGICAL RESPONSE TO VARIOUS CONCENTRATIONS OF CHLORINE

	Parts of Chlorine Per Million Parts of Air
Least detectable odor	3.5
Least amount causing immediate irritation to the throat	15.1
Least amount causing coughing	30.2
Maximum concentration allowable for prolonged exposure	1.0
Maximum concentration allowable for short exposure (½ to 1 hour)	4.0
Dangerous for even short exposure	40 to 60
Rapidly fatal for short exposure	1,000

Fatal Dose: Chlorine is dangerous, for even short exposure, from forty to sixty parts per million. It is rapidly fatal for short exposure 1000 parts per million. In Table IX are given the effects of various concentrations.[150]

Symptoms: The chlorine content of one to 20,000 produced conditions in soldiers such as to render them incapable of fighting, producing a strong dyspnea, cyanosis, and death. Fifteen and one-tenth parts per million cause immediate irritation to the throat and with higher concentrations, irritation of the conjunctiva. The symptoms will vary with the concentration and the time of breathing the gas; bronchitis, or a serious bronchopneumonia may develop. The inhalation of the gas may cause loss of sense of smell, bronchiectasis, gastritis, loss of appetite with loss of weight; headache, giddiness, insomnia, and cardiac disturbances. Many of the ills of city people may, in the future, be attributed to the drinking of the oxides of chlorine in their water supply. There is something very striking when city people leave for the north woods on a vacation, for their general physical condition improves. This improvement may be due to the change of water supply more than to a change of air. Pernice[151] reports the case of a man working in a cellulose factory where he was exposed to chlorine gas frequently. The first time he was exposed to a dense cloud of chlorine gas, which escaped at a pressure of about seven to eight atmospheres, he fainted and had to be removed by fellow workmen. After regaining consciousness, he began to cough violently, expectorated pure blood, and complained of a feeling of tightness in the chest. During the first two days he expectorated clots of blood. After a few weeks following the accident he began to complain of an oppression in the chest; had cardiac disturbances and slept very poorly. About one year later he experienced a similar accident, again coughing violently, expectorating blood and having a severe palpitation with pain in the region of the heart. He was incapacitated for five weeks. He had two more such accidents during the course of several years. He changed his occupation, but the cardiac disturbances did not subside and he often had hemorrhages from the lungs. He was not able to perform any heavy work, and finally had to give

150. HENDERSON and HAGGARD: Noxious Gases, 132, 1927.
151. PERNICE, H.: *Deutsche med. Wchnschr.,* 59:1644, 1933.

up work altogether. His hemoglobin was 59%; red blood cells 2,700,000 and white blood cells 6,600. Roentgenologic examination revealed an enlargement of the heart. The diagnosis was a compensated mitral stenosis, and a severe secondary anemia. The author comes to the conclusion that his disturbance had been caused exclusively by the effect of the chlorine gas. The chlorine inhaled through the lungs attacks the valve of the left heart by dehydration, with the result that this valve shrinks and becomes stenosed. According to Flury-Zernik, chlorine has a dehydrating action; during its dehydration, oxygen is liberated and hydrochloric acid is formed. Lewin explains this condition on the basis of the formation of thrombi followed by the formation of infarcts and processes of shrinkage, with a resulting stenosis of the valvular orifice. The acute effect on the nervous system in severe cases is characterized by a rapidly occurring loss of consciousness. Sometimes it is observed that workmen who are exposed to chlorine gas at first do not complain of any symptoms. Symptoms, and eventually death, occur much later. Brezina[152] reports several such cases. After a chronic exposure to chlorine there may form opacities of the cornea and perforations of the nasal septum. The prognosis of chlorine intoxication is favorable if the victim is taken away rapidly from the contaminated atmosphere. Ninety-five cases of chlorine intoxication were reported in England from 1924 to 1930. Some of these intoxications occur in the artificial silk industry. Jacobsohn[153] reports a case of hyper-susceptibility to very small quantities of chlorine. Ravant and Koang[154] report dermatitis of the hands, arms, face and neck caused by javelle water, and secondary eczematoid lesions of the legs of allergic origin. The patient observed by these authors had been using javelle water shortly before observation. This is interesting because they have found that eczematoid lesions may not only be produced by fungal and bacterial antigens, but also by chemical antigens which in this particular case may be called "javellides."

Postmortem Appearances: Postmortem examinations have

152. Brezina, E.: Die Gewerblichen Vergiftungen und ihre Bekamphfung, Ferdinand Enke, Stuttgart, 1932.
153. Jacobsohn, I.: *Klin. Wchnschr.*, 11:111, 1932.
154. Ravant and Koang: *Bull. Soc. franc. de dermat. et syph.*, 37:655, 1930.

revealed laryngitis, edema of the lungs, and emphysema. Klotz[155] reported the changes found in the lungs of animals dying from chlorine poisoning. Blood coagulates within the dilated pulmonary capillaries. Human blood placed in the atmosphere of one to 1000 of chlorine, coagulates in about fifteen minutes.

Treatment: Remove from the contaminated atmosphere and give fresh air immediately. Treat the symptoms of laryngitis and bronchitis by appropriate therapeutic measures.

Detection: The gas can be detected by its bleaching action on moist litmus paper, or, when it is very dilute, a silver nitrate solution will give a white precipitate insoluble in nitric acid, but soluble in ammonia. Starch iodide paper is turned blue by the liberations of iodine from potassium iodide.

TELLURIUM (Te)
(Atomic Weight 127)

TELLURIUM is found free, or as a telluride, in certain ores of gold, silver, selenium, and iron. Strong acids act on a telluride forming hydrogen-telluride, similar to arsine and hydrogen sulphide. Kobert reports that tellurium and selenium resemble arsenic in their physiological action. In gaseous form they act as powerful hemolytic poisons. In the body they are changed to methyl compounds in part, and give to the breath a garlic odor.

Symptoms: Shie and Deeds[156] found that the early sign of the ingestion of tellurium was the garlic odor of the secretions and excretions, later suppression of saliva, sweat and the acid of the gastric juice. They also found that moderate exposure to fumes and dust for some weeks or months caused a dry mouth, a metallic taste, inhibition of sweat, with a scaly, itching skin, vomiting and somnolence. The occupational history of the individuals working in tellura ferrous ores is very important in arriving at a diagnosis. In animals death is preceded by dyspnea, convulsions and coma, after lethal doses have been administered.

Treatment: Withdraw from the source of contamination; give diaphoretics, laxatives, and diuretics to assist in elimination of the material.

155. KLOTZ, O.: *J. Lab. & Clin. Med.,* 2:889, 1917.
156. U. S. Pub. Health Reports, 35:939, 1920.

Postmortem Appearances: Postmortem appearances are the same as are seen after gastro-intestinal irritations, with the additional fact that there is hemolysis and parenchymatous nephritis.

Detection: The garlic odor of solutions in great dilutions indicates the presence of tellurium and selenium. Materials are precipitated by hydrogen sulphide treated with ammonium sulphide, which dissolves tellurium and selenium, and again precipitated by hydrochloric acid. This leaves the tellurium undissolved. The residue is dissolved by nitric acid, as an acid to be neutralized by potassium hydroxide. Evaporated to dryness, tellurium is recognized by melting with potassium cyanide and dissolving in water, which turns red from potassium cyanotellurid. Biological test: Similarly to arsenic, tellurium and selenium are converted by Penicillium brevicaule to volatile odoriferous compounds, giving garlic odors; selenium, however, has more of a mercaptan odor. Having eliminated arsenic by appropriate tests, one may follow Gosio's method, using crumbs of bread with a culture of the special mold, yielding the garlic odor.

THALLIUM (Tl)
(Atomic weight 204.15)

THALLIUM was discovered by Crookes, by means of the spectroscope in 1861, in selenium residues of the sulphuric acid factory at Tilkerode in the Hartz Mountains, Germany. It was used in 1898 to check the night sweats of tuberculous patients, but was found to be too toxic and was therefore discontinued. Marme[157] was the first to show the presence of this poison in the urine, stool, gall-bladder, milk, secretions of the conjunctival sac, saliva, phlegm of the trachea, gastric juice, and in the fluid of the pericardial sac. Blake[158] reported the action of thallium salts, and Luck gave all the older literature and described the action of thallium in a dissertation delivered at Dorpat in 1891. Its metallic nature was demonstrated by Lamy,[159] of Lille, in 1862, when he isolated it and described its properties. He noticed, during his studies with thallium, that he experienced weakness and pains in the legs which made him

157. MARME: *Gotting, gel. Anzeigen,* 20:397, 1867.
158. BLAKE: *Compt. rend. T.,* 3, 1890.
159. LAMY, A.: *Compt. rend. Acad. d. sc.,* 55:866, 1862.

suspicious of a toxic influence from the metal. This he demonstrated experimentally by giving animals thallium sulphate and producing intestinal and respiratory embarrassment with peripheral paralyses and general weakness.[160] While it was being used for night sweats of tuberculosis it was discovered that these patients were losing their hair.[161] Huchard,[162] Jeanselme,[163] and Guinard,[164] made similar observations.

Sabouraud,[165] used 1% local applications in managing hypertrichosis. He noticed no signs of intoxication even after eighteen months of daily use. If used in larger quantities or in stronger amounts it produces albuminuria, subcutaneous ecchymoses, sialorrhea, and tachycardia. On account of this Sabouraud gave up this preparation in favor of the x-ray. Vassaux[166] used thallium acetate against the night sweats of tuberculous patients. Dixon[167] reported the pharmacology of thallium in 1920. The first response is a relaxation of the smooth muscle of the bronchioles, intestine, and uterus. It acts on the autonomic nervous system, allowing impulses to pass more readily than normal. He believes that the alopecia is produced through the autonomic nervous system, and supports his views by the observations of others who state that the hair of the head is under the trophic control of the internal secretory system through the sympathetic nervous system. His experimental work demonstrated not only a depilatory effect, but also a stimulating influence on hair. Commercially thallium has been used as a rat poison in "Zeliopaste", and in Koremlu cream as a depilatory. It is also used commercially in the dye and glass industries. Rube and Hendriks[168] in 1927, reported severe poisoning among men recovering thallium from the flue dust of sulphuric acid works. One man suffered loss of vision in both eyes, which was unchanged two years later, although he recovered from the other symptoms of thallium poisoning. An unusual occurrence of thallium poisoning was noted by

160. LAMY, A.: Compt. rend. Acad. d. sc., 57:442, 1863.
161. COMBEMALE, F.: Echo méd. du nord., 2:100, 1898.
162. HUCHARD, H.: Bull. Acad. de méd., Paris, 39:572, 1898.
163. JEANSELME, E.: Ann. de dermat. et syph., 9:299, 1898.
164. GUINARD, A. J.: Méd de Paris, 10:572, 1898.
165. SABOURAUD, RAYOND: Clinique, Paris, 7:102, 1912.
166. VASSAUX, L.: L'Acetate de thallium on therapeutique These de Paris, 1898.
167. DIXON, W. E.: Proc. Roy. Soc. Med., 20:77, 1927.
168. RUBE and HENDRICKS: Med. Welt., 1:20, 1927.

Neal, Appelbaum, Gaul and Masselink[169] when seven members of a family affected, with five fatalities, were diagnosed with spectroscope analysis. Atrophy of the optic nerve has been reported by Buschke, Rubenstein, Hendriks, and Stein.[170]

Thallium was introduced as a rat poison in Germany in 1920. In its action, thallium seems definitely to select nervous tissues. In rats it produces slight degenerative changes in the brain. The death of at least four children, and the poisoning of two other children and five adults from eating grain to which thallium chloride had been added, is recorded. A woman poisoned her husband by adding to his food a rat poison containing thallium sulphate. He had been given 30 gm. of thallium sulphate at intervals of about three months.

Several mass misfortunes have occurred in which dosage was miscalculated in the clinical treatment of tinea of the scalp in children.[171] The syndrome has often been very puzzling, even acute abdominal symptoms being simulated, as Ramond[172] reported. Rubenstein[173] has observed encephaliticlike phenomena. There have been reports of polyneuritis,[174] and some with psychic manifestations and kidney involvements.[175] Retrobulbar neuritis was noted by Kaps[176] in a patient who became demented before death, and suicidal attempts have occurred.[177] Mahoney[178] reported three cases of retrobulbar neuritides from the use of a depilatory cream. Two of them improved after the discontinuance of the depilatory. The creams used contained 7.18% thallium acetate.

Lubenau[179] reported an accidental case of poisoning from "Zeliopaste" in a child two years of age, which terminated

169. NEAL, JOSEPHINE, APPELBAUM, E., GAUL, L. E., and MASSELINK, R. J.: *J.A.M.A.*, 105:466, 1935.

170. BUSCHKE, RUBENSTEIN, HENDRIKS, and STEIN: *Am. J. Ophth.*, 15:949, 1932.

171. LYNCH, G. R., and SCOVELL, J. M.: *Lancet*, 2:1340, 1930. MERKEL, H.: *Samml. v. Vergiftungsfallen*, 1:85, 1930.

172. RAMOND, LOUIS: *Presse méd.*, 37:691, 1929.

173. RUBENSTEIN, M. W.: *Arch. Dermat. & Syph.*, 23:477, 1931.

174. SHORT, C. L.: *J.A.M.A.*, 97:101, 1931; WARING, T. P.: *J.A.M.A.*, 97:703, 1931.

175. DEUTSCH, J.: *Samml. v. Vergiftungsfallen*, 1:149, 1930; HEINICHEN, W.: *Samml. v. Vergiftungsfallen*, 2:27, 1931.

176. KAPS, L.: *Wien. klin. Wchnschr.*, 40:967, 1927.

177. GREVING, R., and GAGEL, O.: *Klin. Wchnschr.*, 7:1323, 1928.

178. MAHONEY, W.: *J.A.M.A.*, 98:618, 1932.

179. LUBENEAU: *Ztschr. f. Med.-Beamte, Berl.*, 41:106, 1928.

fatally in forty-eight hours. Thallium was demonstrated in the blood. Haberda[180] reported a homicidal case in which a woman killed her husband by a gradual mixture of "Zeliopaste" in various foods, over a long period of time.

Properties: Specific gravity 11.777 to 11.9. It is a bluish-white metal, softer than lead, malleable and ductile, may be preserved under water. It is soluble in sulphuric and nitric acid, and with difficulty in hydrochloric acid. The carbonate is soluble in about twenty parts of water; the sulphate and phosphate are soluble; the chloride very sparingly soluble; the iodide insoluble in water. Haberda reports that the administration of thallium[181] removes calcium from the bones and produces disturbances of growth, testicular atrophy, changes in the lining of the stomach with serious effects on the nervous system.

Symptoms: According to Buschke,[182] a very important fact is that the point of attack of thallium in chronic poisoning is the vegetative system, which shows here, as in many other cases, synergism between the endocrine and the autonomic systems in the affected organs. This causes the falling out of hair, gray cataract, inhibition of growth and of sexual development, the skeletal disorders, diseases of the thyroid, parathyroid, sex, and suprarenal glands, and other symptoms. It eventually produces a glomerulo-nephritis in the kidneys, swelling of the reticulo-endothelial cells in the liver and spleen, degeneration and hemorrhages in the heart, and deterioration in the central nervous system. Ginsburg and Nixon[183] report eleven cases of poisoning from the use of barley mixed with thallium sulphate. "The first symptoms noticed were a tingling sensation and pains in the hands and feet, followed by severe paroxysmal abdominal pains and vomiting. No diarrhea was observed. Shortly after the first manifestations, weakness of the extremities developed. This weakness did not involve any particular muscle group except that it was more marked peripherally than proximally. Patients were afebrile but with an acceleration of the pulse rate. The blood picture in the first two to five days was normal. The urine showed traces of

180. HABERDA, A.: *Beitr. z. gerichtl. Med.*, 7:1, 1928.
181. *Beitr. z. gerichtl. Med.*, 7:1, 1928.
182. BUSCHKE: *Ergebn. d. allg. Path. u. path. Anat.*, Bd. 25, 1935.
183. GINSBURG, H. M., and NIXON, C. E., *J.A.M.A.*, 98, 1932.

albumin and hyaline casts. In all cases there was a marked stomatitis. Some exhibited a purplish line at the junction of the teeth and gums. Marked salivation was present in all cases. Bleb formation appeared on the lips; the breath was foul. Within two to five days after the onset all patients showed evidence of cerebral involvement manifested by cranial nerve palsies and disturbed sensorium and choreiform or myoclonic movements of the extremities and the head. Among the cranial nerve manifestations, ptosis, strabismus and dilated pupils which reacted feebly to light, were prominent. Falling out of the hair occurred in all these patients at this time." These authors reported more toxic cases when convulsions occurred, which were followed by a marked delirium after which the patient became comatose and died of respiratory failure. About twenty-four to forty-eight hours before death the temperature had risen to 103°F. with pathologic changes in the chest, indicative of a bronchopneumonia or pulmonary edema. Five weeks after the onset, three patients (two children and one adult) had been discharged from the hospital, free from symptoms except for the alopecia. Two male adult patients had evidences of neuritis, showed mental changes, and had traces of thallium in the urine.

In 1909, Cicero[184] spoke of the dangers from its use in depilation of the tinea, and in 1912, Sabouraud[185] mentioned his experiences of excessive salivation, tachycardia, albuminuria and ecchymosis.

In 1899, Richet,[186] after experimental work, reported that thallium as well as lead produced a non-inflammatory keratitis characterized by progressive opacity of the cornea. In 1927, Kaps[187] reported a case where rat poison was given with intent to murder. The man had an alopecia, peripheral neuritis, in addition to failure of vision and retrobulbar neuritis, before dementia and death. In 1928, Buschke[188] and his co-workers reported the experimental production of partial optic atrophy in animals which they considered a new feature. Lillie and Parker[189] report two cases of retrobulbar neuritis due to

184. Cicero, R., and Rayos, X.: Gac. méd de México, 4:499, 1909.
185. Sabouraud, Rayond: Clinique, Paris, 7:102, 1912.
186. Richet, C.: Compt. rend. Soc. de biol., 1:253, 1899.
187. Kaps: Wien. klin. Wchnschr., 40:967, 1927.
188. Buschke, A.: Klin. Wchnschr., 7:1515, 1928.
189. Lillie, W. I., and Parker, H. L.: J.A.M.A., 98:1347, 1932.

thallium poisoning. Swollen, hot and tender lower extremities were observed by Davies and Andrews.[190] Headaches, insomnia, paleness and loss of weight,[191] lacrimation, salivation and deafness,[192] also psychic disturbances,[193] choreiform movements, dermatitis and even fever,[194] have been reported. In both cases the full development of the neuritis in the lower extremities, was characterized by pains, paresthesia, and the appearance of visual symptoms. This same occurrence followed in one of Mahoney's cases; in the other two the visual disturbance antedated the neuritis. In all three cases, however, some visual disturbance persisted after pain and weakness in the legs had disappeared. Rambar[195] reported the death of a nineteen months old child who ate a sandwich made of two layers of bread between which crude thallium sulphate mixed with peanut butter had been spread.

Poisoning by thallium causes swelling of feet and legs, with pains in the joints sometimes suggestive of acute articular rheumatism, colic, vomiting, sleeplessness, hyperesthesia and paresthesia of hands and feet, mental confusion, as well as a striking loss of hair from the head and body. Fourteen children died in Granada, Spain, as a result of a dose ten times larger than should have been given.[196]

According to Teleky, the dose of thallium acetate is 8 mg. to the kilogram of body weight, but only children tolerate the drug, not adults or adolescents. The explanation lies in the changes which occur in the endocrine system after childhood. There was also occasional incontinence of the bladder and rectum, angina-like pains, wasting and weakness, an acidity of the gastric juice, slight nephritis, lymphocytosis, and eosinophilia.[197] These blood changes, according to Buschke,[198] were observed in men who had worked with thallium for some months. Lutz[199] tested all the compounds on the market, except the chloride, which is not soluble in water, and found that all

190. DAVIES, J., and ANDREWS, M.: Brit. M. J., 2:1139, 1927.
191. DIVELLA, M.: Gior. ital di dermat. e sif., 67:291, 1926.
192. GRSHEBIN and SALZMANN: Dermat. Ztschr., 52:105, 1928.
193. RITTER and KARRENBERG: Dermat. Wchnschr., 86:434, 1928.
194. DIVELLA: Arch. f. Dermat. u. Syph., 150:438, 1926.
195. RAMBAR, A. C.: J.A.M.A., 98:1372, 1932.
196. J.A.M.A., 100:678, 1933.
197. GREVING, R., and GAGEL, O.: Klin. Wchnschr., 7:1323, 1928.
198. BUSCHKE, A.: Med. Klin., 24:1042, 1928.
199. LUTZ, G.: Zentralbl. f. Gewerbehyg., 5:172, 1928.

had the same action when injected under the skin. Cramps were a common symptom, and the animals wasted to a third of their original weight.[200] Teleky described thallium intoxication in a factory where thallium was produced. There were forty workmen in this plant. The severest intoxication was observed in a nineteen year old boy who in a few weeks following employment, complained of severe pain in the joints and noticed that his hair began to fall out. Four months following his admission to the factory his eyesight began to fail. Examination of the blood of a number of workmen revealed eosinophilia. The other workmen showed a variety of symptoms, such as pain in the lower extremities, tremor of the eyelids, exaggeration of the patellar reflexes and albuminuria. These symptoms did not disappear when the men were removed from the dangerous environment. In one case there was observed an optic atrophy which could be traced back to thallium. They found changes in the bones, such as rickets and osteomalacia, renal diseases, hepatic disease, and also partial optic atrophy. The red blood cells showed basophilic stippling indicating damage to the bone-marrow. Rubenstein[201] reports the case of a colored boy, seven years of age, who was admitted to the clinic for ringworm of the scalp. He was given 0.16 gm. of thallium acetate orally, and his head was shaved the following day. Several days after the thallium acetate had been administered, he was not able to come to the clinic because of weakness of the knees. Eleven days later, following the administration of the drug, the patient appeared toxic. The blood count was: R.B.C. 4,400,000; W.B.C. 13,400; H.B. 85%; polys, 71%; lymphos, 23%; monos, 6%; temp. 99.6; pulse rate, 120; respiration, 24. The temperature ranged between 99.6 and 104. He was given sodium thiosulphate intravenously, also chloral hydrate and sodium bromide by rectum, and codeine was given when necessary. The patient went steadily down hill until finally even cardiac stimulants gave no response. The lungs became congested, the heart failed, and he ultimately died.

Treatment: There is apparently no known certain anti-

200. For a full bibliography see TELEKY, L.: *Wien. med. Wchnschr.,* 78:506, 1928; and BREZINA, E.: Die Gewerblichen Vergiftungen und ihre Bekampfung, 119.

201. RUBENSTEIN, M. W.: *Arch. Dermat. & Syph.,* 23:477, 1931.

dote to the action of thallium. It is a cumulative poison of high toxicity, without taste, smell or other warning properties. Its general use as a rat poison should be forbidden and its use among highly resistant species of rodents should be entrusted only to people who understand its dangerous qualities and who will exercise care in handling it.

Sodium idodide was given in 2 gm. doses. Two patients were given calcium lactate and parathyroid extract. In addition to these, dextrose and salt solutions and other symptomatic therapeutic measures were used as indicated.

The best treatment is to wash out the stomach with four grains of calcium sulphide to a pint of water until the washing water fails to give tests for thallium. Give colonic flushings with water containing four grains of calcium sulphide to the pint. Sodium thiosulphate may be given intravenously, 1 gm. twice daily. However, this has not proved successful in the few cases in which it has been used. Cases of poisoning by thallium should be treated in the same manner as mercurial poisoning.

Postmortem Appearances: In the case reported by Rambar[195] postmortem examination showed an acute bilateral bronchopneumonia and a cloudy swelling of the heart, liver and kidneys. Chemical examination for thallium was negative in the brain, lungs, liver, heart and kidneys. Some bile, hair and a piece of vertebra were also examined without a trace of the element. In the case reported by Rubenstein[196] there was a mild encephalitis with a peculiar necrosis of the liver, and an acute nephritis superimposed on the renal tissue showing an old chronic glomerular lesion. The patient showed signs of congenital syphilis. The lung showed a diffuse pulmonary tuberculosis.

Scharrer[202] reported histologically a case of thallium poisoning. The patient died eight months after taking the poison with suicidal intent. In the central nervous system there were found marked changes in the dentate nuclei. There was found in the thoracal segment of the spinal cord a pronounced degeneration of the tract of Goll. Chronic thallium poisoning is characterized by injury of the endocrine glands, peripheral neuritis, and falling out of the hair. Andrews and

202. SCHARRER, E.: *Zentralbl. f. d. ges. Neurol. u. Psychiat.*, 69:358. 1933.

Davies[203] showed that children up to seven and eight years of age withstand the action of thallium well. Older children and adults are more apt to show toxic symptoms. In one of their cases, arthritis and periarthritis of the knee joints were present. The analysis of postmortem made by Ormerod[204] showed that muscles act as the main storehouse for thallium, and that the excretion is mainly by way of the kidneys, but that thallium is also present in all the body secretions. Buschke and Peiser report seven deaths from an overdose of thallium during its therapeutic use. According to the statistical material of Arijewitsch, children of from five to nine years of age tolerate thallium best, whereas among children below that range 44%, and above it 59%, show symptoms of poisoning.

Detection: Hydrochloric acid precipitates from solution not very dilute, thallium chloride, $TlCl$, white and unalterable in the air. Like lead chloride it is slightly soluble in hot water, giving a light yellow precipitate of iodide, TlI, on adding a drop of potassium iodide solution. Hydrogen sulphide precipitates the acetate, but not the acidified solutions of its other salts. Ferrocyanides give a yellow precipitate, $Tl_4Fe(CN)_6$. Chromates precipitate yellow normal chromate; the platinic chloride, pale orange, thallious chloride, Tl_2PtCl_6. Thallium compounds readily impart an intense green color to the flame, and one green line to the spectrum, which is the most delicate test for this material. The flame color and spectrum from small quantities are somewhat evanescent, owing to rapid vaporization.[205]

The Benzidine Test:[206] Upon a piece of paper add one drop of ammonia and one drop of the unknown solution and then one drop of the benzidine test solution (dissolving benzidine by means of heating dilute sulphuric acid and filtering). In the presence of thallium a blue color will develop. Delicate to one in 166,000.

SILVER (Ag)
(Atomic Weight 107.92)

SILVER is of importance chiefly from the standpoint of causing local or general silver gray coloration of the skin, caused by the precipitation of the absorbed silver. This silver

203. ANDREWS, M. C., and DAVIES, J. H. T.: *Brit. M. J.*, 2:1139, 1929.
204. ORMEROD, M. J.: *Canad. M. A. J.*, 19:663, 1928.
205. PRESCOTT and JOHNSON: Qualitative Chem. Analysis, 199, 1915.
206. FEIGL, F.: *Chem. Ztg.*, 44:689, 1920.

may be absorbed through the action of silver nitrate or the organic silver preparations. Care must be exercised in the continuance of applications of the preparations for the nose and throat.* Witthaus[207] reported eight cases of intoxication, five of which were the result of accidents in children. A child of fifteen months died after a stick of lunarcaustic had been swallowed during its medical application. Death occurred in six hours with violent convulsions. A woman fifty-one years of age died in three days from the effects of fifty grains of silver nitrate taken in divided doses. The symptoms were those of an intense gastro-enteritis.

Fatal Dose and Period: Death has resulted from thirty grains. Death occurred in six hours in the case of a child of fifteen months.

Treatment: A teaspoonful of common salt to a pint of water will induce vomiting. Precipitate the silver as the insoluble silver chloride. Continue washing out the stomach until the washings fail to give a precipitate with the salt water. Treat as under corrosive poisons.

Postmortem Appearances: Postmortem appearances of the mouth, esophagus, and stomach will depend upon whether the silver nitrate was taken in solid form or in solution. The stains on the lips and tongue will be bluish-black. The stomach and bowels will show the presence of gastro-intestinal irritant.

Tests: Filter the washings from the stomach lavage, add to the filtrate hydrochloric acid or sodium chloride. In the presence of a soluble salt of silver, a white curdy precipitate will be formed which is easily soluble in ammonium hydroxide, as ammonio-silver chloride. Ammonium hydroxide can be added to the solid residue on the filter paper, and the filtrate can be acidified in nitric acid which will cause a re-precipitate of the silver, if it is present in the solid portion of the washing water or in the vomitus as silver chloride.

VANADIUM (V)
(Atomic Weight 51.4)

DUTTON[208] reported in 1911 a case of vanadium poisoning which resulted from the inhalation of vanadium dust. There was a dry irritating cough with conjunctivitis and

---

* STILLIANS, A. W.: *Arch. Dermat. & Syph.,* 35:67, 1937.
207. WITTHAUS and BECKER: Toxicology, 304, 1911.
208. DUTTON, L. F.: *J.A.M.A.,* 56:1648, 1911.

rhinitis. Anemia is one of the early symptoms. Destruction of red blood cells, loss of appetite, emaciation and pallor, were also noticed. Gastro-intestinal symptoms similar to those seen under arsenic were reported. Vanadium poisoning seems to be a very rare form of poisoning.

CHROMIUM (Cr)
(Atomic Weight 52.1)

CHROMIUM is not found native, but is found in several minerals chiefly as chromic iron or chromite ($FeOCr_2O_3$). It is prepared by the electrolysis of the chloride; by fusing the chloride with potassium or sodium; by ignition of the oxide with carbon, removing the excess of carbon or magnesium by dissolving in nitric acid which does not dissolve metallic chromium. Chromium forms an oxide (Cr_2O_3), which forms salts of chromium, such as chromous chloride ($CrCl_2$), chromium trioxide (CrO_3), and the corresponding acids derived from it are chromic acid (H_2CrO_4) and dichromic acid ($H_2Cr_2O_7$). Chromous oxide (CrO) has not been isolated. The corresponding hydroxide, $Cr(OH)_2$, is made by treating $CrCl_2$ with potassium hydroxide. Chromium has come into importance as an industrial poison on account of the chromic acid being employed in electric plating. It is now used extensively in plating automobile accessories. The chromates of sodium, potassium, and ammonium are used as mordants in dyeing and in the quick method of tanning leather. Chromates are used in the manufacture of paper, wall paper, aniline dyes, explosives, electric batteries, artificial flowers, in the bleaching of oils and fats, in textile printing, and in paints as lead chromate. Potassium bichromate occurs in orange-red crystals used by furniture stainers and in the manufacture of battery fluids. By mistake a Breslau[209] pharmacist used potassium bichromate in the preparing of an ointment for the treatment of scabies. A number of people were severely poisoned and twelve died from using this ointment. The symptoms were burning pain and vomiting, bloody and albuminous urine and anuria. Brieger[210] reported that the poison was found in the blood, urine, feces and gastric contents. The derivatives of chromic

209. *J.A.M.A.*, 73:1590, 1919.
210. BRIEGER: *Ztschr. f. exper. Path. u. Therap.*, Berl., 21:393, 1920-21; URBAN: *Berl. klin. Wchnschr.*, 56:363, 1919; COLDEN: ibid., 365.

acid are decidedly toxic when taken internally, and a number of cases of severe or fatal poisoning (accidental or suicidal) have occurred from this cause. When the dust or the solutions of the dichromate come in contact with the skin, dermatitis and ulcers develop. The dermatitis is seen chiefly among photographers and blue-print makers, who come in contact daily with dilute solutions of potassium dichromate. In the plating industry where chromic acid derivatives are used, perforation of the nasal septum is very common.[211]

Symptoms: When taken internally the compounds of chromium cause a disagreeable taste, vomiting, pain, diarrhea, collapse, unconsciousness, dilated pupils, very slow respiration, and muscular cramps. In addition to acting as gastro-intestinal irritants, they cause nervous symptoms such as headache, stiffness of the back of the neck, and cramps. The blood pressure is abnormally low, in spite of the uremic symptoms. Hemorrhage of the stomach, bronchi, pleura, and endocardium is found in the serious cases. The non-protein nitrogen may rise to 268 mg. during the anuria. Potassium dichromate may cause nephritis.[212]

Chromic salts, such as chromic carbonate and chromic phosphate, are not poisonous to cats whether introduced through the digestive tract or the respiratory system.[213] In view of the enormous increased industrial utilization of chromium, a sharp distinction should be made between chromic salts, which are relatively inert and harmless, and the derivatives of chromic acid, which certainly exhibit toxic properties.[214]

Fatal Dose: Fifteen gm. of potassium dichromate have proved fatal on the tenth day, in a girl twenty-one years of age. Macniven reported a recovery from about three drams, and Philipson reported a recovery from 273 grains.[215]

Fatal Period: Life may be prolonged for ten days, as in

211. BLOOMFIELD, J. J.: Pub. Health Reports, 43:2330, 1928; CARTER, W. W.: M. J. & Rec., 130:125, 1929; SCHWARTZ, L.: Zentralbl. f. Gewerbehyg., 7:232, 1930; WERTHER: Deutsche med. Wchnschr., 56:1098, 1930; PANKHURST, H. J.: Arch. Dermat. & Syph., 12:353, 1925.

212. BERNARD, E.: Bull. et mém. Soc. méd. d. hôp. de Paris, 53:281, 1929.

213. AKATSUKA, K., and FAIRHALL, L. T.: J. Indust. Hyg., 16:1, 1934.

214. FELL, A.: Semaine d. hôp de Paris, 6:364, 1930.

215. MACNIVEN: Lancet, 2:496, 1883; PHILIPSON: Lancet, 1:138, 1892.

the above cited case, or death may occur in forty minutes after taking one ounce of the dichromate.

Treatment: Wash out the stomach. Give sodium chloride and glucose intravenously, and keep the patient on a nitrogen poor diet. Opiates and barbiturates may be given for the pain, cerebral and respiratory stimulants for the depression of the nervous system.

Postmortem Appearances: Postmortem appearances are such as are seen from an irritant poison. There are hemorrhages in the pleura and the endocardium, blood in the bronchi, fatty degeneration of the liver, cloudy swelling of the kidneys, thickening of the bladder wall with softening of the mucous membrane, necrosis of the tonsils and the epiglottis, hemorrhages in the stomach, injection of the small intestine, and degeneration of the kidney epithelia.[216] Pneumoconiosis caused by chromate has been discussed by Lukanin.[217]

Detection: Dry the tissue at a gentle heat in a porcelain dish, char, and then transfer to a muffle furnace maintained at a low red heat. Cool, and completely dissolve the ash in a dilute hydrochloric acid with the aid of gentle heat. Take the hydrochloric acid solutions of the ash completely to dryness two or three times with concentrated nitric acid in order to destroy the hydrochloric acid, and finally dissolve the residue in dilute nitric acid. Neutralize with potassium hydroxide, adding a slight excess, and then add 5 cc. of superoxal (concentrated hydrogen peroxide) and heat. Boil off the excess peroxide. The metal hydroxides precipitated by this treatment retain some of the chromium mechanically; it is necessary to filter and dissolve the residue in dilute nitric acid and again neutralize and oxidize. This oxidation serves to remove every trace of chromium from the insoluble constituents of the ash. The filtrates are combined, neutralized with acetic acid, and a slight excess is added. On adding lead acetate, the chromate is precipitated quantitatively. Dissolve the well washed lead precipitate in hydrochloric acid, transferring the precipitate to the bulk of solution and stirring well. Make the solution of soluble chromate up to a given volume in a volumetric flask. The chromium content may be estimated in a colorimeter against standard potassium chromate, or measured amounts in 50-cc.

216. OLBRYCHT: Leschke, 85, 1934.
217. LUKANIN, W. P.: *Arch. f. Hyg.*, 104:166, 1930.

Nessler tubes may be compared against similar standards. The s-diphenyl carbazide reagent is best prepared by dissolving 0.4 gm. of s-diphenyl carbazide in 30 cc. of glacial acetic acid and diluting to 400 cc. with distilled water. One cubic centimeter of this 0.1% solution of reagent is added to the unknown and to the standard in Nessler tubes, the walls washed down with a little distilled water, the contents mixed thoroughly, allowed to stand fifteen minutes and then diluted to 50 cc. The amounts that could be read with the greatest accuracy were found to be from 0.003 mg. to 0.01 mg. of chromium in a 50-cc. Nessler tube, with 0.007 representing an ideal amount. According to Fairhall[218] this is as accurate a means as any investigated by him. In this colorimetric method, however, one must keep in mind that colors are obtained by other metals with the diphenyl carbazide reagent.

CADMIUM (Cd)
(Atomic Weight 112.41)

CADMIUM is a white metal possessing a bluish tinge with a bright lustre, capable of taking a high polish. It is a soft metal, but harder than zinc or tin; more tenacious than tin; malleable and very ductile, can easily be rolled out into foil or drawn into fine wire, but at 80° C. is very brittle. It may be completely distilled in a current of hydrogen above 80° C., forming silver white crystals.[219] Its boiling point is from 763° C. to 772° C. It melts at 321.6° C. Specific gravity is 8.67. The metal dissolves slowly in a hot dilute hydrochloric or sulphuric acid with evolution of hydrogen. It is capable of taking a high polish and upon this is based its meteoric rise industrially, as a plating metal for rust proofing. It was first used as a coating for piano strings and other musical instruments. Now it has been adopted as a coating for many motor vehicle parts. Because of its relatively high melting point and wear, its application in the future may be greatly extended. In 1934, 2,777,384 pounds were produced in the United States. It is found chiefly as greenockite, (a cadmium sulphide) in Greenland, Scotland, and Pennsylvania. It was found accompanying many zinc ores to the extent of 1% to 3%. The more important compounds of cadmium are the oxides, sulphate, sulphide, chloride, iodide, and bromide. It should not be used in plating where food is

218. AKATSUKA, K., and FAIRHALL, L. T.: *J. Indust. Hyg.*, 16:4, 1934.
219. KAMMERER: *Berichte*, 7:1724, 1874.

handled, as food is dissolved in cadmium in contact with solutions containing .5 to 2.5% of acetic acid.[220]   Hazen[221] reported a serious illness from eating a gelatin dessert which had been allowed to solidify in a tray coated with a metal containing 56% cadmium.

The greatest danger to health is found in the manufacture of cadmium and in the handling of its compounds.   Danger comes from inhalation of the fumes and vapors from the retorts or condensers of the blue powder furnaces in making both cadmium and cadmium oxide and in the bagging and handling of these two materials.   Prodan[222] gives the early history of cadmium poisoning and experimental cadmium poisoning. He fed large doses of cadmium to cats, and found that it induced vomiting, salivation, loss of appetite, followed by loss of weight.   In the consideration of cadmium as an industrial hazard, we have to deal with the poison which enters the body mainly through the respiratory tract and secondly through the gastro-intestinal tract.[222]   Legge[223] reported three cases of poisoning of workers in a paint factory, where ingots of cadmium were melted.   One of these workmen died.   Autopsy on the man showed congestion of the air passages and gastro-intestinal tract, and acute inflammation of the kidneys and spleen.   Several cases of fatal poisoning are reported due to the inhalation of cadmium vapors arising from molten metal.*

Symptoms: The chief symptoms are dryness of the throat, headache, nausea, rapid pulse, passage of brown-colored urine, and the sensation of cold.   Schwartz[224] reported a case of cadmium poisoning in a man employed in a factory melting cadmium, and inhaling the fumes.   The symptoms were vehement coughing and headache.   The following day he had nausea, shivering, pains in the sternal region and difficulty in respiration.

A man, twenty-six years of age, working in a cadmium plating factory for two years was examined December 26, 1934.

220. GRONOVER and WOHNLICH: *Ztschr. f. Untersuch. d. Lebensmitt.*, 53:392, 1927.
221. HAZEN, C. K.:   *Food Ind.*, 6:268, 1934.
222. PRODAN, LEON: *J. Indust. Hyg.*, 14:174, 1932.
223. LEGGE, T. M.:   Ann. Report Chief Insp. Factories for 1923, London, 74, 1924.   And see SCREMIN, L.:   *Boll d. soc. ital di brol. sper.*, 7:670, 1932.   * *Die Gasmaske*, 9:37, 1937.
224. SCHWARTZ, L.:   Gewerbliche Cadmium Vergiftung, *Ztschr. f. Gewerbehyg.*, 36:190, 1930.

He complained of "shakes," pain in the chest, cough, pain in the back, difficulty in breathing, shortness of breath, poor appetite, and pain in the nose. His pulse was 108, blood pressure systolic 102, diastolic 72. As he was exposed to sulphuric and nitric oxide fumes in addition to the cadmium, some of his respiratory trouble might be attributed to the acid fumes.

After exposure to cadmium sulphide dust for twenty-four to thirty-six hours animals vomited, had diarrhea, and occasional salivation. They also had an increased rate of respiration which was dyspneic, and noisy. Cadmium sulphide causes generalized pneumonia and bronchopneumonia accompanied by edema and extensive empyema and atelectasis of a mechanical nature. Dizziness, dyspnea, vomiting, colic, diarrhea, and low pulse are among the first symptoms.

Postmortem Appearances: Prodan reported the autopsy of an engineer who died of cadmium poisoning. Examination showed inflammation of the pharynx, trachea, bronchi, and gastro-intestinal canal, with fatty degeneration of the heart and the liver; hemorrhagic inflammation of the spleen, and acute inflammation of the kidneys.

In the autopsy of cats Prodan found emphysematous patches at the bases; mediastinum was edematous. The lungs of one cat showed a yellow pleural effusion. All organs showed congestion and the liver had a fatty appearance. Microscopical examination revealed edema of the lungs, desquamation of the epithelia of the bronchioles and alveolar ducts and polymorphonuclear leukocyte infiltration in the walls. In the kidneys polymorphonuclear leukocyte infiltration and some early fatty degeneration were also noted. All other organs presented no pathology. In these animals, cadmium was found chemically highest in the lungs, with the liver next, and then the kidneys.

Tests: The cadmium solution may be precipitated by hydrogen sulphide as yellow cadmium sulphide which is insolubule in $(NH_4)_2S_x$ and soluble in hot dilute nitric acid. It is separated with Pb, Bi, and Cu from the remaining metals of the second group. Dilute sulphuric acid with C_2H_5OH removes the lead, and NH_4OH precipitates the bismuth as $Bi(OH)_3$, leaving the copper and cadmium in solution. If copper is present, KCN is added until the solution becomes colorless when the cadmium is detected by the formation of the yellow cadmium sulphide with hydrogen sulphide. By passing in hydrogen sulphide, cadmium alone is precipitated as yellow sulphide, CdS, whereas copper remains in solution as potassium cuprocyanide, $K_4Cu_2(CN)_6$.

The Diphenylcarbazid Test:[225] Upon the addition of an alcohol solution of diphenylcarbazid to a neutral cadmium solution a red-violet precipitate will form or just a red-violet color. The test is not specific for cadmium, as it is given by copper, lead and mercury.

NICKEL (Ni)
(Atomic Weight 58.7)

NICKEL occurs in nature together with cobalt. It is found as millerite, NiS_2; as nickel blende, NiS; as iron nickel blende, NiFeS; as cobalt nickel pyrites, $(NiCoFe)_3S_4$. It is prepared by a number of methods: by reduction, by ignition in CO, by heating the carbonyl, $Ni(CO)_4$, to 200° C. Nickel carbonyl is a gaseous compound of nickel and carbon monoxide which can be condensed by cold into a clear yellow liquid, volatilizing at room temperature, and when heated to 150° C. decomposes with a deposit of metallic nickel and the release of carbon monoxide. Owing to the great volatility of the nickel carbonyl it becomes a source of danger, although the Mond process is usually conducted in a closed apparatus, which prevents serious injury from leakage. Kotzing[226] reports five cases of poisoning which have been observed in the last three years at an Industrial Disease Hospital at Ludwigshaven. Brandes[227] reports a case of poisoning, the symptoms being the same as reported by Armit.[228]

Symptoms: Air containing as much as one part in a thousand of nickel carbonyl is dangerous. The nickel is dissolved by the tissue fluids, taken up by the blood, and has a specific effect on the endothelium of the capillary vessels, causing hemorrhages, especially in the brain and adrenals. Patients complain of pains in the forehead, faintness, nausea, and a feeling of tightness in the chest. There is a troublesome cough with thick

225. FIEGLE, F., and NEUBER, F.: *Ztschr. f. anal. chem.*, Wiesb., 62:378, 1923.

226. KOTZING, K.: *Arch. f. Gewerbepath. u. Gewerbehyg.*, 4:500, 1933.

227. BRANDES, W. W.: *J.A.M.A.*, 101:1204, 1934.

228. ARMIT, H. W.: *J. Hyg.*, 8:565, 1908.

expectoration, dyspnea, raised temperature, and circulatory weakness. The clinical picture according to Kotzing is that of an acute bronchitis or bronchopneumonia. In fatal cases in man, delirium of various types appears. After twelve to thirty-six hours the signs of lung irritation are evident. Death occurs from the fourth to the eleventh day, after exposure.

Postmortem Appearances: Histologic changes in the lungs are quite unusual and correspond more nearly with descriptions of observations in lungs damaged by irritating substances such as phosgene. Brandes found small multiple hemorrhages in the lungs, also degenerative changes and areas of anemic necrosis in the brain. That these changes are due to nickel is indicated by the presence of this metal in the amounts of the tissues analyzed. Armit demonstrated that nickel appeared to be transported in the blood in a condition of colloidal solution. There is edema of the lungs and the liver is enlarged.

Treatment: Treatment consists of inhalations of oxygen to which 5% of carbon dioxide has been added, and a low-fat diet with aperients. When eczema or nickel itch[229] occurs in men working in nickel plating plants, they should be given a change of employment, for they are certain to have other attacks which come on more rapidly than the first and are slower to heal.

Tests: Digest the tissue by the Fresenius and von Babo method as previously described (page 22). Separate the cobalt with nitrosonaphthol precipitation. The nickel remains in the filtrate and can be precipitated with H_2S (after neutralizing with NH_4OH), and its presence confirmed by the usual tests. Quantitatively the nickel may be separated and weighed as NiO, or it can be converted into the sulphate and deposited on platinum as the free metal by the electrical current.

Detection: Upon a filter paper or a porcelain crucible cover, add one drop of the nickel solution and one drop of a 1% solution of dimethylglyoxim in alcohol. An intense red insoluble salt is formed. It is delicate, one to 300,000.

Palladium and platinum give an insoluble yellow precipitate, iron giving a soluble red compound of similar constitution as the nickel compound. The presence of large amounts of

229. DRINKER, FAIRHALL, RAY, and DRINKER: *J. Indust. Hyg.*, 6:307, 1924.

oxidizing agents, such as hydrogen peroxide, halogens, and nitrates, hinders the precipitation of the nickel-dimethylglyoxim.

MANGANESE (Mn)
(Atomic Weight 54.93)

MANGANESE was discovered by Scheele in 1774. It is not found native but is widely diffused, as it accompanies nearly all iron ores. The chief minerals in which it is found are the sulphide in alabandite (MnS), hauserite (MnS$_2$); oxides as pyrolusite (MnO$_2$) braunite (MnO$_2$O$_3$, MnSiO$_3$, MnSIO$_3$), manganite (MnOOH), hausmannite (Mn$_3$O$_4$), franklinite (FeZnMn (FeMn)$_2$O$_4$), psilomelane (MnO$_2$ (+H$_2$O, K$_2$O, or BaO), wad (a mixture of manganese oxides, such as cobalt, copper and lead); as the carbonate in rhodochrosite (MnCO$_3$); as a silicate in tephroite (Mn$_2$SIO$_4$), knebelite (FeMn)$_2$SiO$_4$, heterocline, helvine and rhodonite (MnSiO$_3$ or MnOSiO$_2$); as a phosphate in triplite (RF) RPO$_4$, (—R chiefly representing manganese and iron). The principal use of manganese minerals is in the production of alloys with iron, spiegeleisen and ferromanganese, in the manufacture of steel. It appears to unite with iron in all proportions. It retards the oxidation of iron in operations such as puddling, Bessemerizing, and open-hearth methods of making steel. It also appears to volatilize to some extent in these operations,[230] a possible factor in poisoning. Manganese has a valence of 2, 3, 4, 6, 7 and consequently has a great number of compounds which it may form. Manganous oxide (MnO) represents the only base capable of forming stable salts, manganic oxide (Mn$_2$O$_3$), trimanganese tetraoxide (Mn$_3$O$_4$), manganese peroxide (MnO$_2$), manganese trioxide (MnO$_3$), manganese heptoxide (Mn$_2$O$_7$), and manganese teroxide (MnO$_4$). It forms a large number of salts, of which the manganous salts are derivatives of the trivalent manganese. In the manganates, it produces the derivatives for manganic acid (H$_2$MnO$_4$), which is not known in the free state. Other uses are in the manufacture of dry batteries, chlorine, and oxygen driers for varnish; as a decolorizer for molten glass, to color glass pottery and bricks; and in making paints and enamels, and dyeing calico and linoleum. A small quantity finds use in coloring and grain-

---

230. Hiorns: Steel and Iron, 301, 1903.

ing soaps in the aniline and alizarin factories. Manganese, like silica, appears to be found in all plant and animal tissue. Maumene[231] found it only sparingly in the potato, while in the sugar beet he found it in considerable amounts. In the ash of the tea leaves Maumene found 10% of manganese. Von Schroder[232] found 33% of manganese dioxide in the ash of a ninety year old tree, which had grown on brownstone. Peterson and Skinner[233] report the manganese content of eighty-three representative foods as ranging from 0.028 mg. per liter of milk to 49.9 mg. of bran flakes. In urine, bones and hair, it is found only in traces. It is a normal constituent of the blood of man and animal. Bertrand[234] in 1905 began a series of exact scientific researches on the subject of manganese. These papers deal with the effect of the catalytic action of traces of manganese on the growth of certain molds, plants and bacteria.

Symptoms: I have collected eighty-one signs,[235] symptoms, and conditions reported by various authors. Some of these signs are duplications and could be placed under one heading.

The first consideration in arriving at a diagnosis of chronic managanese poisoning would be an occupational history of having worked in manganese for over three months. Second, a peculiar gait, which occurs in all cases. Third, weakness in the legs, and tremors, 88%. Fourth, mask-like face, 83%. Fifth, impulsive laughter, 70%. Sixth, propulsion and retropulsion, 70%; tremors of the whole body or extremities, 70%. Seventh, monotonous speech, or disturbance of speech, 60%. Eighth, fatigue, 52.9%. Ninth, disturbances in upper extremities. Tenth, increase of tendon reflexes, 50%. Eleventh, all reflexes exaggerated, 50%. Twelfth, sudden onset, 50%. Thirteenth, spastic gait, 46%. Fourteenth, pains in the legs, arms, and back, 36%. Fifteenth, no sensory disturbance. Six-

231. MAUMENE, E.: Compt. rend. T., 98:1056, 1884.

232. VON SCHRODER, J. V.: Tharandter forstliches Jahrbuch erster Suppl. Bd., Dresden, 105, 1878.

233. PETERSON, W. H., and SKINNER, J. T.: J. Nutrition, 4:419, 1931.

234. BERTRAND G.: Compt. rend. Acad. d. sc., 141:1255, 1905; Rev. gen. de Chim., 8:205, 1905; Compt. rend. Cong. de Chim. appl. de Berlin, 1903; de Rome, 1906; de Londres, 1909. BERTRAND, G., and JAVALLIER, M.: Ann. Inst. Pasteur, 26:241, 515, 1912; BERTRAND, G.: Ann. Inst. Pasteur, 26:767, 1912; BERTRAND, G., and SEZERAC, R.: Ann. Inst. Pasteur, 29:178, 1915.

235. McNALLY, W. D.: Indust. Med., 4:11:582, 1935.

teenth, micrographia. Seventeenth, impulsive weeping, 26%. Eighteenth, disturbances of sexual function, 25%. (This probably would be larger in number, but was neglected or omitted entirely in many histories.) All of the other symptoms occurred less than 25%. Kappe* reported loss of weight and stomach disorders from a worker breathing air heavily laden with manganese dust.

Laboratory examination does not aid in the diagnosis unless the examinations are made early or while the patient is still at work. The urine has repeatedly been negative for manganese. Blood normally contains 0.01 to 0.02% of manganese per 100 gm. of blood. Examinations made after the men had been away from the mills for months would not show abnormal amounts of manganese. The blood examination would show variations according to the time of removal from the dusty atmosphere. The erythrocytes might be over 6,000,000 or less than 5,000,000 per cubic mm. Most of the blood counts and other examinations of the blood have been normal. Lymphocytosis occurred in 33.8% of the cases. The blood pressure is normal. The spinal fluid examinations have all failed to show manganese or other abnormalities from histological, biological, and chemical points of view. The feces have shown small amounts of manganese, 2.2 mg. to 7.5 mg. per 100 gm. of sample.

The shortest period of work causing illness was one and a half months and the longest period before the first symptoms occurred was twenty-eight years. Therefore, it seems there is no immunity against this poison although some individuals are particularly susceptible to this type of intoxication since two or three out of every 200 workmen in manganese mills develop the disease. Seemingly, most of the cases occur in young men nineteen to thirty years of age. Liver involvement did not occur in any case. Seelert and others have reported the same findings. The disease develops without involvement of the cranial nerves. Sensory symptoms have been negative in nearly 100% of the cases. Cohen[236] reports sensory disturbances in the lumbar and sacral regions. New symptoms may appear as the disease progresses. Some cases where drowsi-

---

* KAPPE: Arbeitsschutz, 82, 1937.
236. COHEN, G.: *Zentralbl. f. d. ges. Neurol. u. Psychiat.*, 50:155, 1928. And see CRONZIN and DESOILLE: *Paris. méd.*, 26:361, 1936.

ness was reported later developed insomnia. Muscular twitchings or tremors, while reported in 88% of the cases, probably were present at some time in 100% of the cases. Chronic manganese intoxication incapitates one, but does not shorten the span of life. Most authorities state that all cases affected by pneumonia, end fatally. From the few postmortem examinations made, the conditions found were very similar to those seen grossly in silicosis, an extensive connective tissue proliferation in the lung, particularly along the lymphatic channels and along the bronchi.

This condition often simulates Wilson's disease, due to a hepatico-lenticular degeneration. However, this latter condition is characterized by the facts that it affects adolescence and that it usually runs in families. The coarseness of the tremor, the early onset of dysarthria and dysphagia with the characteristic mental symptoms and the very rapid course in the acute cases with fever and emaciation, would tend to favor Wilson's disease. In manganese poisoning, the patients are always well nourished, and the disease comes on suddenly. Fritsche[237] discusses a case of oligophrenia in which a patient showed symptoms referable to the basal ganglia involvement, and states that we should consider manganese among the etiological factors. Some of the cases represent a typical disturbance referable to the pyramidal system,[238] others to a disturbance in the striate body, caused by manganese dust.[239]

237. FRITSCHE, R.: *Arch. Neurol. & Psychiat.*, 35:1, 1935.

238. FLINTZER, H.: *Arch. f. Psychiat.*, 93:84, 1931; BAADER, E. W.: *Arch. f. Gewerbepath. u. Gewerbehyg.*, 4:101, 1933.

239. COUPER: *J. de Chem. med. de. Pharm. et de Toxicol.*, 3 (2nd series): 233, 1837.

VON JAKSCH, R.: *Prag. med. Wchnschr.*, 26:122, 1901; *Wien. klin. Rundschau*, 41, Sonderabdruck, 1901; *Verhandl. d. Gesellsch. deutsch. Naturf. u. Aertze, Leipz.*, 2:44 and 342, 1902, 1903.

VON JAKSCH, R.: Vergiftungen, 1910, Nothnagel, H., Spezielle Pathologie und Therapie, Band 1.

VON JAKSCH, R.: *München. med. Wchnschr.*, 54:969, 1907.

EMBDEN, H.: *Deutsche med. Wchnschr.*, 27:795, 1901.

VON JAKSCH, R.: Vergiftungen, 1910, Nothnagel, H., p. 233.

EDSALL, D. L., and DRINKER, C. K.: Contributions to Medical and Biological Research—dedicated to Sir William Osler, 1:447, 1919.

LEWY, F. H., and TIEFENBACH, L.: *Ztschr. f. d. ges. Neurol. u. Psychiat.*, 71:303, 1921.

DAVIS, G. G., and HUEY, W. B.: *J. Indust. Hyg.*, 3:231, 1921.

WILSON, G.: *Arch. Neurol. & Psychiat.*, 8:332, 1922.

FINDLAY, G. M.: *Brit. J. Exper. Path.*, 5:92, 1924.

The pharmacology of manganese is given in an article by von Oettingen.[240]

Treatment: Charles[241] treated seven cases with liver, obtaining only temporary relief. Electrotherapy, hydrotherapy, potassium iodide and sodium thiosulphate have all been tried. There seems to be little hope for recovery no matter what the treatment.

Postmortem Appearances: The pathology of chronic manganese intoxication has not been entirely elucidated, since only a few autopsies have been performed. We have had to rely upon the results of animal experimentation.

Casamajor, in 1916, performed the first postmortem upon a patient who had suffered from chronic manganese poisoning, dying from pneumonia. In the kidneys he found an interstitial nephritis and the liver showed an extensive biliary cirrhosis. He found that in the brain there was some degeneration of the longitudinal fibers of the pons. Casamajor probably failed completely in recognizing the true pathology. In 1927, Ashizawa[239] reported an autopsy on a case of chronic manganese poisoning. This report is complicated by other pathology caused by caries of the vertebrae and cerebral involvement not due to manganese intoxication. Changes in the central nervous system were found. Marked alterations were found in the putamen and nucleus caudatus, and the degeneration of the large ganglion cells was more pronounced than that of the small. The thin nerve fibers were lessened significantly in the striatum, but the thick fibers remained normal.

Canavan, Cobb and Drinker report an autopsy on a man fifty-five years of age who had been working in a mill where manganese-containing fractions were separated from the ores. The air inhaled by this man carried 10 to 20 mg. of dust per cubic foot, with manganese content of 9 to 12%. Thirteen years after leaving the mill he died of cardiorenal disease. The

GAYLE, F.: J.A.M.A., 85:2008, 1925.

ASHIZAWA, R.: Jap. J. M. Se. Tr., VIII; Internat. Med., Pediat., & Psychiat., 50:173, 1927.

GRUNSTEIN, A. M., and POPOWA, N.: Arch. f. Psychiat., 87:742, 1929.

FLINTZER, H.: Arch. f. Psychiat., Nervenkrankheiten, 93:84, 1931.

BAADER, E. W.: Zentralbl. f. Gewerbehyg., 19:1, 1932.

HILPERT, P.: Med. Welt., 7:522, 1933.

SOURATE, V.: Rev. neurol., 1:678, 1934.

240. VON OETTINGEN, W. F.: Physiol. Rev., 15:175, 1935.

241. CHARLES, J. R.: Brain, 50:30, 1927.

autopsy was confined to the brain, as the abdominal postmortem could not be obtained. Frontal sections of the brain showed greater atrophy of the cortex on the left, and some indistinctness in the basal ganglia. One slice of the brain which included both striate bodies and optic thalami showed atrophy. The decrease in size of the basal ganglia was between 3 mm. and 10 mm. smaller than in a control section. Microscopical examination showed that the cells of the choroid plexus were on the outside of the tufts; they were mostly low and single but occasionally heaped up. Some tufts showed enlarged vessels; some were thrombosed. This pia mater was definitely thickened.

With an elastic stain it was striking to see the disarrangement of the elastic fibrils in many of the vessels.[242]

Baader, in 1933 reported that an autopsy on a man dying from pneumonia showed that the lung contained numerous particles of manganese dust, and there was found an extensive connective tissue proliferation in this organ particularly along the lymphatic channels and along the bronchi.[243] And Schopper, in 1930, reported two autopsies of cases of pneumonia in brownstone miners. He did not report on the pathology of the brain. The findings were the same as given by Baader. Baader found manganese in a man dying of croupy pneumonia.*

Tests: Blood or urine is evaporated to dryness in a silica dish in the presence of sodium carbonate and ashed in an electric muffle. Add sulphuric acid until effervescence ceases, then a few drops of nitric (one to three dilution). Filter, and to the filtrate add five drops of a 2.5% silver nitrate, and 0.3 gm. of crystallized potassium persulphate. Place beaker or test-tube containing the unknown in warm water. In a few minutes a purple color of permanganate appears. Run a blank on all chemicals and dishes used. Make up to 50 cc., compare with a standard permanganate solution containing 0.002 to 0.025 mg. of manganese.[244]

242. CANAVAN, M. M., COBB, S., and DRINKER, C. K.: *Arch. Neurol. & Psychiat.*, 32:501, 1934.
243. BAADER, E. W.: *Arch f. Gewerbepath. u. Gewerbehyg.*, 4:101, 1933; SCHOPPER, W.: *Arch. f. Hyg.*, 104:175, 1930.
* BAADER: *Arrtzlich Sachverstand. Ztg.*, 43:75, 1937.
244. See SUTTON: Volumetric Analysis; BERTRAND, G.: *Bull. Soc. Chim.*, 9 (series IV):361, 1911; or REIMAN, C. K., and MINOT, A. S.: *J. Biol. Chem.*, 45:133, 1920 and 1921, for details.

BARIUM (Ba)
(Atomic Weight 137.4)

BARIUM occurs in nature chiefly as heavyspar ($BaSO_4$), and witherite ($BaCO_3$). Poisoning by barium salts is comparatively rare, in view of the large number of barium meals given for fluoroscopic or roentgen-ray studies. In a review of the literature, twelve deaths from barium carbonate, six deaths from barium chloride and four deaths from barium sulphide poisoning were found. Common salt (NaCl) has been found to contain ponderable amounts of barium chloride as a not infrequent impurity, so that the U. S. Bureau of Chemistry has established as a standard of purity the presence of not more than 0.05% of barium chloride in common salt.[245]

Barium carbonate ($BaCO_3$) occurs native as witherite, a white crystal slightly soluble in water and freely so in acids. It is used alone and also mixed with arsenic trioxide as rat poison, and has been responsible for a number of deaths where it had been administered by mistake for barium sulphate. Witthaus and Becker [246] reported thirty cases of poisoning, with twenty deaths. Of these poisonings, fourteen were by the chloride, ten by the carbonate, four by the nitrate, and two by the acetate. Twenty-two were accidental, three were suicides, one was taken to produce abortion, and in the other three the motive was not stated.

Barium sulphate ($BaSO_4$) is a heavy white crystal, insoluble in water and acids, but slightly soluble in hot concentrated sulphuric acids. It is used in paints, also used extensively in roentgen-ray work as it is cheap, opaque, and harmless. A number of mistakes have been made in the writing and filling of prescriptions, where the soluble barium carbonate and sulphide have been substituted for the sulphate.

I have reported two cases of barium poisoning, one of barium sulphide and one of barium carbonate which had been dispensed in error for barium sulphate.[247] Two similar mishaps were reported in Prague,[248] each taking 50 gm. of the

245. See Service and Regulatory Announcements, No. 13, Bur. of Chemistry, U. S. Dept. of Agriculture.

246. WITTHAUS and BECKER: Medical Jurisprudence, Forensic Medicine and Toxicology, 682, 1911.

247. McNALLY, W. D.: *J.A.M.A.*, 84:1805, 1925.

248. Vienna letter, *J.A.M.A.*, 58:2041, 1912; KRAUSE: *Deutsche med. Wchnschr.*, 48:319, 1912.

carbonate in suspension in water, for roentgen work. Two other cases were reported by Bensaude and Antoine.[249] Ten cases of poisoning by barium sulphide being taken by mistake for barium sulphate have been reported.

Symptoms: Barium poisoning manifests itself by great weakness, salivation and nausea. Vomiting and diarrhea follow. The purging is very violent, and causes severe abdominal pains. At this stage, usually, the victim becomes very cold. There is a catarrhal affection of the conjunctiva, the mucous membrane of the respiratory tract, and the nose. Paralysis of the extremities and finally of the trunk are succeeding developments. The muscles of speech become very weak early in the poisoning, and swallowing is very difficult. Consciousness always remains to the end. Schwartz[250] reported toxic manifestations of barium chloride in a patient with complete heart block.

TABLE X
BARIUM CALCULATED AS BARIUM SULPHIDE

Organ	Gm. per 100 gm. Tissue	Gm. in Total Specimen Received
Bowel (large)	0.0383	0.0283 in 74 gm.
Bowel (small)	0.0320	0.0602 in 188 gm.
Brain	0.0030	0.0109 in 358 gm.
Cecum	0.0168	0.0082 in 48 gm.
Diaphragm	0.0117	0.0112 in 96 gm.
Heart	0.0023	0.0077 in 335 gm.
Kidney (left)	0.0152	0.0208 in 137 gm.
Kidney (right)	0.0135	0.0185 in 137 gm.
Liver	0.0152	0.1266 in 833 gm.
Lung	0.0037	0.0334 in 902 gm.
Pancreas	0.0131	0.0118 in 90 gm.
Spleen	0.0440	0.0054 in 135 gm.
Stomach	0.7976	1.8983 in 238 gm.

Treatment: Treatment usually consists of ingestion of magnesium or sodium sulphate, stomach lavage, hot bags around the abdomen and spine, stimulation with aromatic spirits of ammonia, and strychnine injection.

Therapeutics: All barium salts with the exception of the sulphate are toxic in large quantities. However, when given in

249. BENSAUDE and ANTOINE: *Bull. et mém. Soc. méd. d. hôp. de Paris,* 43:15, 1919; MAYRHOFER and MEIXNER: *Wien. klin. Wchnschr.,* 32:1068, 1919; DRAFFT: *Ztschr. f. Nahrungsmit.-Untersuch. u. Hyg., Wien.,* 42:390, 1921.

250. SCHWARTZ, S. P.: *Am. Heart J.,* 4:612, 1929.

proper doses they exert a marked stimulating action on all muscular tissue, and a gradual sustained rise in blood pressure. A depression may occur, depending on the condition of the organs, and also on the presence of other substances. The elimination of barium takes place mainly through the bowels. Barium chloride has been used medicinally in place of digitalis,[251] with good results, but the irritation of the former on the bowels makes its application very limited.

Fatal Dose: Riley[252] states that 3.8 gm. is the smallest fatal dose of the chloride, although larger doses have been taken without ill effect when prompt treatment followed. Schuchardt[253] had a case in which 3 gm. caused death. Kobert[254] believes that, under certain conditions, 2 gm. would be fatal. The toxic dose he believes to be 0.2 gm., and when larger amounts are tolerated it is chiefly due to the ingestion of a sulphate-rich food which renders some of the barium insoluble. Twenty gm. of barium chloride taken by mistake for magnesium sulphate caused death in five and one-half hours. A chemical examination of the viscera gave the data of Table XI.

TABLE XI

BARIUM CHLORIDE IN VISCERA

Organ	Weight Gm.	Barium Choride free Anhydrous	Barium Sulphate Trans.	Calculated to Barium Choride
Stomach contents	38	0	Trace	Trace
Intestinal contents	25	0	0.019	0.020
Liver	670	0.126	0.088	0.091
Kidney	132	0.050	0.028	0.029
Spleen	58	Trace	0.003	0.003
Lung	335	0.070	0.021	0.022
Brain	500	0	0	0
Blood	15	0.003	0.003	0.003
Total	1,773	0.249	0.162	0.168

Thus, in 1,773 gm. of the organs there was an equivalent of 0.417 mg. of the anhydrous barium chloride. Stern[255] reports that 8.6 gm. of the chloride caused death in nine hours. A man

251. SALANT and KLEITMAN: J. Pharmacol. & Exper. Therap., 20: 247, 1923.

252. RILEY: Toxicology, 50, 1906.

253. SCHUCHARDT: Nach. Machka, Hand. d. gerichtl. Med., 2:174, 1869.

254. KOBERT: Lehrbuch der Intoxikationen, 237, 1906—literature of Ba poison up to 1906.

255. STERN: Ztschr. f. Med.-Beamte, Berl., 9:381, 1896.

recovered from 6.5 gm. of the chloride taken on a full stomach.[256] Aloy and Saloz[257] report two cases of death within ten hours from 30 gm. of barium chloride taken in place of barium sulphate. Krafft[258] gives the lethal dose of barium chloride as 0.09 gm. per kilogram of body weight when taken by mouth.

Intravenous injection of 0.04 gm. in full grown cats of from 3 to 5 kg. killed all in from one to thirty minutes. A dog of 7.8 kg. weight died in twenty-two minutes after the injection of 0.21 gm., given in seven divided doses. Aloy and Cournet[259] determined the minimal lethal dose of this salt to be from 0.01 to 0.015 gm. per kilogram of body weight by injection and 0.09 gm. per kilogram by ingestion. The longest duration of poisoning with death is that reported by Lewin[260] of a person dying in three days from the ingestion of 10 gm. of barium chloride.

Although barium carbonate is insoluble, the hydrochloric acid of the gastric juice changes it to the soluble toxic chloride. From 80 to 100 gm. of barium carbonate taken in a roentgen-ray examination, substituted by a pharmacist for bismuth subnitrate, caused death in thirty-six hours.[261] Adults have recovered from taking 35 gm. of the carbonate.[262] Forty-five gm. caused death in seventeen hours,[263] and from 10 to 12 gm. caused death in thirteen hours.[264] Mayrhofer and Meixner[265] reported a case in which 10 gm. of barium carbonate were found in the stomach of a man who had taken rat poison with suicidal intent. Krafft[258] reported the death of a man who died after eating some cooked beans. The remainder of the food contained granules of a white powder which on analysis proved to be a mixture of the carbonate and sulphate of barium. The

256. BECKER: *Ztschr. f. Med.-Beamte, Berl.*, 24:677, 1911.

257. ALOY, J., and SALOZ: Bull. Soc. Chem., 563, 1912.

258. KRAFFT, K.: *Ztschr. f. Untersuch. d. Nahrungs.-u. Genussmittel, Berl.*, 42:390, 1921.

259. ALOY, J., and COURNET, A.: *J. de pharm. et chim., Par.*, 17:76, 1918; *Chem. Zentralbl.*, 848:1918.

260. GADAMER: Lehrbuch d. chem. Tox., 252, 1908.

261. BENSANDE, R., and ANTOINE, E.: *Bull. et mém. Soc. méd. d. hôp de Paris*, 43:369, 1919.

262. FELLETER: *Pest. med.-chir. Presse, Budapest*, 34:1073, 1892.

263. ALTHOFF: *Med. Klin.*, 20:1426, 1924.

264. WOLFF: *U. D. f. gericht. Med.*, 1:522, 1922.

265. MEIXNER: *Wien. klin. Wchnschr.*, 32:1068, 1919.

possibilities for poisoning were markedly increased by roentgen-ray examinations due to contamination (Krause) of the harmless sulphate with soluble barium salts. In Warsaw, an epidemic of muscular paralýsis resulted from the intoxications due to the adulteration of flour with barium sulphate and carbonate.[266]

Barium sulphide caused ten deaths in cases in which quantities ranging from 38 to 120 gm. had been taken. An eight-ounce guinea-pig was fed one-fourth grain portions of barium sulphide for four successive mornings, with no ill effects. The experimenter[267] then swallowed a dose of proportionate size (61 grains, 120 pounds body weight) with toxic symptoms, but with recovery.

Fatal Period: The shortest time for death in a barium poisoning occurred in ten minutes after the ingestion of 40 gm. of barium sulphide. Thirty gm. of barium nitrate caused death in one hour.[268] Tidy,[269] in 1868, reported one death from 15 gm. in six and one-half hours. Baum[270] reported two deaths. A tailor took a teasponful of barium nitrate for sodium bicarbonate, death occurring in five hours; in another instance, death occurred in thirteen hours. Baum, in the first case, found 0.1293 gm. of barium nitrate in the stomach and contents, 0.0313 gm. in the liver, spleen and kidneys, and 0.005 gm. in the urine; while in the other case, in which life was prolonged for thirteen hours, no barium was found in the viscera.

Thirty gm. of barium acetate given by mistake for sodium ethylsulphate caused death, the time not being given.[271]

Postmortem Appearances: CASE 1. M.P., a Filipino, aged twenty-nine, took four ounces of barium carbonate in a pint of milk. The physician had prescribed barium carbonate in place of barium sulphate. The error was not detected by the pharmacist. Vomiting occurred in a few minutes. The patient was removed to a hospital. The rate of respiration was 30; the pulse, 106. A leukocyte count of 32,400 was obtained. The patient complained of severe abdominal pain, and vomited yellow

266. HIGIER: *Zentralbl. f. Nervenh. u. Psychiat., Coblenz & Leipz.,* 73:337, 1922.

267. STEDAN: *Bull. Pharm.,* 34:40, 1920.

268. GADAMER: Lehrbuch d. Chem. Tox., 252, 1908.

269. TIDY: *M. Press u. Circ.,* 6:447, 1868.

270. BAUM: *Ztschr. f. Med.-Beamte, Berl.,* 9:759, 1896.

271. LEGARDE: *Union med.,* 14:537, 1872.

mucoid material. Diarrhea was present. The patient grew progressively weaker, developing a difficulty in enunciation of words and a paresis of the arms. He died at 3:45 P.M., eight and three-quarter hours after ingestion of the poison. As the cause of the acute illness was not apparent, antidotes were not given for barium. The postmortem did not disclose evidence of corrosion of the mouth. The heart presented a marked parenchymatous degeneration of its myocardium. The lungs were acutely edematous. The liver, spleen, and kidneys presented a parenchymatous degeneration. The pancreas, suprarenals and urinary bladder were without gross changes of note. The gastric mucosa was somewhat hyperemic, with numerous petechiae. The stomach contained a small amount of bile-stained fluid with no characteristic odor. The intestinal mucosa presented no gross changes of note. A chemical examination gave 0.2919 gm. (calculated as barium carbonate) in 139 gm. of stomach, and 0.0219 gm. (calculated as barium carbonate) in 398 gm. of bowel. A box containing a small amount of white powder, said to have been a portion of that taken by the deceased, was examined and found to be barium carbonate.

CASE 2. Mrs. C. F. B., aged fifty-one, took a portion of a mixture containing four ounces of barium sulphide in a pint of buttermilk, at 4:00 A.M., The buttermilk burned and nauseated her so much that she was able to drink only half of the mixture. When seen by a physician at 4:30, she was vomiting and in great pain. Her pulse was rapid and weak. The vomited material had the odor of rotten eggs. The pulse gradually became weaker, death occurring at 7:00 A.M., three hours after taking the barium sulphide. A postmortem examination did not show marks or evidence of external injury or violence. The brain was congested and edematous. When the thoracic and abdominal cavities were opened, the odor of hydrogen sulphide was marked. The lungs, liver, kidneys, and spleen showed a passive congestion. The heart showed some myocardial changes. The bowel and stomach were distended with gas. The upper portion of the small intestine was of a blackish discoloration. A chemical examination of the organs disclosed the presence of barium sulphide. A small amount of powder, said to be a portion of that taken by the deceased, was examined and found to be barium sulphide, dispensed in error by the pharmacist for the harmless barium sulphate. The amounts of barium found in the organs, calculated as barium sulphide, are given in Table X, page 141.

Fühner[272] reports a case of a pharmacist who gave barium chloride by mistake instead of chloral hydrate as a soporific. The man, fifty-five years of age, took one dose and fell ill during the night with violent abdominal pains, diarrhea and vomiting. Having no idea of the poisonous nature of the sedative he was supposed to take, that night he again took a dose, and fell ill, with vomiting, paralysis of the neck muscles, arms, and legs, and died the following day from cardiac paralysis. Postmortem examination showed hemorrhages in the stomach, and hyperemia in the lungs and kidneys. The patient had been given 2.25 gm. of barium chloride per dose, and again within twenty-four hours, making a total of 4.5 gm. causing the death.

Tests: When dilute sulphuric acid is added to a soluble barium salt, a white insoluble barium sulphate is precipitated. Soluble chromates, as K_2CrO_4, precipitate barium chromate, yellow, almost insoluble in water, sparingly soluble in acetic acid, moderately soluble in chromic acid, and readily soluble in hydrochloric and nitric acids. The volatile salts of barium as the chloride or nitrate impart a yellowish-green color to the flame of the Bunsen burner, appearing blue when viewed through a green glass. The spectrum of barium is readily distinguished from the spectra of other metals by the green bands Ba, (alpha, beta and gamma.) Barium carbonate is very stable when heated, requiring a very high heat to decompose it into BaO and CO_2.

Detection: An aliquot portion of the organs is made alkaline and ashed. The residue is dissolved in from 3 to 5 cc. of 10% hydrochloric acid, diluted to 100 cc., and the barium precipitated as the sulphate. The sulphate is filtered and washed free from sulphuric acid. The precipitate is fused with potassium carbonate and the cooled fusion is boiled with about 25 cc. of water and filtered. The filtrate is tested for barium. The precipitate is digested with hydrochloric acid and filtered, the residue washed, and washings added to the original filtrate, and the usual determination for barium made. Linossier[273] found barium in the greatest amount in the bones, in less quantity in the liver, kidneys, brain and cord, and only traces in the lungs,

272. FUHNER: *Sammlung von Vergiftungsfallen*, 1, 1930.
273. LINOSSIER: *Compt. rend. Soc. de biol.*, 4:122, 1887.

muscles, and heart. The distribution per hundred grams is fairly uniform in Table X (page 141), the bowel and stomach containing the largest amounts. A chemical examination of the organs of a man dying nine hours after taking a mouthful of a solution of barium chloride (about 8.6 gm. of crystallized barium chloride) failed to show the presence of barium in the stomach, stomach content, esophagus, and duodenum. The heart and the blood of the heart, with the lungs, contained 0.158 gm. of barium sulphate.

In an attempt to determine the presence of normal barium in organs, the material of eleven cases with negative histories of poisoning was used. The liver, kidney, bowel and brain failed to give the chromate and sulphate tests for barium in 200-gm. samples.

An accidental case of barium sulphide poisoning is reported by Singh.[274]

LEAD (Pb)
(Atomic Weight 206.92. Synonym: Plumbum)

PURE LEAD is almost white, soft, malleable, very slightly ductile, and tarnishes in the air from formation of a film of oxide. Its melting point is 327°C., and it boils at 1540°C. It forms alloys with most metals; lead and tin in various proportions form solder and pewter; lead and arsenic form shot metal; lead and antimony, type metal; lead, bismuth, tin and silver form a fusible alloy melting as low as 45°C.; bell metal consists of tin, copper, lead and zinc.

Lead is found most abundantly as galena, PbS; it also occurs as cerussite, $PbCO_3$; anglesite, $PbSO_4$; pyromorphite, $3Pb_3P_2O_8 PbCl_2$; krokoite, $PbCrO_4$; and in many minerals in combination with arsenic, antimony, and others.

Lead is not soluble in pure water, but the ordinary water served in plumbers' pipes contains enough free oxygen to oxidize a fresh lead surface, which may then form a soluble bicarbonate by the aid of the carbon dioxide present.

Nitric acid is the proper solvent for metallic lead; the lead nitrate formed is readily soluble in water but insoluble in concentrated nitric acid. Dilute sulphuric acid slowly changes the metal to the sulphate with evolution of sulphur dioxide, a portion of the salt being dissolved in the acid, precipitating on the

274. SINGH: *Indian M. Gaz.*, 64:506, 1929.

addition of water. Hydrochloric acid dissolves the metal very slowly—more rapidly when warmed—evolving hydrogen; the chloride formed dissolves in the acid in quantities depending upon conditions of temperature and concentrations.

Pure water, free from air, is without action upon pure lead, but water containing air and carbon dioxide very slowly attacks lead, forming the hydroxide and basic carbonate. This action is promoted by the presence of salts, as ammonium nitrate, nitrite, chloride, etc.; the action seems to be hindered by the presence of sulphates. Carlson[275] reported that galena ore from Federal, Illinois, was soluble to the extent of 2.94% in human gastric juice at 38°C., for ten hours; ore from St. Joseph Lead Company to the extent of 3.32%; while a sample of lead sulphide in his laboratory supply was much more soluble than the other two, dissolving 4.6%. Pelle and Artus[276] report a gingivitis, stomatitis, and dental caries in addition to gastrointestinal symptoms from drinking water containing lead. An epidemic of poisoning due to drinking water containing lead occurred in Leipzig[277] in July, 1930, in newly erected buildings. The pathological blood picture was found in one-third of 2,000 people examined. The lead content of the drinking water supplied to the newly constructed houses amounted to 5.3 mg. per liter in the morning and 3.5 mg. per liter during the day. A serious case was that of a woman, aged forty-one, with diabetes insipidus, who drank ten to twenty liters of water daily, and after four weeks suffered from diarrhea and vomiting. When admitted to the hospital, she showed a blue line on the gums, and a moderate anemia with 75% hemoglobin, 4,300,000 red cells, and 0.4% punctate basophilia. The symptoms quickly disappeared when she ceased drinking the water containing the lead. In a case described by Strotmeyer, drinking water containing 4.5 mg. lead per liter led to a bilateral paralysis of the radial muscles, together with an anemia of 60% hemoglobin, and 0.14% punctate basophilia. Picard[278] observed sixty-six cases of lead poisoning in ten years which could be traced to drinking water. His report shows that lead poisoning due to drinking water constituted a veritable social danger in the region of France

275. Carlson: *Am. J. Physiol.*, 31:151, 1912.
276. Pelle, A., and Artus: *Bull. Acad. de méd., Paris*, 113:54, 1935.
277. Editorial, *J.A.M.A.*, 96:1422, 1931.
278. Picard, R.: *Rev. de méd., Paris*, 51:133, 1934.

in which Picard lived. In all the cases observed the patients had installed, relatively recently, a pump which contained parts made of lead, and rarely the water was derived from lead pipes. The majority of patients presented very severe digestive disturbances which reminded one of intestinal obstruction or appendicitis, ulcer, cholecystitis, or even cancer of the body of the pancreas. The diagnosis in these cases is very difficult because the disease presents itself under various aspects, and the classical signs of lead poisoning in such instances are unfortunately absent and even basophilic stippling cannot usually be observed. Spira[279] reported cases of lead poisoning from tap water.

Fairley[280] found that lead poisoning occurred quite commonly in children in Queensland, Australia; and in Japan infants were poisoned from the use of toilet water containing white lead. Hereditary influences, scarlet fever, congenital lues, and other infections, may act in certain cases as factors, which predispose to lead poisoning and chronic nephritis. Most of the cases of lead poisoning in Queensland children are apparently derived from weathered lead paint on external surfaces, some may arise from the ingestion of fruit and vegetables that have been sprayed with lead arsenate. A number of cases of lead poisoning come from small infants chewing on the framework of their cribs. Fairley thought that the etiological agent in chronic nephritis originated in the lead poisonings in children. Kraft and Kato[281] reported a lead line in growing bones as a sign of lead poisoning in children.[282]

Williams, Schulze, Rothschild, Brown and Smith[283] report a group of forty cases of acute lead poisoning due to the inhalation of lead derived from discarded storage battery casings. In all large cities during the cold months, cases like these appear. In November, 1935, two children died of lead poisoning in Chicago, and several others were poisoned, from the inhalation of

279. SPIRA: *München. med. Wchnschr.*, 79:1003, 1932.
280. FAIRLEY, K. D.: *M. J. Australia*, 1:600, 1934.
281. KRAFT and KATO: *Fortschr. a. d. Geb. d. Röntgenstrahlen*, 46: 249, 1932.
282. See KASAHAN, H., and HEROSHIMER: *Ztschr. f. Kinderh.*, 53: 587, 1932; PARK, E., JACKSON, D., GOODWIN, T. C., and KADJI, R.: *J. Pediat.*, 3:265, 1933.
283. WILLIAMS, H., SCHULZE, W., ROTHSCHILD, H. B., BROWN, A. S., and SMITH, F. R.: *J.A.M.A.*, 100:1485, 1933.

lead from the burning of battery casings in the kitchen stove. Measures should be instituted for the destruction of these battery casings which will eliminate this health hazard; the health authorities in every city should have regulations or ordinances passed causing the destruction of all discarded wood resulting from the salvaging of lead plates from junk dealers, or from storage batteries. The manufacture of tetraethyl lead has caused cases of death and a number of cases of illness. Since the adoption of preventive measures, very few cases of poisoning by this agency have been reported. Gehrmann[284] divides the preventive measures into two classes: (a) those applicable to the workman, and (b) those of the operation. "The methods applicable to the workman comprise a thorough physical examination made with sufficient care to include all the essential details. The history of the workman is of particular interest and any previous exposure to lead is a definite contra-indication to acceptance unless the examiner can assure himself that only an insignificant absorption took place." It is a great risk to the employer to accept a man who has already been leaded. The superintendent should educate the men in personal hygiene. Every worker should be given two suits of clothes, one to be laundered every day. The workmen should not be allowed to consume food in the plants. All workmen should wash their hands and faces before eating, never eating in the plant, unless a special room is provided for that purpose. Each man should be required to report routinely to the physician, whether he feels ill or not, so that routine examinations can be recorded. In the plants the ventilation should be properly designed to reduce the lead content to an absolute minimum. Sweeping should be done by men with masks and never in the presence of other workmen. Frequent determination of the lead count of the air should be made in all parts of the plant so as to reveal the dangerous spots, as 1 or 2 mg. of lead absorbed each day will cause lead poisoning in about a year, while 10 mg. a day will cause plumbism in a few weeks.

Lead poisoning, like silicosis has become a depression disease. It was known for centuries by the early Greek and Roman physicians. Hippocrates[285] was possibly the first of the ancients to recognize lead as the cause of certain symptoms. Aub

284. GEHRMANN, G. H.:   Am. J. Pub. Health, 23:678, 1933.
285. AUB, FAIRHALL, MINOT, and REZNIKOFF: Lead Poisoning, 7, 1926.

and his co-workers in their monograph on "Lead Poisoning," give over 500 references on various phases of lead poisoning. Although lead poisoning has been known for many years, it is only in the last few years that chronic lead poisoning has caused grave concern to the manufacturer. A workman who is laid off because of lack of work, soon finds an attorney who is willing to start suit for him on the grounds of lead poisoning, claiming it to be an occupational disease coming under the Workmen's Compensation Act. Lead poisoning has appeared in every civilized country where lead is mined or used in the arts. The extensive literature of the world shows that lead poisoning is very common. It occurs chiefly in connection with lead pigments, battery plates, painting, plumbing, the printing trades, glazing china and porcelain ware, covering on cables, bearing metals and corrosion resistant alloys, the smelting and refining of lead, and in any industry that uses lead in any step of the process of manufacture. In the automobile industry where solder is used on the metallic bodies, the vapor or molten lead from the blow-torches or the finely divided lead from the sandpaper and buffing wheels[286] are fruitful sources of poisoning. There are over 150 trades which expose the workman to this hazard. Cosmetics containing lead have been responsible for a few cases of poisoning.

There are several factors that predispose to chronic lead poisoning. The young are peculiarly susceptible to the presence of lead. The colored race is more susceptible to lead poisoning than the white race. A colored man, aged thirty-nine years, melting battery plates, noticed in five days after starting work that his appetite began to fail. Then he began to have pains in his knees and wrists and abdomen. These pains were described as being located on the anterior surface of his body. In three months he had to stop this kind of work. His hemoglobin was 78; red blood cells, 3,390,000; white blood cells, 6,400. There was no lead line or basophilic stippling, the urine and stool showed lead in abnormal amounts. Oliver and Hamilton[287] believe that women are much more affected than men. Susceptibility has been found to be one to seven among women and one to thirteen among men in the pottery and allied industries in the

286. DEEN, A. S.: *J. Indust. Hyg.*, 6:245, 1924.
287. HAMILTON, ALICE: Industrial Poisons in the United States, 1929.

United States. Some men are more susceptible to lead than others. Some can work for years without showing effects, while others show symptoms in a few days. Part of this susceptibility can be explained upon the ground of personal habits, carelessness in personal hygiene, poor housing conditions, and chronic alcoholism, and pre-existing pathology caused by diseases earlier in life.

Lead Acetate ($Pb(C_2H_3O_2)_2 . 3H_2O$)—Lead acetate contains not less than 85.31% and not more than 89.57% of $(CH_3 . COO)_2Pb$, corresponding to not less than 99.5% of the hydrated salt, $(CH_3 . COO)_2Pb . 3H_2O$. It is a colorless, shining, transparent substance, crystallizing in monoclinic prisms or plates, or in heavy, white crystalline masses or granular crystals. It has a faintly acetous odor, is efflorescent, and absorbs carbon dioxide on exposure to air. At first it has a sweetish taste, from which its name of sugar of lead is derived, but soon the taste becomes styptic and metallic in character. It is present in pharmaceutic preparations as a pill with opium, a compound suppository with opium, and an ointment. The subacetate, $(Pb(C_2H_3O_2)_2)$ (PbO), is present in liquor plumbi subacetatis, in a dilute form in Goulard's water, and in the compound ointment or Goulard cerate. It is found in lead plaster, lead oleate, and lead ointment, and is present in the official ointment of lead carbonate and in various lead paints.

Lead Sulphate ($PbSO_4$)—Lead sulphate is an insoluble powder which is precipitated when a soluble sulphate is given as an antidote in lead poisoning, or when added to a soluble lead salt. It gives body to some brands of white lead paint and lends weight to white silk.

When lead is melted and vaporized at the higher temperatures to which it is subjected by lead smelters, zinc smelters, brass molders, and workers in type metal, lead pipe, wire solder, and shot, lead suboxide (Pb_2O) is formed on the surface.

The higher oxides, litharge and red lead are frequent sources of plumbism. The salt which is of greatest importance in acute poisoning is lead acetate, while chronic poisoning is most frequently caused by lead carbonate. Wine that has been clarified by lead acetate may contain sufficient lead to cause poisoning. The subacetate of lead present in Goulard's extract has a similar effect as the acetate. Lead chromate, lead oxides, and finely divided metallic lead, while not soluble in water, dissolve in the dilute vegetable acids of food and in the gastric juice, and exert a slowly cumulative poisonous action. All salts of lead are poisonous, no matter whether inhaled or taken by means of the gastro-intestinal tract. The lead carbonate used as a face powder has caused plumbism. The lead in sulphur dyes has been responsible for cases of lead poisoning. I have examined the urine of a number of persons using hair conditioners and found lead as high as 0.44 mg. per liter of urine. To my astonishment not any of these individuals had gastro-intestinal disturbances nor any signs of lead intoxication. The medicinal use of lead washes should be discouraged, as prolonged use is dangerous.

Acute Lead Poisoning.—The patient complains that there is a sweet, then a metallic astringent, taste in the mouth, and a dry throat. Later, within a half-hour, this is followed by an intensive burning and abdominal pain and vomiting, followed by diarrhea, rarely by constipation. The stools are black, from lead sulphide. The urine is scanty, with albumin and casts. The breath is foul, and the tongue is coated. There is headache, and pain and cramps in the legs, with numbness and local palsies which appear within a few hours. The symptoms vary in the acute stage, depending upon whether the acute poisoning has developed from the taking of a lead salt, or whether there has been inhalation of lead from the volatilization of a lead compound, as from the burning of battery boxes as previously mentioned. In these cases an encephalopathy develops. There may be convulsions followed by stupor, and the patient may be unconscious when first seen by the physician. In some cases of acute poisoning the symptoms may resemble, after twenty-four hours, a condition seen in chronic lead poisoning: colic, constipation, anemia, slight weakness of the extensors, and mild cerebral symptoms, all of which under appropriate treatment are completely curable, not causing permanent disability.

Fatal Dose: The fatal dose of lead acetate, and subacetate, and carbonate, for man is not definitely known. However, it is not small. Since recovery has taken place after taking one ounce of the acetate, it would seem that the fatal amount must be larger. In one instance, however, 10 gm. were said to have produced death, while 50 gm. of lead acetate would always prove fatal. Forty to 50 gm. of lead carbonate have caused death. In a small town in Illinois, in December, 1935, two ounces of a prescription which was compounded erroneously containing 2.85% of lead acetate, with sodium iodide, sodium bromide and sodium salicylate, and taken in divided doses for four days caused the death of a fifty-eight year old woman. Lead was found in the organs and bones.

Fatal Period: Witthaus recorded forty-four alleged deaths from acute lead poisoning in 124 cases. Death may occur on the second or third day.

Treatment: With a history of having taken a salt of lead, the stomach should be washed out immediately with a soluble sulphate, as sodium or magnesium sulphate, using 15 gm. to the pint of water, allowing one-half ounce of the magnesium sulphate to remain in the stomach, after the stomach has been thoroughly washed, which would aid in changing it into an insoluble lead sulphate. The patient should be given an intravenous injection of calcium gluconate, 1 gm. in 10 cc. of water. The pain should be controlled by opiates. The patient can be given milk and eggs after the stomach has been thoroughly washed and the half ounce of magnesium sulphate has been given.

Postmortem Appearances: The postmortem examination in acute lead poisoning reveals the pathology seen in death following a gastro-intestinal irritant. The bowel might show a contraction, and the contents would be black from the formation of lead sulphide.

CHRONIC LEAD POISONING
(Synonyms: Plumbism, Saturnine Intoxication)

CHRONIC lead poisoning is seen chiefly in industries that employ lead or its compounds in some process in the manufacture of the commodity which they sell. Subacute and chronic lead poisoning can occur from the ingestion of food or water which contains lead. Crosetti, Lorenzo, and Forgoni[288] reported about 200 cases of subacute poisoning which was due to consumption of flour contaminated by lead used in mending the millstones in the local mill. This type of poisoning is very rare, since many governments prohibit the use

288. CROSETTI, LORENZO, and FORGONI: *Policlin., Roma,* 41:516, 565, 1934.

of millstones which have been repaired by lead. The cause of lead poisoning has already been alluded to from wines, and liquors of all kinds. The lead content of wines varies from a trace to 74.25 mg. of lead per liter of wine. Distilled liquors gave from 0.6 to 52.7 mg. of lead per liter of distilled liquor. Chevallier and Oliver[289] cite an instance of an epidemic of lead poisoning caused by the use of litharge in treating "green" wine. Campbell,[290] and Allden[291] reported cases of lead poisoning occasioned by home-made wine which had dissolved lead from the containers. Vaughan[292] cites instances of lead poisoning after the consumption of "moonshine" whiskey which had evidently been contaminated by the lead in the stills. I have found lead and copper in a large number of samples of "moonshine" which had been submitted by the deputy coroners, in cases where death was due to alcoholism. Toys, chairs, and cribs that have been painted with lead, wallpaper, and cooking utensils which have been soldered with lead, are a potential source of lead poisoning. Absorption has been reported from the use of glazed and enameled ware. In hardening steel wires, a lead bath is used which furnishes a common source of contamination. In tinning material containers with tin, the tin is often mixed with lead, which is attacked by fluids and other substances placed in the containers. Some kinds of silk thread have been weighted with lead, and people who have chewed this thread have been reported poisoned. Outbreaks of lead poisoning have occurred in connection with beer, which was stored in large iron tanks lined with white enamel. The lead glaze was slowly dissolved by the beer.[293] Bech[294] reported a case of poisoning which was traced to the lead foil in which snuff was packed.[295]

Many authors report lead poisoning from retained lead

289. CHEVALLIER and OLIVER: *Ann. d'hyg.*, (1st series) 27:104, 1842.

290. CAMPBELL, D.: *Practitioner*, 37:477, 1886.

291. ALLDEN, G. H.: *Lancet*, 1:728, 1889.

292. VAUGHAN, W. T.: *J.A.M.A.*, 79:966, 1922.

293. REYNOLDS: Account of the Epidemic Outbreak of Arsenical Poisoning Occurring in Beer Drinkers in the North of England and Midland Countries in 1900, *Tr. Med.-Chir. Soc. Edinburgh*, 84:424, 1901; Editorial: An Outbreak of Lead Poisoning Due to Beer, *Lancet*, 5163: 349, 1922.

294. BECH, A.: Serious Lead Poisoning (caused by snuff), *Rev. Hyg. Pref.*, 55:541, 1933.

295. TELEKY: *Deutsche med. Wchnschr.*, 59:723, 1933.

missiles. Missiles which remain in the body after gun-shot injuries, can produce in later years, secondary illness due to mobile lead.

Such a case was reported by Leschke.[296] "A business man, thirty-four years of age, had been wounded in 1918 in the head of the right humerus by a shrapnel bullet. There was no noticeable disability for the next ten years. In the spring of 1928, however, the following disorders appeared: profuse salivation, constipation, flexor cramps of the right index finger after writing for a short time, numbness, and disturbances in visual accommodation. Once, when he was walking, he experienced a cramp of the eyes, which he described as follows: both eyes were suddenly pulled upwards with irresistible force, and he had to return home; the convulsions ceased after one and a half or two hours, during which time he had no power over his eyes. In addition, he complained of headache after mental effort, loss of power to concentrate, and impotence. After mobilization of the lead deposits by administration of 20 gm. of sodium bicarbonate four times a day for three days, punctate basophilia appeared, though previously they had not been detectable. Before mobilization the lead content of the blood was 0.01 mg. per cent, afterwards it was seventeen times as great, 0.175 mg. per cent. Before mobilization the urine was free from lead by the ordinary method of analysis; afterwards it contained 0.17 per liter on one day, and 0.055 mg. per liter on another." Haagen[297] reports a case in which lead poisoning was traced to a gun-shot wound. Wilcox and Caffey[298] reported lead poisoning in infants, from the prolonged use of lead nipple shields. Froboese[299] found that certain toothpastes absorb lead from tinned lead tubes. I made this observation years ago, in a number of proprietary preparations in which the paste had become darkened. The amounts of lead found by Froboese ranged from 0.5 to 357 mg. per 100 gm. of paste.

Chronic lead poisoning has come from men sweeping floors containing lead dust. Mlodenoff[300] reports an outbreak of lead

296. LESCHKE: Clinical Toxicology, 9, 1934.
297. HAAGEN, W. W.: Deutsche Ztschr. f. Chir., 215:39, 1929.
298. WILCOX, H. B.: J.A.M.A., 86:1514, 1924.
299. FROBOESE: Ztschr. f. Untersuch. d. Lebensmitt., 65:176, 1933.
300. MLODENOFF, D.: Presse méd., 1923.

poisoning in Videin, in Bulgaria, in 1923. The source of poisoning which affected 314 persons with thirteen deaths was found to be adulterated red pepper. Red pepper is much used. In this pepper was found 20.5% of red lead and 4.1% of sand, and the analysis showed that each teaspoonful contained about three grains of red lead. Reference has already been made to the Leipzig epidemic. A similar occurrence was reported in Boston which demonstrates the presence of lead in the water supply as a public health problem.[301] It was shown by analysis that, in connection with the poisoning of one child, the water which stood in the lead pipe leading from the street to the house contained 0.0657 parts of lead per 100,000 of standing water, while the running water showed the presence of 0.0314 parts. According to another analysis, it seems that the amount might at times increase, even to 0.1114 parts per 100,000, and the U. S. Public Health Service has decreed that no water is to be used for drinking purposes which contains lead compounds in a quantity greater than what would correspond to half a part of lead per million of water. Lead to the extent of 0.025 parts per 100,000 is sufficient to condemn a potable water, and 0.36 parts per 1,000,000 may be poisonous.

Lead Absorption: Wherever fumes or dust are in the air, absorption can take place by the respiratory tract. In one industry, samples of air taken near a melting pot gave 6.2 mg. of metallic lead per 60 cu. ft. of air. Fortunately, this process was not used all day, but had caused the illness of one workman who was working part time. In another industry, the air contained 0.03 mg. to 0.1 mg. of lead per cubic foot of air breathed by over 100 workmen. Many of these men had lead poisoning. A typical case was that of P.G., thirty-five years of age, examined in July, 1935, who had worked for twelve years in this particular industry, and had a red blood count of 3,780,000, white blood count of 8,150, with 21,712 stipped cells per million red cells. He was again examined on November 9, 1935, and showed a red blood count of 4,350,000, white blood count of 6,100, with 8,000 basophiles per million. The blood pressure varied from 108 to 112 systolic, and was 74 diastolic. Belknap, [301-A] in the examination of eighty-one cases of heavy

301. Editorial: Boston Lead Poisoning Problem, *New England J Med.*, 209:559, 1933.
301-A. BELKNAP, ELSTON L.: *J. Indust. Hyg. & Tox.*, 18:381, 1936.

lead absorption, clinically observed for one to five years, came to the conclusion that there is no definite trend towards increase in systolic and diastolic blood pressure; that all blood pressures were in normal limits for each age group. The urine contained 3.451 mg. of lead per 100 cc. The urine was free from albumin and casts.

Lead poisoning appears more rapidly and intensely by the inspiration of lead-laden air, than by the gastro-intestinal route. Lead given by stomach tube to dogs can be largely recovered in the feces because most of the ingested lead is not absorbed and because the greater portion of the fraction that is absorbed is caught by the liver and re-excreted into the intestinal tract in the bile. Much of the lead that enters the gastro-intestinal tract is not absorbed into the organism, but is either eliminated directly or never passes beyond the liver. From my experience in examination of cases of lead poisoning, I believe that there is greater damage from the respiration route than by the gastro-intestinal route. If men will wear their masks during working periods, the number of cases of chronic lead poisoning will be greatly reduced. Very few cases of lead poisoning are noticed in men handling pig solder and bars of lead, but wherever workmen come in contact with lead carbonate dust, or fumes of lead melting, smelting, or soldering, or in any process that would produce finely divided particles, lead poisoning cases are sure to appear. The U. S. Public Health Service[302] investigated potteries in 1921 and found among 1,809 employed in lead work, a rate of 22.8% with symptoms of lead poisoning. Dangerous amounts of lead dust were found in 28.5% of the rooms tested. Many cases of lead poisoning are seen in men burning off the paint on battle ships. On these ships there is also a process of scraping the paint off structural steel, from which a few cases of poisoning are derived. Some of the most severe cases of lead poisoning I have treated came from the inhalation of lead fumes from the burning of paint from steel beams. Cone, Russel, and Harwood[303] believe lead to be a possible cause of multiple sclerosis. Lead was found in the spinal cord in one typical case of multiple sclerosis. Six cases of the type progressing by exacer-

302. NEWMAN, B. J., McCONNELL, W. J., SPENCER, O. M., and PHILLIPS, F. M.:   J. Indust. Hyg., 3:390, 1921, 1922.
303. CONE, W., RUSSEL, C., and HARWOD, R. U.:   Arch. Neurol. & Psychiat., 31:236-269, 1934.

bation and undergoing remission showed lead in the stools, urine, and cerebrospinal fluid. Calcium stopped the advancing myelitis and caused lead to disappear from the spinal fluid.

Distribution: Aub and his co-workers have demonstrated that lead is distributed to the tissues by the blood, possibly in the form of colloidal phosphates of lead, and deposited in the bone tissues as a tertiary lead phosphate. This combination is sensitive to changes in acidity, particularly to variations caused by such acids as lactic. The sensitiveness of tertiary lead phosphate to changes in hydrogen ion concentration may be an important factor in the frequent development of acute lead intoxication following acute infection or acidosis. They concluded that lead is deposited in the form of the inorganic phosphate rather than as the albuminate as suggested by Sir Thomas Oliver.[304] These workers claim that the phosphates thus formed in the blood stream do not precipitate from the blood serum when present in small amounts, but remain suspended as peptonized or highly dispersed colloidal lead phosphate. When lead in its various combinations enters the system by way of the alimentary tract, it is first deposited in the liver and then quite generally in the body. "Since the skeleton is the only tissue to retain permanently any significant amount of lead, an ever increasing percentage of the total absorbed lead comes to be stored in the bones. While stored in such a deposit the lead is apparently harmless, since the symptoms of plumbism are noted only when lead is generally distributed throughout the organism, as a result either of recent absorption from an external source, or of mobilization of a skeleton store."[305] It is my opinion that, once leaded, always leaded. Even though a man leaves his occupation for several years, lead will still be found in the bones, or can be detected by appropriate tests, after mobilization by such agents as potassium iodide, thyroid, ammonium chloride, or in any condition inducing an acidosis.

Potassium iodide is the drug of choice in making tests for lead in the human body, as we can test for the iodide in the urine and see whether the patient has taken or has been given the iodide as prescribed. Kehoe[305] and his associ-

304. HAMILTON, ALICE: Industrial Poisons in the United States, 1929.

305. AUB,. et. al.: Lead Poisoning, 7, 76, 1926. KEHOE, R. A., THAMANN, F., and CHOLAK, J.: *J. Indust. Hyg.,* 15:257, 1933.

ates have shown that lead is normally found in the excretions of human beings. They have also shown that lead is a normal constituent of nearly all the foods that we eat or drink — eggs contain 0.11 mg. per kilogram. Where small amounts of lead are reported, 0.02 mg. per kilogram of sample, using a colorimetric method as delicate as the one employed by them makes it doubtful whether these facts should be used at the present time, in medicolegal work. The results would cause considerable consternation among the employers if it were shown that every one of the employees was eliminating lead. On the other hand, the employer could show from these facts that lead was a normal constituent of all the foods, and, therefore, meant nothing. I discarded the colorimetric method a long time ago because of the inconsistent results, and believe that only those methods should be used by which the lead can be demonstrated as such—either the Fairhall or the electrolytic method. Extremely small quantities of any poison do not have any great significance in toxicological work. By extremely delicate methods, or by the spectrographic methods, we can find many elements in all parts of the body that previously were thought to be foreign elements. There is a gradual excretion of lead, as is shown by its appearance in the stools and urine of lead workers. Certain conditions in the body favor this elimination. Starvation or an alcoholic debauch or an acute infectious disease, such as influenza or pneumonia, may precipitate an attack of plumbism in a lead worker. Any condition which will withdraw calcium from the bones will also mobilize lead. The metabolism of lead runs parallel with that of calcium.

Legge and Duckering[306] conclude that if the workers breathe no more than 2 mg. of lead during their eight-hour working day, there will rarely be any cases of colic and there will be no palsy or encephalopathy. The lead in the air must be kept down to 5 mg. per 10 cu. m. of air, estimating that a man breathes 4.6 cu. m. of air in eight hours.

Symptoms: The first examination of the patient may show no significant symptoms, while the second examination may reveal signs indicating that the workman should be removed from his particular employment, thereby preventing further deposition of lead from the early stages of chronic lead poison-

306. DUCKERING, G. E.:   Rep. Chief Insp. Factories, 201, 1910.

ing. The first symptoms may show that the patient becomes tired easily, has headaches, loss of appetite, nausea and colic. Many men can work for months and never show these symptoms. Industrial surgeons advise a change of occupation for these men who have been working in lead; and find that when this has been done the men are seldom bothered with any symptoms unless they become sick from some other disease, which might mobilize the lead. The first of the outstanding symptoms is the ashen slate gray color of the complexion; the second, a lead line on the gums; the third, the stippling of the red blood cells, and the fourth, a mild secondary anemia (Table XII). The pale complexion does not parallel the anemia in the worst cases of lead poisoning. The lowest red count was 3,780,000, with 63% hemoglobin. This case also had poor dental hygiene, with a lead line on the gums, stippling of the red blood cells, and a mild secondary anemia.[307]

TABLE XII
SIGNS AND SYMPTOMS OBSERVED IN 400 CASES OF CHRONIC PLUMBISM

1. Fatigue and weakness..	100%	10. Pains in muscles and joints	58%
2. Loss of appetite	100%	11. Nausea and vomiting..	38%
3. Loss of weight	100%	12. Lead line	36%
4. Headaches	91%	13. Nervousness	35%
5. Anemia	90%	14. Exaggerated reflexes ..	26%
6. Pallor, sallow, pale complexion	83%	15. Hypertension	8%
7. Tremors of hands, tongue, eyelids	80%	16. Diarrhea	8%
8. Abdominal pain*	68%	17. Nephritis	7%
9. Constipation	68%	18. Dizziness	7%
		19. Gastric ulcers*	4%
		20. Duodenal ulcers	2%

* The above data were obtained from workmen having exposures from six weeks to thirty-one years. A history of colic was obtained from the men, which was not seen at the time of examination. In the majority of the cases of gastric and duodenal ulcers the histories revealed gastro-intestinal disturbances before lead exposure.

The patient may complain of loss of appetite and the vomiting of any solid food eaten, especially at breakfast. Very few complain of a sweetish and metallic taste in chronic poisoning. Many continue to complain of loss of strength and that they tire easily. At some time or other, they complain of headache. There may be dizziness, insomnia, and some develop encephalopatic conditions and mental affections. A tremor of the eyelids, and tongue, and a coarse tremor of the fingers

307. AUB, et al.: Lead Poisoning, 7, 1926.

may be noticed. The blood may show a normal hemoglobin, and in less than half of the cases a basophilic degeneration will be found. Arteriosclerosis and hypertension are not symptoms to be relied upon.

In my 400 cases I have found 8% with hypertension. (See Table XII.) Mayers reported she was unable to find any evidence that lead played an important part in arteriosclerosis and hypertension when compared to a group of men in the same social and economic class. Belknap, in the examination of

TABLE XIII

BLOOD PRESSURES OF 438 MEN INDUSTRIALLY EMPLOYED

No.	Age	Systolic	Diastolic	No.	Age	Systolic	Diastolic
2	18	118-130	78-96	12	43	118-197	62-110
3	19	110-130	70-80	9	44	130-240	90-140
3	20	140-158	82-110	13	45	90-210	50-110
13	21	76-170	50-96	17	46	100-230	70-114
8	22	120-175	80-100	11	47	114-166	76-110
8	23	126-158	68-96	11	48	130-172	78-110
6	24	120-180	80-90	16	49	120-182	70-114
4	25	134-180	88-100	16	50	106-190	80-130
10	26	124-160	80-108	12	51	128-170	76-130
6	27	138-180	80-180	10	52	130-180	76-120
11	28	130-160	75-100	12	53	140-162	76-120
12	29	120-156	60-106	12	54	134-210	70-115
7	30	114-162	80-102	7	55	119-188	74-120
7	31	122-170	76-100	8	56	140-210	80-170
9	32	92-175	60-100	8	57	146-184	70-100
4	33	138-160	80-100	7	58	108-189	76-90
13	34	106-165	70-100	8	59	130-185	70-110
9	35	110-170	78-100	7	60	150-190	44-104
14	36	118-174	62-100	4	61	150-230	78-120
6	37	128-170	70-100	6	62	130-220	76-150
17	38	108-200	76-124	1	63	162	98
10	39	100-150	68-100	2	64	146-210	80-100
14	40	105-180	64-112	2	65	140-180	80-100
13	41	104-186	60-106	2	67	130-159	100-100
15	42	134-200	85-130	1	68	168	90

eighty-one cases of heavy lead absorption observed from one to five years, states that there is no significant trend toward increase in systolic or diastolic blood pressure in men who have had exposures of five to twenty years. Teleky states that during colic an increased blood pressure with remissions and exacerbations for one to four days has been noticed, and then a fall below normal. I have included in Table XIII a list of blood pressures of 438 persons who were industrially employed but not in lead.

I found in 1.59% of this group, systolic pressures of 200 to

TABLE XIV
BLOOD PRESSURES OF 114 PERSONS EMPLOYED IN OFFICES

No.	Age	Systolic	Diastolic	No.	Age	Systolic	Diastolic
1	19	130	85	3	37	112-158	80-90
3	21	117-142	64-96	1	38	112	80
3	22	122-130	80-84	3	39	118-160	80-95
4	23	108-136	32-94	3	40	116-134	72-88
6	24	97-160	56-80	4	41	104-138	86-88
6	25	110-132	70-82	3	42	100-122	70-80
6	26	100-138	68-88	2	43	128-140	78-90
4	27	137-115	70-92	4	44	122-134	72-90
3	28	94-130	58-75	3	45	120-134	78-90
3	29	122-130	80-86	2	46	124-136	76-82
5	30	115-152	60-92	2	47	104-182	66-112
6	31	110-130	60-92	2	49	96-235	56-110
10	32	98-136	68-88	1	51	130	85
8	33	110-160	70-100	1	54	174	100
3	34	104-125	74-88	1	56	195	102
5	35	112-170	74-98	1	59	158	82
2	36	118-148	50-74				

240; in 0.68%, pressures of 190 to 200; in 3.42%, pressures of 180 to 190; in 6.25%, pressures of 170 to 180; in 10.04%, pressures of 160 to 170; in 17.95%, pressures of 150 to 160. These men were employed from two to fifty years, and their ages ranged from twenty to sixty-eight years. For comparison I have taken the blood pressures of 114 persons employed in offices

TABLE XV
BLOOD PRESSURES OF 280 MEN ENGAGED IN THE MANUFACTURE OF LEAD PRODUCTS

No.	Age	Systolic	Diastolic	No.	Age	Systolic	Diastolic
3	19	112-144	70-90	6	40	124-138	86-98
12	20	110-140	68-95	6	41	120-160	80-100
6	21	110-130	55-80	8	42	110-148	70-104
22	22	110-162	68-96	5	43	116-140	70-92
11	23	110-154	70-98	9	44	86-212	60-135
12	24	104-140	64-96	9	45	110-220	70-140
9	25	114-144	68-99	3	46	122-150	90-104
12	26	118-150	70-100	4	47	120-160	80-118
8	27	114-126	75-86	3	48	122-160	88-120
17	28	110-152	62-98	1	49	128	76
8	29	110-160	72-100	8	50	115-168	70-88
18	30	110-150	60-88	1	51	132	90
3	31	120-130	75-92	4	52	116-198	72-110
10	32	110-162	70-98	2	53	120-130	70-80
10	33	110-155	68-116	1	54	132	84
7	34	112-166	68-110	3	55	135-160	80-100
5	35	110-145	72-80	3	56	125-148	70-80
9	36	116-152	76-94	2	57	135-150	80-85
7	37	110-158	76-104	1	58	170	100
5	38	120-140	76-95	1	61	154	96
5	39	120-140	78-95	1	68	160	94

(Table XIV) who had systolic pressures ranging from 94 to
235, with ages from nineteen to fifty-nine years. Fourteen per
cent had pressures of 140 or over.

In Table XV, I have included the blood pressures of 280
men engaged in the manufacture of lead products and find
10.9% with pressures 140 or over, and 1.1% with blood pressures
of 154 to 170 in ages of fifty-eight to sixty-eight years. Compar-

TABLE XVI

BLOOD PRESSURES OF MEN ENGAGED IN THE MANUFACTURE OF
LEAD PRODUCTS FOR 15 YEARS OR OVER

Age	Blood Pressure	Years Em- ployed	Occupation	Age	Blood Pressure	Years Em- ployed	Occupation
40	124-86	15	Die Casting	46	122-90	20	Printer
40	124-86	15	Die Casting	44	130-88	21	Setting Molds
41	130-88	15	Assembling transformers	55	135-80	22	Wire Cleaner
42	132-98	15	Die Casting	39	120-85	24	Color Maker
45	118-80	15	Linotype	42	130-88	24	Setting Molds
58	170-100	15	Melting Pot				
30	126-88	16	Assembling	44	130-88	24	Setting Molds
30	126-88	16	Assembling				
39	134-95	16	Plating Dept.	47	120-85	24	Color Mixer
32	125-78	17	Galvanizer	52	138-87	24	Monotype Operator
36	128-80	17	Monotype Operator	41	160-100	25	Color Mixer
38	120-84	17	Die Casting	43	132-92	25	Assembling
41	138-80	17	Foreman, Finish Dept.	47	125-80	25	Color Mixer
				44	212-135	30	Printer
44	126-84	17	Die Casting	46	140-90	30	Color Mixer
47	155-118	17	Breaking	52	160-110	30	Die Casting
53	130-70	17	Plating	47	160-80	32	Color Mixer
32	110-72	18	Composing Room	50	122-78	32	Transmitter Dept.
38	140-95	18	Color Mix- er's Helper	53	120-80	32	Foreman, Color Dept.
44	158-98	18	Laborer, metal	56	125-80	32	Linotype Operator
45	130-82	20	Foreman, Plating Dept.	52	198-120	38	Printer
				68	160-94	50	Brass Molder

ing this with Table XIV, it will be noted that 28.99% not working in lead have the same range of blood pressure. (American
Experience Table of Mortality Life Expectancy Chart gives a
blood pressure of 140 as hypertension for all ages.)

As shown in Table XVI the blood pressures of forty men
working in lead for fifteen years or over ranged from 110 to 212
systolic with 70 to 135 diastolic, of which number 26.8% had
pressures over 140. A man sixty-eight years of age who worked
in lead for fifty years had a pressure of 160/94.

In another group (Table XVII) I have included the blood pressures of ninety-three applicants for insurance who had systolic pressures ranging from 118 to 190. Thirty per cent had pressures of 140 or over.

TABLE XVII

BLOOD PRESSURES OF 93 APPLICANTS FOR INSURANCE NOT
WORKING IN LEAD

Age	Occupation	Systo-lic	Di-astolic	Age	Occupation	Systo-lic	Di-astolic
19	Repairman	119	76	47	Farmhand	139	88
22	Pressman	122	82	47	Steel Labor	138	92
24	Machinist	120	85	47	P. W. A.	128	86
24	Truck Driver	120	80	47	Carpenter	190	130
26	Freight Handler	129	88	47	Hostler	128	82
26	Waiter	154	100	47	Laborer	166	96
28	Express Helper	118	80	48	Doorman	170	58
29	Vulcanizer	128	80	48	Cook	134	84
29	Grinder	122	85	48	Electrical	136	88
31	P. W. A.	118	78	48	Carpet Layer	129	86
31	Mechanic	126	78	49	Yard Foreman	150	100
32	Pumpman	130	84	49	Janitor	152	90
32	Laundress	125	82	49	Handyman	178	115
33	Decorator	119	80	49	Machinist	190	115
33	Farmer	124	78	50	Roofer	136	84
34	Motorman	134	82	50	Laborer	162	96
35	Garment Worker	120	92	50	Machinist	190	115
36	Punch Press	126	84	50	Laborer	180	84
36	Janitor	132	90	51	Peddler	135	86
36	Electrician	129	83	51	Laborer, P. W. A.	138	90
37	Machinist	166	92	51	Chemist	136	86
38	Police	134	86	51	Trucking	116	78
38	Mill Worker	128	85	51	Foreman	188	72
38	Laundress	140	80	52	Electrical	132	82
39	Bricklayer	130	82	52	Farmer	133	88
39	Laborer	128	82	52	Carpenter	140	92
39	Cab Driver	128	84	52	Cement Worker	140	88
39	Electrician	128	80	53	Laborer	175	108
39	Sta. Engineer	130	82	54	Laborer	180	112
40	Engineer	130	82	54	Soap Works	178	115
40	W. P. A.	134	76	55	Upholsterer	152	94
41	Meat Cutter	129	78	55	Undertaker	140	90
42	Baggageman	136	85	56	Engineer	135	84
42	Cook	139	90	56	Woodwork	152	95
42	Machinist	125	80	57	Mover	142	92
43	Paper Factory	138	90	57	Peddler	138	88
43	Local Coal Yard	130	86	57	Tanner	125	80
43	Structural Steel	138	85	57	Polisher & Buffer	138	82
43	Roofer	133	82	58	Section Boss	142	90
43	Fireman	128	80	59	Janitor	145	92
44	Pressman	170	80	59	Plasterer	132	90
44	Landscaper	138	96	59	Contractor	139	93
44	Laborer	132	82	59	Farmer	160	100
44	Carpenter	134	82	60	Farmer	176	98
45	Butcher	143	88	61	Carpenter	134	90
46	Driver	129	86	63	P. W. A.	105	78
47	P. W. A.	138	94				

TABLE XVIII
Blood Pressures of 293 Men Industrially Employed

Age	Years of Service	Blood Pressures	Occupation	Age	Years of Service	Blood Pressures	Occupation
19	1	156-50	Machinist	27	7	140-84	Milling Machine
20	1	120-84	Core Maker	27	7	154-74	Draftsman
20	1	126-80	Foundry Laborer	27	10	124-78	Draftsman
20	1	140-82	Clerk	28	5	148-82	Engineer
21	3	148-70	Machinist	28	5	138-84	Grinder
21	2	140-84	Machinist	28	12	132-84	Machinist
21	1	114-68	Assembler	28	7	138-80	Machinist
21	1	144-94	Timekeeper	28	6	124-80	Machinist
22	1	136-84	Assembling	28	7	132-80	Machinist
22	3	120-80	Grinder	28	12	128-78	Machinist
22	3	116-76	Boring Mill	28	12	124-84	Machinist
22	3	142-74	Assembler	28	2	128-78	Core Maker
22	1	140-90	Stenographer	28	12	118-70	Core Maker
23	2	120-70	Drill Press	28	7	150-88	Machinist
23	1	130-70	Machinist	28	12	134-70	Accounting
23	2	150-80	Machinist	29	4	150-70	Machinist
23	1	134-70	Draftsman	29	7	142-80	Foreman
24	2	150-86	Machinist	29	7	128-84	Drill Press
24	1	130-70	Repair Man	29	14	134-80	Machinist
24	4	126-78	Machinist	29	4	118-80	Draftsman
24	3	140-80	Milling Machine	29	7	140-64	Accountant
24	1	130-74	Machinist	29	3	130-78	Draftsman
24	2	120-78	Radial Drill	30	10	126-80	Molder
24	2	148-96	Assembler	30	10	130-80	Grinder
24	2	132-70	Draftsman	30	8	130-90	Grinder
25	10	154-84	Machinist	30	10	132-80	Machinist
25	6	160-90	Truck Driver	30	9	126-74	Assembler
25	9	146-70	Machinist	30	12	140-92	Machinist
25	9	140-84	Machinist	30	5	126-80	Draftsman
25	3	138-78	Lathe Operator	30	15	120-80	Designer
25	1	136-92	Drill Press	31	11	160-90	Machinist
25	2	138-82	Lathe Operator	31	2	120-80	Core Maker
25	5	124-78	Core Maker	31	8	138-80	Grinder
25	2	160-90	Clerk	31	12	150-80	Machinist
25	7	138-88	Clerk	31	8	136-80	Machinist
26	2	136-84	Assembling	31	15	144-80	Machinist
26	6	126-80	Machinist	31	1	110-70	Foundry
26	8	142-88	Core Maker	31	7	130-96	Machinist
26	11	132-76	Machinist	32	16	130-80	Machinist
26	10	136-74	Machinist	32	15	140-84	Machinist
26	2	136-84	Accountant	32	16	110-70	Machinist
26	8	140-76	Accountant	32	10	126-70	Trucking
27	5	142-84	Machinist	32	13	124-76	Machinist
27	9	140-86	Machinist	32	14	150-85	Maintenance
27	11	122-76	Machinist	32	16	156-78	Office Worker
27	1	128-84	Machinist	32	10	130-74	Draftsman
27	5	122-80	Machinist	33	16	120-84	Accountant
27	8	124-86	Coremaker	33	15	164-88	Engineer
27	8	130-78	Machinist	33	16	122-76	Tool Maker
				33	12	150-88	Machinist
				33	1	124-94	Laborer
				33	12	122-76	Draftsman

TABLE XVIII—Cont.

BLOOD PRESSURES OF 293 MEN INDUSTRIALLY EMPLOYED

Age	Years of Service	Blood Pressures	Occupation	Age	Years of Service	Blood Pressures	Occupation
34	20	138-84	Machinist	40	17	106-60	Machinist
34	18	134-80	Machinist	40	16	124-80	Machinist
34	16	136-84	Machinist	40	20	144-84	Machinist
34	2	124-78	Machinist	40	10	134-94	Machinist
34	15	106-64	Foundry	40	20	214-136	Machinist
34	16	126-82	Sales Engineer	41	20	164-80	Machinist
				41	18	136-86	Machinist
35	12	130-70	Assembler	41	20	146-96	Machine Foreman
35	15	160-90	Carpenter				
35	5	120-80	Machinist	41	20	120-75	Molder
35	8	146-80	Boring Mill	41	20	154-88	Draftsman
35	12	110-65	Repair Man	42	21	120-70	Machinist
35	8	108-68	Draftsman	42	15	140-90	Machinist
36	10	130-80	Inspector	42	22	124-80	Machinist
36	2	130-76	Machinist	42	22	140-80	Crane Operator
36	15	130-78	Machinist				
36	14	136-90	Machinist	42	15	160-80	Machinist
36	21	124-70	Machinist	42	20	126-80	Milling Machine
36	12	126-78	Machinist				
36	12	122-72	Assembler	42	25	180-128	Machinist
36	21	132-76	Machinist	42	16	122-80	Molder
36	8	158-90	Draftsman	42	20	124-76	Machinist
37	5	118-76	Machinist	43	13	134-88	Molder
37	20	172-114	Machinist	43	12	124-76	Machinist
37	18	130-74	Core Maker	43	15	160-80	Inspector
37	22	116-80	Machinist	43	20	140-86	Machinist
37	15	150-94	Machinist	43	15	128-80	Machinist
37	15	128-80	Draftsman	43	25	124-70	Machinist
38	10	168-90	Shipper	43	4	180-100	Grinder
38	15	132-90	Machinist	43	18	134-84	Machinist
38	4	142-80	Machinist	43	22	130-90	Milling Machine
38	10	138-80	Machinist				
38	15	150-80	Machinist	43	21	142-88	Draftsman
38	18	124-80	Machinist	44	15	134-100	Machinist
38	2	138-80	Laborer	44	24	120-70	Machinist
38	17	154-110	Machinist	44	28	200-120	Machinist
38	7	122-84	Machinist	44	10	130-70	Machinist
38	11	132-90	Machinist	44	11	145-84	Machinist
38	12	122-78	Machinist	44	8	150-80	Grinder
38	9	150-90	Service Man	44	21	138-84	Machinist
38	20	140-94	Machinist	44	28	128-88	Machinist
39	17	132-86	Machinist	44	9	140-84	Machinist
39	25	122-76	Laborer	44	20	124-80	Machinist
39	18	128-92	Grinder	44	31	116-78	Molder
39	20	140-60	Machinist	44	20	132-100	Draftsman
39	20	170-100	Machinist	45	31	126-80	Core Maker
39	22	110-70	Grinder	45	19	150-80	Machinist
39	12	120-70	Lathe Operator	45	19	136-84	Lathe Operator
39	25	144-84	Machinist	45	20	148-82	Core Maker
39	2	124-90	Assembler	45	29	94-58	Machinist
39	20	136-86	Machinist	45	20	132-90	Milling Machine
39	15	124-90	Core Maker				

TABLE XVIII—Cont.
Blood Pressures of 293 Men Industrially Employed

Age	Years of Service	Blood Pressures	Occupation	Age	Years of Service	Blood Pressures	Occupation
45	25	124-86	Machinist	51	20	160-60	Foundry
45	26	146-88	Machine Foreman	51	2	120-80	Laborer
45	25	150-94	Machinist	51	30	166-94	Laborer
45	11	158-106	Machinist	52	38	100-60	Machinist
45	30	156-76	Machine Foreman	52	30	130-80	Machinist
45	7	120-70	Sales Engineer	52	25	138-82	Foreman
46	28	138-90	Machinist	52	30	188-100	Assembling
46	20	132-90	Inspector	52	14	120-88	Chipper
46	25	180-120	Machinist	53	30	134-82	Lathe Operator
46	26	150-110	Machinist	53	26	162-90	Laborer
46	26	160-100	Molder	53	40	170-130	Machinist
46	12	166-100	Planer	53	30	160-90	Carpenter
47	25	144-88	Machinist	53	33	136-86	Machinist
47	21	164-90	Foundry	53	33	150-94	Molder
47	21	140-88	Chipper	53	7	150-100	Tool Room
47	25	126-90	Machinist	53	20	124-90	Machinist
47	18	148-86	Machinist	54	17	176-128	Foundry
47	26	138-84	Laborer	54	30	110-70	Machinist
47	30	134-82	Machinist	54	17	150-86	Foundry
47	15	190-104	Chipper	54	36	160-80	Machinist
47	8	138-84	Clerk	54	30	142-80	Machinist
48	22	128-78	Machinist	54	20	150-80	Machinist
48	30	118-80	Machinist	55	32	154-88	Machinist
48	26	168-100	Machinist	55	2	154-86	Fireman
48	31	120-82	Lathe Operator	56	36	148-70	Machinist
48	32	120-80	Machinist	56	14	168-90	Laborer
48	26	168-90	Machinist	56	33	175-100	Molder
48	22	162-90	Machinist	56	40	150-100	Foreman
48	10	154-90	Machinist	56	35	168-94	Molder
48	15	160-104	Machinist	56	30	150-86	Machinist
48	20	124-80	Milling Machine	57	40	160-80	Machinist
49	27	162-70	Machinist	57	40	142-90	Tool Maker
49	6	140-80	Grinder	57	20	160-100	Laborer
49	17	140-98	Core Maker	57	20	172-104	Molder
49	25	180-98	Machinist	58	30	140-86	Machinist
49	35	138-88	Foundry	58	14	150-90	Carpenter
49	22	114-80	Cupola Tender	58	10	152-82	Tool Room
49	25	126-86	Machinist	58	38	112-70	Draftsman
49	24	140-76	Inspector	59	20	144-88	Molder
50	35	136-94	Machinist	60	35	220-110	Molder
50	12	184-90	Machinist	62	40	180-110	Watchman
50	35	160-80	Assembler	62	35	134-70	Assembler
50	35	104-70	Machinist	62	40	214-120	Blacksmith
51	25	116-70	Electrician	64	4	145-80	Milling Machine
51	35	128-80	Machinist	66	45	110-70	Cupola Tender
51	30	134-80	Machinist	68	45	210-84	Machinist
51	26	150-90	Machinist	70	38	230-110	Molder

In Table XVIII (pp. 166-168), I have included the blood pressures of 293 men industrially employed but not in lead. Of this number 44% had pressures of 140 or over.

In Table XIX, below, I have given the pressures of 120 men engaged in the manufacture of lead products and found some interesting data. For instance, one man who worked in lead for over forty years had a systolic pressure of 140/90. Of the 119 men, 7.50% had systolic pressures of 150 to 160; 5.04% had pressures from 160 to 170; 1.68% had pressures from 170 to 180 and 0.83% had pressures from 180 to 190. In other words only 15.11% of those working in lead from one to forty years had pressures from 150 to 190, while in 20.63% not employed in lead, there was the same range of blood pressures. Taking this range from Table XIII (438 men) 28.66% had blood pressures in the same degree; 30% of the men working in lead in Table XIX had pressures of 140 or over, while in Table XVIII 44% of the workmen industrially employed but not in lead, of

TABLE XIX

BLOOD PRESSURES OF 120 MEN ENGAGED IN THE MANUFACTURE OF LEAD PRODUCTS

Age	Years of Service	Blood Pressure	Age	Years of Service	Blood Pressure
21	1	114-76	27	4	120-70
22	2	130-70	27	4	108-60
23	1	126-86	27	6	124-68
23	1	124-74	27	10	138-78
23	2	124-60	27	11	112-78
23	3	126-70	28	1	126-80
23	3	150-100	28	1	140-80
24	1	114-76	28	2	128-70
24	2	112-60	28	3	130-78
24	2	110-70	28	3	110-60
24	2	124-90	28	4	118-64
24	3	110-68	28	5	114-70
24	3	116-70	28	6	112-68
24	3	138-76	29	1	116-76
25	1	114-70	29	2	126-90
25	2	130-74	29	3	118-70
25	3	128-78	29	4	114-80
25	3	166-90	29	7	104-74
26	1	150-78	29	8	124-88
26	2	104-50	30	9	114-70
26	3	114-78	30	11	144-76
26	3	120-76	30	12	132-74
26	3	160-76	31	4	126-78
26	4	120-76	31	8	120-60
26	4	120-68	31	11	112-60
27	2	110-64	31	12	126-84
27	3	128-86	31	14	108-70

TABLE XIX—Cont.

BLOOD PRESSURES OF 120 MEN ENGAGED IN THE MANUFACTURE
OF LEAD PRODUCTS

Age	Years of Service	Blood Pressure	Age	Years of Service	Blood Pressure
32	1	140-80	40	12	126-80
32	1	124-76	40	13	122-90
32	3	130-78	40	16	122-80
32	4	176-100	41	3	90-60
32	7	154-80	41	10	150-84
32	8	120-88	41	13	136-80
32	8	128-70	41	16	156-100
32	10	156-88	42	1	120-78
33	3	138-78	42	4	120-70
33	6	140-90	42	4	120-70
34	2	110-60	42	15	160-100
34	1	130-76	43	7	166-112
34	7	126-80	44	2	114-70
35	14	154-90	44	15	146-84
35	14	124-76	45	4	130-64
36	1	120-76	45	4	132-80
36	2	138-80	45	7	148-60
37	2	134-80	46	3	110-60
37	2	142-84	46	16	146-90
37	2	112-60	47	4	140-78
37	4	136-80	48	6	144-60
37	8	160-76	48	8	132-80
37	8	160-76	48	8	144-90
37	11	140-76	48	9	114-70
37	12	130-80	48	15	160-110
37	14	144-90	48	21	158-90
38	6	112-68	48	21	158-90
38	6	144-100	49	14	190-110
38	8	138-90	49	18	160-90
39	3	114-66	50	8	130-84
39	6	114-50	51	19	146-90
39	6	120-70	52	4	174-110
40	3	148-90	55	40	140-90

the same social and economic class had pressures of 140 or over. From this data I believe I am safe in stating that in American practice in the manufacture of lead products, it can no longer be contended that lead causes high blood pressure. At a conference in July, 1937, on lead poisoning, held in New York City under the auspices of the New York Tuberculosis and Health Association and Cornell University Medical College, it was decided there is no relationship of hypertension to lead poisoning.

The best way to make a diagnosis of lead poisoning where only one symptom may appear, is to have the stools and urine examined for the presence of lead. McCord, Holden, and Johnston report that "in lead exposed persons, the detection of basophilic-containing red cells in percentages in excess of

1.5%, and particularly in excess of 2%, suggests lead absorption and the possibility of approaching clinical lead poisoning."[308] The air should always be examined whenever a suspicion of lead poisoning is entertained. One to 1.5 mg. of lead in the amount of air breathed by a workman in a normal working-day is the figure at which lead poisoning may arise. It is well established that the majority of persons exposed to much higher amounts, such as 4 to 8 mg., may not develop this disease even after years of exposure.

Kehoe, Thamann, and Cholak[309] demonstrated that lead is a natural constituent of soil and vegetation as well as of animal and human tissues. It is now apparent that lead occurs regularly in the feces and in the urine of normal healthy persons, in many parts of the world. These authors found 0.01 mg. of lead in 215 gm. of corn stalk; 0.04 mg. in 99.40 gm. of wheat; 0.03 mg. of lead in 411.70 gm. of pork sausage; and that the soil contained from 0.8 to 0.22 mg. per 50 gm. of soil. These same authors found: "that the normal adult American excretes lead at a rate of from 0.02 to 0.08 mg. per liter of urine, and at a rate of from 0.03 to 0.1 mg. per gram of ash in the feces; that the lead intake of the food of selected subjects was approximately equivalent to the lead content of their feces, which fact may be taken as evidence, not only of the passage of the great proportion of ingested lead through the alimentary tract, unabsorbed, but also of the predominant source of the lead which is absorbed and excreted by normal persons (the daily intake of lead in the food ranges from 0.16 to 0.28 mg.); that normal persons whose lead metabolism is followed for prolonged periods show no evidence of lead accumulation, but appear to have established an equilibrium with their environment, in which excretion of lead keeps pace with absorption; that two persons, of widely varying age and weight, apparently normal shortly before their deaths, showed considerable amounts of lead in their tissues, in approximate relationship to their respective weights, approximately 135 mg. of lead having been present in the body of the adult; that the oral administration to a human subject, of 1 mg. and 5 mg. of lead chloride daily for two respective short

308. McCord, C. P., Holden, F. R., and Johnston, Jan.: *Indust. Med.*, 4:184, 1935.

309. Kehoe, R. A., Thamann, F., and Cholak, J.: *J. Indust. Hyg.*, 15:273, 1933.

periods resulted in the elimination of the greater portion of
the lead, unabsorbed, and in the absorption of amounts averaging slightly less than 0.5 mg. daily for the former dosage, and
approximately 1 mg. daily for the latter; and, that such
amounts of absorbed lead are sufficient to produce a measurable increase in the rate of urinary lead excretion, during the
period of active absorption, and for a time thereafter."

The lead line, or Burtonian line, consisting of fine granules
of pigment situated within the tissue of the gums about a
millimeter from the border of the teeth cannot be well seen
by the naked eye, and a careful examination of the margin
gums must be made with a hand lens after food particles and
pus have been carefully wiped away with a cotton applicator.
It appears chiefly around infected or pyorrheic teeth, and is
seldom seen in the lead worker who takes good care of his
teeth. Mistakes have been made by the inexperienced examiner in diagnosing lead poisoning in colored people. About
one-quarter of an inch below the margin of the gums, nearly
all colored people have a dark blue line, which has caused
some confusion. The lead line may appear in the gums after
medication with potassium iodide where it has not previously
been noted. Such a case was seen in L.L., a young woman,
who had a red blood count of 4,000,000, a white blood count
of 10,000 and an 80% hemoglobin, with occasional stippled
red cells. An unexplained anemia was soon accounted for
by the occupational history of this young woman, for she
had been working with a soldering iron. A twenty-four hour
specimen of urine was taken, with instructions for a second
twenty-four hour specimen after the administration of 30
grains of iodide had been given, in three doses. The nurse
continued administering the iodide until 330 grains had been
taken, which mobilized the lead in sufficient quantities to
cause a lead colic and produce a lead line. Her hemoglobin
dropped to 65%, she had a red blood count of 3,280,000 with
40 to 50 basophiles per high power field. The lead line is an
indication of absorption and does not mean intoxication, and
may be entirely absent in people showing symptoms of intoxication. A laxity in caring for the teeth markedly increases the development of fine granules in the gums. This
is said to be due to the formation of lead sulphide. The
absorption of other heavy metal poisons can cause a similar

marking in people with a poor denture. The stippling of the red cells does not always occur in lead poisoning, although in many cases the basophilic granules of the red cells indicate the presence of lead within the body.

Symptoms: Evidence has been presented that measurable quantities of lead are excreted in the urine and feces of persons with and without a history of industrial exposure to lead compounds. Leake and his associates in the U. S. Public Health Service verified this report.[310] "The appearance of lead in both the urine and the feces of students shows that some degree of lead absorption is normal for everybody. That the matter has been previously overlooked is no doubt due to inadequate analytical methods, rather than to any recent and abrupt changes in the quantity of general exposure to lead compounds or the influences of selected localities." Studies which are now being made show that infants and young children taken at random from among hospital patients are excreting small amounts of lead.

Fukushima and Matsumoto[311] found 298 cases of lead poisoning in infants ranging from eight months to one year, which was caused by a white face powder used by the nursing mothers. The most common symptoms noticed by the mothers at the beginning were vomiting, green diarrhea, bad humor, paleness, slight fever, emaciation, no appetite, nervousness, and inactivity. Of these cases 94.3% had the constant symptom of vomiting. In four cases the eyesight was weak, and in eleven cases the patients were blind. Teething is delayed in this disease; in 12.3% the teeth did not appear through the gums until one year old. In 83.3% the teeth turned black at the neck, and in one case lead-rims appeared. Nervous symptoms were positive in 87.2% of the cases, and in the majority they appeared in the initial stage of the disease. Of the patients 72.8% had convulsions. A grinding of the teeth was heard in 29.5%, and trembling of the arms was found in 17.7% of the cases. Twitching of the face and limbs was apparent in 27.5%. Paralysis of the upper and lower limbs was positive in only 2% of the cases, an exceedingly small amount. The finger-nails turned black in 54.8% of the cases.

310. LEAKE, J. P., et al.:   Bull. 163, U. S. Pub. Health Service, 1926.
311. FUKUSHIMA, M., and MATSUMOTO, H.:   *Orient J. Dis. Infants,* 121, 295, March, 1928.

In 199 cases diarrhea was present, and in 79 cases constipation was observed. In 196 cases the stool was greenish-black, which is peculiar to this disease. In the majority of cases an examination of the urine showed it to be clear and acid in reaction, containing acetone, albumin, indican, and urobilinogen. Basophilic granulation of the red blood corpuscles was found. The spinal fluid was cloudy in 15.6%, and in 72.1% it was of a yellowish-blue color. In 98.6% the albumin was increased. In seventy-one cases examined, it was discovered that the mothers of the infant patients had used a powder which contained lead. In ten cases the mothers alone had used the white face powder which contained the lead. In forty-five cases both the mothers and the infants had used the same kind of white powder. In one case the toys of the infant had been colored with lead paint.

Kasahara and Schun[312] found that, owing to the wide use of toilet powder containing lead in Japan, cases of lead poisoning arise because of the transferring of lead to the infant in breast feeding. The lead content of the mother's milk was found to vary from traces to 0.8 mg. per liter. Frazzetto[313] studied twenty-five cases of lead poisoning in which arthritic symptoms were apparent, which suggests a relationship between the two.

Diagnosis: In a case of chronic poisoning with acute exacerbations due to an infectious disease, or acidosis, a few of the following symptoms would be elicited: Abdominal pain, arthritis, constipation, gastric disturbances, a bad taste, especially in the morning, loss of appetite, headache, disturbed sleep, loss of strength, especially in the muscles most used, slight tremors of the tongue, lips and fingers, and loss of weight. A hypertension and nephritis are noted in some cases. The former is seldom found in workmen under sixty years of age. These symptoms may accompany those previously described as anemia, basophilic stippling, lead line and pallor of the skin. Nephritis is found in only a few of the cases. The blood pressure seldom runs over 140 systolic. In the consideration of nephritis the examining physician must keep in mind that many of these men consume large quantities of alcohol and have led a hard rugged life. The mere

312. KASAHARA and SCHUN: Ztschr. f. Kinderh., Berl., 55:576, 1933.
313. FRAZZETTO, S.: Med. d. lavoro., 25:335, 1934.

finding of albumin in the urine has no significance, as it is found in the same types of workmen who have never worked in lead. The individual who is suffering from a lead colic may have a slight transient albuminuria which clears up when the protein intake is reduced. A contracted kidney is the after effect of the arteriosclerosis and an increased blood pressure, or, with high blood pressure due to the arteriosclerosis, the changes do not result from lead poisoning. A contracted kidney with a low blood pressure is found many times in individuals who have not absorbed lead and who fail to show abnormal lead in the organs. However, if young men with an hereditary high blood pressure start to work in a lead factory the pressure may be elevated, so a family background should be considered in deciding whether the lead was a factor in causing the hypertension.

Symptoms: Colic is an outstanding symptom; it occurred in about 90% of the cases that I have examined. These attacks occur mostly with constipation. I have never seen a true lead colic with a diarrhea. Tenderness in the region of the appendix has occasionally caused surgeons to operate upon an individual, with the appendix found to be normal after removal. As an aid in the differential diagnosis, one must consider the acute abdomen in the absence of a lymphocytosis. The liver may be affected, and a jaundice may be another complication. In my series of 400 cases (page 161) ulcers were found only ten times. Five were operated upon, normal appendices being removed. There is no reliable data showing the number of ulcers appearing in office people for comparison. Ulcer cannot be said to be diagnostic of lead poisoning, because many thousands of people have ulcers who are not industrially employed, as physicians, doctors, and office people. Clonic spasms are seen occasionally in patients who fail to be relieved medicinally. That these may be of a neurotic nature must be considered. The fact that a man has had colics does not prevent him from returning to the same type of work at the cessation of the attack, for a number of these men seem to develop a certain resistance against lead and may not have another attack for many years.

Crosetti, Lorenzo and Forgoni report that ulcerative gastric or duodenal processes were not observed. The roentgenologic examination was always negative. In their series of cases, the intestinal syndrome was especially tenacious, the colics and obstipation yielding only to antispastics, not to enemas or laxatives, which points to a spastic condition of the smooth musculature cooperating with an excitation of the lowest sympathetic nerve, which is an intestinal inhibitor.[314] Enlargement of the liver was present in many of the cases, with jaundice of varying degrees. The intensity of the jaundice reactions was always parallel to the toxic syndrome.

Crawford[315] described a case of a four year old child who when seen gave a history of frequent attacks of intestinal colic associated with vomiting. The child was living in a painted wooden house and was a nail biter. Examination revealed a patient who was sallow, with a foul breath. There was no lead line on the teeth. The abdomen was somewhat distended, but showed no rigidity or tenderness. Albumin and lead were found in the urine. The condition improved under treatment. One and one-half months later there was a recurrence of vomiting and abdominal pain and the urine contained a moderate amount of albumin and some reducing agent. Over a week later the patient developed pains and weakness in the lower limbs, and in the evening had three cerebral seizures. Sometime later a complete extensive paralysis of both feet developed. Three days later the child became comatose. The urine was dark in color and hematoporphyrine could be detected spectroscopically. Four days later the blood picture was 4,470,000 R. B. C., 12,200 W. B. C., and hemoglobin, 75%. There was no basophilic stippling. The hematoporphyrine persisted in the urine, but only a small quantity of lead could be found. Ultimately, the child died of bronchial pneumonia.

Vigliana[316] calls attention to the fact that there is a lead parotitis. Animals which have been poisoned with lead have shown extensive changes of the thyroid gland; still a relation between lead poisoning and Basedow's disease has always been denied. The author reported six cases of lead poisoning complicated by hyperthyroidism; in all cases he observed the presence of a struma, exophthalmos, tachycardia, increased

314. CROSETTI, LORENZO, and FORGONI: *Policlin., Roma,* 41: 516, 1934.

315. CRAWFORD, H.:   *M. J. Australia,* 1: 589, 1933.

316. VIGLIANA, E.:   Lead Poisoning, *Arch. f. Gewerbepaph. u. Gewerbehyg.,* 5: 18, 1934.

BMR, tremors, diarrhea, and a nervous and psychic irritability and monocytosis. In reviewing 2,500 cases of lead poisoning, the author has selected five persons who gave a previous history of lead poisoning. An important fact that the author stresses is that hyperthyroidism occurs usually in the remission periods of lead poisoning and that it develops gradually, and in two cases the onset of hyperthyroidism was followed by a severe exacerbation of the lead poisoning. The small number of cases which this author reports, I believe, should be considered incidental—as in the lake region around Chicago we have a large number of cases of thyroidism and yet I have seen but very few who were leaded.

Lehmann[317] says that basophilic stippling cannot be regarded as specific for lead poisoning, inasmuch as a series of other harmless stimuli play on the hematopoietic tissues causing an appearance of basophilic stippling which cannot be differentiated from that seen in lead poisoning. The clinical picture should be considered with the appearance of the stippling, before the diagnosis. The author and other investigators have injected into rabbits and guinea pigs, intraperitoneally, sand, coal and other foreign particles, and have found regularly stippled cells such as are seen in lead poisoning. The appearance of basophilic stippling may be considered as the result of bone-marrow stimulation. Guinea pigs which have been made to inhale benzene have responded with polychromatophilia and basophilia of the erythrocytes.

The figures supplied by P. Schmidt's data show that granulated erythrocytes proportionately 100 to 1,000,000 are quite normal, while figures from 100 to 300 per 1,000,000 are signs of danger, and that 500 to 1000 per million are of greatest diagnostic value. These figures are not in agreement with McCord, who finds that the stippled cells run parallel with the basophilic aggregation. However, it is a well known fact that the number of basophilic cells varies from day to day. The mere reporting of the presence of basophilic cells is insufficient; the laboratory should report so many cells per million red cells. Winkler* states that numbers below 300 per million were termed negative, as positive, in the sense of provocation by potassium iodide double that number. Out of 100 con-

317. LEHMANN, H.: *Arch. f. Hyg.*, 111:49, 1934.
* WINKLER: *Wien. med. Klin.*, 33:637, 1937.

trol patients 4% showed an increase over the limit, 6% after administration of potassium iodide. (The presence of basophilic substance in immature red cells is also caused by benzol, toluol, xylol, chlorinated hydrocarbons such as carbon tetrachloride, and lead.) Poppitz[318] found stipple cells in cases of tuberculosis. Litzner[319] reports a case of kidney atrophy which had never been exposed to lead, yet it presented a characteristic picture of basophilic stippling. Even in normal individuals there are cases which show stippled cells, as has been reported by Lane,[320] who examined 223 individuals in London and Manchester. The author, however, does not mean to infer that examination of the blood smear is useless in the early diagnosis of lead poisoning, but these findings should only be considered as one of the symptoms of lead poisoning. Normal blood, not associated with any of the above toxic agents, may contain a few stippled red cells. These cells may be found in some chronic diseases such as pernicious anemia and the leukemias. These disturbances must be ruled out and the proportion of the red stippled cells must be large enough to show that the blood is abnormal. McCord states that "polychromasia (polychromatophilia), punctate stippling and reticulations are but different manifestations of one phenomenon —the presence of basophilic substance. The exact form of this basophilic substance existing in the unaltered blood is little known." Krafka[321] experimented with leading guinea pigs and found that the quantitative estimates of reticulocyte numbers, punctiphilia, polychromatophilia and normoblasts must be used with caution in attempts to establish a prognosis in lead poisoning, since at the very time that the lead is in action the counts may be very low.

Ziewagel[322] states that the blood of normal human adults contains an average of 1% basophilic erythrocytes. In the absence of other pathology an amount exceeding 1.5% in workmen exposed to lead indicated lead absorption. In early lead poisoning, without clinical manifestation, the per cent ranges from 1.5% to 4.0%, with occasional findings up to 20%. Too much stress has been placed in the past upon the de-

318. POPPITZ: Inaug. Dissert., Med. Fakultät, Leipzig, 1931.
319. LITZNER: *Med. Klin.*, 3, 1931.
320. LANE, R. E.: *J. Indust. Hyg.*; 13:276, 1931.
321. KRAFKA, JOSEPH, JR.: *J. Indust. Hyg.*, 17:13, 1935.
322. ZIEWAGEL, K.: *Folia haemat.*, 486:7, 1930.

termination of stippled cells, losing sight of the fact that this is just another manifestation of polychromatophilia consisting of a change in the staining capacity of the red cells. Normally-shaped red cells as well as poikilocytes which take the acid components from staining mixtures, are tinged with methylene blue, or eosinhematoxylin, the color varying from an eosin red to a pure violet. Many stains have been recommended for this purpose. Some laboratory men use Loeffler's alkaline methylene blue after good fixation, or Wright's, Jones', or McCord stains. With the first two stains normal red cells appear pale yellow, while polychromatophiles appear green to blue. The basophilic granulation has been studied by Lazanis,[323] Grawitz,[324] Nägeli, and many others. Rosin and Biber state they have observed basophilic granules in the erythrocytes of healthy individuals. Grawitz succeeded in producing this change in mice by overheating the animals. Janein[325] observed this change in a patient recovering from a bothriocephalus anemia. Nägeli regards it as a sign of regeneration, basing his opinion on Pappenhein's demonstration of basophilic stippling cells from normal blood marrow, and on Engel's and Schmietts report of finding these cells in embryonic blood. Basophilic forms are best revealed in laked cells. Jones[326] recommended fixing one-half of the blood smear, leaving the remaining half to be laked. In this manner it becomes possible to compare readily the numbers on a percentage basis of the total number of erythrocytes in the fixed and stained portion of the slide, with the basophilic-containing cells appearing in the unfixed portion below. The Sussmann-Weindel stain recommended by Jones has proved in five out of six lots quite unreliable, due to impurities in the toluidine blue which is one constituent of the stain. The Sussmann-Weindel stain advocated by Jones is quite satisfactory when its several ingredients are pure, as follows: toluidine blue 0.5 gm.; methylene blue solution (Loeffler's) 5 cc.; distilled water 100 cc. McCord claims that more consistent results were obtained with Manson's methylene blue

323. LAZANIS, ASKANAZY, and PLEHN: *Deutsche med. Wchnschr.*, No. 28-30, 1899.

324. GRAWITZ: *Deutsche med. Wchnschr.*, No. 36, 1899; No. 9, 1900.

325. JANEIN: *Berl. klin. Wchnschr.*, 38:901, 1901.

326. JONES, R. R.: Pub. Health Report 48:1011, 1933; *J.A.M.A.*, 104:195, 1935.

stain than with the stain recommended by Jones, since the toluidine blue does not seem to be uniform and has caused considerable trouble. The sodium borate is dissolved in boiling distilled water, and to this is added the methylene blue. After filtering, this stain is ready for use and provides a satisfactory, stable, and uniform stain for at least two weeks. After longer periods, a precipitate may appear, gradually, which interferes with the interpretation of the results. Manson's methylene blue is made as follows: borax, 0.4 gm.; boiling distilled water, 100 cc.; and methylene blue 2 gm. A uniform smear is made upon a slide, allowing the slide to dry one to three hours. "If permitted to become excessively dry, that is longer than twelve hours, some of the basophilic-containing cells will not lend themselves to aggregation of their basophilic material. On the other hand, insufficient drying facilitates removal of cells during the staining period. Ordinarily the optimum time lies between one and three hours. Under peculiar industrial conditions, involving high temperatures and low humidity or conversely high humidity, special consideration for the drying period may be required. After drying, one half of the slide is overlaid by a strip of filter paper, as set for by Jones, and cautiously there is applied with a pipet or dropper the minimum amount of methyl alcohol C.P. (methanol, wood alcohol) required to moisten the filter paper until it clings to this slide. This is allowed to dry until the filter paper becomes loose. The slide is now immersed in a Coplin staining jar containing the Manson stain for approximately ten minutes. The time is of minor importance, since a readable stain may be had in two minutes. After staining, it is necessary to wash the slides through three or four rinses of distilled water. In some cities tap water may be safely used for this purpose. Air drying of the slides is recommended. An oil immersion objective is provided, and a 10 X ocular, which is fitted with a Whipple grid. The average field in a good preparation contains approximately 150 red blood cells. Before counting, the slide should be examined for an area showing suitable distribution of the red cells." In the unfixed portion of the slide, customarily ten consecutive fields in two parallel rows are counted, making a total of twenty fields, but in the more evenly distributed slide twenty consecutive fields. Then moving to the fixed portion of the slide, five correspondingly appropriate fields are counted. The basophilic aggregations are then expressed as a percentage of the latter. Thus, if in the twenty fields counted in the unfixed portion of the slide there were found seventy-six basophilic aggregations, and if in the five fields of the fixed portion 1,000 red blood cells (or 4,000 in twenty fields), the obvious percentage is 1.9 (McCord). Lead exposed persons whose blood contains basophilic red cells in excess, and particularly in excess of 2%, at once suggest lead absorption and the possibility of approaching lead poisoning. "The chief value of this test is as a mark of lead absorption and early lead poisoning. As lead poisoning progresses to extended chronicity, the worth of the procedure diminishes." Teleky[327] is of the opinion that "stippling is more intense in early than in late severe plumbism." In my experience I found it in only 47% of the cases in which lead was demonstrated in the urine beyond the normal amount. Badham[328] states that "if punctate basophilia of the red cells is found in a worker in this State, in the absence of signs of a primary anemia or of a good cause for a secondary anemia (or even in their presence if the number of basophile cells is large), one is entitled to assume that it has arisen from a lead intake and to proceed to investigate the industrial conditions and the lead excretions of the patient." In 1927 Badham and Taylor published their findings with regard to the average lead excretion of the inhabitants of Sydney—0.02 mg. per liter. This figure was about the same as that of Weyrauch and Litzner for the German people, and a little lower than the figure found by Fretwurst and Hertz in Hamburg. Francis, working for the English Departmental Committee on tetraethyl lead in 1930, found that the average for normal London inhabitants was 0.049 mg. per liter, and for country people 0.023 mg. All these are much smaller than the amounts found by Kehoe and Thamann in students, which averaged 0.08 mg. per liter. "In lead poisoning one expects to find between 0.10 and 0.30 mg. per liter, but occasionally lead excreted is quite low and may not exceed the normal figure."

An increased leukocyte count has been found in the

327. TELEKY: Quoted by SCHOENFELD, J.: Zur. Frühdiagnose der Bleivergiftung, *Zentralbl. f. Gewerbehyg.*, 9:3, 1921.
328. BADHAM, C.: *M. J. Australia*, 816, December 16, 1933.

majority of cases, due to infected tonsils or infected teeth, occurring simultaneously with the presence of lead. In one case coming under my observation a man had very bad teeth and hypertrophied tonsils, with a marked swelling in the right hand and wrist. This painful condition of the right hand I attributed to his infected teeth and tonsils, and not to the mobile lead which was present in abnormal amounts. Pain with a high leukocyte count has led some surgeons to believe that they were dealing with an acute abdomen. In 1934 I saw five such cases; in one case the patient died five days following an operation for appendicitis. Material was submitted to me for examination and showed the presence of lead in the kidney, the bowel, the lung and the bones. The appendix was examined by two pathologists and was found to be normal.

Leschke says that the basophile granulation is not identical with the polychromasia and the vitally stainable network of the reticulocytes. The punctate basophilia are a sign of a qualitatively changed cell regeneration. (Schmidt-Kehl.)

In about three-quarters of the cases, the white cells show a relative increase in the lymphocytes, which, moreover, often present an irregular, fringed, or protruding edge to the cytoplasm. Another important finding in the blood in chronic cases is a marked increase in the large mononuclear cells in abnormal numbers in supposedly chronic carbon monoxide poisoning, and Brullowa found that they were present after inhalations of air containing from 0.2 to 0.3% of benzene.

Litzner[329] recently reported eight cases of contracted kidney in which lead poisoning could be ruled out but which showed an increase of stippled cells in the blood, and points out the danger of depending on the presence of these cells in the diagnosis of chronic lead poisoning in such a condition. Lehmann quotes R. E. Lane's article[330] in which he states that some 33.3% of normal students showed stippled cells in proportions from 100 up to 2000 per million reds, while no less than 58% of laborers not exposed to lead showed the same. Kojranski, from an investigation of the Moscow type workers, found punctate basophilia in 13.3%; blue line of the gums in 5.5%; colic in 2.1%, and paresis in 1.7% of the cases. Out of total of 1600 men employed in white lead industries during sixteen months,

329. LEHMANN, H.: Arch. f. Hyg., 111:49, 1933.
330. LANE, R. E.: J. Indust. Hyg., 13:276, 1931.

388 cases were found, or one case of poisoning in four exposed.[331]

The lead content of the blood is increased in lead poisoning. The blood shows 0.05 to 0.35 mg. of lead per 100 cc. in an average case of lead poisoning. The urine shows from 0.07 mg. upwards. The amount of lead excreted per day in the urine will be in excess of 0.1 mg. The same figures apply for the stool, 0.1 mg. and over.

The clinical signs of lead poisoning are chiefly a weakness and continued fatigue; increased lack of appetite; constipation; muscular weakness, especially of the extensors of the right hand; tremors of the eye, tongue, and mouth. Paralysis of the radial nerve and colic are late symptoms of the already fully developed picture of severe lead intoxication. The blue line of the gums occurs in less than 40% of the cases, indicating that lead absorption has taken place, and there may be no other symptoms of lead poisoning. It occurs chiefly in those with poor dental hygiene. The lead colic originates in a spasm of the intestinal muscles and vessels. In the denervated gut, lead causes an increase of the tonus, with simultaneous inhibition of the motility, the changes being characteristic of the typical spastic constipation of lead poisoned persons.[332] The violent pains are localized mostly in the parts below the navel, and are often in the region of the appendix. In contrast to the pains of appendicitis and peritonitis, those of lead colic are often soothed by firm pressure of the hands upon the abdomen, while appendicitis and peritonitis are not so relieved. Pickett, Nachman and Levitt* reported a case where the flat x-ray plate of the abdomen, taken a number of hours after onset of lead colic, gave the characteristic roentgenogram of intestinal obstruction. The patient died sixty hours after operation. An analysis of the liver revealed 0.6 mg. of lead per 100 gm., 108 mg. per 100 gm. of kidney. During the attacks of colic the pulse frequently falls to fifty, forty, or even twenty beats per minute, whereas the blood pressure, like the blood sugar, rises with a later decrease. Jaundice is seen occasionally.

Vascular spasm is noted by the paleness of the skin, slow pulse, and spasms of the retinal arteries which may lead to sudden transitory or permanent blindness, contracted kidney, and

331. Bull. 85, U. S. Dept. Commerce and Labor, Washington, D. C., 1911; HAMILTON: *J.A.M.A.*, 59:777, 1912.
332. AUB and SMITH.   * *Illinois M. J.*, 71:442, 1937.

changes in the brain vessels which cause an encephalopathy as well as an immediate poisonous effect on the nerve membranes. The contracted kidney which may cause the encephalopathy, may also cause gangrene of the extremities.[333] Netzler reported lead encephalitis from an acute infection.* There is suprarenal insufficiency and arterial hypotension.[334] Schnitter, among fifty-nine cases of lead poisoning, found only four with a pressure of more than 140 mm. Hg., and three of over 130 mm., as compared to twenty-eight with normal blood pressures and twenty-two with subnormal blood pressures of only 80 to 100 mm.

A hypertension can not be considered diagnostic of lead poisoning. It is found so commonly in the industrially employed people that it loses its significance. In most cases where found, it is probably only a complication, as some of these patients would have had high blood pressure whether or not they had ever worked with lead. (See pp. 161-170.)

Vigdortchik[335] found that Teleky,[336] in the Handbuch published in 1928, says: "The blood pressure of the old-stagers is often above normal"; and Chajes in his textbook on industrial hygiene similarly states: "As regards the vascular system there is observed a more or less severe arteriosclerosis as the outstanding complaint, accompanied by an increase in blood pressure."[337]

Chajes summarizes the principal conclusions of his work as the following:

1. Prolonged influence of lead increases the blood pressure. This is expressed in a higher percentage of prehypertonia and marked hypertonia cases, and in the higher value of blood pressure in each age group.

2. Work involving inhalation of metallic lead dust creates a greater predisposition to hypertonia than is found in other lead works.

3. Nephrosclerosis is not necessarily a companion of lead

333. Schwarz, L.: Zentralbl. f. Gewerbehyg., 9:253, 1932. Gerbid, H.: Zentralbl. f. Gewerbehyg., 10:65, 1933.
    * Netzler: California & West. Med., 46:289, 306, 1937.
    334. Chillia, A.: Folia med., 19:139, 1933.
    335. Vigdortchik: J. Indust. Hyg., 17:1, 1935.
    336. Teleky, L.: Vergiftungen durch Blei Handbuch d. soz. Hyg., Vol. 2, Gewerbehyg. und Gewerbekrankheiten, Berlin, 1928.
    337. Chajes: Grundriss der Berufskunde und Berufshygiene, Berlin, 1929.

hypertonia; in most cases hypertonia is accompanied by no kidney modifications, although work with lead undoubtedly predisposes to some kidney trouble in general, and to nephrosclerosis in particular. Such kidney modifications in lead cases occur about three times as often as in non-lead cases.

In animal experiments contracted kidney cannot be produced even after the lead has acted for years. A contracted kidney was reported in a rather severe case of lead poisoning in New South Wales.[338] Among sixty cases, Seiser and Litzner found it only once. In that case the kidney did not excrete lead, although the lead level of the blood was high.

Teleky measured the angle between the forearm and the hand with the latter extended as far as possible, comparing the right with the left. He found that it was seldom possible to detect weakness of the extensor after poisoning of short duration, but that it was frequently the only sign of damage after lead absorption for a longer time, especially in cases in which the lead absorption took place so slowly that other morbid appearances were not visible. There is a paralysis of the forearm, beginning with the common extensors of the fingers (third and fourth fingers), then paralysis of the other extensors, and finally of the thumb extensors and the muscles of the forearm. This form of paralysis is found particularly in hand workers. And there is a paralysis of the biceps, brachialis, and deltoids, and the shoulder muscles may be involved, while the triceps is not. This occurs in men painting, or shoveling dry lead pigments. Paralysis of the bladder and rectum does not occur in lead poisoning, an important finding from the point of view of differential diagnosis. Lead encephalitis results from damage to the brain vessels, which may cause lead to pass even into the cerebrospinal fluid. The first symptoms may appear at an early stage: nervous excitability and exhaustion, sleeplessness, headache, tremor of eye and mouth muscles, and of the fingers. This is followed by paralysis of brain nerves, paresis of the motor nerves of the eyes, the abductors and facial nerves, changes of the pupillar width and reaction, nystagmus, lowering of the upper limit of audibility and hearing by bone conduction. Terminally, mental changes occur: decrease in the intellectual and concentrating powers, weakening of memory, initiative and attention; hallucinations, irrational speech, ex-

338. Badham and Taylor.

citement, delirium, or apathy up to the stage of stupor. At the beginning of the encephalopathy, the patients often lapse into unconsciousness, and have epileptiform fits and deliria. Convulsions may occur, and death may ensue in two or three days. The majority of cases recover, with mental deterioration.

Paul as early as 1860 pointed out the damage to the germ cells, with abortion and sterility of lead workers.

In the diagnosis of chronic lead poisoning, all of the classical symptoms will not be found. The classic clinical picture includes anemia, anorexia, a blue line of the gums, local paralysis, especially of the right forearm, lead in the urine, colic with constipation, joint pains, and disorders of the central nervous system, but not every one of these is essential to the diagnosis. There is no arthritis.

The basophilic stippling found in the early cases of poisoning may not be seen in the chronic cases, unless the individual has an infectious disease and develops an acidosis from some intercurrent disease. Its diagnostic significance has been greatly exaggerated.[339] The same is true of the blue line in chronic cases, which may appear in only 36% of the cases. A case history is essential, as in most of the cases typical symptoms can be caused by other conditions such as disturbances of the digestive system, vomiting after eating, anorexia, constipation, and anemia. The pallor or sallowness of the skin, and metallic taste, especially in the morning, should warn the physician that he is probably dealing with a patient who is absorbing lead. The lead line is never seen when all the teeth have been extracted.

Treatment: The aim of the plant superintendent should be to keep the incidence of lead poisoning at a minimum. Dust is the most dangerous source of lead poisoning. The conversion of every dry process to a wet process would decrease the hazard. Adequate hoods should be placed over pots of molten metal and solder, so that the lead oxide which forms on the surface of the metal cannot be blown into the room in which the men are working. Many manufacturers require the workmen to change to clean clothes every day. The men should be educated in personal hygiene, the superintendent seeing that they wash their hands and faces before eating lunch, and also that they do not eat in the same room in which they work.

339. VAUGHAN, LINENTHAL: J.A.M.A., 62:1796, 1914; and OLIVER.

A physical examination of prospective workmen should remove anyone having digestive disturbances, and those having any degree of anemia, or showing evidence of nephritis, or cardiac disturbances. Frequent examination should be made periodically to check on loss of weight, loss of appetite, whether there is anemia, pallor, lead line, basophilic stippling, or any other symptom of active lead intoxication. The men should be compelled to undergo these examinations whether they desire them or not, for frequently the symptoms appear without any warning to the patient.

Melsens[340] was the first to mention the use of potassium iodide for the excretion of lead stored within the body. Parkes[341] reported the finding of lead in the urine after administration of potassium iodide, when it had not been excreted by this route before treatment. I found this lead excretion to be greatest on the second day. I have found in some cases that the amount of lead excreted in the second twenty-four hour specimen was increased to ten times that found before the administration of the iodide. The amount I use is far in excess of that recommended by others; I give thirty grains three times a day. If this is given longer than one day, acute attacks of plumbism are very apt to occur because of the mobility of a toxic quantity of lead in the blood. The administration of large doses of iodide was for a specific purpose: so that the chemist could demonstrate that the iodide had been given in the collection of the second specimen. I do not use potassium iodide for the treatment of lead poisoning. De-leading can be accomplished by a diet which contains very little calcium. In the experimental work of Aub, Fairhall, Minot, Reznikoff[342] the following diet proved satisfactory: meat, liver, potatoes, rice, tomatoes, canned corn (cooked without milk), bananas, apples (peeled), tea and coffee without milk, butter fat (prepared by melting butter in hot water and skimming off the butter fat), bread (prepared without milk, such as salt-free nephritic bread or sodium bicarbonate biscuits or crackers), sugar, salt, and pepper. With phosphoric acid the authors found they could mobilize lead effectually. The phosphoric acid is placed in water and sweetened; the taste is somewhat similar to lemon-

340. MELSENS: *Compt. rend. Acad. d. sc.*, 1840.
341. PARKES, E. A.: *Brit. & For. Med. Clin. Rev.*, 9: 522, 1853.
342. AUB, et al.: Lead Poisoning, 225, 1926.

ade. Doses of 20 cc. of the dilute acid should be given in a glass
of water every hour about ten times daily for several weeks. If
acidosis becomes too severe, and loss of appetite, headache, and
general malaise give evidence that the limits of tolerance of the
patient have been overstepped, that medication must be reduced. One gm. of ammonium chloride given in a glass of
water ten times a day will also produce an acidosis.[343] Ammonium chloride has increased the average excretion of lead three
fold. Sodium bicarbonate given 20 to 40 gm. a day produces
an effect similar to that of potassium iodide.

Aub and his associates recommend in the case of colic,
where the diagnosis of an acute surgical abdomen has been
ruled out, to give cathartics, using one ounce of magnesium
sulphate. The pain can be relieved by the application of local
pressure, heat, and moisture on the abdomen.

For the treatment of palsy give calcium gluconate, 1 gm.
dissolved in 10 cc. of water intravenously. The patient can be
given calcium gluconate wafers one every hour during the day,
which assist in immobilizing the lead. An encephalopathy
should be treated by methods aiming to fix the lead. I formerly
used thiosulphate intravenously, but have found that calcium
gluconate gives better results. The calcium gluconate should
be given slowly, covering a period of five to ten minutes. If
given rapidly the patient becomes very flushed, complains of
being warm, and causes the physician a great deal of worry;
if it is given slowly, however, none of these untoward results
will appear. I have used sodium tetrathionate on a large number of cases with better results than with the calcium preparations; injections of colloidal sulphur do not give as good results.
The treatment of lead paralysis should consist of massage, electrotherapy, and salicylates.

Postmortem Appearances: Patients who have had lead
poisoning and die from it or another disease complicating lead
poisoning, show an absence of subcutaneous fat. An examination of the mouth usually shows poor denture, with pyorrhea,
and a dark line on the gingiva near the border of the diseased
gums. Sections of this show microscopically that the lead line
is composed of smaller black granules lying in the connective
tissue at the base of the epithelium. A similar black discoloration in the mucosa of the colon and in the lower portion of

343. HALDANE, J. B. S.: *J. Physiol.*, 55:263, 1921.

the small intestine, first observed by Tanquerel,[344] is sometimes seen. Maier[345] reported that finding hemorrhages in the gastrointestinal tract contributed to this list of changes: a fatty degeneration of the secretory cells, enlargement of arteries, venous stasis, and circumscribed areas of softening. Jores[346] reported that he was able to produce gastric and intestinal ulcers in dogs by the administration of lead. These are significant because of the frequent occurrence of ulcers in lead intoxication, and may suggest a method of investigating the mechanism by which such lesions are produced. Ulcers have been reported in lead intoxication, but as statistics have not been properly controlled concerning the incidence of ulcer in the same type of men doing hard work away from lead dust, it cannot be stated at this time that lead is a contributing factor. Lead that enters the system by way of the mouth is removed by the liver. It has been reported as producing a cirrhosis of the liver. Since many of the workers in lead are large consumers of alcohol, the cirrhosis of the liver in plumbism may be caused by the alcohol instead of the lead. The opinion of most pathologists is that postmortem examination of the liver reveals no changes characteristic for lead. The lead also has no specific effect on the heart.

Picard[347] found only one case of nephritis in sixty-six cases investigated, two cases with mental symptoms, and two cases of optic neuritis. The majority presented disturbances of the digestive tract which reminded one of intestinal obstructions, appendicitis, cholecystitis and even cancer of the body of the pancreas. The marked asthenia is suggestive of a suprarenal insufficiency. Hypotension was marked in all cases. Strong[348] reported meningitis in a nineteen months old child, caused by lead poisoning. Kato[349] gives a resume of Japanese contributions to the diagnosis of lead meningitis in infants. There are two cases on record in which definite evidence of congenital lead poisoning was obtained. Lead was found in the organs of the new-born infants and in the placenta.[349]

344. TANQUEREL DES PLANCHES, L.:   Traites des maladies de plomb, ou saturnines, Paris, 1839.
345. MAIER, R.:   Virchow's Arch. f. path. Anat., 90: 455, 1882.
346. JORES, L.:   Beitr. z. path. Anat. u. z. allg. Path., 31: 183, 1902.
347. PICARD: Rev. de méd., Paris, 51: 133, 1934.
348. STRONG: Arch. Pediat., 37: 532, 1920.
349. KATO, R.: Am. J. Dis. Child., 44: 569, 1932. Symposium Section, Intern. Med. Dig., 30: 6, 1937.

The chronic nephritis caused by lead presents the picture of a secondarily contracted kidney. Legge and Goadby maintain that the changes found in the kidney have never been traced directly to lead, and are probably due to alcohol. The experimental work of a great many pathologists has not yet succeeded in establishing lead as a causative of nephritis. Many animals (dogs and rabbits) used in my experiments showed the same condition in the control division as those which were given lead for eight months. There is no evidence up to the present time that lead can cause a chronic interstitial nephritis. Hassin[350] reported that he saw marked proliferation of fibrous tissue and blood vessels in the pia-arachnoid space, especially near the cerebellum, optic chiasma, and temporal lobe; and infiltration by lymphocytes and plasma cells in the relatively acute cases. From his observations Hassin concluded that "lead encephalopathy contrasts sharply with infiltrative, infectious encephalitis. In plumbism, the meninges, the base of the brain, the cerebellum, the optic chiasma, and the temporal lobe are involved, while epidemic encephalitis affects chiefly the mid-brain." The occurrence of a type of amyotrophic lateral sclerosis in lead poisoning makes a study of the pathology of the spinal cord of value. Gross changes have never been observed, but many microscopic alterations have been found.[351] Therefore, in cases of atrophic paralysis, the lesion is probably amyotrophic in character and may perhaps include some sclerosis of the lateral columns. The peripheral neuritis seen in lead poisoning has been attributed, by some authors, to cord lesions. However, the consensus seems to confirm the peripheral location of the lesion and is based upon the observation of very distinct changes in the peripheral nerves themselves. Atrophy of the muscles has been observed in most cases of chronic lead poisoning. Most investigators who have examined the muscles agree with Messing (quoted by Aub) that the lesion is a chronic, degenerative, parenchymatous myositis, with fibrous tissue replacement, and that the changes are not merely secondary atrophy following nerve lesions, but are caused directly by the action of lead. The spleen shows no changes that could be attributed to chronic lead poisoning. The storage of lead in the bones appears to have no effect upon their

350. HASSIN, G. B.:   Arch. Neurol. & Psychiat., 6:268, 1921.
351. AUB, et al.:   Lead Poisoning, 1926.

structure. X-ray pictures of the tibia, femur, humerus and ribs removed from a man who had died of pneumonia, and who was exposed to lead for many years, failed to show any changes, although the bones contained from 1 to 4 mg. of lead per 100 gm. of bones. There is no evidence of changes in the lungs, salivary glands, or glands of internal secretion. The eye is the only sense organ in which lesions have been found in lead poisoning. Various pathological changes such as retinal hemorrhages and acute neuro-retinitis, characterized by swollen, hyperemic discs have frequently been observed. Optic atrophy has been described by Hutton and Mosso.[352] From examination of considerable pathological material submitted to me there was nothing characteristic that could be definitely stated as due to lead. The changes found in the various organs could have been present long before the individual started his work in lead.

Tests: I use the Fairhall method[353] for the quantitative estimate of lead. This method depends upon the complete destruction of the organic matter by ashing and the extraction of the ash by the hydrochloric acid and hot water from which the lead is precipitated as lead sulphide. The precipitate of lead sulphide after filtering is washed with boiled distilled water and dissolved in from 2 to 5 cc. of concentrated nitric acid; then boiled to expel H_2S, the excess of which is neutralized with sodium hydroxide and acidified with acetic acid. An excess of potassium chromate is added (usually 1 cc. of a 10% potassium chromate solution) and the solution is boiled for a few minutes; the precipitated lead chromate is allowed to stand over night before filtering. The precipitate of lead chromate is filtered through a small filter paper, and washed with warm water in order to remove traces of potassium chromate (wash water should be tested with diphenyl carbazid until there is no further pink obtained, showing the absence of chromate in the wash water), and should be washed as completely as possible from the filter paper into the flask, the flask being labelled "before" and "after," so as to distinguish the specimens — "before" meaning before the administration of potassium iodide to the patient. The filter paper should be washed with 5 cc. of a dilu-

352. Hutton, R. M.: Provincial Bd. of Health of Ontario, Toronto, 1923. Mosso, G.: *Minerva med.*, 7:930, 1927.
353. Fairhall, L.: *J. Indust. Hyg.*, 4:9, 1922.

tion of one-to-one hydrochloric acid, followed at once with warm water so as to remove the least trace of chromic acid. The lead is estimated by adding an excess of potassium iodide (1 cc. 10% sol. of KI) and titrating the iodine liberated by the action of the chromic acid with 0.005 normal sodium thiosulphate solution (using a starch indicator). One cc. of the standard sodium thiosulphate solution is equivalent to 0.3451 mg. of lead.

Boyd and De[354] for very small amounts used direct ashing, but for larger amounts acidulated the sample with acetic acid and electrolytically deposited the lead on a platinum electrode. They added 1 cc. of glacial acetic acid per 100 cc. of urine and electrolyzed the solution for three and one-half hours, using a current of 0.35 amperes. The deposit on the platinum electrode is removed by treatment with pure acetic acid and the solution dried on the water-bath, adding a few drops of sodium chloride solution to increase the bulk. The residue was used for the analysis. Standard plates were first prepared showing the line intensities obtained from various known amounts of lead. They used dilutions of lead acetate which were dried out directly on the water-bath, adding first a little sodium chloride to increase the bulk. This residue was transferred to a suitably prepared H. S. brand graphite electrode, and the arc struck, using a current of four amperes at 220 volts. The time of exposure was thirty seconds. The plates used were Ilford Isozenith, speed 700. To guard against the impurities in the electrodes, preliminary blank spectrographic examinations were carried out, using a more powerful current and a longer exposure. The R. V. lines (Twyman) of lead are invariably present with 0.0001 mg. In many cases they found the lines to persist up to 0.00001 mg. while occasionally they have detected them in 0.000001 mg.[354]

Harwood and Brophy[355] give the most convenient characteristic test for minute quantities of lead in the "triple nitrate" test of Behrene and Kley.[356] This test has been adapted to biological materials by Fairhall,[357] who pointed out its applications in the study of lead poisoning. Weller and Christen-

354. Boyd, T. C., and De, N. K.: *Indian J. M. Research*, 21:109, 1933. For the colorimetric dithizone method see "Methods of Analysis" A.O.A.C., p. 375, 4th ed., 1935.

355. Harwood, R. U., and Brophy, Doris: *J. Indust. Hyg.*, 16:25, 1934.

356. Behrene, H., and Kley, P. D. C.: Leipzig, 3rd ed., 28, 1915.

357. Fairhall, L. T.: *J. Biol. Chem.*, 57:455, 1923.

sen[358] have modified this method in order to make it more applicable to cerebrospinal fluid. After complete destruction of the organic matter in the biological material, lead is precipitated as the sulphide and under controlled conditions, a few drops of 2% cupric acetate are added. (This carries down the lead by entrainment.) After careful washing of the precipitate the lead sulphide is dissolved in a few drops of concentrated nitric acid. A drop of this solution is evaporated to dryness on a microscope slide; minute quantities of sodium acetate and acetic acid and a small crystal of potassium nitrate are added. Lead, if present, crystallizes out as characteristic dark brown squares and cubes of potassium-copper lead hexanitrite, $K_2CuPb(NO_2)_6$. Berg[359] favored hydrogen sulphide catalyzed by a trace of copper sulphate. The method is similar to the Fairhall method. The addition of a small drop of 2% cupric acetate serves to carry down the lead sulphide by entrainment. Any traces of inorganic salts are removed by careful washing of the precipitate. This is accomplished by using 0.01 normal hydrochloric acid, saturated with hydrogen sulphide, which has been used in place of the distilled water.

Seiser, Necke, and Müller[360] recommend the destruction of organic matter in the presence of 5% by volume of concentrated sulphuric acid in a muffle with a maximum temperature of about 500° C., as it has been found that there was no loss of lead if the temperature did not exceed 500° C. If there were any carbon particles present they were removed by digestion with sulphuric acid in a Kjeldahl flask, with occasional drop-wise addition of concentrated nitric acid.

Fretwurst and Hertz,[361] described a method for the detection of lead in the urine and feces by which 0.01 mg. of lead may be detected.

Normal Lead: Pfrieme[362] reported finding in the teeth of man the normal lead content of 0.065 mg. to 0.24 mg. per 3 gm., the ages varying from one and a half to eighty-six years.

358. WELLER, C. V., and CHRISTENSEN, A. D. The Human Cerebrospinal Fluid, (Hoeber), 466, 1924.

359. BERG, R.: The Human Cerebrospinal Fluid, 198:420, 1928. Der Nachweis winziger Bleispuren in organischen Substanzen, 1928.

360. SEISER, A., NECKLE, A., and MÜLLER, H.: Ztschr. f. ang. Chemie, Berl., 42:96, 1929.

361. FRETWURST, FRITZ, and HERTZ: Arch. f. Hyg., 104:315, 1930.

362. PFRIEME, F.: Arch. f. Hyg., 111:232, 1934.

In cases of lead poisoning the ash varied from 0.22 to 0.55 mg. In various wild and domestic animals, lead was also found in the teeth. Weyrauch and Müller found in 3 gm. of ashed vertebrae from 0.05 to 0.27 mg. of lead.[363] The quantity increased with the age of the person. The upper limit of the normal lead content among non-lead workers is generally accepted as about 0.25 mg. of lead in 3 gm. of ashed vertebrae.

Barth[364] reported that the bones of adults who had never worked in lead industries or suffered from lead poisoning, and of infants one day to four months old, were analyzed for lead by the micro-method of P. Schmidt. In 3 gm. of infant bone 0.01 to 0.04 mg. lead was found. With increasing age amounts varying from 0.02 to 0.065 in youth to 0.08 to 0.19 in old age were detected. The bone-marrow always contained no less lead than the solid bone. No difference was found in people living in villages without central water piping and those in cities where lead pipes were used. The lead was probably absorbed in the food from time to time. Tompsett[365] states that the femora and tibiae contain much higher concentrations of lead than ribs and vertebrae, the ribs containing 4.0 to 17.5; vertebrae, 3.4 to 16.5; femur, 18.2 to 108.3; tibia, 15.3 to 96.5 mg. of lead per kilogram of fresh bone.

Weyrauch, Necke, and Müller[366] found that with advancing age the lead content of the bones increased proportionately to the years. They fed a goat various lead salts during a period of several months. The animal received in three months, a total intake of 460 gm. of lead salts, and it steadily gained in weight, and apparently showed no symptoms. It seems the goat is rather resistant to lead poisoning. Of blood from this animal 520 cc. yielded 240 cc. of serum and 280 cc. of clot. The serum contained 0.05 mg. of lead; the clot 0.85 mg. of lead, which makes one assume that lead adheres mostly to the blood corpuscles, and particularly the leukocytes. From the analysis of the body of the goat it was found that the bones, kidney, liver, brain, spleen, and pancreas were able to store lead. In the kidney, the lead is particularly confined to the cortex. In

363. WEYRAUCH, F., and MÜLLER, H.: Ztschr. f. Hyg. u. Infektionskr., 115:216, 1933.
364. BARTH, E.: Arch. Path., 281, 1931.
365. TOMPSETT, S. L.: J. Biochem., 30:345, 1936.
366. WEYRAUCH, F., NECKE, A., and MÜLLER, H.: Ztschr. f. Hyg. u. Infektionskr., 116:28, 1935.

cases where sudden changes of metabolism are brought about, lead patients may often have severe relapses.

Normal urine will always show traces by colorimetric methods, while the electrolytic and Fairhall methods will often fail to show traces of lead. Millet found 0.05 mg. per liter, and Seiser and Litzner found 0.001 to 0.005 mg. per liter. Kehoe and his associates found 0.017 to 0.087 mg. per liter in normal individuals. The daily intake of only 1 or 2 mg. of lead produces a lead intoxication after some months, and 10 mg. produces symptoms after some weeks. When the urine contains an average of 0.1 mg. or over per liter of urine, the patient is suffering from lead poisoning. After administration of potassium iodide this amount may be increased to 15 mg., but more often is under 0.6 mg. per liter. Schmidt[367] has given a comparative spectrographic and colorimetric determination in body fluids and organs. For estimation of lead in blood, urine and feces see Schmidt.[368] For distribution of lead in organisms, especially in the bones, see Dauchworth.[369]

Peipers[370] observed a case of chronic lead poisoning, which was complicated by a duodenal ulcer. The case refers to a man forty-six years of age, who had worked with lead for ten years. Schiff[371] reported in chronic plumbism, non-characteristic pains, due to hyperacidity, and a duodenal ulcer. These authors have come to the same conclusion I have already alluded to, that the simultaneous presence of an ulcer and lead intoxication in general is merely an accidental one, but in this case there seems to exist a relation between the two conditions. Behrend and Baumann[372] have found that, on injecting radioactive lead into animals, the distribution of the metal among the organs can be studied by placing tissue sections on photographic plates. With this method new investigations were made in the attempt to confirm the various opinions expressed by writers in the past concerning the distribution of the metal within the organism. They found as a result of their observations that if

367. SCHMIDT, P.: *Deutsche med. Wchnschr.*, 54:50, 1928.
368. SCHMIDT, P.: Arbeiterschutz, No. 7, 132, 1928; for distribution see also FAIRHALL: *M. J. Australia*, 1:216, 1929.
369. DAUCHWORTH, E., JURGENS: *Arch. de Pharm.*, 266: 492, 1928.
370. PEIPERS, A.: *Deutsche med. Wchnschr.*, 59:254, 1933.
371. SCHIFF, W.: *Klin. Wchnschr.*, 387, 1919.
372. BEHREND, B., and BAUMANN, A.: *Ztschr. f. d. ges. exper. Med.*, 92:241, 1934.

larger amounts of lead are used, the distribution differs if a large portion of the metal is retained in the liver and spleen.

In the investigation of the source of chronic poisoning, an examination of the air of the industrial work rooms should always be made. The Greenburg-Smith impinger apparatus is used for the collection of samples of lead, distilled water being used in the collecting flasks. The lead is determined by the Fairhall method, using all the reagents and the distilled water from one of the impinger flasks as a control. In one industry the air contained 0.03 to 0.5 mg. of lead per 10 cu. ft. of air, close to men working with blast lamps and small bars of solder. Isbell and Bloomfield[373] found 0.09 mg. per 10 cu. ft. of air in congested street centers. The finding of lead in the air we breathe and in all of our food accounts for the presence of lead in the excretions of people not exposed to it industrially.[374] Litzner and Weyrauch[375] consider the lead content of the blood a fairly reliable measure of the degree of lead intoxication. The lead content of 0.01 mg. per cent to 0.03 mg. per cent did not cause symptoms. When the lead content was above 0.04 mg. symptoms could be detected. The examination of the urine is more often used to show absorption and fixation of lead. Lead poisoning does not result from the lead stored in the bones and organs, but from the lead in the circulating blood,[375] the concentration and duration of which determine the symptoms of the poisoning. A low concentration circulating for a long time finally produces the same symptoms of poisoning as a larger amount circulating for a short time.

In a recent survey (May, 1936) of a factory, made by the author, thirty-two men gave blood counts from 3,800,000 to 5,100,000 red cells; 5,400 to 13,800 white cells; hemoglobin 58% to 100%. Not one of the smears gave evidence of basophilic stippling. The urine gave 0.03 mg. to 0.39 mg. per 1000 cc. There were no subjective symptoms of lead poisoning.

Respirators to prevent lead inhalation must pass government inspection at a humidity of 40-70%, relative humidity 25°

373. ISBELL, H. S., and BLOOMFIELD, J. J.: J. Indust. Hyg., 15:144, 1933.

374. LITZNER and WEYRAUCH: Med. Klin., 29:381, 1933.

375. LITZNER and WEYRAUCH: Med. Klin., 29:381, 1933. For hazards of contaminated fruits and vegetables see Editorial, J.A.M.A., 108: 1178, 1937; and 109:135, 1937; also HANZLIK, P. J.: Scient. Month., 44: 435, 1937.

C., a continuous flow of 32 liters per minute with a test suspension of 15±5 mg. per cu. m. of lead as lead oxide fume produced by the decomposition of lead tetraethyl, sample period of two 156-minute periods, the test suspension containing not to exceed 1.5 mg.

The following chart will be useful to the industrial surgeon, in keeping a record of his lead cases (Chart I):

CHART I
INDUSTRIAL HYGIENE — PLUMBISM

Name.................................... Address...........................Date............

Age...........................Sex.......................................

Home ....
          Congested   House   Apartment   Light   Dampness   Heating

Habits (Alcohol, Tobacco, etc.)...

Previous Unemployment Causes ....

Previous Industrial History

Names of Employers	Addresses of Employers	Industry	Occupation	Date Began Work	Date Stopped Work
1.					
2.					
3.					

Present Occupation

    Hours ....
          Day   Night   Overtime   Noontime   Per Week   Steadiness   Seasons

Hazards...........................(Use Key)

    Protection
        Hoods...........Drafts...........type...........Masks...........Are Floors and
        Machines Vacuumed...........Lunchroom...........Washrooms...........
        Water Fountains (Foot pedal or hand type).....................Medical
        Inspection (How often)...
        Change of Occupation ....

History
    Abdominal operations, especially appendicitis...........................
    Breathing dust containing lead ....
    Breathing lead fumes or vapors...
    Paleness, weakness, dyspepsia...
    Rheumatism ....
    Sore throat or tonsillitis...
    Loss of weight...
    Weakness of arms or legs...
    Paralysis of arms or legs...
    Headache ....
    Constipation ....
    Diseased teeth and gums...
    Loss of appetite ....
    Dizziness, "nervousness"...
    Staggering spells ....
    Confusion ....

Insomnia ....
Memory defective...
Chronic bronchitis...
Insanity, or detention for peculiar actions.................................

Present Symptoms

Abdominal pain (especially colic)...
Dyspepsia ....
Constipation ....
Poor appetite ....
Headache ....
Backache ....
Rheumatism, etc. ....
Weakness (general or local)...
Mental depression, "Neurasthenia"......................................
Dizziness ....
Nervousness ....
Poor sleep ....

Physical Signs

Premature aging ....
Pallor (especially about mouth and lower face).................
Excessive sweating ....
Ocular palsies ....
Tremors (tongue, lips, chin, hands)......................................
Incoordination (fingers, arms)..
Grip strength weak (dynamometer).....................................
Strength of wrist extension (weak).......................................
Wrist drop ....
Reflexes usually decreased (knee jerks, wrists, elbows, cremasteric)

Ataxia ....
Arteriosclerosis (radial, brachial, temporal)........................
Abnormal blood pressure (systolic) but subject to wide variations....

Teeth and gum diseases (look for "lead line").....................
Acne, dermatitis ....
Gouty signs (ears, great toe joints, palms, other joints)........
Edema of ankles...
Dropsy ....
Encephalopathy ....

Laboratory Tests

Blood

Hb.............R.B.C................Color Index.............. W.B.C..............
Differential (white) ....
Anemia (secondary) ....
Basophilia (especially to be looked for during colic). How
many per million..

Urine

Albumin ....
Lead in milligrams per 1,000 cc. (volumetric not colorimetric
method) ....
Casts ....
Red corpuscles ....
Findings for chronic (interstitial) nephritis.................

Wassermann (Blood) ....

X-ray (of joints involved)..

Key: A—Assembling battery plates, T—Testing, M—Mixing pastes,
ML—Melting, WS—Wire stripping, SW—Sweeper.

MERCURY (Hg)

(Atomic Weight 200. Synonyms: Quicksilver, Hydrargyrum)

METALLIC mercury is used in thermometers, barometers, manometers, mercury vapor lamps, electric interrupters, and in the preparation of the large number of its compounds. Poisoning may occur in the mining of metallic mercury. Most of our mercury occurs as the harmless sulphide, cinnabar, but a few mines have an admixture of native quicksilver. Occasionally, a case occurs in the metallurgy of mercury when old-fashioned furnaces are used, or when the condensers which collect the mercury from the furnaces are being cleaned out. Unusually dangerous jobs are those of repairing, with a torch, the high-frequency induction furnaces or mercury boilers. Death from industrial mercurialism is very rare. One case has been reported from the vapors escaping from a high-frequency induction furnace with a mercury seal.[376]

Properties: Mercury has a specific gravity of 13.5953. Its melting (freezing) point is—38.85°C. Its boiling point is 357.33° C. at 760 mm. It is the only metal which is a liquid at ordinary temperatures. It is white when pure, with a slightly bluish tinge, and having a brilliant silvery lustre. It is slightly volatile even at —13° C.[377] The principal ore of mercury is cinnabar (HgS), red, found in California, Illyria, Spain, China, Ural, and some other localities. The free metal is sometimes found in small globules in rocks containing the ore. It is also found amalgamated with gold and silver, and as mercuric iodide and mercurous chloride. It is prepared by roasting with a regulated supply of air, lime may be added to the ore, and the mercury is then distilled. The U. S. Pharmacopeia, XI, mercury contains not less than 99.5% of mercury. The U.S.P. preparations are: hydrargyri chloridum corrosivum (corrosive mercuric chloride); hydrargyri chloridum mite (mild mercurous chloride); hydrargyri iodidum flavum (yellow mercurous iodide); hydrargyri iodidum rubrum (red mercuric iodide); hydrargyri oxidum flavum (yellow mercuric oxide); hydrargyri salicylas (mercuric salicylate); hydrarygrum (mercury); hydrargyrum ammoniatum (ammoniated mercury); hydrarg-

376. JORDAN, L., and BARROWS, W. P.: *J. Indust. & Eng. Chem.,* 16:898, 1924.
    377. REGNAULT: *C. R.,* 93:308, 1881.

yrum cum creta (mercury with chalk); unguentum hydrargyri ammoniati (ointment of ammoniated mercury); unguentum hydrargyri fortius (stronger mercurial ointment); unguentum hydrargyri mite (mild mercurial ointment); unguentum hydrargyri oxidi flavi (ointment of yellow mecuric oxide.)

Mercury can be reduced to a finely divided state by shaking with sugar, grease, chalk, turpentine, ether, etc. The metal is used therapeutically in the pure state to remove obstruction from the bowels mechanically, with no injurious consequences unless retained for a number of days. Taylor[378] reports a case, in which, after retention for nine days, there was some salivation, all the metal not being expelled until the fourteenth day.

In England, a girl took four and a half ounces of liquid mercury as an abortive, and suffered from mercurial tremors, but did not abort.[379] External applications of blue ointment have caused death.[380] Welander [381] reported two deaths resulting from his method of mercurial treatment, which consists in wearing flannel sacks smeared with mercurial ointment upon the breast or back. Mercurial poisoning has been reported in dentists working with amalgam fillings.[382] The slow absorption of the mercury from these fillings may cause fatigue, restlessness, irritation, headache, disturbed sleep, excessive flow of saliva, inflammation of the gums, loosening of the teeth, inflammation of the throat and ulcers of the mucous membranes. Sonder and Sweeney report that the claims for mercury

378. TAYLOR, A.:   On Poisons, 351, 1875.

379. GIBBS: Lancet, 1:339, 1873.

380. CRAMPTON: Tr. Ass. King's and Queen's Coll. of Phys., Ireland, 4:91, 1824; Lancet, 2:108, 1845; Pharm. J. & Tr., 2nd series, 9:395, 1868; 80 to 90 boys, one death.   LEIBLINGER: Wien. med. Wchnschr., 19:1595, 1869.   LOWE: Brit. M. J., 1:188, 1882; BRAUS: Deutsche med. Wchnschr., 13:593, 1887; two deaths.   VIRCHOW: Berl. klin Wchnschr., 24:252, 1887; SACKUR, ibid., 29:618, 1892; LETOUX: These Paris, 44, 1893; LEWIN: Berl. klin. Wchnschr., 32:310, 1895; two deaths.   EICHORST: Med. Klin., 1:80, 1905; München. med. Wchnschr., 54:1282, 1907; STEIN: Med. Martiale, 96; ex. Ann. d'hyg., 4th series, 9:278, 1909; one death.

381. WELANDER: ibid., 40:257, 1897.

382. Present status of mercury from amalgam fillings: HOFFMAN, K. H.:   Aertzl. Rundschau, München, 38:51, 1928; STERNER, RAINER: Alleged Danger of Mercury Amalgam Fillings, Ztschr. f. Stomatol., 25: 201, 1927; ATRON, J.: Amalgam Filling and Mercury Poisoning, Deutsche Monatschr. f. Zahnh., Leipz., 45:433, 1927;   SCHREIBER, E.: Mercury Poisoning from Amalgam Fillings of Teeth, Ztschr. f. Stomatol., 25:203, 1927;   FLEISCHMANN, P.: Poisoning from Small Amounts of Mercury, Especially in Dental Fillings, Deutsche med. Wchnschr., 54:304, 1928.

poisoning either as a vapor or a solution, from the standard amalgams through the air or food taken in the mouth, are not justified.[383] However, clinical evidence with proper control is not available to verify the correctness of their conclusions. Stock[384] found that concentrations of from 0.001 to 0.01 mg. mercury to the cubic meter of air were sufficient to cause mercury poisoning of himself and associates. He also reported a chronic mercurial poisoning in which the removal of twenty-four amalgam fillings caused immediate improvement in a Marbery professor. Hertz[385] observed fifty persons, thirty-five of whom had amalgam fillings and fifteen had none. Of the thirty-five he found thirty-four excreted mercury in the urine and feces, and of the fifteen he found eleven excreting mercury. He observed thirteen actively engaged in dentistry, all of whom were excreting mercury, but not in sufficient amount to indicate mercurial poisoning. Fleischmann[386] reports on fifty-one individuals; thirty-seven had copper amalgam fillings, and from thirty mercury was demonstrated in the mouth outside the fillings. Of the fourteen having pure "silver" amalgams, only one showed mercury. Fuhner,[387] discussing Stock's paper, gives the impression that, with the daily excretion of a few hundredths of a mg. of mercury, no signs of chronic poisoning have been observed, but with excretions of a few tenths of a mg. such signs have appeared, and that it would be exceptionally rare for silver amalgams to give off mercury in these quantities. The experiments of Washburn[388] show conclusively that mercury vapor is not to be expected from amalgam fillings which are kept moist. However, there may be a question on the possibility of vapor being given off from the dry fillings in the mouths of those who breathe through the mouth or sleep with the mouth open.

Williams and Schram report the accidental acute mercurial poisoning of thirty-two workmen.*

383. SONDER, W., SWEENEY, W. T.: Dental Cosmos, Phila., 73:1145, 1931.
384. STOCK: Berlin letters, J.A.M.A., 87:685, 1926; Med. Klin., Nos. 24, 29 and 30, 1928.
385. HERTZ, A.: Berl. klin. Wchnschr., 8:541, 1929; abst. J.A.M.A., 1929.
386. FLEISCHMANN, Berlin letter, J.A.M.A., 90:1056, 1928.
387. FUHNER: Berlin letter, J.A.M.A., 89:388, 1927.
388. WASHBURN, BRUN, and HICKES: J. Med. Research, Bost., 2:483, 1929.
* WILLIAMS, J. E., and SCHRAM, C. F. N.: Acute Mercurial Poisoning, Indust. Med., 6:9:490, 1937.

CORROSIVE SUBLIMATE (HgCl₂)
(Molecular Weight 268.86)

CORROSIVE sublimate, bichloride of mercury, mercuric chloride, and hydrargyri chloridium corrosivum, contains not less than 99.5% of mercuric chloride. It occurs as heavy, colorless, odorless rhombic crystals or crystalline masses, or a white powder. One gm. of corrosive sublimate is soluble in 13.5 cc. of water, in 3.8 cc. of alcohol, in about 12 cc. of glycerin, and in 22 cc. of ether, at 25° C. One gm. is soluble in 2.1 cc. of boiling water, and in 1.6 cc. of boiling alcohol. The salt fuses to a colorless liquid at about 265° C., and at about 300° C. volatilizes as a dense, white vapor. An aqueous solution of corrosive mercuric chloride (one in twenty) is acid to litmus paper, but becomes neutral upon the addition of sodium chloride. It sublimes at 180° F. (82.2° C.) and is deposited in needles, in octahedra, or in stellate aggregation of crystalline plates. It has no odor, but has an acrid metallic taste. Mercuric chloride forms definite insoluble compounds with matter, such as albumin, and is fatal to low forms of animal and vegetable life. In antiseptic surgery it is extensively employed as a bactericide in irrigating solutions of one to 4000 or even one to 1000 of water. Its use in surgery began about 1880, and cases of poisoning began to appear from that time on. In Macon, Georgia, in 1910, a banker took a tablet of bichloride of mercury, mistaking it for a salicylate. The papers led the public to believe that bichloride of mercury was a satisfactory poison for self destruction. This caused an enormous increase in cases in Cook County, Illinois, and probably in other parts of the United States. From the average of one to two cases of bichloride of mercury poisoning, the number of cases jumped to forty or fifty per year. The majority of these cases died. Most of them were deliberate attempts at suicide, a few were accidental. To prevent this latter type of poisoning, drug manufacturers were urged to produce a blue tablet with irregular corrugated sides, so that one would be warned in the dark, as well as in the light, that he was dealing with an unusual drug. The outgrowth of this was the introduction of the U. S. P. toxitabellae hydrargyri chloridi corrosivi (poisonous tablets of corrosive mercuric chloride). They are dispensed in a blue-colored angular form, with the bottle stamped "Poison," each tablet weighing about 1 gm. and containing about 0.5 gm. each of corrosive sublimate and common salt.

In the Berlin-Westend Hospital during the years 1912 to 1925, 250 cases of poisoning with medicants and chemicals were reported, of which ten were suicides due to bichloride of mercury, two were due to mercuric cyanide, and one was due to mercury. In Cook County (Illinois) in 1936, six died from mercuric chloride.

Symptoms: The symptoms of acute poisoning from corrosive sublimate vary with the amount of mercury absorbed, and upon the degree of dispersion. They usually appear within a few minutes after taking the poison. The immediate effects are due to coagulation, irritation, and superficial corrosive action. The patient may experience, in a few minutes, a burning sensation in the throat, an astringent metallic taste, salivation, great thirst, abdominal distress, and pain. Vomiting occurs usually within five minutes, the vomitus being colored blue if the U. S. P. tablets were taken, or bloody mucous shreds may appear in the vomitus. There is a gray, ashy discoloration of the mouth and pharynx, with edema of the glottis. The inflammation of the throat may involve the larynx, and in acute poisoning the pharynx may cause asphyxia. Within a half-hour a white coating may form on the shrivelled lining of the mouth, which usually ulcerates and causes annoyance to the patient.

In seventeen cases out of twenty-one, vomiting occurred in two minutes to one-half hour after ingestion.[389] The urine is scanty or suppressed. Temperature may be febrile or subnormal. There may be a cold clammy sweat, with weak irregular pulse. Diarrhea usually sets in within two hours, the stool being liquid and blood-stained. Within thirty-six hours mucous patches may be found in the stool, as large as half of one's hand; within seventy-two hours, salivation, stomatitis, glossitis, and gingivitis, with severe pains over the entire abdomen, may occur. Anuria occurs usually on the third day. A typical case illustrating the progress of bichloride of mercury poisoning is that of a man forty-eight years of age, American, white, who on November 6, 1929, was given a prescription for thirty-two one-fourth-grain calomel tablets. He had the prescription filled at his usual pharmacy, rated high from the standpoint of

389. JOHNSTONE, B. I.: *Canad. M. A. J.,* 24:500, 1931.

accuracy in compounding prescriptions. At the close of the day's work, he decided to take a couple of the tablets. After four of the tablets had been taken by the patient he noticed an irritation and burning in his throat and mouth. Nausea, vomiting and diarrhea soon appeared. Within forty-five minutes from the time of taking the tablets, his physician arrived to find him vomiting every few seconds, his skin being moist and cyanotic. He complained of burning pain in the stomach, throat and mouth, and of a metallic taste in the mouth. The tablets which had been taken, as dispensed by the druggist, were found to be seven-and-a-half-grain tablets of bichloride of mercury instead of calomel. The whites of two eggs and a glass of milk were given to the patient, but these were promptly expelled. His condition became acute and he was removed to a hospital. Hot packs and colonic flushings were given to eliminate the mercury. The whites of eggs and milk were again tried, but the patient was unable to retain them. The vomitus and stool contained bright red blood, and there was an immediate oliguria, only 370 cc. of urine being passed in the first twenty-four hours. On the third day I was called in consultation on the case, and ordered gastric lavages every eight hours. One-half gm. of sodium thiosulphate was given twice in twenty-four hours for ten doses. On the fourth night the patient became very nervous and lapsed into a state of semiconsciousness. In his wakeful moments he talked incoherently. On the fifth day, however, his condition improved. On the soft palate there was an erosion due to the corrosive action of the bichloride of mercury. The gingival margins of the gums were darkened, and the salivation caused a burning of the skin below the mouth. The water used for the gastric lavages and colonic flushings contained eight grains of calcium sulphide per liter of water. Two gm. of potassium acetate in water were given twice daily for the first week, and all of the water that the patient was given to drink during his illness contained 2 gm. of sodium bicarbonate to each six ounces.

The patient remained in the hospital thirty-seven days. He had lost twenty-five pounds in weight, and had a mild secondary anemia. Mercury was found in the urine up to and including the twelfth day, also in the gastric lavage up to the sixteenth day, and in the colonic flushings up to the twenty-sixth day. Urinary analysis showed albumin in the greatest amount on the third, fourth, and fifth days of his illness, and remained present until the time of his death over a year later. On the fourth day his non-protein nitrogen was 82, and on the fourteenth day 104, when it gradually decreased, until, on the one-hundred and sixty-first day, it was 30. The urea nitrogen on the fourth day was 78, and on the fourteenth day 92, which was the highest point reached, after which it gradually returned to normal. The creatinine was 8.6 on the fourth day and 8.9 on the fourteenth day when it rapidly dropped to normal. The normal non-protein nitrogen is 25 to 35, urea nitrogen is 12 to 14, creatinine nitrogen is 0.5, and creatine nitrogen is 1.0.

In another case the non-protein nitrogen on the fourth day was 127.6 mg. per 100 cc., and on the eighth day was 206.9 mg. per 100 cc. of blood. This case was a cyanide of mercury poisoning, ending fatally on the eighth day after admittance to the hospital, although given the same treatment as the preceding case which made a complete recovery. All the cases showing a bloody diarrhea have an anemia with a red count as low as 2,225,000. The first case had a red count of 3,630,000 on the sixth day, 75% hemoglobin and 12,050 w. B. C. The second case, on the second day, showed a red count of 4,730,000 and a white count of 30,100.

Marchand, Smith and Church found, in one case, 300 mg. of non-protein nitrogen, 7.8 mg. creatinine and 8.6 mg. uric acid per 100 cc. of blood. There was a greater loss of blood in their case than in the one reported above. If the non-protein nitrogen continues to increase after the fourth day, the prognosis is very grave. The non-protein nitrogen may be used as a guide to the condition of the patient, this condition being directly proportional to the mg. of non-protein nitrogen found per 100 cc. The blood chemistry is much easier to determine than a quantitative mercury, although the decrease in the amount of mercury in the secretions can be easily shown by the Reinsch test. The temperature of the patient is practically normal, and the pulse rate is elevated, usually above 100 per minute. Edema is seldom present in these cases, although it has been reported. This may be accounted for by the removal of considerable water and salt from the body, due to the violent diarrhea. From an investigation of over 150 cases, I have come to the conclusion that if the anuria begins after the fourth day, the prognosis is more favorable than where the mercury acts as a diuretic. Hayman and Priestly[390] found an urea nitrogen 247 mg. on the nineteenth day of treatment.

Hull and Monte[391] studied the case records of 302 people who had taken bichloride of mercury. There were seventy-two deaths, a mortality of 23.8%. About one-half of the patients did not develop any signs of mercury poisoning. It frequently happens that patients give a history of having taken bichloride of mercury to win over someone with whom they are in love. I saw a number of similar cases where absolutely no mercury was found in the urine or stool, which might imply that these authors disregarded those cases without symptoms, and gave the true mortality of mercury as approximately 50%. They gave the mortality in severe cases as 90%. Of ninety-six patients who took the poison undissolved, twelve died, a mortality of 12.5%. Of forty patients who dissolved the salt before taking, thirteen died, a mortality of 32.5%. No recoveries occurred in patients whose blood non-protein nitrogen exceeded 190 mg. per cent, or whose creatinine was above 5 mg. per cent. In this series, they report that the different methods of treatment employed had no effect on the mortality. Porter and Simons[392] report a study of forty-six cases. One patient secreted no urine for 192 hours, the anuria having immediately followed the taking of the mercury. Recovery occurred despite the fact that a blood creatinine of 12.2 mg. per 100 cc. was reached before diuresis was established. In their series they report a leucocyte count of above 20,000 per cm. and a red cell count of 5,-000,000 or more. In the majority of the patients examined by me, the red cell count was below normal.

Fatal Dose: Sansum[393] found that 4 mg. of bichloride of mercury given intravenously per kilogram produced death without anuria, while 5 mg. per kilogram produced anuria before death. These amounts would be between four and five grains respectively. For man, 70 mg. per 150 lbs. have caused death.

Recovery has taken place from thirty grains, as in the case cited. Recovery has followed the administration of 192.6

390. HAYMAN and PRIESTLEY: *Am. J. Sc.*, 176:510, 1928.
391. HULL, E., and MONTE, L. A.: *South. M. J.*, 27:918, 1934.
392. PORTER, W. B., and SIMONS, C. E.: *Am. J. M. Sc.*, 188:375, 1934.
393. SANSUM: *J.A.M.A.*, 70:825, 1918.

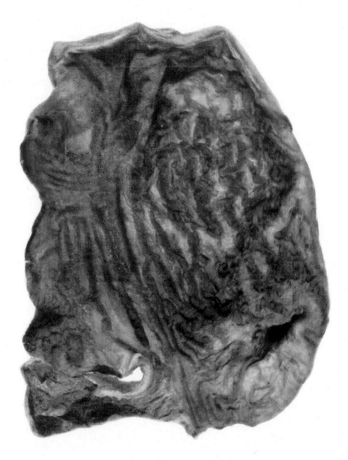

Stomach from case of sublimate poisoning
(McNally)

grains in alcoholic solution.[394] After prompt treatment by gastric lavage, milk and eggs, an emetic should be given. The less soluble the mercury compound, the lower the toxicity. Occasionally individuals are found who succumb to an exceedingly smaller amount of a mercury preparation than can be tolerated by the normal individual. Death has occurred from administration of ammoniated mercury, mercuric nitrate, and mercuric cyanide.

A dose of 10 mg. of mercurochrome per kilogram of body weight by intravenous injection is fatal to rabbits. As this is only about twice the dose per kilogram given to man, the margin of safety does not seem to be very wide.

Fatal Period: Death has occured within a few hours, but life is usually prolonged from five to twelve days. One case is reported of a woman suicide, aged thirty, who lived for twenty-five days after taking a single dose of the bichloride. I have seen a case of recovery in one week from 100 grains of the bichloride.

Treatment: Remove the poison from the stomach as quickly as possible, by means of a gastric lavage containing one teaspoonful of sodium bicarbonate in water. If it is an attempted suicide, it may be necessary to restrain the patient.

Berger, Applebaum, and Young[395] report the analysis of 163 cases of mercury poisoning. Cecostomy was performed in nine cases. In three, cecostomy was done on the fourth day after ingestion. All the patients died. Three patients were operated on fifteen, nineteen, and nineteen and one-half hours respectively after ingestion. All three recovered. After recovery, stomatitis, pharyngitis, esophagitis, and gastritis of varying intensity were present. Ulcerative gangrenous stomatitis was frequently observed in the late cases. The chief condition was the gangrenous colitis. In this series, three principal causes of death were given: (1) shock, and hemorrhage; (2) renal damage before the sixth day after the ingestion; (3) gangrenous colitis from the sixth to the twelfth day after ingestion (i.e. later than the renal damage). Hashinger and Simon[396] report

394. ARMSTRONG: *Med. News,* 50: 67, 1887.

395. BERGER, S. S., APPLEBAUM, H. S., and YOUNG, A. M.: *J.A.M.A.,* 98: 700, 1932.

396. HASHINGER, E. H., and SIMON, J. F.: *J. Lab. & Clin. Med.,* 20: 231, 1934.

the successful treatment of a case of mercurial poisoning with transfusion.

In one instance 100 grains of bichloride of mercury had been taken in a carbonated beverage. I saw the patient within five minutes and was unable to introduce the stomach tube. Two policemen arrived within another five minutes, and with their aid the stomach tube was introduced. The major portion of the tablets was removed, both by the vomiting of the patient and the washing out of the stomach. The patient should drink, or should be given, a quart of milk containing two raw eggs, and be made to evacuate it. Remove the cream from the top of the bottle before using the milk, as fats dissolve mercury salts more quickly and aid in the absorption. The physician should carry animal charcoal in his medicine bag. Relatives should be advised to administer milk and eggs, and after the arrival of the physician the patient can be removed to a hospital. The stomach should again be washed out with a pint of water containing three tablespoons of charcoal with 20 gm. of magnesium sulphate. One gm. of charcoal binds 180 mg. of bichloride of mercury. After this treatment gastric lavages should be given every four hours and colonic flushings every eight hours, the water containing eight grains of calcium sulphide per liter of water. One gm. of sodium thiosulphate is given intravenously twice the first day and once each day afterwards. The colonic flushings and the gastric lavages with the sulphide are continued until the Reinsch test fails to show mercury. Two gm. of potassium acetate in water are given twice daily for the first week. All the water the patient is given to drink should contain 5 gm. of sodium bicarbonate to each six ounces. If there has been considerable vomiting the chlorine impoverishment of the blood will be overcome by the intravenous injection of a normal saline solution with 5% of glucose. Sodium chloride can be given with sodium bicarbonate by mouth, which many times has stopped the vomiting. Sodium bicarbonate may be given intravenously in a 20% solution, if the patient lapses into unconsciousness. This prevents a loss of chloride and acidosis whereby non-protein nitrogen of the blood begins to decrease.

Young and Taylor[397] came to the conclusion that in large

397. YOUNG and TAYLOR: *J. Pharmacol. & Exper. Therap.*, 42:185, 1931.

and repeated doses sodium thiosulphate did not decrease tissue injury, nor did it influence the rise of the non-protein nitrogen in the poisoned animals. Haskell, Henderson, and Hamilton[398] report negative results with thiosulphate. Sodium hydrosulphite has proved to be unsatisfactory.[399] Rosenthal[400] recommends the intravenous use of sodium formaldehyde sulphoxylate, giving 10 gm. in 200 cc. of distilled water, the injection to be repeated four to six hours later in severe cases. Brown and Kolmer[401] were unsuccessful in their endeavor to corroborate the results obtained by Rosenthal with sodium formaldehyde sulphoxylate in mercurial poisoning. The authors report that sulphoxylate apparently has no direct curative action on kidneys which have already been damaged by the poison. Sulphoxylate is primarily a reducing substance and is effective and more pronounced when administered by mouth early and in sufficiently large doses. Intravenous injections are probably of no benefit if the administration by mouth has been delayed and the poison has been absorbed from the stomach. Therefore, if given early by mouth, sodium formaldehyde sulphoxylate is a valuable substance in the treatment of mercurial poisoning.

Burmeister and McNally[402] found that within a few minutes after the administration of mercury it can be detected chemically in the blood of animals poisoned with mercuric chloride, and that irrevocable damage to the kidneys takes place rapidly; the action is instantaneous when the mercury is in the circulating blood. One does not wonder that the therapeutic efforts in so many cases of acute mercurial poisoning have failed. However, a great percentage of cases will recover if, after a gastric lavage and the administration of milk and eggs, the physician will give intravenous injections of sodium bicarbonate, which increases the blood chlorides, and in turn diminishes the nitrogen retention, thereby improving the general condition. Morphine may be given after the stomach has been thoroughly washed out, and orange juice may be

398. HASKELL, HENDERSON and HAMILTON: J.A.M.A., 1808, 1925.
399. BOND, W. R., and GRAY, E. W.:   J.A.M.A., 92:23, 1919.
400. ROSENTHAL: Pub. Health Reports, 48:52, 1933.
401. BROWN, H. and KOLMER, J. A.:   J. Pharmacol. & Exper. Therap., 52:462, 1934.
402. BURMEISTER, W. H., and McNALLY, W. D.:   J. Med. Research. Bost., 36:87:1917.

given daily. Milk and eggs should be given as soon as the vomiting has been controlled. The amount of feedings should be small, beginning with a half of a glass of milk given every two hours. Colonic flushings with eight grains of calcium sulphide should be continued until there is no further test for mercury.

Blaidsell[403] reports the use of large doses of thiosulphate in ten acute cases of mercurial poisoning without a fatality.

Postmortem Examination: The changes in the organs seen at autopsy in a case of death caused by a mercurial, vary according to the length of duration of its action. The greatest alterations in the tissues are seen in the alimentary tract and in the kidneys. In some cases there are no changes in the mouth, in others an ulceration develops. The lips, tongue, and buccal mucous membranes are red and swollen; these may be of a gray-white or slate color, the lesions varying with the concentration of the preparation taken. When a powder is taken and not washed down immediately, the greatest changes are noted. When tablets are taken and immediately washed down, there may be no changes in the mouth. In cases of long duration most of the lesions will have disappeared. The gums may be softened and darkened, the teeth loosened, with an extensive gingivitis and pyorrhea. The salivary and lymphatic glands in the mouth may be inflamed and ulcerated. The lesions found in the stomach vary with the strength of the poison taken, and are mainly those of corrosion. I have seen eight stomachs that contained a dark tarry mass resembling cases of sulphuric acid. Several hundred other cases showed only a reddened mucous membrane. Only a few stomachs showed the gray color that is freely shown in textbooks. Mucous membrane of the esophagus and the pyloric opening may be softened and easily detached. The corrosion may extend to the muscular coat and deeper. I have never seen a perforation of the stomach or the duodenum. The bowel may be hyperemic throughout. The lesions such as are found in the stomach, may extend into the duodenum. The damage may be more extensive in the cecum than in other parts of the large bowel. The mucosa may show a peculiar intense inflammatory condition, usually hemorrhagic, in which the necrotic surface layer is welded together with the fibrinous

403. BLAIDSELL: *Maine M. J.*, 23:3, 1932.

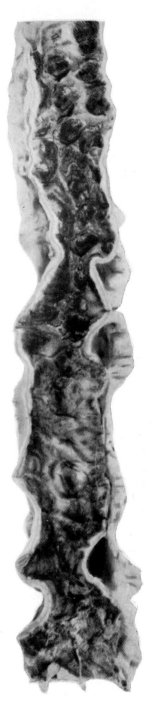

Corrosion of the bowel from bichloride of
mercury poisoning (McNally)

tissue in a membrane-like film, similar to that seen in diphtheritic enteritis. This particular enteritis and hemorrhagic colitis, probably caused by the mercury which is absorbed, is re-excreted through the mucosa of the intestine. Similarly you may find ulceration in the sigmoid flexure of the colon. The mucous membrane may be reddened and detached in shreds, or may show evidence of desquamative ulcerative scars, while the sub-mucosa may be reddened and show evidence of hemorrhage. Intestinal lesions do not show in all cases, but are more marked where there has been an extensive diarrhea, and colitis. The kidneys are usually pale and swollen. On sectioning, yellow and white spots and streaks are found, which are produced by deposits of amorphous nodular granules or masses of calcium carbonate and phosphate in the convoluted tubules, both in the epithelium and in the lumina of the tubes. These deposits can be removed by dilute sulphuric acid while being examined under the microscope. These deposits do not form in all cases of bichloride of mercury poisoning, as I have examined sections from a large number of kidneys which failed to show calcium deposits. Sections of the kidneys may show acute parenchymatous nephritis, necrosis, and fatty degeneration of the epithelium, and may also show the presence of casts in the tubules. These lesions are usually confined to the convoluted tubules. Glomerulitis has been reported. The liver shows no marked lesions, but where life has been prolonged for several days it becomes pale and anemic, and fatty degeneration may be noted. Ecchymosis of the endocardium, and degeneration of the heart muscle may be noted, but aside from a hyperemia, the other organs may show no changes. In the studies of Burmeister and McNally, mercury was found in the blood a few minutes after ingestion, and had caused degenerative changes in the kidney. When the poison has been absorbed through an application to the skin, or absorbed from the uterus and vagina in attempted cases of abortion, the most pronounced lesions are those in the digestive tract.

CHRONIC MERCURY POISONING

THIS type of poisoning occurs among operatives in quicksilver mines, mirror makers, thermometer and barometer makers, and among workers in factories making bulbs, and furs, and in hatteries*; in the absorption of mercury and salts of mercury by inunction. Chronic mercury poisoning is characterized chiefly by nervous phenomena, tremors, psychic inability, and restlessness. There may be complaints of colicky pains and diarrhea. There may be very little impairment of the kidneys. Lymphocytosis has been reported, as some others have stated, in the diagnosis of mercurialism. The same conditions that are found in acute poisoning where life has been prolonged for a week or so, are found in chronic mercurial poisoning if the poison has been swallowed. The gums are inflamed, the teeth become loose and may fall out; muscular tremors, and psychic inability also occur. There is an excessive flow of saliva. The patient complains of a metallic taste in the mouth, there is loss of appetite, and weakness with night sweats. The patient has a peculiar sallow color. Albumin is usually present in the urine, from traces to moderate amounts. The attention of the examiner may be called to the intention tremor. This tremor is first seen in the hands and may be later followed by marked shaking of the whole body, beginning with the arms and progressing through the whole trunk. The gait may be staggering and uncertain, as seen in Parkinson's disease or in manganese poisoning, but can be distinguished from the latter in which there is no mental irritability, excitability, or embarrassment. If not removed from the source of poisoning, and if medication and the therapeutic application have not been stopped, the patient will become anemic with loss of weight and appetite. The urine contains the greatest amount of albumin in the first stages. The symptoms vary slightly from those evident from working with inorganic salts or organic compounds, in the inhalation of the vapors during purification, or in the industrial use of mercury. The inhalation of the vapors of mercury seems to cause the nervous symptoms to predominate, whereas if the mercury is absorbed through the gastro-intestinal tract the intestinal and renal symptoms are more prominent. Most of the patients have a lymphocytosis of from 30 to 60%.[404] Berinski, of the Berlin Department of Health,[405] brought out

* GELMAN and DEIRZ: *J. Indust. Hyg. & Tox.*, 19:215, 1937. BLOOMFIELD and DALLAVALLE: *Am. J. Pub. Health*, 27:167, 1937.

404. LUDDICKE: *Berl. klin. Wchnschr.*, 9, 1928.

405. BERINSKI: *Deutsche med. Wchnschr.*, 25:1060, 1931; No. 4, 10:455, 1931; *En. Rundschau*, 45, 1928; 35,1935.

the fact that human beings who have never come in contact with mercury may excrete 0.0001 mg. a day, and that many important foodstuffs contain traces of mercury. Those who are working with mercury daily may show an excretion as high as 100 mg. per day. Anyone handling dimethyl and diethyl mercury may have symptoms referable to the nervous and circulatory systems. The diagnosis is always established by the chemical examination of the excreta. Protection against mercury vapors can be afforded by the use of the canister gas mask as described by Yant and Traubert.[406] The efficiency of this canister is tested by placing a small piece of selenium sulphide test paper in the face piece, or suspending it in the breathing tube. If the canister allows the mercury vapor to pass through, the test paper will be turned black. Adler[407] reported five cases of chronic mercurial poisoning in the felt hat industry. These cases showed marked salivation. There was no diarrhea, the palsy beginning in the upper extremities and gradually involving the entire muscular system. There was no disturbance in swallowing or mastication. Four had exaggerated knee-jerk, while the ankle clonus was absent in all. In one, there was a distinct blue line on the gum margin.

Tests: 1. Sublimate Test: The suspected solid is thoroughly dried, mixed with dry sodium carbonate, and heated gently in a reduction tube. Mirror-like rings form on the inside of the tube. When this portion is cooled, it is examined under the microscope. Minute, shiny spheres of metallic mercury may be seen. If some of these mirror-like rings are allowed to vaporize in the presence of iodine, a yellow and later red mercuric iodide will be formed.

2. Hydrogen Sulphide Test: Pass hydrogen sulphide through a weakly acidulated solution of the solid. A black precipitate of mercuric sulphide will be formed. From mercuric salts there are formed, first, a white precipitate soluble in acids, and secondly, excess of the mercuric salts; on further additions of the gas, the precipitate becomes yellow-orange, then brown, and finally black. Mercuric sulphide is insoluble in dilute nitric acid, insoluble in hydrochloric acid, soluble in

406. YANT, W. P., and TRAUBERT, C. E.: Report of Investigations, Bur. of Mines, R. I., 3187, October, 1932; NORLANDER, B.: Selenium Sulphide, a new Detector for Mercury Vapor, *Indust. & Eng. Chem.,* 19:518, 1927.

407. ADLER: *Med. News,* 59:186, 1891.

chlorine, nitro-hydrochloric acid, and insoluble in ammonium sulphide except when KOH or NaOH is present.

3. Reinsch Test.[408] This test is an exceedingly useful and simple method for the detection of arsenic, mercury and antimony. For clinical use the rapidity with which this test can be conducted makes it of great value to the physician. Although it is a qualitative test, using the tube with a capillary constriction as devised by the author, the relative quantity of the arsenic or mercury present can be readily determined by weighing the constricted portion with and without the sublimed metal. A few grains of the unknown powder or 25 gm. of tissue are put in a porcelain dish, adding arsenic, free hydrochloric acid and water and bringing it to a thin consistency, except in the case of fluids like urine, to which a piece of pure copper foil one-eighth inch wide is added (this foil, having been previously tested with the hydrochloric acid as a blank). This mixture is boiled for five minutes, or until the substance under examination is thoroughly disintegrated. The supernatant fluid is decanted from the copper foil which is washed with distilled water, then removed to a clean beaker and washed with alcohol and ether. The copper foil is placed in a tube similar to that devised by the author (Fig. 4, page 27). This tube can be drawn out of any clear glass which is free from bubbles or defects. It is a small piece of tubing about five and one-half inches in length and three-eighths inches in diameter, drawn out in a fine capillary, the capillary measuring from one to one and one-half inches in length, leaving a short arm of about one and one-half inches and a long arm of about three inches, making a total length of about seven inches depending upon the constricted portion. Around the capillary constricted portion a piece of filter paper that has been dipped in cold water is wound. In the long arm of the tube is placed the strip of copper foil. In the presence of much mercury this foil will be silvery-gray, but mercury may be present even when it is invisible to the naked eye. The long arm of the tube is closed with the thumb and the short arm held with the thumb and finger of the other hand. Heat is applied beneath the copper foil until the glass becomes red. Mercury volatilizes very easily, thus making it necessary to use this amount of heat, as arsenic, antimony or bismuth may be pres-

408. *J. f. prakt. Chem., Leipz.,* 24:244, 1841.

sent. If mercury is present, it will be deposited on the constricted portion of the tube and can be identified under the microscope as shiny spheres. If only a few spheres of mercury are seen, it can be substantiated by the sublimate test by adding a minute fragment of iodine which gives the yellow, and then later the red, mercuric chloride. The copper may have deposits of antimony, bismuth, silver or platinum, or may be colored by any unoxidized sulphur, but none of these will give the spherical globules as noted above. Wormley,[409] using capillary reduction tubes of peculiar construction, has obtained characteristic globules from 1/500,000 grain of corrosive sublimate; under ordinary manipulation 1/100,000 grain is nearer to the limit of delicacy. With practice, it becomes an exceedingly delicate test. The mercury can be separated as the sulphide in the Fresenius and von Babo process as previously described (page 22). After conversion to the nitrate, take up with hydrochloric acid to get rid of the excess nitric acid, dissolve in water, and immerse a thin strip of gold or platinum (which can be connected to two dry cells or used with the Brown apparatus) and the mercury is deposited on the gold electrode. The gold is washed in water, alcohol and ether, weighed on a delicate balance, heated to volatilize the mercury, and re-weighed. The loss represents the amount of mercury present.

The electrolytic method of Booth and Schrieber[410] is used on urine, the volume being reduced about one-third or one-fourth and the test conducted in a small beaker of about 75 cc. capacity. The current from an ordinary dry cell (about one volt) is allowed to flow through the specimen to be tested for fifteen minutes, a platinum wire being used for the anode and bright copper strip for the cathode. The mercury, if present, is deposited as a silvery metallic film on the copper. The method is delicate and reliable and does not require preliminary digestion. The sensitivity of the test is increased by concentrating the specimen by evaporation. The method has been modified from that originally given by Booth and Schrieber, approximately 25 cc. of the specimen to be tested being used in a small evaporating dish instead of a few drops in a tissue culture slide as recommended by Booth and Schrieber, and also a strip of

409. WORMLEY: Micro-Chemistry of Poisons, 350, 1885.
410. BOOTH and SCHRIEBER: *J. Am. Chem. Soc.*, 47:2625, 1925.

copper several mm. in width being employed for the cathode in place of a fine copper wire. The method is economical, dispensing with the use of the large quantities of chemicals, and there are no disagreeable fumes.[411]

In its earlier stages, chronic poisoning is difficult to diagnose, as the symptoms closely resemble those met with in neurasthenia, but recourse should be had to examination of the urine and feces, which contain small quantities of mercury if poisoning by that metal is in question. The air of the room should also be tested, using the colorimetric method with diphenylcarbazide, which permits of the detection of 7×10^{-6} mg. of mercury. The presence of only a few thousandths of a mg. of mercury per cubic meter of air can give rise to chronic mercurial poisoning. Stock and his associates[412] describe a method which depends upon the electrolytic deposition of the mercury on a copper wire from a solution containing mercury as the chloride. After the electrolysis, the wire and its deposit are dried and heated. The mercury distills off and is collected in a capillary. It is finally collected together into a tiny globule, the size of which is measured under the microscope. To determine the mercury in urine, feces, etc., the mercury is precipitated together with about 20 mg. of added copper by introducing hydrogen sulphide into the hydrochloric acid solution, the mixture of copper sulphide and mercury sulphide is transformed to chloride, and the solution (not over 20 cc.) is electrolyzed. The method appears to be extremely sensitive and remarkaby accurate. Biancalani[413] recommends heating the urine with dilute sulphuric acid and iron filings. The filings are removed, dried, placed in a test-tube, and heated so that the mercury vapors liberated are deposited on strips of filter paper coated with cuprous iodide. In the presence of mercury the surface of the paper turns red. Control tests made on urine show that 0.005 mg. mercuric chloride can be detected by this method. This reaction may also be used for detecting mercury on skins previously treated with mercury salts or ointments. In the electrolysis of mercury, using a current of one-to-ten or one-to-fifteen volts with a gold cathode

411. STELLING, O.: Svenska chem. tidning., 41:80, 1929.
412. STOCK, ALFRED; LUX, HERMAN; CUCUEL, FRIEDRICH; GERSTNER, FRANZ: Ztschr. f. ang. Chemie, Berl., 44:200, 1931.
413. BIANCALANI, G.: Bol. Soc. ital. biol. sper., 7:1421, 1932.

and a platinum anode of 15 to 20 mm., mercury must be present in the form of the bichloride.[414]

In experimental work, Hesse[415] recommends strontium thioacetate to counteract the effects of the administration of mercuric chloride to animals.[416] Müller[417] recommends the determination of mercury in air with an absorption tube of 50 cm. length; 3.9 to 1050 10^{-6} gm. of mercury per cubic meter can be detected. Observations were carried out in different laboratories and compared with the results of chemical analysis. (Stock's method.) The latter gives much lower results than the physical procedure which requires only five minutes.[418] The diphenylcarbazide colorimetric method was found to be simple and rapid but gave accurate readings up to 0.2 gamma only when the solution was a clear solution of mercury chloride. Heavy metals, acids, free chlorine and salts of the light metals had to be removed; this separation is the source of many errors.

Majer[418] found that mercury in air must be concentrated before it can be determined chemically. By combining the mercury vapors with gaseous chlorine or bromine and concentrating the mercury salt caught in solution, Majer was not able to prevent large losses during evaporation. The adsorption of mercury on metallic gold was incomplete, for other vapors contained in air, inactivated the gold surface; from air containing 10-30 gamma mercury per cubic meter only the third adsorption tube, containing gold, deposited mercury; carefully filtered air, containing 400 gamma mercury per cubic meter, deposited 90% to 95% of its mercury vapor in the first adsorption tube. The most satisfactory concentration occurred when air passed through U-tubes (10 to 20 mm. in diameter and 25 cm. long), immersed in liquid air for nine hours, at a rate of 250 to 500 cc. per minute. The tubes were removed from the liquid air, the carbon dioxide melted, and 2 to 3 cc. water remained in them. The tubes were filled with chlorine gas and

414. *Biochem. Ztschr., Berl.*, 223:86, 1930; Chem. Abst., Am. Chem. Soc., 24:47, 1932; BROWN, D., KAYSER, F., and SIFRAS, J.; *Bull. Soc. chim. biol.*, 12:504, 1930.

415. HESSE, E.: *Arch. f. exper. Path. u. Pharmakol.*, 144:327, 1929.

416. See also HASKELL, and FORBES, C. A.: 23:3023, 1929.

417. MÜLLER, KURT: *Ztschr. f. phys. chemie*, 65:739, 1930.

418. MAJER, VLADIMIR: *Chem. Listy*, 28:169, 1934; and 28:228, 1934.

allowed to stand undisturbed. After the contents were placed in a 5-cc. test-tube, the U-tubes were washed three times with 0.5 cc. of chlorine water. The mercury was then precipitated on an iron wire plated with a copper film, and was determined micrometrically. About 1.5 liters of liquid air were required for the procedure. By using micro-methods, Majer determined 0.01 gamma mercury by precipitating the mercury on an iron wire from solutions containing copper salts. A volume of less than 5 cc. was necessary, but by electrolyzing the solution volumes of 20 cc. could be used. The wire plated with mercury was placed in a glass tube (with one end drawn into a 0.1 mm. capillary 8 cm. long) sealed at the wide end and distilled. In a capillary of these dimensions, the water vapors formed a column 1 to 2 mm. long and served as a stopper before the mercury distillate entered the capillary. Under these conditions, the mercury coalesced into a single drop, and after washing with alcohol on a glass slide, the diameter was measured under a microscope at 190-360 magnification. If many drops formed, they were coalesced by heating the capillary in a micro-flame, or washed with alcohol into a Jorgensen counting chamber. The drops entered the markings and were easily measured under the microscope. As many as sixty-six drops were measured with a smaller average error than if the mercury had been in the form of a single drop. Stock and Zimmerman[419] show that in one instance 53 gamma mercury was retained for the first few days; this, on the basis of a man's weight, would amount to 6 mg. mercury, since about 40 mg. mercury would have passed the man's lungs during that time, by far the largest amount of mercury breathed in leaving the body in the expired air. The absorbed mercury leaves the body very slowly, so that even after five weeks one-fourth of it is still present. In the estimation of mercury, the liquid should be equivalent to a 1.5 N hydrochloric acid and should contain sufficient $CuSO_4$ to give 10 mg. copper. The copper and mercury sulphide precipitate is centrifuged and redissolved in a small volume (10 to 20 cc.) with chlorine; the chlorine is again driven off with carbon dioxide and the solution once more treated with hydrogen sulphide. After warming and centrifuging, the residue is again dissolved with chlorine

    419. STOCK, A., and ZIMMERMAN, W.: *Biochem. Ztschr., Berl.,* 216:243, 1929.

and the excess is driven off with carbon dioxide. Any precipitated sulphur is filtered off. To the clear filtrate in a 25-cc. volumetric flask is added 2 to 3 gm. of finely powdered ammonium oxalate; this is warmed to 35° C. until the resulting solution is clear. The mercury is precipitated on a copper wire (heated and reduced with methyl alcohol) and determined colorimetrically with diphenylcarbazide.

CALOMEL (HgCl)

(Molecular Weight 236.07. Synonyms: Mercurous Chloride, Calomel, Subchloride of Mercury)

CALOMEL occurs as a heavy, white, impalpable powder, becoming yellowish-white when triturated with strong pressure. It is odorless, and is stable in the air, and gradually darkens when exposed to light. It is insoluble in water, in alcohol, in ether ,and in cold dilute acids. In the U. S. P., XI, the dose is 0.15 gm., or 2½ grains. Owing to the difficulty with which calomel is placed in solution, few cases of poisoning are reported. A physician prescribed twenty grains of calomel for a two year old child. There was marked salivation and diarrhea, and the child died within twenty-four hours. Runeberg[420] reported a fatal case in which three hypodermic injections of 1½ grains each were given in one month. Calomel is converted into mercuric chloride by nitrohydrochloric acid and chlorine water, and probably to a slight extent also by hydrochloric acid and alkaline chlorides. It is changed to oxide or reduced by the alkaline bases and carbonates. Prolonged exposure to sunlight changes it to metallic mercury and mercuric chloride.

ARSENIC (As)

(Atomic Weight 75. Synonyms: Arsenum, Arsenicum)

ARSENIC is very widely distributed geographically. It is found as arsenic trioxide; as an alloy with other metals, as $FeAs_2$, $NiAs$, $CoNiAs_2$; as realgar, As_2S_2; orpiment, As_2S_3; arsenical pyrites, $FeAsFeS_2$; as an arsenate, in cobalt bloom, $Co_3(AsO_4)_2$; and in a great variety of minerals.

Arsenic poisoning may occur in any metallurgical process, owing to the frequent contamination of various ores with

420. RUNEBERG: *Deutsche med. Wchnschr.*, 15:4, 1889.

arsenic. In the lead works of Colorado and the copper works of Montana, the ores contain a large amount of arsenic, which is volatilized in the furnaces and carried into the flues and deposited in the funnels as white arsenic. The handling of these deposits for the purification of this arsenic by sublimation may prove a source of arsenical poisoning, if the men are not equipped with masks. Perforation of the nasal septum has been reported in men handling arsenic trioxide.

In industry, the greatest trouble seems to be the lesions of the skin and the troublesome irritation of the conjunctiva, as well as the lining of the mouth, nose and air passages. The handling of any solid compound of arsenic is attended with a great variety of skin lesions, from a mild inflammation to more profound changes such as eczema and melanosis, which may develop into ulceration, or hyperkeratosis. In some industries large quantities of arsenic are handled without cases of poisoning developing. Arsenic trioxide is used to decolorize clarified glass, for the bronzing of metals, and in the form of lead arsenite for the preparation of white enamel. It is used for the preservation of skins, furs, and rugs. The preservation of rugs should be under the same restriction as wallpaper in regard to the arsenic content, and with the present amount of arsenic, seven to ten grains per fifty-four square feet, it will be interesting to see if any cases of mild chronic arsenical poisoning develop. The permissible limit of arsenic in wallpaper is 1/10 grain per square yard. Sodium arsenate and other arsenic preparations are used as mordants in cotton printing, and in the manufacture of various insecticides containing arsenic, as Schweinfurt's green and lead arsenate. Small amounts of arsine are evolved in the pickling of iron. Symptoms of lead poisoning may develop following the long exposure to lead arsenate as a spray. Arsenical lesions may follow the use of arsenical insecticides.[421] Cases of poisoning have been observed in aviators from the inhalation of arsenic-containing poisons, scattered from airplanes in a fight against various types of insect pests. Arsine, which has caused a few deaths, and many cases of illness, will be considered separately.

Elementary arsenic, when first isolated is a brittle, crystalline steel-gray solid, having a metallic lustre, which is soon

421. BAADER, E. W.: Zentralbl. f. Gewerbehyg., N. S., 4:385, 1927; DORLE and ZIEGLER: Ztschr. f. klin. Med., 112:237, 1930.

lost on exposure to air. It has a specific gravity of 5.727 at 14°C., it volatilizes in an atmosphere of coal gas without melting at 450°C., and is slowly oxidized in moist air at ordinary temperature; when heated in the air it burns with a bluish flame and becomes white arsenous anhydride, As_2O_3. It is insoluble in pure water; is readily attacked by dry chlorine and bromine on contact, and by iodine with the aid of heat. Nitric acid oxidizes it, first to arsenic trioxide, As_2O_3, and then to H_3AsO_4. The metal is used with lead in the manufacture of shot. A number of flypapers containing sodium salts of arsenic, have been responsible for cases of murder and suicide.

The following case illustrates the use of flypaper as a source of arsenic. T.M., a boy seventeen years of age, on December 18, 1930, complained of a sore throat, great thirst, vomiting, diarrhea, pain in the abdomen, and inability to hold water or food upon his stomach, had pain in the calves of his legs, and was unable to walk. He was sent to a hospital on January 16, 1931, where his case was diagnosed as polyneuritis of toxic origin. The boy was given ten grains of thiosulphate, three times a day and after a time gradually improved. He was sent home on March 3, 1931. Three or four days later he had a repetition of the symptoms noted on December 18, and died. The examination of the organs showed that death was due to arsenical poisoning.

At the trial of a Mrs. T. S. it was developed that she had poisoned her husband, a boarder, and a nephew, for the insurance they carried, by administering an aqueous solution of arsenical flypaper. Conviction followed. An examination of the organs gave the following:

	T.M.		T.S.		T.L.	
	Wt.	Mg. As_2O_3	Wt.	Mg. As_2O_3	Wt.	Mg. As_2O_3
Part of:						
Brain	1325	1.060				
Lung	670	0.536				
Heart	225	0.180			270	.81
Stomach	207	0.205	201	0.754	250	0.50
Liver	1313	14.77	533	6.663	570	28.5
Spleen	155	0.124	138	0.591	140	0.49
Kidney	281	3.83	292	2.92	302	1.88
Bowel	1255	1.883			390	.0683

In England, frequent cases of arsenical poisoning have been produced in the manufacture of products for washing sheep. These substances contain arsenous acid, which is incorporated in the dust and acts on the skin and mucous membrane, causing a hyperkeratosis and catarrh of the respiratory passages. Three cases developed epitheliomatous lesions. In 1928, a workman, who had worked for the last nine years with emerald green, died of arsenical poisoning.

A symposium on insecticides, in affiliation with the eighty-fifth meeting of the American Chemical Society, in March, 1933, uncovered many interesting facts relative to the use of arsenic compounds as insecticides. The origin of the insecticide industry was traced back to 1860, when a green paint made from arsenic and copper was diverted from its intended use on shutters, to a poison for the potato beetle which was proving troublesome at that time. Since then the employment of arsenicals as insecticides has developed into an important industry.[422]

In 1900, in England and Wales, more than 6,000 persons were made ill, and seventy killed, by the consumption of beer which contained traces of arsenic.[423]

In 1906, the United States Food and Drug Act limited the arsenic residue on apples to the equivalent of 1/100 grain of arsenic trioxide per pound of fruit. The regulation was not enforced until 1927. This led to successful experimentations in washing fruit to keep the arsenic within the specified bounds. The arsenic content of fruit is carefully checked by State and Federal laboratories.

In 1933, the Department of Agriculture made a further ruling which restricted the arsenic content of apples and other fruit to 0.014 grains per pound. In the Oregon Experiment Stations, Corvallis, Oregon, several years' experience has shown that hydrochloric acid is probably the most generally satisfactory solvent for the spray residues.[424] A 1% solution of this acid is strong enough to remove both arsenic and lead to within the amount permitted, irrespective of the arsenical coat, providing no wax has been formed on the fruit and no oil has been used after the early cover sprays. Where waxy or oily residues are present, alkaline washes such as NaOH, Na_2CO_3, Na_3PO_4, Na_2SIO_3, have proved effective for the removal of arsenical spray. Ingerson found that the heavy

422. MEYER, C. N.: *Indust. & Eng. Chem.*, 25:624, 1933.
423. WHITE, W. B.: *Indust. & Eng. Chem.*, 25:622, 1933.
424. *Indust. & Eng. Chem.*, 25:617, 1933.

rains in late August and September cause no significant reduction in the amount of arsenic adhering to apples sprayed with lead arsenate. The smooth skin varieties of apples retain less arsenic than the rough skinned varieties.[425] Addition of lime to lead arsenate sprays facilitates removal of the arsenic. Kohn-Abrest[426] found that the average food in France contained various proportions of arsenic, but the doses are too small to be toxic and therefore are not of any significance in medicine. The origin of this arsenic can be traced back to its use as an insecticide on food plants.

Arsenic compounds are used more by suicides and by the secret homicide, than any other poison with the possible exception of carbon monoxide. In 1936 in Cook County (Illinois) seven people died of arsenic compounds. During the latter part of the seventeenth century and early in the eighteenth century, the use of arsenic as an agent of secret poisoning became very common in Italy and France. La Spara, in 1659, gave arsenic to young women who wished to be rid of their husbands. At a latter period Toffana carried on a similar traffic at Naples. She was credited with the poisoning of nearly 600 people. Frau von der Linden,[427] during the course of fourteen years in Leyden, poisoned seventy persons of whom twenty-four died, including her father, mother and son.

In Chicago, Illinois, on October 17, 1923, I was called to see in consultation, a Mr. K. who was alleged to have been suffering from alcoholism. From the physical examination of Mr. K., and a chemical examination of the hair, stool and urine, I made a diagnosis of arsenical poisoning. Mrs. Tillie K. was arrested and after questioning confessed she had given to her husband a powder furnished by her cousin. Investigation revealed that she had poisoned over twenty people. Thirteen bodies of her relatives which were exhumed, gave evidence of arsenical poisoning. Two of her victims, who were her husbands, Mrs. K. told they were going to die, and ordered her mourning apparel and brought it in to show them how she was going to be attired. Mrs. K. was given a life sentence.

425. INGERSON, H. G.: *Penn. State Hort. Ass. News,* 9: 1:37, 1932.

426. KOHN-ABREST: Les Science et La Vie, Paris, December, 1920; J. 2:16, 1921.

427. *Am. J. M. Sc.,* 118:614, 1886; *Zaaijer Vrtljsch. f. ger. Med. m. f.* 44:249, 1886.

In 1919, I reported statistics[428] gathered during a period of thirteen years showing that seventy-four different kinds of poisons were instrumental in causing the death of 2,118 persons. In this group fifty-six deaths were caused by arsenic trioxide, fifty-five by Paris green, and thirty-eight by "rough-on-rats." (Some of the preparations contained arsenic trioxide and barium carbonate.) Kuttner[429] reports six cases of arsenical poisoning due to wallpaper. Harding[430] records a group of cases of chronic poisoning among the nurses at an asylum, traced to green baize curtains which were found to contain a large amount of arsenic.

Paris green which is used as an insecticide in gardens has, been a source of poisoning from the eating of cabbage. Arsenic is found in pigments such as Scheele's green (copper arsenite), $CuHASO_3$, which contains 52.8% of arsenous acid. Paris green (copper aceto arsenite, Schweinfurt's green) contains 50% of arsenic. It is used to eliminate the Colorado beetle which destroys the potato plant; it is also used on the tobacco plant. This latter use accounts for the finding by investigators of arsenic in smoking and chewing tobaccos.[431]

I have found arsenic in the soil of old cemeteries in and around Chicago. Most of the arsenic I believe, came from the former use of arsenic-containing embalming fluids. The soil being removed from one grave close to another grave containing a body that had been embalmed with arsenic would impregnate the surrounding soil to such an extent that when a new grave was dug adjacently the arsenic laden soil would be scattered around.

Dorle and Ziegler report an intoxication in people handling substances used for the extinction of parasites in the vineyard. Tropp and Ranch[432] report a mass poisoning by arsenic following the drinking of wine aboard a ship. These authors state that the first instance of this sort of poisoning was reported in the literature in 1808, when 500 persons drank wine which contained arsenic. Fifteen out of the 500 people died. Schwartz reported six men of a crew on a French boat as being poisoned with arsenic by consuming wine which contained from 3 mg. to

428. McNally, W. D.: Med. Rec., February 1, 1919.
429. Kuttner: Berl. klin. Wchnschr., 69:2122, 1912.
430. Harding: Lancet, 1:525, 1892.
431. Remington, R. E.: J. Am. Chem. Soc., 49:1410, 1927.
432. Tropp, C., and Ranch, G.: Dermat. Wchnschr., 95:1023, 1932.

12 mg. of arsenic per liter of wine. The men drank daily one liter of wine. A review of the most recent literature of this phase of arsenical poisoning is given by this author.[433]

Arsenic can be administered in a great variety of ways. It may be given in capsules, added to medicine that has already been prescribed by a physician, or it may be given in soups, cooked cereal, candy, and cake. Paris green has been given in coffee, table salt, and in sugar, intentionally and accidentally. In a Vienna restaurant some apfelstrudel was spread with arsenic instead of sugar. Two persons died from this accident, and several others experienced vomiting and diarrhea. In 1931 a homicidal mass intoxication occurred when a revengeful worker poisoned fifty-three of his fellow workers by introducing arsenic into their coffee.

Medicinal Uses: Arsenic has been used for years in the treatment of chorea, neuralgia, and the various rheumatic and arthritic diseases. It is used extensively internally and externally in chronic non-parasitic skin diseases and to improve the condition of the skin and hair. It is used widely in the treatment of ricketts, osteomyelitis, leukemias, and anemias. The use of the inorganic arsenic has been largely replaced by the organic arsenicals. It is a constituent of many proprietary preparations which are employed as tonics in cachectic conditions. Occasionally a theory in a murder case is advanced that the amount of arsenic found was due to a medicinal administration. The usual prescription for arsenic in the solid form is from one-sixtieth to one-thirtieth grain per capsule or tablet, and when the residue in a solid form in the stomach exceeds that amount, the supposition of the arsenic having been given as a therapeutic measure can be negatived. Arsenic is not accumulative in the stomach, and the existence of more than one-half grain of unabsorbed arsenic cannot be explained on the theory of its introduction as a medicine. In the majority of cases of poisoning by arsenic which I have examined, I have found weighable quantities of arsenic in the liver, kidneys, stomach, and other organs of the cadaver. Occasionally the amounts found were very small, but these along with the symptoms, the postmortem appearances, and the history of having been given something causing these symptoms, would strengthen the case for or against the medi-

433. SCHWARTZ, L.: *Neue Deutchen klin.*, 7:35, 1931.

cinal administration of the arsenic. Arsenic may be introduced as an impurity in a medicine, but this is highly improbable today with our efficient laboratory control of the drugs and chemicals used in pharmacy. These preparations might have to be given in pound quantities in order to obtain a lethal dose of the arsenic, which shows the absurdity of such an administration.

In the United States Pharmacopeia, XI, arsenic is found in combination as arsenic trioxide, arsenous iodide, arsphena-mine, neoarsphenamine, and as Fowler's solution (liquor potassi arsenitis). In the National Formulary preparations, it is found as Clemens' solution of arsenic, solution of gold and arsenous bromide, Pearson's solution of sodium arsenate containing 0.1% of dried arsenate. There are stronger pills of iron, quinine, strychnine arsenate; mild pills of iron, quinine, strychnine arsenate. In the New and Nonofficial remedies of the American Medical Association, sulpharsphenamine, silver arsphenamine, and stovarsol are listed.

ARSENIC TRIOXIDE (As_2O_3)
(Synonyms: Arsenic, Arsenous Oxide, White Arsenic)

UNITED States Pharmacopeia, XI, arsenic trioxide, contains not less than 99% arsenic trioxide. It is a white, odorless powder of irregular masses of two varieties: one amorphous, transparent, and colorless like glass; the other, crystalline, opaque, and white, resembling porcelain. Frequently the same piece has an opaque white outer crust enclosing the glassy variety. Contact with moist air gradually changes the glass-like into the white opaque variety. The average dose of arsenic is one-thirtieth grain, or 2 mg. For the liquid 1% preparations, two to three drops three times daily are given. The usual method for the administration is to establish a tolerance by beginning with small doses and gradually increasing them until some local manifestation of poisoning appears, such as colicky pains, nausea, or puffiness of the eyes.

Arsenic trioxide is soluble one part in 100 parts of water at 25°C; fifteen parts in boiling water, and sparingly soluble in 94.7% alcohol. While it is sparingly soluble in water this does not prevent it from being suspended in liquid foods such as milk, beer, coffee, or placed in cereals and cakes, as above mentioned. Since the arsenic trioxide varies in form, the solubility will vary with the form used, but a fluid ounce of cold water will dissolve one-half to three-quarters of a grain. Although the specific gravity of the crystalline arsenic trioxide is high, 3.699 to 3.86, it does not sink when thrown upon water. A portion of the powder floats upon the surface of the water, forming a film consisting of particles of the crystals buoyed up by the adherent air. Gmelin[434] reported that one part of the oxide if digested with eighty parts of water for several days at ordinary temperature, will go into solution 11.11 parts per 1,000. The peculiar properties of the arsenic trioxide floating upon the surface of liquids would prevent its use in this manner unless it were mixed with an opaque preparation, such as an antacid which was being given to correct the hyperacidity of the stomach, and the milky appearance of the liquid and floating particles would not be so apt to attract the attention as being an unusual condition. If arsenic trioxide is boiled for one-half hour in contact with an excess of the solid in a flask fitted with a reflux condenser, 100 cc. would dissolve 8.0112 parts from porcelainous arsenic in lumps; 9.6092 from the crystalline arsenic; and 15.3785 from freshly prepared crystals.[435]

TABLE XX
SOLUBILITY OF ARSENIC TRIOXIDE

100 Parts of Alcohol Dissolved	Alcohol of 56%	Alcohol of 79%	Alcohol of 86%	Absolute Alcohol
Crystallized arsenic, at 15° (59° F.)	1.680	1.430	0.715	0.025
at the boiling point	4.895	4.551	3.197	3.402
Vitreous oxide, at 15°, (59° F.)	0.504	0.540		1.060

The presence of fats and oils would affect the solubility of the arsenic in an attempted homicide case, and would account for the delayed symptoms seen in some murder cases. The question of the solubility of the oxide in alcohol occasionally appears in murder trials, and the expert must be able to state the solubility in varying degrees of alcohol. If the arsenic has been given in beer, wine, or whiskey, the solubility

434. GMELIN: Handbuch. d. chem., Cavendish Soc. Transl., 4:257, 1850.

435. WITTHAUS and BECKER: Medical Jurisprudence, Forensic Medicine and Toxicology, IV:407, 1911.

in that particular brand of alcoholic beverage should be reported. There is a great difference in the solubility of the crystalline oxide and the vitreous oxide at the same temperature and the same percentage of alcohol, as is shown in Table XX.

It is seldom that the expert finds undissolved arsenic trioxide in crystalline form. However, with Paris green I have recovered as high as 45 gm. of this preparation from the stomach contents in a case of suicide.

Symptoms: The time of the appearance of symptoms of arsenical poison depends upon the form in which it was taken, whether food was in the stomach, and whether this food contained materials that would retard the solubility of the arsenic. If the poison has been administered in solution upon an empty stomach the symptoms are sure to appear within ten minutes.

The first symptoms of acute arsenical poisoning are those of a violent irritant, producing an inflammation of the gastrointestinal tract. If death occurs within twenty-four hours, there may be added to these symptoms, or occurring independently, collapse and coma, due to the involvement of the central nervous system. The patient complains of an excruciating pain in the pit of the stomach. There may be sensations of nausea, preceding or accompanying the pain; a feeling of dryness, burning, and irritation in the mouth; persistent or forcible vomiting. The patient is unable to support the blandest drinks; the vomitus may be a rice-water-like fluid containing mucus, bile, or even streaked with blood. A continuation of the vomiting and abdominal pains is followed by a profuse diarrhea and painful tenesmus. The picture at this time looks like cholera and can be distinguished by a chemical examination of the excreta. Occasionally there is an obstinate constipation.[436] The urine may be scanty or suppressed, containing bloody albuminous material. The patient is completely exhausted, his pulse is feeble, frequent, and irregular. He has an anxious face, sunken eyes, cold and clammy skin. There is a marked dehydration, due to the excessive vomiting and diarrhea. Cramps in the legs and restlessness may be accompanied by clonic and tonic spasms, or followed by a

436. As seen in the Baker case: McNALLY, W. D.: *J. Am. Chem. Soc.,* 39:826, 1917.

general paralysis. Death usually occurs from exhaustion as the result of the profound and prolonged gastro-enteritis. All of these symptoms may be present or a few may be absent, as in the nervous and cerebral type of poisoning, when the symptoms of the central nervous system predominate. In this type of poisoning there may be prostration, stupor, paralysis, collapse, and death in coma. Occasionally cases of poisoning are seen that go through the regular course of symptoms as given above, but show improvement on the third or fourth day. One or two days later the pulse becomes weak and thread-like, failure of circulation is noted, an anuresis gradually develops, and the patient dies from collapse. Many of these people retain full consciousness until the end. There is usually a pronounced fall in the blood pressure, as the result of watery diarrhea, which occurs as one of the early symptoms.

In subacute poisoning, the above symptoms may appear in a milder form, except that a violent diarrhea may remain for weeks. This type of poisoning occurs from the gradual administration of small doses of arsenic, and is usually the method of choice of the secret murderer. The symptoms for the first twenty-four hours may be very much like those described under acute poisoning, the patients being able to get up and walk around, showing slight improvement, until the next dose of arsenic is given, when they have a repetition of symptoms, which makes them believe they have eaten contaminated food. The patients will complain of loss of appetite, fainting sensations, nausea, dry throat, retching, shooting pains in the stomach and bowels, and a persistent diarrhea. Suspecting the food at home, they refuse to eat. If a patient is confined to his bed for days or weeks, a secret poisoner may give him one large dose of the poison, so as to be relieved of further care of the victim. This occurred in the Baker case. After Baker had been ill for six weeks he was given a dose of poison which ended his life in a few hours. The Clugston case at Bushnell, Illinois, was a similar one. The wife and a Dr. C. W. A. conspired for the insurance of Clugston. Their neighbors were led to believe he had typhoid fever. Mrs. Clugston gave her husband powdered glass in the forepart of July, which however, did not kill him. In August, she repeated the dose of powdered glass and then finally resorted to arsenic. After several weeks of illness, a three-grain capsule of arsenic was administered to Clugston at 1:30 A.M. and he died before 7:00 o'clock that same morning. A postmortem examination did not sustain the typhoid fever theory, and the organs were examined for poison. A piece of glass was found in the appendix of the man, and arsenic was found in all of the organs. Mrs. Clugston and her paramour were given life sentences.

Subacute poisoning was resorted to by Tillie K., who poisoned twenty people, seven of whom recovered. She administered the poison to her relatives in soup and candy. To her last husband she gave small amounts of arsenic in soup over a period of weeks. He had vomiting, abdominal tenderness, tenesmus, scanty and albuminous urine, with a copper color to the palms and soles, and a marked keratosis. On account of his nervousness and muscular pains, his family physician was led to believe that it was a case of alcoholism. When I saw the patient after removal to a hospital, I noticed a garlic odor upon his breath. The excretions and hair were examined and the case was diagnosed as a chronic arsenical poisoning, which led to an investigation, resulting in a life sentence for Tillie K. A twenty-four-hour specimen from K. gave 0.00079 gm. of arsenic, calculated as arsenic trioxide. A polyneuritis is frequently seen in chronic arsenical poisoning. The hair, toe-nails and finger-nails in these cases should always be examined for the presence of arsenic. After the symptoms of acute poisoning have subsided to appropriate treatment, symptoms due to the chronic inflammation of the peripheral nerves may appear.

The skin may be marked by a great variety of lesions in addition to that of herpes, as reported in the Clugston case, and one may also find a general redness, petechial hemorrhages, roseola, eczema, and icterus. There may be puffiness under the eyes, and the conjunctiva may be congested. Occasionally there is a delirium, loss of consciousness, and death in convulsions, as reported in Merbach's case. There may be remission or complete suppression of the symptoms, with a reappearance a day or two later, and which points strongly to a second administration of the poison. MacLagen[437] reports a case in which the patient having been taken to a hospital

437. MacLagen: *London & Edinburgh M. J. A. Chem. Sc.*, 16:15, 1853.

improved somewhat and had ceased to vomit. Vomiting, however, reappeared on the fourth day, and the patient died on the seventh day.

The temperature, in both acute and subacute arsenical poisoning, does not vary much from the normal; except that during the period when there is a bloody diarrhea, the temperature is apt to be above normal. Violent delirium and convulsions are reported in a few cases.[438] Cases with delirium and convulsions occur rarely. With the organic arsenicals, however, this condition has been reported a few times. In one of the victims in the K. case (already cited) there was a fever, leukocytosis, with a very severe sore throat. It was thought that the patient had a streptococcus infection of the throat and frequent cultures were made. He died four or five days after removal to a hospital. The death certificate gave streptococcus infection as the cause of death. However, a few months later his body was exhumed and I found that death was due to arsenical poisoning. Pain in the mouth and pharynx has been observed by others.[439] Disturbances of vision and hearing have been observed by a number of physicians where arsenic has been applied to cancers of the skin and uterus. The symptoms are the same as by mouth with the added local effects. Whether the poison is taken by mouth or introduced through the skin or the orifices of the body, death usually occurs from exhaustion and heart failure, in collapse, or in coma, or from paralysis of the central nervous system, according to the type of intoxication which predominates, whether it is gastro-enteric or cerebrospinal. Death may occur in some cases from asphyxia, where difficulty of respiration was one of the outstanding symptoms. In arriving at a diagnosis of poisoning, one must largely depend upon the chemical findings of arsenic in excretions, hair, nails, or in the autopsy material. The symptoms are taken up one by one by the lawyer for the defense, who asks the expert if vomiting is not caused by an infectious fever, appendicitis, or some other disease. The great majority of over 200 cases of arsenical poisonings which I have seen or examined, showed symptoms as given under acute arsenical poisoning.

438. FOSTER: *Lancet*, 2:305, 1840; THOMPSON: *Northwestern Med. Soc.*, 8:89, 1851.

439. *Schaeffer-Nelson's North Lancet*, 8:145, 1853, POWELL: *Westminster Hosp. Reports*, 5:215, 1889.

A man taking Fowler's solution for several weeks, five drops three times a day, developed numbness and pain in his arms. His skin was dry and scaly, with a brownish pigmentation in spots. The deep reflexes were diminished in both arms, the patellar reflexes were absent, and the patient showed different mental depressions. The patient's hemoglobin was 55%; red blood count, 3,030,000; white blood count 4,300 with 15% eosinophiles. A study of the morphology of the red blood cells showed a slight anisocytosis and poikilocytosis. The icterus index was four. The Kahn test was negative. The urine was negative except for a few hyaline casts. The man had a marked peripheral neuritis, due to ingestion of Fowler's solution. When seen three months later, his peripheral neuritis had improved somewhat, but was still giving him a great deal of discomfort.

Peripheral neuritis and polyneuritis in the K. case referred to above, were still present after one year.

In arriving at a differential diagnosis before a chemical examination has been made, one could distinguish from the mercurials: by the absence of salivation and pain in the mouth; from the corrosives: by the lack of swelling of the mouth, lips, and corrosion of the mucous membrane; from carbolic acid: by the odor of carbolic acid. Symptoms of gastro-enteritis are caused by eating foods such as sausage, fish, cheese, beans, and ice cream which contain decomposed products and various bacteria, such as the paratyphoid group (B. paratyphosus, or B. enteritidis) and bacillus botulinus.

In poisoning by foods, a number of persons are usually attacked, and one should suspect a certain food as the cause. In 1914, in Chicago, Illinois, at a banquet given in honor of Archbishop M., over 100 people were poisoned by partaking of a soup which contained arsenic, placed there by a cook, who was never apprehended. In one quart of soup I found 1.227 gm. of arsenic trioxide. A young woman who was disappointed in love sent her sweetheart a box of fudge. The fudge was passed around to other people working in the same office, and all became very ill. An examination of the candy revealed the presence of ground glass and arsenic trioxide.

An acute abdomen might be mistaken for a case of poisoning. However, a careful history will reveal that the same food and drink were consumed by others without ill effects. When there is a peritonitis as a result of a ruptured gangrenous appendix, there is usually a history of pain for a few hours or days prior to nausea, vomiting, and great thirst. The chief point of observation during life is localization of the pain; the lower quadrant in case of appendicitis, whereas, in arsenical poisoning the pain is located in the region of the stomach. An operation during life, or an autopsy after death, of course would remove all doubt as to the cause of illness.

In many cases of arsenical poisoning a fall in blood pressure is noted. In animal experiments it has been proved that vasodilatation is most conspicuous in the pancreatic area and that the blood pressure drops, even when the intestines are tied off so that the muscular walls are dilated. The arsenic would act upon the intestines, no matter whether it was given per mouth or intravenously. There seems to be a capillary paralysis with great permeability which results in the production of an exudation through the connective tissues. This causes the epithelium to become raised and thrown off in shreds or false membranes. This exudation is excreted into the lumen of the bowel and largely coagulates. The distention, as well as the circulatory changes, cause increased peristalsis and watery diarrhea. The shreds of mucous membrane are coagulated and give rise to the evacuation, characteristic of the white watery stool. Boehn and Pistorius[440] report this condition as always seen in Asiatic cholera, and as best differentiated by a chemical examination and history. Occasionally there is a nephritis. Absorption may occur from the intact skin by the use of cosmetics containing arsenic. Arsenic may be found in all of the excretions, urine, feces, sweat, milk, epithelium of the skin, hair and nails. The excretion usually begins in two to eight hours after administration, but lasts for a much longer time, from three to ten days. In one case of poisoning I found arsenic in the urine thirty days after the last administration of sodium arsenite. Sanger[441] found arsenic in the urine of cases of poisoning by wallpaper for a period as long as 140 days.

Fatal Dose: To state the fatal dose one must know the solubility of the particular preparation, also the conditions and manner of administration. A nurse in a hospital gave a child

440. BOEHN and PISTORIUS: *Arch. f. exper. Path. u. Pharmacol.*, 16:188, 1882.
441. HILLS, W. B.: *Boston M. & S. J.*, 131:455, 1894.

seven years of age, 5 cc. of Fowler's solution in place of five minims, with fatal results. This would be equivalent to 0.77 grains of arsenic trioxide, calculated from the amount of potassium arsenite. The symptoms were typical of acute arsenical poisoning. A chemical examination of the organs showed that the stomach contained .0015 gm., the liver .008 gm., the kidney .0024 gm., and the bowel and content .0010 gm. of arsenic per 100 gm. of sample.

The lethal dose is usually placed as 2.7 to 3.1 grains. Rouyer and Feltz[442] found that absorption by dogs, of 0.0025 gm. calculated as arsenic per kilo (0.021 grains per pound) always causes death. Taking this into consideration, the fatal dose for a man weighing 150 pounds should be 2.7 to 3.15 grains. Hoffman, Husemann, Kobert, and Seidel, state the fatal dose to be one-half grain to three grains. Brian, Chaude and Buoid place three-quarters to one and one-half grains as the fatal dose.

Fatal Period: In my experiences in acute poisoning, death occurred in from thirty minutes to twenty-four hours, although a case reported by Dr. Iliff[443] shows that a woman took a glassful of a saturated solution, fell directly and died instantly without a struggle.

The symptoms have been delayed as long as six hours, death occurring two hours after the first symptoms.[444] The symptoms may be delayed in a person under the influence of alcohol, or because the solution of the arsenic was interfered with by an albuminous or fatty substance in the stomach. A man, D. L., took two ounces of Fowler's solution and died within four hours. In the subacute cases the fatal period may not occur for several weeks, as in the Baker case above referred to.

Treatment: Recovery is possible from three grains or more. However, where poor health is present, it would be possible to cause death with a much smaller dose.

If vomiting is not already present, an emetic mixture of a teaspoonful of mustard and a tablespoonful of salt in a tumbler of warm water may be given. Then the stomach should be washed out immediately, preferably with colloidal ferric hy-

442. Rouyer and Feltz: *Gaz. d. hôp., Paris,* **76,** 1:962, 1875.
443. Iliff: *Lancet,* 2:432, 1845.
444. Fox: *Lancet,* 2:503, 1848; and *Virchows Arch. f. path. Anat.,* 47:524, 1869.

droxide suspension, as this antidote may delay absorption of the arsenic through adsorption. This antidote can be prepared by adding magnesium oxide to a tincture of ferric chloride, or a solution of ferric sulphate. There has been some doubt cast upon the antidotal properties by De Buscher, in 1902,[445] and McGuigan,[446] who found that this antidote at its best postpones death but for a few hours. Its administration, however, can do no harm, and if it delays absorption it gives time to wash out the stomach repeatedly. Wash out the stomach with a tea-spoonful of activated charcoal in a pint of water. Thiosulphate should be given intravenously, fifteen grains in 10 cc. of water, repeating in four hours. Give colonic flushings of four grains of calcium sulphide to a pint of water. If the diarrhea is so pronounced as to cause dehydration of the patient, hypodermoclysis should be resorted to, giving 1000 cc. of physiological salt solution, with 5% glucose, or 5% saline intravenously by the drop method. In extreme weakness, give 100 cc. of a 50% glucose solution intravenously in place of the former. The patient should be treated symptomatically, giving caffeine with sodium benzoate, or strychnine, as the occasion may require.

Postmortem Appearances: The postmortem appearances will vary according to the duration of the case, and whether death occurred in a few hours, or after several days. If the individual had been sick for a number of days there will be a marked emaciation, and the skin may be cyanosed, particularly that of the hands and feet. Putrefactive changes in the body are usually delayed. The pathological changes are those usually seen in poisons that are local irritants of the stomach and bowels, and if the patient lives for a number of hours, there may be seen fatty changes in the heart, liver, and kidneys. The mouth, pharynx and esophagus may show no changes whatever. However, the repeated acts of vomiting bring up the poison from the stomach, which may cause inflammatory changes, or even ulceration.

Ecchymosis has frequently been observed between the endocardium and the muscle of the left ventricle in cases which have been rapidly fatal. Congestion of the lungs with subpleural ecchymosis and occasionally edema are noted. Grossly, there appear to be no changes in the brain or its membranes.

445. DE BUSCHER: *Arch. Inst. Pharmacol.*, 10:415, 1902.
446. McGUIGAN: *J. Pharmacol. & Exper. Therap.*, 21:65, 1923.

There may be a hyperemia of the meninges, with effusion of the ventricles. The postmortem examination occasionally reveals a dilatation and paralysis of the capillaries of the entire gastro-intestinal tract. The mucosa varies from a pink to a dark red; the epithelium is occasionally necrotic, and in shreds. However, in many cases of arsenical poisoning there were no such changes. Fatty degeneration may be found in the liver and kidneys.

In the examination of the stomach, Paris green or some other brightly colored combination may be noted. The color of the stomach is not uniform; it may be light red, bright or brownish-red. The redness may appear in spots or patches (see Plate), more frequently, however, toward the greater end and chiefly on the prominence of the rugae. Occasionally, petechial hemorrhages may be seen scattered over the entire mucous membrane, or at the striations, stretching in curved lines between the cardiac and pyloric openings. The mucous lining of the stomach may be covered with extravasations of blood. Occasionally if the arsenic has been in a solid form, the lining of the stomach may be covered with a tough mucus, in which particles of the poison may be found. Sections of the mucous membrane may show injection of the vessels and octahedral crystals of the undissolved arsenic. The pathological changes found in the bowel are similar to those found in the stomach. The inflammation occurs in patches, while other parts of the bowel may be practically normal in appearance. The hyperemia varies greatly in degree and does not necessarily increase with the duration of the poison. In the large bowel there may be patches of denuded epithelium, hemorrhages, and the colon may be contracted. The gall-bladder is rarely empty, while the urinary bladder is nearly always so. Petechial hemorrhages have been found in the muscles of the left ventricle in cases which have been rapidly fatal. The heart muscle may show beginning fatty degeneration. The blood may not show any important changes and is usually dark.

Chronic Arsenical Poisoning: In this type of poisoning the most characteristic symptoms can be attributed to the changes in the nervous system and in the skin. The diagnosis may be somewhat difficult, as the symptoms may be obscure, or resemble those produced by chronic lead poisoning. The old-time practitioner used to describe the condition as one of

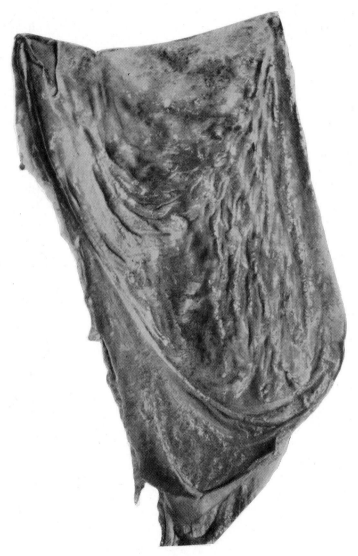

Hemorrhages in the lining of the stomach in
arsenic poisoning

"walking typhoid." There is anemia, loss of appetite, loss of weight, and a general feeling of weakness. The organic arsenicals used so effectively as amebicides occasionally show individual sensitivity, characterized by severe peripheral neuritis, toxic erythema, severe enough to be considered as dermatitis exfoliativa. This occurred in 5.6% of 232 cases treated with acetarsone.[447] If the arsenic is taken through the respiratory tract as arsenical fumes or dust, the patients may complain of a chronic rhinitis, and there may be ulcerations of the septum and a chronic bronchitis. Men working in Paris green may have perforations of the septum similar to those seen in men working with the arsenic trioxide. This is not seen in men working in lead arsenate. These cases never show an exfoliative dermatitis. Where the arsenicals are in contact with a moist skin, various degrees of inflammation with ulceration are seen. These clear up easily and the men return to the same type of work. There is a mild gastro-enteritis with cramps and recurrent attacks of diarrhea. This type of poisoning may be the result of small quantities of arsenic administered with criminal intent, or may be of industrial origin, or from contaminated air or food. Tattersall and Reynolds[448] report the history of 4,000 individuals who were poisoned, 300 ending fatally. Two hundred ninety-six patients were carefully examined and presented the following symptoms, which are enumerated in descending order of frequency:

234	paralysis
228	sensory disturbances
107	skin eruptions
106	rhinitis and lacrimation
68	melanosis
39	gastro-intestinal symptoms
10	edema
9	psychic disturbances

The nervous disturbances were explained on the basis of an inflammatory degenerative nervous process, causing arsenical neuritis. This may be caused by a too intensive medication, or in one very sensitive to the arsenic, such as the case described above (page 232) in which the individual had taken Fowler's solution for several weeks. It is manifested in the

447. Brown, Philip W.: J.A.M.A., 105:1319, 1935.

448. Tattersall and Reynolds: Leschke, Clinical Toxicology, 65, 1934.

form of a tingling, tickling sensation, decrease of the sensation of temperature, and other paresthesia, hyperesthesia, and anesthesia. This is followed by violent pains in the hands and feet which may radiate upwards, visual and auditory disturbances, dizziness, headache, and disturbances of taste and smell. The patient becomes increasingly weaker; there occur tremors, cramps, and paralysis, whereby the reflexes are eliminated; there occur also spasms and ataxia. The sexual power is also markedly decreased. In the majority of the cases, paralysis begins in the legs, involving the hands a few days later. The paralysis involves mostly the extensor muscles of the feet and hands bilaterally, being contrary to lead intoxications in which the paralysis is apt to involve first the extensor muscles of the right forearm, mostly unilateral, and rarely involving the muscles of the feet. This paralysis involving the extensor muscles, leads to an atrophy of musculature, with flexion contractures. In chronic arsenical poisoning there may be pigmentative melanosis, cancer, rhinitis, lacrimation, and catarrhal involvement of the pharynx, larynx, trachea, and bronchi. Franseen and Taylor[449] reported nine cases of cancer. The gastro-intestinal symptoms are milder in character than those seen in acute intoxication and may continue for a longer time. There is a loss of appetite, nausea, vomiting, and diarrhea, associated with colicky pains. The bone-marrow function is exhausted, and not only secondary anemia is produced, but occasionally also a pernicious or aplastic anemia. Insomnia, forgetfulness, vertigo, and soon loss of power of concentration, are common complaints. The chief and most aggravating complaint of the patients is the peripheral neuritis, numbness, and tingling of the hands and feet. Some motor changes are usually detectable at this stage. The muscles of the forearms and hands are sometimes paralyzed, giving rise to a wrist drop, this condition seldom occurring in the absence of lower limb involvement. Mr. K. (page 223) had a peripheral neuritis with a marked ataxia simulating tabes dorsalis, a hyperkeratosis, and bronze pigmentation of the skin. The pigmentation had a copper bronze hue on the soles and the palms.

In the Clugston case there was an erythema and herpes labialis. There is a tendency for the hair to fall out and the

449. FRANSEEN, C. C., and TAYLOR, G. W.: *J. Indust. Hyg.*, 17, 1935.

nails to become brittle and ridged. One should look for the white bands seen across the nails, following acute arsenical poisoning. The skin lesions just described, when associated with diarrhea and digestive disturbances, may confuse one with Addison's disease. However, in chronic arsenical poisoning, there will be a neuritis or polyneuritis. The finding of arsenic in the hair, nails, and urine should indicate arsenic as the causative agent.

Treatment: The patient should be removed from the source of contact, and placed in a hospital, as the ingestion of arsenic might be at home. The patient can be given fifteen grains of sodium thiosulphate in water, three times a day, and fifteen grains in 10 cc. of water, intravenously three times a week. He should be placed on a mild diet, increasing the food gradually, with much rest and plenty of fresh air. The symptoms may continue for many months in spite of all treatment. It was necessary for K. (page 223) to use crutches for nine months, and it was over a year before he recovered from the polyneuritis. The damage done to the liver, kidneys, and muscular tissues may lead to a fatal termination.

Arsenical Applications: Arsenic Eating: While in Europe, in 1925, I investigated arsenic eaters in lower Austria. The late Professor Ipsen, of Innsbruck, informed me he had heard of such individuals, but in his forty years of experience, had never seen a case. He put me in touch with the superintendent of the poor, a man, who had lived in that neighborhood some sixty years, and who also informed me he had never seen people having the habit of eating arsenic. Dr. Ipsen gave me samples of arsenic which he said the people might have taken and which caused but very slight symptoms of poisoning. I found this arsenic to be of a vitreous form, a type that I had fed to dogs in several grains without causing death, but which when ground and put in a solution caused illness and death of the animals. In Vienna I inquired of Dr. H. Jansch if he had ever seen any cases of arsenic eaters and he replied he had not, but that Kobert in his book mentioned that people in America were in the habit of taking arsenic to improve their complexion. Arsenic is used externally and internally to improve the nutrition of the skin and hair, and in non-parasitic chronic skin diseases, but this is not to be considered as arsenic eating, as the continued use of arsenic without medical supervision for these conditions leads to chronic arsenical poisoning. Harding[450] began with one-sixtieth grain (0.001 gm.) of arsenic trioxide thrice daily after meals and gradually increased the dose to 1.2 grains (0.08 gm.), which he found unendurably toxic. Even one-grain (0.065 gm.) doses could only be taken with dry foodstuffs. With soups or beverages at the meal it caused immediate pain in the abdomen and later loosening of the bowels.

As early as 1844 toxicologists recognized the difference in the absorption of poisons. Christison said: "the situations where arsenic is met with in largest quantity are the liver." The rate of absorption is modified by the condition of the body, whether it is taken upon an empty stomach, whether the poison was in solution or in solid form, and, from the definition given earlier in the text, all poisons to produce their specific effects, must be absorbed. As chemical methods become more refined, the distribution of various poisons can be more thoroughly traced than in the past. The form of the poison has a great influence on its absorption and consequent distribution. Scolosuboff,[451] experimenting with sodium arsenite, found that the brain contained three times as much arsenic as the liver. In another experiment he found that the brain contained, per 100 gm. of tissue, just double the amount of arsenic contained in the muscles, as pointed out in a previous publication. (See Baker case, page 229). Scolosuboff was dealing with a form of the poison seldom seen by toxicologists, thus explaining why many thousands of analyses made of the human organs have failed to confirm Scolosuboff's work.

Arsenic pentoxide, As_2O_5, is deliquescent, soluble in water, forming H_3AsO_4. It is an irritant poison, similar to arsenic trioxide. It is used in medicine in combination. It forms a brick-red precipitate with silver nitrate and should be reduced to arsenous acid by an addition of sulphur dioxide and the latter removed by carbon dioxide before the introduction of hydrogen sulphide.

Distribution: In most of the cases of toxicological interest, the arsenic has been taken or administered by mouth. It is chiefly with the absorption from the alimentary tract that it becomes of forensic interest. The expert may be called upon

450. HARDING: *London Lancet*, 1:288, 1914.
451. SCOLOSUBOFF: *Bull. Soc. chim., Paris*, 24:125, 1875.

to testify in cases regarding death from the intravenous administration of an organic arsenical or from illness caused by the inhalation of arsenic dust, or from the continual use of some pigment or paint containing very small amounts of arsenic trioxide. A case of interest along this line, is one from Decatur, Illinois, where it was claimed that a man painting for five days with an iron paint containing .074% calculated as arsenic trioxide, acquired an exfoliative dermatitis. A negative Gutzeit was obtained for arsenic in the filtrate of three samples of dried pigment boiled with N/10 sodium hydroxide and 0.5% hydrochloric acid and distilled water. However, a large number of men using this same paint during the same time, and for longer periods, failed to show any effects of arsenical intoxication. Many cases of exfoliative dermatitis occur in people who never worked with arsenic, or never had taken it internally. When arsenic is taken into the stomach in solution it can be detected in the blood in a few minutes, and consequently changes again in the gastro-intestinal tract with the attending symptoms seen in the typical acute poisoning. Because of its irritant action, it disappears sooner from the gastro-intestinal tract than from the liver or other parenchymatous organs. The arsenic will nearly always be found in the liver, when it is not present in the stomach or bowel. In several cases that have been reported, where arsenic was absorbed otherwise than by the alimentary canal, the poison was found in the stomach in six, and in two of these it was detected in the liver. In death by salvarsan or neosalvarsan the stomach may contain less than one part per million, or may contain a weighable amount, as 0.13 mg. arsenic trioxide per 100 gm. in nearly all of these cases, the liver will show the presence of arsenic. I have had three cases of salvarsan poisoning in which the liver showed only traces, and the kidney showed a weighable amount. The bowel and content show very little arsenic where life has been prolonged for three or four days. There is a fatty degeneration of the liver cells which is more marked with organic than with inorganic compounds. There are degenerative changes in the kidneys, capillaries, and blood. Where life has been prolonged for several days and where comparable analytical results were obtained, they indicate, so far as they go, that the distribution is more nearly equal in cases which are of long duration than in those which are more rapidly fatal.

CASE No. 1, a male, thirty-eight years of age, died four and one-half hours after taking an unknown quantity of arsenic; in this case the stomach was not emptied. The autopsy and analysis were made nine days after death. One hundred gm. of tissue from the stomach walls contained 0.0249 gm. of arsenum; large intestine 0.0262; liver, 0.0144; stomach contents, 0.8926; small intestine, 0.0134; kidneys, 0.0175; heart, 0.0065; pancreas, 0.0095; lung, 0.0021; gall-bladder, 0.0042; brain, 0.0002.

CASE No. 2, male sixteen years old, died three weeks from first dose, and ten days from second dose. The early symptoms were a gastro-enteric disturbance; later, numbness and tenderness in the extremities led up to feeble muscles, complete paralysis, and death. The analysis was made eighteen hours after death. For 100 gm. of tissue, the spinal cord contained 0.0011 gm. of arsenum; blood, 0.0005; stomach walls, 0.0005; stomach contents, 0.0005; kidneys, 0.0016; spleen, 0.0013; urine, 0.0017.

CASE No. 3, a male, forty-two years old, died in twenty-four hours. For 100 gm. of sample, the liver contained 0.00087 gm. of arsenum; the kidneys, 0.00264 and 0.00023; stomach, 0.00013; bowel, 0.000132; and heart, 0.00594.

CASE No. 4, a male, fifty-two years old, died within four days. The stomach contained no arsenic; kidneys contained 0.00013 gm.; liver contained 0.0052; heart contained one-tenth part per million; brain contained none; cord, none.

The liver, spleen, and kidneys uniformly contain a greater proportion of arsenic than an equal weight of muscle or brain and this preponderance, in some cases at least, tends to diminish as life is prolonged. The quantity of arsenic trioxide in the liver at death probably never exceeds 0.2 gm. if indeed it ever reaches that amount. The largest quantity actually found has been 2.77 grains (0.18 gm.) in a homicidal case in which death was supposed to have occurred in twenty-six hours after the administration of the first dose. From these analyses it has been calculated that the liver reaches its maximum at seven and a half hours after the ingestion of the poison. I have examined a number of bodies that had been buried for some time, and have included in Table XXI the analyses showing how much arsenic existed in the organs at death. This cannot always be determined by the expert because there is a certain amount of postmortem migration. Where the bodies had been buried a long time and the organs were not present, I have included in the analyses, the skeletal structure.

Leibowitz[452] established the distribution of arsenic in the bodies of rabbits throughout the duration of the effects, from the poisoning to the death changes. The poison is detectable at an early stage in the kidneys. It enters the bones in relatively large amounts soon after poisoning, increasing up to the fifth day and from then on decreasing slowly. It is found in the hair after five to six days and increases slowly, until finally about one-sixth of the total arsenic absorbed is found there. Arsenic is taken up by the bones in a manner very similar to lead, the quantity being greater in chronic than in acute poisoning. In chronic poisoning, it is possible to find arsenic in the bones when the organs fail to show it.

Brouardel[453] came to the conclusion that "arsenic accumulates very sensibly in the spongy tissues of bones and becomes fixed in such manner that its presence can be detected, in the bones of the skull or vertebrae particularly, some time after every trace has disappeared from those organs, such as the liver, in which it is localized in greater amount."

In the case of J. DeL. (87—page 255) there was copious vomiting. The physician called was unable to introduce the stomach pump, and at autopsy many crystals of white arsenic were found in the stomach. Weight for weight in cases where death occurs early, more arsenic would be found in the intestine than in the stomach. I have made a number of analyses where the bodies had been buried for several months to many years.

Arsenic is not stored in the body to the same extent as lead, and that there is some accumulation is very evident from the number of analyses showing the presence of arsenic in the secretions several months after the removal of the person from the source of contaminated air. It is not known definitely whether arsenic enters into combination with the elements of the tissues to form a new compound which may be difficult to eliminate, or if it is stored in the form in which it is introduced. However, we know from the examination of the urine, hair, and

452. LEIBOWITZ, T.: *Schweiz. med. Wchnschr.*, 64:947, 1934.
453. BROUARDEL: *Ann. d'hyg.*, 3rd series, 31:486; *Bull. Acad. de méd., Paris*, 2nd series, 22, 4:53, 1889.

TABLE XXI
Arsenic Found in Exhumed Bodies Calculated as As_2O_3 †

	32 F.K.	33 W.S.	34 J.M.	35 J.B.
Skull				
Sternum		16 gm. 0.00118	0.00165	5 ppm
Ribs		19 gm. 0.00026	0.00273	1 ppm
Humerus (Prox.)	0.00013	1 ppm	0.00013	
Humerus (Shaft)		1 ppm	1 ppm	
Humerus (Dist.)	0.00027	2 ppm		
Radius (Prox.)				
Radius (Dist.)			1 ppm	
Femur (Prox.)		1 ppm	0.00056	10 ppm
Femur (Shaft)		5 ppm	2 ppm	
Femur (Dist.)		1 ppm	0.00049	5 ppm
Vertebrae (Lumbar)		100 gm. 0.00041	0.0030	0.00181
Bones of Hand				
Bones of Wrist			5 ppm	
Ulna			0.00056	1 ppm
Ulna Shaft			2 ppm	2 ppm
Hair	0.000264		0.00139	
Dry Matter from region of Liver	0.00062	0.0049	0.0010	0.0010
Muscle (Deltoid)	0.00058			
Muscle (Psoas)				
Muscle (Intercostal)				
Muscle of Thigh				
Brain				
Lungs				
Heart	0.00059			
Stomach	0.00013			
Bowel	0.00013			
Liver	0.00087			
Kidney (1)	0.00236			
Kidney (2)	0.0026		0.00231*	
Spleen				
Pancreas				
Urinary Bladder				
Prostate				
Scapula				
Soil over grave	negative			
Soil of cemetery away from grave				
Soil over body		0.0026		

*Region of left kidney, Dry Material.
†Analysis of 100 gm. unless otherwise stated.

TABLE XXI—Cont.

ARSENIC FOUND IN EXHUMED BODIES CALCULATED AS As_2O_3

	36 M.M.	Child 37 S.S.	61 Courtney Case	28 M.S.
Skull	....	0.0005	50% Arsenic used in hardening compound	
Sternum	0.0016	......	......	......
Ribs	0.0079	0.0079	0.1250	0.00078
Humerus (Prox.)	4 ppm	0.00026	......	......
Humerus (Shaft)	......	......	......	......
Humerus (Dist.)	......	......	......	......
Radius (Prox.)	......	......	......	......
Radius (Dist.)	......	......	......	......
Femur (Prox.)	......	0.00026	0.4424	0.4424
Femur (Shaft)	3 ppm	......	0.0473	0.0473
Femur (Dist.)	2 ppm	......	......	......
Vertebrae (Lumbar)	......	......	......	......
Bones of Hand	......	0.00079	......	......
Bones of Wrist	......	......	......	......
Ulna	......	......	......	......
Ulna Shaft	......	......	......	......
Hair	0.00139	......	......	0.0211
Dry Matter from region of Liver	0.0079	......	......	......
Muscle (Deltoid)	......	......	......	......
Muscle (Psoas)	......	......	......	0.00079
Muscle (Intercostal)	......	......	0.211	0.00025
Muscle of Thigh	......	......	0.3432	......
Brain	......	......	......	0.00013
Lungs	......	......	0.1346	0.00064
Heart	......	......	......	0.00132
Stomach	......	......	......	0.00264
Bowel	......	......	......	0.00052
Liver	......	......	......	0.0052
Kidney (1)	......	......	......	0.00052(rt)
Kidney (2)	......	......	......	0.00052(lt)
Spleen	......	......	......	0.00264
Pancreas	......	......	......	......
Urinary Bladder	......	......	......	1 ppm
Prostate	......	......	......	0.0005
Scapula	......	......	......	......
Soil over grave	......	......	*	5 ppm
Soil of cemetery away from grave	......	......	**	......
Soil over body	......	0.0003	***	......

*Soil over rough box buried 19 yrs., 0.0011.

**Soil from top of grave, 0.005. Soil 4 ft. away 28 inches below surface 0.0016; below rough box, 0.0063.

***Adipocere from inguinal region and over crest of ileum, 0.4693. After burial whole body was bathed in solution of arsenic during the wet season.

nails of those who have had repeated small doses, that the arsenic is not all eliminated in a few days. From the analysis of material in Table XXI showing the findings at autopsies, it is quite evident that bony tissues retain some of the arsenic. It is possible that arsenic replaces some of the phosphate with an arsenate in a similar manner to lead. From the experiments with formaldehyde, mercury, and other poisons, I believe arsenic would be found in the urine within a short time after administration. With our delicate methods of detection of arsenic it is certain that we would find arsenic within the first half hour.

Taylor quotes a case of Geoghegan's[454] in which no arsenic was found in the small quantity of urine passed up to the fourteenth hour, and that passed from fourteen to thirty-six hours yielded only faint traces. The peculiarity of arsenic is that when it is administered in small quantities over a period of time, we find arsenic in the urine, feces, hair, and nails for a longer period of time than when one massive dose is given, as illustrated in the case previously mentioned where I failed to find it in the urine after thirty days from adminis-tration. Cases have been reported where arsenic was found ninety-three days after ingestion in non-fatal cases where one dose was said to have been taken. Carter quotes a case from Gubler,[455] who found arsenic in the hair eight months after poisoning. In one case 6.02 gm. of hair and nails gave .0001 mg. of arsenic trioxide in a chronic case of poisoning, with polyneuritis. In another case 11.8 gm. of hair and toe-nails gave .012 mg. of arsenic trioxide in an exhumed body, buried for one year. In a body buried for about seven years 7.7 gm. of hair and nails gave .002 mg. of arsenic trioxide. Eulenberg[456] found arsenic in the hair of an ex-employee in a Schweinfurth green factory two years after he had stopped employment.

Almquist and Welander[457] found weighable quantities of arsenic in the urine of patients up to sixty days after the discontinuance of the treatment, and qualitatively detectable quantities up to seven months. The amount eliminated by the urine would be no indication of just how much had been taken

454. TAYLOR: Poisons, 3rd Am. ed., 38, 1875.
455. Liverpool. Med.-Chir. J., 10:137, 1890.
456. EULENBERG: Schad. u. Gift. Gasen, 411, 1865.
457. ALMQUIST and WELANDER: Ergebn. d. Physiol., 2:115, 1923; Arch. int. de Pharmakol., 15:399, 1905.

per mouth. The expert can say that this represents only a portion of the arsenic taken by mouth. Almquist and Welander analyzed the urine of a psoriasis patient under treatment by intravenous arsenical injections. With a daily administration of 0.02 mg. of arsenic trioxide, the day's urine contained from 0.0033 to 0.014 mg. of arsenic trioxide, an elimination by this channel from 16.5% to 70% of the intake. Failure to detect arsenic in the urine by Gutzeit or Marsh test does not mean that elimination is complete, because it may still be eliminated

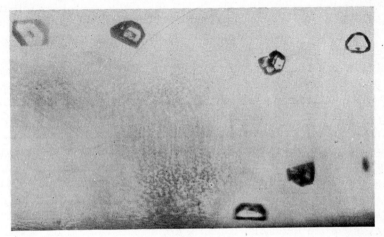

FIG. 13.
Arsenic Trioxide (Reinsch Test)

in the feces. Arsenic is thrown off by the bile and gall-bladder as seen in case 87 (page 255). In this case I found arsenic equivalent to 4.2 mg. of arsenic trioxide in the bile and gallbladder. Arsenic is eliminated in perspiration; is found in mother's milk, in the serum of vesication, and in the skin. In the hair of J. M. (34) I found 1.39 mg. of arsenic trioxide per 100 gm. after burial for two years. Care should be exercised in interpreting the results of arsenic found in the hair unless the soil around and above the coffin had been examined for its presence. Death may occur in two weeks from arsenical poisoning after the administration of one large dose, and arsenic may be found in mere traces, as one part per million, in the soft parts, whereas in the hair, nails, and bones it will be found in definite amounts. Elimination from the bones takes place much more slowly than from the soft parts in cases of poisoning where very small doses had been taken or given.

In the manufacture and handling of Paris green men may have laryngitis, bronchitis, and huskiness of the voice, which disappear as soon as they are removed from the source of the poison. Perspiration collecting freely at the point where the skin is bare, as at the wrist end of gloves, may produce redness and ulceration when the deposition of the arsenical green comes in contact with the skin. The same is true when a mask is worn. At the edge of the mask where there is perspiration, there will be areas of erythema, and ulceration. There may be redness and swelling of the eyelids, conjunctivitis, coryza, and erythema of the body with brownish pigmentation. This pigmentation usually appears on the face and neck. In one case it appeared only on the left leg below the knee. This same man had disturbance of hearing and frequent bleeding from the nose, during a four-year period of working in lead arsenate and Paris green. Medical directors of industrial concerns reported never seeing a case of exfoliative dermatitis appearing in men working with Paris green, lead arsenate, or Scheele's green. Perforation of the nasal septum occurs in workmen with Paris green the same as with arsenic trioxide. There is a great turnover of labor in this industry because men do not like the itching, burning sensation following the work in arsenic dust. However, in one industrial concern, a man has worked for seventeen years without any symptoms of chronic arsenical poisoning. He has had a perforated septum and occasionally develops an irritation of the hands where perspiration has acted upon the arsenic compounds. When perforation occurs in these workers the cartilage is seen flush with the swollen edge of the mucosa which becomes edematous and crusted. After the loss of the cartilage, spontaneous healing occurs within a few months. During the time the crusts are forming in the nose, the laborer is apt to breathe through his mouth, thus causing an irritation of the throat and larynx, and soreness of the tongue with excessive salivation. When removed from the dusty work, the laryngitis and pharyngitis clear up. All of the symptoms seem to be local and systemic poisoning does not occur. With lead arsenate the perforation of the septum does not occur as with workers in Paris green or Scheele's green. In industrial workers in arsenic, the palms and soles are moist and there may be papular or vesicular eruptions and infections in these lesions, which lead to ulceration. Hyperkeratosis may occur in the palms and soles, as when the arsenic is taken by mouth in the subacute or chronic poisoning. The typical skin affections caused by long-continued absorption of arsenic consist of patches of scleroderma or warts or horny patches with diffuse brown or grayish pigmentation—melanoderma. Arsenic in small quantities may cause formation of epithelial growths. This was advanced by Hutchinson[458] in 1887, and a number of authors have brought forth cases of arsenical keratoma epithelioma following the protracted administration of arsenic compounds.

Men working in Paris green and Scheele's green have their clothing laundered every day so as to eliminate a chance of absorption through the skin, and in industrial plants are directed to take shower baths and to wash their faces and hands thoroughly before eating. Plant foremen find it difficult to keep masks on workers.

Scheele's green, cupric arsenite, $CuHAsO_3$, is a pale green powder, and contains 52.8% arsenous acid.

Paris green, Schweinfurth green, emerald green, mitis green, mineral green is cupric-metarsenite, with the formula $(C_2H_3O_2)_2Cu\ 3Cu\ (AsO_2)_2$, containing 25.07% of copper and 44.35% of arsenic. It is a bright green crystalline powder, insoluble in water, but decomposed by prolonged boiling. It is readily attacked by alkaline solutions with separation of cupric oxide, and then reduced to cuprous oxide, the solution then containing an alkaline arsenite. Mineral acids and strong acetic acid decompose it completely, removing all of the copper and liberating arsenious acid. An enormous amount of this compound is used in the eradication of the Colorado beetle found on potato plants. It is also used on tobacco plants, and accounts for the arsenic found in the finished tobacco. I have had a number of cases of suicide by its use, and one murder case, where it was given in coffee.

Of the arsenic sulphides, realgar (As_2S_2), and orpiment (As_2S_3), the first occurs in ruby-red crystals containing 70% of arsenic; the second, containing 60%, is a yellow powder which, by mistake has sometimes been substituted for the harmless vegetable tumeric. The action is similar to that which

458. HUTCHINSON: Quoted by NUT, BIGGE, and PYE-SMITH: *Lancet*, 2:210, 1913.

is characteristic of white arsenic, when it is taken by mouth.

Normal Arsenic: Fordyce, Rosen and Myers'[459] work must be read for the question of normal arsenic in the body. Billeter and Marfurt[460] examined organs and tissues of many bodies, from new-born infants to men of seventy years. They came to the conclusion that arsenic is always present and increases progressively with age. They have established that the body of an adult contains in round numbers, one ten-millionth of its weight in arsenic. The arsenic of the body is usually attributed to food because of chemical treatment in manufacture, taken up by plants from soil, or present in sea food. Headden[461] reported that our virgin soils contain from 2.5 parts per million, and underlying marl four to fifteen parts per million, and that crops on such soils, and animals that fed on such crops, contain arsenic. Bertrand,[462] in a review of French literature, cites the amounts present in various foods and concludes that arsenic is a constant constituent of plants and animals. Remington[463] has examined a large number of brands of manufactured tobacco, in the form of pipe tobacco, cigars, cigarettes, and chewing tobacco, and has found arsenic to be invariably present in quantities many times greater than those cited as permitted in foods.

Remington's method for the separation and estimation of arsenic is a micro-Marsh method which is capable of separation and estimation by comparing quantities as small as one micro-milligram, or one part in ten million on a 10-gm. sample. His method is similar to that used in our laboratory. Organic matter is destroyed by wet combustion. The digestion is started on the water-bath with nitric acid, the sample being moistened with water to prevent ignition. When largely liquefied, 10 cc. of sulphuric acid is added and the digestion continued, first on the water-bath and later on an air-bath with a temperature of 200° in the bath. Nitric acid is added as needed from time to time to keep the space beneath the cover glass continuously filled with brown fumes. The material is never permitted to char, and oxidizing conditions are always present. When the digestion is complete, the cover glass is removed and nitric acid

459. FORDYCE, ROSEN and MYERS: *Arch. Int. Med.,* 31:739, 1923.
460. BILLETER and MARFURT: *Helv. Chim. Acta.,* 6:258, 771, 780, 1923.
461. HEADDEN: Proc. Colorado Scientific Soc., 9:345, 1910.
462. BERTRAND: *Bull. Soc. Hyg. Aliment.,* 8:49, 1920.
463. REMINGTON, R. E.: *J. Am. Chem. Soc.,* 49:1410, 1927.

is eliminated by repeated additions of water, and heating until a drop of the solution gives no color with diphenylamine reagent. Prior to introduction into the Marsh apparatus the solution is diluted to about 25 cc., heated to boiling, and a small crystal of stannous chloride added to insure that the arsenic is in the trivalent state. The generator is started with sufficient one-to-four sulphuric acid to cover the zinc, and allowed to run until action has died down to a practically constant rate and the flame is between 1 and 2 mm. in size, after which the sample is run in at a rate so as not appreciably to increase the flow of gas. Marshing is continued for a half-hour after the remainder of the sample has been introduced. Carefully controlled blank determinations were made from time to time on all reagents. This is important because the best arsenic-free zinc obtainable gives a distinct mirror under the conditions of the experiment.

Billeter maintains that the last traces of organic matter are not destroyed by wet combustion, and follows it by an alkaline nitrate fusion. I have found that occasionally a sample will froth in the generator, suggesting the possibility of some organic matter still unacted upon. The amounts recovered are too large to be estimated by comparison with standard mirrors without introducing a large factor, so that the mirrors are dissolved in a standard iodine solution and titrated according to the method of Billeter. The portion of the tube containing the mirror is cut off, dropped into a glass-stoppered 100-cc. flask, and 25 cc. of 0.002 N iodine solution added, following by 2 cc. of 1% sodium bicarbonate. The stopper is then inserted, and covered with a few drops of potassium iodide solution, and the neck of the flask covered with an inverted test-tube to prevent evaporation of the sealing fluid. Solutions of such large mirrors as those obtained is very slow, requiring sometimes as long as twenty-four hours. After solution is complete, the stopper and neck of the flask are rinsed, and the excess of iodine is titrated with 0.002 N thiosulphate solution. Samples of American smoking and plug tobacco have been examined for arsenic, and found to contain from six to thirty parts per million, or from 0.05 to 0.27 grain of arsenic trioxide per pound. Bertrand reported arsenic in various vegetable and food substances, peas containing 0.04 parts per million of arsenic. Cox[464]

464. Cox: *Analyst*, 50:3, 1925.

found arsenic in fish up to three parts per million. Approximately half of the arsenic in pipe tobacco is evolved in the smoke, and about half that in plug tobacco is soluble in water.

In the following table giving the analysis of an exhumed body, M.S., it will be noted that the liver gives ten times as much arsenic per 100 gm. as the kidney. The urinary bladder contained only two parts per million, and the brain contained the least arsenic of any of the other organs.

In this examination the arsenic trioxide calculated to the whole organ for the liver, both kidneys, stomach, brain, spleen, heart, bowel and psoas muscle gave a total of 1.908 grains of arsenic trioxide. This patient was probably given arsenic daily,

TABLE XXII
ARSENIC TRIOXIDE IN ORGANS OF EXHUMED BODY

Organ	Wt. of Part.	As_2O_3 per 100 Grams.
Kidney, (right)	156	.00052
Kidney, (left)	178	.00052
Liver	452	.00528
Stomach	172	.00264
Brain	380	.000066
Spleen	163	.00264
Heart	291	.00132
Bowel	315	.00052
Psoas muscle	107	.00079
Urinary bladder	52	2 parts per million.
Prostate	23	.0005
Ribs	66	.00787
Intercostal muscle	62	.00258
Hair	5	.0211
Soil from grave		
Soil-water soluble .... Neg.	Total soil .... 5 parts per million.	

so he cannot be used as an example of finding arsenic in the stomach after several weeks of illness. The literature contains reference to the finding of arsenic in the body a number of days after the supposed administration of arsenic. Finding it in very small amounts, as a few parts per million, would not be unusual since all of the food that we eat contains a small amount of arsenic. It frequently happens that in subacute poisoning there may be a uniform distribution of arsenic in all of the organs, and where the stomach contains more than is usually found with this uniform distribution, it would indicate that the arsenic had been given in the last few hours of life. In Table XXIII, I have tabulated a few findings showing the distribution of the poison in the various organs.

Van Italle, in determining the period of time during which

arsenic was administered in chronic poisoning, uses a method which consists of clipping a sample of hair close to the scalp, cutting it into successive lengths of 6 to 8 cm. and determining the arsenic content of each portion.* The maximum arsenic content indicates the period during which the poison was administered. The rate of hair growth may be taken as 1.5 cm. per month. The method is quite satisfactory in the case of women with long hair.

Tests for Arsenic: A great many special methods have been devised for the detection of arsenic in various materials. For the presence of arsenic in biological material, the Fresenius and von Babo method where the organic matter is destroyed by the use of concentrated hydrochloric acid and potassium chlorate, is used. The filtered solution is partially neutralized and saturated with arsenic-free hydrogen sulphide, which precipitates arsenic, antimony, tin, copper, bismuth and cadmium. This precipitate, after thorough washing with water, is washed with a hot mixture of equal parts of ammonia and yellow ammonium sulphide. The filtrate is warmed and poured over the precipitate again, so as not to give too large a volume of the extract. Repeat this extraction several times, finally washing the filter paper with a few cc. of ammonia and yellow ammonium sulphide. In the precipitate will be found antimony, tin and copper. Evaporate the solution to dryness upon the steam-bath. Moisten the residue with fuming nitric acid and again evaporate. Add 3 gm. of a mixture of 2 gm. of sodium nitrate and 1 gm. of sodium carbonate. This mixture is dried upon the steam-bath, and small portions of it are introduced into a porcelain crucible containing a little fused sodium nitrate heated to redness. After a final addition, heat the crucible, adding a little more sodium nitrate until the fused mass is colorless. In the presence of copper the melt is gray or grayish-black from copper oxide. Allow the fused mass to cool, dissolve with hot water, and wash into a flask. Add a little sodium carbonate to decompose the quantity of sodium stannate that might be in solution, and then filter. The filtrate contains any arsenic present as sodium arsenate (Na_2HAsO_4). The arsenic present may be examined by the Marsh-Berzelius, Fresenius-von Babo, Reinsch, Bettendorff, or Gutzeit method. If the arsenic is in a solid form it may be examined under the micro-

* VAN ITALLE, L.: *Pharm. Weekblad.* 74, 206-9, 1937.

TABLE XXIII

HUMAN BODY POSTMORTEMS MADE WITHIN 24 HOURS AFTER DEATH; ARSENIC FOUND PER 100 GRAMS OF TISSUE CALCULATED AS As_2O_3

No.	Stomach and Contents	Spleen	Liver	Kidneys	Bowel	Heart
1 M.N.	158 gm. .00021	......	.00040	280 gm. .00030	......	......
2 B.D.	136 gm. .0179	......	.0050	207 gm. .00429	......	......
3 U.W.M.	411 gm. .09851	......	422 gm. .00177	(1) 92 gm. .00085 (2) 103 gm. .00362	......	......
4 J.M.	100 gm. .0162	......	100 gm. .0017	(1) .00118 (2) .00132	......	......
5 A.G.	.01320	......	.02059	(1) .00507 (2) .0040	.01452	......
6 W.N.	.0137	......	.0074	.0063	......	......
7 V.M.	.0846	......	.0034	(1) .00269 (2) .0026	.0053	.00169
8 S.S.	.01584	......	.00528	.00462	.00106	......
9 H.G.	.0256	.0062	.0053	(1) .0042 (2) .0042	......	......
10 J.McG.	.0552	.0159	.0050	(1) .0251 (2) .0177	......	......
11 H.H.	.0640	......	.0022	.0010	.0872	......
17 W.K.	.0038	......	.0030	....	.0048	......
20 V.M.	.00267	......	.00007	....	......	......
21 D.Z.	.0347	......	.0008	.0013	......	......
24 J.R.	.00158	......	.00593	....	......	......
26 C.W.	.5 ppm	......	.00105	(1) .00125 (2) .00422	1.2 ppm	......
27 H.D.	.00158	.00137	.00211	.00184	sm. .00013	......
30 A.E.	.00026	......	.0037	....	......	......
40 L.Z.	.0052	......	.0010	(1) .0008 (2) .0006	.0018	......
41 T.M.	.0044	......	......	....	......	......

Remarks:
No. 2—B.D.: brain, .000245.
No. 4—J.M.: 95 gm. of stomach washings containing Paris green contained 4.8442 gm. calculated as As_2O_3.
No. 7—V.M.: lung, .0026.
No. 21—D.Z.: given white arsenic containing 99.8% As_2O_3.
No. 26—C.W.: pancreas, 0.5 ppm.
No. 27—H.D.: esophagus, negative.
No. 41—T.M.: stomach-washing 95 cc. gave .00752 Paris green.

TABLE XXIII—Cont.

HUMAN BODY POSTMORTEMS MADE WITHIN 24 HOURS AFTER DEATH; ARSENIC FOUND PER 100 GRAMS OF TISSUE CALCULATED AS As_2O_3

No.	Stomach and Contents	Spleen	Liver	Kidneys	Bowel	Heart
46 J.N.	negative	......	.0007	.0010	.0003	......
47 K.P.	.00039	......	.0046	.0036	......	......
48 S.K.	.0892	......	.0054	.0084	......	......
49 M.T.	.0720	......	.0220	.0032	.044	.0004
50 F.P.	.0028	......	.0022	110 gm. of composite samp. .0029	......	......
51 A.B.	.0066	......	.0072	.0306	.0018	....:
52 F.K.	.0051	.0021	.0072	.0020	.0022	.0010
54 M.K.	.0042	......	.0020	......	.0042	.0010
55 J.P.D.	.0020	.0012	.0078	.0006	.0070	.0008
57 S.S.	.0120	......	.0104	.0020	.0160 .2240	......
58 L.C.	.00369	.0100	.00753	.0021	.01161	......
68 C.K.	.00052 .00059	......	.00294	.0021	.01180	......
70 M.L.	.040923	.00198	.0211	.0165	.01320	.05225
72 W.L.	.0022	......	......	......	......	......
W.L. — Took arsenic at 11:00 A.M.; died at 9:00 next morning.						
73 I.S.	.00233	......	.0105	.0032	.0013	.0016
76 F.A.	.00174	......	.00396	.00693.	.00093	......
78 G.S.	.027363	......	.02244	.002475	.00792	......
83 D.C.	.00183	.00035	.00132	(1) .00184 (2) .0011	.00052	.00046
85 E.L.B.	.00066	.00139	.00171	.00211	......	......
87 J.DeL.	.02485	......	.0144	(1) .0093 (2) .00828	.0262	.0065

No. 50—F.P.: fly-paper fluid poisoning—18 months of age.
No. 54—M.K.: fingers, .0038; lungs, .0012; radius—ulna, .0020;
No. 55—J.P.D.: lung, .0006.   No. 57—S.S.: mesentery, .0080.
No. 68—C.K.: Paris green poisoning. Fat 1 ppm.; blood, .00019.
No. 70—M.L.: muscle, .06468; pancreas, .0132; lungs, .00528; 7.8 gm. hair gave .0079; blood and embalming fluid .00420.
No. 83—D.C.: 40 gm. spinal cord—0.5 ppm.; 1.25 ppm. Urine, .0005; blood, .00015; pancreas, .00039; lung, .0001.   No. 85—E.L.B.: blood, .00066.
No. 87—J. DeL.: brain, .00026. Took 4 oz. of Fowler's solution (unknown amount of As_2O_3) and died within 4 hours. Undissolved particles of As_2O_3 in stomach content caused bloody particles. Lung, .0021; pancreas, .00925; duodenum, .0134; colon, .0262; gall-bladder, .0042.

scope to see whether it exists as octahedral crystals or in amorphous form. Arsenic trioxide sublimes at a temperature of 208° C., and octahedral and tetrahedral crystals will be formed.

Some of the white powder is placed in a hard glass tube which is covered with a cover glass and the arsenic heated. Octahedral crystals will be found upon the cover glass and upon the sides of the subliming tube. This forms a separation from other white substances like corrosive sublimate, or oxalic acid.

Reduction Test: The reduction test is applicable to any solid compound of arsenic, including Paris green, the sulphide, and the arsenites. Take a small amount of the unknown, place it in the bulb of the reduction tube, cover with sodium carbonate and potassium cyanide. Upon heating, the arsenic compound is reduced to metallic arsenic, which is deposited in the form of a mirror. The potassium cyanide changes to potassium cyanate, or potassim sulphocyanate.

In the Fresenius and von Babo method the oxide and the sulphide are placed in a boat with a mixture of three parts of dry sodium carbonate and one part of pure potassium cyanide. This boat is placed in a hard glass ignition tube, and heated in a stream of carbon dioxide dried by means of arsenic-free sulphuric acid. A mirror will appear on the cooler part of the tube if arsenic is present.

The Bettendorff arsenic test has been modified by King and Brown.[465] In their modification the presence of mercury chloride makes the Bettendorff test more delicate than the Gutzeit or Marsh test. These authors found that Bettendorff's test, if made in the presence of mercury chloride, will detect arsenic in 10 cc. of 0.00001 M arsenic trioxide dissolved in concentrated hydrochloric acid. The faint brown color appears in about ten minutes. When, in addition to saturated stannous chloride, enough mercuric chloride to produce a concentration of 0.00001 M is added to solutions of arsenic trioxide in concentrated hydrochloric acid, colorations appear immediately when concentrations of arsenic trioxide are as low as 0.00001 M, and in one minute with concentrations as small as 0.0000001 M with respect to arsenic trioxide. The presence of mercuric chloride

465. KING, W. B., and BROWN, F. E.: *Indust. & Eng. Chem., Analytical Ed.*, 5: 168, 1933.

hastens the appearance of the coloration due to arsenic in Bettendorff's test, after boiling with potassium chlorate. Concentrated stannous chloride solution precipitates metallic arsenic from arsenious acid cold and from arsenic acid with heat or after long standing. A very nearly saturated solution of stannous chloride was prepared by dissolving 453 gm. of $SnCl_2 . 2H_2O$ in 250 cc. of hot concentrated hydrochloric acid. After cooling, strips of metallic tin were added to prevent oxidation. Solutions of mecuric chloride and arsenic trioxide were prepared by diluting 0.1 M stock solution in volumetric apparatus. "When the excess of stannous chloride is added to a solution of arsenic compound in a high concentration of hydrochloric acid, a brown colloidal suspension of arsenic appears. If the concentration of arsenic is sufficiently great the suspension changes to a black precipitate." The addition of enough mercuric chloride to make its concentration 0.00001 M before the addition of stannous chloride hastens the appearance of the coloration, increases the sensitivity of Bettendorff's test ten to one-hundred fold, and enables the test to be made in a lower concentration of hydrochloric acid. Mercuric chloride in 0.00001 M solutions does not produce turbidity when stannous chloride is added. In the presence of mercuric chloride Betendorff's test will detect a smaller quantity of arsenic than the Gutzeit or Marsh test.

Reinsch Test: (See under tests for mercury, page 214): Always heat the copper foil in the subliming tube, as arsenic may be present even when the foil does not show darkening. Antimony, mercury, bismuth, gold, platinum, and sulphides will darken the copper foil. The Reinsch test does not work if an oxidizing agent is present, such as nitric acid, chlorates and manganese dioxide. Under their action the copper is dissolved and the formation of an arsenical coating is prevented. The test is delicate to 1/50,000 of a grain of arsenic trioxide.

Marsh Test: In the case of vomited matter the material should be spread in a thin layer on a plate or a large dish and a careful search made for grains of white arsenic, Paris green, or yellow sulphide of arsenic. A portion can be examined using the Gutzeit or Marsh test. A small sample of 25 gm. of tissue can be used or, if the arsenic appears to be small, use 100 gm. of sample, which is placed in a casserole or may be put in an evaporating dish with 20 cc. of nitric acid. Warm for a few minutes over a Bunsen flame. Allow to stand for two hours on a water-bath, stirring occasionally. The mass gradually becomes yellow to orange in color. Add 3 cc. of concentrated sulphuric acid, which has been previously tested for the presence of arsenic, stirring vigorously, watching the temperature to see that it does not exceed 180° C. The mass will gradually become tar-like when 6 cc. more of nitric acid are added drop by drop. The temperature may now be raised to 200° C. for fifteen minutes. Add sulphuric acid, drop by drop, on the edge of the casserole to free traces of nitric acid. Heat until all traces of nitric acid have been expelled and a carbonaceous residue remains. Arsenic now exists as arsenic acid which is readily soluble in water. Boil and filter. Repeat the extraction with boiled water three times, making up to a definite volume, either 100 or 250 cc. Add a measured volume to the Marsh apparatus after the apparatus is free from air and the Marsh tube is heated to redness. In the preparation of the Marsh tests, zinc is placed in a Woulff bottle for generating hydrogen, and sulphuric acid is added through a Squibb funnel. Three dilutions of sulphuric acid are used for the evolution of hydrogen. We begin with acid number one, and as the gas becomes weaker we add number two or three. These are prepared as follows:

No. 1 Acid 180 cc.   C. P. H_2SO_4 in 1000 cc. H_2O.
No. 2 Acid 260 cc.   C. P. H_2SO_4 in 1000 cc. H_2O.
No. 3 Acid 425 cc.   C. P. H_2SO_4 in 1000 cc. H_2O.

The gas is finally condensed through a wash bottle containing lead acetate, and through a dry tube containing calcium chloride, which is held in the tube between plugs of glass wool and then through a hard glass tube of the McNally type, about 50 cm. long, which has a constricted area about 5 cm. long, the end of the constricted area being 15 cm. from the tip end. It has an outside diameter of 5 cm. Its attachment to the calcium chloride tube is 7 to 8 cm. beyond the constricted area, and the tube is drawn out to a tip to make a jet for the burning of the hydrogen gas. The tube which passes through an asbestos box (Fig. 14) is heated red hot about an inch away from the beginning of the constricted area. To prevent the tube from getting too hot or melting, I cover the heated area with a small piece of wire gauze. The hydrogen gas which is liberated at the tip of the McNally tube is tested in a test-tube before applying the heat for the presence of oxygen. After the apparatus has been found to be oxygen-free by no further explosion being caused in the test-tube of gas, the jet may be lighted and heat applied in the asbestos box. After the apparatus has run for fifteen minutes, and there is no mirror appearing on the constricted portion, the chemicals may be considered practically arsenic free. Blanks should, however, be run using the same amount of acids and zinc as is used in the test of the unknown. An aliquot part of the solution as prepared above with nitric and sulphuric acid digestion is poured into the Squibb funnel and allowed to drop slowly into the Woulff bottle. As the evolution of the gas becomes weaker, add some of number two or three sulphuric acid as prepared above. The constricted area

FIG. 14.
Marsh Apparatus

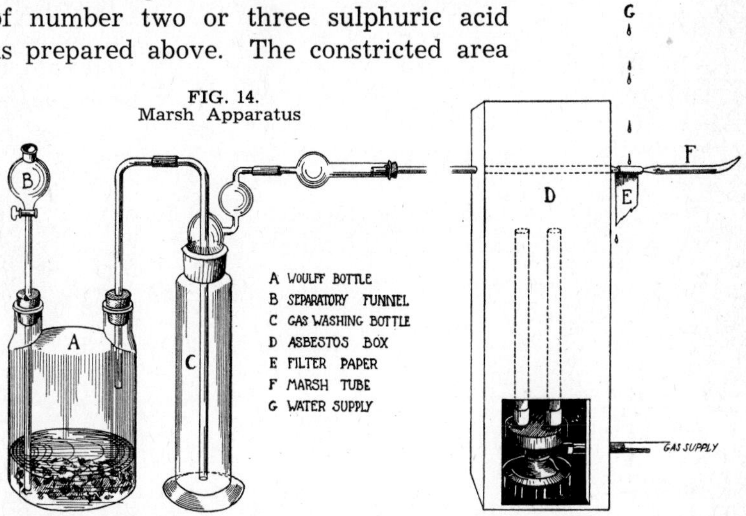

A WOULFF BOTTLE
B SEPARATORY FUNNEL
C GAS WASHING BOTTLE
D ASBESTOS BOX
E FILTER PAPER
F MARSH TUBE
G WATER SUPPLY

of the McNally-Marsh tube is refrigerated by a piece of filter paper upon which cold water is dripping continuously. The strip of filter paper can be made small, and the arsenic mirror condensed for a better comparison with the controls. If antimony is present, a similar deposit may be noticed. The difference between it and that of the arsenic mirror is that the film of antimony is more tin-like in lustre and is deposited closer to the flame. Antimony may be deposited before or on both sides of the flame, the gas being decomposed considerably below a red heat. Arsine decomposes in the absence of air at 450° C. allowing the arsenical mirror which does not melt, to be drawn along the McNally tube. The antimony mirror will melt to minute globules at 432°C. By vaporization in a current of air, a white amorphous coating is obtained, insoluble in water, soluble in hydrochloric acid, and giving reactions for antimonous oxide. By vaporizing a stream of arsenic, a garlic odor is noted, while with antimony there is no odor. Further, with arsenic as seen in the Reinsch tube by slow vaporization in a current of air a deposit of octahedral and tetrahedral crystals is obtained, forming a white coating, soluble in water and giving the reactions for arsenous oxide. The constricted area can be cut off with a sharp file, dried, weighed, and the arsenical stain can be removed by a warm solution of chlorinated lime or liquor sodae chlorinatae, U. S. P., X, while the antimony is insoluble, or soluble with difficulty, in these reagents. This tube is washed with water, alcohol, and ether, is dried in the oven, cooled in the desiccator, and weighed again. The difference between the original weight A, and B, the second weight, gives C, the metallic arsenic in the aliquot portion of the sample. Multiply this arsenic by 1.3201, the product being the amount of arsenic trioxide in that portion of the sample. By calculation, the amount of arsenic in the total organ or sample can be determined. The foregoing test is described as a quantitative test; other portions of the solution may be used for qualitative tests for arsenic.

In the qualitative test for arsenic previously described, the spot is of a steel-gray to black lustre. The arsenic spot dissolves in a solution of sodium hypochlorite, whereas the antimony does not. The arsenic is then warmed with a drop of ammonium sulphide, forming yellow spots, soluble in ammonium carbonate, insoluble in hydrochloric acid. Antimony may give a white precipitate with the nitric acid, but gives no further changes with ammonium molybdate. Magnesia mixture is added to the solution of the mirror or spots in nitric acid. A white crystalline precipitate of magnesium ammonium arsenate, $MgNH_4AsO_4$, is yielded. The crystals of arsenous oxide obtained from the Reinsch test or from the oxidation of the mirror from the Marsh test, when dissolved in water and treated with ammonium silver nitrate, form the yellow silver arsenite, or, with ammonium copper sulphate, form the green copper arsenite. The Marsh test if conducted as above described, is capable of detecting 1/5000 of a grain of arsenic trioxide.

Lachele[466] has described a method for the determination of

466. LACHELE, C. E.: *Indust. & Eng. Chem., Analytical Ed.*, No. 6, 4:256, 1934.

arsenic by estimating the evolved arsine deposited upon a mercuric bromide impregnated diaphragm. It is applicable for estimating minute quantities of arsenic in the presence of impurities such as iron, tin, antimony, or reducible sulphur and phosphorous compounds. The reagents used are as follows:

Hydrochloric acid: dilute 50 cc. of 35% arsenic-free hydrochloric acid to 100 cc. with water.

Stannous chloride solution: dissolve 40 gm. of arsenic-free $SnCl_2.H_2O$ in concentrated hydrochloric acid and make up to 100 cc. with the same strength acid.

Mercuric bromide paper: carefully selected filter sheets (similar to S & S No. 589 black ribbon paper for weight and texture) are soaked one hour in a saturated alcoholic solution of mercuric bromide. After sensitizing, remove sheets, dry by means of an air blast, and cut in disks of the same diameter as the diaphragm tube. Avoid touching the sensitized disks with the hands as far as possible. Disks should not be used when more than five or six days old.

Zinc: cut arsenic-free zinc in pieces about 1 cm. in length. Activate the pieces by covering with hydrochloric acid (one to three) containing about 2 cc. of special stannous chloride solution for each 100 cc. of acid. Allow the action to continue for fifteen minutes, and wash well with distilled water.

Potassium iodide solution: dissolve 15 gm. of potassium iodide in water and dilute to 100 cc.

Ferrous ammonium sulphate: use this substance or ferrous sulphate crystals free from arsenic.

Cuprous chloride solution: dissolve 15 gm. of cuprous chloride in 100 cc. of one-to-one hydrochloric acid.

Cadmium iodide solution: dissolve 20 gm. of cadmium iodide in water and dilute to 100 cc.

Standard arsenic solution: dissolve 1 gm. of arsenic trioxide in 25 cc. of 20% sodium hydroxide. Saturate the solution with carbon dioxide and dilute to one liter with recently boiled water. One cc. of this solution contains 1 mg. of arsenic trioxide. Dilute 40 cc. of this solution to one liter, diluting 50 cc. of the resulting solution to one liter. One cc. of this latter solution contains 0.002 mg. of arsenic trioxide and is used to prepare stains. Prepare fresh dilute solutions frequently.

For the apparatus the author makes use of an Erlenmeyer flask connected by a two-hole stopper to a Liebig or Allihn condenser (Fig. 15). A gas, such as nitrogen or hydrogen, is introduced through a tube extending below the surface of the contents of the flask. The upper end of the condenser is packed with absorbent cotton, the lower half of which is saturated with cuprous chloride solution which acts as a scrubber to remove impurities evolved from the actions of the acid, zinc, or material under investigation, from phosphine, hydrogen sulphide, and arsine. Two thick-walled tubes of the same diameter with ground-glass joints are held together by an outside sleeve of Gooch rubber tubing, so that a chamber is formed. This chamber, which has a diameter that will accommodate a sensitized diaphragm of a size sufficient to combine with all the arsine, is fitted to the condenser. The impregnated paper is fited between the two ground joints as pictured in the figure.

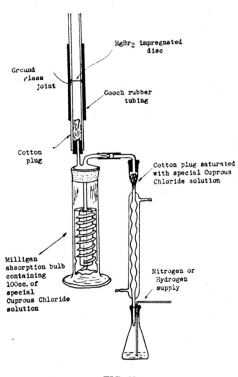

FIG. 15.
Lachele Apparatus for Arsenic

An aliquot part of the sample as prepared under the Marsh test is placed in a 1000-cc. Erlenmeyer flask with enough distilled water to make about 200 cc. of solution. Then 2 gm. to 3 gm. of solid ferrous ammonium sulphate, or ferrous sulphate, ten to fifteen drops of stannous chloride solution, and 50 cc. of one-to-one hydrochloric acid are added. Just before connecting to the condenser, introduce two or three pieces of activated zinc. A continual stream of nitrogen is kept flowing through the system to carry all the traces of evolved arsine through the scrubber cotton to the paper diaphragm impregnated with mercuric bromide. The content of the flask is boiled until all the arsine is evolved, which usually requires about fifteen minutes. When the reaction is complete, the disc is removed and developed in cadmium iodide solution. This fixes the stain more permanently to light and water than does potassium iodide, and changes the color from yellow to brown. The disc is allowed to remain in the iodide solution until all traces of red mercuric iodide, which forms immediately, have been dissolved. The excess reagent is removed from the disc by washing with water and then alcohol, and the disc is then dried between blotters. When dry, the stains are compared with the standards. The standards are prepared in a similar manner to the unknown in steps of 0.0025 mg. of arsenic trioxide, keeping them free from excess light exposure. The stains have a tendency to bleach slightly with age, and it is desirable to prepare fresh standards frequently, especially in the approximate range of the unknown.

Gosio's Arsenic Fungus Test:[467] If a mold, penicillium brevicaule, grows on arsenical substances an intense garlicky odor is formed, probably due to diethyl arsine. In this test 1/1,000,000 gm. of arsenic can be detected. Tellurium compounds also evolve a volatile substance which has a garlic odor. With selenium compounds an offensive odor like that of mercaptan is given off. Antimony, bismuth, phosphorus, and sulphur do not produce gas with any garlic-like odor. The test is prevented by mineral acids, which may be neutralized with sodium or with an excess of tartaric and citric acid. If the material contains 0.01 mg. of arsenic, the garlic odor may remain for weeks.

Gutzeit Test: Prepare the sample as under the Marsh test making a solution up to a definite volume, 50 to 100 cc. The method I use is that found in Methods of Analysis of the Association of Official Agricultural Chemists.[468]

Determination: Introduce 20 cc. of the solution (or, if the quantity of arsenic is large, an aliquot containing approximately 0.03 mg. of arsenious oxide), prepared as directed, into the generator of the apparatus. (Fig. 15, page 262.) The generator used is a two-ounce wide-mouthed ground glass bottle which

467. *Arch. ital de biol.*, 18:253, 1892.
468. Page 370, 1935.

is connected to a glass tube one centimeter long, which contains lead acetate paper rolled into a coil. This tube is connected by means of a second narrow ground-glass tube, 3 mm. in diameter and 12 cm. in length, containing a strip of the mercuric bromide paper. Add 20 cc. of the dilute sulphuric acid, or 20 cc. of the dilute hydrochloric acid. If the total volume is less than 40 cc., dilute to that volume with water and add 4 cc. of the 20% potassium iodide solution. Heat to about 90°C., add three drops of the stannous chloride solution, and heat for ten minutes. Cool the generator and its contents, first in air and then in a pan containing water and ice, to a temperature of about 5° C., add approximately 1 gm. of the stick zinc, and connect the entire apparatus as described. Keep the generator in ice water for fifteen minutes, remove from the bath, and allow the evolution of gas to proceed for an hour longer. Remove the sensitized paper and compare the stain with similar stains produced under like conditions with known quantities of arsenic, using portions of the standard arsenic solution containing 0.001, 0.002, 0.005, 0.010, 0.015, 0.025, and 0.30 mg. of arsenious oxide (As_2O_3), and adding water and sulphuric or hydrochloric acid in such quantities as to maintain the same volume and acid strength as in the determination.

Conduct a blank test on the reagents alone; correct the result of any arsenic found. The blank should not exceed 0.001 mg.

Use the following reagents, as given in the Official and Tentative Methods of Analysis of the Association of Official Agricultural Chemists:

(a) Strong nitric acid: arsenic-free and containing not less than 67% nitric acid (HNO_3).

(b) Concentrated sulphuric acid: arsenic-free and containing not less than 93% sulphuric acid (H_2SO_4).

(c) Dilute sulphuric acid: dilute one volume of the arsenic-free concentrated acid with four volumes of water.

(d) Dilute hydrochloric acid: dilute one volume of arsenic-free, strong hydrochloric acid with three volumes of water.

(e) Zinc: break arsenic-free stick zinc into pieces approximately 1 cm. in length.

(f) Lead acetate paper: soak heavy filter paper in 20% lead acetate solution, dry, cut into pieces 4.5 cm. by 0.6 cm.

(g) Lead acetate cotton: soak absorbent cotton in 5% lead acetate solution.

(h) Mercuric bromide paper: cut heavy close-textured drafting paper (similar to Whatman's cold pressed) into strips exactly 2.5 mm. wide and approximately 12 cm. long. Soak for an hour in a 5% solution of mercuric bromide in 95% alcohol, squeeze out the excess solution, and dry on a glass rod. Cut off the ends of the strips before using.

(i) Potassium iodide solution: dissolve 20 gm. of potassium iodide in water and dilute to 100 cc.

(j) Stannous chloride solution: dissolve 40 gm. of arsenic-free stannous chloride crystals in sufficiently strong hydrochloric acid to make 100 cc.

(k) Standard arsenic solution: dissolve 1 gm. of arsenious oxide in 25 cc. of 20% sodium hydroxide solution, add about 375 cc. of air-free water, acidify with the dilute sulphuric acid, and dilute to one liter with air-free water. One cc. of this solution contains 1 mg. of arsenious oxide (As_2O_3).

Dilute 20 cc. of this solution to one liter. Make 50 cc. of the diluted solution to one liter and use to prepare the standard stains. Each cc. of the latter solution contains 0.001 mg. of arsenous oxide (As_2O_3). Prepare the dilute solutions immediately before use.

Various electrolytic methods have been recommended. The simplest known is that described by Mai and Hurt.[469] The sample is prepared as under the Marsh test and introduced in the apparatus as shown in Fig. 16. The advantages of the electrolytic detection of arsenic are, first, the avoidance of traces of arsenic that sometimes come from zinc in the Marsh test, and, second, the fact that destruction of organic matter is often unnecessary. This latter has been shown to be the case in the examination of beer worts and malt extracts for arsenic. To reduce arsenic acid and its salts, a few drops of zinc sulphate solution should be added to the sulphuric acid acting as the electrolyte. The cathode is said to have a higher tension and the hydrogen to be very active. A is the reduction tube and B a bulb tube with five or six bulbs containing 0.01 N silver nitrate solution. A and B are connected by a small tube containing pieces of pumice stone saturated with an alkaline lead solution, or glass wool, to retain any traces of hydrogen sulphide. Anode a and cathode e are lead strips 1 to 2 mm. thick. Their

469. MAI, C., and HURT, H.: Ztschr. f. Untersuch. d. Nahrungs.-u. Genussmittel, Berl., 9:193, 1905.

upper ends about 5 mm. thick are luted into glass tubes *b* which pass through the stopper of the U-tube and are tight. The dropping funnel *d* holds about 25 cc., and its capillary end dips about 2 cm. into the solution to be electrolyzed. Tube *c* for the escape of oxygen from the anode chamber, contains a little water. Fill U-tube to the mark with 12% arsenic-free sulphuric acid and bulb tube *B* with 10 cc. of 0.01 N silver nitrate solution. Turn on the current and keep at two to three amperes. If the silver nitrate solution remains unchanged after

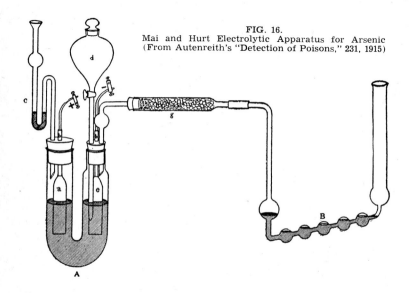

FIG. 16.
Mai and Hurt Electrolytic Apparatus for Arsenic
(From Autenreith's "Detection of Poisons," 231, 1915)

hydrogen has been running for one hour, the lead cathode and sulphuric acid are arsenic free. Without stopping the current, introduce from the dropping funnel the solution to be tested for arsenic, the quantity of which should not be more than 10 cc. Add this solution as slowly as possible, and wash the last traces in with a little water. If the solution contains arsenic, or arsenic acid, the silver nitrate solution will become dark in a few minutes and the reaction will be at an end in three hours. Pour the contents of the bulb tube through a small asbestos filter, wash with 3 to 4 cc. of water, and titrate the excess of 0.01 N silver nitrate with 0.01 N potassium sulphocyanate according to Volhard's method. One thousand cc. of 0.01 N silver nitrate are equivalent to 0.00125 gm. of arsenic.

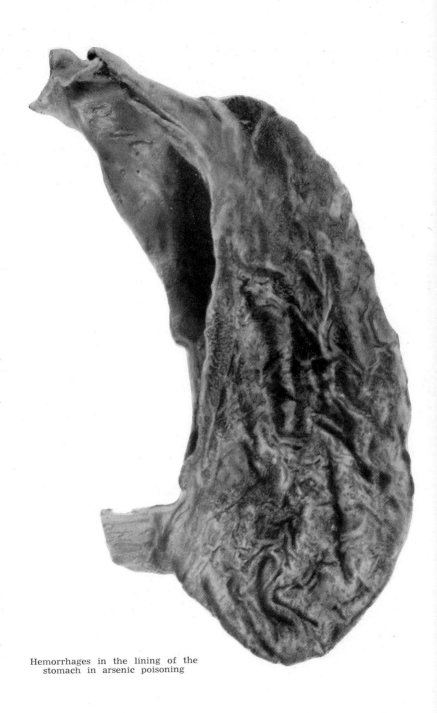

Hemorrhages in the lining of the
stomach in arsenic poisoning

ORGANIC ARSENICALS

IN THIS group there are included: cacodyl, 2As (C_3H_2), a poisonous, volatile, colorless liquid with a strong garlic odor; cacodylic acid, As (CH_3)$_2$ O_2H, a white crystalline substance, soluble, odorless, and comparatively non-poisonous although it contains 54% of arsenum; calcium-cacodylate, which contains about 45% of arsenum in the form of cacodylic acid and is free from arsenite, arsenate, and mono-methyl arsenate; iron-caco‧ dylate, Fe (CH_3) $_2AsO_2$)$_3$, a ferric salt of cacodylic acid containing about 42% of arsenum; and arrhenal, neo-arsykodile, arsynal which is disodium-methylarsenate, $CH_3.AsO. (ONa)_2$. Its arsenic content is 25.68% when crystallized. It is a white, odorless, water-soluble crystal. Arsenoferratin, sodium arsenoferri-albuminate is a compound of arsenic with ferri-albuminic acid. It contains ferric iron in an organic arsenical equivalent to 5% metallic iron and 0.06% arsenum. Arsenotrifferin is an iron arsenoparanucleate containing 16% of iron, 0.1% of arsenum, and 2.5% of phosphorus, all in organic combination. Arsindiphenylchlorid,[470] As(C_6H_5)$_2$Cl, a "sneezing gas"; arsinmethyldichlorid, As.CH_3.Cl_2, and arsinethyldichlorid, As-C_2H_5.Cl_2[471] were used alone and together in the late World War for filling explosive shells.

Sodium cacodylate, sodium dimethylarsenate, "arsykodile," (CH_3)$_2AsO.ONa.3H_2O$, is a white crystal or granular powder, with a faint odor of garlic, deliquescent, very soluble in water or alcohol. When anhydrous it contains 35% of arsenum. Sodium cacodylate occasionally causes poisoning when given in too large a dose intravenously. Very few instances of poisoning by other substances are seen as they have been entirely supplanted by the arsphenamine group. Their elimination and distribution are similar to arsphenamines and will be taken up later.

Detection: The cacodylates may be isolated from the tissues by the method of Vitali.[472] Take an aliquot portion of the finely divided tissue with water, acidify with tartaric or hydrochloric acid, and evaporate to dryness. Extract this residue two or three times with 90% alcohol, filter, distill off the alcohol from the filtrate and use the watery residue for further pro-

470. NORRIS: *J.A.M.A.*, 71:1823, 1918.
471. *J.A.M.A.*, 71:1825, 1918.
472. VITALI: *Boll. chim. farm.*, 40:657, 1901; 42:641, 1903.

cedures. Place the watery residue in a Kjehldal flask and heat with concentrated sulphuric acid or a crystal of potassium sulphate and two or three crystals of potassium permanganate, adding more of the potassium permanganate, if necessary, to complete the oxidation. Dilute the mixture, filter, neutralize as usual, and precipitate the arsenic with hydrogen sulphide.

Arsanilic acid is derived from arsenic acid, $AsO.(OH)_3$, by substituting anilin for one hydroxyl. Other compounds are made by similar substitution with anilin derivatives. Arsacetin is a white crystal, odorless, tasteless, and water soluble. It is not decomposed by heating for an hour at 130° C., and its solutions are stable even when boiled. It gives no reaction of arsenous or arsenic acid, and is less toxic than sodium arsanilate or sodium para-amidophenylarsenic acid. This latter, sold under trade names "Atoxyl" and "Soamin," is a white, odorless, water-soluble crystal with an arsenic content of 23% to 30%. If given by mouth, atoxyl is decomposed by the gastric acids, and poisoning may result. It is best given hypodermically in doses of .02 to .2 gm. (1/3 to 3 grains) every other day, increasing to single doses of .65 gm. (10 grains). Schlecht[473] reported a fatal case in a man who had taken 2.4 gm. in four hypodermic injections within eight days, and died on the second day after the last injection, with edema of the lungs and paralytic phenomena. The autopsy revealed such cardiac and hepatic degenerations as are seen in arsenic poisoning. Most of it is eliminated by the urine, unchanged. Some is found in the feces. The cadaver of a poisoned animal[474] showed inorganic arsenic in liver, kidneys, lungs, bile, blood, spleen, muscles, brain, and hair.

Tests: After prolonged boiling the Reinsch test will show the presence of arsenic. After the tissues have been destroyed by sulphuric or nitric acid, the resulting solution responds to the Marsh and Gutzeit test. With silver nitrate it does not yield the red arsenate of silver, but a white precipitate of silver arsanilate soluble in nitric acid or ammonia. It can be detected by the electrolytic method. For the quantitative determination prepare as for a Marsh test using the electrolytic apparatus described by Thorpe:* an electrolytic cell with a perforated cone made of thin lead foil as cathode and a strip of platinum

473. SCHLECHT: *München. med. Wchnschr.*, 56:972, 1909.
474. *Bull. Soc. pharm., Bordeaux*, 20:443, 1908.
* *Proc. Chem. Soc.*, 19:183, 1903.

foil as anode. The cathode is suspended in the cathode chamber by a platinum wire fused in the glass stopper.

CARBARSONE

P-CARBAMINO-PHENYL arsenic acid ($H_2O_3As . C_6H_4NH-CONH_2$) has a theoretical arsenic content of 28.85%. It appears as a white, crystalline, odorless solid, stable in air, and having a slightly acid taste, practically insoluble in water but soluble in carbonate or bicarbonate solutions; amebicidal in vitro at one to 4,000. Although no damage to the optic tract has been observed with therapeutic doses, the possibility of such injury should be kept in mind in its further clinical use. In its use in amebiasis, the average adult is given 0.25 gm. twice daily after meals for ten days. A large dose should be planned only on the basis of body weight, and the dosage for children should be determined accordingly. It should not be administered in amebic hepatitis or in the presence of liver or kidney damage. Epstein,[475] reported a woman aged fifty-five who died from an overdose of carbarsone.

TRYPARSAMIDE

TRYPARSAMIDE is a white, odorless, crystalline powder, freely soluble in water, and under ordinary conditions is uniform. The dried salt should contain, by analysis, not less than 25.1% nor more than 25.5% of arsenic (As), and not less than 9.25% nor more than 9.6% of nitrogen (N). It is used for intravenous injection in connection with other medication for the treatment of syphilis of the central nervous system. It has caused urticarial reactions and mild dermatitis and jaundice. Patients complain occasionally of dizziness, ringing of the ears, or a feeling of being dazed. It should not be given by mouth with nephritis. There is no difficulty in the administration of this compound if instructions are followed. The eyes should be examined before the administration of this preparation, since ocular disturbances occur occasionally from the administration. Some of these might already have been present due to the infection. The patient complains that his vision is blurred. At times bright flashes appear before the eyes, at other times dark spots. Treatment at such a time should be stopped until the condition clears up. However, I have given tryparsa-

475. EPSTEIN, E.: *J.A.M.A.*, 106:767, 1936.

mide in cases where a diplopia was present which cleared up during the course of treatment.

ARSPHENAMIN

ARSPHENAMIN (U. S.), salvarsan (Germany), arsenoben-zol (France), diarsenol (Canada), arsaminol (Japan), correspond to 31.57% arsenum in a trivalent form. Neo-arsphenamin (U.S.), neosalvarsan (Germany), neodiarsanol (Canada), neokharsivan (England), novarsenobenzol (France), nearsaminol (Japan) are a combination of arsphenamine with sodium formaldehyde sulphoxylate mixed with inert inorganic salts. Three parts of neo-arsphenamin are about equal in arsenic content to two parts of arsphenamin. It has about 20% of arsenum. Silver arsphenamin is sold in closed tubes to exclude air. The arsenic content is about 22%, the silver about 14%.

These compounds have a much less toxic effect on animals than mineral arsenicals. Since the introduction of arsphenamin by Ehrlich, in 1909, I have seen numerous cases of poisoning and deaths. If they are introduced in too large doses, the impurities are responsible for the untoward action. The organic arsenicals such as arsphenamin and its derivatives liberate trivalent arsenic slowly while they are stored in the tissues and by this mechanism the substance exerts its action over a long period of time on the invading organism.

Properties: It is a pale-yellow, odorless powder, micro-crystalline, hygroscopic, decomposing readily in air, dissolving in water freely, imparting an acid reaction. When sodium hydroxide solution is added in the proportion of two molecules to one, the free base is precipitated. On further addition, aided by shaking, the precipitate redissolves in the strongly alkaline fluid. Arsphenamin may be marketed officially only in sealed colorless glass ampoules containing an inert gas. It is useful in the treatment of syphilis, and is also recommended for other spirochetal diseases, such as frambesia and relapsing fever. It is usually given intravenously. It should never be given in its acid solution, hence at the time of administration the dose is neutralized with normal sodium hydroxide by a careful technique, which redissolves in alkaline excess the basic precipitate. The sealed ampoules should not be opened unless used immediately, as oxidation sets in very rapidly. Any solution that remains after injection should be discarded at once.

Dosage: The dose varies according to age, sex, and condition of the patient. As the first dose 0.15 gm. is given, increasing gradually to 0.6 gm. Many of the fatalities which I have seen were due to an administration of 0.9 gm. Death occurred after the third or fourth administration of this dose. Because of the numerous accidents which have taken place with this preparation, it has been supplanted by neo-arsphenamin. Following an injection the patient should be allowed to rest before leaving an office or a clinic. In the treatment of syphilis some mercurial or bismuth adjuvant is given as a follow-up course.

Fatal Dose: Roth[476] showed that the minimal lethal dose given to rabbits or rats intravenously averaged 0.1 to 0.15 gm. per kilo, which is equivalent to 7 to 10.5 gm. for a man weighing 70 kilos (150 pounds). Corlett[477] collected reports of 126 deaths from its use in such a number of cases as to rate the mortality one death to 18,000 injections. This estimate is high, as is shown in the following figures of Levedde:

Year	Number of Injections	Deaths
1910	50,000	16
1911	800,000	92
1912	1,280,000	66
1913	2,000,000	37

The majority of deaths are due to a developing hemorrhagic encephalitis or myelitis which is caused by arsphenamin. Careless manipulation by the physician may lead to the formation of organic arsenicals of high toxicity. The toxicity of the substance is greatly influenced by the manner of preparation at the time of injection. The shaking of the substance may render it very toxic. Biological tests are resorted to in determining the safety of the drug before it is marketed. In fixing the standard of toxicity permissible, the U. S. Public Health Service requires that 75% of the rats shall tolerate a dose of 50 to 100 mg. per kilogram of bodyweight. Toxic effects occasionally encountered were ascribed to the compound p. oxyphenylarsenoxid ("arsenoxid") formed by oxidation changes on exposure to air. Most of the untoward results following the use of arsphenamin have been due to too large a dose, or too rapid injection.

476. ROTH: Bull. 113, U. S. Hyg. Lab., Washington, 10, 1918; Reprint 688, Pub. Health Reports, 1990, 1921.
477. CORLETT: *J.A.M.A.*, 61:961, 1913.

Toxic reactions are manifested by vertigo, taste and smell. Most serious reactions which may become fatal are seen, such as in dermatitis exfoliativa, jaundice, syphilis, and gangrene. Occasionally, infiltration about the vein, either of blood or blood plus the solution of the salvarsan, will cause pain which may remain for several days, leaving a lump which may be present for months. Such accidents cause thrombosis, and phlebitis; they are not common, but may happen with the best of operators. If the injection has been given too rapidly, the patient may show signs of distress, such as dyspnea and redness of the face. These usually cause considerable concern to the physician but soon pass off. Death has occurred within a few minutes after the administration of arsphenamin and neo-arsphenamin. A patient may take three or four doses and become ill with nausea and dysentery.

In a series of forty-two fatal cases which I have collected, twenty-eight occurred following the fourth dose. Nephritis, local paralysis, loss of hearing and sight due to the neuritis of the auditory and optic nerves have been reported. Luithlen[478] reported the contra-indications, which include tuberculosis, chronic alcoholism, nicotinism, plumbism, severe gastro-intestinal and nervous diseases, and pregnancy. Studying 274 fatalities, including forty-one in non-syphilitics, from injections of arsphenamin he concluded that the prompt primary symptoms were due to the whole organic arsenical. Fatal results have befallen feeble patients, especially those subject to diseases of the heart and vessels, fetid bronchitis, and advanced nervous syphilis.

Symptoms: The symptoms following the injections of arsphenamin have been classified by Martin[479] as, first, slight untoward incidents in those whose tolerance is normal: vertigo, palpitations, nausea, disturbances of taste and smell; second, reactions in syndromes of discomfort and incapacity ascribed to allergy or acquired susceptibility or to toxicity of the solution; third, grave reactions, sometimes fatal, such as dermatitis exfoliativa, jaundice, hermorrhages, encephalitis, gangrene; and fourth, accidents such as thrombosis, phlebitis, or infiltrations about the vein.

Occasionally just at the time or after receiving an intra-

478. LUITHLEN: *Ztschr. f. exper. Path. u. Therap., Berl.*, 13:495, 1914.
479. MARTIN: *J.A.M.A.*, 74:1218, 1920.

venous injection the patient may have a crisis of redness of face, dyspnea, distress, precordial pain, or it may take the form of chill and fever. These reactions may be slight and pass off within ten minutes, or they may end fatally. Gordon and Feldman,[480] and Roch[481] found six cases of syphilitic meningitis after arsphenamine injections. The adverse arsenical results can be explained on the ground that the patient has small individual eliminative powers for arsenical preparations—liver injury of any kind manifested by jaundice whether it be due to syphilis, cirrhosis, cancer, hepatitis, cholecystitis or cholelithiasis; focal infections, infected teeth, tonsils, sinuses, or asthmatic conditions; acute febrile infections, acute or chronic nephritis, arteriosclerosis, pernicious anemia. To explain them a theory has been advanced that they are due to precipitates in the blood which may result in pulmonary embolism. Berman[482] regarded these precipitates as compounds of protein due to increased protein content in certain syphilitics, and designated them as nitritoid crises. In the immediate or nitritoid types the reaction is similar to vaso-paresis and the milder grades of nitrite action. The symptoms begin during or immediately after the injection, and usually start with an erythema on the upper chest, which soon extends to the face and neck; it is followed by a sense of constriction in the chest and fullness in the head; dilation of the pupils; congested conjunctiva; coughing, rapid pulse, and backache. In a study of these cases Schamberg, Tokuda, and Kolmer[483] discovered that these precipitates were formed only when acid solutions of arsphenamin were added to serum, plasma, or defibrinated blood. Alkaline solutions of arsphenamin, that did not produce them in serum, did in some cases cause the immediate reactions when injected intravenously. Variations in alkalinity might explain varying reactions of the patients. Accidents from the administration of arsphenamin are very few, since this preparation is given chiefly in clinics where it is properly prepared. Epinephrin given intravenously has proved helpful as a prophylactic. One-tenth mg. of atropine has been used with good results, when the salvarsan is given in fractions an hour apart.

480. GORDON and FELDMAN: *J.A.M.A.*, 83:1310, 1924.
481. ROCH: Abst., *J.A.M.A.*, 82:1482, 1924.
482. BERMAN: *Arch. Int. Med.*, 22:127, 1918.
483. SCHAMBERG, TOKUDA, and KOLMER: *Arch. Dermat. & Syph.*, 3:263, 1921; also SCHAMBERG, KOLMER, and RAIZISS: *Ibid.*, 1:235, 1920.

The early toxic reactions are quite common, and start in from one to four hours with a chill and febrile symptoms, headache, nausea, vomiting, and diarrhea.

Rabbits weighing 1,600 to 2,500 gm. were given several intravenous injections of 0.1 to 0.6 gm, of novarsenobenzene.

TABLE XXIV
Distribution of Arsenic in Organs in Deaths Attributed to Arsphenamin and Neo-Arsphenamin
AS_2O_3 per 100 Grams of Tissue

No.	Stomach	Liver	Kidney	Comments
1.	.00039	.0052	.0001	trace in the heart
2.	trace	trace	trace	trace in the urine, less than 1 ppm.
3.	.0001	.0052	.0001	
4.		.0243	.0229	Bowel and content 2 ppm. Died in office after injection.
5.		.0078	.0016	
6.	2ppm	3ppm		Bowel and content 1 ppm. Died three days after .9 gm. arsphenamin was injected.
7.	.0005		.0013	Bowel 0.00211. Woman was given two shots of 0.4 gm. of neo-salvarsan eight days apart. Died two days after the last injection. Blood contained 0.00132 As_2O_3.
8.		.0033	(.0052 lt. (.0042 rt.	Brain less than 1 ppm; heart 1 ppm.
9.	.0001	.0002	.0001	Bowel 1 ppm; patient died three days after 0.9 gm. had been administered.
10.	.0001	.00036	.0128	Bowel 2 ppm; urine before death 100 cc. contained .0042; urine after death thirty-six hours later contained 0.0006.
11.	2 ppm	.0013	.0001	This man had three shots of .6 gm., and died after the fourth injection, had an enlarged thymus.
12.	1 ppm	.004.. (.0087(139 gm.) (.0089(130 gm.)	.0004	Bowel .0004. Patient was given .6 gm. neo-salvarsan on March 8, and again on March 12, dying on March 17.

Sclerosis of the glomeruli was produced in those which did not die immediately, and sometimes hepatic lesions. Other effects were relatively unimportant.[484]

Distribution and Elimination: In cases dying from the administration of salvarsan and neo-salvarson, I have found that elimination is very slow, as is noted in the last case. The

484. Pasteur Vallery-Radot, Gilbrin, E. Gauthier-Villars: *Comp. rend. Soc. de biol.,* 119:833, 1935.

patient was given the last dose on March 12, dying at 1:30 A.M. on March 17, five days later. The chemical examination disclosed an unusualy large amount of arsenic in both of the kidneys, 0.0087 gm. arsenic trioxide in one, and 0.0089 gm. in the other. Traces of arsenic have been found in the urine within one-half hour after a dose of arsphenamin, and usually disappeared after one or two weeks. Shephard[485] found arsphenamin in the urine 111 days after having taken neo-salvarsan. Watson[486] states that he found traces of arsenic in the urine fifteen months after a course of ten injections of novarsobenzol.

Postmortem Appearances: Pearce and Brown[487] showed that fatal doses of arsenic trioxide and of the organic arsenicals cause kidney lesions which are separable into two extreme groups. In one would be the red kidney of arsenic trioxide, congestion, hemorrhage, and capillary changes with only slight tubular necrosis. The other would be a pale kidney showing that tubular nephritis has dominated the congestion. Grossly in many of the cases there will be little seen in the examination of the liver, kidneys, stomach and bowel.

NEO-ARSPHENAMIN

NEO-ARSPHENAMIN (U. S.), neosalvarsan, "914" (Germany), neo-diarsenol (Canada), neokharsivan (England), novarsenobenzol (France), and neo-arsaminol (Japan), is a combination of arsphenamin with sodium formaldehyde sulphoxylate mixed with inert inorganic salts. It is an orange-yellow unstable powder, changing rapidly in air to a dark brown color. Neo-arsphenamin is less stable both in the ampoule and in solution than arsphenamin and sulpharsphenamin. An accident to the ampoule will lead to oxidation of the drug. Solutions of neo-arsphenamin oxidize very rapidly on standing. The same precaution should be used in the administration of neo-arsphenamin as with arsphenamin. Arsphenamin reactions have been described and discussed in detail by Cole and Ireland.[488] Because of its comparative safety neo-arsphenamin is the better product to use in the office. One should begin with small doses to obtain the tolerance of the

485. SHEPHARD: *Lancet*, 1922.
486. WATSON, C.: *Lancet*, 1922.
487. PEARCE and BROWN: *Proc. Nat. Acad. Sc.*, 1:463, 1915.
488. COLE, N. H.: *J.A.M.A.*, 97:897, 1931; IRELAND, F. A.: *Am. J. Syph.*, 16:22, 1932.

patient. Ampoules of sterile, cool, double-distilled water are used to make the solution. Untoward reactions are seldom seen. From my experience, I believe that 0.9 gm. of either of these two preparations should be used only in exceptional cases. The maximum dose for women should be 0.45 gm., and for men 0.6 gm. With ordinary care and with elimination of those having contra-indications, few mishaps will occur.

Fatal Dose: Roth[489] proved that variation in individual susceptibility is quite marked, that toxicity closely parallels the arsenic content, and that neo-arsphenamin is less toxic than arsphenamin. The minimal lethal dose for rabbits and rats averaged from 0.13 to 0.2 gm. per kilo, which is equivalent to 9 to 14 gm. for a man weighing 70 kilos (150 pounds). Much smaller amounts have caused death, as in the case of M.D. (87), where 0.6 gm. of salvarsan was given, and, after the second dose, death occurred within four days. In this case mercury was used in conjunction with arsenic. The toxicity is practically the same as that of arsphenamin, differing, however, in degree and in the lower frequency of alarming reactions at the time of administration. The research of Schamberg, Kolmer and Raiziss[490] demonstrated that the difference of toxicity is proportionally greater than that of the arsenic content.

Delayed Symptoms: Some cases have been reported where the symptoms appeared several days after the third or fourth injection. In such cases jaundice is usually the outstanding symptom. Milian treated sixty cases of this kind in which the jaundice had appeared several weeks after the arsenical course had ceased. Arsenic and mercury are given in the course of treatment, and there is no doubt but that the mercury has some effect on the untoward action of the arsphenamin. A fatal case of jaundice in a woman after a single dose of 0.122 gm. of neo-arsphenamin was reported by Hyman.[491] I have seen a number of cases in which death occurred after a dose of 0.9 gm. of arsphenamin and neo-arsphenamin had been administered. A series of delayed poisonings has been reported by Strathy, Smith and Hannah.[492] The toxic symptoms developed after an interval averaging forty-three days from the last treatment

489. ROTH: Bull. 113, U. S. Hyg. Lab., Washington, 34-40, 1918.
490. SCHAMBERG, KOLMER, and RAIZISS: *Am. J. M. Sc.*, 160:188, 1920.
491. HYMAN: *New York Med. J.*, 112:496, 1920.
492. STRATHY, SMITH, and HANNAH: *Lancet*, 1:80, 1920.

with neo-arsphenamin. Jaundice was present in all of the eight fatalities, and in thirty-nine of the non-fatal cases. Exfoliative dermatitis was noted in eight cases. The medication consisted of intensive doses of neo-arsphenamin intravenously and of mercurial oil intramuscularly each once a week for seven or eight weeks. Most of the necropsies showed nephritis and hepatic atrophy. This emphasizes the fact that the administration of large doses of neo-arsphenamin and mercury produces more after effects. It can be explained on the grounds that the kidney is damaged by the massive doses of mercury, and becomes unable to eliminate the arsenic as it does when the neo-arsphenamin is given alone. It is better to give a course of neo-arsphenamin and then follow up by a course of mercury or bismuth.

Elimination: Elimination is the same as that reported under arsphenamin.

Postmortem Appearances: Postmortem appearances are the same as those seen under arsphenamin. Kolmer and Lucke[493] found that the histologic changes included vascular injury, cellular degenerations, and necrosis. They involved the nervous and circulatory organs, the liver, lungs, kidneys, spleen, and suprarenals.

SODIUM ARSPHENAMIN

SODIUM DIARSENOL: In this preparation the arsphenamin has been neutralized in advance, thus dispensing with the addition of sodium hydroxide at the time of administration. It causes the chain of symptoms as given under arsphenamin.

SILVER ARSPHENAMIN

ARGENTUM ARSPHENAMINA: Silver arsphenamin is a combination of sodium arsphenamin and silver, containing 20% of arsenic and about 15% of silver. It is claimed that this preparation continues in solution in the blood and body fluids for a long time.[494] In the treatment of syphilis it is given in 0.1 gm. to 0.3 gm. at intervals of twenty-four hours to four days. Many authors claim that it does not offer any definite advantages over arsphenamin. On account of this preparation being

493. KOLMER and LUCKE: Arch. Dermat. & Syph., 3:483, 515, 1921.
494. KOLLE and RITZ: Deutsche med. Wchnschr., 45:481, 1919;
KOLLE and RITZ: Zentralbl. Biochem. u. Biophys., 21:240, 1919.

used much less than the other arsphenamins, little has been reported upon its toxicity. A few after-effects have been mentioned, as icterus and argyria. A few patients so treated had mild headache, chill, nausea, vomiting, and gastric disturbances.

SULPHARSPHENAMIN

DISODIUM - diamino - dihydroxy - arseno - benzen - n - dimethylene-sulphonate, mixed with inert salt to an arsenic content of 19 to 24%. It is an orange-yellow powder, readily soluble in water, yielding a yellow acid solution. Combes[495] reports the case of a man fifty-four years of age who had beginning tabes. The Wassermann was four plus. He had been treated with a saturated solution of potassium iodide, 4 cc. three times a day and mercurial inunctions. Later he was given bismuth and sulpharsphenamin. Treatments were started on June 4 and continued through July and August. September 9 a blood transfusion was made which, however, failed to give results, the patient soon dying. No autopsy was permitted.

Methods of Determination: Lehman's Method:[496] After the sample has been digested, add to the solution very cautiously, while still hot, dilute hydrochloric acid to precipitate silver chloride. Through a tared asbestos Gooch crucible filter off the silver chloride, wash, dry, and weigh. From the weight of chloride, which should be about 15%, the filtrate is used for the determination of the arsenic content which should be about 20%.

Weigh out accurately about 0.2 gm. of the substance and transfer to a 200-cc. Erlenmeyer flask. Add 1 gm. of powdered potassium permanganate and 5 cc. of dilute sulphuric acid and let it stand for ten minutes, covered with a watch glass or a glass stopper. Rotate the flask frequently. Add 2 cc. of concentrated sulphuric acid in several additions until 10 cc. of acid has been added, rotating the flask after each addition. When there is no longer any reaction, add about 5 cc. to 7 cc. hydrogen peroxide solution, which should be sufficient to dissolve the brown precipitate. Dilute the liquid with 25 cc. of distilled water and boil over gauze carefully for ten minutes, to remove the excess hydrogen peroxide. To prevent the formation of a brownish coloration, if the evaporation has been car-

495. COMBES, F. C.: *Arch. Dermat. & Syph.*, 15:194, 1927.
496. LEHMAN: *Apoth. Ztg.*, 27:545, 1912.

ried too far to remove the excess, the last trace of hydrogen peroxide can be removed by the addition of a drop of 1% solution of potassium permanganate, clearing up the pink color by adding a small amount of oxalic acid solution. After diluting with 50 cc. more of distilled water, the solution is cooled and 2.5 gm. of potassium iodide are added. The flask is stoppered tightly and allowed to stand in a cool place for one hour. Finally, the free iodine is titrated with $N/10$ sodium thiosulphate volumetric solution. One cc. of $N/10$ sodium thiosulphate solution is equivalent to 0.003748 gm. of arsenum.

Robertson's Method: Robertson[497] has a two-hour method in which the substance is oxidized with a mixture of nitric and sulphuric acids, and then freed from nitrous compounds by use of ammonium sulphate, reduced with hydriodic acid and titrated with standard iodine.

Hiramatsu[498] bases the determination of salvarsan on osmic acid changes which produce a black discoloration when mixed with arsenic. The shading is proportional to the amount of salvarsan present. In aqueous solution salvarsan may be discovered by merely adding three drops of a 1% osmic acid solution in 0.1 cc. A quantity of 0.0005 mg. of neoarsaminol can be detected in this manner. For determining salvarsan quantities in the blood, 0.1 cc. of blood is diluted in 0.3 cc. distilled water, adding 20% sulphosalicylic acid, and then filtering. Three drops of a 1% osmic acid solution are added to the filtered mixture. Such a specimen is compared with one containing neoarsaminol. As little as 0.002 mg. can be detected. The test may be used on the cerebrospinal fluid.

Estimation: Arsphenamin and neo-arsphenamin may be extracted from the tissues by the method described under sodium cacodylate, or by diluting with acidified alcohol. After filtration and evaporation of the alcohol, the residue is submitted to digestion with ammonium persulphate or arsenic acid. The arsenic then is determined by the same method as for the estimation of inorganic arsenic. Or use the official method,* digesting 0.2 gm. of the sample with 10 gm. of K_2SO_4, 0.3 gm. of starch, and 20 cc. of H_2SO_4. Then estimate with standard iodine after neutralization.

497. ROBERTSON: *J. Am. Chem. Soc.*, 43:182, 1921.
498. HIRAMATSU, TSURUKICHI: *Sei-I-Kwai M. J.*, 48:7, 5.
* Methods of Analysis, A.O.A.C., 591, 1936.

COPPER (Cu)
(Atomic Weight 63.6. Synonym: Cuprum)

COPPER has specific gravity, 8.914; melted, 8.921; natural crystals, 8.94; rolled and hammered sheet, 8.952 to 8.958. Its melting point is 1080.5°C. It is a red metal, but thin sheets transmit a greenish-blue light. It is found native in various parts of the world, and especially in the region of Lake Superior. It is found chiefly as sulphides in enormous quantities in Montana, Colorado, Chile, and Spain; as a carbonate in Arizona.

In 1934 there was 1,478,640,000 pounds of copper produced in the mines, 488,454,107 at smelters, 466,058,360 at refineries. In 1933 there was 25,436,881 pounds of copper hydrous, copper sulphate, or blue stone, produced in the United States. Copper industrially is used in electrical wires, in automobiles, buildings, home equipment, ammunition, and miscellaneous other uses.

In spite of the enormous uses of copper we seldom have cases of poisoning. Copper salts, such as the sulphates, are occasionally used for homicidal purposes. Poisoning from copper is rarely accidental except through the formation of the sub-acetate (verdigris) on poorly cleaned copper pipes or vessels. Copper salts have been used to impart a lively green color to pickled cucumbers, spinach, peas, and beans. Some authors believe that it forms an insoluble non-poisonous compound with chlorophyl. However, the investigation of the United States Department of Agriculture led to the conviction that copper sulphate used for the greening of vegetables is injurious.[499] The Department regards as adulterated all foods so treated, and forbids their importation or shipment by interstate commerce. This action was based on the report of the Referee Board of Consulting Scientific Experts.[500]

Symptoms: When a soluble salt of copper has been taken, there is a metallic taste, a sensation of burning, vomiting, diarrhea, extreme weakness, and inability to hold water or milk upon the stomach for a number of hours. The breathing is difficult, there is an intense thirst, cold perspiration, and severe headache. The vomitus is colored green or blue and may be

---

499. Food Inspection Decision, December 26, 1912, Washington, D. C.
500. Report No. 97, U. S. Dept. of Agriculture, 1913, *J.A.M.A.*, January, 1934, p. 132.

blood-tinged.   Headache, exhaustion, and giddiness occasionally occur among brass grinders.

Chronic poisoning may result from the absorption of small
amounts of copper from copper vessels that are not kept clean
or in foods that contain amounts in excess of that necessary to
color them.   The symptoms of chronic copper poisoning may
consist of anemia, loss of appetite, nausea, vomiting, colic, and
diarrhea.

Mallory and his associates[501] reported the relation of chronic copper poisoning to a disease known as hemochromatosis or
bronzed diabetes.   The disease is characterized by cirrhosis of
the liver, diabetes mellitus, and brown pigmentation of the
skin, liver, and pancreas.   Mallory[502] found that copper inhaled
in the form of dust or swallowed is dangerous to life, unless its
action is exceedingly slow.   Copper is widely distributed in the
animal and vegetable kingdom, and is found in all the tissues
of the body.   Small amounts do not harm, but larger amounts
as copper dust or the absorption of copper salts over a long period are regarded as dangerous.   Mallory from animal experimentation explained the pigmented cirrhosis of the liver on
the ground that copper dust caused a hemolysis of the red blood
cells as its chief action.   Some of the hemoglobin from the destroyed corpuscles is eliminated by the kidney.   Some of it is
distributed in the liver and pancreas as hemofuscin.

E. H. Funk and H. St. Claire[503] reported a case of hemochromatosis without diabetes in which the liver contained 331.8
mg. of copper.   Less than 1 mg. of copper was found in the
spleen.   They found, in the liver of a person not working in
metals, 9 mg. per kilo and not less than 1 mg. per kilo.

Andrianoff[504] reported experimental cirrhosis of the liver
caused by the presence of copper in food.[505]

Tests: W. Gerlach,[506] found in the examination of the liver
in seven healthy people, 3 to 13 gamma.   The copper content of
the liver varies in the fetal period between 15 gamma and 250
gamma.   At the end of the first year the liver contains more

501. *J. Med. Research, Balt.*, 42:461, 1921.
502. *Arch. Int. Med.*, 37:366, 1926.
503. *Arch. Int. Med.*, 45:37, 1930.
504. ANDRIANOFF: *Schweiz. med. Wchnschr.*, 60:421, 1930.
505. See also OSHIMA, F., and SEIBERT, P.: *Beitr. z. path. Anat. u.
z. allg. Path.*, 84:106, 1930.
506. *Virchows Arch. f. path Anat.*, 294:171, 1934.

copper than in adult life (20 gamma). Placenta tissue contains from 1 to 10 gamma, the average in liver cirrhosis equals 28.3 gamma, while in T. Bc. the average content equals 15.4 gamma. The spleen is poor in copper, average 2.6 gamma, the limit being 1 to 10 gamma. The lungs show 2.5 gamma, both in fetus and adult; the kidneys 2.98 gamma in adult, in fetus it is 3.84. The copper content of the heart, brain, pancreas, skin, and bones is between 1 and 0.6 gamma copper.

J. M. Inonye and F. B. Flinn[507] recommend for the determination of copper in biologic material the following: The sample is weighed and dried, then ashed in a fused quartz or porcelain dish. Concentrated nitric acid is added and this taken to dryness. Nitric acid is again added and then diluted to 100 to 150 cc. with water. Digest on the electric plate for about one hour, and filter through an ashless filter paper (9 to 12.5 cm.). The insoluble residue is treated in a fused quartz crucible with 1 cc. concentrated nitric acid, ignited, diluted with water, and filtered. This is repeated. To the combined filtrates, add a few drops of concentrated sulphuric acid, to keep the iron present in solution, and any precipitated sulphates are removed by filtration. Evaporate to about 200 cc. and transfer to a 250-cc. beaker. The copper is deposited from this solution electrolytically. The cathode is a platinum gauze (52 mesh, height 2 in., diameter 1 in.). The anode is a platinum spiral. Clean the electrodes with concentrated nitric acid, wash with water and redistilled alcohol, and ignite to insure a surface free from organic matter.

The electrodes are fastened by means of aluminum screws to a bar of pure aluminum and placed in the copper solution. A current of three volts and 1.5 amperes is used for five or six such cells and allowed to run over night. In the morning the level of the solution is raised and run for twenty minutes to test the completeness of the deposition. The gauze is washed quickly with water and alcohol, and removed before turning off the current. It is then dried and weighed.

Check by dissolving the copper from the electrode in nitric acid, and heating. Treat this solution with ammonia water until a blue color is produced. Then glacial acetic acid is added until the blue color disappears, plus 1 cc. in excess. An excess of potassium iodide (1 to 2 cc. of 25%) is added, and the liber-

507. *J. Lab. & Clin. Med.*, 16:49, 1920.

ated iodine titrated with 0.005 N thiosulphate solution using starch as an indicator. At the same time a control titration is run, using a solution of copper nitrate, obtained by the electro-deposition of the copper from a known quantity of copper sulphate. The accuracy is 0.02 mg.

E. Cherbuliez and S. Anabacher[508] recommend separation of the copper as the sulphide. Dissolve the copper sulphide with nitric acid, evaporating to dryness, and take up with water and titrate with nitrosa-chromotropic acid, 1 cc. of which equals 10.1 gamma of copper. This reagent is prepared as follows:

Dissolve in a small amount of water 1.8 dioxy, 2 nitrosa, 3.6 naphtholindisulfonic acid (nitrosachromotropic acid), 0.37 g. sodium chromotropate (Kahlbaum). Add 1 cc. N/2 sodium carbonate (212 gm. in liter) 0.5, 0.6 cc. N/2 sodium nitrite (138 gm. $NaNO_2$ in liter) and dilute acetic acid in excess. Stand twenty-four hours, filter, and add Na_2CO_3 to weak alkalinity. Dilute to 100 cc. Take 34 cc. and dilute to one liter with water and 50 cc. ethyl alcohol. This solution is brown. With copper a permanganate color is obtained; 1 cc. equals 10.1 gamma copper.

After separation the copper may be determined volumetrically by reduction with grape sugar and subsequent titration with ferric chloride and permanganate, iodimetric-determination after precipitation as cuprous iodide. The last method is based on the fact that when potassium iodide is mixed with a salt of copper in acid solution cuprous iodide is precipitated as a dirty white powder and iodine is set free. The free iodine can be titrated with thiosulphate and starched. Each cc. of an entio sulphate is 0.006357 gm. of copper.

Copper also may be determined colorimetrically using a potassium ferrocyanide, which gives a purple brown color with very dilute solutions of copper. One part of copper in a neutral solution containing ammonium nitrate can be detected in 2,500,-000 parts of water.[509] The delicacy of the micro-chemical test for copper with mercuriammonium thiocyanate in the presence of other metals was described by Korenman and Lukashevich.*

508. *Virchows Arch. f. path. Anat.*, 278, 1930.

509. See also INOUYE, J. M., and FLINN, F. B.: *J. Lab. & Clin. Med.*, 16:49, 1930; SPRINGER, J. W.: *Ztschr. f. Untersuch. d. Lebensmitt*, 58:651, 1929; KLEINMANN, H., and KLINKE, J.: *Virchows Arch. f. path. Anat.*, 275:422, 1930; CALLAN, T., and HENDERSON, J. A. R., *Analyst*, 54:650, 1929; PRING, M. E., and SPENCER, J. F.: *Analyst*, 54:509, 1929.

   * KORENMAN, I. M., and LUKASHEVICH, E. N.:   C. A. 31:2959, 1937, also C. A. 28, 429.

BISMUTH (Bi)
(Atomic Weight 208.1)

BISMUTH has a specific gravity of 9.7474, a melting point of 269.22° C. It vaporizes at 1700° C. It is a hard, brittle, reddish-white lustrous metal, and forms beautiful rhombohedral crystals. Alloys of bismuth with other metals give compounds of remarkably low melting points, an alloy of: Bi two, tin one, and lead one, parts by weight, melts at 93.7°C.[510]

Few cases of poisoning by bismuth are seen by the toxicologist. Stomatitis and other forms of bismuth poisoning have been observed since the use of bismuth salts in the treatment of lues. Blum[511] states that stomatitis appears to be most frequently observed, although gastro-intestinal, renal, and hepatic lesions have been observed. Toxic symptoms have been observed after the application of bismuth subnitrate to varicose ulcers, burns, etc.; this forms a soluble albuminate in contact with a raw surface. Black patches on the gums, tongue, and enteritis, and albuminuria have been reported. Eggenberger has published a fatal case in a child seven years of age, and Reich and Matsuoka have recorded fatal cases in which renal lesions were found at the autopsies. Poisoning by bismuth carbonate is much more rare than with the subnitrate. A case is recorded[512] in which symptoms of grave stomatitis and nephritis were observed after one intramuscular injection of bismuth. This is a very rare condition. Beck,[513] in a series of 1800 patients treated with a bismuth paste, reports the treatment without a single fatality. Pigmentation of the gums would be early evidence of poisoning by bismuth.

Elimination: Elimination is mainly by the gastro-intestinal tract and kidneys.

Postmortem Appearances: There will be found brownish-purple patches on the tongue, the lining of the mouth and throat. The teeth are loose, and the gums spongy, with a blue line more diffuse than that seen in lead poisoning. In a necropsy upon an individual dying six weeks after an ingestion of three ounces of bismuth-vaseline paste, Mayer and Baehr[514]

510. PRESCOTT and JOHNSON: Qualitative Chemical Analysis, 100, 1915.
511. BLUM, PAUL: Paris méd., July 29, 1922, p. 105.
512. Bull. et mém. Soc. méd. d hôp. de Paris, February, 1927.
513. BECK: J.A.M.A., 67:21, 1916.
514. MAYER and BAEHR: Surg., Gynec. & Obst., 15:309, 1912.

found the mucosa of the small intestine to show areas of inflammation and necrosis. The steel-gray color studied with a lens was seen to be stippled with fine black points. The large intestine was coated with a greenish-black membrane, while underneath there were ulceration and necrosis. The liver cells showed cloudy swelling and disintegration. The lumina of the kidneys were choked with cellular debris.

Fatal Dose: Death has followed a dose of two drams of a bismuth salt. Recovery has taken place from as large a dose as six drams.

Tests: Bismuth, if present, will be found in the Reinsch test. If the tissues have been digested according to the Fresenius and von Babo method, a black precipitate will be obtained with hydrogen sulphide. This precipitate is dissolved in hot nitrohydrochloric acid, and, poured into an excess of water, a white precipitate of bismuth oxychloride is obtained.

ANTIMONY (Sb)
(Atomic Weight 120.4. Synonym: Stibium)

ANTIMONY is a lustrous, silver-white, brittle, and readily pulverizable metal. It tarnishes but little in dry air and oxidizes slowly in moist air, forming a blackish-gray mixture of antimony and antimonous oxide. At a red heat it burns in the air or in oxygen with incandescence, forming white inodorous vapors of antimonous oxide. It has a melting point of 630°C. and a boiling point between 1090°C. and 1450°C. It occurs native in considerable quantities in northern Queensland, Australia, as stibnite; as valentinite; in many other minerals, usually as a double sulphide. It is used as an alloy in type metal, Brittania metal, brass, and bell metal. In the printers' trade the type contains from about 3% to 16% antimony in lead. It is also used in the compounding of rubber, with golden and crimson sulphides of antimony, which act partly as accelerators of vulcanization and partly as dyes to make red-brown rubber. Where it accompanies lead, it would be difficult to discover a case of antimonial poisoning, because the symptoms of lead poisoning are much the same, except where skin lesions appear.

Antimony resembles arsenic in its action, having an irritating effect on the skin and mucous membranes, causing eczema and other forms of dermatitis, and inflammation of the lining of the mouth, nose, and throat. Miller found that some of the cheaper gray enameled cooking utensils contributed antimony to various foods.[515] Acid substances such as cider and cranberries dissolved out from 3 to 14 mg., spinach 10 mg., and even fresh milk acquired 3 mg. It is used in the manufacture of storage battery plates, which, like printers' type, are made of an alloy of antimony and lead. Selisky[516] reported 200 cases, including some relapses, of industrial dermatitis in men who were using antimony salts as a mordant in dyeing cloth or who handled the dyed cloth. The lesions are described as a pustular necrotic dermatitis commencing usually as a folliculitis and ending in an atrophic scar. Seitz[517] found that foundries no longer use a metal containing arsenic as an impurity, but in the foundry the antimony which, next to lead, is the chief component of the dust, is an important factor in gastro-intestinal poisoning. The blood picture in experiments on animals with antimony, showed a reduction of neutrophiles, an increase in small lymphocytes, and an initial decrease in red blood cells, followed by an increase. Rambousek[518] refers to a workman in Hamburg engaged in pulverizing pure antimony who was attacked with vomiting lasting several days, and in another case nose-bleeding and vomiting were noted as following the crushing of antimony ore.

Antimony Trichloride: Antimony trichloride occurs as a strong solution of the chloride in hydrochloric acid; it is employed in the arts as a bronzing liquid, and as a constituent of many furniture polishes.

Antimony Chloride: Death has occurred from two ounces, and recovery has followed the administration of one ounce. A woman forty years of age died in less than two hours; a chemical examination showed the presence of eight grains of antimony and 1/10 grain of arsenic.

Tartar Emetic: Tartar emetic contains not less than 98.5% of $K(SbO)C_4H_4O_6.\frac{1}{2}H_2O$. It consists of colorless, odorless, transparent crystals of the rhombic system, or a white granular powder; the crystals effloresce upon exposure to air. It is made by the action of a boiling solution of cream of tartar upon antimony trioxide. It has fallen out of use as an emetic, its

515. MILLER: *J. Home Economics*: 8:561, 1916.
516. SELISKY, A. B.: *Dermat. Wchnschr.*, 86:723, 1928; Abst. *J. Indust. Hyg.*, 11:125, 1929.
517. SEITZ, A.: *Arch. f. Hyg.*, 94:284, 1924.
518. RAMBOUSEK: Industrial Poisoning, 146, 1913.

action being too slow and too depressing. The emetic dose is 0.03 gm. It is employed mainly as a depressant expectorant in the first stages of acute bronchitis, often in the form of Wine of Antimony, 1 cc. equal to 4 mg. (1/15 gm.) It also enters into a number of compound expectorants, such as Mistura Glycyrrhizae and Compound Syrup of Squill.

Symptoms: The symptoms produced are similar to those produced by arsenic, vomiting always being an outstanding feature. Cases have been reported where no vomiting occurred for an hour. In a case in which drowsiness and powerlessness came on early, they were succeeded by tetanic spasms, the other symptoms also being present, and later persistent enteritis, with loss of hair on recovery. A study of a large number of typesetters[519] working with an alloy containing lead 75%, antimony 20%, and tin 5%, showed that typical lead poisoning was rare, but frequently a syndrome existed, marked by mental and muscular weakness, nervousness, neuralgia, insomnia, vertigo, headache, nausea, vomiting, and constipation.

Fatal Dose: Recovery has followed a dose of 170 grains.[520] A healthy woman, aged twenty-five years, took the minimum medicinal dose, 1½ grains, without effect, but a similar dose twenty-four hours later excited violent purging and vomiting, with death in thirty-six hours.[521]. A child died from the administration of three-fourths grain.[522]

Fatal Period: Death has occurred in seven hours. Taylor reported the death of a child in three-quarters of an hour. Life may be prolonged after the toxic dose for several days.

Treatment: The chemical antidotes are eggs, milk, and tannic acid. If vomiting is not induced, the stomach should be thoroughly washed out with a solution of tannic acid or tea. Treat symptomatically, giving morphine hypodermically.

Postmortem Appearances: Postmortem appearances may not show anything characteristic. The pathology closely resembles that seen under arsenic. Byth[523] described a case in which there was destructive ulceration of the membrane of the epiglottis and of the adjacent parts, exposing the muscular fi-

519. STRUMPF and ZABEL: Ztschr. f. exper. Path. u. Pharmakol., 63: 242, 1910.
520. CARPENTER: Med. Rec., N. Y., 24:401, 1875.
521. BEAU: Bull. gén. de thérap., 51:231, 1856.
522. TAYLOR: Guy's Hosp. Rep., 3rd series, 3:369, 1857.
523. BLYTH: Poisons, Their Effects and Detection, 4th ed., 609, 1906.

bers of the pharynx. Cook[524] found the gastric membrane was almost black from congestion. In cases of chronic poisoning inflammation of the kidneys and liver is usually found. Saikowski[525] reported that there was fatty degeneration of the liver, kidneys, heart, and muscular tissue of the diaphragm, and gastric follicles in the chronic form, and that it is a constant effect of the prolonged action of tartaric emetic, and probably also exists in some degree in all cases. As secondary appearances congestion of the dura mater, effusions into the arachnoid and ventricles, and congestion of the cerebral vessels may be noted.

Tests: Antimony may be found in the urine and in all of the organs of the body, as well as in the bones, skin, and hair. In making the Reinsch test for the presence of mercury and arsenic, antimony may be found. Its identification by this method is not as easy as the other two metals. The copper foil may be covered with a film of metallic antimony, with coloring from a black to violet hue. Upon heating the foil in the tube as described under the Reinsch test, the white substance, which is usually amorphous, will sometimes show crystals as previously described under tests for arsenic. (See page 253.) The antimony trioxide is dissolved in weak tartaric acid, and an orange-red precipitate is obtained by passing hydrogen sulphide after acidification with hydrochloric acid. Again the film of antimony on copper may be identified by boiling in a weak solution of potassium hydroxide, removing the strip at intervals to expose it to the air. If the solution of antimony thus made is acidified with hydrochloric acid, it will yield an orange-red precipitate with hydrogen sulphide. A distinct violet-colored deposit on the copper can be obtained from one drop of a solution containing 1/20,000 grain of tartar emetic, or 1/50,000 of a grain of antimony trioxide.

Marsh Test: This test is the same as given under arsenic (see page 257). If antimony be present, the gaseous terhydride will be formed, which has not the garlic-like odor of arsenic terhydride. Its flame produces a black spot on cold porcelain, while a metallic mirror forms in the delivery tube if that be heated by Berzelius' method. These spots are often mistaken for the similar deposits made by arsenic. The antimony deposit is insoluble, while arsenic dissolves when treated with a so-

524. Cook: *Lancet*, 1:860, 1883.
525. Saikowski: *Arch. f. path. Anat. (etc.), Berl.*, 24:73, 1865.

lution of chlorinated lime or chlorinated soda. Yellow ammonium sulphide dissolves both, but on evaporation the solution of antimony sulphide leaves an orange-red spot, soluble in strong hydrochloric acid, but insoluble in ammonia. The corresponding arsenic sulphide is yellow, insoluble in hydrochloric acid, but soluble in ammonia. If the gas generated from the Marsh apparatus is passed into a solution of silver nitrate, there is a black deposit of silver antimonid, Ag_3Sb. Antimonous sulphide is insoluble in ammonium carbonate in distinction from arsenic, slowly soluble in boiling solution of the fixed alkali carbonate in distinction from tin, soluble in hot moderately concentrated hydrochloric acid in distinction from arsenic. If arsenic is also present, it remains in solution and, by filtration, we can separate the two. The filtrate can be tested for arsenic. The antimony in the precipitate may be separated from the silver by dissolving in boiling weak hydrochloric acid. When filtered again and treated with hydrogen sulphide, the filtrate gives orange-red antimony sulphide. With this method, 1/200 grain of antimony trioxide can be detected.

Antimonic compounds are reduced to antimonous compounds by HI, and by $SnCl_2$, the antimony not being further reduced. Antimonic and antimonous compounds are reduced to the metallic state by lead, tin, bismuth, copper, cadmium, iron, zinc, and magnesium; but in the presence of dilute acids and metals which evolve hydrogen the antimony is still further reduced to stibine. Iron in the presence of platinum (iron platinum wire couple) precipitates the antimony from acid solutions as SbO; 0.000012 gm. can be detected.[526] Some of the suspected liquid can be put into a platinum crucible and acidified with hydrochloric acid. Upon immersing a strip of pure zinc, the antimony is at once deposited on the platinum as a black stain, which can be removed later by nitric acid or by simple heat. Arsenic will not cause a similar deposit. The stain can be removed by nitric acid, evaporated with dilute ammonium sulphide, when an orange-red color will be produced, due to the formation of antimony trisulphide. In two minutes a brown stain will appear when the solution holds but 1/10,000 grain of antimony, a definite reaction showing in a quarter of an hour when the amount is only 1/20,000.[527]

526. RIDEAL, C. N.: 51:292, 1885.
527. FRESENIUS: Qualitative Analysis, American Ed., 361, 1921.

Detection: Digest the tissue by the Fresenius and von Babo method. After neutralization of the filtrate, pass in hydrogen sulphide, which will precipitate the antimony as the sulphide. Wash the precipitate and then treat with strong nitric acid, and evaporate to dryness. A small quantity of a strong solution of potassium hydroxide is added to the residue, it is filtered, evaporated to dryness, and fused. The potassium antimonate in this fluid is boiled with a solution of tartaric acid, acidulated with hydrochloric acid, filtered, and saturated with hydrogen sulphide gas. The orange-red antimonic sulphide thus obtained is washed on a Gooch filter, dried in a water-oven, and the free sulphur and residual moisture, which are always present, expelled by heating in an atmosphere of dry carbon dioxide. Of this residue, which has been converted to the black sulphide, the Sb_2S_3 is multiplied by 0.7169 and gives the metallic antimony. The Gutzeit method may be used for the estimation of antimony in a manner similar to that described under arsenic. (See page 263.) Dissolve 2,3060 gm. of pure recrystallized tartar emetic in a liter of water. This solution contains 1.0 mg. of antimonious oxide per cc. From the stock solution, various dilutions can be made.

"Mickey Finn" powders (tartaric emetic) added to beer by disgruntled waiters who had not received sufficient tips from customers, have been responsible for a number of cases of poisoning. In several cases investigated the powders contained 1 gm. of tartaric emetic.

TIN (Sn)
(Atomic Weight 119.0. Synonym: Stannous)

VERY few cases of poisoning have been reported as caused by tin. Tin has a specific gravity of 7.293; it has a melting point of 231.68°C., and boils between 1450°C. and 1600°C. It does not distill in a vacuum at a red heat. It is a silver white metal, and does not tarnish readily in pure air. At a red heat it decomposes steam with evolution of hydrogen; at a white heat it burns in the air with a dazzling white light, forming stannic oxide, SnO_3. Tin forms alloys with many metals. Bronze consists of copper and tin; brass frequently contains from 2 to 5% of tin; solder consists of lead and tin. The only use of tin in industry causing ill effects is the use of tetrachloride of tin in weighting silk. Tin tetrachloride was examined by Pedley in order to discover whether its use in silk mills would be harm-ful.[528] He found that concentration as high as 3 mg. per liter is well tolerated by guinea pigs even when there is daily exposure for a period of months. Nothing more than a transient irritation of nose and eyes was noted. The symptoms observed in a man who worked a number of years with tin tetrachloride were irritation of the throat, chilliness, particularly in the morning, and anemia. Traces of tin were found in both the urine and stool. Eight and one-half parts per million in air caused coughing in men, and it was found that mice died after an exposure of ten minutes to 1 mg. per liter. Salant[529] fed tin tartrate and chloride to cats, 20 mg. per kilo of body weight, daily, for three months without harmful effects. However, moderately large doses, 30 to 50 mg. per kilo fed for two and one-half months caused loss of weight.

Symptoms: No chronic cases of industrial poisoning by tin, aside from that reported by Pedley, have been recorded. Tin salts act as gastro-intestinal irritants, causing sometimes a metallic taste, usually nausea, vomiting, abdominal pain, diarrhea, cyanosis, and collapse. Luff and Metcalfe[530] reported four cases of poisoning due to eating tinned cherries, the strongly acid juice in the can showing 3.2 grains of malate of tin to the fluid ounce.

Treatment: Wash out the stomach with a solution of sodium bicarbonate, a teaspoonful to a pint of water, followed by bland demulcent drinks, and treat symptomatically.

Quantitative Estimation: Alkali hydroxides and carbonates precipitate from solutions of stannous salts, stannous hydroxide, white, readily soluble in excess of the fixed alkali hydroxides, and insoluble in water, ammonium hydroxide and the alkali carbonates, in distinction from antimony. Hydrosulphuric acid and soluble sulphides precipitate from solutions of stannous salts dark brown hydrated stannous sulphide, insoluble in dilute, but soluble in moderately concentrated hydrochloric acid. This is readily dissolved by oxidation with the alkali supersulphides, the yellow sulphides, forming thiostannates from which acids precipitate the yellow stannic sulphide.

Determination: For the qualitative estimation of tin use

528. PEDLEY, F. G.:   J. Indust. Hyg., 6:28, 70, 1924.
529. SALANT: J. Indust. Hyg., 2:72, 1920.
530. LUFF and METCALFE: Brit. M. J., 1:833, 1890.

the tentative methods for tin.[531] Weigh out about 100 gm. of organs, put them into an 800-cc. Kjeldahl flask and add 100 cc. of strong nitric acid. Place over a water-bath until the following day, heat can be applied gently. Add 25 to 50 cc. of concentrated sulphuric acid, adding a little at a time so that it does not boil out of the flask. Heat until white fumes are generated. Cool, and add 5 to 10 cc. of strong nitric acid, and heat as before. Repeat the addition of nitric acid until the solution remains clear after the nitric acid is boiled off and fumes of sulphur trioxide appear. Add 200 cc. of water to the digested sample and transfer to a 600-cc. beaker. Rinse the Kjeldahl flask with three portions of boiling water, making a total volume of approximately 400 cc. Cool, and add strong ammonium hydroxide until just alkaline, then 5 cc. of strong hydrochloric acid or 5 cc. of dilute sulphuric acid (one-to-three) for each 100 cc. of solution. Place the beaker, covered, on a hot plate; heat to about 95° C. and pass in a slow stream of hydrogen sulphide for an hour. Digest at 95° C. for an hour and allow to stand a half-hour longer. Filter, and wash the precipitate of tin sulphide alternately with three portions each of wash solution (100 cc. of saturated ammonium acetate solution, 50 cc. of glacial acetic acid, and 850 cc. of water) and hot water. Transfer the filter and precipitate to a 50-cc. beaker, add 10 to 20 cc. of ammonium polysulphide, heat to boiling, and filter. Repeat the digestion with ammonium polysulphide, and the filtration twice, and then wash the filter with hot water. Acidify the combined filtrate and washings with dilute acetic acid (one-to-nine), digest on a hot plate for an hour, allow to stand overnight, and filter through a double 11-cm. filter. Wash alternately with two portions each of the wash solution and hot water and dry thoroughly in a weighed porcelain crucible. Ignite over a Bunsen flame, very gently at first to burn off filter paper and to convert the sulphide to oxide; then partly cover the crucible and heat strongly over a large Bunsen or Meeker burner. (Stannic sulphide must be roasted gently to the oxide, which may be heated strongly without loss by volatilization.) Weigh as stannic oxide and calculate to metallic tin, using the factor 0.7877. The tin sulphide may be dissolved in hydrochloric acid and potassium chlorate, the excess of chlorine dispelled by sheet aluminum and titrated with .01 N iodine solution.

531. Methods of Analysis, A.O.A.C., 396, 1935.

IRON (Fe)
(Atomic Weight 55.9. Synonym: Ferrum)

POISONING by salts of iron is very rare. Ferric chloride is said to have been the means of causing four cases of homicidal poisoning in Martinique.[532] Ferrous sulphate ($FeSO_4$ $7H_2O$) commonly known as "copperas" and "green vitriol" was used unsuccessfully in an attempt at suicide when a woman took two ounces on an empty stomach.[533] Functional nervous disturbances soon appeared, but subsided in a day or two, while diarrhea and abdominal pain marked the course of a subacute gastro-enteritis which lasted for nearly a month.

Fatal Dose: Death has been reported after five weeks from a dose of the chloride equal to one and one-half ounces of the tincture of iron. A man aged seventy-two years recovered from the effects of three ounces of the tincture.[534]

Treatment: Wash out the stomach with sodium bicarbonate. The gastro-enteric symptoms should be controlled by the use of opiates.

Postmortem Appearances: In one of the Martinique cases, a greenish-black fur-like mud covered the tongue, esophagus, and stomach; swelling, congestion, and ecchymotic points were the changes noted in the liver and kidneys, and hyperemia marked the brain and its membranes.

Tests: Potassium ferrocyanide precipitates ferrous salts as potassium ferrous ferrocyanide, $K_2FeFe(CN)_6$, bluish-white, insoluble in acids, transposed by alkalis. This is converted into Prussian-blue immediately by oxidizing agents. With ferric salts, ferric ferrocyanide, $Fe(Fe(CN)_6)_3$, Prussian-blue is formed, insoluble in acids, decomposed by alkalis. If the reagent be added in strong excess the precipitate is partially dissolved to a blue liquid. Strong acids should not be present, as they color the reagent blue. The ferrocyanides are transposed by KOH and decomposed by fusion with $NaNO_3$ and $NaCO_3$, the iron being obtained as Fe_2O_3. Potassium ferricyanide precipitates from dilute solutions of ferrous salts ferrous ferricyanide, $Fe_3(Fe(CN)_6)_2$, (Turnbull's blue), dark blue, insoluble in acids, transposed by alkali hydroxides; with ferric salts no precipitate is obtained, but the solution is colored brown or green.

532. BERENGER-FERRAUD, and PORTE: *Ann. d'hyg.*, 1:312, 508, 1879.
533. HALL: *New York Med. J.*, 38:401, 1883.
534. BLYTH: Poisons, Their Effects and Detection, 4th ed., 698, 1906.

This is a very important reagent for the detection of the presence of even traces of ferrous salts in the presence of ferric salts. Potassium thiocyanate gives no reaction with ferrous salts; with ferric salts the blood-red ferric thiocyanate, $Fe(CNS)_3$, is formed. This is an exceedingly delicate test. According to Wagner,[535] one part of iron, as ferric salt, may be detected in 1,600,000 parts of water. Ferrous salts with dimethyl glyoxalin added, and then made alkaline with ammonia, give a more or less intensive red color in the presence of iron. This is delicate to one part in 1,250,000. The tissues can be digested according to the Fresenius and von Babo method, and ashed. The ash is treated with dilute sulphuric acid, and the solution tested with ammonium sulphide or potassium ferrocyanide. As all tissues contain iron, the analyst must make due allowance for the normal iron present.

ZINC (Zn)
(Atomic Weight 65.38)

ZINC has a specific gravity of 7.142. Its melting point is from 418.5°C. to 419.44°C.; it has a boiling point of 907°C. It is a bluish-white metal, retaining its lustre in dry air, but slightly tarnishing in moist air or in water. When heated to the boiling point with abundant excess of air it burns with a bluish-white flame to zinc oxide. It is more malleable at 100° to 150°C. than at other temperatures, and at that temperature may be drawn into wire or rolled into sheets. At 205°C. it is so brittle that it may be easily powdered in a mortar. Zinc is found as calamine ($ZnCo_3$), as zinc blende (ZnS); it is also associated with many other metals in numerous ores.

Industrial zinc poisoning is caused mostly by the finely divided and freshly sublimated zinc oxide powder, which is formed in the smelting of zinc and in brass foundries. It is in this connection that zinc becomes of importance. Poisoning by the compounds of zinc is very rare in the United States, most of the poisonings having been reported from Great Britain. Zinc chloride was responsible for most of the cases, zinc sulphate being responsible for about half as many.

Zinc ores contain lead, iron, cadmium, and small amounts of arsenic. In 1929 there was an output of primary metallic zinc from domestic ores producing 612,136 short tons. This

535. WAGNER, Z.: 20:350, 1881.

dropped down to 207,248 short tons in 1932, but is now gradually on the increase, 355,366 short tons being produced in 1934. It is used in the manufacture of German and silver white metal; in the manufacture of zinc oxide (zinc white), in the rubber and paint industry, and in the making of salts of zinc. It is used as a substitute for lead in paints and enamels, and in the manufacture of oil cloth, and in soldering flux.

The cases of zinc poisoning that I have examined have been accidental and suicidal from the taking of soldering fluid containing hydrochloric acid and zinc chloride. Zinc stearate used as a dusting powder has caused toxic symptoms in children from the inhalation of the powder. A child one year old died suddenly after inhaling zinc stearate. A chemical examination of the lungs failed to show the presence of zinc stearate. Two rabbits were given daily 0.15 gm. of zinc stearate per mouth, for ten days without ill effects. Zinc sulphate has been taken in mistake for Epsom salts. The cooking of food in galvanized iron vessels may dissolve enough zinc to cause poisoning. Apples cooked in a galvanized iron vessel caused illness of 200 people, a few minutes after eating the applesauce.[536] The chief complaints were dizziness, sickness, colic, tightness of the throat, and diarrhea. An examination of the stewed apples showed the presence of 1.62 gm. of hydrated zinc sulphate per pound of apples. Salant and his co-workers[537] fed zinc acetate and malate daily for four months to rats and cats with no untoward results. However, when introduced into the circulation directly, it caused depression of the heart, and affected the muscle of the intestine, besides causing glycosuria and albuminuria. Foods should not be stored, cooked or transported in zinc vessels, as illness may occur from the continued absorption of the zinc.

Normal Zinc: Zinc is found normally in the tissues of the human body and in plants. Since it is a common constituent of all foods, it will be found in all the excretions of an ordinary mixed diet. Drinker, Fehnel and Marsh[538] found an average excretion of 10.7 mg. of zinc per day. One subject, following ingestion of a meal especially rich in zinc, excreted 200 mg. of

536. *Brit. M. J.*, February 3, 1923.

537. SALANT: *J. Biol. Chem.*, 34:463, 1918.

538. DRINKER, K., FEHNEL, J., and MARSH, M.: *J. Biol. Chem.*, 72:375, 1927.

zinc on the next day. Such figures as these, coupled with animal experiments on feeding non-caustic zinc compounds, and with observations upon men working in zinc plants and showing zinc excretion averaging 48 mg. a day, make it obvious that the ingestion of zinc is of no great importance. A zinc compound when taken by mouth might be changed to zinc chloride in the stomach, causing nausea, and would be of greater concern. Some foods especially rich in zinc are yeast, which contains 414.8 mg. of zinc per kilo; oysters, 26 to 2,298 mg. per kilo; bran, 139.2 mg. per kilo; corn, 25.2 mg. per kilo; and gelatin, 27.4 mg. per kilo. These figures are taken from Lutz's review[539] of the normal occurrence of zinc in biological materials. Common sources of zinc are cereals, milk, and eggs of which each yolk gives an average of 1 mg. zinc. The milk from cows contains on an average 4.2 mg. of zinc per kilo.[540]

Elimination and Distribution: Ghigliotto[541] reported the results of examining the viscera of twenty-two victims of accidental death and found that the content of zinc oxide varied between 0.0015% and 0.0028% of organic tissue. He found it constantly in the human and bovine fetus. Giaya[542] made determinations of zinc contained in human viscera from seven subjects, aged three months to seventy years, and also the human fetus. Zinc was constantly present, the proportion increasing with age. His experiments convinced him that zinc was not significantly toxic up to 0.05 gm. per kilo of viscera weight. De Gramont[543] proved that zinc could be detected in all tissues. Zinc is a constant constituent of the urine and feces of all people, since it is a constant constituent of all the foods they eat. Zinc is found normally in water in amounts from 0.9 to 50 parts per million. Bartow and Weigle[544] found that when zinc was administered as high as 100 parts per million, no appreciable ill effects were noted. These authors state that water supplies carried through and coming in contact with galvanized pipes, may contain other harmful substances, such as cadmium and zinc, which are sometimes present in the zinc used for galvanizing.

539. LUTZ, R.: *J. Indust. Hyg.*, 8:177, 1926.
540. BIRCKNER: *J. Biol. Chem.*, 38:191, 1919.
541. GHIGLIOTTO: *Ann. fals*, 12:2, 1919.
542. GIAYA: *Compt. rend. Acad. d. sc.*, 170:906, 1920.
543. DE GRAMONT: *Compt. rend. Acad. d. sc.*, 170:1037, 1920.
544. BARTOW and WEIGLE: *Indust. & Eng. Chem.*, 24:463, 1932.

Anderson, Reinhard and Hammel[545] conclude that chlorination reduces the attack of water upon zinc and is thus advantageous rather than the reverse. Lothian and Ward[546] previously came to the same conclusion.

The human liver contains from 10 to 76 mg. of zinc per kilo; kidney, 19.5 to 49 mg.; spleen, 10 to 12.7 mg.; lung, 6.1 to 7.1 mg.; heart, 12.6 to 15.6 mg.; muscle, 25.6 to 36 mg.; uterus, 32 mg. per kilo, and human hair, 9 mg. per kilogram. Abnormal amounts of zinc may enter and leave the body for years without causing symptoms or evidence which can be detected clinically or by laboratory examinations significant of gastro-intestinal, kidney, or other damage.

Zinc chloride ($ZnCl_2$) is a white deliquescent solid, very soluble in water, used as a disinfectant and as a caustic in medicine. It has caused death when applied to wounded surfaces.[547] In solution zinc chloride is used as an escharotic on granulations, cancerous tumors, and ulcers. It has been applied as paste by cancer quacks. It is a constituent of the Tilton quack cure for cancer. Blyth[548] mentions a fatal case in which the external application to the breast produced general symptoms of poisoning by zinc.

Zinc sulphate ($ZnSO_4$), or "white vitriol," is a white, crystalline solid, very soluble in water, and sparingly soluble in dilute alcohol. It closely resembles magnesium sulphate, and several instances of poisoning have been reported when it has been taken in mistake for this cathartic. Zinc sulphate is an emetic, has an action similar to copper, is less irritating, and is practically as efficient. It is given in doses of 1 to 2 gm. in a glass of water. There is a period of slight depression and nausea, in the absence of harmful irritation. It finds use as an astringent antiseptic solution for conjunctivitis and chronic gonorrheal diseases, and other cathartic conditions.

Symptoms: Zinc chloride is more of a corrosive than the sulphate, and causes gastro-intestinal symptoms, such as pain

545. ANDERSON, E., REINHARD, E., and HAMMEL, W.: Quoted by DRINKER and FAIRHALL, Pub. Health Reports, 32:48, 1933.

546. LOTHIAN and WARD: J. Roy. Army Med. Corps, 39:163, 1922.

547. STIMSON: Phila. M. News, 42:572, 1883; NICHOLS: Boston M. & S. J., 115:343, 1886; BUTTERSACK: Monatschr. f. Geburtsh. u. Gynäk., 29:11, 1909.

548. BLYTH, A. W.: Poisons, Their Effects and Detection, 4th ed., 690, 1906.

in the mouth, throat, and stomach. Violent vomiting begins immediately, particularly if the stomach contains food. There is severe thirst, followed by purging with tenesmus and bloody stools. In those cases which die in a short time the prostration is great, while in those cases where life is prolonged there may be more or less complete remission of all symptoms, then a recurrence of the pain, and vomiting which in some cases may continue obstinately for several days. The patient becomes emaciated and finally dies of exhaustion, as seen with cases of arsenical poisoning. In the case reported by Willis[549] death occurred in eight and one-half hours, and the condition resembled that of a narcotic poisoning. McCord and Kelker[550] report that handling wet wood treated with fungicide and fire-resistant material causes dematoses from tar, and, in addition, multiple lesions on fingers, hands, forearms, and legs ascribed to the presence of zinc chloride which becomes more concentrated by evaporation.

The sulphate does not act as a corrosive, but more as an irritant. After swallowing this salt, there is persistent vomiting, pain in the mouth, throat and stomach, with salivation and diarrhea. Schwartze and Alsberg[551] state that the efficient emetic concentration is 3,000 parts of zinc per million.

Fatal Dose: Death has taken place from one and one-half ounces. Zinc chloride has caused death secondarily after several weeks, from the administration of six grains. Recovery has taken place after a dose of one ounce, from the action of zinc sulphate. Death occurred in two hours in a woman fifty-two years of age from the effects of Burnett's solution.[552] Crosse[553] reports the case of a man sixty-two years of age who died in four and a half hours after swallowing two ounces of soldering fluid. I examined the organs of a man forty-eight years of age who died in three hours from taking an unknown quantity of soldering flux containing zinc chloride, which was in a half-pint "Bourbon Whiskey" flask. Two hundred cc. of the eight ounces had been removed from the bottle from which the deceased drank. It is not known whether he drank the full amount

549. WILLIS: *Assoc. J. J.*, 2:743, 1855.
550. McCORD, C. P., and KELKER: *J.A.M.A.*, 76:7, 1917.
551. SCHWARTZE, E. W., and ALSBERG, C.: *J. Pharmacol. & Exper. Therap.*, 21:1, February, 1923.
552. BRUNTON: *Glasgow M. J.*, 5th series, 514, 1869.
553. CROSSE: *Brit. M. J.*, 2:820, 1883.

or not. A man fifty years of age died in two hours after having taken about 125 gm. (four ounces) of a mixture of sulphates of zinc and magnesium containing 75% of the former.[554]

Treatment: The stomach should be promptly washed out with water containing sodium bicarbonate. Opiates may be given to allay pain and stop the diarrhea. Intravenous injection of 100 cc. of 50% glucose should be given.

Postmortem Examination: Postmortem examination will show severe corrosion of the gastro-intestinal canal. The mucous membrane of the mouth, fauces, and esophagus is deprived of epithelium and is white, opaque, and swollen. The mucous membrane of the stomach is softened and disintegrated at the cardia; is particularly toughened at the greater curvature and greatly corrugated toward the pylorus. Its color varies from gray to purple-black. The vessels are engorged with blood, the smaller capillaries as well as the larger vessels. Occasionally, there may be ulceration, seen in the upper part of the small bowel, it being congested and inflamed, and sometimes it has been found thinned and eroded. The stomach has been found ulcerated and perforated, but in one instance the immediate cause of death was found in the constriction of the pylorus. The postmortem findings are not characteristic, and could be confused with other corrosives.[555]

Industrial Zinc Poisoning: Zinc is not a poison in the usual sense of the word. We have seen from the foregoing that some compounds of zinc are caustic and irritant, and that certain other compounds of zinc such as zinc stearate may do harm, but this is more on account of the zinc content. Textbooks on toxicology have held for many years that zinc was a poison, and in so doing lose sight of the fact that many of the ores in which zinc is found also contain substances that are definitely poisonous, such as lead, arsenic, and cadmium, as Fairhall and Drink-

554. BUCHNER: *Friedreich's Bl. f. gerichtl. Med., Nürnb.*, 33:255, 1882.

555. ABT, I. A., WOODWARD, C. W., and LEECH, PAUL N.: Danger of Zinc Stearate Dusting Powders, *J.A.M.A.*, 83:120, 1924; *J.A.M.A.*, 84:750, 1925. MIDDLETON, R. H.: *Atlantic, M. J.*, 29:307, 1926. SCHLAEPPER, K.: Death Following Inhalation of Zinc Stearate, *Am. J. Dis. Child.*, 31:474, 1926. IGLESIAS, M. S.: Zinc Chloride Poisoning, *Gac. méd de México*, 61:9, 1930. BERTRAND, G., and BEAUZMONT, Y.: Zinc Content of Animal Bodies According to Age; Influence of Milk Diet, *Bull. Soc. chem. biol.*, 12:741, 1930; *Ann. Inst. Pasteur*, 45:247, 1930.

er previously mentioned. We must look at zinc in an entirely different light. There is a large amount of experimental evidence showing that zinc is not toxic, and that ill health associated industrially with zinc is due to the toxic impurities mentioned above. Batchelor, Fehnel, Thomson and Drinker[556] found that their careful, detailed clinical laboratory studies on twenty-four workmen exposed for from two to thirty-five years to dust, zinc oxide, zinc sulphide, or finely divided metallic zinc, poor in lead and cadmium, revealed no acute or chronic illness attributed to zinc. Dusty atmospheres of both the chloride and sulphate of zinc cause perforation of the nasal septum in workmen. They found that these men inhaled 0.30 mg. of zinc per cubic foot of air in the bag-shaking room; 1 mg. per cubic foot in the bag-house; 0.136 mg. per cubic foot in the packing-house; 2.04 mg. per cubic foot two feet away from the furnace, and 0.176 mg., six feet away from the furnace. One man, forty years of age, who had worked for ten and a half years in this industry showed a blood picture of 82% hemoglobin, 5,270,000 red blood cells, 10,000 white blood cells, 17 small lymphocytes, 4 large lymphocytes, and 2 basophiles. They found on examination that the urine contained from 0.3 to 1.38 mg. of zinc per 100 cc.; the feces 27.63 mg. in a twenty-four hour specimen, and the blood .466 mg. per 100 cc. In a second sample of stool there were found 54.31 mg. The normal excretion of zinc in the urine is from 0.75 to 1.75 mg. per twenty-four hours. They found that zinc in the feces may be increased from 12 to 70 mg. in twenty-four hours by eating oysters. "In general there is no correlation at all between the dustiness of the job and the amount of zinc excreted in the urine."[557] It is apparent, however, from our investigation that for years abnormal amounts of zinc may enter and leave the body without causing symptoms or showing any evidence which can be detected by laboratory or clinical examination. The fact should be stressed that the increased zinc in the urine and feces of zinc workers represents increased amounts of a normal urinary constituent and not the presence of a metal abnormal to cells and to the metabolic process. These findings have been confirmed by Heller and Burke.[558]

556. BATCHELOR, R. P., FEHNEL, J. W., THOMSON, R. M., and DRINKER, K. R.: J. Indust. Hyg., 8:322, 1926.
557. McCORD, C. P.: Am. J. Pub. Health, 16:274, 1926.
558. HELLER, V. G., and BURKE, A. D.: J. Biol. Chem., 74:85, 1927; abstr., J.A.M.A., 89:1282, 1927.

From my examination of a large number of men who had been engaged in galvanizing, and in melting zinc, I have been unable to find the existence of any chronic diseases. In one instance, I found that all the symptoms could be attributed to lead, and in another case to cadmium.

Metal Fume Fever: The metal fume fever is found in workmen engaged in brass foundries, in the smelting of zinc and other metals, giving rise to the same symptoms. Lehmann[559] noted that the course of the disturbance did not resemble an intoxication by a metallic compound, but rather an infection by bacteria or the injection of foreign protein, since there is a sudden chill followed by a rise of temperature and the attacks result in a temporary immunity. These fumes caused a protein poisoning from the resorbtion of the products of cells lining the aveoli of the lungs, which cells have been killed by the action of the zinc oxide. Lehmann was unable to explain why it was not possible to produce the same symptoms by insufflation of ordinary zinc oxide powder. Drinker showed that freshly formed oxide particles such as occur in fumes from heated zinc are not yet agglomerated and so pass easily through the air passages. Metal fume fever is never caused except by the freshly formed fumes from heated metal. Drinker, Thomson and Finn[560] connect the temporary immunity which is familiar to brass founders with the leucocytosis, which is a defensive mechanism. The symptoms of metal fume fever come on a few hours after exposure, very rarely in the foundry, more often after the man has reached home. Chilling of the body is often the exciting cause, and the cases are always more numerous in the winter. This may be partly due to poor ventilation. The actual chill is preceded by a feeling of dryness in the throat, with cough, a sense of lassitude and oppression in the chest, sometimes nausea, and rarely vomiting. The chill is followed by sweating and general weakness which disappears by morning, and the man usually goes back to work. The temperature rarely goes over 101°. These authors found that metal-fume chills follow the inhalation also of freshly precipitated magnesium oxide.

Tests: Several methods have been described for the deter-

559. LEHMANN, K. B.: *Arch. f. Hyg.*, 28:291, 1897.
560. DRINKER, P., THOMSON, R. M., and FINN, J. L.: *J. Indust. Hyg.*, 9:187, 1927.

mination of zinc.[561] The ashing may be carried on at 450° C. with absolute safety, ashing to a soft char. Extract this with 10 to 20 cc. of hydrochloric acid and hot water. The filter paper and char are returned to the oven for incineration. Extract this ash as before, having a combined extract of about 100 cc. per 100 gm. of sample. The iron and copper must be removed. Sodium, potassium, and calcium lead to high values in titration. In the case of urine, the solution should have a volume of 25 cc. containing 10 to 15 cc. of a one-to-one hydrochloric acid. Cool, and add to the solution an excess of cupferron (ammonium nitrosophenyl hydroxylamine) dissolved in water. The iron is found as a red precipitate, and the copper a dirty red gray. The iron is completely precipitated when white crystals of the cupferron reagent are noticed on further addition of the reagent. Shake thoroughly until the colloid is coagulated. The filtrate is a greenish color. Partly neutralize with sodium hydroxide and finally ammonium acetate. To this solution is finally added 5 mg. copper as copper nitrate, and the solution is diluted to a volume of 150 cc. The precipitate is washed with cold water and finally with hot alcohol to remove organic material. The funnels are then returned to their original flasks and the precipitates washed with hot water once, and then alternately with concentrated hydrochloric and nitric acid until completely dissolved. Evaporate to dryness and add 1 cc. sulphuric acid, and 2 cc. of nitric acid and heat until the remaining traces of organic material have been completely oxidized, and the excess of sulphuric acid has been fumed off. Dissolve the residue in 5 cc. of one-to-one hydrochloric acid, cool, and add 25 cc. of water and saturate the cold solution with hydrogen sulphide gas. Filter. Evaporate the filtrate to dryness. Remove the iron by boiling to the ferric condition with bromine. Cool. Precipitate iron as phosphate by sodium phosphate, and neutralize with ammonium acetate. Dissolve the precipitate, add 1 cc. of sulphuric acid (one-to-two) and 2 cc. of nitric acid, and heat till the remaining traces of organic material have been completely oxidized and the excess of sulphuric acid fumed off. Dissolve the residue in 5 cc. of one-to-one hydrochloric acid, cool, add 25 cc. of water, and saturate the cold solution with hydrogen sulphide gas. Filter. Evaporate the filtrate to dryness. As traces of cal-

561. FAIRHALL: *J. Indust. Hyg.*, 8:165, 1926.

cium interfere with the micro-method of zinc estimation, it will be found advisable as a routine procedure to reprecipitate the zinc and copper sulphides in all cases where this method is applied. In the analysis of bones for zinc, calcium phosphate will occasionally slowly precipitate from the cold solution saturated with hydrogen sulphide gas. It is therefore advisable to filter at once after saturation, wash and dissolve the sulphide precipitate, and reprecipitate the zinc and copper.

Titration Method: "Zinc chloride reacts in hydrochloric acid solution with potassium ferrocyanide giving a precipitate of zinc ferrocyanide. By using an indicator which will react with the excess of potassium ferrocyanide, the amount of ferrocyanide required by the zinc may be determined. The indicator which has been found to be most suitable at low concentrations of zinc is uranium acetate. It is used externally and the titration followed on a porcelain spot plate. The successful application of this method of zinc estimation lies, therefore, in the adoption of uniform conditions throughout. Temperature and concentration are factors that must not be varied if the greatest accuracy is to be obtained. Prepare a solution of potassium ferrocyanide having an equivalent value of 1 mg. of zinc per cubic centimeter (3.464 gm. of crystalline potassium ferrocyanide, $K_4Fe(CN)_6.3H_2O$, per liter of solution). The solution should stand for twenty-four to forty-eight hours and be filtered out. If prepared from pure salt and stored in the dark, the solution is less apt to change. Its zinc value is obtained by the analysis of a standard zinc chloride solution to dryness, add exactly 5 cc. of one-to-one hydrochloric acid and 20 cc. of water. For small amounts of zinc, reduce the volumes to 1 to 2 cc. of hydrochloric acid and 4 to 8 cc. of water. Heat to the boiling point and titrate with ferrocyanide, using a spot plate and uranium acetate as an external indicator. The solution should not be allowed to become cooled appreciably during the titration, and the lapse of time required for color development in the indicator should be uniform. Blank experiments using the same volumes of acid and of water and the same temperature of titration will establish the indicator allowance which must be deducted."

Turbidity Method: "For amounts of zinc which lie between those conveniently determined and the extremely small amounts determinable by the Lutz method, a range of from 0.05

mg. to 2 mg., the turbidimetric method is most satisfactory. This method consists in comparing the turbidity produced by potassium ferrocyanide with a given amount of zinc solution, with that similarly produced with various amounts of a standard solution of zinc. Nessler tubes having optical glass bottoms and supporting a column of liquid of approximately 17 mm. by 210 mm. are best suited for comparison, and some care must be used in selecting good light and a dead black background for best results. Experience has shown that the most suitable range of standards is from 0.05 mg. of zinc to 0.55 mg. and that especially accurate readings can be made over the range, 0.15 to 0.35 mg. of zinc. Dissolve the zinc chloride residue carefully in 10 cc. of N/10 sulphuric acid, evaporate to dryness, and carefully fume off the excess of acid. Dissolve the residue of zinc sulphate in 5 cc. of N/10 sulphuric acid and make the volume up to exactly 25 cc. with distilled water in a volumetric flask. Transfer various known amounts of this solution to Nessler tubes and arrange a set of zinc sulphate standards in Nessler tubes ranging from 0.05 mg. to 0.55 mg. of zinc. Zinc sulphate is used as the standard, as it gives somewhat sharper readings than zinc chloride. In order to adjust the degree of salt concentration add phenolphthalein indicator to each tube and determine the required for the most acid tube—usually the unknown—and then add a similar amount of alkali to every other tube in the set. Titrate each tube to neutrality with N/10 sulphuric acid and add one drop excess of sulphuric acid. In this way each tube will have a similar salt content and degree of acidity. Add 1 cc. of a cold saturated solution of sulphurous acid to each tube, dilute to about 45 cc., add 1 cc. of 2% (freshly prepared) potassium ferrocyanide solution, dilute to the mark, and shake thoroughly. The sulphurous acid prevents any oxidation and hence any greenish coloration that would be likely to interfere with the readings. Set the tubes aside in a dark place for twenty minutes in order to allow the full turbidity to develop. In comparing the turbidities, avoid direct sunlight and make the readings against a dull black background."

Micro-method: For quantities of zinc below 0.05 mg. the only accurate procedure is that developed by Lutz.[562] In this method the iron may be removed by the phosphate precipita-

562. LUTZ, R. E.: *J. Indust. Hyg.*, 7:273, 1925.

tion method with practically as much facility as by the cupferron method, since but small volumes of solution are
involved. The zinc residue obtained is free from traces of
calcium, magnesium, copper, or the alkali metals. Use nothing but No. 40 Whatman filter paper throughout, as other
grades of filter paper contain appreciable amounts of zinc.
The detection of zinc by this method is facilitated by using
30 to 40 mm. filter paper and micro-funnels and micro-flasks.
Evaporate the zinc chloride residue carefully to the point at
which the last drop of liquid is vaporized by breathing on it.
This will leave sufficient acid in the residue to insure complete
solution. Adjust the volume accurately to 5 or 10 cc. and
use convenient aliquot parts of this for the actual estimation
of the zinc. Into Nessler tubes similar to those used for the
turbidimetric method, introduce 15 to 20 cc. more of alcohol,
mix the contents of the tubes, add 1 to 2 cc. of urobilin solution, adjust to the 50-cc. mark, and again carefully shake the
tubes. If illuminated by a carbon or iron arc-lamp against
a dark background a greenish fluorescence will be noted. The
depth of the fluorescence is proportional to the amount of zinc
and is strikingly apparent in amounts as low as 0.001 to 0.002
mg. of zinc. With the aid of standard tubes containing known
amounts of zinc, it is, therefore, possible to estimate small
quantities of zinc very closely. "The fluorescence with
amounts of zinc as low as 0.005 mg. was destroyed in the
presence of many substances, and the permanence of the
color was affected by impurities present in the reagents or
the solvent. Commercial 95% ethyl alcohol was used as the
solvent. In order to remove impurities that imparted a yellow
color to alkaline solutions, it was distilled over lime. Recovered
alcohol was found to accumulate impurities (probably aldehydes) which caused the fluorescence with urobilin and zinc
salts to fade appreciably in a short time, thus making consistent readings difficult or impossible. Careful purification
of recovered alcohol by repeated distillation was found to be
essential in order to obtain consistent results. A large excess
of ammonia or ammonium salts was found to have a decided
depreciatory effect on the fluorescence." For zinc in foods, after
precipitation as a sulphide, dissolve in hydrochloric acid and
bromine water. Boil off excess bromine, add iron chloride and
sodium acetate solutions to precipitate the phosphates. Add

H_2S to filtrate, filter off the ZnO. Then ZnO x .8034 = Metallic zinc.

MAGNESIUM SULPHATE ($MgSO_4 . 7H_2O$)
(Magnesii Sulfas; Molecular Weight 246.49)

MAGNESIUM sulphate occurs as small, colorless crystals, usually needle-like, with a cooling, saline, and bitter taste. It effloresces in warm, dry air. One gram of magnesium sulphate is soluble in 0.8 cc. of water and in about 1.1 of glycerine, at 25°C. One gram of the salt is soluble in about 0.2 cc. of boiling water. It is sparingly soluble in alcohol at 25°C. (U.S.P., XI).

Although this substance is extensively used as a laxative, and is used widely by the laity for the reduction of swelling due to trauma and arthritis, etc., very few cases of poisoning have been reported. Magnesium sulphate is employed as a laxative in doses of 2 to 10 gm., and as a hydragogue cathartic in doses of 10 to 15 gm.

Meltzer and Auer[563] after intravenous injections of magnesium sulphate induced general anesthesia and relaxation of the abdominal walls. Repeated doses paralyzed the skeletal muscles and the reflexes, and abolished respiration. The margin of safety was too small for a general anesthetic, one of the earliest effects being, in some cases, respiratory paralysis. When intravascular injection is used, it produces severe and immediate, often fatal, depression of the heart and central nervous system. After absorption, and with parenteral administration, the excretion occurs by the kidneys,[564] only a small part from the large intestine. Ten cc. of a 20% magnesium chloride injected into the intestine, with the stomach tied off, produces death by respiratory paralysis in about twenty-five minutes. When administered to rabbits by mouth, even very large doses are not fatal. The intramuscular or intravenous injection of magnesium salts or sulphates into dogs causes the appearance of hyaline casts in the urine. Gates and Meltzer found no other casts, albumen, or other signs of nephritis. It has been found to control the convulsions of tetanus, and as locally anesthetic by subcutaneous injection.[565]

563. MELTZER and AUER: *Am. Med.*, 10:916, 1905; *Med. Rec.*, 68:965, 1905; *Am. J. Physiol.*, 14:366, 1905-6; *J. Exper. Med.*, 23:641, 1916.
564. MELTZER and LUCAS: *J. Exper. Med.*, May 25, 1907.
565. MENDEL and BENEDICT: *Am. J. Physiol.*, 25:1, 1909-10.

Boos[566] in observing ten cases noted that six were fatal; in only one was there active purging, and in five there was no purging whatever. The paralysis of the bowel with enteritis called for laparotomy in two cases. Vomiting occurred in five. The urine was scanty in all, and in some was suppressed. There was paralysis of the respiratory and motor nerves, and of the reflexes; two had convulsions.

Treatment: Wash out the stomach with lime water, giving calcium chloride and calcium gluconate intravenously. The physician should be prepared to combat failure of respiration by artificial respiration, together with physostigmine (0.5 to 1 mg. hypodermically) or calcium chloride (50 cc. of 2%, intramuscular; or 0.02% in normal saline, intravenous, to 600 cc).

Postmortem Appearances: Curtis[567] reported a case of death following hypodermoclysis of magnesium sulphate, using 310 cc. of a 4% solution of pure magnesium sulphate as an aid to the nitrous oxide-oxygen anesthesia. Death occurred sixty hours after operation, following a period of marked prostration. Postmortem examination showed intense jaundice, extensive acute fatty changes in the liver, marked cloudy swelling of the parenchymatous organs, and multiple petechial hemorrhages of the pleura, pericardium, and endocardium. The lining of the stomach and bowels was unchanged.

THORIUM (Th)
(Molecular Weight 232.12)

THE nitrate of thorium is markedly astringent, precipitating proteins and coagulating blood. It is not used as a contrast medium in roentgen work, because of the dangerous action. A fatality due to acute toxemia was studied by Weld.[568] A fatality occurred in a woman, aged fifty-five, following the use of thorium nitrate as a pyelographic medium carefully introduced by catheterization, to the pelvis of the kidney. At the end of six hours she was suddenly seized with nausea, vertigo, and weakness. She grew rapidly worse, with marked vomiting and prostration, dying nine hours after the pyelogram. Autopsy revealed general arterial sclerosis, some atrophy of the kidney, edema of the lungs, and fatty changes in the liver.

566. Boos: *J.A.M.A.*, 55, 1910.
567. Curtis: *J.A.M.A.*, 77:1492, 1921.
568. Weld: *J. Urol.*, 2:415, 1919.

GASEOUS POISONS

THE inspired air contains 20.96 volume per cent of oxygen, 79% of nitrogen and argon, and 0.004% of carbon dioxide, with minute traces of hydrogen, xenon, krypton, neon, and variable amounts of ammonia and ozone, in addition to floating particles and micro-organisms. The expired air contains 16.3 volume per cent of oxygen, 79.5% nitrogen, and 4.10% of carbon dioxide. These figures for the composition of inspired and expired air refer to dry air at a temperature of 0°C. and 760 mm. Under normal circumstances inspired air contains a variable amount of aqueous vapor and has a variable temperature corresponding with the time of year. When awake a man takes in 350 cc. of oxygen, and gives out 300 cc. of carbon dioxide per kilo per hour. With the tidal air of 500 cc. and respiratory rate of 17, the total pulmonary ventilation during the hour would be 500 x 17 x 60 = 510,000 cc. per hour.[569]

The volume of air that a man breathes is the principal physiological factor in determining the amount absorbed of any gas or vapor mixed with the air. Oxygen alone supports human life; the inhalation of any other gas is followed by suffocation—that is, by suspended animation due to obstruction of blood aeration. The volume of air breathed varies according to whether the individual is sitting down, walking, sleeping, working, or undergoing strenuous exercise. Under these various conditions the man breathes so many liters and parts of air per minute.[570] "Respiration is the volume of air which is inspired and expired in one minute. It is expressed in liters at the prevailing temperature and barometer. It is most accurately measured by means of a mouthpiece or mask, fitted with very light valves of mica or rubber so that the stream of air to or from the mouth passes through some measuring apparatus. The changes in the volume of air in the lung are brought about through movements of the diaphragm and ribs. The volume of air breathed by a normal man at any time is dependent upon, and is the mathematical product of, two conditions or sets of conditions: (1) the amount of oxygen he is consuming and the amount of carbon dioxide he is producing, and (2) the ratio of ventilation to oxidation, the dilution fac-

569. STARLING: *Principles of Human Physiology,* 1052, 1915.
570. HENDERSON and HAGGARD: Noxious Gases, Monograph Series, No. 35, 1927.

tor, at which his breathing is set. In fact, leaving aside for the moment certain details and assuming a constant dilution ratio, the volume of air breathed per minute by healthy men is within moderate variations proportional to the respiratory exchange in the ratio of 25 to 1 or 100 to 4 for carbon dioxide and 20 to 1 or 100 to 5 for oxygen. In other words, the inspired air contains 21% of oxygen while the expired air has lost 5% of oxygen and gained 4% of carbon dioxide. These relations hold true with very slight changes alike when a man is lying in complete rest or when walking, and when the volume of breathing and the oxygen consumption and carbon dioxide elimination are doubled. Even when he works fairly hard and they are multiplied several fold, the volume of breathing so nearly keeps pace with the combustion going on in the body that the carbon dioxide in the expired air only rises to about 5%. But the relation is disturbed by very vigorous exercise; and especially in men with poor training any considerable exertion causes heavy panting so that the elimination of carbon dioxide rises out of proportion to the oxygen absorbed, and the volume of breathing increases out of proportion to the gaseous exchange." The relation of the volume of carbon dioxide produced to the volume of oxygen consumed, i.e., CO_2/O_2, is called the respiratory quotient.

A liter of oxygen consumed in the body produces an amount of energy which, expressed in heat units, is always very close to 4.8 calories for one on the ordinary American diet. On a diet of pure fat it would be 4.69 calories per liter of oxygen, and on one wholly of carbohydrates 5.05 calories per liter.

Not all of the air breathed reaches the lungs. Some of this air does not go beyond the mouth, windpipe, and bronchi, and this air takes little or no part in the respiratory exchange, being expired almost unchanged.

"When a low concentration of a gas of high solubility in blood, such as ethyl ether, is inhaled in air, nearly all of it that reaches the lungs at first is absorbed, but the mixed expired air still contains approximately 33% as much of the gas as the inspired air." This amount comes from the air referred to above. "Since the dead space is about 33% of each breath, the volume of air which actually enters the lungs is about 66% of the volume of respiration. For this same reason, the air in the lungs has a concentration of carbon dioxide which is about one and one-half times the concentration in the mixed expired air. It is this lung air primarily which is kept at a nearly uniform composition by variations in the volume of respiration."

"Even the deepest possible expiration leaves in the lungs about one and one-half liters of air, the so-called residual volume. An ordinary expiration leaves in them perhaps as much more. This supplemental air, plus the residual, together constitute the so-called stationary air. The tidal air of quiet breathing is 0.3 to 0.6 liter of which, as we have seen, only two-thirds reach the lungs; the other third not penetrating beyond the dead space and therefore not participating to any considerable degree in the respiratory exchange."

This changes our conception, somewhat, of the absorption of various gases, as we usually have figured in the past that if a man breathes one liter of carbon dioxide air he is getting all of the carbon dioxide. However, if only two-thirds of it enters into the respiratory exchange, this must be taken into consideration in figuring how much gas an individual is receiving into his lungs over a definite period. The temperature and humidity are more important than the carbon dioxide content.[571] From Winslow's experiments in rebreathed stale air, containing twenty parts of carbon dioxide, no discomfort was noted if the temperature was not allowed to rise. In a second experiment he found warm stale air, or fresh air if warmed, produced distinct and clearly marked physiologic reactions. At a temperature of 75°F. with 50% relative humidity the rectal temperature was 2°C. higher and at 86°F. with 80% humidity was 0.5°C. higher with the pulse increased five to twelve beats.

Gases differ widely in their mode of action. Some, like nitrogen, merely exclude the oxygen of the air from the lungs, and the blood is then gradually exhausted of its oxygen. Life is restored in such cases when efforts to produce artificial respiration are not too long delayed and are sufficiently protracted. It may take an hour or more of persistent effort to revive a patient, and the rules laid down for the resuscitation of the drowned are applicable. Other gases, such as carbon monoxide, deprive the blood of its property of

571. WINSLOW, C. E. A.: *Am. J. Pub. Health,* 7:827, 1917.

absorbing oxygen. They act directly upon the blood corpuscles and are specific poisons. Such gases greatly retard or even prevent reoxygenation. Still other gases, like hydrogen sulphide, entering the system by absorption through the air cells of the lungs, pass rapidly into the circulation and produce effects on special organs or on parts of the nervous system. The only gases supposed to be purely negative in their action are nitrogen and hydrogen. To these the recently discovered argon may be added. There are no direct experiments on its inhalation. It is present in the air to the extent of nearly 1% without producing ill effects. Truly poisonous gases, even though present in much smaller quantity than this, seriously affect the organism. We are thus led to the assumption that argon is as passive in this as in all other respects. Since hydrogen when breathed with oxygen in atmospheric proportion has been found to produce narcotism, it should not, perhaps, be classed with nitrogen.[572]

Experiments made on rats confined in a space in which they could live in air without inconvenience for three hours showed the relative periods in which certain gases proved fatal.[573] Thus pure nitrous oxide killed in twenty-five seconds; pure hydrogen, in nine minutes, pure carbon dioxide, in eight seconds. Since experiments conducted by the Committee of the Medico-Chirurgical Society showed that the heart's action continued for eight minutes and twenty seconds under a complete deprivation of air, the above results indicate the truly poisonous action of vapors and gases, a conclusion substantiated by other facts.[574] (Several of the gases, such as carbon dioxide, methyl chloride, sulphur dioxide, and ammonia, have been treated under refrigerants and will not be repeated in this chapter.)

CARBON MONOXIDE (CO)

CARBON monoxide is one of the most important poisons associated with human life and industry. It is outdistanced by only one other poison, grain alcohol. With the kindling of the first fire man came in contact with carbon monoxide, the most subtle of poisons. The effects of carbon monoxide were known in antiquity. Aristotle, nearly 300

572. TAYLOR: Medical Jurisprudence, 11th Am. ed., 439, 1892.
573. NORRIS: Brit. M. J., 2:401, 1873.
574. TAYLOR: Medical Jurisprudence, 11th Am. ed. 493, 1892.

years B.C., observed that "men suffer from heaviness of the head and often die from coal gas." Lewin,[575] in his exhaustive monograph on carbon monoxide, gives many instances of poisoning by this agency, showing that it had been a frequent cause of death by accident, by suicide, and as means of punishment and torture. In 68 A.D. Seneca, after a number of attempts at suicide, finally "ended his life by breathing the vapor of charcoal." Hannibal (247-183 B.C.) put the inhabitants of Nuceria to death by "coal vapors."

The number of deaths from illuminating gas has been steadily dropping in the last few years due to the more extended use of electricity as a means of illumination, and also due to the use of natural gas, which does not contain

TABLE XXV

DEATHS DUE TO CARBON MONOXIDE POISONING IN COOK COUNTY, ILLINOIS

1917	1918	1919	1920	1921	1922	1923	1924
470	470	518	386	237	214	361	412
1925	1926	1927	1928	1929	1930	1931	1932
320	403	375	398	237	310	323	188
1933	1934	1935	1936				
128	143	74*	80				

* Of this 74, 46 were due to auto gas.

carbon monoxide. However, this gas is usually mixed with other gases containing carbon monoxide. Natural gas is practically odorless and therefore lacks the property of indicating significant leakage by the sense of smell, the means most widely used by gas employees and consumers for detecting leaks of the more odorous types of fuel gases. Sayers, Fieldner, Yant, Leitch and Pearce[576] recommend the use of ethyl mercaptan, to detect leaks in natural gas distribution systems. In the survey at each city the entire sendout to the distributing system was odorized for several days with comparatively low concentrations at the start, 7.7 to 9.3 pounds of ethyl mercaptan per million cubic feet of gas, for indicating house leaks, and then increased to high concentrations, 31.0 to 46.5 pounds per million cubic feet of gas for several days to indicate underground leaks.

Carbon monoxide when pure is nearly insoluble in water.

575. LEWIN, L.: Die Kohlenoxydvergiftung, Berlin, 3, 1920.

576. SAYERS, R. R., FIELDNER, A. C., YANT, W. P., LEITCH, R. D., and PEARCE, S. J.: Dept. of Commerce, U. S. Bureau of Mines, R. I., 3007, 1930.

It is a colorless, tasteless, and practically odorless gas, this latter physical property making it dangerous as a source of poisoning. The density compared to air is 0.967.[577] It can be compressed into a liquid and a solid. It has a coefficient of solubility of 0.0243 at 15° C. It burns with a blue flame, two volumes of carbon monoxide uniting with one volume of oxygen to form two volumes of carbon dioxide: $CO+2O=CO_2$. Under the ultra-violet rays carbon monoxide becomes formic acid. The alkaline hydroxides change it to the formates: $CO +KOH=HCO_2K$. Carbon monoxide unites with chlorine forming phosgene, which was used as a toxic war gas and has also caused industrial poisonings.

Carbon monoxide is produced at the electrodes or from the charges of electric furnaces. In electric furnaces having limestone linings the carbon dioxide is reduced to carbon monoxide at the heated electrodes; the gas escapes unburned, producing characteristic symptoms. The most common sources of carbon monoxide, with the exception of its marked formation during a severe lightning storm, are stoves, grates, salamanders, domestic and industrial furnaces, distillation of oil, gas engines, fumes from explosions, burning x-ray films, smouldering ashes and mine coal, and natural and artificial gases. It is formed whenever incomplete combustion of carbon occurs, such as fumes on besooted surfaces and low burning oil lamps. Using an intermittent aspirator to imitate the smoking of tobacco, I found that carbon monoxide from the inhaled smoke of cigarettes was from 0.01 to 0.26% of the tobacco and paper consumed; from cigars, 0.027 to 0.15%, and from pipe tobacco 0.027%.

The atmosphere contained 1% carbon monoxide after a dust explosion in a coal mine, while immediately after an experimental explosion as much as 8% has been found. The proportion of carbon monoxide differs greatly in domestic and industrial gases, varying from 2% to 30%; in coal gas 4% to 10%; 30% in water gas, and 20% to 30% in producer gas. The gas from a blast-furnace stack averages 28%; Bessemer furnace gas, 25%; and gas from a cupola, 17%. Lime-kiln gases, waste gases from ammonia soda processes, and gases left in the track of explosions in coal-pits contain

577. NICLOUX: L'Oxyde de Carbone et L'Intoxication Oxycarbonique, 24, 1925.

from 1.25% to 2.5%.[578] Wood gas made by the Wilkinson process was found to contain 33.75%, while the commercial gas served to the consumer and made by mixing of gases from wood, coal, and naphtha contained 11.25%.[579] Almost all illuminating gas contains a large proportion of water gas, so that when the gas is discharged into an inhabited space it becomes exceedingly dangerous. An atmosphere containing 0.2% is capable of destroying life.[580] Natural gas does not contain carbon monoxide, but the products of combustion do contain carbon monoxide. The composition of natural gas is as follows:

Methane	40.6
Ethane	7.6
Carbon dioxide	24.2
Nitrogen	27.6

The average carbon monoxide content of exhaust gas from 101 cars of all makes was found by the Bureau of Mines to be 7%. Ciampolini, of the Division of Industrial Hygiene, tested, in 1932, the blood of forty-two garage workers for carbon monoxide and found twenty-eight that were positive.[581] Wilson and his colleagues[582] demonstrated carbon monoxide in the blood of fourteen traffic policemen, in six of whom the amount ran from 20% to 30% carbon monoxide hemoglobin (HbCO). Owens[583] states that the exhaust from heavy oil engines, such as Diesel engines, contains a lower proportion of carbon monoxide than that coming from petrol engines. The safe limit for carbon monoxide in the air is given by Haldane,[584] who studied conditions in the London Underground Railway, as 0.01% for continuous exposure. On the other hand, Henderson[585] and his colleagues allowed as much as 0.04%, since it was supposed that nobody would remain in that atmosphere for more than three-quarters of an hour and

578. HERMAN, DOUGLAS: Notes on Poisoning by Carbonic Oxid, J. Soc. Chem. Indust., 15:857, 1896.

579. DOREMUS, C. A.: Wilkinson's Process of the Manufacture of Illuminating Gas from Wood, J. Am. Chem. Soc., 2:449, 1880.

580. HALDANE: J. Physiol., 18:430-462, 1895.

581. CIAMPOLINI, E.: J. Indust. Hyg., 6:102, 1924.

582. WILSON, E. D.: J.A.M.A., 87:319, 1926.

583. OWENS, J. S.: Lancet, 154-155, January 21, 1933.

584. HALDANE, J. S.: Brit. M. J., 2:16, 1930.

585. HENDERSON, Y., HAGGARD, H. W., TEAGUE, M. C., PRINCE, A. L., and WUNDERLICH, R.: J. Indust. Hyg., 3:79, 1921.

in that time would suffer nothing worse than a frontal headache at such a concentration of carbon monoxide.

Bloomfield and Isbell[586] reported that the average of 141 tests made in city streets at parking hours of traffic showed a contamination of 0.8 part of carbon monoxide per 10,000 parts of air. Only 20% of all the street samples had more than one part of carbon monoxide in 10,000 parts of air. Samples taken inside of auto-buses yielded even lower concentrations of carbon monoxide gas. Of 102 tests made in twenty-seven garages of the fourteen cities visited, the average carbon monoxide content was found to be 2.1 parts in 10,000. More than half of the samples (59%) contained over one part carbon monoxide, and 18% of all the samples contained over four parts of this gas in 10,000 parts of air.

Yant and Sayers,[587] state that "men while at rest have often been exposed all day to small amounts of carbon monoxide without ill effects, but on walking home in the open air, have experienced severe symptoms, even to unconsciousness." In a personal communication to the author, Yant states that, during his work in connection with the ventilation of the Holland Tunnels, persons were subjected to various concentrations of carbon monoxide, and later put through an exercising period to bring out latent symptoms. This exercising consisted of hopping for a distance of forty to fifty feet. On several occasions, eight to twelve persons suddenly collapsed and became unconscious, after hopping. In some instances the persons collapsed while observations such as taking of pulse were being made. In all instances the individuals had reported that they were all right, and were without apparent symptoms at the end of the test period.

In human experiments it took from ten to eleven hours to reduce a 35% saturation to 5%. An unusual case was reported by Nicloux and Nerson[588] in which oxygen was administered: a saturation of 41.3% was reduced to 25.4% in one hour; to 8.4% in four and a half hours; and to only a trace after twenty-three and a half hours. Oxygen inhalations were given during the whole period.

586. BLOOMFIELD, J. J., and ISBELL, H. S.:   Pub. Health Reports, Reprint No. 1217, March, 1928.

587. YANT, W. P., and SAYERS, R. R.:   Report of Investigations, U. S. Bureau of Mines, R. I., 2476:2, 1923.

588. NICLOUX, M., NERSON, H.: Compt. rend. Soc. de biol., 92:174, 1925.

Farmer and Crittendon[589] studied fourteen mill operatives, who were, daily, during a working period of eight hours, breathing air containing small amounts of carbon monoxide. They found that the blood saturation was 6% to 7%, varying somewhat with the type of employment. These operatives returned to the plant the following day after a rest period of sixteen hours, their blood still showing an average of 2% saturation.

Sayers, Yant, Levy and Fulton[590] made experiments, and at the conclusion of their investigation, in which six men were exposed four to seven hours daily over a period of sixty-eight days to gasoline exhaust gas-air mixtures containing two, three, and four parts of carbon monoxide per 10,000 parts of air, they found there was a distinct increase in the hemoglobin accompanied by an increase in the red blood cells, the most important changes occurring in the leukocytes. Exposure to two parts of carbon monoxide in 10,000 parts of air caused some subjects at rest or exercising mildly to experience slight but not discomforting symptoms in approximately two hours, and distinct frontal headaches of a discomforting nature in three and one-half to four hours. No symptoms of any type were experienced in more than 50% of the exposures, and no occipital headaches occurred in any subjects even after six and one-half hours' exposure. The blood attained 20% carbon monoxide hemoglobin in three and one-fourth to four and one-fourth hours, and 25% in five to six hours, depending on the person and whether he was at rest or exercising mildly.

In 1933, there were 58,900 unexplained automobile accidents in which cars driven off the roadway for no apparent reason killed 3,260 persons and injured 53,240. Tests were made and it was concluded that 7% of motor vehicles when in operation contain enough carbon monoxide to cause collapse of occupants. At least 60% of the automobiles tested contained measurable quantities of the gas when in operation. It is possible for a dangerous concentration of carbon monoxide to accumulate within a car which is following another at the usual trailing distance. The gas may enter the trailing car whether its windows are open or shut.[591] I believe that most of the gases

589. FARMER, C. J., and CRITTENDON: J. Indust. Hyg., 11:329, 1929.
590. SAYERS, R. R., YANT, W. P., LEVY, E., and FULTON, W. B.:   Pub. Health Bull. No. 186, U. S. Treasury Dept., 1929.
591. Science News Letter, 173, March, 1934.

come from beneath the hood, as was previously mentioned.

An interesting case occurred in July, 1934, when a young man, W. P. G., of Des Moines, Iowa, was driving a Chevrolet truck in which the exhaust gas was emitted below the driver's seat. The patient became sick at his stomach, felt weak, especially in the legs, began to have dizzy spells, was drowsy, and had a fever. Following this he had severe headaches in the occipital region, and a stiffness of the neck. He continued to drive his truck for two weeks, when his headache became so severe and he felt so weak and drowsy that he was unable to accomplish all of his usual duties. He then consulted a physician who advised him to remain in bed for a month and a half. Ten months following the accident he still complained of stiffness of the neck, loss of memory, pains about the heart, vague abdominal pains; a case of neuro-circulatory asthenia.

Harbitz[592] describes an instance of wholesale poisoning from exhaust gas. Of a party of seven adults and six children, on a pleasure trip in a motor boat, nine developed symptoms of carbon monoxide poisoning while all were sitting on the open deck back of the cabin, and two who went to lie down in the cabin, died. A leak in the "sound deadener" allowed the exhaust gas to escape and accumulate in the cabin. The high sidewalk back of the cabin helped to retain the escaping gas. The boat was twenty-two feet long and eight feet wide, and the door of the cabin stood open. A child aged seven was the first to feel the effect, half an hour after starting.

Crank Case Gas Analysis:

No. 1. From crank case, motor racing:

Carbon monoxide .... 0.9%, or 90 parts per 10,000 of air.
Carbon dioxide.................... 2.9%, or 290 parts per 10,000 of air.
Oxygen ....16.5%, or 1650 parts per 10,000 of air.

No. 2. From crank case, motor idling:

Carbon monoxide .... 1.4%, or 140 parts per 10,000 of air.
Carbon dioxide.................... 4.0%, or 400 parts per 10,000 of air.
Oxygen ....15.1%, or 1510 parts per 10,000 of air.

No. 3. From exhaust, no dilution:

Carbon monoxide .... 4.0%, or 400 parts per 10,000 of air.
Carbon dioxide....................12.1%, or 1210 parts per 10,000 of air.
Oxygen .... 0.2%, or 20 parts per 10,000 of air.

The average composition of the exhaust gas by volume of twenty-three cars in this country is shown as follows:

592. HARBITZ, F.: *Norsk. mag. f. laegevidensk.*, 85:47, 1924; J.A.M.A., 82:508, 1924.

Carbon dioxide	8.6
Oxygen	2.3
Carbon monoxide	6.3
Methane	0.9
Hydrogen	3.0
Nitrogen	78.6

The blue flame at the surface of the fire in grates and blast furnaces shows the presence of carbon monoxide. Much escapes unburned. In furnaces with forced drafts the blue flame is often seen at the top burner in the superheaters of the air supply. It is, therefore, a constant constituent of the products of combustion of carbonaceous materials, and, while the poisonous action of charcoal, coke, and coal vapors is in part due to carbon dioxide, it is due mainly to this poisonous gas. Quantities of this gas accumulate above the fire in hot air furnaces and stoves. So much, indeed, that on opening the door the inrush of air will form an explosive mixture which, igniting, may produce serious accidents. The common construction of dampers is that they shall be loose enough to allow a constant draft to the chimney. Notwithstanding this, it frequently happens that a down draft fills the room with the products of combustion to a poisonous extent. A large proportion of the accidents that happen yearly is due to the leaving off of stove lids. The presence of any carbon monoxide in the atmosphere is due either to the faulty construction of the furnace, or to the action of the heated plates on the organic dust with which they are generally covered.[593] Notwithstanding all attempts to render furnaces gas-tight, their lacking of this is seen in the rapid tarnishing of silverware as soon as the furnace is lighted; by the occasional escape of furnace gas, detectable by its odor, or of smoke, which pervades the home. The general malaise and headaches during the winter months are undoubtedly due in many instances to the presence of this gas. Enormous quantities of carbon monoxide are daily produced in the manufacture of illuminating gas, producer gas, and water gas. In the city of Chicago, during 1935, there were 3,724 miles of pipe used for the transportation of 117,000,000 cubic feet of gas per day, having the average composition of 2.8% carbon monoxide. The proportion of carbon monoxide differs greatly in domestic and

593. REMSEN: Nat. Bd. of Health Bull., Washington, D. C., No. 52, 2:857, 1881; GOTTSCHALK, J.: Mengen und einege Bemerkungen zu der sogenannten Lufheizungsfrage.

industrial gases, varying between 4% and 30%; in coal gas 4% to 10%; 30% in water gas; and 20% to 30% in producer gas. The exhaust of an automobile may have from 1.5% to 16% of carbon monoxide.

The greatest percentage of carbon monoxide asphyxiation is through the medium of illuminating gas, which has the characteristic odor of the hydrocarbons accompanying the carbon monoxide gas. The familiar odor does not prevent many accidental poisonings, as the odor may not be perceived by those in deep sleep, or by a person with a defective sense of smell.

It has been suggested that ethylene (C_2H_4), which is very poisonous to plants, might be the real cause of asphyxiation.[594] Using a mixture containing 50% of ethylene, which is six

TABLE XXVI

ASPHYXIATION IN COOK COUNTY

1916	Carbon Monoxide Per Cent	Water Heaters	Acci-dental	Undeter-mined	Sui-cides	Homi-cides	Totals
				Deaths			
Jan.	23.9	1	16	9	23	5	54
Feb.	26.4	1	13	7	13	0	34
March	24.1	0	18	7	21	0	46
April	23.9	0	19	8	19	0	36
May	27.2	2	14	8	23	0	47
June	26.2	2	11	2	12	4	31
July	23.0	0	5	12	20	4	41
Aug.	24.2	0	5	4	12	0	21
Sept.	22.4	0	13	8	26	3	50
Oct.	22.6	0	23	9	17	1	50
Nov.	29.1	0	7	5	20	0	32
Dec.	31.0	0	14	6	13	2	35

Undoubtedly many of the "undetermined" cases were suicides, the evidence being inadequate to warrant a verdict of suicide.

times that found in illuminating gas distributed to homes, the author was unable to show other than a narcotic action upon mice and rats. In lethal percentages of illuminating gas, Smith, McMillan and Mack[595] summarize the following: (1) Male rats succumb more quickly than females. (2) Young adult rats die more quickly than older animals. (3) Pregnancy greatly reduces the lethal interval. (4) Potent metabolic stimulants decrease the lethal interval by as much as one half.

It is commonly believed that during the winter months the percentage of carbon monoxide increases, and that this is the chief reason for more deaths from gas poisoning. The per-

594. MATTHEWS: Physiological Chemistry, 495, 1915.
595. SMITH, E., McMILLAN, E., MACK, L.: J. Indust. Hyg., 17:18, 1935.

TABLE XXVII
Total Gas Asphyxiation Cases for the Seventeen Years from 1905 to 1921 inclusive

Asphyxiation by gas	Acci- dental	Undeter- mined	Indus- trial	Water Heaters	Sui- cide	Homi- cide	Totals
1905	59	55			83	7	204
1906	87	36			59	5	187
1907	76	61			74	1	212
1908	85	75			115	3	278
1909	102	81			107	12	302
1910	127	65	10	4	116	7	329
1911	103	66	4	7	115	2	297
1912	110	61	11	10	153	9	354
1913	148	64		1	163	3	379
1914	103	78	3	3	200	5	392
1915	126	93	5	17	242	6	489
1916	160	92	6	6	219	18	501
1917	167	85	10	3	193	12	470
1918	196	80	11	7	168	17	479
1919	222	56	11	11	207	11	518
1920	199	41	5	11	127	3	386
1921	194	43	1	8	168	5	419

centage of carbon monoxide does not, however, increase in winter. (Table XXVI). The majority of deaths from carbon monoxide are due to the inhalation of illuminating gas. Table XXVII shows how deaths from this poison increased from 1905 to 1921. During 1920 there was a decided decrease in deaths from asphyxiation.

From the records of death from carbon monoxide poisonings during 1918 and 1919, the author found fifty-two causes for

TABLE XXVIII
Causes for the Inhalation of the Gas

	1918	1919
1. Open jet, cause of its being open unknown	86	133
2. Open burner of gas plate or range	48	44
3. Open burner of range, vessel boiling over	24	20
4. Deceased intoxicated	19	
5. Disconnected hose	17	29
6. Defective fixture	14	5
7. Lighted gas heater	10	6
8. Coal stove gas	8	1
9. Hot-water heater	7	11
10. Gas heater	6	6
11. Defective rubber hose	5	14
12. Automobile motor running in closed garage	5	2
13. Clothing hanging on fixture	5	
14. Wind blew out light	4	3
15. Coke gas from furnace	4	3
16. Disconnected pipe	4	2
17. Broken supply pipe	4	1
18. Gas frozen	4	

the inhalation of the gas. In Table XXVIII there have been enumerated some of the causes, where they have produced three or more deaths. The chief cause was "open jet, cause of its being open unknown;" the next was "open burner of gas plate or range," and the third, "the boiling over of water from a vessel, putting out the flame."

The following is a typical analysis of gas from a city main:

		Per cent
	Carbon dioxide	1.2
	Illuminants	2.2
	Carbon monoxide	3.0
CHICAGO:	Oxygen	0.4
	Hydrogen	24.8
	Ethane	7.0
	Methane	55.2
	Nitrogen	6.2

The average carbon monoxide content of the gas supplied to the city of Chicago for the year 1935 was 2.8% by volume.

Table XXIX shows where the deaths occurred, the majority having taken place in homes:

TABLE XXIX
WHERE GAS CASES OCCURRED

	1918	1919
Gas cases in homes	263	272
Gas cases in hotels	10	17
Gas cases in plants and factories	12	8
Gas cases in garages	5	2
Gas cases on street (in wells)	3	
Gas cases in railroad yards	1	
Gas cases in clubs	....	1
In city	275	289
Outside of city	19	11
Accidental and undetermined cases (male)	215	215
Accidental and undetermined cases (female)	79	85
Children fifteen years or under	7	28
Deceased seventy years or over	47	45

Action: Carbon monoxide may be freely respired, its presence in air is not manifested by either irritation to the air passages or by its affecting the sense of smell as is noted with sulphur dioxide gas used in mechanical refrigeration. However, the moment carbon monoxide comes in contact with the blood, by diffusion, it unites with the red pigment of the blood corpuscles, forming a definite compound; carbon monoxide acts like 220 volumes of oxygen. The corpuscles are not dead. All they need is oxygen under sufficient tension to displace the carbon monoxide. Hill and Barcroft[596] have demonstrated that carbon monoxide combines more readily with unsaturated oxyhemoglobin than with hemoglobin. Hemoglobin will take up more carbon monoxide at a given tension if a little oxygen is present than if oxygen is completely absent. In Barcroft's experiments with carbon monoxide poisoning, he found that an animal at rest could breathe an atmosphere containing a low percentage of CO and yet the hemoglobin in the spleen pulp remains perfectly free from the gas although the blood in general circulation reaches a 20% saturation. It is evident that during this period the blood must pass from the arteries to the veins by some other route than through the pulp. During exercise, on the other hand, the hemoglobin of the pulp became charged with CO in the space of five minutes. The spleen therefore appears to be a place where a reserve of red blood corpuscles may be stored until some emergency arises demanding an increased oxygen transportation. Hufner[597] found that 1 gm. of carbon monoxide hemoglobin contains 1.338 cc. of carbon monoxide, computed at 0° C. and 760 mm. pressure. The oxygen absorbed from the air is normally taken up by the blood in the form of a loose chemical combination with the red coloring-matter (hemoglobin) of the corpuscles, and in this form it is carried to the tissues in which it is used. Oxygen and carbon monoxide combine chemically with hemoglobin in equal molecular proportions, and, therefore, in equal volumes, the oxygen combination readily liberating its oxygen, while the carbon monoxide is relatively stable. Haldane believes that all the effects can be referred to lack of oxygen, the symptoms increasing with the saturation of the blood with carbon monoxide. Mice were kept alive on exposure to 200 to 300 times the fatal dose of carbon monoxide in the presence of oxygen under high pressure (one to two atmospheres). Mosso repeated Haldane's experiment, using monkeys instead of mice, with the same result. The blood corpuscles are not changed in form, though those found in the liver are, after a time, somewhat modified. Nicloux[598] has shown that the red blood cells, even when saturated with carbon monoxide, are not devitalized at all, but are ready to resume functioning when supplied with

596. HILL: *Biochem. J.*, 7:471; BARCROFT: *Biochem. J.*, 7:481, 1914.
597. HUFNER: *Arch. f. Physiol.*, 130, 1894.
598. NICLOUX: *Presse méd.*, 29:701, 1921; *Medicine*, 3:913, 1922.

oxygen. The gas causes the blood to assume a color varying from violet to cherry-red and both blood and foam are readily distinguished from normal arterial blood. Blood containing carbon monoxide hemoglobin may be deprived of the gas by submitting the blood to diminished pressure, or by passing the oxygen or air through it for a considerable length of time.

From observations on human beings some claim that this change may take place in a few hours, while others state in from four to six. Out of forty-three consecutive gas cases received at the Cook County Hospital, of Chicago, 34% were examined within one-half hour from the time the patients were removed from the source of exposure, carbon monoxide being found in all of these; in 30% the exact time was not known, but was greater than one-half hour, 27% being positive and 3% negative. Twenty to forty minutes elapsed in 14%, 12% gave positive tests and 2% negative; 10% were examined in three hours, all being positive; in another 10% five hours elapsed, all were positive, and in 2% after twelve hours all were positive.

It is claimed that the carbon monoxide may be in part changed by oxidation into carbon dioxide within the body.[603] Others, among them Gaglio, claim that this oxidation does not take place, but that the carbon monoxide is voided, quantitatively, unchanged.[599] Carbon monoxide when injected into the abdomen or swallowed, dissolved in water, also produces poisonous effects the same as when inspired. The blood is, however, never fully saturated and some of the gas may diffuse from the corpuscles into all the tissues; indeed, it has been shown by Fehling to pass from the mother to the fetus. This raises the question of whether a corpse may not absorb the gas from the atmosphere and thus give indications of carbon monoxide poisoning when death has been due to other causes. The experiments of Strassmann and Schulz[600] have demonstrated that carbon monoxide may penetrate by diffusion all parts of the cadaver, with sufficiently long exposures in air containing carbon monoxide. Schulze believes carbon monoxide is a tissue poison.*

599. Re the elimination of carbon monoxide, consult L. DE SAINT-MARTIN: Recherches sur le mode d'elimination de l'oxyde de carbone, Compt. rend. Acad. d. sc., 112:1232, 1891; 115:825, 1892.

600. STRASSMANN and SCHULZ: Berl. klin. Wchnschr., 41:1233, 1904; WACHHOLZ and LIMBURGER: Vrtljschr. f. gerichtl. Med., Berl., 3F., 23:223, 1902. * Klin. Wchnschr., 16:427, 1937.

The question as to whether carbon monoxide has any direct action upon the nervous system has been the subject of much dispute. The inhalation of oxygen with at least 20% of carbon monoxide seems to affect the nervous system, since violent disturbances of the system with cramps and total paralysis of the limbs appear within the first minute of inhalation, while the blood could certainly not have become sufficiently saturated with the gas by that time to produce such symptoms. Kobert, Geppert, and others strongly incline to the belief in an action upon the nervous system, both of the peripheral nerves and of the ganglion-cells of the brain, from the symptoms produced and the pathologic appearances, and they extend the poisonous action of the gas to the production of a degeneration of the muscles and glands.[601] Haggard has demonstrated that this gas has no direct toxic action upon nervous tissue.

People nearest doors or windows in a room into which illuminating gas is escaping suffer the least, and those nearest the floor the most.

CASE No. 1. December 22, 1906, E. F. and a woman went to a rooming house at 4:00 P.M. At 5:00 P.M. the landlady noticed the odor of gas coming from the room. As no one responded when she knocked at the door, entrance was gained through the transom. The man was found dead. The woman, still breathing, was removed to a hospital, where she recovered. The woman was on the inside of the bed, near a window. A gas heater was found in the room with two burners still lighted, and three unlighted burners from which the gas was escaping.

CASE No. 2. February 12, 1915, C. W. and roommate were found in a room unconscious from gas escaping from a defective hose on a gas heater. The roommate, who was nearer to the window, recovered.

CASE No. 3. March 16, 1916, F. M. A. died from gas escaping from a defective heater. The roommate on the inside of the bed nearer the window recovered.

CASE No. 4. Stevens[602] reports the case of a seven weeks old baby dying of carbon monoxide poisoning, having a satura-

601. KOBERT: *Lehrbuch*, 2:871, 1906; also KOBERT: Practical Toxicology (English Trans., L. H. Friedburg, New York) 1897; HAGGARD, H. W.: *Am. J. Physiol.*, 60:244, 1922: MEYER, A.: *Ztschr. f. d. ges. Neurol. u. Psychiat.*, 100:201, 1926.

602. STEVENS, A. M.: *J.A.M.A.*, 86:1201, 1926.

tion in the blood of 18%. In the baby's bedroom a small leak was found in a gas fixture. The mother who had been in the bedroom almost constantly was poisoned only enough to suffer from headache.

The next two cases—also the author's—illustrate the homicidal use of carbon monoxide.

CASE No. 5. December 14, 1916, Mrs. B. turned on the gas, killing her two children. Her husband had committed suicide the previous day. The woman was found to be insane and was committed to an asylum.

CASE No. 6. June 26, 1917, a mother killed her baby with gas, attempting suicide. She was held for murder.

Lethal Dose: Since the poisonous action of this gas was noticed in 1802 by Guyton de Morveau and submitted to personal experiment by Sir Humphry Davy, a large number of experiments have been made on men and animals and observations recorded from the results of accidents. It would appear from these that about 0.8 gm. (twelve grains) of carbon monoxide is fatal to a man of 70 kilos (154 lbs.), 11.5 mg. per kilo being fatal to rabbits. From this it would appear to be less poisonous than hydrocyanic acid. Nevertheless, extremely small portions when breathed produce unmistakable symptoms of poisoning. According to Gruber, 0.02% is the limit of toxicity, while at 0.05% symptoms were clearly observable.[603]

Exposure to a contaminated atmosphere for two or three minutes may cause serious illness. Burrell[604] found that exposure for twenty minutes to air containing 0.25% of carbon monoxide made him sick for eight hours after the exposure. Air containing as little as 0.1% of carbon monoxide when breathed for several hours produced headache and vomiting with some members of the Bureau of Mines while others were not affected. An exposure of ten minutes in a cellar has killed a person.[605] Two men in a cooper shop fire in Chicago, June 7, 1917, went into the burning building to recover their tools. In thirty minutes both were found dead. Examination of the blood showed death due to carbon monoxide asphyxiation.

603. GRUBER, MAX: Ueber den Nachweis und die Giftigkeit des Kohlenoxyds, und sein Vorkommen in Wohräumen, *Arch. f. Hyg.*, 1:145, 1883.

604. BURRELL and SEIBERT: Miners' Circ. 14, Dept. of Interior, U. S. Bureau of Mines, Washington, D. C., 1914.

605. COULLAUD: *Ann. d'hyg.*, s. 4, 12:490, 1909.

It is especially noticeable that all animals do not behave alike. In some, as birds and chickens, convulsions or cramps are caused, while this effect is not noticed in mice or rabbits. Gruber found that rabbits behaved abnormally in an atmosphere containing between 0.07 and 0.08%. As soon as the quantity reaches 0.1% the poisonous effect is produced, while with 1% the toxic action is rapid. Gruber breathed air containing 0.021 to 0.024% of carbon monoxide for over three hours without experiencing any unpleasant sensations. He states that the blood of the entire body is capable of containing one liter of oxygen or one liter of carbon monoxide. The quantity of carbon monoxide breathed by him amounted in total to 300 cc., but being distributed over a considerable length of time did not produce poisonous effects. Frogs placed by him in an atmosphere of pure carbon monoxide lived over ten hours. Worms survive many hours' exposure to this gas.[606]

The rapidity of the action has been established by many observations. Birds die instantly in an atmosphere containing 5%, while dogs, rabbits, and other animals are killed in times varying from a minute or so to half an hour, according to the amount of this gas in the atmosphere.[607]

The speed with which carbon monoxide acts is illustrated by a case given by Sonnenschein of a chemist, who, at a single breath of an atmosphere laden with this gas, fell backward as if struck by lightning. After a quarter of an hour's serious symptoms he recovered through timely aid.[608]

Henderson and Haggard,[609] from their studies, have arrived at a standard for calculating the toxic action of carbon monoxide which refers to the concentration of the gas and the time of exposure to it. When the time of exposure in hours multiplied by the concentration of CO in parts per 10,000 of air equals three there is no perceptible physiologic effect; when it equals six, there is a just perceptible effect; when it equals nine, headache and nausea are induced; and when it equals fifteen or more the conditions are dangerous to life.

606. JORDON, H., and SCHWARZ, B.: *Arch. f. d. ges. Physiol.*, 185: 311, 1920.

607. WOODMAN and TIDY: Forensic Medicine and Toxicology, Phila., 485, 1877.

608. SONNENSCHEIN, F. L.: *Handb. d. ger. chemie, Berl.*, 288, 1869.

609. HENDERSON and HAGGARD: *J. Indust. & Eng. Chem.*, 14:229, 1922.

Duration: In the majority of cases the victims are found dead or die a short time afterward. Fishbein[610] reports a patient living five days; Long and Wicki,[611] thirty-six days; Sibelius,[612] three months. The author has examined the blood of several patients who lived two days and one who lived four days after exposure to illuminating gas. Recovery is usually complete within a week, but after-effects may persist for weeks and months. O'Malley[613] reports a case of a woman who, poisoned by illuminating gas, did not regain her mental faculties for three months. He refers also to a case cited by Brouardel of a physician poisoned by carbon monoxide, who lost his memory, this amnesia lasting eighteen months, at the end of which time he fully recovered.

There are only a few references in toxicologic literature to homicidal poisoning unaccompanied by simultaneous suicide by illuminating gas, or gases containing carbon monoxide.

Carbon monoxide poisoning may be of interest in civil cases, for instance, under conditions in which death is a form of chronic poisoning and the results amount to criminal negligence on the part of another.

One of my early cases, the first to go to a higher court in Illinois, illustrates this point. In the estate of Catchman Olsen vs. City of Chicago,[614] the widow was given a verdict of $3500, the death of Olsen having been proved to be due to a leaky gas pipe in one of the repair shops of the city. When an insurance policy is involved it is of the utmost importance to show the presence of carbon monoxide by chemical examination, and to prove whether the case is a murder, a suicide, or an accident, as a policy may be void in the case of a suicide. The origin of the poisonous gas may usually be found from the surroundings, as an open gas jet or a leak in the feed pipes. A loose-fitting stopcock may be opened by careless persons throwing their wraps over a wall gas-bracket or over a gas fixture suspended from the ceiling. Several cases of such carelessness were investigated by the Coroner's Office of Cook County, Illinois,

610. FISHBEIN, MORRIS: Illuminating Gas Poisoning, *J.A.M.A.*, 60: 737, 1913.

611. LONG and WICKI: *Rev. méd. de la Suisse Rom.*, 22:172, 1902.

612. SIBELIUS: *Ztschr. f. klin. Med.*, 49:111, 1903.

613. O'MALLEY: *Am. J. M. Sc.*, 145:865, 1913.

614. *Olsen* vs *City of Chicago*, Decision on Review, 697, Book 2, Case 262, 1914.

during 1916. At inquests it is frequently desirable to distinguish between poisoning by coal gas, illuminating gas, or other sources. At the present time there are no efficient analytic methods by which we can distinguish illuminating gas poisoning from that due to coal fumes. Wachholz[615] has suggested that the presence of hydrocyanic acid in the blood, and Cruz[616] that the presence of hydrocarbons in the blood gases would identify the source of the carbon monoxide as being illuminating gas. An investigation of the room for the source of the carbon monoxide will give more definite results than a chemical examination of the blood gases.

In one case investigated a medical student had been overcome by carbon monoxide from a smoking oil stove on which he was cooking his meals. The room, free from gas fixtures, was covered with soot. In three different instances a closed stove-pipe damper caused the coal gas fumes to enter the room and produce death by carbon monoxide gas.

Two or more persons may be exposed to a contaminated atmosphere; one or more may die, while the others recover. Three young physicians in Melbourne, after playing tennis, went to bathe in a shower bath, in which the water was heated by a gas burner. After a half hour a messenger found one dead and two unconscious.[617]

On January 5, 1917, three men were found unconscious in a room. One of the three died, the other two recovered. A stovepipe had parted from a hard coal burner, allowing the carbon monoxide to escape into the room. The blood of the man who died was 45% saturated with carbon monoxide.

The time required to eliminate completely carbon monoxide by respirations of pure air has not been determined definitely. It varies greatly with different persons, the carbon monoxide hemoglobin apparently not being in all cases under sufficient tension with oxygen to liberate readily the carbon monoxide. Henderson[618] states that carbon monoxide is practically eliminated in three or four hours. The experiments of Michel[619] tend to show that it does not exceed a few hours;

615. WACHHOLZ: *Ztschr. f. Med.-Beamte, Berl.*, 9:400, 1896.
616. CRUZ: *Ann. d'hyg.*, Series 3, 385, 1898.
617. Australian letter, *Lancet*, 2:1102, 1911; see also DARLING: *M. J. Australia*, 2:191, 1918.
618. HENDERSON, Y.: *J.A.M.A.*, 68:580, 1916.
619. MICHEL: *Vrtljschr. f. gerichtl. Med., Berl.*, 14:36, 1897.

Koch[620] states that he has found it after ten hours; Pouchet[621] after sixty hours; Fishbein after five days; Wachholz[622] after seven days. In specimens of blood submitted to me from two cases ending fatally in two days, and one of four days' duration, I was able to detect carbon monoxide hemoglobin. I have had over 100 cases of over four hours' standing, in which carbon monoxide could be detected by definite color tests and the palladous chloride method. In a large number of my cases of gas poisoning, with clear histories of attempted or consummated suicide by means of illuminating gas, the blood failed to show the presence of carbon monoxide after the respiration of pure air and oxygen for a few hours. Blood from suicides who died within a half-hour after being discovered in a gas-filled room contained as high as 13.6% of carbon monoxide by volume. Blood from other cases in which life was prolonged for a few hours contained from traces to 5.5% carbon monoxide.

The compound of carbon monoxide hemoglobin can be dissociated by hydrogen and carbon dioxide as well as with oxygen. Gaglio[623] demonstrated that carbon monoxide inhaled by an animal may be recovered from the expired air with a loss of only 2.8%, due to experimental conditions. The odor of illuminating gas has frequently been noticed in the expired air of patients after being taken to a hospital. Nicloux states that he has found carbon monoxide in normal blood of dogs and in human blood. The amount found in the blood of dogs living in Paris varied from 0.08% to 0.18%. Buckmaster and Gardner[624] failed to find carbon monoxide in the blood of cats. Carbon monoxide has been found to be present in the blood of smokers.

Symptoms: The diagnosis of carbon monoxide is often very easy, sometimes difficult and never positive unless a chemical examination of the blood has been made. The symptoms may simulate many other conditions. The reason for this is chiefly in the rate of absorption and the extent of the combination of the hemoglobin with the gas. When the volume of breathing is increased by muscular exertion the absorption of gas is pro-

620. Koch: Diss., Greifswald, 1892.
621. Pouchet: *Ann. d'hyg.*, 30:361, 1888.
622. Wachholz: *Vrtljschr. f. gerichtl. Med., Berl*, 23:231, 1902.
623. Gaglio: *Arch. f. exper. Path. u. Pharmakol.*, 22:235, 1887.
624. Buckmaster and Gardner: *J. Physiol.*, 41:60, 1910; *Proc. Roy. Soc. Med.*, 81:516, 1909.

portionally increased. The smaller or younger the individual the quicker the saturation of the blood by carbon monoxide. In the resting stage the volume of breathing varies between individuals as a function of the surface area of their bodies. Small individuals succumb to carbon monoxide more rapidly than large individuals, for the volume of their respiration is greater in relation to the volume of their blood. This fact is made of practical use in the examination of the air of mines when mice or canaries are carried into the vitiated air as living signals of dangerous amounts of gas. Men breathing the same atmosphere have about twenty times as long a stay in the contaminated air as the small animals before getting into a like condition, as men have one-twentieth the skin surface of the small animal per unit of body weight.

Unless accidental, pure carbon monoxide poisoning is rarely met with in the human subject, but since many of the gaseous mixtures contain a high proportion of the gas, the other gases being of a less toxic character, we may fairly assume the symptoms in these cases to be due to carbon monoxide. A large number of experiments on animals made to breathe carbon monoxide, diluted with either oxygen or air, have resulted in showing that the blood pressure is at first considerably increased as the result of the stimulation of the vasomotor center. A benumbing of this center is then shown by the decrease of the pressure and a distention of the blood-vessels. Apoplexy may result from the first stage. More or less extended patches of bright color, especially on the anterior portion of the body, make their appearance and are distinctly different from the violet-red patches that appear, postmortem, especially on the dependent portions of cadavers. The pulse becomes slower when the blood pressure rises, and a violent beating of the heart is experienced.[625] Subsequently the pulse becomes frequent, but small. Breathing is deep and difficult, and, as a result of deficient oxygenation, a diminished production of carbon dioxide occurs.[626] Respiration ceases when the respiratory center is paralyzed, but the stage of stimulation is protracted. The muscular system is very generally affected, in which case the extremities may fail to perform their func-

625. HAGGARD: *Am. J. Physiol.,* 56:390, 1921.
626. HENDERSON and HAGGARD: *J. Pharmacol. & Exper. Therap.,* 16:11, 1920.

tions for many days, or special muscles or muscle groups become paralyzed and afterward degenerate. Sensation to pain may be absent or remain suspended for a long time. The onset of symptoms may be sudden, but usually there are warning sensations, as headache, throbbing of the temples, ringing in the ears, faintness, dizziness, and vomiting. The face becomes red, and there is loss of memory, vertigo, fainting, anesthesia, and loss of all spontaneous power of movement. The heart action is at first violent, then weak, slow, and arrested. The body temperature is lowered.

The recovery is sometimes rapid. Men working around gas mains, in ditches, will be affected, but when taken into the air or given a drink of whiskey or other stimulant speedily recover and return to work. As a rule, however, there is a slow return to consciousness, with more or less prolonged headache, nausea, and weakness. Symptoms may continue for several days. Where the gas has been inhaled for a considerable length of time, the red patches on the skin will remain for quite a while. The paralysis and anesthesia begin in the lower extremities and rise to the trunk. The loss of power and sensibility is frequently shown by the severe burns received by a person falling on a gas or other stove or a brazier. Loss of consciousness is often sudden. At other times there is a slowly increasing drowsiness. There is a great similarity in the symptoms to those of drunkenness. Recovery may in some cases follow a protracted sojourn in a not too poisonous atmosphere, while others, after an hour or two of inhalation, cannot be brought to life. While most have no remembrance of symptoms, many claim to have suffered greatly. Death follows from paralysis of the respiratory apparatus.[627] When the gas itself does not kill, apoplexy or softening of the brain may follow. Pneumonia not infrequently follows the intoxication. According to Becker and Schwerin, the sequelae divide themselves into four groups: (1) primary gangrene[628] with blisters and decubitus; (2) primary hemorrhages, as of the lungs, apoplexy, and the like; (3) a persistent distention of the capillaries and other vessels in which the symptoms are shown in the skin, red nose,

627. LOGAN: *J. State Med.*, 28:306, 1920.

628. RATHERY, R., and GOURNAY, J. J.: *Bull. et mém. Soc. méd. d. hôp. de Paris*, 48:486; BRIGGS: *J.A.M.A.*, 73:678, 1919; GIRAULT and RICHARD: *Presse méd.*, 52:30, 1922.

red spots not unlike those caused by frost-bite; (4) a deep seated disturbance of the regeneration of all organs, especially of the vascular walls and the ganglion cells of the nervous system, evidenced by secondary hemorrhages, idiocy, imbecility, chorea, ascending paralysis, etc. Indeed, the results of this variety of poisoning are manifold, reminding one of diseases of the brain, spinal cord, lungs, kidneys, liver and skin.

Hofmann[629] reports that serological experiments were conducted on rabbits which were exposed six hours daily for nine months to the action of an atmosphere containing 0.01, 0.03 and 0.09% carbon monoxide, and on dogs which breathed 0.05% carbon monoxide daily for five and one-half months. Dogs reacted noticeably to 0.05% carbon monoxide and rabbits showed no changes in their general condition. Yant, Chornyak, Schrenk, Patty and Sayers[630] studied the neuropathology produced in dogs by fatal exposures of twenty to thirty minutes to 0.6% carbon monoxide in air by volume. The brain, as a whole, showed a severe perivascular and perineuronal edema. The circulatory changes are characterized by dilatation, stasis, perivascular hemorrhage, and edema. Edema is diffuse and severe. It is both perineuronal and perivascular. There is a marked difference in the susceptibility of the nerve cells to oxygen deprivation. The cells of the cortex, corpus striatum, dorsal motor nucleus of the vagus, and the dorsal sensory areas of the medulla, are the most sensitve. The nucleus ruber, nuclei of the oculomotor, trochlear, abducens, and facial nerve, and the large polygonal cells in the reticular formation of the medulla are the least susceptible. There are two general types of degenerative changes in the nerve cells following asphyxia: (a) some become shrunken and stain diffusely, (b) others show varying degrees of chromatolysis. Carbon monoxide produces a diffuse degenerative change throughout the entire brain. In this type of asphyxia the most serious effect apears to be edema of the dorsal motor nucleus of the vagus and the adjacent area in the medulla oblongata.

The same authors report the neuropathology found after exposure to carbon monoxide air mixtures which caused death in about eight to fifteen hours. A profound state of asphyxia

629. HOFMANN, P.: *Ztschr. f. Hyg. u. Infektionskr.*, 116:177, 1934.
630. YANT, W. P., CHORNYAK, J., SCHRENK, H. H., PATTY, F. A., and SAYERS, R. R.: Pub. Health Bull. No. 211, August, 1934.

was maintained for the greater portion of the exposure period and death occurred at the end of the period. They came to the following conclusions:

1. Prolonged severe anoxemia resulting from exposure to carbon monoxide produces a diffuse degenerative change in the brain.

2. The circulatory changes are characterized by marked dilatation, stasis, perivascular hemorrhage, and edema. This stasis is complete, as is seen from the degeneration of the red blood cells in some of the extremely dilated vessels.

3. Edema is diffuse and severe. It is both perineuronal and perivascular. The edema is especially severe in the medullary substance.

4. There is a marked difference in the susceptibility of the nerve cells to oxygen deprivation. The cells of the cortex, corpus striatum, the visceral motor nuclei, as the vagus and nucleus ambiguus, the dorsal sensory areas of the medulla, and the Purkinje cells of the cerebellum are the most sensitive. The nucleus ruber, the somatic motor nuclei, and the large polygonal cells (motor type) in the reticular formation of the medulla are the least susceptible. In general, throughout the entire brain, the large polygonal-shaped cells containing well developed Nissl granules show the least damage. The small sensory cells and the smaller types of cells as seen in the corpus striatum, the olives, and in the visceral motor nuclei, showed the most severe damage.

5. There are two general types of degenerative changes in the neurons: (a) some become shrunken, "wavy" and stain diffusely; (b) others show varying degrees of chromatolysis. In the extremes of both types where the cell was completely destroyed only a small fragment was left.

6. In carbon monoxide asphyxia the most serious effects as to life appear to be edema, hemorrhages, and degenerative changes in the visceral motor nuclei, as the dorsal motor nucleus of the vagus nerve, the nucleus ambiguus, and the adjacent area in the medulla oblongata.

7. The degenerative nerve cell changes, especially in parts of the cortex and the corpus striatum, were a great deal more severe when death occurred after an eight to fifteen hour period of severe anoxemia than when death occurred after a twenty to thirty minute period.

In a third paper, in the same studies, the report deals with the neuropathology, particularly the tissue reaction and chronic lesions the authors found in dogs killed sixteen to 165 days after a continuous exposure of thirteen to nineteen hours to carbon monoxide air mixtures which produced and maintained a profound state of asphyxia for the greater portion of the exposure period and a moribund state at the end of the period. The principal lesions and tissue reactions found are as follows:

1. An extensive proliferation of both neuroglia and endothelium.

2. Large cystic areas were found in the medullary substance of the brain. There was a marked cellular reaction in these areas consisting of phagocytic neuroglial ("granule") cells. These cells were large and filled with fat.

3. The proliferation of the endothelium was found at the sites of hemorrhages, collapsed vessels, and in vessels that were extremely dilated and contained fragmented blood cells.

4. Some of the nerve cells were fragmented and invaded by neuronophagocytic cells. In the edematous areas many of the nerve cells showed chromatolysis, shrinkage and dark staining. These areas were similar in appearance to those seen immediately after exposure to carbon monoxide. In general the nerve cells in the deepest layer of the cortex adjacent to the medullary substances showed the most severe damage. Many cells, especially in the upper layers of the cortex, and most of the cells throughout the brain stem had completely recovered.

5. There were focal areas of myelin degeneration throughout the entire nervous system, including the peripheral nerves.

6. Lesions and tissue reactions were most severe in the two dogs killed sixty-two to sixty-five days, respectively, after the exposure as compared with seven dogs killed sixteen to thirty-one days after exposure and one dog killed 165 days after exposure. It was not positively ascertained whether this difference in degree was the result of greater susceptibility, or a more severe exposure, or whether the degenerative changes were progressive for the sixty-two to sixty-five day period.

In the fourth paper they reported the study of the neuropathology resulting from comparatively rapid asphyxia by atmospheres deficient in oxygen. The findings in all these dogs were similar to lesions due to carbon monoxide poisoning but varied in degrees. In the case of dogs killed by atmospheres deficient in oxygen after eleven and fourteen minutes exposure, the period was too short to produce very extensive morphological changes in the nerve cells, but the circulatory changes were present. They summarize their work as follows:

1. The circulatory changes in the dog were characterized by dilatation, stasis involving the entire capillary system, and perivascular hemorrhages.

2. There is a marked difference in the susceptibility of the nerve cells to oxygen deprivation. The cells of the cortex, especially those in the outer granular layer, thalamus, sensory and correlation centers throughout the brain stem and the visceral efferent nuclei, are the most sensitive. The nucleus ruber, nuclei of the oculomotor, trochlear, abducens, and facial nerve, the large polygonal-shaped cells in the reticular formation and the anterior horn motor cells are the least susceptible in the dog.

3. The circulatory changes in the rate were limited mostly to the large perforating cerebral vessels. There was no congestion in the meninges, and the capillaries throughout the cortex showed no remarkable changes.

4. There is a marked difference in the reactions of the nerve cells of the rat as compared with those of the dog. The cerebrum of the rat, with the exception of some large cells in the olfactory cortex and large polygonal-shaped cells in the mon-olfactory cortex, showed no damage. The motor type of cells, which are least susceptible in the dog are much more susceptible to oxygen deprivation in the rat.

5. There are two general types of degenerative changes in the nerve cells following asphyxia; some become shrunken and stain diffusely; others show varying degrees of chromatolysis.

6. There is a definite and remarkable difference in the susceptibility of nerve cells in the same brain and in the same type of cells in different species, as the dog and rat.

7. These observations on the differences in the reaction of dogs and rats to atmospheres deficient in oxygen are in general alinement with the current neurological views on cerebral mechanisms.[631] These observations also reveal the serious

631. LASHLEY, K. S.: (1) Studies of Cerebral Function in Learning, *Psychobiol.*, 2:55-128, 1920; (2) The Effects of Long Continued Practice upon Cerebral Localization, *J. Comp. Psychol.*, 1:453-468, 1921; (3)

difficulties that are encountered in formulating theories on cerebral mechanisms in human behavior from data obtained from rats.

In the fifth paper they reported the blood chemistry changes in dogs asphyxiated by exposure to atmospheres deficient in oxygen which caused death in less than thirty minutes. This study was made not only to ascertain the changes attending asphyxia by insufficient atmospheric oxygen but also for comparison with a similar study of the changes attending asphyxia by carbon monoxide. The purpose of the comparison was to ascertain if the changes were peculiar to each type of asphyxia or if they were identical and due entirely to anoxemia.

1. There was a marked hyperglycemia and hyperuricemia; the non-protein nitrogen and urea increased slightly; the total and preformed creatinine remained practically normal; and the inorganic phosphorus increased.

2. There was a decrease in the hydrogen-ion concentration and a marked decrease in the carbon dioxide capacity of the plasma, and the carbon dioxide content of the blood.

3. The oxygen saturation of the arterial blood at death ranged from 1.3% to 8%.

4. The red blood cells increased in one case, but showed no significant change in two. The white blood cells and the polymorphonuclears increased, while the lymphocytes decreased.

The sixth paper deals with the blood chemistry of dogs after comparatively rapid carbon monoxide asphyxia under conditions which caused death in twenty to thirty minutes. They found a large percentage increase in the uric acid, which is probably due to the fact that since uric acid is oxidized to allantoin in the dog, inhibition of oxidation would tend to prevent complete oxidation and cause a building up of uric acid.

1. None of the chemical changes found in dogs is thought to be of a nature that would be readily corrected when the anoxemia is relieved by treatment with oxygen or a mixture of 5% to 7% carbon dioxide in oxygen. It is therefore apparent that the changes found are not primarily responsible

The Motor Areas, *Brain*, 44:255-285, 1921; (4) Vicarious Function of the Visual Areas, *Am. J. Physiol.*, 59:44-67, 1922; (5) The Retention of Motor Habits After Destruction of the so-called "Motor Areas" in Primates, *Arch. Neurol. & Psychiat.*, 12:249-276, 1924. And see HERRICK, C. J.: Brains of Rats and Men, 1926.

for the failure of moribund cases of carbon monoxide poisoning to respond to such treatment.

2. There was a marked hyperglycemia and hyperuricemia; the non-protein nitrogen and urea increased slightly; the total and preformed creatinine remained practically normal; and the inorganic phosphorus increased.

3. There was an increase in the hydrogen-ion concentration, and a marked decrease in the carbon dioxide capacity of the plasma, and a lesser though a distinct decrease in the carbon dioxide content of the blood. The oxygen saturation of the venous blood at death ranged from 0.0 to 5.6 cc. in 100 cc. of blood.

4. The carbon monoxide saturation at death varied from 83% to 90%.

5. The blood counts showed a slight but insignificant tendency toward an increase in hemoglobin, red blood cells, white blood cells and polymorphonuclears. The lymphocytes showed a slight decrease. No significant change occurred in the number of endothelials and eosinophils.

6. The blood chemistry findings were similar to those previously found for the same degree of asphyxia produced by exposure of dogs to an atmosphere deficient in oxygen.

Chronic Carbon Monoxide Poisoning: Chronic poisoning by carbon monoxide has received the attention of many observers in recent years. There is very good evidence of this form. Accumulated cases show that it is the result of being in a constantly contaminated atmosphere. The symptoms are described as an alteration in the digestion, diminished vigor, gray color of the skin, coated tongue, loss of memory, diminution of the psychic powers, and occasional convulsions. The pathologic findings at autopsies have shown, in some cases, fatty degeneration; in others, pernicious anemia. Bect and Fort[632] reported two cases of chronic carbon monoxide poisoning with a blood picture simulating a pernicious anemia. Forbes,[633] quoting Dr. Geo. G. Davis, former Chief Surgeon of the Illinois Steel Company, reports that in investigating carbon monoxide poisoning in blast furnace workers, he fails to find evidence of anemia resulting from frequent exposure to carbon monoxide; 64.1% of the red blood cell counts were over

632. Bect, H. G., and Fort, W.: *Am. J. Clin. M.*, 3:437, 1934.
633. Forbes: *J. Indust. Hyg.*, No. 1, 3:13, 1921.

5,000,000, 2.2% were over 6,000,000, and none was under 4,000,000.

Brandt[634] reports a number of workers with chronic carbon monoxide poisoning who had symptoms as headache, loss of appetite, fatigue, palpitation of the heart, reduction of visual acuity and of sexual potency. In two cases the complaints reached serious proportions. In the case of a chemist there was a condition of excitement with confusion which led to his commitment to an institution for mental disease. The right pupil was irregular in shape. Encephalography showed shrinking and distortion of the right lateral ventricle. A girl employed in a kitchen where there was a leaky stove, showed decided loss in weight, reduction of efficiency, headache, vertigo, and increased thirst. Pilman[635] gives a detailed report of the examinations of thirty-six men working in an atmosphere containing an excess of carbon monoxide. Eight had vascular dilatation in the fundus. Only two had normal visual fields, and contraction first appearing for color and later for form; and repeated examinations demonstrated the progressive tendency of the visual field changes. Amblyopia was reported from the inhalation of carbon monoxide gas by Murray.[636] Forbes, Cobb, and Fremont-Smith[637] demonstrated that carbon monoxide causes a marked rise in cerebrospinal fluid pressure, and concluded that the carbon monoxide headache is closely associated with congestion and possibly with edema. The fibers of the optic nerve apparently are not especially susceptible to the action of carbon monoxide. The earliest and most constant sign of carbon monoxide intoxication is congestion of the retinal veins and hyperemia of the optic disk. These generally disappear, but the literature shows a number of serious permanent visual effects.

A stoker,[638] aged sixty-two years, fell into a tank containing coal gases. He inhaled the gas and fell from a height of half a meter to the bottom, where he lay unconscious for some minutes before rescue. He regained consciousness, but

634. BRANDT, A.: *Arch. f. Gewerbepath. u. Gewerbehyg.*, 5:433, 1934.

635. PILMAN, H.: Abstr. from *Sovet. vestnik. oftal.*, 4:433, 1934, in *Am. J. Ophth.*, 17:1191, 1934.

636. MURRAY, W. R.: *Minnesota Med.*, 9:561, 1926.

637. FORBES, COBB, and FREMONT-SMITH: *Arch. Neurol. & Psychiat.*, 11:264, 1924.

638. *Am. J. Ophth.*, 1924.

complained of disturbance of sight. When he left the hospital his sight was sufficiently restored to enable him to shave himself on the following day. He lost his sight the next day. No traces of injury on the head or face in the vicinity of the eyes were seen. Movement of the eyes was satisfactory in every direction. The pupils were equal, their reaction good in all respects, the media were clear and transparent, the papilla sound. In the eye ground a minor discoloration was seen, but the blood vessels of the retina did not show any aberration in respect to their course and their repletion of blood. The patient perceived movements of the hand with both eyes, his sensibility to light and localization of light were good. He could count fingers from a distance of one and one-half meters. His vision gradually increased and after a few weeks became normal. Another case is reported of total blindness for eight days. The author stated that a hemorrhage or softening either of the visual radiations or of the cortex, itself, has in his cases caused bilateral blindness, and hemianopsia.

Lindemann reports blindness from gases of dynamite.[639] Grinker[640] reports the case of a woman fifty-eight years of age who was found unconscious in a gas-filled room on October 18, 1924. She regained consciousness after a few hours in a hospital, where she had daily emesis, and was apparently physically normal and revealed no motor disturbances until six months later. Then her orientation gradually became poor, she became apathetic, did not speak, and acted queerly. She was sent to a hospital for mental diseases. It was found that the pupils reacted to light and accommodation, the reflexes were equal and normal, and the plantar response was in flexion. She lay motionless and rigid, with a mask-like face. The palpebral fissures were widely opened, and winking was frequent. The left nasolabial fold was deeper than the right. There was no paralysis. Muscle tone was greatly increased in the arms, and the legs were slightly stiff. The patient presented catatonic symptoms, the legs returning slowly to a position of rest. On standing she fell backward, and the gait was small-stepped, without swinging of the arms. She answered questions only

639. LINDEMANN, K.: Ztschr. f. Augenh., 61:72, 1927. And FEJIR, J.: Wien. klin. Wchnschr., 27:216, 1924; Am. J. Ophth., 7:522, 1924.
640. GRINKER, R. R.: J. Nerv. & Ment. Dis., 64:18, 1926.

after long pauses, with great difficulty, and finally became mute. The rigor increased markedly, especially in the left arm. On December 21, death occurred, with pulmonary edema. On examination of the brain grossly in coronal section, symmetrical yellow-brown, necrotic areas were seen in the globus pallidus. They extended from the anterior tip to the center of the ganglia. Dorsally they reached to the dorsal border of the pallidus and lay against the internal capsule.

Ziemke[641] reported a case of carbon monoxide poisoning and death from the inhalation of burning acetylene in a closed room. Postmortem revealed a subacute carbon monoxide poisoning. In the brain there were found symmetrical foci of softening lenticular nuclei, and almost all of the brain sections showed punctate hemorrhages about the size of a pinhead. Microscopically there were found the typical lesions of subacute carbon monoxide poisoning referable to the blood vessels, that is to say granular and in part homogenous calcifications in the media. Vermeylen[642] states that in the majority of cases mental disturbances are seen in acute cases of carbon monoxide poisoning. His case gives reference to a slow intoxication which for a long time remained undetected. The patient had to be guided like a child. On questioning he answered with "I don't know." His wife stated that for a few days her husband had had a bizarre attitude. The most outstanding changes were a mental inertia and a marked amnesia. The patient improved and ultimately returned to work.

The number of deaths caused by the inhalation of carbon monoxide from automobile exhausts in closed garages is increasing. The author reported sixty-three deaths from carbon monoxide poisoning in private garages during six years in Chicago alone.[643] Early reports of death or poisoning from gas engines were referred to as "gasoline fumes" or "petromortis." Only after pathologic and chemical investigations was the true cause of death determined, for the postmortem appearance and chemical proof of carbon monoxide poisoning were well known long before the advent of the automobile. Longhurst[644] reported a death from petrol poisoning. Blumen-

641. ZIEMKE, E.: Deutsche Ztschr. f. d. ges. gerichtl. Med., 20: 503, 1933.
642. VERMEYLEN, G.: J. belge de neurol. et de psychiat., 33: 595, 1933.
643. McNALLY, W. D.: Arch. Path., 5: 43, 1928.
644. LONGHURST: J. Roy. Army Med. Corps, 13: 584, 1909.

shen[645] reported four deaths from automobile fumes. Johnson[646] reported forty-two poisonings, but no deaths from fumes of a gasoline engine in a sewer. Foote[647] reported three poisonings, but no deaths, in the hold of a submarine. The author reported that the exhaust gases of automobiles, as a source of poisoning, contained from 1.16 to 6.62% carbon monoxide.[648]

Briggs[649] reported the illness of two men and one death from the exhaust of a motor boat pouring into a cabin; the estimated time of exposure was fifteen minutes. Barclay[650] also reported deaths from carbon monoxide on a motor launch. Homan[651] reported the illness of twenty persons in a closed auto truck[652] twenty minutes after the car was started. Twelve men, found unconscious, were laid out on the road, and an effort was made to revive them. A boy, aged 17, died. Two people seated near an engine in an excursion boat[653] were killed by the exhaust. Hitchcock[654] reported three fatal cases of poisoning in a garage and a fourth with slow recovery. "Fourteen months after the accident an anterograde amnesia was still present, some emotional disturbance and some depression." Logan[655] reported carbon monoxide poisoning from the exhaust in closed motor vehicles, such as cars, lorries and ambulances used at the front in the World War. Logan briefly alludes to the death of men returning in ambulances from the front in English, French, and Italian armies. Ciampolini,[656] Kranenburg,[657] Henderson,[658] Yant,[659] and Hayhurst[660] report the dangers of exhaust gases from automobiles. Yant, Jacobs and Berger[661] give the percentages of carbon monoxide in the air

645. BLUMENSHEN: *Med. Rec.*, 93:342, 1918.
646. JOHNSON, J. W.: *Canad. M. A. J.*, 3:118, 1917.
647. FOOTE: *U. S. Nav. M. Bull.*, 10:681, 1916.
648. McNALLY, W. D.: *J.A.M.A.*, 69:1586, 1917.
649. BRIGGS, J. E.: *J.A.M.A.*, 73:678, 1919.
650. BARCLAY: *New Zealand M. J.*, 7:42, 1909.
651. HOMAN: *Lancet*, 1:1334, 1920.
652. *J.A.M.A.*, 83:284, 1924.
653. *Brit. M. J.*, 1:338, 1924.
654. HITCHCOCK, C. W.: *J.A.M.A.*, 71:257, 1918.
655. LOGAN: *J. State Med.*, 28:306, 1920.
656. CIAMPOLINI: *J. Indust. Hyg.*, 6:102, 1924.
657. KRANENBERG: *Nederl. tijdschr. v. geneesk.*, 78:1794, 1924; 79:509, 1925.
658. HENDERSON: *Progres med.*, 40:332, 1924.
659. YANT: *J. Indust. & Eng. Chem.*, 16:1047, 1924.
660. HAYHURST, E. R.: *Am. J. Pub. Health*, 16:218, 1926.
661. YANT, JACOBS; BERGER: *J. Indust. & Eng. Chem.*, 16:1047, 1924.

of a closed garage of 2,950 cubic feet capacity in which the engine of a five-passenger car was running at 200 revolutions per minute. In twenty-five minutes the air contained 1.31%, in sixty minutes, 2.10%.

Kranenburg investigated 157 public garages and found 0.10% carbon monoxide in the air ten feet from the exhausts of running motors, white at thirty feet he found none. In garages in which the air was contaminated to the extent of 0.2%, almost all of the workers complained of headache. Forty workers from thirty-one different garages submitted to blood tests, and in 69.5% of these carbon monoxide hemoglobin was found. The author found in his report of sixty-three cases of poisoning, that fifty-nine of the deaths were accidental and four were undetermined as to whether accidental or homicidal; fifty-one, or 80.95%, of the patients had insurance ranging from $200 to $100,000; over half of the policies were for $3,000 or less, three were for $5,000, one was for $6,000, one was for $34,000, and one for $100,000. Eleven, or 17.46%, were repairing their cars, while the others were found sitting at the wheel with the engine running.

The Bureau of Census,[662] reported 3,572 deaths in 1931, 3,352 in 1932, and 3,543 in 1933 from carbon monoxide poisoning.

Rossiter[663] claims that in New York City there is an average of about three deaths a day from this gas; in 1925 there were 1,009 deaths, 388 of which were suicides; in 1926, 1,190 deaths, with 371 suicides. In Cook County, Illinois, over a period of sixteen years there were 6,031 deaths, with 2,509 suicides; in one year there were 518 cases, 272 due to gas stoves. In the Pittsburgh District, the number of cases is not high due to the fact that natural gas is used, which contains no carbon monoxide; during the last five years there were 183 deaths, forty-six due to exhaust gas. In Rossiter's 2,000 cases he claims he has never seen a case of pneumonia. "Tuberculosis is not so often attributed to gassing directly, but it is claimed that the irritation from the inhaled gas opens inroads for infection of the lungs, or that a pre-existing condition is aggravated."

662. Provisional Summary of Mortality Statistics in U. S. A., Bureau of Census, Washington, D. C.

663. ROSSITER, F. S.: Address at Twenty-Fourth Annual Convention of International Claim Association, Atlantic City N. J., 1933.

Engel[664] shows the composition of smoke from blast furnace gas to be as follows:

Carbon monoxide	25%
Carbon dioxide	12%
Oxygen	6%
Hydrogen	2%
Nitrogen	55%

Engel, with twelve years experience in industrial work, examined 1,200 cases of gassing, had no deaths, no complications, and no sequelae following mild or severe gassing. All of his cases were acute, no case of chronic poisoning has ever been reported to him. His illness records for the past two years show that among blast-furnace employees there was less time lost due to pulmonary disease than among other lines of employment.

The exhaust gas from internal combustion engines contains carbon monoxide in percentages ranging from a fraction of 1% to 7%, or even higher. The variation depends upon the proportion of air and gasoline in the mixture burned; the carbon monoxide increases with increase in the proportion of gasoline, that is with a rich mixture. "A rough estimate of the volume of carbon monoxide that an automobile may produce is one cubic foot (twenty-eight liters) per minute per twenty horse power. This is sufficient to render the atmosphere of a single car garage deadly within five minutes, if the engine is run while the garage doors are closed."[665]

Carbon monoxide combines with the hemoglobin of the blood to the exclusion of oxygen. Animals (amphioxus and leptocephalus) which have no hemoglobin are quite normal in 80% carbon monoxide and 20% oxygen. Nerve cells of the chick in a drop of serum grow normally in such an atmosphere. A mouse can tolerate a high percentage of carbon monoxide if the pressure of oxygen is also increased. The toxic action of carbon monoxide can be explained through the anoxemia resulting from the conversion of oxyhemoglobin to carbon monoxide hemoglobin, and the resulting asphyxia.

Carbon monoxide displaces oxygen from hemoglobin, and in turn oxygen may displace carbon monoxide from its com-

664. ENGEL, R. C.: *J. Indust. Hyg.*, 7:122, 1925.

665. HENDERSON and HAGGARD: Noxious Gases, Monograph Series, No. 35, 1927.

bination. Red corpuscles, in which the hemoglobin has been joined to carbon monoxide and then freed from the combination by means of oxygen, are not injured; they are capable of transporting oxygen as if they had never been exposed to the other gas. But so long as the combination with carbon monoxide continues they are incapable of fulfilling their respiratory function.

The reaction between oxygen, carbon monoxide and hemoglobin is reversible, as expressed by the following equation:

$$HbO_2 + CO \rightleftharpoons HbCO + O_2$$

Stadie and Martin[666] report that an increase of carbon dioxide in the blood decreased the affinity of hemoglobin for carbon monoxide as compared with its affinity for oxygen.

"The average man at rest has a pulmonary ventilation of approximately five liters of air per minute. This assumes a volume of respiration of 7.5 liters a minute and a dead space of 33%. Now five liters of air holding 0.07% of carbon monoxide would represent 0.0035 liter (3.5 cc.) of the gas, so that 0.21 liter (3.5 x 60=210 cc.) at most would come in contact with the blood during the course of one hour. The total volume of blood in the body of an average adult is about five liters and has the capacity to hold approximately one liter of oxygen. Each thousandth of a liter of carbon monoxide that is absorbed into the blood decreases the oxygen capacity by an equivalent amount, that is 0.1%. At the end of one hour the maximum amount by which, under these conditions, the oxygen capacity can be replaced by carbon monoxide, would be 21%; an amount sufficient to elicit only slight symptoms of anoxemia."[667] Less than the amount of carbon monoxide thus estimated would be combined in the blood, for as the absorption continues the rate falls farther and farther short of total absorption. The reason for this reaction approaches equilibrium, the balance of pressure between the oxygen and carbon monoxide in the blood and their attractions for hemoglobin shift automatically and progressively until at equilibrium carbon monoxide is displaced by oxygen in amount each minute equal to that in which oxygen is displaced by carbon monoxide.

666. STADIE and MARTIN: *J. Clin. Research*, 2:77, 1925.
667. HENDERSON and HAGGARD: Noxious Gases, Monograph Series, No. 35, 1927.

Exercise causes an increase in the respiratory rate, and the absorption of carbon monoxide is proportionately accelerated. "A rough, but useful rule is that one-half the carbon monoxide inhaled is absorbed during the early stages of exposure. (By 'inhaled' is meant the total volume of respiration per minute and not only the pulmonary ventilation, which is the volume of respiration minus the allowance for dead space.") Frequently an expert is asked who dies first, an adult or a child. The answer to this would be if both were at rest and exposed to the same concentration of carbon monoxide, the smaller and younger, the individual with the more active metabolism, would absorb carbon monoxide and tend to approach saturation the more rapidly, with an earlier death. In such cases it is the relation of the respiration to the size of the body and its volume of blood which influences the rate at which oxygen is displaced by carbon monoxide. Smaller individuals, therefore, succumb to carbon monoxide more rapidly than large individuals, for the volume of their respiration is greater in relation to their volume of blood. This comparison finds its extreme expression, and a very practical application, in the rate of saturation as between men on the one hand and such small animals as the mouse and canary on the other. In mine rescue operations the animals are carried into vitiated air as indicators of the presence of carbon monoxide. When the mouse can no longer maintain its equilibrium, or the canary falls off its perch, this gives the rescuers warning that they are breathing a dangerous concentration of carbon monoxide, for men have only about one-twentieth the skin surface of the small animal per unit of body weight, so twenty times as long a stay in the atmosphere will bring them into the same condition.

The symptoms resulting from the inhalation of carbon monoxide depend upon the degree of anoxemia, that is the extent of combination of the hemoglobin with the gas. Table XXX gives the average physiological response to the various percentages of saturation of the hemoglobin with carbon monoxide.

Haines, Karasek, and Apfelbach,[668] in their investigations of the effects of carbon monoxide, found that workmen exposed

668. HAINES, KARASEK, and APFELBACH: Report of (Illinois) Commission on Occupational Diseases, 89, 1911.

frequently to the gas in metallurgical establishments in a large majority of cases developed a considerable increase of red blood corpuscles above the normal, the number in one case examined reaching 9,000,000. The amount of hemoglobin was also usually above normal. These investigators attribute the increase in red cells and hemoglobin to a protective effort on the part of the system. The same investigators also found that workmen frequently exposed to carbon monoxide in metallurgical establishments showed more or less muscular weakness, as was demonstrated by tests with a hand dynamometer, a comparison being made with an equal number of workmen of the same social grade employed in industrial establishments in which they were not exposed to the gas.

TABLE XXX
PERCENTAGE SATURATION OF THE BLOOD WITH CARBON MONOXIDE AND CORRESPONDING PHYSIOLOGICAL EFFECTS

Per Cent of Hemoglobin in Combination with Carbon Monoxide	Physiological Effect
10	No appreciable effect except shortness of breath on vigorous muscular exertion.
20	No appreciable effect in most cases except short wind even on moderate exertion; slight headache in some cases.
30	Decided headache; irritable; easily fatigued; judgment disturbed.
40-50	Headache, confusion, collapse and fainting on exertion.
60-70	Unconsciousness; respiratory failure and death if exposure is long continued.
80	Rapidly fatal.
Over 80	Immediately fatal.

Gruber[669] has shown, along with others, that carbon monoxide is not a cumulative poison, but that when inhaled in very small quantities it disappears from the blood. In cases of chronic poisoning the blood does not serve for diagnosis. This is not the case, however, in acute poisoning, where a timely examination of the blood taken from the patient as soon

669. GRUBER: Arch. f. Hyg., 1:145, 1883. And see also SEDGWICK, W. T., and NICHOLAS, W. R.: A Study of the Poisonous Effects of Coal and Water Gas, Sixth Annual Report of the State Board of Health and Charity of Massachusetts, 1885; HENDERSON: J.A.M.A., 67:580, 1916; HALDANE: J. Physiol., 18:201, 1895.

as possible will indicate the poisonous effect of carbon monoxide and lead to the adoption of proper methods of resuscitation. As a further aid to diagnosis, the comatose condition, low temperature, absence of odor of alcohol, loud snoring, and bright red appearance of the face would lead one to suspect gas poisoning, especially if the body were found in a closed room or in a confined space with indications of gas poisoning more or less apparent. As a further diagnosis the urine is found to contain a reducing substance, generally glycuronic acid, and in many cases there is albuminuria. Red patches or spots upon the surface of the skin are characteristic. Legry and Lermoyes,[670] have shown that the blood in the cerebrospinal fluid may reveal carbon monoxide long after it has disappeared from the blood-stream.

Litten found glycosuria in 70% of cases of carbon monoxide poisoning. While the glycosuria may last three or four days, it generally disappears before the end of the second day and is therefore frequently missed as urine examinations are not made until twenty-four to forty-eight hours afterward. The author found glycosuria present in about 20% of the cases of carbon monoxide poisoning admitted to the County hospital. This is not peculiar to the action of carbon monoxide, but follows asphyxia from other causes, and is the result of the pouring out of adrenalin into the circulation under the stimulus of asphyxia and the resultant increased supply of blood sugar from the liver under the stimulus of the adrenalin. The glycosuria may be indirectly due to anoxemia. In the acute state, a diagnosis of food poisoning, strychnine poisoning, diabetes, and alcoholism have been made in cases of carbon monoxide poisoning. The symptoms are so varied that a physician is reminded of diseases of the brain, spinal cord, lungs, kidneys, liver and skin.

Mayers, Rivkin and Krasnow[671] have shown the effect of pure carbon monoxide, illuminating gas, and automobile gas on the fragility of the red blood cells. When normal blood was exposed to purse carbon monoxide gas under laboratory conditions, there was no increase in the fragility of the red blood cells. Normal blood exposed to both illuminating gas and automobile exhaust gas, under the same laboratory conditions,

670. Legry and Lermoyes: *Presse méd.*, 28:816, 1920.

671. Mayers, May R., Rivkin, Helen, and Krasnow, Frances: *J. Indust. Hyg.*, 12:300, 1930.

showed a tendency to a somewhat increased hemolysis of the red cells. The increase in hemolysis due to automobile exhaust gas is slightly less than that produced by illuminating gas. The hemolyzing effect of these gases would seem, therefore, to be due to the presence of other toxic constituents rather than to their carbon monoxide content.

Treatment: The person must be removed from the poisonous atmosphere and into the fresh air and artificial respiration introduced as soon as possible. The patient should be taken to a hospital where the elimination of carbon monoxide can be hastened. The Fire Department in many large cities has equipment to give inhalations of oxygen and carbon dioxide. Drinker and Shaughnessy[672] recommend the use of 7% carbon dioxide and 93% oxygen for the first five to twenty minutes.

Carbon Dioxide Treatment: Murphy and Drinker[673] came to the conclusion that a 5% mixture gave no stimulation, while a 10% mixture gave some response. Ten per cent carbon dioxide is more effectual in the treatment of certain degrees of carbon monoxide asphyxia than is the 5% mixture; and artificial respiration should be administered to patients who are breathing but who are not suffering from severe grades of asphyxia. In these persons a brief period of artificial respiration will induce conditions favorable to the stimulation of breathing by the carbon dioxide in the inhalation mixtures. Henderson[674] reports that with dogs given oxygen plus carbon dioxide, the carbon monoxide hemoglobin is reduced below 10% in twenty minutes, while with inhalation of air it takes 140 minutes to accomplish the same result. Methylene blue is not an antidote for carbon monoxide. The results from the carbon dioxide and oxygen treatment are excellent, and where it is available all other methods are superfluous.

In cases of carbon monoxide poisoning, or in asphyxia from other causes, such as drowning, reliance has been placed in some quarters on the use of the pulmotor. This is nothing more than an apparatus for inducing artificial respiration by mechanical means. Concerning its use it is to be said that it is probably no more efficient than are other means, properly ap-

672. DRINKER, C. K., and SHAUGHNESSY, T. J.:   *J. Indust. Hyg.*, 11: 301, 1929.
673. MURPHY, D. P., and DRINKER, C. K.: *J. Indust. Hyg.*, 12: 92, 1930.
674. HENDERSON, Y.:   *Brit. M. J.*, 1: 41, 1926.

plied, of bringing about artificial respiration and, further, the time spent in trying to obtain the apparatus would much better be employed in careful and strenuous manipulations by the most approved methods in the endeavor to produce renewed respiration, as the elements of time and prompt action are essential to the resuscitation of the individual overcome.[675]

The gas mask perfected and used by the U. S. Army[675] should be a part of the equipment of ambulances and every piece of fire apparatus, so that firemen who are forced to enter burning buildings may have protection against noxious fumes.

The principal features as given by Dewey are:

1. Canister of metal containing both neutral-

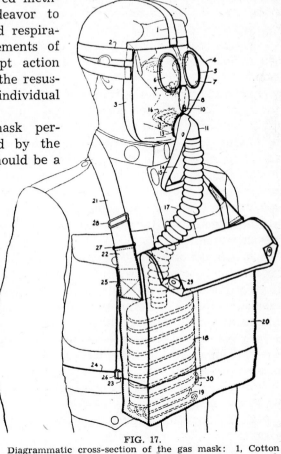

FIG. 17.

Diagrammatic cross-section of the gas mask: 1, Cotton tape; 2, elastic tape; 3, binder; 4, face-piece; 5, eye cup; 6, lens; 7, lens washer; 8, nose spring; 9, nose pad; 10, nose rivet; 11, die casting; 12, die casting nut; 13, die casting washer; 14, flutter valve; 15, flutter guard; 16, mouthpiece; 17, hose; 18, canister; 19, spring; 20, knapsack; 21, shoulder strap; 22, large loop chape; 23, small loop chape; 24, body cord; 25, eyelet; 26, small loop; 27, large loop; 28, center bar slide; 29, "Lift the dot" fastener; 30, grommet

izing and absorptive chemicals and a smoke filter. The air to be breathed passes through an inlet valve and through chemicals and smoke filter.

675. DEWEY: *J. Indust. & Eng. Chem.*, 11:185, 1919.

2. A flexible rubber hose through which the purified air passes from the canister to the face-piece.

3. A face-piece effectively covering the eyes, cheeks, lower forehead, nose, mouth, and chin, provided with eye-pieces permitting vision and a harness to hold the face-piece in place when wearing the mask.

4. An exhalation valve which affords easy discharge of exhaled air and at the same time instantly closes upon inspiration.

5. A knapsack slung from the neck or shoulder, in which the mask and canister are carried. In the box respirator type manufactured, the inhaled air, passing through the canister and hose, went directly into the mouth through a rubber mouthpiece, which in this manner offered protection to the lungs in the event of the failure of the fit of the face-piece or of damage to the face-piece. At the time the mask was provided with a spring and rubber device which closed off the air passage through the nose and compelled breathing entirely through the mouth.

It is also worth while to enumerate a few of the principal requirements to be fulfilled by a respirator:

1. It must successfully remove all gas fumes or smoke from the air to which a man is exposed, and must do this for the maximum of time for which the man is liable to be on duty.

2. It must be reasonably comfortable to the wearer.

3. The fit of the face-piece around the face must be a perfect gas-tight joint.

4. The material of the face-piece must be substantially impermeable to all noxious gases.

5. The eyepieces must be strong and provide for good vision.

6. The complete equipment must have durability, for all personal equipment of a man in the field receives extremely hard usage.

7. The resistance to flow of air through the various parts must be kept at a low figure in order that the efficiency of the individual may not be too much reduced.

8. It must be of minimum weight and bulk.

The points mentioned indicate but few of the severe requirements which had to be met during the course of production.

The canister filled with hopcalite (MnO_2 50%, CuO 30%, Co_2O_3 15%) acts as a catalyst, oxidizing the carbon monoxide readily, when the contaminated air has been dried by passing over calcium chloride.[676] The efficiency and life of the canister depend upon the life of the drying agent.   When the canister has gained more than 35 gm. above the original weight, it should be withdrawn, as it then fails to act as a catalyst.   The higher the temperature the longer the life of the canister, as the hopcalite is less sensitive to water vapor at high temperatures.

Workmen around blast furnaces are always exposed to carbon monoxide poisoning.[677]   After passing the gas through the washers, where it is freed from its suspended matter, it is usually invisible and practically odorless.   The men working around the blast furnaces receive some warning (odor and dusts) of its presence when it escapes, while those working in places where the washed gas is being used fail to recognize the presence of the carbon monoxide.   The gas mask with the hopcalite would prevent many asphyxiations in these workers.

Postmortem Appearances: Poisoning by a small amount of carbon monoxide may produce very few changes, or if the patient lives for a number of hours after exposure, only a careful examination of the blood will reveal the presence of the gas.   Where the blood is well saturated with the gas, the surface of the body is cherry-red.   The eyes are closed and the countenance usually composed.   The dependent parts at the surface of the body are of deeper red than other parts.   There are frequently bright red patches upon the thighs and the front of the trunk and neck.   The most characteristic change is the bright cherry-red blood, usually fluid and coagulating slowly, present in the arteries, veins, and all of the tissues. Blood of cats gassed with carbon monoxide showed no constant change of coagulation time.[678]   The brightness of the carbon monoxide hemoglobin may be masked by carbon di-

676. LAMB, BRAY, and FRAZIER: *J. Indust. & Eng. Chem.,* 12:213, 1920; see also ROGERS, PIGGOT, BAHLKE, and JENNINGS: *J. Am. Chem. Soc.,* 43:1973, 1921; and MERRILL and SCALIONE: *J. Am. Chem. Soc.,* 43: 1982, 1921 (who advise catalysts of mixtures of metallic oxides), and LAMB, SCALIONE, and EDGAR: *J. Am. Chem. Soc.,* 44:738, 1922.

677. WATKINS: Tech. Paper 156, 1917, U. S. Bureau of Mines; FORBES: *J. Indust. Hyg.,* 3:11, 1921.

678. FORBES and HOMPE: *J. Indust. Hyg.,* 3:213, 1921.

oxide from the fumes of coal gas or from the smoke of burning wood or other combustible material. When death occurs rapidly from cyanide poisoning, the blood is also bright red, but the color is not as permanent as in gas poisoning, changing to blue on exposure to air. If the gas poisoning be prolonged, small hemorrhages are present in the pleural cavities, with pulmonary edema and bright red froth in the air passages. The gastric and intestinal mucosa may also have small punctiform hemorrhages. Occasionally, rather large hemorrhages are met in the great omentum and in the leptomeninges under conditions difficult to explain, except under carbon monoxide poisoning. The hemorrhages in the omentum are as large as the open hand.[679] The hemorrhages in the brain are never in sufficient degree to cause compression. A very character-istic change in prolonged carbon monoxide poisoning is the occurrence of punctiform hemorrhages and softening in the cortex and central nuclei of the brain, notably in the two internal segments of the lenticular nucleus.[680] Gunther des-cribes a hemorrhage and necrotic myositis occurring eight days after carbon monoxide poisoning. The kidneys may show fatty degeneration and necrosis in the convoluted tubules. Where life has been prolonged, the skin may show herpes, blebs, and pemphigus followed by gangrene.[681] Polycythemia and leukocytosis are quite regularly present, though a mild chronic poisoning may induce an anemia. Czoniczer[682] has shown the presence of uricacidemia in carbon monoxide poisoning. Glycosuria is present in about 20% of the cases of gas poisoning, including those that die of carbon monoxide and those that recover.

Stevenson[683] reports a case where the condition of the viscera was phenomenal, the rosy hue being visible after seventeen months. This is also the case with blood, which a great many observers say retains its color for several years, observations which McNally confirmed by his experiments.

679. LeCount, E. R.:   Personal Communication.
680. Kolisko: *Beitr. z. gerichtl. Med.,* 2, 1914; Photakis, B. A.: Anatomical Changes in the Central Nervous System Following Carbon Monoxide Poisoning, *Vrtljschr. f. gerichtl. Med., Berl.,* 62:42, 1921.
681. Mott: *Brit. M. J.,* 1:637, 1917; Hill and Semerak: *J.A.M.A.,* 71:644, 1918.
682. Czoniczer: *München. med. Wchnschr.,* 67:1121, 1920.
683. Stevenson: *Guy's Hosp. Rep.,* 46:223, 1889.

Otto[684] states that Landois was able to detect carbon monoxide in the body of a woman eighteen months after death. The blood retained its red color notwithstanding the fact that the body had undergone extreme putrefaction. Otto himself preserved the blood for two years by keeping it in a closed vessel.

Pathology: The pathology of carbon monoxide is explained by oxygen starvation, transient or prolonged. If it is prolonged there will be in some cases, permanent damage to certain elements of the body, the cells of the central nervous system being the most vulnerable. The sequelae of severe gassing are usually abnormalities of cerebal or spinal function, and the anatomical changes are found in the central nervous system chiefly. The lesions in the central nervous system are primarily vascular, with degenerative changes caused by lack of nutrition. A marked hyperemia of the cerebral vessels seems to be the first effect of the anoxemia. Lewin[685] found such a hyperemia in forty-eight out of sixty-four autopsies, in the brain and in the meninges, very severe in fourteen, and often accompanied by edema. Janossy[686] reported fibrous myositis after illuminating gas poisoning.

Forbes, Cobb, and Fremont-Smith[637] have repeatedly shown in animal experiments and in man that a rise in intracranial blood pressure occurs under the influence of carbon monoxide, a rise which they attribute to the increased congestion and edema. According to Weimann[687] the characteristic pathology of sudden severe gassing with carbon monoxide is an intense congestion of the entire cerebrum and its membranes, more marked than that which follows strangulation or drowning, and while in the latter case the congestion is venous, in carbon monoxide asphyxia it involves both veins and arteries, so that the cut surface of the brain looks as if stained in eosin. Lungs, spleen, and myocardium are also intensely congested.

The nutritive changes (cell degeneration, necrosis, subsequent softening) vary in intensity according to the adequacy

684. OTTO: Anleitung zur Ausmittelung der Gifte, 7th ed., Braunschweig, 262, 1896.

685. LEWIN, L.: Die Kohlenoxydvergiftung, Berlin, 1920.

686. JANOSSY, J.: *München. med. Wchnschr.*, 72:905, 1929.

687. WEIMANN, W.: *Ztschr. f. d. ges. Neurol. u. Psychiat.*, 105:213, 1926.

or inadequacy of the blood supply, and are typically most marked in the lenticular nucleus of the corpus striatum, particularly the pallidal region, as first described by Klebs in 1865 and since confirmed by many others, Polchen,[688] Hill and Semerak,[688] Photakis[680] and Grinker.[640]

Other foci of degeneration may be found scattered widely through the cerebrum,[689] and their varied localization accounts for the wide variation in symptoms which have been described as following the severer types of carbon monoxide asphyxia. Strecker, Taft and Willey[690] found a diffuse infiltration of the white matter of the cerebrum with proliferation of glia elements and endothelial cells, a condition of myelinopathy. Hemorrhage may occur in practically every organ or tissue as a result of the high blood pressure and of the dilatation and weakening of the vessel walls. Hemorrhage may occur in the brain after quite an interval of time, but should be traced to the weakening of the vascular wall by carbon monoxide or perhaps to a resulting thrombosis.[691] The greater vulnerability of alcoholics to carbon monoxide asphyxia is attributed to pre-existing vascular condition.[692] The same explanation is given for the severity of the lesions in the middle-aged and elderly as compared with the youthful.

Lewin described hemorrhage from the lungs, from the uterus with premature expulsion of the fetus, and from the stomach and intestines. In one of his cases there were bloody stools, ten or twelve times in twenty-four hours for a fortnight or more, and he quotes a case described by Greidenberg in which acute carbon monoxide poisoning was followed by bloody diarrhea appearing eighteen days later and increasing up to death. Strassmann[693] found hemorrhage into the musculature of the heart; Günther[694] found a "hemorrhagic polymyositis;" and

688. POLCHEN: Berl. klin. Wchnschr., 19:396, 1882; HILL, E., and SEMERAK, C. B.: J.A.M.A., 71:644, 1918.

689. WILSON, G., and WINKELMANN, N. W.: Arch. Neurol. & Psychiat., 13:191, 1925.

690. STRECKER, E. A., TAFT, A. E., and WILLEY, G. F.: Arch. Neurol. & Psychiat., 17:552, 1927.

691. HEDINGER, E.: Virchows Arch. f. path. Anat., 246:412, 1923.

692. CLAUDE, H.: Progrès méd., 19:265, 1913; Tr. Internat. Cong. Med., 1913, (London, 1914), sec. II, part 2, p. 343.

693. STRASSMANN, G.: Vrtljschr. f. gerichtl. Med., Berl., series 3, 58:50, 1919.

694. GÜNTHER, H.: Ztschr. f. klin. Med., Berl., 92:41, 1921; abst., J.A.M.A., 78:396, 1922.

Braun[695] attributed the pain in the muscles and the skin lesions following carbon monoxide inhalation to hemorrhages. According to Lewin the kidneys are rarely involved in carbon monoxide poisoning. Sandall found no abnormality in the heart in 85% of cases in which tachycardia had been a definite symptom. Walters [696] found that inhalation of carbon monoxide depresses the rate of metabolism with a parallel lowering of temperature, and Mikami[697] found in fatal gassing a fall in oxygen and carbon dioxide content of the blood, together with an increase in blood sugar.

Abnormal moisture in the lungs is a common feature of acute gassing,[698] and death is often due to edema of the lungs or to pneumonia.[699] In some cases it is a deglutination pneumonia because the patient has vomited before recovering consciousness. According to Strassmann edema is found in cases of rapid death, edema with foci of inflammation in those surviving some thirty-six hours, and pneumonia in those who live several days. Or a pneumonia may develop some weeks after the accident. Sandall[700] studying the late effects of carbon monoxide asphyxia, found in 46% of his cases evidence of emphysema of chronic bronchitis, or both, but no evidence that pulmonary tuberculosis is a sequel.

Recovery from severe gassing depends on several factors. It is more likely to be incomplete, to be followed by some permanent disturbance, if the rescue from the poisoned atmosphere is delayed, and if there is pre-existing disease, especially disease of the blood vessels and of the respiratory tract.[701] The great majority of victims of carbon monoxide asphyxia recover without any lasting symptoms, but there are exceptional cases in which structural damage has occurred, usually as a result of slow and prolonged asphyxia. Many observers found that the patients having had carbon monoxide poisoning have a dulled mentality with a loss of memory and will power. (See the case

695. BRAUN, A.: *München. med. Wchnschr.*, 72:13, 1925.

696. WALTERS, F. M.: *Am. J. Physiol.*, 80:140, 1927.

697. MIKAMI, S.: *Tohuku J. Exper. Med.*, 8:237, 1927, abstr., *J. Indust. Hyg.*, 10:88, 1928.

698. DRINKER, C. K., and CANNON, W. B.: *J. Indust. Hyg.*, 4:463, 1922.

699. OLIVER, T.: *Lancet*, 1:1768, 1907; HATTON, W. A.: *Brit. M. J.*, 1:1164, 1911; LAMPE; quoted by DRINKER and CANNON, ref. 698.

700. SANDALL, T. E.: *Lancet*, 2:857, 1922.

701. HAMILTON, ALICE: *Industrial Toxicology*, 131, 1934.

of W. P. G., truck driver, of Des Moines, Iowa, page 317).

Hitchcock[702] and O'Malley[703] state that characteristic sequels of accidental gas poisonings in English collieries, and gassings in garages have been described in this country with similar symptoms. Haldane considers loss of memory and lack of judgment as definite symptoms of carbon monoxide asphyxia, both while the victim is under its influence and after his recovery. Epileptoid convulsions may be a symptom, not of the early stage, but of the stage of recovery.[704] Pineas,[705] Borman[706] and Grinker[640] have all described cases showing the symptom-complex which was called by Kleist "psychomotor apraxia," and the last attributes it to diffuse cerebral lesions, while the Parkinsonism, which was also present in a case of Grinker's, was held to be of pallidal origin. A picture of disseminated sclerosis was presented by a patient of Becker's,[707] and by one of Beck's.[707]

The symptoms of brain involvement may come on sometime after the accident, in the form either of an apoplectic seizure or of an increasing psychosis.[708] Attacks of headache and dizziness may persist for many weeks after recovery from severe symptoms, or there may be tremors, or pains in the cardiac region,[709] or abdominal pain, which are possibly functional in origin,[700] perhaps caused by hemorrhage and pressure. Blindness, complete or incomplete, transient or permanent, is an accompaniment or a sequel to carbon monoxide poisoning. Neuroretinitis with subsequent optic atrophy has been described by Wilmer,[710], Brose,[711] and Abt and Witt.[712] In other cases no change in eye-ground is found and the lesion is assumed to be central in origin.

Mankowsky attributed the polyneuritis that follows car-

702. HITCHCOCK, C. W.:   *J.A.M.A.,* 71:257, 1928.
703. O'MALLEY, M.:   *J.A.M.A.,* 59:1540, 1912.
704. HILLER, F.:   *Ztschr. f. d. ges. Neurol. u. Psychiat.,* 93:594, 524.
705. PINEAS, H.:   *Ztschr. f. d. ges. Neurol. u. Psychiat.,* 93:36, 1924.
706. BORMAN, M. C.:   *Am. J. Psychiat.,* 6:135, 1926; abstr., *J.A.M.A.,* 87:1769, 1926.
707. BECKER, E.:   *Arch. Neurol. Path. Lab. Lond. County Asyl. Claybury, Lond.,* 3:246, 1907. BECK, H. G.:   *Clin. Med.,* 5:1088, 1927.
708. QUENSEL: *Arch. f. Psychiat.,* 35:612, 1902.
709. KLEBS, E.:   *Virchows Arch. f. path. Anat.,* 32:450, 1865.
710. WILMER, W. H.:   *Am. J. Ophth.,* 4:73, 1921.
711. BROSE, L. D.:   *Arch. Ophth.,* 28:402, 1899.
712. ABT, I. A., and WITT, D. B.:   *M. Clin. North America,* 5:1645, 1921.

bon monoxide asphyxia in some cases, to hemorrhages compressing the nerves, causing infiltration of the epineurium and perineurium with ischemia, the symptoms ceasing as the exudate is absorbed.[713] Wilson and Winkelman found both polyneuritis and involvement of the cortex, or of the globus pallidus, or of both, as shown by exaggeration of the deep reflexes. Cardiac symptoms are not at all unusual immediately after severe gassing, and they may be long continued or even permanent, pointing to a myocarditis or even atheroma of the coronaries as a sequel.

Palpitation of the heart, breathlessness on exertion, and precordial pain are fairly common complaints.

Men with chronic bronchitis or asthma resist the effect of gas very badly, and the course of carbon monoxide poisoning is unfavorably influenced by alcoholism, obesity, and chronic disease of the heart, while chronic vascular disease increases decidedly the damage done to the basal ganglia. Sayers was unable to produce anemia in monkeys, dogs, rabbits, and guinea pigs, even after several hundred exposures repeated almost daily.[714]

Loewy[715] reported a case in a man thirty-six years old who had been a furnace man for twelve years. He was greatly troubled with dizziness, on looking down. He would be quite free from it when on a vacation in the country. He staggered to the right when standing with his eyes shut, there was nystagmus and a clouding of the lens along the margin. The blood was normal except for a white count of 12,000. Loewy had three other cases of dizziness, which he attributed to over-irritability of the labyrinth caused by this gas, and these also cleared up on leaving work.

Baader[716] also saw a case of labyrinth disturbance in chronic carbon monoxide poisoning.

The cases of profound anemia with marked nervous symptoms and cardiac disturbances which have been attributed to chronic carbon monoxide poisoning are practically all of nonindustrial origin. Pernicious anemia due to atrophic gastritis

713. MANKOWSKY, B. N.: Deutsche Ztschr. f. Nervenh., 109:84, 1929; abstr., J.A.M.A., 93:1513, 1929.
714. U. S. Pub. Health Bull. 186, March, 1929.
715. LOEWY, L.: Zentralbl. f. Gewerbehyg., 3:153, 1926.
716. BAADER, E. W.: Gewerbekrankheiten Klinische Grundlagen der 22 meldepflichtigen Berufskrankheiten, Berlin, 1931.

caused by exposure to carbon dioxide which interfered with the formation of the intrinsic factor of hydrochloric acid was reported by Bergh and Grill.

The late Dr. E. R. LeCount in a personal communication said:

1. A dilated heart does not arise from carbon monoxide poisoning without coma of some hours duration.

2. Carbon monoxide gas does not kill in this interval in the absence of coma or unconsciousness at or immediately after inhalation.

3. Carbon monoxide poisoning does not cause heart disease such as myocarditis or valvular disease.

4. No worth while studies of the human heart have ever been made after death in the absence of coma preceding death.

Gürich noted changes of heart muscle in poison with illuminating gas.[717] Gunther mentions an acute interstitial myocarditis following acute gas poisoning. Kroetz reports necrosis of heart muscle. Electrocardiographic variations may be severe and last for many months. Acute coronary thrombosis usually appears twenty-four to seventy-two hours after the gas inhalation. Three fatal cases are reported.

Tests: Carbon monoxide may be detected in the air through the absorbent power of a solution of cuprous chloride in an excess of hydrochloric acid or an excess of ammonia. In either liquid it is completely absorbed. When large quantities exist, the diminution of the volume of the air passed through this reagent may be observed, but generally large volumes of the air have to be drawn through the solution, and the presence of the gas determined either by heating the solution to boiling, which causes its expulsion passing the gas into a brick-red solution of palladous chloride, whereby a black precipitate of metallic palladium is produced

$$(PdCl_2 + CO + H_2O = CO_2 + 2HCl + Pd)$$

I was able to detect the carbon monoxide generated by the burning of a smokeless fuel by the former method, absorbing the gas in cuprous chloride solution, and afterward expelling it. Tests were applied, and the gas found to burn with a pale blue flame.

Care must be taken in using the palladium solution to exclude the presence of hydrogen sulphide, ammonium sul-

717. Gürich: *München. men. Wchnschr.*, 72:2194, 1925; *J.A.M.A.*, 86:455, 1926.

phide, ozone, or hydrogen.   Carbon monoxide may be burned
to carbon dioxide, but this method is open to error through the
presence of hydrocarbons.

Gruber[718] prefers to absorb carbon monoxide from air by
blood, using Fodor's[719] method modified.   From 10 to 20 liters
of the suspected air are shaken with slightly diluted blood for
fifteen minutes.   The blood is then placed in a small flask and
heated to boiling.   Air, purified by being passed through a solution of palladous chloride, is drawn through the heated blood
and is conducted through solutions of lead acetate, dilute sulphuric acid, and finally palladous chloride.   A black precipitate may be caused by hydrogen sulphide and ammonium sulphide, so these gases must be excluded.   Fodor claims to be able
to detect one part of carbon monoxide in 20,000 parts of air, in
which he is corroborated by Gruber.   Marsh-gas and other hydrocarbons do not interfere with the test as thus conducted.
The test indicates quantities of carbon monoxide below the
limit of toxicity.   The quantity of palladium reduced may be
determined by dissolving it in aqua regia and titrating with potassium iodide.   Desgrez and Labat[720] employ strips of filter
paper saturated with a 10% solution of palladous chloride for
the detection of carbon monoxide in the air, the depth of darkening of the sensitive paper giving a clue to the relative amount
present.

Vogel[721] uses diluted blood solution and examines the spectrum.   Thus, by shaking diluted blood with from 100 to 200 cc.
of air and examining by the spectroscope, 2.5% may be detected. This represents a highly poisonous quantity.   For lesser
quantities 20 liters of air may be shaken with 10 cc. blood, which
is then tested according to Fodor's method.   The wash-water
from the bottle in which the air was shaken may be used for the
spectroscopic examination, whereby 1% to 0.05% of carbon
monoxide is detectable.

This latter test has the advantage of enabling the experimenter to submit the blood to further tests, yet of preserving

718. GRUBER: *Arch. f. Hyg.*, 1:145, 1883.

719. FODOR: *Deutsche Vrtljschr. f. öff. Gsndhtspflg., Brnschwg.*,
12:377, 1880.

720. DESGREZ and LABAT: *Ann. chim. et. anal. chim. appl.*, 1:294,
1919.

721. VOGEL: *Ber. d. deutsch. chem. Gesellsch., Berl.*, 10:796, 1877;
11:235, 1878.

the wash-water with its characteristic action in the spectroscope, in a sealed tube as an exhibit. Carbon monoxide hemoglobin imparts to blood a characteristic pink color, even when only a small proportion of the gas is present. Five-tenths cc. of the unknown sample of blood and a like amount of normal blood are diluted to 100 cc. in a cylinder. The normal blood will have a buff-yellow tint and the sample, if it contains carbon-monoxide, will have a pink color. In testing for carbon monoxide in a contaminated atmosphere, a tube or cylinder containing the diluted normal blood is taken to the place where the air is to be examined. The normal blood is poured out into another tube, so that the air takes the place of the blood. The normal blood is then added to the tube, corked and shaken for about ten minutes. If the air contains carbon monoxide, a distinct pink color of the carbon monoxide hemoglobin will be noticed when the comparison is made with the original buff-colored blood.

Gas analysis apparatus of various types may be used for the analysis of larger quantities of carbon monoxide.[722] Hoover recommends[723] the use of hoolamite (a mixture of fuming sulphuric acid, iodine pentoxide, and pumice stone) for the detection of carbon monoxide. This reagent gives a green color, varying in depth with the concentration of the carbon monoxide.

Hempel[724] exposed mice to a contaminated atmosphere and examined their blood spectroscopically. By this means he was able to detect 0.5% of carbon monoxide, though his results are disputed by Gruber.

Wolf[725] has also given directions concerning the detection of this gas. For poisonous quantities, especially in the air of mines and other closed places, use is made of its physiologic action. A cage containing several varieties of warm-blooded animals is hung in the suspected atmosphere; if they die and the blood shows the presence of carbon monoxide, the test is definite. White mice are preferable to gray, first, because they are accustomed to captivity, and, second, because the color of

722. DENIS, L. M.; EDGAR, C. G.: *J. Am. Chem. Soc.*, 19:859, 1897.

723. HOOVER: *J. Indust. & Eng. Chem.*, 13:770, 1921; KALETA, T.. *Chem. Ztg.*, 46:430, 1922; KATZ and BLOOMFIELD: *J. Indust. & Eng. Chem.*, 14:304, 1922.

724. HEMPEL: *Ztschr. f. anal. Chem., Wiesb.*, 18:399, 1879.

725. WOLF, C. H.: *Pharm. Ztschr.*, 268, 1880; *Chem. Centralbl.*, 51: 773, 1880.

the blood is clearly visible in the ears, nose, and eyes, the last being especially brilliant. Burrell[726] claims that canaries are more sensitive to carbon monoxide, 0.2% causing distress in one and a half minutes, and they will fall from the perch in five minutes.

Detection of Carbon Monoxide in Blood: Since the discovery by Hoppe-Seyler in 1862 of the spectrum of oxyhemoglobin, and in 1864 and 1865 of the spectrum of carbon monoxide hemoglobin, and its irreducible character, no toxicologic analysis of the blood has been considered complete without this test being applied. In forensic medicine it was first applied in 1867.

Blood taken from persons or animals poisoned by carbon monoxide shows a characteristic absorption spectrum closely resembling that of oxyhemoglobin. The absorption occurs between the D and E lines chiefly, and is apparent through the appearance of two absorption bands of nearly equal intensity and width. The one near D coincides almost exactly with that of oxyhemoglobin of the same position; the space between it and the band toward F is considerably wider than that between the two bands of the oxyhemoglobin spectrum (See No. 7, Plate).

When more than 27% of the blood coloring-matter has been saturated by carbon monoxide, the addition to the blood of reducing agents, as a drop or two of a solution of crystallized ammonium sulphide, does not convert the spectrum into one of reduced hemoglobin. The character of this spectrum is that of a single band beginning on the D line and occupying a little more than half of the space to the E line (See No. 3, Plate). A solution of ferrous sulphate in ammonium tartrate may be substituted for the ammonium sulphide.[727]

The spectroscopic examination may be made by the use of an ordinary spectroscope, or, in a more refined manner, especially on very small quantities of blood, with the microspectroscope. The single prism spectroscope has an adjustable slit which is provided with a micrometer set-screw so that a particular width of opening may be accurately determined. Two

726. BURRELL: Tech. Paper 11, U. S. Bureau of Mines, Washington, D. C., 1912; BURRELL, SEIBERT, and ROBERTSON: Tech. Paper 62, U. S. Bureau of Mines, 12, 1914.

727. HOPPE-SEYLER: *Physiologische Chemie*, 384, 1877; *Med. Chem. Untersuch.*, 1:202, 1866; PREYER, W.: Die Blutkrystalle, Jena, 1871.

burners placed on an adjustable stand supply white light, the one directly to the spectroscope, the other through a comparison prism attached to one-half of the slit. The blood contained in the test-tube is placed in the path of the rays from the first

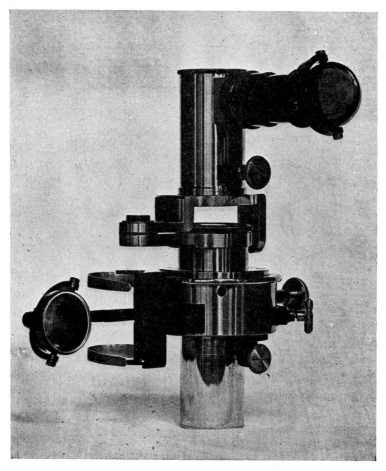

FIG. 18.
The Microspectroscope for the Detection of
Small Amounts of CO in Blood

mentioned lamp. The lamps are provided with tin casings which allow the light to pass through small windows cut in them. The position of any absorption bands is determined by the illuminated scale of the spectroscope. Recently methods have been used whereby photographs of the blood spectrum may be taken, with precautions to exclude optical illusions.[728]

Dilution of the blood is advisable. Dreser[729] has made use of this method for the quantitative determination of carbon monoxide in blood. About one-third of the hemoglobin of the blood remains unconverted into carbon monoxide hemoglobin at the time of death under the toxic action of this gas on man and animals. Since some claim that carbon monoxide blood loses its characteristics when exposed to the air for the week, it is always advisable to seal up a specimen of the blood at the time of the autopsy. Such blood retains its character for years.

Many prefer to extract the gas from the blood and measure and identify it. For this purpose 100 cc. of the blood are introduced into the spacious receiver of a mercurial air-pump. The extraction of the gas is begun by the exhaustion of the blood by the action of a solution of glacial acetic acid saturated with sodium chloride and preferably boiled, and then application of heat to about 50°C. By the use of proper absorbents carbon dioxide and oxygen are removed, and the carbon monoxide can be measured by its absorption in cuprous chloride solution. This solution may be caused to yield up its content of carbon monoxide by the addition to it of an excess of potassium hydroxide. The gas, if in sufficient quantity, may be ignited and seen to burn with a blue flame.

The following additional tests are of importance because of their simplicity:

. Blood rich in carbon monoxide when boiled yields a brick-red mass; ordinary blood becomes brown-black.

To 10 cc. of 2% solution of a blood strongly charged with carbon monoxide, add 2 cc. of yellow ammonium sulphide and 0.2 cc. of 30% acetic acid; a bright red appears, while normal blood yields a green, precipitate. (Katagama.)

When blood is added to diluted hydrogen sulphide water drop by drop, it produces a bright red precipitate when carbon monoxide is present, otherwise a bright green. (Salkowski.)

Normal blood when shaken with one or two volumes of a solution of sodium hydroxide of 1.3 specific gravity becomes black, in thin layers dark greenish brown; carbon monoxide blood remains red and appears like red lead or cinnabar.

728. BIDER, G.: *Arch. d. Pharm.*, 130:609, 1892.

729. DRESER, A. H.: *Arch. f. exper. Path. u. Pharmacol.*, 25:119, 1891.

A mixture of calcium chloride and sodium hydroxide produces a beautiful carmine-red color if carbon monoxide is present, while normal blood becomes brown. (Eulenberg.)

A reducing agent, as ammonium sulphide, alkaline stannous chloride solution, or a ferrous salt, changes the color of normal blood almost to black, while carbon monoxide blood retains its red color. Two cc. of carbon monoxide blood with an equal quantity of water and three drops of a one-third saturated solution of copper sulphate when mixed produce a brick-red precipitate, while normal blood yields a greenish-brown one. (Zaleski.)

When four or five volumes of lead acetate are added to one of carbon monoxide blood and thoroughly shaken for about a minute, it retains its red color; normal blood, under like circumstances, becomes dark. The differences increase by keeping, being visible for a week or two even in open test-tubes. (Rubner.)

When 10 cc. of blood are mixed with 15 cc. of 20% potassium ferrocyanide solution and 2 cc. of moderately strong acetic acid (one volume of glacial acetic acid to two volumes of water), a solid coagulum gradually results; if normal, the coagulum is black-brown, but when the blood contains carbon monoxide, bright red. (Wetzel.)

Blood diluted one part to four with water and shaken with three times its volume of a 1% tannin solution becomes in twenty-four hours of a gray tint when normal, but is carmine-red when carbon monoxide is present. This color still persists in tubes the author has kept for over twenty years.

Carbon monoxide may be found in exhumed bodies a number of months after burial. In one specimen of blood submitted by Dr. L. Hektoen, where the body had been buried for over a year, I was able to demonstrate the presence of carbon monoxide. Lagnna presents a case of a woman who had died as the result of this poisoning, but an inference was made that she had been killed by strangulation, and probably by her own husband. Therefore, the cadaver was ordered to be exhumed and the case was to be reinvestigated. The material to be examined consisted of the liquid content of the pleural and peritoneal cavity, and also the liquid obtained from the spinal canal. These portions were found by chemical spectroscopic examination to contain carbon monoxide. In this particular case the presence of carbon monoxide was detected after 210 days.

The experiments of Strassman and Schulz[730] have demonstrated that carbon monoxide may penetrate by diffusion all parts of the cadaver, with sufficiently long exposure in air containing carbon monoxide. Wiethold[731] found carbon monoxide many months after burial. Blumenstock found it after

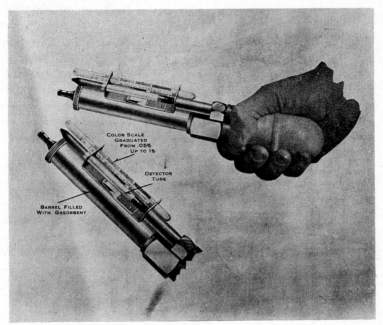

FIG. 19.
Carbon Monoxide Detector
(Mine Safety Appliance Company)

fourteen days. Raestrup, in one case where the body was in a frozen condition after sixty-nine days, found it by tannic acid test. Strassman found carbon monoxide spectroscopically three months after death. McNally found carbon monoxide in the blood of an embalmed body twelve months after burial. Sodium citrate has no effect upon the chemical spectroscopic tests for carbon monoxide.[732]

730. STRASSMAN and SCHULZ: *Berl. klin. Wchnschr.*, 4:1233, 1904; WACHHOLZ and LIMBURGER: *Vrtljschr. f. gerichtl. Med., Berl.*, 3F., 23: 233, 1902.

731. WIETHOLD, F.: *Deutsche Ztschr. f. d. ges. gerichtl. Med.*, 14:30, 1929.

732. *Wien. klin. Wchnschr.*, 41, 1928.

The Mine Safety Appliance Company manufactures an instrument that quickly determines the presence of carbon monoxide in the air. It determines as low as 0.05% carbon monoxide. The detector tube is filled with an activated iodine pentoxide and sealed. The ends of this tube are broken and inserted into the apparatus shown in Fig. 19. A bulb is squeezed a required number of times, forcing the air through the detector tube through a barrel filled with "gas absorbent," a preparation which removes any material which may affect the reading. The pentoxide changes color, from a grayish-white to a shade of green that varies with the amount of carbon monoxide present. The color is compared with a color scale mounted beside the detector tube and graduated to read the concentration up to 1% carbon monoxide. Under ordinary circumstances the color soon fades on standing, permitting the re-use for several tests. This instrument will be found useful in testing the air in manholes, sewers, garages, foundries, coal and metal mines, and in any operation that uses carbon monoxide gas as a source of heat.

Hanson and Hastings[733] report the analyses of the blood for carbon monoxide saturation made on a group of non-smokers and on a group who smoked cigarettes or pipes. In the first group the average saturation was 1.5%, whereas in the group of smokers it was from 3.0 to 4.0. After an interval of twelve hours without smoking, the percentage saturation in one subject fell from 4.1 to 2.0, where it remained after another six hours' abstinence.

Quantitative Methods: Haldane's[734] Quantitative Method: For carbon monoxide, this yields satisfactory results with fresh blood, but with dark-colored blood from cadavers, the colors are hard to match with a Duboscq colorimeter, the results obtained being far too high compared with the palladous chloride method.

For the quantitative estimation of carbon monoxide in air and in blood, the method of Nicloux,[735] or that of Fodor,[736] is

733. HANSON, H. B., and HASTINGS, A. B.: *J.A.M.A.*, 100:1481, 1933.
734. HALDANE: *J. Physiol.*, 18:430, 1895; 20:521, 1896.
735. NICLOUX: *Compt. rend. Acad. d. sc.*, 126:746, 1898; *Bull. Soc. Chem. biol.*, 2:171, 1920; Micro-method for Estimating CO, *Bull. Soc. Chem. biol.*, 3:286, 1921.
736. FODOR: *Deutsche Vrtljschr. f. öff, Gsndhtspflg., Brnschwg.*, 12:377, 1880.

preferred to that of Haldane, especially with blood from cadavers which may not be of a bright cherry-red. The method of Nicloux is based on the action of the oxidation of carbon monoxide by iodic acid and the determination of the liberated iodine with a standard solution of thiosulphate. In a form of apparatus devised by Seidell,[737] the carbon dioxide liberated may also be determined. The reaction may be expressed by the equation: $I_2O_5 + 5CO = 5CO_2 + I_2$.

The method of Fodor is based on the reduction of palladous chloride by carbon monoxide. The reaction is expressed by the equation: $PdCl_2 + CO = Pd + 2HCl + CO_2$. For the examination of the blood, 5 cc. are diluted with 20 cc. of water in a large test-tube of 80 cc. capacity; a small piece of sodium hydroxide is then added to aid in the expulsion of carbon monoxide. A tube containing 10 cc. of palladous chloride precedes the tube containing the blood to remove the carbon monoxide from the laboratory air. A third U-tube following the tube containing the blood contains a solution of lead acetate and a fourth tube contains dilute sulphuric acid. The chain of tubes is completed by the addition of three U-tubes containing a solution of palladous chloride. (The commercial salt is dissolved in hydrochloric acid, with the addition of nitric acid, evaporated to dryness on the water-bath, moistened with hydrochloric acid, dried, taken up with a small amount of water and again dried to free it from excess acid. The residue is then made up to volume so that 500 cc. will contain 1 gm.) The test-tube containing the blood is heated in a water-bath to 90°C., while a gentle current of air, previously drawn through the tube of palladous chloride is conducted through the chain of tubes at the rate of 300 cc. per hour for four hours. If carbon monoxide is present, the palladous chloride is reduced, and a black precipitate of palladium will be deposited. The reduced palladium is collected on a filter paper, washed with water, and dissolved in hot nitrohydrochloric acid. The U-tubes after washing with water will have a small amount of palladium adhering to the sides. This can be dissolved in the hot nitrohydrochloric acid and added to that dissolved from the filter paper. The solution is evaporated on the hot water-bath, and taken up with strong hydrochloric acid three or four times to remove all traces of nitric acid. The residue

737. SEIDELL: *J. Indust. & Eng. Chem.*, 4:321, 1914.

is dissolved in water and titrated with a solution of potassium iodide containing 1.486 gm. to the liter. The diluted palladium chloride solution is heated on the water-bath before each addition of the potassium iodide solution. A brown precipitate of palladous iodide is filtered off, and the operation is repeated until the addition of potassium iodide fails to produce a brown cloudiness. Each cubic centimeter of the potassium iodide solution represents 0.1 cc. of carbon monoxide. In case the blood contains only a small amount of carbon monoxide, as is demonstrated by the tannic acid and other color tests, 20 cc. of the blood are used in a small Erlenmeyer flask. When it is desired to report the saturation of the blood after obtaining the percentage of carbon monoxide by volume, one can use the relation x : 20, since a saturated blood will hold in combination 20% by volume of carbon monoxide.[738]

Method of Van Slyke and Salvesen: The principle of this method[739] is to set free the oxygen and carbon monoxide from their combination with hemoglobin in the blood by addition of ferricyanide and then to remove both gases with the help of a Torricellian vacuum in the apparatus devised by Van Slyke for determining the carbon dioxide combining power of the plasma. The oxygen is absorbed in the apparatus by alkaline pyrogallate and the volume of residual carbon monoxide is measured directly at atmospheric pressure, a correction being made for the small and constant amount of nitrogen gas dissolved by the blood. From the recent work of O'Brien and Parker,[740] who absorbed the carbon monoxide in a solution of ammoniacal cuprous chloride and thus determined this gas directly, it is evident that the amount of carbon monoxide dissolved in the blood-serum, used in the test, is so small that there is little to be gained by making a correction for this factor, as is done by Van Slyke in his method for oxygen of the blood and by Stadie for methemoglobin.

The blood-gas apparatus is prepared by introducing into

738. FLORENTIN and VANDENBERGER: Compt. rend. Acad. d. sc., 172: 391, 1921; NICLOUX, M.: Bull. Soc. Chem. biol., 2:171, 1920; and 3:286, 1921.

739. J. Biol. Chem., 40:103, 1919.

740. O'BRIEN and PARKER: J. Biol. Chem., 1:289, 1922. And see NICLOUX (Refs. 735 and 738); HARTRIDGE: J. Physiol., 53:77, 1921; HILL: Bio-Chem. J., 15:577, 1921; and SAYERS and YANT: J.A.M.A., 78:1745, 1922.

it five drops of redistilled caprylic alcohol and 6 cc. of ammonium solution made by diluting 4 cc. of concentrated ammonia to a liter. If saponin powder is available, as much is added to the 6 cc. of ammonia, while in the cup of the apparatus, as will stick to the end of a glass rod (approximately 1 mg. per cc.). After the ammonia is introduced into the 5 cc. chamber of the apparatus, the latter is evacuated and the air is extracted from the ammonia solution by shaking for about fifteen seconds. The extracted air is expelled, and the extraction repeated to make sure that no air is left in the solution. Finally, about 2 cc. of the air free ammonia are forced up into the cup of the apparatus. The oxalated blood is now thoroughly stirred with a rod to assure even distribution of the corpuscles, and a 2-cc. sample is drawn into a pipet and run under the ammonia in the cup of the apparatus. (The lower delivery mark of the pipet should be 3 or 4 cm. above the tip, as a pipet calibrated for complete delivery would be inconvenient for placing the entire sample of blood below the layer of ammonia.) The blood is now run from the cup into the 50-cc. chamber, the ammonia layer following the blood and washing it in. A few additional drops of the air-free ammonia may if necessary be added from a dropper to make the washing complete.

The blood and ammonia in the chamber are mixed and allowed to stand until the blood is completely laked. This requires about thirty seconds when saponin is present and five minutes when it is not. After laking is complete, 0.4 cc. of a saturated potassium ferricyanide solution is introduced to set free the oxygen and carbon monoxide combined with the hemoglobin. (This ferricyanide solution is made by dissolving 40 gm. of the salt in 100 cc. of water and is made air-free by boiling or shaking in an evacuated flask and is kept in a buret under a layer of paraffin oil 2 or 3 cm. thick to exclude air.) The apparatus is now evacuated by lowering the leveling bulb until only a few drops of mercury remain above the lower stop-cock, and is shaken, preferably with a rotary motion, to whirl the blood in a thin layer around the wall of the chamber. If the blood was completely laked before the cyanide was added, extraction of the gases may be completed by half a minute of efficient shaking. The extracted solution may be drawn into the bulb of the apparatus below the lower cock and the extracted gas measured over mercury. When the reading of the volume of the gas mixture, consisting of oxygen, carbon monoxide, and a little nitrogen, is constant, a solution of alkaline pyrogallate (prepared by dissolving 10 gm. of pyrogallic acid in 200 cc. of strong potassium hydroxide, consisting of 160 gm. KOH dissolved in 130 cc. of water) is introduced into the cup of the apparatus, is covered by a thin layer of paraffin oil, and is allowed to flow slowly down into the inner wall of the graduated part of the apparatus. A little suction is produced during this part of the procedure by lowering the leveling bulb slightly. The absorption of the oxygen is quite rapid and is completed in less than one minute; the reading is taken and the pyrogallate solution introduced once more until a constant reading is obtained. The gas is then measured under the conditions of prevailing pressure and temperature. As the solution is very dark and it is a little difficult to get good reading of the meniscus, a new meniscus is produced by letting water flow down after the pyrogallate solution; the water floats on top of the fluid and one may obtain readings to about 0.002 cc. The apparatus is washed out twice with dilute ammonia solution after each determination.

Calculation: The gas measured is reduced to standard conditions by the use of the factor

$$X = \frac{B}{760} (100.8 - 0.27t)(V - 0.136 + \propto t)$$

in which

B equals the observed barometric pressure;

t equals the observed temperature at which the analysis and readings were made;

V represents the actual reading in mm., of the gas in the pipet, and

X expresses the cubic centimeters of CO reduced to 0°C. temperature and 760 mm. pressure.

If 2 cc. of blood have been used, as directed in the test, the values of this factor may be found in the following table, (Table XXXI), the result then being expressed in cubic centimeters of CO per 100 cc. of blood, from which amount the nitrogen correction, 1.2 cc. is subtracted.

The tannic acid method as described by Wetzel's qualitative test has been modified and adapted to a quantitative test by the Bureau of Mines, and is now known as the pyrotannic acid method. The specimen of blood suspected to contain carbon monoxide hemoglobin is, after chemical treatment, compared to a set of standards ranging from 0 to 100% saturation. These can be prepared by the chemist or can be purchased from a supply house. One-cc. solutions of oxyhemo-

TABLE XXXI
FACTORS USED TO REDUCE TO STANDARD CONDITIONS CO IN 100 cc. OF BLOOD

Temperature C.	Factor by which observed gas volume is multiplied in order to give CO in 100 cc. of blood
15°	$46.5 \times \frac{B}{760}$
16°	$46.3 \times \frac{B}{760}$
17°	$46.0 \times \frac{B}{760}$
18°	$45.8 \times \frac{B}{760}$
19°	$45.6 \times \frac{B}{760}$
20°	$45.4 \times \frac{B}{760}$
21°	$45.1 \times \frac{B}{760}$
22°	$44.9 \times \frac{B}{760}$
23°	$44.7 \times \frac{B}{760}$
24°	$44.4 \times \frac{B}{760}$
25°	$44.2 \times \frac{B}{760}$
26°	$44.0 \times \frac{B}{760}$
27°	$43.7 \times \frac{B}{760}$
28°	$43.5 \times \frac{B}{760}$
29°	$43.3 \times \frac{B}{760}$
30°	$43.1 \times \frac{B}{760}$

globin and carbon monoxide mixtures are made. The concentration of HbCO varies from 0 to 100% in steps of 10. These solutions are contained in a test-tube, approximately five-sixteenths of an inch inside diameter, of clear, thin glass. To each standard thus prepared is added 1 cc. of a mixture consisting of equal parts of a strictly fresh solution of 2% tannic acid. If standards are for immediate use, pyrogallic acid should also be added, after which the tube is inverted twice to insure thorough mixing. The tube should be sealed immediately by pouring a little melted paraffin on top of the content while the tube is immersed in cold water as a caution against overheating. This temporary seal will exclude the air until the walls of the tube become dry, when a tight, permanent seal can be made by placing a disk of cardboard on top of the paraffin and filling the remainder of the tube with ordinary sealing wax. Care should be taken to exclude all air. Standards thus prepared develop their full color in thirty minutes and, if properly sealed and kept in a cool place, will retain their permanence for one or two weeks, not changing enough to interfere with accuracy of determination.

For the quantitative determination of carbon monoxide there is required:

(a) A set of color standards, prepared either from blood or pigments, to represent the color of blood having varying known amounts of HbCO (as 0, 10, 20, 30, etc.). The standards are contained in small clear test-tubes, five-sixteenths inch in diameter, and having a volume of 2 cc. which may be arranged in a suitable rack with spaces between for interposing tubes of similar size that contain the blood samples for analysis.

(b) Small test-tubes (of the same size and glass as those used for the standards) in which to prepare specimens for analysis.

(c) Dilution pipet. The dilution may be made by using a 0.1-cc. pipet for measuring the blood into the required volume of water or by having a dilution pipet, with capillary stem that holds 0.1 cc. and a bulb above which has a total volume of 2 cc., thus making a dilution of one in twenty, which seems to be the most suitable blood concentration.

(d) Spring hemospast or blood lancet for making a small wound in the finger or other convenient place from which the blood may be obtained.

(e) Small watch glass or spot plate for catching the blood as it flows from the wound. This is not essential, as the blood may be drawn up directly from the head over the wound. However, the spot plate is convenient where two or more specimens are desired from the same wound, as for air analysis.

(f) Piece of one-fourth inch rubber hose ten inches long, or a similar band of rubber for wrapping the finger, beginning at the base and proceeding toward the tip in order to force the blood out if it does not flow freely when the sample is being taken.

(g) Mixture of equal parts by weight of tannic and pyrogallic acids either solid or in solution. If in solid form it may be prepared in capsules or tablets, or, if it is in powder form, it may be kept in a bottle as in the equipment used by the Bureau of Mines, with a measuring spoon holding approximately 0.04 gm., which is the amount found to be the most suitable for 2 cc. of a one-in-twenty blood solution. If less blood solution is used, the amount of the acids must be decreased correspondingly.

(h) Bottle of water (preferably, but not necessarily distilled if clean tap water is available) for making the blood dilutions.

All of this apparatus can be arranged in a compact pocket case, 7⅞ by 4 by 2¼ inches, and can be kept in readiness for immediate use.

The following procedure is based on the apparatus described, but it may be modified to suit blood apparatus and facilities at hand, as suggested before:

A small puncture wound (approximately 2 mm. deep) is made with the hemospast in the tip of the finger of the victim, or suspected victim, of CO poisoning, and several drops of blood are caught on the spot plate or drawn directly into the pipet. If the blood does not flow freely, the finger is wrapped with the rubber hose, beginning at the base and progressing toward the tip. Massaging the finger also aids the flow. (If death has intervened, it may be difficult to obtain liquid blood, but this usually can be done during embalming.) When the blood has been procured, it is quickly drawn into the stem of the pipet to the 0.1-cc. mark. The pipet is then held horizontally, and any blood on the exterior of the top is removed. The tip is raised slightly to allow a little of the blood to flow into the diluting bulb, and by inserting it quickly into the bottle of water and using suction at the same time, it can be filled to the 2-cc. mark to give proper dilution. The blood solution is then discharged into one of the test-tubes, a little of the solution being drawn back once or twice into the pipet to wash out any adhering concentrated blood. To eliminate possible clotting, the entire procedure of obtaining the blood specimen should be as rapid as possible. If it is desired to take more

than one sample, the pipet can be rinsed out with a little
dilution water, care being taken to blow the capillary stem free
from water and to dry the tip of the pipet before the next
sample is obtained.

Immediately after the blood solution has been discharged
into the test-tube, approximately 0.04 gm. of the tannic-
pyrogallic acid mixture is added by the spoon, capsule or solution method, and the tube is inverted several times to insure
thorough mixing with the reagents. The tube is then placed
in the rack and allowed to stand fifteen minutes at room
temperature (if particles of the solid acids settle out, the tube
should be inverted several more times) at the end of which
period it is compared with the standards by interposing it
between them until the standard is found which most nearly
matches it. If CO is indicated, the tube should be allowed to
stand fifteen minutes longer and another reading made. The
latter reading should be taken as the more accurate. The
percentage of HbCO, or what is designated as "blood saturation," is estimated from the value of that standard.

The observations are best made in daylight, but not in
direct sunlight. The observer should stand with his back to the
light, viewing the tubes by reflections, and should change their
position several times to note any difference due merely to
unequal lighting effect. Observations may be made after
several hours without serious loss of accuracy, although this
is advisable only in case of necessity.[741]

Martinek and Marti[742] have modified Teague's[743] method of
iodine-pentoxide for the determination of carbon monoxide in
the air and blood. This method depends on the oxidation of
carbon monoxide to carbon dioxide by iodine-pentoxide, and
the accurate determination of the liberated iodine. It is based
on the following reaction:

$$I_2O_5 + 5CO = I_2 + 5CO_2$$

The sample of gas to be analyzed is passed into the apparatus from a 500-cc. Thoerner gas bottle W, by displacement with
saturated salt solution, and the apparatus is then washed with
3½ liters of air. The washing requires about forty-five minutes.

741. SAYERS, R. R.: *Tice's Practice of Medicine*, 8:130, 1931.
742. MARTINEK, M. J., and MARTI, W. C.: *Am. J. Pub. Health*, 19:
293, 1929.
743. TEAGUE, M. C.: *J. Indust. & Eng. Chem.*, 20:10, 1920.

The liberated iodine is then titrated with N/200 sodium thio-sulphate solution, using a micro-burette.

TABLE XXXII

VOLUME OF GAS PER MILLION VOLUMES OF AIR (CC. GAS PER CUBIC METER OF AIR) *

Substance	Fatal with 5-10 Min. Exposure	Dangerous (toxic) ½-1 Hr. Exposure	Endurable ½-1 Hour Exposure
Mustard gas	20	15	1
Phosgene	50	25	1
Chlorine	500	50	5
Arsine	300	60	20
Prussic acid	200	100	50
Nitrous fumes	500	100	50
Hydrogen sulphide	800	400	200
Phosphine	1,000	400	100
Carbon disulphide	2,000	1,000	500
Sulphur dioxide	3,000	400	100
Hydrochloric acid	3,000	1,000	100
Ammonia	5,000	2,500	250
Carbon monoxide	5,000	2,000	1,000
Benzene	20,000	7,500	3,000
Chloroform	25,000	15,000	5,000
Petrol	30,000	20,000	15,000
Carbon tetrachloride	50,000	25,000	10,000
Carbon dioxide	90,000	50,000	30,000
Acetylene	500,000	250,000	100,000
Ethylene (in O_2)	950,000	800,000	500,000

* From LESCHKE: Clinical Toxicology, p. 156, 1934.

Sequelae of Carbon Monoxide: Schillito, Drinker and Shaughnessy[744] report that Glaister and Logan[745] made sweeping statements of severe nervous and mental sequelae following acute or chronic carbon monoxide exposure. Sayers and Davenport[746] cited from the literature cases showing after-effects. Schillito examined the records of seven state institutions that serve the New York City area. Of the patients there, thirty-nine were poisoned during the ten-year period, 1925-1935, while four were poisoned either before or after this period. In the same period there were more than 21,000 carbon monoxide exposures in the same area. There were thirty-nine cases of psychoses due to carbon monoxide poisoning. (An

744. SCHILLITO, F. H., DRINKER, C. K., and SHAUGHNESSY, T. J.: J.A.M.A., 106: 669, 1936.
745. GLAISTER, J., and LOGAN, D. D.: Gas Poisoning in Mining and Other Industries, William Wood & Company, 1914.
746. SAYERS, R. R., and DAVENPORT, S. J.: Review of Carbon Monoxide Poisoning, U. S. Pub. Health Bull. 195, 1930.

additional group of four cases, in which poisoning occurred either before or after the ten-year period, is not included in these tabulations concerning the incidence of sequelae.) The ratio of carbon monoxide psychoses to all other psychoses gives the incidence percentage of 0.05%, or roughly one carbon monoxide case to 2,000 other psychoses. From these facts it appears that one case in 500 acute exposures later showed nervous or mental symptoms. The average age of forty-three patients was fifty-three years. The youngest was twenty and the oldest eighty-three.

Onset of Sequelae of Carbon Monoxide Poisoning: These symptoms consist of headache, dizziness, and perhaps, gastric distress with nausea. It has been quite conclusively demonstrated by Forbes, Cobb, and Fremont-Smith[747] that these symptoms are due to cerebral edema induced by the poisoning. The exact time of the onset of symptoms of nervous and mental sequelae in carbon monoxide poisoning is variable. Two classes are seen: (1) those cases with the onset of symptoms within one week, and (2) those of from one to three weeks.

The Typical Psychosis Following Carbon Monoxide Poisoning: A psychosis, most usually temporary in character, was the most common manifestation of the after-effects of carbon monoxide poisoning. It was marked by confusion and bewilderment, combined with a loss of memory. The events occurring at the time of the accident were forgotten. Such symptoms as hallucinations and delusions were absent. At the time there was an overactivity of short duration. Improvement was usually noted by three months after the accident. I have had a case of a truck driver who was overcome by carbon monoxide and who suffered confusion and bewilderment and hallucinations for six months afterwards. A year later the man was still unable to work.

Amnesia in some form was the most regular feature of the psychosis following carbon monoxide poisoning. It usually consists of defects in memory. One case showed an auditory aphasia. The least apparent lesion was marked by increased reflexes. From these minimal symptoms the case graded upward to well advanced Parkinsonism, with increased reflexes,

---

747. FORBES, H. S., COBB, S., and FREMONT-SMITH, F.: Cerebral Edema and Headache Following CO Asphyxia, *Arch. Neurol. & Psychiat.*, 2:264, 1924.

slow movement, lack of coordination, fixed facies, and scanning speech. Occasional hemiplegias and paraplegias have been encountered.

In addition to these changes denoting muscular hypertonia, and indicating basal ganglion lesions, muscle atrophies and skin hyperesthesias were found. The two-year period following the individual's exposure to carbon monoxide is arbitrarily designated as the period beyond which signs and symptoms are considered permanent. Of the forty-three patients, twenty-three recovered, eleven died, and nine suffered permanent effects.

From the investigation by Schillito and associates in covering the after effects in 21,000 cases of acute carbon monoxide poisoning, they believe that the prognosis as to sequelae is not alarming. A clear period of from seven to twenty days preceded the onset of symptoms in one-third of the cases. In the remainder of the cases the symptoms started immediately following the poisoning.

"Mental sequelae consisted of confusion psychosis, with disorientation, lack of judgment, and amnesia. Motor overactivity and aphasia were much less common. Hallucinations, delusions or convulsions played no difficult part." Nervous sequelae consisted of signs varying from slightly increased deep reflexes to well advanced Parkinsonism. Sensory disturbances, such as skin anesthesia and peripheral motor neuritides, were also encountered. All of these cases showed improvement, but the final result depended on the degree of initial damage.

Wolff[748] reported atasia and abasia and perseveration following carbon monoxide poisoning. McGurn[749] mentions more than 100 neurological and other symptomatological conditions as well as two cases of a syndrome not unlike that of multiple sclerosis. Makay,[750] after a review of the literature on the clinical and experimental aspects of carbon monoxide poisoning, stated that the nervous system is the seat of highly variable and complicated degenerative changes, and that these changes are the result of functional and organic vascular disturbances dependent on anoxemia. Poelchen[751] is of the opinion

748. WOLFF, H. G.: J. Neurol. & Psychopath., 7-8:1926, 1929.
749. McGURN: Med. Rec., 91:149, 1917.
750. MAKAY, R. P.:   J.A.M.A., 94:1733, 1930.
751. POELCHEN: Berl. klin. Wchnschr., 5:19, 396, 1882.

that people who have suffered carbon monoxide poisoning sooner or later show signs of mental deterioration. He describes the case of a woman who lay unconscious for two days as a result of carbon monoxide poisoning, but who apparently recovered fully and was able to attend to her household duties for more than two weeks. She then suffered a relapse, her limbs became more or less rigid, her power of speech was almost completely lost, and there was a marked mental apathy. Less than four weeks after the accident, she died of paralysis of the bowels. Lewin mentions a case of severe gassing in which there was an apparent recovery in thirty-six hours except for headache, but twenty days after the accident the man had a relapse with increasing paralysis of the limbs which became complete on the twenty-fourth day and resulted in death the day following. Another victim was up and about for five or six days after the accident, when he was seized with convulsions followed by paralysis of the jaw, and death. This is of the greatest importance to those who testify before the Industrial Board in deciding upon compensation, as many of these people claim latent effects of carbon monoxide poisoning. Schultz[752] reported a case of carbon monoxide poisoning in a twenty-six year old man, who had attempted suicide by turning on the gas. He regained consciousness on the second day and had a spastic gait. The pupils were equal and round, and reacted to light and accommodation. The patellar and ankle reflexes were exaggerated, and there was a bilateral ankle clonus. The Babinski sign was positive on both sides, and a very marked positive Oppenheim sign was determined. The fundi were normal, speech was muffled, and on the tip of the tongue a large biting wound was found. The blood picture showed a leukocytosis and a shift to the left. The residual nitrogen of the blood was 58.8 mg. per cent. There was at first an albuminuria, which subsided. Lumbar puncture yielded a normal spinal fluid. After four days the patient started to urinate spontaneously, improved markedly, and the spastic gait became less pronounced. After a lapse of two months, only the Babinski sign was found to be positive, and the above described skin lesions had been converted into necrotic areas. The author has reported another case in which paralysis of the lower extremities and a partial paralysis of the nerves of the

752. Schultz, E. G.: *Deutsche Ztschr. f. Nervenh.*, 127:222, 1932.

right hand, with urinary retention for four days, and the formation of a muscle hematoma in the right forearm, and skin and tissue necrosis, occurred. The patient recovered in three months.[753]

SATURATED HYDROCARBONS
METHANE ($CH_4 = 16$)
(Synonyms: "Marsh-gas;" "Light Carburetted Hydrogen;" "Firedamp")

METHANE is the chief constituent of natural gas, and large quantities of it are also obtained in coke-oven gas and in the off gases from cracking higher hydrocarbons.[754] In mines it is called "firedamp". Methane is a relatively inert gas, so far as its chemical activity is concerned.

The uses of the gas are chiefly for domestic fires and lighting by mantle systems, iron works, and glass works. "Firedamp" is ever present in certain mines. In the Wilkes-Barre anthracite region there is a constant outflow of gas that is piped to the surface and burns the year round. Accidents are frequent, and visitors are dissuaded from entering the mines. The gas mixes readily with air, owing to its lightness (specific gravity, 0.5596), and forms an explosive mixture as soon as it amounts to one-eighteenth of the volume of the air. Fortunately, the mixture does not ignite readily. Electrolytic gas—hydrogen and oxygen—ignites at 674°C., marsh-gas and oxygen, at 656°C.[755] The force of explosion of the latter is 557 pounds per square inch, while marsh-gas with air gives 210 pounds per square inch. The miner's safety lamp indicates by the "corpse light", or faint blue flame extending in the gauze cylinder, the presence

753. For sequelae of carbon monoxide poisoning see: PETRI, E.: Centralbl. f. allg. Path. u. path. Anat., 40:385, 1927; WEIMAN, W.: Ztschr. f. d. ges. Neurol. u. Psychiat., 105:213, 1926; MEYER, A.: Klin. Wchnschr., 6:145, 1927; MEYER, A.: Ztschr. f. d. ges. Neurol. u. Psychiat., 112:187, 1928; ALTSCHUL, R.: Ztschr. f. d. ges. Neurol. u. Psychiat., 111:442, 1927; FERRARO, A., and MORRISON, L. R.: Psychiatric Quart., 2:506, 1928; LEPPMANN, F.: Deutsche Ztschr. f. d. ges. gerichtl. Med., 12:121, 1928; GRUNSTEIN, A. M., and POPOWA, N.: Arch. f. Psychiat., 85:283, 1928; BOURGUIGNON, G., and DESILLE, H.: Rev. neurol., 1:360, 1927; MATTAUSCHEK, E.: Wien. med. Wchnschr., 77:1239, 1927.

754. STORCH, H. H.: U. S. Bureau of Mines, Inf. Circ. 6549, 1932.

755. MAYER, VICTOR: Ber. d. deutsche chem. Gesellsch., Berl., 22:428, 1893; FREYER, and MAYER, V.: Ztschr. f. phys. Chemie, 11:28, 1893; MITSCHERLICH, A.: Ber. d. deutsche chem. Gesellsch., Berl., 26:160, 428, 1893.

of the gas before the proportion reaches the explosive stage.

As the gas has no odor, the miner is never warned of its presence by the sense of smell. It is only slightly soluble in water. It burns with a pale, illuminating, smokeless flame. In burning it yields watery vapor and carbon dioxide—"after-damp." It forms a large proportion of illuminating gas, and is present in "water-gas," "producers gas," etc.

Though generally considered an indifferent gas,[756] it has slight toxic properties. When mixed with air, it greatly reduces the proportion of oxygen; 45% marsh-gas with air leaves 11.5% oxygen and 43.5% nitrogen, while 70% reduces the oxygen to 6.3% and the nitrogen to 23.7%. Haldane's experiments may be briefly put in tabular form, and the gas thus compared with other gaseous mixtures:

TABLE XXXIII
Physiological Response of Man to Common Gases

Carbon Monoxide (CO).		Carbon Dioxide (CO_2).		Firedamp or Methane (CH_4).		Oxygen (O).	
Percentage present in air.	Effects on man	Percentage present in air.	Effects on man	Percentage present in air.	Effects on man	Percentage present, remainder being N.	Effects on man
0.05	After half an hour or more, giddiness on exertion.	3.5	Breathing deeper.	5.5	Nil.	17.3	Nil.
0.1	After half an hour or more, inability to walk.	6.0	Marked panting.	45.0	Breathing slightly deeper.	12.0	Breathing slightly deeper.
0.2	After half an hour or more, loss of consciousness and perhaps death.	10.0	Severe distress.	70.0	Life endangered.	9.0	Breathing deeper and more frequent. Face bluish.
1.0	After a few minutes, loss of consciousness and final death.	15.0	Partial loss of consciousness.			5.0	Loss of consciousness and final death.
		25.0	Final death.			0.0	Death with convulsions.

While toxicologically it has little interest, from the fearful loss of life it annually causes through explosions in mines and as the result of escaping street gas, it has a very important forensic bearing.

756. Hermann, L.: Lehrbuch der exper. Toxikologie, Berlin, 275, 1874.

The extensive experiments relative to explosions in mines are closely related to the numerous explosions that have occurred in various cities since the introduction of steam heating and electric lighting, explosions resulting in the loss of many lives and of much property. Among these may be mentioned the serious one that took place some time since in Boston, where, during the construction of the underground road, a leak occurred followed by a disastrous explosion, causing extensive wreckage and great loss of life.

In the experiments of Mason and Wheeler[757] on the propagation of the flame in mixtures of methane and air, the speed of the flame was about 60 mg. per second and was of short duration.[758]

The higher homologues of this series, C_nH_{2n+2}, are to be found in petroleum and are collected in the first distillates when cooled to a sufficiently low temperature. Other still higher members occur, as gasoline, naphtha, etc. They have highly anesthetic properties, and have been used for such. Several boys were detected in Philadelphia who climbed the lamp posts, dipped rags in the naphtha of the reservoirs, and inhaled the vapors. They became mildly intoxicated. The effect was similar to that of liquor taken internally.[759]

Tests: Ambeler[760] described a method in which the hydrogen and carbon monoxide are oxidized by means of cupric oxide at about 300°C. The resulting carbon dioxide is removed and the methane is determined by burning with oxygen in the presence of platinum wire at bright yellow heat.

For the evolution of methane detecting devices for coal mines, see Ilsley and Hooker.[761]

757. MASON and WHEELER: *J. Chem. Soc.*, 117:36, 1920.

758. PAYMAN: *J. Chem. Soc.*, 117:48, 1920; WHEELER: *J. Chem. Soc.*, 117:903, 1920; SMITH and HAMON: U. S. Bureau of Mines Tech. Paper, 190:46, 1918; SEIBER and HARPSTER: U. S. Bureau of Mines Tech. Paper, 185, 1918.

759. *Am. Gas-light J.*, 67:774, 1897.

760. AMBELER: *Analyst*, 56:635, 1931.

761. ILSLEY, L. C., and HOOKER, A. B.: U. S. Bureau of Mines, Inf. Circ. 6733, June, 1933.

For more complete information on gas analysis, consult: "The Chemists' Handbook (American Gas Association, 420 Lexington Ave., New York); "Gas Analysis, by DENNIS and NICHOLS (MacMillan); U. S. Bureau of Mines Bulletin 197: "Sampling and Examination of Mine Gases and Natural Gases," and Technical Paper No. 320: "Orsat Gas Apparatus for Gas Analysis"; and "Unitized Gas Analysis Apparatus", *Indust. & Eng. Chem., Analytical Ed.*, 6:72, 1934.

UNSATURATED HYDROCARBONS
ACETYLENE
$(C_2H_2 = 26)$

THIS gas, present in a very small proportion in illuminating and in oil gas, has acquired importance through the manufacture of calcium carbide by the aid of the electric furnace by the Wilson process.[762]   When wetted with water, calcium carbide changes to slaked lime and evolves acetylene. This ignites readily and burns with a brilliant but smoky flame. When burned from a properly constructed jet, it gives a very white light of greater intensity than any other known gas. Acetylene is an endothermic compound.   When a little fulminate of mercury is exploded in it, it detonates with violence, being decomposed into carbon and hydrogen.   (Berthelot.) Mixed with a proper proportion of oxygen and ignited in an open mortar, it shatters the vessel. (Victor Meyer.) Mixed with air it also forms a violent explosive. Cyanogen compounds are formed as the result.   It unites with metals, forming acetylides, that of copper being the best known. These are also explosives.   Acetylene may be liquefied at 0° C. under 26.05 atmospheres pressure.   It is said to be the lightest liquid known, and has a high coefficient of expansion.   It is considered more explosive than the gas.   In some countries liquid acetylene is classed as an explosive.   The gas has an odor of geranium, and is agreeable when pure.   (Moissan.)   Its escape into the air is usually detected because of the impurities.   It is a product of all incomplete combustions of hydrocarbons, and is, therefore, found when lamps or gas-jets are allowed to burn with an insufficient air supply.   The characteristic odor of a Bunsen burner which has "retreated" or of an oil- or gas-stove heated room is due mainly to acetylene.   It is also an intermediate product in the combustion of olefiant gas and it escapes unburned in the use of illuminating gas. (Lewes.) It is absorbed by water in sufficient quantity to impart a strong smell to the water and to yield precipitates with either ammoniacal cuprous chloride or silver nitrate.

Very little was known of its physiologic action until recently, when experiments with large quantities showed that a considerable amount may be present in air without causing ill

762. ROSEMANN: The Mineral Industry; COWLES, A. H.: 75 *et seq.*, 1898; also FRANK and WEIL.

effects.[763] Dogs can inhale 20% pure acetylene for one hour without any other apparent supply of air; 40% caused stupor, coma, vomiting, and deep low breathing. The impurities of the gas are the chief causes of the toxicity. In the manufacture of acetylene gas from calcium carbide and water it usually contains hydrogen sulphide, phosphine (Pontoppidan[764] reports a case of poisoning from acetylene, in which the symptoms indicated phosphoreted hydrogen poisoning. Acetylene gas not infrequently contains sufficient of this impurity to cause toxic effects.) 0.04%, and carbon dioxide, carbon monoxide 0.5%, carbon disulphide 0.5%. If carbon disulphide were present in abnormally large amounts, then the sulphur dioxide by combustion would be irritating to the mucous membrane. In two cases of poisoning[765] the patients were in a deep comatose condition, associated with slow breathing, vomiting, cyanotic face, small, fast and irregular pulse, wide and expressionless pupils. After inhalation of oxygen both men improved. One patient after an hour became very restless, had hallucinations, waved arms, and sometimes would burst into hard laughter. Both men in two hours fell into a deep sleep. Upon awakening, dizziness, headache, restlessness, and a depressed feeling were noted, which disappeared in several hours.[766]

The combination[767] with hemoglobin claimed to take place, as with carbon monoxide and with nitric oxide, to form a bright red compound which becomes gas-free by the action of reducing agents, is denied by recent observers.

From experiments upon blood, acetylene has been found to behave as an indifferent gas.[768]

Tests: Acetylene may be estimated in illuminating gas and in air mixtures[769] by means of Ilosva's reagent[770] which gives an immediate red precipitate of copper acetylide, upon

763. GREHANT, N.: Sur la toxicitie de l'acetylene, Compt. rend., 121:564, 1895; BROCINER, L.: Compt. rend., 121:774, 1895.

764. Ugesk. f. laeger, 83:1222, 1921.

765. NICOL: München. med. Wchnschr., 63:193, 1916.

766. BETTINK: Utrecht Pharm. Weekblad, 54:513, 1917.

767. LIEBREICH and BRISTOW: Ber. d. deutsch. Chem. Gesellsch., 1:220, 1868.

768. HERMANN, L.: Lehrbuch der exper. Toxikologie, Berlin, 115, 1874.

769. ARNOLD, MOLLENY, and ZIMMERMAN: Ber. d. deutsch. chem. Gesellsch., 53:1034, 1920.

770. Ber. d. deutsch. chem. Gesellsch., 32:2698, 1899.

shaking the solution with a portion of the confined gas. (This reagent is prepared by dissolving 1 gm. of cupric nitrate $(Cu(NO_3)_25H_2O)$ in a 50-cc. flask with a little water, adding 4 cc. of ammonium hydrate and then 3 gm. of hydroxylamin hydrochloride and making the mixture up to 50 cc. with water.) Fill a three-liter separatory funnel with illuminating gas; place about 20 cc. of the reagent in the funnel, and shake frequently during one hour. Transfer to a beaker and dilute with ammonia water to prevent air oxidation; filter and wash well. Place the precipitate with the filter in a crucible with a little concentrated nitric acid, heat, and weigh the copper oxide. The calculation assumes that $(Cu_2C_2H_2)O$ is formed.

$x = 100$ g. $(1+0.00366t)$ 760/vp., in which

$x =$ per cent C_2H_2, $V =$ vol., p. $=$ barometric pressure

$t =$ temperature, and g. is the weight of the CuO.

Willstätter and Maschmann[771] filter the copper salt obtained as above on a long-fibred asbestos suction filter, and wash to remove excess of ammonia. When wash-water remains pink on the addition of one drop of 0.1 normal $KMnO_4$, the precipitate is dissolved on the filter with 25 cc. of acidified ferric sulphate (100 gm. ferric sulphate, 200 gm. H_2SO_4, make up to one liter). The filtrate is titrated with N/10 $KMnO_4$ according to the equation:

$$C_2Cu_2 + Fe_2(SO_4)_3 + H_2SO_4 = 2FeSO_4 + 2CuSO_4 + C_2H_2.[722]$$

ETHYLENE ($C_2H_4 = 28$)
(Synonyms: Olefiant Gas, Heavy Carburetted Hydrogen)

THIS is a constant constituent of gas obtained by the destructive distillation of wood, coal, or oils. The "illuminants" of ordinary illuminating gas consist of a mixture of ethylene, propylene, and higher homologues, with which are also mixed members of other series, as benzene, naphthalene, etc. It has a pleasant odor, is slightly soluble in water, and unites directly with chlorine or bromine. The action of this gas, and also of the other gases of this group, is that of a weak narcotic. Gases of this category are now made by the destructive distillation of oil, and are then compressed in iron cylinders. These supply the gas for the Pintsch system of lighting.

771. WILLSTATTER and MASCHMANN: *Ber. d. deutsch. chem. Gessellsch.*, 53:939, 1920.

772. MULLER: *Bull. Soc. Chem.*, 27:69, 1920.

Ethylene in dilutions as high as one part in 2,000,000 will noticeably accelerate the coloring of black green lemons.[773] For commercial practice on citrus fruits one part to 5,000 to 10,000 parts of air seem to give most satisfactory results. Ordinary citrus fruit will color in two to five days under this treatment and will soften sufficiently for satisfactory packing. Tomatoes and bananas seem to improve their color when exposed to ethylene. Ethylene has also been used for removing the hulls from walnuts; treatment with ethylene causes the hulls to become friable so that they are readily removed by the various hulling devices.

Ethylene used with fruits is often called a coloring process, which is a misnomer because the substance does not add color but destroys chlorophyl and leaves the natural color of the fruit in place. Chase states that the ethylene, in the dilutions used in this process is absolutely harmless to workers.

When ethylene was first introduced[774] as an anesthetic numerous serious complications followed its use. One of the complications was the presence of carbon monoxide as an impurity in the gas. Walker and Alley[775] report a fatality in a white man thirty-nine years of age who was given ethylene anesthesia for the reduction of a fracture. When the anesthesia was withdrawn the pulse began to thin out and became imperceptible. Immediately inhalations of oxygen and 10% carbon dioxide were given as a restorative. The man died. The authors reported three cases of blood examinations, revealing the presence of carbon monoxide.

Harvey[776] uses castor oil plants to detect ethylene in the air, claiming that in air atmosphere containing as little as 0.00001% C_2H_4 will cause the petoiles of the leaves to drop or the lamina to fold down.

The gas is also said to be poisonous to sweet pea seedlings and carnations.

Beyond their narcotic action the other gases of this group have slight interest here.[777]

773. CHACE, E. M.: *Am. J. Pub. Health,* 24:1152, 1934.

774. SHERMAN, W. O., SWINDLER, M., and McELROY, W. S.: *J.A.M.A.,* 86:1765, 1926.

775. WALKER, B. S., and ALLEY: *Anesth. & Analg.,* 8:227, 1929.

776. HARVEY: *J. Roy. Hort. Soc.,* 40:300, 1914.

777. MAHSOFF and EGLOFF: A Review of the Chemical and Physical Properties of Ethylene, *J. Physiol. Chem.,* 23:65, 1919.

ETHYLENE DICHLORIDE (CH₂Cl—CH₂Cl)

ETHYLENE DICHLORIDE, the first known of the ethylene-halogen compounds, was discovered in 1795 by Dutch chemists who named it "Dutch liquid," CH_2Cl-CH_2Cl. It is not to be confused with dichlorethylene, from which it differs chemically as well as pharmacologically, especially in its action on the eye. Ethylene dichloride was first used as an anesthetic[778] in 1848 and 1849.[779] In 1887, Du Bois and Roux[780] discovered that it caused corneal opacities, which was a factor in its being discarded. The maximum dose is stated as 1 cc. for a single dose and 3 cc. per day. Today ethylene dichloride is used commercially chiefly as a solvent; in cleaning fluids and lacquers it has a wide and increasing application. It has been used to kill moths and weevils, the latter in the fumigation of grain and flour. The inhalation of ethylene dichloride is an important problem in industrial hygiene. It is strange that in spite of its extensive commercial use, no cases of ethylene dichloride poisoning after oral ingestion have apparently been reported. Sayers, Yant, Waite and Patty,[781] stated that ethylene dichloride has been cited as a stimulant for sprouting potatoes. A case of fatal poisoning is reported by Hueper and Smith[782] in a man sixty-three years of age who accidentally drank upon an empty stomach two ounces of ethylene dichloride which he had mistaken for gin and had mixed with orange juice and ginger ale. Two hours later he began to feel nauseated and faint, and started to vomit during the hour. When he arrived at the hospital, five hours after the accident, he appeared dazed and distressed and was unable to stand. He vomited a liquid that resembled milk, which had been given him three hours before. On physical examination the blood pressure was 152/84. The lips were slightly cyanosed. The face was cool and moist. The pupils were dilated and equal. The odor of the breath resembled that of chloroform. The tongue had a heavy yellow coating. The upper pharynx was injected. The heart

778. NUNNELEY, T., SIMPSON, N., and SNOW: *Providence M. & S. J.,* 98:1849.

779. EULENBERG, H.: *Haudb. d. Gewerbehyg.,* 401, 1876.

780. DU BOIS, R., and ROUX, L.: *Compt. rend. Acad. d. sc.,* 104: 1869, 1887.

781. SAYERS, R. R., YANT, W. P., WAITE, C. P., and PATTY, F. A.: Pub. Health Report, 45:225, 1930.

782. HUEPER, W. C., and SMITH, C.: *Am. J. M. Sc.,* 189:778, 1935.

sounds were distant. A blood count taken eight hours after the accident showed erythrocytes, 5,260,000; leukocytes, 11,800; 86% neutrophils, 11% lymphocytes, 3% monocytes; no reticulocytes; no abnormality of erythrocytes. He died twenty-two hours after taking the ethylene dichloride.

Postmortem: A pathological diagnosis gave hemorrhagic colitis; nephrosis with calcifications of the tubular epithelium and tubular and vascular elastic membranes; fatty degeneration and passive congestion of the liver, passive congestion of the spleen and lungs; multiple perivascular hemorrhages of the brain; chronic myocarditis and myositis due to trichinosis.

Parnas in 1888[783] Faravelli,[784] Erdmann,[785] Bullot in 1896,[786] and Steindorff,[787] in 1922, observed during the course of extensive experimentation with ethylene dichloride that this substance, when inhaled or injected subcutaneously or intravenously, caused a temporary, white, blue-white opacity of the cornea in various animals. These opacities they found, cleared up from the periphery after several months, and were due to an infiltration of the cornea by lymphocytes and connective tissue cells. Joachimoglu[788] found that ethylene dichloride has about the same anesthetizing effect as chloroform, but that its hemolytic action is only half as strong as that of the latter substance. Kistler and Luckhardt[789] found that dogs given ethylene dichloride either by stomach tube or by intravenous injection, did not die immediately. They passed through a stage characterized by depression, general sickness, emaciation, anorexia, lack of thirst, dyspnea, tarry stools and corneal opacities lasting several weeks, before they gradually recovered. The postmortem findings typical of all dogs that died from the effects of the poisoning were delay of rigor mortis by several hours, bloody discharge from mouth and nostrils, edema of the lung, subserous hemorrhages of the heart, hyperemia of the liver, brownish discoloration of the liquid blood, hemorrhages into

783. PARNAS, M.: Action des inhalations du chlorure d'ethylene pur sur l'oeil, *ibid*, 921.

784. FARAVELLI, F.: *Arch. per le sc. med.*, 16:79, 1892.

785. ERDMANN: Ueber Auhenveraenderungen durch Aethylenchlorid., *Klin. Monatsbl. f. Augenh.*, 50:370, 1912.

786. BULLOT: *Zentralbl. f. prakt. Augenheilk.*, 21:124, 1897.

787. STEINDORFF, K.: *Arch. f. Ophth.*, 109:252, 1922.

788. JOACHIMOGLU, G.: *Berl. klin. Wchnschr.*, 58:147, 1921.

789. KISTLER, G. H., and LUCKHARDT, A. B.: *Anesth. & Analg.*, 8:65, 1929.

the mesentery and intestinal lumen, albumin and bile pigments in the urine. Sayers, Yant, Waite, and Patty noted similar symptoms and postmortem findings. Ploetz[790] stated that ethylene dichloride had a hemolytic effect and Plagge[791] noted that this substance inhibited fermentation of yeast. The appearance of large amounts of albumin and sugar in the urine and the occurrence of extensive tubular necrosis with calcifications resembling those seen in mercury bichloride poisoning indicated that the kidney is the excretory organ of this substance or its decomposition product, which is presumably acid. The hemorrhagic condition of the mucosa of the colon, on the other hand, was most likely the result of the toxic action of the ethylene dichloride exerted upon the intestinal mucosa during the process of absorption.

ETHYLENE CHLORHYDRINE

MIDDLETON[792] reported a fatal case of poisoning by ethylene chlorhydrine in two men, a burner, and his laborer, who were employed in the repair of a still in which ethylene chlorhydrine was present. It boils at about 124°C. The period of exposure of the man fatally poisoned was only about a quarter as long as that of the one who recovered. It seems certain that in the fatal case most of the poison was absorbed through the skin when mopping up the water which contained the ethylene chlorhydrine in solution.

ILLUMINATING GAS

THE composition of this gas has varied from time to time in the last ten years, depending upon its introduction into various localities. As the methods of manufacture differ and are continually changing, it is difficult to give an average analysis. Four or five varieties are delivered to consumers in New York. In Chicago two grades of gas are distributed —on the North and Northwest side straight water-gas, and on the South side a mixture of two-thirds water-gas and one-third coal gas. All observers agree, however, in ascribing its poisonous properties to the carbon monoxide it contains. Street gas deprived of carbon monoxide is not destructive to

790. PLOETZ, W.: *Biochem. Ztschr.*, 103:242, 1920.
791. PLAGGE, H.: Aethens and Aethylens, *Biochem. Ztschr.*, 118: 129, 1921.
792. MIDDLETON, E. L.: *J. Indust. Hyg.*, 12:265, 1930.

mice, though 11% be present in air (Gruber) and the air breathed for hours. Though stupefied, they recover promptly. Animals live in marsh-gas or hydrogen if supplied with sufficient oxygen. (Freitag.)

Fortunately, the intense odor of street gas enables it to be detected long before the proportion of carbon monoxide in the air reaches the toxic limit. Tidy claims one part in 12,000 of air—certainly one in 8000; Soyka, 0.01 to 0.02%, when the carbon monoxide would be only 0.004%; Gruber and others give the toxic limit of carbon monoxide as 0.02%. The volume of gas lost to manufacturers by leakage is large—generally not far from 10%.[793]

The retentive power of the soil on the odoriferous constituents of gas was accurately demonstrated in a long series of experiments, and many investigations bearing upon the subject of the escape of gas into dwellings through the soil were made by workers in Pettenkofer's laboratory.[794]

A similar and complete study concerning the permeation of gas, and a series of experiments bearing on the subject of the escape of gas into dwellings, have determined that it is greater in winter than in summer, and that the liability of poisoning is in correspondence thereto.[795]

Numerous accidents occurred throughout the United States in February, 1936, due to the extreme cold experienced. Gas mains were broken, permitting dangerous quantities of gas to enter homes and streets. In Albany, New York, numerous fires were caused by the escaping gas. In other cities deaths were reported, due to the effects of carbon monoxide.

Cobelli gives the details of a case where a mother and two daughters were fatally poisoned.[796] A father, mother, and a daughter were overcome in Berlin, by gas leaking from a pipe at a distance of twenty to thirty-five meters.[797] Numerous

793. WEYL, T.: Hyg., der chem. Gross-Indus., Jena, 1896.

794. VON PETTENKOFER, MAX: Populäre Vorträge, 1:89, 1877; BIEFEL, R., and POLECK, T.: Ueber Kohlendunst und Leuchtgasvergiftung, Ztschr. f. Biol., 16:312, 1880.

795. WELITSCHOKOWSKY: Experimentelle Untersuchungen ueber die Verbreitung des Leuchtgases un des Kohlenoxides im Erdboden, Arch. f. Hyg., 1:210, 1883; SUDERKOFF, A.: Arch. f. Hyg., 5:166, 1886.

796. COBELLI: Vergiftung der Familie Caini durch Leuchtgas, Ztschr. f. Biol., 12:420, 1876.

797. JACOBS: Berl. klin. Wchnschr., 2:322, 1874.

experiments and many observations in cases of death from this kind of poisoning show that the toxic atmosphere may contain an insufficient quantity of gas to form an explosive mixture. It needs one volume of gas to twelve of air to explode. In greater proportion, as one to four, there is no explosion, but the gas takes fire.[798]

Street gas deprived of odor has poisonous properties nearly like those of water-gas or charcoal fumes. Indeed, a differential diagnosis between poisoning by illuminating gas and that by charcoal fumes is difficult to establish, even if the blood shows the characteristic carbon monoxide spectrum. This, however, has been attempted.[799]

When symptoms of carbon monoxide are present in marked degree, illuminating gas is indicated. Sooty appearance of the mouth and nostrils tends to show charcoal fumes. Circumstantial evidence is more valuable than the pathologic appearances. Comparative experiments on animals are given by Biefel and Poleck.[800]

Symptoms: Symptoms are the same as described under carbon monoxide.

HYDROGEN SULPHIDE ($H_2S = 34$)
(Synonym: Sulphuretted Hydrogen)

THIS colorless, transparent gas, possessing the smell of rotten eggs, is found naturally in volcanic regions and impregnating many spring waters. It is quite soluble in water, that of mean temperature dissolving 3.23 times its bulk of the gas. It is a product of the putrefaction of organic substances containing sulphur, and is, therefore, always found where vegetable or animal matter is undergoing decay, as in cesspools, sewers,[801] privy vaults, and tannery vats.[802]

Yant[803] states the principal sources of hydrogen sulphide which are reported from the standpoint of health are gypsum

798. BIEFEL, R., and POLECK, T.: ref. 794; SONNENSCHEIN, F. L.: Handb. d. ger. Med., 296, 1869; SCHUTT: Vrtljschr. f. gerichtl. Med., Berl., 3rd. series, 7: 162, 1896.

799. DEICHSTETTER, J.: Friedreich's Bl. f. gerichtl. Med., Nürnb., 74: 35, 1896.

800. BIELFEL, R., and POLECK, T.: Ztschr. f. Biol., 16: 312, 1880.

801. KLEIN, W.: Deutsche Ztschr. f. d. ges gerichtl. Med., 1: 288, 1922.

802. TAUSS: Zentralbl. f. Gewerbehyg., 1: 74, 1920.

803. YANT, W. P.: Am. J. Pub. Health, 20: 398, 1930.

mines and wells, caissons and tunnels, natural gas, production and refining of petroleum, sewers and other places where organic material is decomposing in confined places, blasting with a black powder and other explosives in heavy sulphide ore, gas manufacture and low temperature carbonization of coal, and manufacture of chemicals, dyes and pigments. The gas is often present also in the water of some mineral springs, in rock fissure gases, and volcanic gases. The gas encountered in the production of oil from certain fields is known now to contain as much as 10% to 12% by volume of hydrogen sulphide, and 50% to 75% is found in refinery gases. It has also been found that a concentration of as little as 0.005% to 0.01% will cause a conjunctivitis popularly known as "gas eyes."

This gas is also generated by the decomposition of organic matter by anaerobic bacteria in deep lakes and ponds, tainting the water or coming to the surface and tainting the atmosphere, where its presence is indicated by the discoloration caused upon dwellings painted with white lead. Many of the small estuaries receiving the sewage of towns become defiled with this gas, being little more than open sewers. From such sources the gas is frequently discharged in considerable quantities, and is carried by the shifting winds in different directions. It is formed spontaneously whenever a soluble sulphate remains in contact with decaying organic matter with deficiency of air; directly by the union of sulphur and hydrogen; indirectly by the action of acids on the sulphide of the metals, generally ferrous sulphide. In certain mines it is found occasionally as an occluded gas in coal seams or places where there is decomposition in the presence of water.[804] It is usual to prepare it in the laboratory from ferrous sulphide and an acid. The gas is rarely pure. It is set free when sulphur is heated with damp wood, charcoal, tallow or paraffin wax. Its intense odor enables it to be recognized when present in minute quantities, one part in 10,000 being easily noted. It is slightly heavier than the air, its specific gravity being 1.1912.

The solution in water gradually changes, depositing white sulphur. The gas is decomposed by heat into its elements. It

804. KOBER, G. M., and HANSON, W. C.: Diseases of Occupation and Vocational Hygiene, Phila., P. Blakiston's Son and Co., 47, 620.

is combustible, burns with a blue flame, producing water and sulphur dioxide, or, if the air is limited, some sulphur is deposited. It is decomposed in the presence of moisture by sulphur dioxide.

It explodes when mixed with half its volume of oxygen and ignited, with a deposition of sulphur; but two volumes of hydrogen sulphide and three of oxygen yield sulphur dioxide on explosion. It is one of the products of putrefactive processes in the body, especially in the intestine, and leads to auto-intoxication, Wells[805] asserting that as much as 66 mg. may be present in each 100 gm. of normal colon contents.

The gas was first examined by Rouelle[806] in 1777. He was the first to make a systematic study of the compound of much importance. In Paris numerous accidental deaths due to the gases from the sewers were investigated. During the next few years Dupuytren, Thenard, and Barruel,[807] by chemical analyses, proved the presence of hydrogen sulphide in the sewers, and this gas was associated with the accidents and believed to be the cause of many of them. Thenard and Dupuytren also began to experiment with hydrogen sulphide and found that 0.066% of hydrogen sulphide was fatal for a greenfinch, 0.125% fatal for dogs, and 0.4% for a horse.

Thenard mentions Magendie[808] as having injected hydrogen sulphide into the venous system of animals. He found that some of the gas was liberated in the lungs but that a greater part was carried in solution in the arterial blood for a certain time, and that it affected the red color of the blood. In 1836 D'Arcet[809] reported the death of three young men from gas liberated from defective sewer connections. Taylor[810] stated that the symptoms of poisoning were marked, and that a number of men died from hydrogen sulphide during the building of the tunnel under the Thames river. The affection ceased only when the tunnel was completed and ventilation was established.

805. WELLS: Chemical Pathology, Phila., 590, 1920; and see HAGGARD: J. Biol. Chem., 49:519, 1921.

806. ROUELLE, M.: J. de méd., 39:449, 1777.

807. DUPUYTREN, M.: Rapport sur une espec de mephitisme des fosses d'aisance, produite par les gas azote, J. de méd., 11:187, 1806.

808. MAGENDIE, M.: cited by THENARD, in CHIMIE, 4, 1827.

809. D'ARCET and BRACONNOT: Ann. d'hyg., 16:24, 1836.

810. TAYLOR, A. S.: Manual of Medical Jurisprudence, 486, 1897.

In 1857 Bernard[811] injected hydrogen sulphide solution into venous blood and proved that hydrogen sulphide was eliminated through the lungs, as determined by the blackening of lead acetate when exposed to the exhaled air. Bernard also found that an animal could often be revived by being given artifical respiration.

In 1898 Harnack[812] demonstrated that when hemoglobin was made oxygen-free by saturation with carbon dioxide, as by Hoppe-Seyler and others, hydrogen sulphide had no action, but if the blood were not so saturated with carbon dioxide, the dark red color with characteristic absorption bands was formed. This spectrum consisted of a band between C and D, extending from λ610 to λ625.

A theory of hydrogen sulphide action, advanced by Diakonow[813] and supported by Pohl,[814] was that a reaction between hydrogen sulphide and the sodium bicarbonate of the blood plasma occurred whereby sodium sulphide was formed. Pohl believed that the sodium sulphide was carried in the blood. Haggard,[815] in his studies, definitely disproved this theory. He stated that "it appears that not only does hydrogen sulphide fail to form sodium sulphide when acting upon blood or plasma, but a portion of the gas is actually destroyed." Haggard believes that the products of oxidation combine, in part, with the sodium of the plasma. The oxygen is withdrawn from the corpuscles at such a rate that normally the hydrogen sulphide produced during digestion and absorption of sulphides, etc., is amply taken care of, and poisoning does not result.

In 1865 Eulenberg[816] subjected animals to toxic doses of hydrogen sulphide. He determined that 0.1% of hydrogen sulphide was fatal for cats, rabbits, and doves within a short time. Young animals appeared to succumb to 0.05%. Biefel and Poleck,[817] some years later found that a rabbit died within

811. BERNARD, CLAUDE: *Arch. gén. de méd., Par.,* 5th series, 9:129. 1867.

812. HARNACK, E.: *Ztschr. f. physiol. Chem.,* 26:558, 1898, 1899.

813. DIAKONOW: Transl. and abstr. by HOPPE-SEYLER in *Med. Chem. Untersuch.,* 71:251, 1866.

814. POHL, J.: *Arch. f. exper. Path. u. Pharmakol.,* 22:1, 1886.

815. HAGGARD, H. W.: *J. Biol. Chem.,* 49:519, 1921.

816. EULENBERG, H.: Die Lehre von den Schädlichen und giftigen Gazen, 260, 1865.

817. BIEFEL, R., and POLECK, T.: *Ztschr. f. Biol.,* 16:279, 1880.

seventy-five minutes when exposed to 0.05% of hydrogen sulphide, and concluded that 0.01% was without effect. In 1884 Smirnow[818] reported that in his experiments he was unable to find the spectroscopic changes in the blood of animals poisoned by hydrogen sulphide, as reported by other investigators. Smirnow states that 0.3% of hydrogen sulphide quickly kills small animals, while 0.2% may cause death, and that 0.1% to 0.15% may be endured for a considerable period.

Wigglesworth[819] reported two cases of insanity caused by inhalation of hydrogen sulphide. They were characterized by great muscular excitement. One case recovered after five months. Lehmann[820] subjected men to varying concentrations of hydrogen sulphide, ranging from 0.01% to 0.05%, and observed severe poisoning. Symptoms were discomfort, depression, loss of appetite, pulmonary disturbances, gastric troubles, debility, and eventually icterus. In 1908 Haibe[821] reported an interesting study of cases of chronic poisoning due to hydrogen sulphide occurring in the gas industry. Seven deaths were caused by hepatogenic function, while in those cases that recovered anemia was a constant finding. In 1911 Sir Thomas Oliver[822] investigated the sulphur mines of Sicily and reported a number of deaths, eleven due to hydrogen sulphide poisoning. One boy was unconscious for several days, and on recovery had lost his speech. In an experimental study on the effects of hydrogen sulphide upon animals (canary birds, white rats, guinea pigs, dogs, and goats), and upon men by Sayers, Mitchell, and Yant,[823] it was found that as low a concentration as 0.005% would cause toxic symptoms and on continued exposure covering a number of days, with a concentration of 0.02%, death occurred. Hydrogen sulphide in such low percentage is often found in certain industries.[824]

Symptoms: Hydrogen sulphide by its direct action on

818. SMIRNOW, L.: *Centralbl. f. d. med. Weissench.,* 37:641, 1884.
819. WIGGLESWORTH, J.: *Brit. M. J.,* 2:124, 1892.
820. LEHMANN, K. B.: *Arch. f. Hyg.,* 14:135, 1892.
821. HAIBE, A.: *Bull. Acad. roy. de méd de Belgique,* 22:535, 1908.
822. OLIVER, SIR THOMAS: *Brit. M. J.,* 2:12, 1911.
823. SAYERS, R. R., MITCHELL, C. W., and YANT, W. P.: Report of Investigations, Ser. No. 2491, June, 1923, U. S. Bureaus of Mines, Dept. of Interior.
824. For the cumulative effects of hydrogen sulphide see *Med. du Trav.,* January, 1935, pp. 1-26; March, 1935, pp. 68-75; May, 1935, pp. 103-122.

tissues induces the phenomena of local inflammation and, therefore, is classified as an irritant gas. Breathed in its pure state this gas is immediately fatal. It acts upon all animals through all tissues, especially the lungs. If somewhat diluted it produces nausea, giddiness, cold skin, labored breathing, irregular action of the heart, transient auricular fibrillation as noted in one case,[825] pains in the stomach, and death by coma or in violent convulsions, with tetanus and even delirium. In greater dilution sleepiness will be produced, the continued respiration of the gas proving fatal, sensibility not being restored. In exceedingly dilute conditions it sometimes occasions febrile symptoms somewhat resembling typhoid. Fatal edema of the lungs can be produced experimentally in animals by exposing them for many hours to a concentration of hydrogen sulphide (500 parts per million) insufficient to cause marked general symptoms.[826] In man, also, an occasional fatality occurs from one to three days after the subsidence of acute symptoms, and is due to edema of the lungs. As the result of exposure to this gas there is an irritating conjunctivitis, in which, on more serious cases, the surface of the cornea appears as if eroded and this is accompanied by characteristic vascular changes, perversions of sight, and, in rare instances, ulceration. Hydrogen sulphide is oxidized when brought into contact with blood in which the hemoglobin contains oxygen; the blood is proportionately reduced and the hydrogen sulphide destroyed. Only an insignificant deoxidation of the blood in the body is caused by hydrogen sulphide, even when an immediately fatal amount is inhaled, and this reduction does not contribute appreciably to the toxic action of the gas. Hydrogen sulphide gas does not result in the formation of hemoglobin compounds. Some of the hydrogen sulphide that is liberated in the blood is oxidized probably to sulphuric acid (and related acids) which are immediately neutralized to the non-toxic sodium salts.

The entire systemic action of hydrogen sulphide is on the nervous system. In very low concentrations the action of the gas is, in general, that of mild depression, both physical and mental. In concentrations of approximately 1,000 parts per million and over in the air breathed, the action passes from

825. ROBINSON: *J.A.M.A.*, 66:1611, 1916.
826. HAGGARD, H. W.: *J. Indust. Hyg.*, 7:114, 1925.

depression to the stimulation which characterizes the acute forms of poisoning. Hydrogen sulphide is to the highest degree a non-cumulative poison; the response of respiration to inhalation of the gas is immediate, and proportional to the concentration breathed. Respired air containing less than 1,000 parts per million (0.1%) has a negligible influence on respiration. Above this concentration active hyperpnea increases and soon terminates in respiratory failure. With a concentration of 1,500 parts per million (0.15%) the course of events is the same except that the reaction is more intense. With concentrations of 2,000 parts per million (0.2%) and over there is little preliminary hyperpnea, and breathing is paralyzed after a breath or two of the contaminated air.

Asphyxia develops as a result of the paralysis of breathing induced by high concentrations of hydrogen sulphide. The heart, however, continues to beat for several minutes after respiration has ceased. If the subject can be induced to breathe by artificial means, or if artificial respiration is maintained until the hydrogen sulphide in the blood is oxidized, normal respiration soon becomes re-established and the subject suffers little serious consequence. Rats may be given concentrations of hydrogen sulphide that cause paralysis of breathing and in another minute artificial respiration is induced and normal respiration is re-established. The Bureau of Mines at Pittsburgh, Pennsylvania, had a novel experiment illustrating this point by having rats under a glass Bell jar, overcoming them with hydrogen sulphide, and then restoring them by artificial respiration. "The action of hydrogen sulphide is not limited to any one part of the nervous system. In severe poisoning convulsions, muscular rigidity, and jactitation form a characteristic part of the general picture but contribute little toward the fatal outcome. The heart is slowed by the action of hydrogen sulphide, which is probably exerted through the vagus nerve. In spite of the cardiac slowing, the action of the heart continues otherwise unimpaired for several minutes after respiration has failed in the more acute forms of poisoning. A profuse flow of saliva and cold perspiration may follow exposure to concentrations of the gas insufficient to produce the more acute forms of poisoning. Concentration of hydrogen sulphide as low as 100 parts per million (0.01%) may cause local irritation and depression of the nervous system, not unlike that following a prolonged course of bromides" (without acneiform eruption).

Teleky[827] saw a number of poisonings in a chemical factory where hydrogen sulphide escaped from pipes. The gas escaped in a large quantity, and the man who happened to be in the vicinity was not in time to get away but fell unconscious to the floor. A second workman was also exposed and every attempt at resuscitation failed, whereas the first workman recovered in a few days. Teleky also noticed hydrogen sulphide poisoning in a few workmen who had been working in

TABLE XXXIV

THE TOXIC CONCENTRATIONS OF HYDROGEN SULPHIDE

Concentration of Hydrogen Sulphide in Air			
Mg. per Liter	Parts per Million	Per Cent	Symptomatology
0.14-0.21	100-150	0.01-0.15	Symptoms of local irritation after many hours of exposure.
0.28-0.42	200-300	0.02-0.03	Causes local irritation if inhaled for one hour and slight general symptoms if inhaled longer.
0.70-0.97	500-700	0.05-0.07	Causes local irritation and slight systemic symptoms within one hour. May cause death after exposure of several hours.
1.0	900	0.09	Causes systemic symptoms in less than thirty minutes. May cause death in less than one hour.
1.7	1500	0.15	Causes death after fifteen to thirty minutes of exposure.
2.0	1,800 and over	0.18 and over	Causes almost immediate death through paralysis of breathing.

a sewer. Most of them had time to escape, but one of them was found dead. A series of intoxications have been observed in the artificial silk industry. Cases of conjunctivitis have also been seen in a coal mine. Hydrogen sulphide was emitted from an accumulator room in sufficient quantities to cause poisoning in a man and his wife, which occurred during the changing of the batteries when many droplets of acid, which were present, reacted with the sulphur content in the material of the wall, producing hydrogen sulphide.

827. TELEKY: *Deutsche med. Wchnschr.*, 57:1026, 1931.

Jaensch reported hydrogen sulphide poisoning in cane sugar factories and in the artificial silk industry.[828] Intoxications have also been observed in certain sulphur bath resorts in the Black Sea, and also in sulphur factories which produce hydrogen sulphide as a side product, and also in the sulphur mines of Japan.

Treatment: The eye irritation is usually improved by goggles. Protection against the inhalation of hydrogen sulphide is provided by suitable masks which can be obtained from supply houses. Air-tight goggles, either alone or as part of a mask equipment, give satisfactory protection if properly and conscientiously used. Workmen, in all types of work, whether zinc, lead, or gases, object to wearing goggles because of the clouding with moisture, and they complain that an irritation and inflammation appear where the goggles rest tightly against the skin.

When the air of a building is contaminated by hydrogen sulphide, forced ventilation or some other means of rapidly changing the air may be employed to reduce the dangers of poisoning. Artificial respiration is instituted immediately. In every instance it should be given by the Schafer, or prone pressure, method, without interruption until the patient continues to breathe. The same method as given under carbon monoxide, giving 5% carbon dioxide and oxygen should be instituted. As this is not always available, artificial respiration should be started immediately.

Tests: Littlefield, Yant and Berger[829] have described a detector for quantitative estimation of low concentrations of hydrogen sulphide, which will indicate hydrogen sulphide in the range of 0.0025% to 0.05%, and is simple enough for the average laborer to obtain accurate results after reading a few directions. It was apparent from their tests with the different kinds of granules, such as silver cyanide coatings on activated alumina and lead acetate on activated alumina, on silica gel, and on sea sand, that the absorptive properties of the carrier granule were important. A hydrogen sulphide detector based on a color change reaction on the surface of sensitized granules placed in a glass tube through which the atmosphere to be

828. JAENSCH, P. A.: *Arch. f. Gewerbepath. u. Gewerbehyg.*, **1:397**, 1930.

829. LITTLEFIELD, J. B., YANT, W. P., and BERGER, L. B.: U. S. Bureau of Mines, Dept. of Interior, R. I. 3276, June, 1935.

examined is aspirated by means of a rubber bulb or hand pump is described. The amount of hydrogen sulphide is indicated by the distance the black color change travels in the column of granules for a constant sample volume, or by the volume of sample required to produce a standard length of travel. A granule prepared by coating twenty to twenty-four mesh granules of activated aluminum oxide with silver cyanide or lead acetate was found satisfactory for estimating hydrogen sulphide in the range of 0.0025% to 0.05% by volume in air. The function of the detector was examined at temperatures of —22° to +25° and found to be satisfactory. Detector tubes filled with silver cyanide coated granules retained their sensitivity and usefulness after eighteen months' storage and ageing in ordinary laboratory daylight.

Horne and Shirey[830] describe an apparatus for the detection of hydrogen sulphide in gases. This is a method for the quantitative removal and determination of hydrogen sulphide from gases obtained in the experimental cracking of crude shale oil. The mixed gases coming from the gasoline condenser are immediately passed through the absorber, and the hydrogen sulphide alone is quantitatively extracted.

Lapin and Hein[831] describe a colorimetric method for the determination of hydrogen sulphide in water. To 200 cc. of the water to be tested, 5 cc. of the phospho-tungstic reagent are added, and after thorough mixing, 3.5 cc. of a 4/N sodium hydroxide solution are added. The resulting blue solution is compared colorimetrically after three minutes with a known standard. It is to be borne in mind that the phospho-tungstic reagent is not specific for hydrogen sulphide and, therefore, a blue solution will be obtained also with a series of other substances such as urea, alloxan, alloxantin, tyrosin, phloroglucin, resorcin, thymol, o-oxychinolin, tannin, and also vitamin **B,** but the sensitivity of the reagent against hydrogen sulphide is much higher than with any of the mentioned compounds. By means of a standard table it is easy to determine the quantity of hydrogen sulphide in water at any given place.

Magnanimis found in animals a congestion of the glomerulus and destruction of the tubular epithelium of the kidneys.

830. Horne, J. W., and Shirey, W. B.: Report of Investigations, U. S. Bureau of Mines, R. I. 3135, October, 1931.

831. Lapin, L. N., and Hein, V. O.: Ztschr. f. Hyg. u. Infektionskr., 114: 605, 1933.

Malossi found fatty degeneration and a deposition of calcium in the pyramid.

SEWER GAS

THE poisonous effects of the air of sewers, cesspools, and privy vaults are due to hydrogen sulphide, ammonium sulphide, other undetermined gases, and to carbon dioxide and nitrogen. In many instances the asphyxiation is due solely to want of oxygen. The greatest danger is due to the presence of the sulphides. Paris sewer air gave on analysis in 100 parts: oxygen, 13.79; nitrogen, 81.21; carbon dioxide, 2.01; hydrogen sulphide, 2.99.[832]

TABLE XXXV

POISONOUS AND EXPLOSIVE GASES FOUND IN MANHOLES

Gas	Source
Ammonia, explosive	Refrigerating plants.
Benzol, explosive	Motor vehicles, storage tanks.
Carbon dioxide, non-explosive	Products of combustion, sewer gas.
Carbon monoxide, explosive	Manufactured fuel gas, flue gas, products of combustion, exhaust gas from motors.
Ethane, explosive	Natural gas, manufactured fuel gas.
Gasoline, explosive	Motor vehicles, storage tanks.
Hydrogen, explosive	Artificial fuel gases, electrolysis of water.
Hydrogen sulphide, explosive	Sewer gas, coal gas.
Methane, explosive	Natural gas, manufactured gas, sewer gas.
Sulphur dioxide, non-explosive	Burning insulation.
Unsaturated hydrocarbons, explosive	Manufactured fuel gases.

According to French ordinances, five kilos of ferrous sulphate are to be added to each cubic meter of night-soil. The mass must be well stirred to expel gas. Many accidents result from not taking this precaution. In entering such an atmosphere a wet sponge should be worn or one of the types of the respirator mentioned under carbon monoxide poisoning.

Gas hazards in sewers and sewage-treatment plants are those due to inflammable and poisonous gases and to oxygen deficiency.[833] The inflammable or poisonous gases usually

832. TAYLOR: Medical Jurisprudence, 12th. Am. ed., 486, 1897.
833. SAYERS, R. R.: U. S. Pub. Health Reports, Reprint No. 1612, February, 1934.

found in treatment plants are methane, hydrogen, carbon dioxide, and possibly carbon monoxide, and hydrogen sulphide.

It will be noted from a study of Table XXXVII that the oxygen varies from 0 to 1.2%, carbon dioxide from 3% to 30%, hydrogen sulphide from 0 to 0.1%, hydrogen from 0 to 8.2%, methane from 63% to 84.2%. Jones[834] calls attention especially to the explosion hazards and gives four factors as essential. Katz, in his paper on gas hazards in street manholes,[835] states the principal gases found as in Table XXXV.

Barr and Buchanan[836] report the production of excessive hydrogen sulphide in sewage disposal plants with consequent disintegration of the concrete.

Jones, Campbell and Goodwin[837] report a survey of explosion and poisoning hazards in 10,831 of the 17,000 manholes in Boston, Massachusetts, and twenty-nine contiguous towns which was continued during 1932. The composition of the samples varied over the following range:

TABLE XXXVI
COMPOSITION OF GASES FROM MANHOLES (BOSTON)

Constituents	Per Cent by Volume
Carbon dioxide	0.0 to 8.3
Illuminants	0.0 to 2.5
Oxygen	3.7 to 20.9
Hydrogen	0.0 to 44.1
Carbon monoxide	0.0 to 3.4
Methane-ethane	0.1 to 25.4
Gasoline vapor	0.0 to 0.1
Nitrogen	19.5 to 85.6

The three types of contamination found were:

Manufactured gas from leaks in gas mains, services, and other sources, and included hydrogen, carbon monoxide, illuminants, methane, and ethane;

"Soil" gases from organic material in the soil;

Gases containing abnormally high percentages of carbon

834. JONES, G. W.: Explosions and Hazards in Sewage Works Operation, 1933.

835. KATZ, S. H., MEITER, E. G., and BLOOMFIELD, J. J.: Report of Investigations, U. S. Bureau of Mines, Serial No. 2710, October, 1925, p. 20.

836. BARR, W. N., and BUCHANAN, R. E.: Bull. 26, Engineering Exper. Sta., Ames, Iowa, January, 1912.

837. JONES, G. W., CAMPBELL, J., and GOODWIN, F. M.: Report of Investigations, U. S. Bureau of Mines, R. I. 3213, June, 1933, p. 17.

dioxide, varying amounts of methane, and low percentages of oxygen, and heavy hydrocarbon vapors reported as gasoline.

To avoid poisoning, air should be blown into the manhole before workmen enter, or masks which offer protection against the gases should be worn. In preliminary inspections never use the candle or lantern test, as an explosion may occur.

TABLE XXXVII

COMPOSITION AND INFLAMMABLE LIMITS
(IN PER CENT) OF GASES FROM SEWAGE
SLUDGE DIGESTION TANKS

SOURCE	IMHOFF TANKS				RANGE
	Lower Compartment		Upper Compartment		
Sample number	h	i	j	k	
Reference	(3)	(3)	(3)	(3)	
Carbon dioxide	11.8	9.6	20.0	23.4	3.3—29.4
Oxygen	1.2	1.0			0.0— 1.2
Hydrogen sulphide	0.0	0.0			0.0— 0.1
Hydrogen	4.6	0.0	1.8	1.7	0.0— 8.2
Methane	70.2	66.1	70.0	67.5	63.0—84.2
Nitrogen	12.2	23.3	8.2	7.4	2.9—23.3
Inflammable Limit:					
Lower	6.55	7.80	7.55	7.80	5.30—8.30
Upper	18.45	19.25	18.45	18.50	16.00—19.25

SOURCE	IMHOFF TANK		SEPTIC TANK		IMHOFF TANKS			
					Foaming		Non-Foaming	
Sample number	a	b	c		d	e	f	g
Reference	(1)	(1)	(2)	(2)	(2)	(2)	(2)	(2)
Carbon dioxide	4.4	5.2	13.6	17.0	19.8	29.4	3.3	28.5
Oxygen	0.6	0.5	0.0	0.0	0.3	0.0	0.0	0.0
Hydrogen sulphide	0.0	0.0	0.0	0.0	0.1	0.0	0.0	0.0
Hydrogen	7.9	8.2	3.5	0.0	0.0	0.0	0.0	0.0
Methane	84.2	82.8	72.5	78.0	68.7	66.6	78.2	63.0
Nitrogen	2.9	3.3	10.4	5.0	11.2	3.9	18.5	8.5
Inflammable Limit:								
Lower	5.30	5.30	6.55	6.70	7.40	7.80	6.40	8.30
Upper	16.00	16.10	17.90	16.65	18.25	18.35	16.85	19.15

References:

(1) Gas from Imhoff Tank, by C. C. MOMMON, Eng. News, 71: 760, 9114.

(2) Some Observations on Sewage Tank Gases, by A. M. BUSWELL and S. I. STRICKHOUSER, Indust. & Eng. Chem., 18:407, 1926

(3) Results of Sewage Treatment, by H. E. BABBITT and H. E. SCHLENZ, Univ. Illinois Bull. No. 198, 88 and 92, 1929.

NITROGEN

NITROGEN has a molecular weight of 28.08. Its vapor density is 14. At —123.8°C. under a pressure of 42.1 atmospheres, it condenses to a liquid. Its boiling point is —194.4°C. Liquid nitrogen is colorless. It kills by excluding air from the lungs, but it is not poisonous. Nitrogen does not burn or support combustion. It is very inert, not attacking other free elements. Its simplest combinations are NH_3, H_2O, NO, N_2O_3, NO_2, and N_2O_5.

NITROUS OXIDE (N_2O)
(Molecular Weight, 44.08)

NITROUS OXIDE becomes a colorless liquid at 0° under pressure of three atmospheres, melts at —99°C. and boils at —92°C. It is a simple asphyxiant, when inhaled without oxygen. It is a colorless gas, with a slight sweetish smell and taste. When breathed it acts as an anesthetic of short duration, and is used in dentistry for that purpose. It has also been used in minor operations. Nitrous oxide is called "laughing gas." Water dissolves its own bulk. It supports combustion, but not life. It is eliminated from the blood unchanged. Nitrous oxide has a specific gravity of 1.53. It becomes liquid at +7°C. and 40 atmospheres pressure; it solidifies at —102°C. at normal pressure. It is sold in a liquid state in wrought-iron containers, and is used from these as an anesthetic. It is prepared for this purpose by heating ammonium nitrate, and must be carefully purified, usually by passing through ferrous sulphate to remove nitric oxide and ammonia, through sodium hydrate solution to remove chlorine and its oxides, carbon dioxide, sulphur dioxide, and hydrogen sulphide.[838] Lehmann found that 0.0017 to 0.008% by volume of nitrous oxide can be tolerated for hours, while 0.0106 to 0.0177% by volume is more dangerous. Hamilton records 1,389 cases of poisoning by nitrogen oxide, in which there were twenty-eight deaths.[839] It is decomposed by heat completely at 900°C. into nitrogen and oxygen. When passed over red-hot iron, N and Fe_2O_3 are formed. It is formed by: heating ammonium nitrate in a retort from 170° to 260°; NH_4-$NO_3=N_2O+2H_2O$; by passing NO through a solution of SO_2; by action of HNO_3, specific gravity 1.42, diluted with an equal

838. HART and MARSHALL: *Brit. Dent. J., Lond.*, 35:77, 1914.
839. See also SCHWARZ, F.: *Beihefte z. Med. Klin.*, 25:9, 187, 1929.

volume of water, upon metallic zinc; a mixture of five parts of
HNO_3, specific gravity 1.3, is heated to boiling:

$$2HNO_3 + 4SnCl_2 + 8HCl = 4SnCl_4 + N_2O + 5H_2O$$

Nitrous oxide falls into the class of simple asphyxiants
because it does not support life.

Symptoms: When breathed in a small quantity, nitrous
oxide produces a delicious tingling sensation and tends to
induce laughter, from which its names "paradise gas" and
"laughing gas" are derived. Persons differ greatly in their
actions when under its influence. Some take the gas quickly
and are very abusive, swear, curse, and become unruly, but
after recovering from the effects of the gas they fail to remember what had taken place. By covering the nose and mouth with
a respirator and keeping the patient's head slightly forward,
breathing is made easy, and unconsciousness speedy; the tint
of the skin is inclined to turn blue, but not livid; insensibility
is complete, and recovery is rapid. The use of the gas for prolonged surgical operations is growing, since there is rarely any
subsequent vomiting. It is frequently given before ether to
patients who are undergoing a surgical operation. The brain
is first paralyzed, then the center of sensation of pain. The
action then extends to the spinal cord, medulla oblongata, and
finally to the heart. Asphyxia follows prolonged inhalation
without oxygen. The blood pressure is augmented, and, therefore, it is dangerous to use where there is a weakened vascular
system. Arterial blood shaken with the gas becomes dark,
while venous blood, though shaken, does not darken. It does
not combine with the blood, but the erythrocytes decrease
25% on the average under nitrous oxide and oxygen anestheti-
zation[840] for one-half hour. The hydrogen ion concentration
is increased in the blood, spinal fluid, and bile, with a progressive decrease in the alkaline reserve of the blood.

Crile[841] had over 1,500 cases without a death. The death
rate is about one in 100,000. Considering the short interval of
time that nitrous oxide is inhaled, and the large dilution with
air and oxygen, also slight amounts of gaseous impurities
present, there should be no poisonous effects. Death during
the administration has not been due to poisonous action of the
gas, but to asphyxia or some other cause.

840. Casto: *Dental Cosmos*, 59:415, 1917.
841. Crile: *J.A.M.A.*, 67:1830, 1916.

NITROGEN DIOXIDE (PEROXIDE) (NO_2)
(Molecular Weight—46.04)

THE melting point of nitrogen dioxide (peroxide) is —10°C., and it boils at 21.64°C. Below —10° it is a white crystalline solid. Between —10° and 21.64° it is a liquid, nearly colorless at —9°C., yellow at 0°. At 21.64°C., it is orange, growing nearly black as the temperature rises. The gas does not support combustion of ordinary fuels, and is poisonous when inhaled. It dissolves in water, forming a greenish-blue solution containing nitrous and nitric acids. With an aqueous solution of a fixed alkali, a nitrate and nitrite are formed:

$$2NO_2 + 2KOH = KNO_2 + KNO_3 + H_2O$$

In whatever molecular form the dioxide is inhaled, it is at once altered to that corresponding to body temperature. At 40°C. approximately 30% of the dioxide is in the form of NO_2, and 70% is N_2O_4. It is in this proportion that the gases act upon the respiratory tract. Nitrogen dioxide in the form of N_2O_4 reacts with water to produce nitric and nitrous acid:

$$N_2O_4 + H_2O = HNO_3 + HNO_2$$

The dioxide in the form of NO_2 reacts with water and oxygen from the air to produce nitric acid and nitric oxide:

$$3NO_2 + H_2O = HNO_3 + NO$$

The decomposition of 1 mg. of nitrogen peroxide reaching the respiratory tract yields 0.55 mg. of nitrous acid and 0.98 mg. of nitric acid. As above mentioned, in the presence of an alkali the neutralization results in the formation of nitrites and nitrates, chiefly the sodium salts, when inhaled. The nitrates when absorbed into the blood stream in the small amounts such as result from the gas have no particular effect, but the nitrites when absorbed show definite reactions. For each milligram of the dioxide acting upon the respiratory tract, 0.75 mg. of sodium nitrite is formed. If thirty-nine parts per million of nitrogen dioxide were inhaled during one hour it would result in the absorption of approximately 20 mg. of sodium nitrite. This would have the same effect as sodium nitrite when swallowed. In large amounts, the nitrite changes hemoglobin to methemoglobin. Men frequently exposed to low concentrations of nitric fumes acquire a tolerance to sodium nitrite which prevents symptoms following its absorption. The first effect of the gas may be only that of bronchial irritation. Later the patient may complain of dizziness, headache, and extreme weakness. Several hours after exposure, difficulty in breathing is noted, and the patient is drowned in his own secretions. The lungs become markedly edematous, death may occur within twenty-four hours or be delayed for several days. A number of patients in the Cleveland Clinic after the accident (see page 408) drove their cars home and died within thirty-six hours of the time of the inhalation of the fumes. The blood of these victims was very dark in color, and I found that it contained carbon monoxide and cyanide.

A typical case, that of J.K., a tunnel worker, is cited. He worked for a number of years where dynamite was used as the explosive. On several occasions he received an overdose of the gas, and on August 4, 1935, was treated by a physician for bronchitis. On October 8, 1935, he inhaled more smoke than usual and was unable to return to work the following day. Four days later he saw a physician, who took an x-ray of his chest, saying it was negative. However, ten days from the onset he became acutely ill and was sent to a hospital. There was a marked dyspnea, and an uncontrollable cough. The patient spat up more than a pint of heavy yellowish fluid, which separated into two layers; one layer was watery and green, while the other had two inches of yellowish green fluid with a putrid odor. His temperature at this time was 103.8°. X-ray pictures were taken, and a diagnosis of bronchopneumonia was made. He became steadily worse; pulse was 144, temperature 104.4°, respiration 26 and blood pressure 128/80. The red blood count was 5,000,000, hemoglobin 92%, and the white blood count 19,900; neutrophiles, 83%; small mononuclears, 10; large mononuclears, 4; transitional, 2, eosinophiles, 1; on October 24, his white blood count ran up to 31,200. The urine showed a small amount of albumin, occasional hyaline, and granular casts. The examination of his chest revealed a condition such as is seen in bronchopneumonia. The patient recovered.

The gases inhaled in tunnels under construction always contain carbon monoxide from the explosion of burning dynamite and I believe these men inhale more of the nitric oxide fumes than they would otherwise, as the carbon monoxide makes them somewhat "dopey".

The term "nitrous fumes" should be eliminated from all

textbooks, as there is a great confusion with nitrous oxide, and those unacquainted with the chemistry of these oxides say that "nitrous fumes" are non-toxic because they have in mind the gas used as an anesthetic.

Fumes from nitric acid in contact with organic matter produce an abundance of nitrogen dioxide. An accident in Milwaukee, where a carboy of nitric acid broke, was responsible for the death of several firemen inhaling these fumes. Such fumes arise from metal etching, photographing, and in the dipping of copper and brass in nitric acid.

People exposed to nitric oxide fumes may die shortly after inhaling the dense fumes, or death may be delayed thirty-six to forty-eight hours. Sometimes apparent recovery may be seen with pneumonia developing after several days, as in the case of J.K., above cited.

Autopsy shows that there may be intense congestion in the gastro-intestinal tract, sometimes with hemorrhage, and congestion of the meninges, or even of the cerebrum, perhaps with punctate hemorrhages. The lungs are markedly edematous, and appear very much like those seen in persons dying from influenza. The blood is thick and tarry and coagulates rapidly. Where death occurs suddenly and the blood is examined early, its alkalinity will be found diminished. It turns red when diluted with water, and may show the oxyhemoglobin spectrum.[842] Methemoglobin has been found by Wood,[843] and Heubner and Meier[844] showed the action of the nitrites which are formed in the blood and which produce the characteristic vasodepressant effect. Müller[845] has shown an actual destruction of erythrocytes following nitric oxide fumes with jaundice, with an accompanying increase of bile pigments, in blood and urine. There is no doubt that men who have been gassed several times are more sensitive to the inhalation of gases evolved from explosives, and should not be returned to work with a risk of being gassed again. Where the gas is light, men do not develop any of the sequelae mentioned above, and can continue work indefinitely. I have seen a

842. McNally, W. D.: Gaseous Poisons, in Legal Medicine and Toxicology, Peterson, Haines and Webster, 2:343, 1923.

843. Wood, F. C., and Fitzhugh, T.: *Arch. Int. Med.*, 44:882, 1929.

844. Heubner, W., and Meier, R.: *Zentralbl. f. Gewerbehyg.*, N. S. 3:395, 1926.

845. Müller, J.: *München med. Wchnschr.*, 72:1860, 1925.

number of instances where they have worked for several years. Where recovery occurs after a severe gassing, they still complain of headache, sleeplessness, inability to lie down at night, loss of appetite and gradual loss of strength. Welch[846] has seen a number of these cases recover.

Schwarz,[847] discusses briefly poisoning by nitric fumes and refers to an accident in a Cleveland Clinic, where the poisoning occurred as the result of the burning of x-ray films which were composed of nitrocellulose. The oxidation products which were found were certain inert nitrogen gases, carbon dioxide, nitrous fumes, and particularly nitrogen tetroxide, (N_2O_4), carbon monoxide, and hydrogen cyanide, (HCn).*

He also states that in industry nitric fumes are found, especially with the interaction of concentrated nitric acid on metals. It is not, however, popularly known as yet that nitric fumes, carbon monoxide, and hydrogen cyanide may form in various proportions from the burning of explosives and during explosions. Schürsler[848] describes a case of poisoning from a solution of nitrosylsulphuric acid in sulphuric acid gas caused by the breaking of a carboy of fuming nitric acid. Worthy of note was an 8,000,000 erythrocyte count and detection of the methemoglobin spectrum in the blood. The case pursued a favorable course.

The diagnosis of these poisonings is usually difficult because of the alarming symptoms that set in as a rule after a few hours following exposure (pulmonary edema).

Postmortem: Postmortem findings include injection of the trachea and bronchial passages, and a marked edema of the lungs. The lung picture is similar to that seen in persons dying from influenza. A marked hyperemia is noted in the liver and kidneys.

Accidents more severe in nature than those occurring in tunnels or mines occur from the burning of nitrocellulose. I have seen forty-eight cases of varying degrees of poisoning, with three deaths (exclusive of cases seen at the Cleveland Clinic).

846. WELCH, G. A.: *J. Indust. Hyg.,* 2:238, 1920, 1921.
847. SCHWARZ, F.: *Beheifte z. Med. Klin.,* 25:187, 1929.
* HOLSTE: (*Zentralbl. f. Gewerbehyg.,* 23:183, 196) gives a review of the literature.
848. SCHÜRSLER: *Samml. v. Vergiftungsfällen, Vol.* 6:123-124, 1935.

Treatment: If seen early the patient should be given inhalations of oxygen. The oxygen is passed through a bottle containing 2 gm. of ammonium carbonate to one and a half ounces of water. The oxygen is introduced by means of two catheters placed in the nose. (If the patient is very restless it may be necessary to strap the hands so he does not pull the tubes from the nose.) When the lungs are highly edematous, the patient should be given an ampoule of salyrgan daily and 100 cc. of a 50% glucose solution intravenously. After the first few hours the inhalation of oxygen may be given by the tent method. It is not necessary to resort to blood-letting and venesection, as the salyrgan, in most of the cases, gives wonderful results.

Ebright[849] described a condition of those working with nitroglycerine and its derivatives, in which he discusses the physiological action of the nitrites. Laws[850] says that the headache following the increased action of the heart may be preceded by complete loss of vision, and that the patient may reach a maniacal state. Ebright describes a case of a patient who became wild, and irrational, and finally ran around shouting and hitting his head against trees, walls, and other objects, and had to be forcibly restrained. In a later observation Laws found that all those who work with nitroglycerine have large families, and that sooner or later these men are troubled with a tachycardia on exertion. New men working in nitroglycerin are very susceptible. The warm weather greatly enhances the incidence and severity of the symptoms. After one has worked for three or four days a rather high degree of immunity is established which persists as long as he remains at work. After an absence of a few days the immunity is generally lost and the man will experience the usual toxic symptoms. This type of headache is characteristic. It is a throbbing headache which begins in the forehead and moves toward the occiput, where it remains up to several days. The patient often feels restless and tosses around in bed. He may be nauseated and vomit, and may have diarrhea. Alcohol enhances the toxic symptoms by relaxing the blood vessels. Thus a man exposed to nitroglycerine the whole day may bring on a

849. Ebright, G. E.: *J.A.M.A.*, 62:201, 1914.
850. Laws, C. E.: *J.A.M.A.*, March 5, 1910, p. 793.

headache by simply taking a cocktail. Ebright observed a case of a man who handled between a ton and a ton and a half of dynamite, who was told that alcohol was a good remedy for headache, and drank a considerable portion of it. He developed into an acute maniac and before he could be restrained shot and wounded his friend and killed a bystander.

Gaisbäch[851] calls attention to the possibility of intoxication following the liberation of carbon monoxide and nitrous fumes near the oven, if certain rugs (linoleum imitation such as "triolin") are used. Wirth[852] believes that death occurs more rapidly after the inhalation of gas mixtures, and more rapidly than after the inhalation of lethal concentrations of the individual gases. Anson and Mirsky[853] have come to the conclusion that nitric oxide forms a loose combination with methemoglobin and not with hemoglobin as is usually believed. They also found that nitric oxide methemoglobin is about 1,000 times as strong an acid as methemoglobin.

TABLE XXXVIII

PHYSIOLOGICAL RESPONSE TO VARIOUS CONCENTRATIONS OF NITRIC ACID

Dose Mg. per liter of air	Symptoms
.1	Nothing abnormal.
.2	Irritating action.
.3 - .5	Can be tolerated only for a short period.
.5	Kills a cat in four hours.
.9 and over	Kills all animals in one to three hours.

Hamilton found in the year 1916, 1,389 cases of intoxication caused by "nitrous" fumes, in the explosive industry. In Germany there were twenty-four deaths from 1914 to 1918. In England there were, in the ten years from 1914 to 1924, 137 cases of severe intoxications, twenty-two of which ended fatally. The toxicity of NO and NO_2 has been studied by Lehmann and Hasegawa.[854] They have determined the toxic dose in animals (the toxic doses are evaluated as total nitric acid). (Table XXXVIII.)

851. GAISBACH, F.: Wien. klin. Wchnschr., 44:937, 1931.
852. WIRTH, W.: Arch. f. exper. Path. u. Pharmakol., 157:264, 1930.
853. ANSON, L. M., and MIRSKY, A. E.: J. Physiol., 60:100, 1925.
854. LEHMANN and HASEGAWA: Arch. f. Hyg., 68:323, 1913.

Lehmann also determined the toxicity in human beings and found as follows:

TABLE XXXIX

PHYSIOLOGICAL RESPONSE OF HUMAN BEINGS TO NITRIC ACID

Dose Mg. per liter of air	Symptoms
2.	Causes an irritation of the respiratory passages.
.3 - .4	Dangerous dose.
.5	Tolerated only for a short period.

Twenty-five cases of poisoning by nitrous fumes were seen at a casualty station at Moscow.[855] The period of incapacity from work was from three to six days, and for the more serious cases two to six weeks.

Feil calls attention to the fact that the nitrogen oxides, besides their irritating and corrosive action possess also a slightly narcotic and anesthetic power. Therefore the defense reflexes and cough are inhibited, and the exposed workman may not realize the danger to which he is exposed.

The fumes of nitric oxide and nitrogen dioxide are found in those industries in which nitric acid is used, as in the preparation of acids, such as nitric, sulphuric, picric, and chromic; and in the production of toluene, metallic nitrates, methyl nitrate, celluloid, and nitro-cellulose (gun-powder), collodion, Prussian-red, English-red, etc. Nitric acid is also used in such industries as metal works, jewelry, metal testing, manufacture of imitation pearls, engraving, manufacture of artificial leather, telegraphy, and explosive industries (nitroglycerine, dynamite, etc.) and in industries which use nitric oxide compounds such as nitrates, nitro-cellulose, artificial silk, photography films, celluloid, smokeless powders, nitrobenzene, and aniline. It may also be found in industries which do not use nitric acid, such as the preparation of nitric oxide by the Haber process and the electric current process. Some men are peculiarly susceptible to these fumes, which may be due to the fact that they consume considerable quantities of alcohol, have tuberculosis, or are advanced in age, or have been subjected to a condition which decreases the resistance of the body, as, after such a condition, they are more apt to show symptoms.

855. *Med. du Trav.*, 6:196, 1934.

The clinical group is divided into the acute and chronic form of poisoning. The acute form is in turn divided into:

1. The severe form in which the period of irritation is followed by a latent period, following which the onset is sudden, the course stormy, and the outcome usually fatal.

2. The fulminating form, which is so rapid that no anatomical changes are produced. In this form Feil believes that the toxic gas acts directly on the respiratory center.

3. The acute mild form, which is characterized by moderately severe manifestations of bronchitis and pulmonary congestion. This form is seen usually in "muckers," miners and tunnel workers. The condition usually appears after two or three days.

Occasionally, a tunnel worker may be seen who complains of disturbance of the gastro-intestinal tract, who has vomiting, colic, diarrhea and pain in the abdomen. For several days these men are unable to eat, however, after alkalinization the vomiting usually stops and they return to normal condition. Most of the "muckers" are men who indulge in alcohol, and after leaving work they have severe headaches, and dizziness which they sometimes attribute to poor alcoholic beverages they had consumed. The chronic form is characterized by mild bronchitis, anemia, general weakness, loss of strength, all of the symptoms being the result of the debilitating action of the "nitrous" fumes on the lungs and blood. There is restlessness and inability to sleep. These men find sleeping easier in a rocking chair than in a bed.

The introduction of the acetate film eliminates the danger of burning x-ray films.

NITRIC OXIDE (NO)
(Molecular Weight 30.04)

UNDER pressure of one atmosphere, nitric oxide is liquefied at —153.6°C.; under 71.2 atmospheres, at 93.5°C.; and it solidifies at —167°C. The odor and taste are unknown, because it is immediately converted into nitrogen dioxide on exposure to air. It is not found free in nature. It is formed by the reduction of nitric acid by means of ferrous sulphate previously acidulated with sulphuric acid, by the action of cold nitric acid, specific gravity 1.2, upon metallic copper;

unless great care be used other oxides of nitrogen are produced. Sulphur dioxide is passed into slightly warmed HNO_3, specific gravity 1.15, and the excess of sulphur dioxide removed by passing through water. According to Emich a strictly pure nitric oxide is made by treating mercury with a mixture of sulphuric and nitric acids.

It is soluble in about ten volumes of water and in five volumes of nitric acid, specific gravity 1.3. One hundred volumes of sulphuric acid, specific gravity 1.84, and 1.50, dissolve 3.5 and 1.7 volumes respectively.[856] It is soluble in carbon disulphide and alcohol.

Lange - Guess Test for Powder Stains: When a small firearm is discharged there is a backward movement of gas and particles of the explosive, which are blown upon the skin of the person holding the weapon. A paraffin cast or a paper pulp mold can be made of the hand and the inner surface tested for the presence of nitrates and nitrites. Add from a small pipet a drop of a sulphanilic and alpha naphthylamin reagent. A red color will develop in the presence of nitrites. This test is delicate to one in 5,000,000.[857] The reagents are prepared as follows:

1. Ten gm. of sulphanilic are dissolved in 1,000 cc. of a 30% acetic acid;

2. Three gm. of alpha naphthylamin are heated with 700 cc. of distilled water and the clear solution decanted from the blue-violet residue. To the clear solution 300 cc. of acetic acid are added.

Nitrites may also be identified by a 0.1% solution of 1:8 naphthylendiamin in 10% acetic acid. A drop of this reagent will give an orange-red color precipitate with nitrites.[858]

MUSTARD GAS
(Synonym: Yperite)

THE use of the toxic shells has been divided into three periods by Goss.[859] During the first period, May, 1915, to July, 1916, only lacrimatory shells were used; while these lacrimators had considerable harassing power, no deaths

856. Lunge: *Ber. d. deutsch. chem. Gesellsch.*, 18:1391, 1885.

857. Greiss, P.: *Ber. d. deutsch. chem. Gesellsch.*, 12:427, 1879; Blom, J.: *Ber. d. deutsch. chem. Gesellsch.*, 59:121, 1926.

858. Agmar, A. de: *Ber. d. deutsch. chem. Gesellsch.*, 7:315, 1874.

859. Goss: *J. Indust. & Eng. Chem.*, 2:829, 1919.

were reported. Lethal shells came into use July, 1916. In addition to the lacrimators, shells were employed containing phosgene, diphosgene, and chlorpicrin. The third period began with the appearance of mustard gas at Ypres, July 12, 1917.

Thiodiglycolchloride, B. B. dichlorethylsulphide, $(CH_2\text{-}ClCH_2)_2S$, commonly known after July, 1917, as "mustard gas," was first made by Victor Meyer in 1882. It is a heavy oily fluid, specific gravity 1.274 at 20°C.,[860] sinking below water and not miscible with it; light straw color, pink or brown; of neutral reaction; having a sweetish ethereal odor but slightly suggestive of sulphur compounds; soluble in alcohol and other organic solvents. It boils at 217°C. with decomposition; crystallizes in long prisms at 0° C.[861] Adams and Williamson[862] found that the freezing-point ranges from 13.9°C. at one megabar to 38.9°C. at 1800 megabars. The latent heat of melting is twenty-five calories per gram, and the freezing point lowering content is 6.5°C. (1 mol. solute per 1000 gm. of solvent.) The peculiar property of the gas to volatilize and recondense with variations of temperature explains its persistence about the bombarded areas.

Symptoms: When this chemical comes in contact with the skin, red patches will appear which develop into blisters. Inhalation of 12 mg. per minute leads to fatal destruction of the lungs. There is but slight lacrimation. The damage to the eyes consists of suppuration, and destruction of the conjunctiva, cornea, and, indeed, of the entire eye. A concentration of only 0.1 to 0.2 cc. of mustard gas per cubic meter of air can produce serious injury to the mucous membrane, and a concentration of 1 to 3 cc. per cubic meter is fatal. After the first few hours of exposure there is a feeling of depression with no anorexia, some vomiting, and diarrhea. Prolonged exposure to small concentrations causes laryngitis and loss of voice sufficient to incapacitate men. After eight to twelve hours the pulse is slow and irregular, the respirations irregular and labored, with frequent coughing, and profuse salivary and nasal discharge. In severe cases bronchitis and pneumonia may

    860. SMITH: *J. Pharmacol. & Exper. Therap.*, 13:1, 1919; POPE, W. J.: *J. Soc. Chem. Indust.*, 38:344, 1919.
    861. *Ber. d. deutsch. chem. Gesellsch.*, 19:3260, 1919.
    862. ADAMS and WILLIAMSON: *J. Wash. Acad. Sc.*, 9:30, 1919.

develop after thirty-six hours. Fair-haired people are more sensitive to mustard gas, and the white man is more sensitive to it than the negro. The gas passes more slowly through rubber than it does through uniforms (suits and underwear), waterproofs, and leather. It penetrates these in thirty minutes. Lewisite has a smaller penetrating power. It was found during the World War that the best protection

TABLE XL

Toxicity of Various Gases and Vapors

Volumes of Gas per Million Volumes of Air (cc. gas per cm. of air)*

Substance	Fatal with 5 to 10 minutes exposure	Dangerous (toxic) one-half to one hour exposure	Endurable one-half to one hour
Mustard gas	20	15	1
Phosgene	50	25	1
Chlorine	500	50	5
Arsine	300	60	20
Prussic acid	200	100	50
Nitrous fumes	500	100	50
Hydrogen sulphide	800	400	200
Phosphine	1,000	400	100
Carbon disulphide	2,000	1,000	500
Sulphur dioxide	3,000	400	100
Hydrochloric acid	3,000	1,000	100
Ammonia	5,000	2,500	250
Carbon monoxide	5,000	2,000	1,000
Benzene	20,000	7,500	3,000
Chloroform	25,000	15,000	5,000
Petrol	30,000	20,000	15,000
Carbon tetrachloride	50,000	25,000	10,000
Carbon dioxide	90,000	50,000	30,000
Acetylene	500,000	250,000	100,000
Ethylene (in O_2)	950,000	800,000	500,000

* From Leschke: Clinical Toxicology, p. 156, 1934.

against this gas was to enclose the whole body, including the head, in a cloth which had been previously soaked in a bleaching solution of potassium permanganate. The best protection is afforded by the use of a suitable gas mask. To prevent skin erosions, chlorite of lime may be applied to the skin, either as a paste or dry. This may also be scattered over the cloth to neutralize the effects of this gas which had condensed on grass or foliage. Patients who have been exposed to mustard gas should have the skin bathed for one or two hours in Dakin's or Carrel's solution. The eyes can be washed with a 1% solution of sodium bicarbonate, or treated as given under tear gas[863] (see page 423). Table XL gives the toxicity of various gases and vapors.

Pathology: An examination of the internal organs offers nothing of a specific nature. The respiratory lesions are proportionate to the concentration and length of exposure. In the mildest cases a superficial degeneration and necrosis of the epithelium of the mucous membrane are obtained, with congestion and edema. Warthin and Weller[864] described a deep necrosis of the mucosa of the respiratory tract, with the formation of a diphtheric membrane in the anterior nares, pharynx, larynx, and upper portions of the trachea. The lungs show extreme passive congestion, the cut surface is dark crimson, rather dry as a rule, apparently pneumonic. Sections show that the condition is a mixed pneumonia, hemorrhagic, and in some necrotic. In milder cases there is an intense engorgement of the capillaries, with desquamation of the vesicated endothelium with catarrhal exudate. Bronchioles show desquamated epithelium and leukocytes. Later, when the pneumonia spreads, vessels become choked with leukocytes and red blood cells. Large patches or whole lobes become hepatized and lung tissue undergoes necrosis. The kidneys show some cloudy swelling. The stomach frequently shows a hemorrhagic gastritis.

Gilchrist[865] analyzed the condition of 6,980 cases of mustard gas, showing parts of the body affected. In the research laboratory there were fifty-eight dogs in the series given mustard gas. Of these, forty were killed at intervals varying from the actual time of recovery to eight months after recovery. Eighteen died or were killed at intervals of from one week to nine months after recovery. Forty-six of the fifty-eight dogs studied appeared normal in the gross. Of the remaining twelve, one had pneumonia. The others showed such lesions as congestion, hemorrhage, edema, atelectasis, and emphysema. As in the case of phosgene, nearly all the gross lesions appeared in dogs that died.

863. McNally, W. D.:   *J.A.M.A.,* 98:45, 1932.

864. Warthin and Weller: See Flury: *Ztschr. f. d. ges. exper. Med.,* 13:367, 1921; Heitzman: *Ztschr. f. d. ges. exper. Med.,* 13:484, 1921.

865. Gilchrist, H. L.:   A Comparative Study of World War Casualties from Gas and Other Weapons, Chemical Warfare School, Edgewood Arsenal, Maryland, 1928.

From experimental work on rabbits, Koontz[866] came to the conclusion that animals gassed with phosgene, mustard, and lewisite are not more susceptible to tuberculosis than are control animals inoculated at the same time with the same dose of bacilli. Elliot[867] reported: "It is very gratifying to be able to state that gas does not seem to have stirred up tuberculosis to any great extent. It was feared that most of the cases would develop into tuberculosis, but few have."

Meade[868] in 1922 summarized the histories of over 3,000 persons examined by the War Risk Insurance Bureau in Kansas City. As a result of his work he made the following statement: "I now believe that we can say to the public upon the best authority (which is based upon universal observation) that a man is no more liable to tuberculosis as a result of gassing than is a man who has never been gassed." The same conclusion was reached by Morris,[869] Meakins and Priestly,[870] Dennis,[871] Cowen,[872] Berghoff[873] Sandall[874] and Miller.[875]

Treatment: The treatment consists chiefly of removing the gas, and washing with Dakin's or Carrel's solution, or the application of chloride of lime. Williams [876] recommends an ointment containing zinc oxide 45%, linseed oil 30%, lard 10%, neutral wool fat 15%. Ointment is for preventive purposes and has little healing value. It can be used with advantage in the armpits, crotch, hands, and feet. Frequent change of clothing and bathing with Dakin's solution are recommended until all symptoms of the gas are removed.

There is an apparent increased susceptibility of the patient to influenza, bronchitis, pneumonia, tuberculosis, chronic eczema, itching, and desquamative dermatitis and pigmentation.

Tests: Muntsch[877] states that, in a series of investiga-

866. KOONTZ, A. R.: *Arch. Int. Med.*, 39:833, 1927.
867. ELLIOT, T. R.: *Brit. J. Surg.*, 3:234, 1915, 1916.
868. MEADE, R. H.: *J. Missouri M. A.*, 19:385, 1922.
869. MORRIS, R. S.: Contrib. to Med. and Biol. Research, dedicated to Sir William Osler, 2:1138, 1919.
870. MEAKINS, J. C., and PRIESTLEY, J. G.: *Canad. M. A. J.*, 9:968, 1919.
871. DENNIS, C. E.: *M. J. Australia*, 2:372, 1919.
872. COWEN, S. O.: *M. J. Australia*, 2:369, 1919.
873. BERGHOFF, R. S.: *Arch. Int. Med.*, 24:678, 1919.
874. SANDALL, T. E.: *Lancet*, 2:857, 1922.
875. MILLER, J. A.: *Am. Rev. Tuberc.*, 3:337, 1919.
876. WILLIAMS. *J. Am. Pharm. Assoc.*, 8:824, 1919.
877. MUNTSCH: *Deutsche med. Wchnschr.*, 57:233, 1931.

tions, the investigators were able to demonstrate bronchiectasis and bronchiolectasis by means of bronchography with lipiodol. They found these changes in former soldiers who had been gassed and who after the war had suffered chronically from asthma. As to the relationship between tuberculosis and chronic gas poisoning, he states that gas poisoning may be considered to be etiologically related to pulmonary tuberculosis. It has been found that in 70,552 gas poisonings there have been 103 cases of tuberculosis, seventy-eight of which were gassed with some unknown substance, sixty-five with mustard gas, twenty-two with phosgene, and eight with chlorine. From these figures it seems that there is no relation between tuberculosis and gas poisoning.

In England in 1920 there were 19,000 men incapacitated and subjected to compensation, about 12% of the cases were due to gas poisoning. Of the gas poisoned soldiers in the American army 2.9% have died, and 20.5% still receive compensation, while in 44.6% there was no claim for compensation.

PHOSGENE (COCl₂)
(Molecular Weight 98.91)

PHOSGENE is a colorless gas of the specific gravity of 1.42, which fumes in moist air as a result of partial conversion into hydrochloric acid. This gas was discovered by J. Davy in 1811. At ordinary temperature it is a gas possessing a very pungent odor, reminding one of foul hay. It was one of the most dangerous war gases, and was used extensively during the World War.

Leschke[878] states that out of 11,000,000 war victims, about 30,000 deaths were due to gas poisoning. Inhalation of air containing phosgene causes immediate irritative phenomena of the respiration, coughing, and a sensation of tightness and constriction in the chest. Two to 5 cc. in a cubic meter of air are dangerous to life, if the time of exposure is prolonged; 5 to 10 cc. per cubic meter lead to serious irritation of the eyes and the respiratory organs; 20 to 25 cc. after an exposure of only a few minutes cause serious pneumonia.

In the early stages of poisoning by this gas, there are nausea, retching, and vomiting. Leschke reported an accident in Hamburg in May, 1928, caused by the release of about

878. LESHKE: *München. med. Wchnschr.*, 79: 673, 1932.

eight cubic meters of phosgene by the bursting of a phosgene tank. Over 300 people became ill, and ten died. He reports the case of two young people who were exposed to gas while rowing on a canal. A physician was called because of an irritating cough and a feeling of oppression in the chest. He could find nothing wrong, but after three hours a rapidly increasing dyspnea developed. One of the patients died four and a half hours after inhalation.

Poisoning by this gas causes great irritation of the mucous membranes, burning of the eyes and throat, cough and provocation to vomit. Respiration becomes more and more rapid, forced and stertorous, and the face becomes cyanosed. Moist rales are heard over the whole lung on account of the edema. In serious cases, death occurs by suffocation. The victim is drowned in his own blood plasma. The lungs are greatly inflated, from four to six times their normal volume. The irritation of the bronchial mucosa is caused by the decomposition of the phosgene into hydrochloric acid and carbonic acid.

Four-fifths of the deaths occur in the first twenty-four hours, very few die after the third day.

Postmortem Appearances: Where death occurred within twenty-four hours, the trachea is moderately congested, and this congestion becomes more marked in the smaller bronchial branches. There is pulmonary edema, rupture of air-vesicles, concentration of the blood and thrombosis. The lungs are usually large, heavy, boggy, edematous, and dusky red. Patches of emphysema alternate with areas of collapse. On cut-section frothy blood exudes from the lungs. The pleural cavities usually contain varying quantities of clear or blood-stained effusion. In patients dying later than the third day the lungs may be quite dry but bronchopneumonia or pleurisy is usually seen. The kidneys are usually enlarged and congested. The blood exhibits definite changes, the hemoglobin percentage rising as high as 140%, with a corresponding increase in the red cell count.

Treatment: The person should be immediately removed from the contaminated atmosphere and placed in a hospital, where oxygen inhalations can be given, the oxygen bubbling through a solution of ammonium carbonate. The patient should be kept at absolute rest; and the application of external heat is important. If the cyanosis is marked, 500 cc. of blood may be withdrawn, or salyrgan given as recommended under nitric oxide poisoning. The irritating cough may be lessened by the administration of dilaudid or codeine. Treat symptomatically, giving digitalis if necessary to strengthen the heart.

TABLE XLI

PHYSIOLOGICAL RESPONSE TO VARIOUS CONCENTRATIONS OF PHOSGENE

	Parts of Phosgene per millions parts of air.
Least detectable odor*	5.6
Least amount required to cause immediate irritation of the eyes*	4.0
Least amount required to cause immediate irritation of the throat*	3.1
Least amount required to cause coughing*	4.8
Maximum concen. allowable for prolonged exposure*	1.0
Dangerous for even short exposure*	25
Rapidly fatal	over 25

* U. S. Department of Interior, Bureau of Mines, Technical Paper, 248, 1921.

Tests: Yant, Olsen, Storch, Littlefield, and Scheflan[879] recommend the sample of air to be led through two simple absorption tubes of the petticoat bubbler type in series, each of which contains 25 cc. of the phosgene absorbent, based on the reaction of aniline in aqueous solution with phosgene (1:3) to form an s-diphenylurea, $COCl_2 + 4C_6H_5NH_2 = CO(NHC_6H_5)_2 + 2C_6H_5NH_2.HCl$. This has been found to give quantitative results for small amounts of phosgene in air. In preparing the absorption solution an excess of aniline is kept in a bottle of distilled water for a week, with occasional shaking; then phosgene is passed through the solution until a permanent precipitate of diphenylurea is formed, and the mixture is kept ready for use. When a determination is to be made some of the solution is filtered several times through a Gooch crucible, and 25-cc. portions are placed in each of the bubblers. After the measured volume of sample is passed through the bubblers it is allowed to stand two hours and the aniline reagent is then filtered through a weighed Gooch. Any precipitate which adheres to the sides of the bubblers is

879. YANT, W. P., OLSEN, J. C., STORCH, H. H., LITTLEFIELD, J. B., and SCHEFLAN, L.: *Indust. & Eng. Chem., Anal. Ed.*, 8:20, 1936. MATUSZAK, M. P.: *Indust. & Eng. Chem., Anal. Ed.*, 6:457, 1934.

dissolved in warm alcohol and evaporated almost to dryness in a small beaker on a steam bath; several cubic centimeters of water are added and the evaporation is continued until there is no longer an odor of alcohol. This additional precipitate is then washed (with thorough policing) into the Gooch crucible and the entire precipitate is washed thoroughly with a solution of 1/N hydrochloric acid saturated with pure diphenylurea; the precipitate is then aerated several minutes, and finally dried at 70° to 80° C. to constant weight.

The diphenylurea is extracted from the Gooch by washing with several portions of boiling ethyl alcohol, and the crucible is again dried at 70° to 80° C. to constant weight. The alcoholic extracts are dried in tared weighing bottles, first to dryness at room temperature, and then to constant weight at 70° to 80° C. These final weights are used in calculating the phosgene content of the gas.

At a room temperature of 23° C. and the usual barometric pressure at this location of 740 mm. of mercury, 1 mg. of diphenylurea is equivalent to 0.1175 cc. of phosgene. This value may be calculated in parts of phosgene per million parts of air by volume as follows:

$$1 \text{ mg. of diphenylurea} = \frac{\text{volume of sample in liters}}{0.1175 \times 1000} \text{ p.p.m.}$$

Matuszak[879] describes an iodometric determination of phosgene.

TEAR GAS (CHLORACETOPHENONE)

TEAR GAS is a common name for chloracetophenone ($C_6H_5COCH_2Cl$), which was first prepared in 1887 but was of no importance until used in chemical warfare. It is a white or gray crystalline solid, having a sweet aromatic odor like locust blossoms. It is a stable compound having a melting point of 59° and a boiling point of 247° C. It has a specific gravity of 1.334 at 0° C. The vapor pressure is low, being 0.0028 at 0° C. The compound is insoluble in water but very soluble in organic solvents. During the World War it was used in shells, hand grenades, candles, the four-inch Stokes mortar and air bombs.

Lacrimation is produced by a concentration of 0.003 mg. per liter. Vedder[880] reports that when men are exposed to the

880. VEDDER, E. B.: The Medical Aspects of Chemical Warfare, Baltimore, Williams and Wilkins Company, 170, 1925.

action of chloracetophenone they complain of irritation of the eyes, lacrimation, and burning of the more tender portions of the skin. In some cases there is a tendency toward increased salivation and irritation of the throat. In low concentration for a long period or in high concentration for short periods men were unable to open their eyes for twenty-four hours. It has comparatively little effect on the skin of either man or animal. When applied in excess to the human skin, there is a burning sensation, slight rubefaction, and sometimes small vesicles appear. This inflammation subsides in about seven days. Hanzlik and Farr[881] found that chloracetophenone gave a mild urticarial rash, moderate swelling, and edema with little or no necrosis.

Aside from its use as a war gas, accidents have happened from the use of a fountain pen "anti-bandit gun" accidentally discharging the tear gas into the faces of children. I have seen a number of these accidents such as:[882]

B. K., a boy, four years of age, while playing with a fountain pen gun in which the charge contained in a 38-caliber shell consisted of chloracetophenone in ethyl acetate as a solvent, accidentally discharged it against the palm of his left hand, causing a burn 1.5 cm. in diameter; the face, forehead, and eyelids were superficially burned. There was an intense photophobia, and the right eye was swollen shut when Dr. Leroy Thompson, to whom I am indebted for the history, arrived approximately forty minutes after the accident. The examination of the eyes was difficult owing to photophobia, profuse lacrimation, and swelling. Therefore petrolatum was wiped into the eyes, and the patient was taken to St. Luke's Hospital for further examination and treatment.

The examination made in the hospital with the assistance of lid retractors showed a mild conjunctivitis in the right eye involving both bulbar and palpebral areas. The cornea appeared to be clear. The examination of the left eye disclosed a second degree burn involving the bulbar and palpebral conjunctivae which seemed to be almost circumcorneal and much more severe in the lower quadrant. The cornea was steamy and partially opaque, but there was no breaking down of the epithelial layer.

881. Hanzlik and Farr: *J. Pharmacol. & Exper. Therap.*, 14:221, 1919.

882. McNally, W. D.: *J.A.M.A.*, 98:45, 1932.

White's ointment and atropine were used, and zinc oxide was smeared over the face and eyelids as a protective healing dressing. The following morning, approximately twelve hours after the accident, an examination was made. It was found that the right eye was closed completely, with a very marked swelling of both upper and lower lids. This condition was much worse in the left eye and on the left side on the face. It was necessary to use forcible traction on the lids with the lid retractor to obtain even a glimpse of the cornea. I recommended the use of 0.4 gm. sodium sulphite in a mixture of 75% glycerine and 25% water, the sulphite first being dissolved in the water. The condition gradually improved, and on the eleventh day the patient had recovered sufficiently to be removed to his home.

All burns of the skin caused by chloracetophenone should be promptly washed with a 4% solution of sodium sulphite in a 50% alcoholic solution (one part alcohol and one part water). In the absence of sodium sulphite, glycerine or alcohol may be used, as the prompt removal of the chloracetophenone will prevent several days of distress. For the eyes the author recommends that 0.4 gm. of sodium sulphite be dissolved in 25 cc. of water and 75 cc. of glycerine. This may be applied on cotton or a few drops introduced to the lid.

ARSINE (AsH_3)
(Hydrogen Arsenide. Synonyms: Arsenic Trihydrate, Arsonia, Arsine, Arsenous Hydride)

ARSINE is formed by the action of nascent hydrogen on reducible arsenical compounds. It is an exceedingly poisonous gas, colorless, has an odor of garlic, and burns with the production of water and arsenic trioxide:

$$2AsH_3 + 3O_2 = As_2O_3 + 3H_2O$$

When it is mixed with air and ignites, it explodes and burns with a somewhat luminous and slightly bluish flame. If present in considerable quantity, a white powder may be observed settling on a piece of black paper placed beneath the flame, if oxidation is prevented, lustrous black and brown-black spots of metallic arsenic are deposited on the porcelain surfaces:

$$4AsH_3 + 3O_2 = As_4 + 6H_2O$$

During the Marsh test, this gas is generated and is decomposed by the heated tube, leaving a black ring of the metallic element condensed on the tube. Arsine has a reducing action upon a solution of silver nitrate, precipitating silver, leaving arsenous acid and free nitric acid in solution. Filter off the silver, neutralize the filtrate with a few drops of very dilute ammonium hydroxide solution, and a yellow precipitate of silver arsenite (Ag_3AsO_3) will appear. It is the most deadly of inorganic compounds of arsenic, 0.1% to 1% of arsine in the air being fatal. Smaller concentrations may cause death in a short period of time.

Arsine intoxication is relatively frequent, because arsine is often present as an impurity in acids and metals such as zinc, copper, and cadmium. I have found it in the air in the pickling of iron and steel. A multiple neuritis has been reported from the inhalation of arsine generated in this process.[883] Legge reported seven cases in 1902, the acid containing 0.035% arsenic or 350 parts per million. Three cases, one of them fatal, occurred in the Puget Sound Navy Yard; here the acid contained 0.05% arsenic or 500 parts per million. Epidemics of poisoning with arsine occurred during the World War in two Italian submarines and one English, and in each the gas was traced to the storage batteries. It was found that the acid had eaten into the lead grids, which had, as is usually the case, some arsenic contaminating the antimony.

Cases have been reported in the production of zinc salts, and in chemical factories from the cleaning of the acid residues in tanks, the residues being removed by means of buckets made of iron. In the production of aniline dyes and coal-tar drugs by the reduction of nitrobenzene to aniline by nascent hydrogen, arsine may be liberated from impurities in the metal or acid used to make hydrogen. During the World War, a number of cases of poisoning occurred from arsine generated from storage batteries in submarines. The lead-antimony grids of the batteries contained 0.02% of arsine.

Ferrosilicon has often been the cause of arsine poisoning. A number of deaths have been reported among steerage passengers on ships carrying cargoes of ferrosilicon. One case was observed in a sailor who slept in the vicinity of the material. A few days later he complained of pain in the chest, headache, and vomiting. His wife had similar symptoms and died a few days later. Postmortem examination revealed a reddish dis-

883. MUEHLBERGER, C. W., LOEVENHERT, A. S., and O'MALLEY, T. S.: *J. Indust. Hyg.*, 10:137, 1928.

coloration of the gray substance of the brain, punctate hemorrhages of the heart muscle and lungs. The spleen and liver
were hyperemic, and the gastric mucosa was blackish and emanated an odor of garlic.[884]

Any zinc containing arsenic, when treated with acid would
liberate arsine. Leymann and Weber[885] claimed that the symptoms of men cleaning out vats containing sulphuric acid, are
not always due to arsine; that in thirteen cases of poisoning,
four were due to nitrous fumes, seven to inhalation of arsine,
and one to inhalation of benzol. In two cases, autopsies were
performed and no form of arsine poisoning was found. These
authors rightfully mention that in the cleaning of vats containing sulphuric acid, we ought to consider fumes other than arsine, as sulphuric acid is apt to contain nitric acid which, when
brought in contact with other substances, would cause the nitric
acid to give off nitrous fumes.

Symptoms: The symptoms of acute arsine poisoning result
from the hemolysis of the red blood cells, which occurs without
the formation of methemoglobin. In mild cases, headache and
nausea may be the first symptoms. Jaundice develops from the
formation of an excess of bile pigment from the liberated hemoglobin. The red cells and hemoglobin are low. Many of the
fatal cases show edema of the lungs. There may be constriction
of the chest, excitement and fear, cold, pressure and pain in
the pit of the stomach, with symptoms of gastro-enteritis as in
acute arsenical poisoning.

Dibbren[886] observed a case of poisoning of a man working
in cadmium. The first symptom recorded was the appearance
of pain in the abdomen. The patient complained of headache,
. nausea, and pain in the upper part of the abdomen, and was
confined to bed. The urine became bloody and he showed a distinct jaundice. He complained of pain in all of the bones of the
body. Upon admission to a hospital he was found to be in a
poor state of nutrition; he was icteric and slightly cyanotic.
The pupils reacted to light and accommodation. There was no
involvement of the cranial nerves. The pulse was small, soft
and rapid. His hemoglobin was 28%; R.B.C's 980,000; color index 1.47; W.B.C's 250,000; myelocytes, 25%; immature forms,

884. See also HAMILTON, ALICE: *Chem. Trade J.*, 65:365, 1919.
885. LEYMANN and WEBER: *Zentralbl. f. Gewerbehyg.*, 7:154, 1930.
886. DIBBREN: *Med. Clin.*, 28:1170, 1932.

23%; polys, 40% and lymphos, 2%. The red blood cells were hyperchromatic and showed basophilic stippling, moderate polychromatophilia, mild anisocytosis, schizocytes, Cabot rings, but no poikilocytosis. Diazo reaction of serum was positive. Alkaline reserve according to Van Slyke's method was 17. The patient died two hours after admission to the hospital before a blood transfusion could be made. Postmortem examination showed yellow staining of almost all of the organs, including the cerebrospinal fluid. The lungs showed pleuritic involvement and adhesions; the spleen was enlarged and the surface appeared to be hyperemic. The liver showed brownish discoloration, and the gall-bladder was filled with reddish brown bile. Chemical examination of parts of the organs showed an average arsenic content of 184 mg. per cent. The condition was unquestionably due to arsine, and the authors attribute this to an impurity of the cadmium which was used in the factory. At first it was believed that the condition may have been a myeloid leukemia superimposed on arsenic intoxication, but this diagnosis had to be discarded because of the pronounced degenerative changes in the plasma and nuclei of the leukocytes. The authors assumed that the frequently introduced doses of arsine had exerted a stimulus on the bone marrow causing a leukocytosis.

Spaeth and Soika[887] reported a case of poisoning where a man used concentrated sulphuric acid instead of acidulated water, which, upon cadmium, gave off arsine. Two hours after inhaling vapors given off in this process he complained of nausea, violent headache, vomiting, and some of the vomitus contained blood. The stools were bloody. He was seen two days later by the authors, who found there were no disturbances referable to the nervous system. The urine was found to contain 3% of albumin but no sugar. The sediment contained a few epithelial casts. The urine was dark brown, and the blood serum was about the same color. The blood findings showed: hemoglobin 57%; R.B.C's 2,380,000; leukocytes, 32,000; eosinophiles, 1%; polys, 84%; lymphos, 13%; monos, 1.5%; hemolysis occurred at 0.52% to 0.48% NaCl. The stools at first were thin and bloody. A diagnosis of arsine intoxication was given, this being made on the basis of the onset occurring two hours after exposure, with a severe gastro-intestinal disturbance, a

887. SPAETH, H., and SOIKA, G. G.: Med. Klin., 27:1388, 1931.

hemoglobinuria and jaundice. At first, cadmium intoxication was suspected. The patient's stomach was washed out and he was given charcoal. Vomiting stopped, but the patient began to belch violently. On the second day following admission to the hospital he began to complain of pain in the region of the liver. On the fourth day he became somewhat stuporous and showed tremors of the hands. On the fifth day he was in deep coma; his heart failed, and he expired on the sixth day.

Postmortem: The tissues of the heart, liver, and kidneys showed fatty degeneration.[888] In a case of inhalation of gas studied by Delepine,[888] chemical examination of 200 gm. of liver showed the presence of 0.01 mg. of arsenic.

Postmortem examination (Spaeth and Soika's Case[887]) showed a yellow discoloration of all of the organs. On the gastric mucosa there was evidence of small hemorrhages, which were also present in the ascending colon and in the sigmoid. The liver was somewhat swollen and showed some fatty degeneration. The spleen was enlarged, soft, and dark red. The kidneys were dark red, and showed cloudy swelling. There was an intravascular hemolysis and a formation of methemoglobin. The kidneys showed a marked degree of nephrosis, and all of the uriniferous tubules were filled with blood. In places there was a leukocytic infiltration. In the small intestine the villi were destroyed and there was an inflammatory infiltration. There were masses between the liver cords, a fatty degeneration, with a biliary pigment in the liver cells. Grossly, no pathology was noted in the brain or heart. Arsenic was found in the organs. Labes,[889] found that the greatest damage in arsine intoxication is due to hemolysis, which is caused by the oxidation of arsine to elementary colloidal arsenic, which in turn destroys the red cells. Meyer and Hubner* observed an acute case of poisoning in which the skin appeared a faded red. From the nose and mouth of the cadaver a dark green material exuded.

The destruction of the red cells and the formation of methemoglobin cause more or less an icterus or bronzing of the skin. The color may vary from a yellow brown to a yellow green. The gums have a murky blue appearance.

888. GLAISHER, G.: Edenberg, Livingston, 1908. DELEPINE: *J. Indust. Hyg.*, 1:356, 1919.

889. LABES: *Deutsche med. Wchnschr.*, 51, 1926.

* MEYER and HUBNER: ELSE PETRI, *Pathalogischen und Histologie der Vergiftung*, 1930.

REFRIGERANTS

ONE of the great and pressing problems that has confronted man from early times has been that of the conservation and preservation of food supplies. In the time of plenty an attempt was made to preserve food to have available at a future date. One of the early methods was that of air drying by means of the heat of the sun. Later, a more rapid method was developed by the use of fire and smoke. Then, gradually, a method of preservation by means of salt, sugar, spices, and chemical preservatives appeared. As the population began to centralize in large cities, foods had to be transported long distances. In order that these could be transported and then kept for a period of time at a destination, the great canning and cold storage industries developed. The cold storage industry made use of mechanical refrigeration, using ammonia and carbon dioxide to reduce temperatures. In the home, ice which had been cut during the winter was utilized during the warm months as a source of refrigeration, but as state and local health authorities began to examine the ice they found that some of it had been cut from rivers and lakes which were contaminated. In consequence, the artificial ice industry developed at this time, and the price of ice was grealty increased. Engineers were urged to develop mechanical devices, using chemicals as refrigerants, after the Federal government passed the Pure Food and Drug Act on June 21, 1906, curtailing the use of food chemically preserved. Prior to that time we had been eating large amounts of boric acid, formaldehye, and other preservatives in our food. The engineers, in their first efforts to produce mechanical methods of refrigeration, used a light grade of gasoline. This was discontinued on account of the fire hazard. Later, ammonia, carbon dioxide, sulphur dioxide, methyl bromide, methyl chloride, ethyl bromide, and ethyl chloride came into use. The rapid development of the industry concerned in the manufacture and sale of devices for use in household refrigeration has given the authorities insufficient opportunity to accumulate enough knowledge necessary for general protection. Little was known regarding the health, and fire and explosion hazards of the material used as a refrigeration medium. All of the substances commonly used in the production of refrigeration are more or less toxic. More interest was shown in the fire hazard of the refrigerant than in the health hazards, until a large number of cases of illness occurred in Chicago.

One classification based upon the fire hazard would be the inflammable refrigerants, as ethane, propane, butane, dichlormethane, dichlorethylene, dichlorodifluoromethane, methylchloride, ethyl chloride, and ammonia, and the non-inflammable refrigerants as carbon dioxide and sulphur dioxide.

The danger attendant in the use of any refrigerant in hotels, theaters and apartments, increases rapidly with the amount of the chemical used, and the manner in which it is distributed. All refrigerating systems in practical use depend upon the repeated gasification and condensation of a material, which is called the refrigerant. In most installations the refrigerant is confined under pressure. Household refrigerants may be either of the pressure or the absorption type. In the former, a motor is required, whence came the name "electrical refrigeration." In the latter, heat is most commonly supplied by a gas burner. Most of the mechanical refrigerants in the home are of the first type. Refrigeration depends upon the well known physical principle that liquids and fluids pass into a gaseous state and take up heat from the space in which they are enclosed.

METHYL CHLORIDE

THE narcotic action of methyl chloride was investigated in 1879, and has been known for over fifty years. Poisoning by methyl chloride has been so infrequent that textbooks on toxicology and legal medicine either mention it briefly or fail to record the toxic properties of the gas. I have had occasion to investigate ninety-eight cases. The first case of methyl chloride poisoning which came to my attention occurred August 10, 1928, in two apartments in the same building, when four people were exposed to the gas from a leaky connection to a multiple system. Three of them died. On December 10, 1935, four persons were poisoned by gas escaping from a hole in the condenser pipe attached to a unit located in the basement of an apartment building. One of these, G. R., died from the effects of the gas. This case was one of the most unusual that I have observed. The man, after inhaling the gas, drove his automobile several blocks to a hospital. After entering the hospital he became unconscious and expired. The postmortem appearances

and the symptoms were similar to the cases described later.
Van der Kloot[890] reported a case of illness due to methyl
chloride poisoning. Eulenberg,[891] in 1876, working with pigeons,
reported the toxic action of methyl chloride. Exposure to the
gas produced difficulty in breathing and dilatation of the pupils, and caused the birds to stagger and fall. Removal from exposure was followed by recovery. Kionka,[892] in 1900, reported
the narcotic action of methyl chloride as one-fourth that of
chloroform. Gerbis[893] appears to have been the first to report
accidental poisoning from this gas in 1914. The patients were
two machinists affected while repairing an ice machine. One of
these, a man aged fifty-two had had a similar attack the year
before which lasted eight days. He suffered from nausea,
vomiting, restlessness, coma, dyspnea, and a decided diminution in vision, which cleared up later. The second machinist,
aged sixty-three, working in the same factory, had sixteen
hours of unbroken sleep following exposure to methyl chloride.
He had the same symptoms as the other man, with the addition of severe headaches. Recovery was not complete till fourteen days later.

Roth[894] reported ten cases of poisoning in which the chief
symptoms were drowsiness, nausea, vomiting, headache, tired
feeling, followed by sleeplessness. Roth concludes from his
observations that poisoning occurs not only by inhalation of a
large amount at one time, but in susceptible individuals the
same symptoms may appear from inhaling smaller amounts
over a period of days. Schwartz[895] reported a similar number of
cases of poisoning, with one death. The methyl chloride in
this as well as in the preceding cases was inhaled during the
repair or installation of ice machines. The outstanding symptoms in all of Schwartz's cases were fatigue, headache, dizziness,
apathy, cyanosis, loss of appetite, and weakness of the legs. The
patients, at first drowsy, later developed insomnia. The symptoms became increasingly severe for several days until they
reached their maximum. They gradually cleared up in from

890. VAN DER KLOOT, ALBERT: *Illinois M. J.*, 45:508, 1934.
891. EULENBERG: Hand. d. Gewerbehyg. f. Hyg., 1876.
892. KIONKA: *Arch. internat. de pharmacod.*, 7:475, 1900.
893. GERBIS: *München med. Wchnschr.*, 61:879, 1914.
894. ROTH: *Schweiz. Ztschr. f. Unfallh.*, 17:169, 1923.
895. SCHWARTZ: *Deutsche Ztschr. f. d. ges. gerichtl. Med.*, 7:278, 1926.

one to two weeks, when all but one of the men returned to their employment without any after-effects. This patient, a man of forty-nine years, died four days after the onset of the

TABLE XLII

PHYSICAL AND CHEMICAL PROPERTIES OF METHYL CHLORIDE COMPOUND WITH GASOLINE AND AMMONIA

	Methyl Chloride	Gasoline	Ammonia
Formula	CH_3Cl	C_5H_{12} to C_9H_{20}.	NH_3
Molecular Weight	50.49	72-128	17
Sp. Gr. (air=1) 0°C. 760 mm. Hg	1.782	3-4	0.59
Relative Rate of Diffusion (air=1)	0.749	0.577 to 0.50	1.301
Boiling Point	−23.7°C. (−10.66°F.)	36-130°C. (96.8-266°F.)	−33.35°C. (−28.0°F.)
Critical Temperature	143.2°C. (289.8°F.)		130°C. (266°F.)
Critical Pressure	73 Atm.		115 Atm.
Vapor Pressure 20° C.	4.83 Atm. (71 Lb. absolute)		124 lb.
Cu. ft. per lb. 20° C.	7.45	4.43-3.32	22.52
Apparent Ignition Temperature	632°C. (1169.6°F.)	280°C. (536°F.)	
Heat of Combustion	846 BTU per cu. ft. 5505 cal/G	4740 BTU per cu. ft. 10,000 cal/G	462 BTU per cu. ft. 5332 cal/G
Heat of Formation	448 cal/G		699 cal/G
Explosive Range per cent by Vol.	8.1-17.2	1.4-6.0	16-25.5
Cu. ft. of air to burn 1 cu. ft. of gas	11.35-4.81	70.44-15.66	5.25-2.92
Per Cent Gas in Air for Combustion (Combining proportions)	12.3		21.74
Explosion Press. in bomb, lb. per sq. in.	69	100	50
Time of Development of Pressure (seconds)	0.110	0.026	0.175

symptoms. He had had a similar but lighter exposure three weeks previous, which left him very nervous. His condition was not realized as serious until he became unconscious and developed convulsions. At that time a physician was called, and the patient was removed to a hospital, where he died. In the spring of 1927, Baker[896] reported twenty-one cases of methyl chloride poisoning at Evansville, Indiana, among the employees of a factory manufacturing refrigerators. The symptoms were drowsiness, vertigo, visual disturbances, staggering gait, anorexia and ptosis; later insomnia, and fine tremors of the extremities developed. Slight nausea occurred in about half of the patients. In all cases the symptoms subsided very slowly with no deaths resulting.

Methyl chloride, CH_3Cl, is non-corrosive, liquefacient, colorless, and transparent in both the gaseous and liquid states. It was discovered in 1835 by Dumas and Peigot. Although manufactured in Europe in small quantities since 1875, it was not available in quantities in the United States until 1920. It has a sweet ethereal odor somewhat resembling chloroform. It has a molecular weight of 50.49. The density of the liquid is 0.998 at —24.09°C. The boiling point is —24.09°C. at 750 mm. barometric pressure. The melting point is —91.5°C. The density of the gas compared to air is 1.7824. A liter weighs 2.3045 gm. The ignition temperature is 632°C.

The Underwriters' Laboratories report that "methyl chloride is a moderate flammable refrigerant. Its general fire hazard is very much less than gasoline. When confined in the refrigeration unit the fire hazard of methyl chloride is small."[897] It burns with a greenish flame. One part of water dissolves four volumes of methyl chloride; absolute alcohol, thirty-five volumes; acetic acid, forty volumes. One hundred parts of the gas contain 23.76 parts of carbon, 5.94 parts hydrogen and 70.30 parts chlorine.

Methyl chloride possesses some antiseptic properties when used as a preservative for biological products.[898] There is a decrease of oxidation during methyl chloride anesthesia, and the narcosis is attributed to the decrease in catalase.[899] The more chlorine introduced into the methane molecule the more effective it becomes in decreasing the catalase. It exerts a paralyzing effect upon the nervous system. It has no effect upon the cornea of the eye of the dog.[900] Plotz reports that the hemolytic

896. BAKER, H. M.:   J.A.M.A., 88:1137, 1927.
897. Underwriters Laboratories Report on the Fire Hazards of Methyl Chloride as a Refrigerant, August 26, 1926.
898. SALKOWSKI, E.:   Biochem. Ztschr., 107:191, 1920.
899. BURGE and BURGE: J. Biol. Chem., 41:307, 1920.
900. PLOTZ, W.:   Biochem. Ztschr., 203:243, 1920.

activity of the homologous series of the chlorine derivatives of methane is proportional to the increasing molecular weight, particularly the entrance of the chlorine into the molecule. Buxson[901] mentions a preparation containing seven parts of methyl chloride, ten parts of ethyl chloride, and one part of ethyl bromide, "large doses of which cause death by setting up powerful contractions of the diaphragm with arrest of the respiration, while the heart still beats strongly."

In nearly all of the cases a tentative diagnosis of food poisoning was made. In two instances, strychnine poisoning was considered, and in five children affected together, metal poisoning was first suspected. Two other cases were initially diagnosed as mushroom poisoning. The possibility of poisoning by methyl chloride first came up in connection with four cases in August, 1928, because of the known exposure to methyl chloride and an observed similarity to methyl alcohol poisoning. In three cases occurring in February, 1929, a probable diagnosis of methyl chloride poisoning was made on the symptoms and known exposure to methyl chloride, but no positive confirmatory evidence could be obtained. When three acute cases came to the attention of Kegel, McNally and Pope[902] in the latter part of June, 1929, accumulated observations of previous suspected cases of methyl chloride poisoning, together with definite knowledge of exposure in this instance, convinced the authors of the etiologic relationship of methyl chloride. Intensive laboratory studies were made, and as a result the authors became certain that they were dealing with a specific poison.

Toxicological studies on animals have been made by the United States Health Service.[903]

Two women patients complained after one year of spasm of the esophagus. X-ray and physical examinations did not reveal anything unusual. Mr. C. C., seen four years later had only the complaint, "I am very nervous." All severe cases of methyl chloride poisoning complain of nervousness for over a year. Some complain for months of not being able to talk coherently and an inability to remember things that have happened recently. Among the complications which affect chiefly

901. BUXSON: Anesthetics, 5th ed., 315, 1914.
902. KEGEL, A. H., McNALLY, W. D., and POPE, A. S.: J.A.M.A., 93, 1929.
903. U. S. Pub. Health Service Bull. 185, 1929.

the nervous system are ataxia, insomnia, vertigo, and dim vission.[904]

Birch[905] reported that methyl chloride can cause both acute and chronic poisoning, depending on whether the exposure is one large dose or continued small doses, as from a leak. The literature of reported cases of poisoning is reviewed. Then an account is given of a case arising from exposure for some forty-five minutes to a high concentration of methyl chloride vapor from a leak in a refrigerating machine. The man experienced severe vomiting, and was admitted to the hospital looking ill and dehydrated. He made an uneventful recovery.

Symptoms: The onset is generally marked by progressive drowsiness, mental confusion, stupor, weakness, nausea, pain in the abdomen, and vomiting. In the more severe types there are convulsions and cyanosis alternating with coma; later delirium and restlessness develop. Most patients show muscular tremors and hiccup during the acute stages. Although six of the patients complained of severe headache for the first few days, this was not usually recalled until they were convalescent, and several were certain they did not have headaches at any time. On account of their mental disturbance, several were referred to psychiatrists for diagnosis. Eleven complained of amblyopia and vertigo, which in many cases persisted after they had otherwise clinically recovered.

The pupils were widely dilated and reacted sluggishly to light. Occasionally a slight strabismus, nystagmus or ptosis was noted. The pulse, temperature and respiration were all increased. In adults the pulse sometimes went as high as 150, and the respiration 32 per minute. In some of the children the pulse reached 164, and in one child the respiration was 56. Anuria, which sometimes lasted as long as forty-eight hours, was usually present. About thirty-six hours after exposure to methyl chloride there generally occurs a rise in temperature, reaching as high as 104° F. in non-fatal cases, and in two instances the temperatures just before death were 107 and 107.4. Prolonged coma is of common occurrence, occasionally lasting as long as from thirty-six to seventy-two hours, with recovery. Death is always preceded by severe convulsions, usually tonic,

904. Gorham, A. P.: *Brit. M. J.*, 1:529, 1934.
905. Birch, C. A.: *Lancet*, February 2, p. 259, 1935; *J. Indust. Hyg.*, May, 1935.

and accompanied by profound cyanosis. During the spasms, marked opisthotonos was noticed. The immediate cause of death appeared to be respiratory paralysis.

The blood picture in nearly all of the patients examined was suggestive of primary anemia. Table XLIII gives the minimum and maximum range in the series, including cases of varying degrees of poisoning. The icterus index on the blood of the one patient tested, taken three days after onset, was 13.4 (normal 4 to 6). On the same specimen the van den Bergh test at that time was 2.2 (normal, from 0.1 to 0.5). Six days later the blood specimen of this patient had a normal icterus index and the direct van den Bergh time was much delayed (the indirect was within the lower limit of normal). Blood films from the same patients three days after onset showed practically no reticulocytes, while films made six days later showed beginning regeneration of red blood cells. Blood films from the same patients taken three days after onset showed marked achromia, with considerable variation in size and shape of the red blood cells and a number of fragmented cells.

Hemoglobin observations of 80 and 85% in two patients had dropped to 56 and 60%, respectively, in the next two days. A red blood cell count of 4,400,000 in one of the patients on admission fell two days later to 3,100,000, and in another from 4,-400,000 to 3,200,000 in three days. The white blood count averaged about 16,000 on the third day of illness. All showed a definite leukocytosis.

TABLE XLIII
MINIMUM AND MAXIMUM BLOOD CHANGES

Hemoglobin	From 50 to 90%
Red blood cells	From 3,100,000 to 4,990,000
White blood cells	From 8,500 to 22,200
Polymorphonuclear neutrophils	From 60 to 89%
Eosinophils	From 2 to 6%
Small lymphocytes	From 16 to 35%
Large mononuclears and transitionals	From 3 to 4%
Basophils	From 0 to 1%

Spinal puncture was made on five patients. In three instances the fluid was under increased pressure. In one case it was cloudy, and in another gave a positive test for globulin. In all instances the cellular content was normal. The blood pressure was significantly lowered in nearly all cases in which it was taken. Readings of 84 systolic and 46 diastolic and 84 systolic and 40 diastolic were obtained on two patients. The most commonly observed pressure was about 100 systolic and 60 diastolic.

Anuria of some degree was the rule during the acute stage of poisoning, and suppression lasting from thirty-six to forty-eight hours occasionally occurred. Incontinence was common during early convalescence. The urine was acid in reaction until rendered alkaline therapeutically. Of the eleven patients tested in the acute stage, eight had acetone and four diacetic acid in the urine. More or less albumin was present in approximately one-half of our cases. Granular or hyaline casts were found in the urine of eight patients; white blood cells were present in six, and a few red blood cells were present in five instances. Formic acid, which Baker[906] found in the urine of nearly all his patients, was present in the urine of only three of our patients on whom the test was made early. Quantitative analysis of two of these gave 6.8 and 9.8 mg. of formic acid per hundred cubic centimeters of the sample.

The diagnosis is based on the symptoms and physical observations previously noted, together with the presence of formates and acetone in the urine and a history of exposure to the gas. The peculiar musty, sweetish odor of the breath when the patient is first seen, and the odor of acetone about the patient, are further aids in the diagnosis. A gradual onset of two days or more, with drowsiness and mental confusion, is an outstanding syndrome. In all cases showing these suggestive symptoms, possible recent exposure to methyl chloride should be investigated.

Treatment: The patient should be removed at once to a hospital. An alkaline balance should be established by giving sodium bicarbonate by mouth. If unable to swallow, the patient should be given a solution of 5% dextrose and 3% sodium bicarbonate in the form of a rectal drip as indicated. Ringer's (Ringer's solution: sodium chloride, 9 gm; calcium chloride, 0.24 gm.; potassium chloride, 0.42 gm.; sodium bicarbonate, 0.3 gm.; distilled water, 1,000 cc.), or Fisher's solution, 500 cc. intravenously, will reduce acidosis and combat dehydration. Inhalations of oxygen should be given from the start. If the patient resists taking the oxygen, the arms and hands may be restrained and the oxygen introduced through the nasal passages

906. BAKER, H. M.: *J.A.M.A.*, 88:1137, 1927.

or by means of an "H. & H." inhalator. The administration of oxygen should be continued until the peculiar "cadaveric blood" odor of the breath and acetone-like odor have disappeared. Convulsions may be allayed by potassium bromide in a dosage of one drachm (4 gm.) to four ounces (120 cc.) of water, administered as a retention enema. Under no conditions should chloral or chloroform be given. If stimulation is needed, caffeine with

TABLE XLIV
SUMMARY OF INSPECTIONS MADE IN 1929

Number Investigated	No. Leaks	No. Leaks Before Invest.	No. SO₂ Leaks	No. of Other Leaks	Illness	Deaths
214	43	70	28	6	40	10

Location of Leaks:

Evaporator	13
Compressor	10
Broken pipes	2
Coupling	17
Syphon	2
Coils	2
Gasket	2
Total	48
Multiple Units	152
Single Units	38

Leaks:

Sulphur dioxide	82
Methyl chloride	77
Ammonia	10
Ethyl chloride	1
Methyl chloride and sulphur dioxide	17
Isobutane	3
	190

Ammonia investigations............55 (by Fire Department)

Leaks:

Single Unit	8
Multiple	41
	49

From November 1928 to November 1929, 205 people were made ill, with 10 deaths; 879 persons were driven from their homes. The number of leaks reported, including those reported by the Fire and Health Departments, was 539.

sodium benzoate may be used. For a weak, rapid heart, one ampoule of digifolin every four hours is indicated until the pulse and temperature are normal and the acute nervous symptoms have disappeared. The convalescent treatment should be supportive and aimed to combat the anemia. Success of treatment depends on early recognition of the cause of illness, prompt removal of the patient from exposure, and rapid elimination of the gas from the system. From tests on blood and tissues it appears that methyl chloride as such is quickly eliminated after the patient is removed from exposure, and the progressive symptoms in the more severe cases are due to continued injury from the oxidation products of the gas until they are eliminated, and to degeneration of nerve cells.[907]

Methyl chloride, used as a refrigerant, now contains 1% acrolein. Upon escape of this refrigerant into a room acrolein serves as a warning agent. Sulphur dioxide added to methyl chloride has proved to be inefficient as a warning agent, since, in the Reynick case, the system contained sulphur dioxide.

Tests: Air containing methyl chloride is admitted through the side arm of the glass T where it mixes with fuel gas (natural gas free of chlorine) and is burned at the top of the glass burner.[908] Cubes of ammonium carbonate are stacked on a screen and placed around the base of the burner tip. This permits secondary air for the flame to pass up through the cubes and become laden with ammonia. The products of combustion then pass up the T and the chlorine products are deposited. After the test the funnel tube and the T tube are washed into a beaker, and the chloride determined by Volhard's method. With this type of apparatus checks may be obtained within 10% when using a three cubic foot sample of gas containing 0.01% methyl chloride. If the air contains 8.2% to 18.7% the flame would furnish a source of ignition and the sample would have to be reduced. From the amount of chlorine obtained by analysis the concentration of the methyl chloride can be calculated.[909]

907. Mechanical refrigeration is supplied through the single unit designed primarily for the home, and the multiple unit system designed for use where a large number of apartments are in one building. The multiple unit may have twenty-five iceboxes, or four times that number connected to one compressor. The compressors are usually located in the basement and are without adequate means of ventilation to take the gas away from an escaping refrigerator in the case of an accident. They have a distinct disadvantage. If anything happens to the unit in an apartment, the whole amount of the refrigerant, 150 pounds, may escape into the apartment. In 1929, the city of Chicago attempted to restrict the amount of a refrigerant to two pounds, because of the many accidents.

908. See Chem. Abst., Vol. 22, p. 1608. Gas Chemists' Handbook, American Gas Assoc.

909. See articles by YANT, SCHRENK and YANT: Indust. Chem. Analyst, Vol. 4: 259, ed. of 1932.

SULPHUR DIOXIDE (SO₂)
(Molecular Weight 64. Synonym: Sulphurous Acid)

SULPHUR DIOXIDE, SO₂, is a colorless gas with a specific gravity of 2.23. (For other properties see Table XLV.) It arises from the combustion of sulphur. It is an irritant irrespirable gas, relatively non-toxic, as compared to carbon monoxide or oxides of nitrogen. There is very little danger from sulphur dioxide poisoning, as the fumes are so irritating that the victim is compelled to seek air at once. In extreme cases[910] of very high concentrations, when the victim cannot retire from the fumes, death may result from respiratory spasms and asphyxia. Ordinarily, however, workmen exposed for some time to a mild degree of sulphur dioxide poisoning complain of headache, anorexia, spasmodic cough, sneezing, hemoptysis, bronchitis, constriction of chest, gastro-intestinal disorders, conjunctivitis, smarting of eyes, lacrimation, and anemia. For these symptoms workmen soon acquire tolerance. The inhalation of large quantities of sulphur dioxide produces ulceration of the mucous membrane.

Sulphur dioxide is produced in large quantities in the refining of petroleum. It is decomposed by sunlight into sulphur dioxide and free sulphur, thus producing part of the haze over large cities. It frequently contaminates the air near metallurgic works, destroying vegetation. It is found in nature in the vicinity of volcanoes. The Selby Smelter Commission made a thorough investigation of the effect of various concentrations of sulphur dioxide on the senses of a number of persons.[911] The average results of these tests are given in Table XLV.[912]

Sulphur dioxide is present in the air of cities and towns where coal containing sulphur is used for fuel. The choking sensation is due to this gas found in tunnels and underground railways where the ventilation is inadequate. It is used as a refrigerant, in the bleaching of paper, and in the manufacture of sulphuric acid by the Chamber process. Poisoning has occurred from the improper purification of illuminating gas, as

---

910. THOMPSON, D. G.: The Occupational Diseases, D. Appleton and Company, New York, 360, 1914.

911. HOLMES, FRANKLIN, and GOULD: Report of the Selby Smelter Commission, U. S. Bureau of Mines, Bull 98, p. 172, 1915.

912. HENDERSON and HAGGARD: Noxious Gases, Monograph Series.

in the accident in Mount Vernon, New York, in 1897, where the whole population suffered from the suffocating fumes of this gas. It is condensible to a clear liquid at —18°C., and is solid at —76°C. The liquid has a specific gravity of 1.45 at —20°C., and boils at —8°C.

The gas is very soluble, water absorbing 43.5 times its volume, and forming sulphurous acid, H_2SO_3. Sulphur candles and liquid sulphur dioxide are much used in domestic disinfection. The gas extinguishes flame even in the presence of much air. In two instances I have seen death from the inhalation of sulphur dioxide from the sulphur candle. Sulphur dioxide under pressure in a liquefied state is used as a refrig-

TABLE XLV
PHYSIOLOGICAL RESPONSE TO VARIOUS CONCENTRATIONS OF SO₂

	Parts of SO₂ per million parts of air.
Least detectable odor*	3 to 5
Least amount causing irritation to the eyes*	20
Least amount causing immediate irritation to the throat*	8 to 12
Least amount causing coughing*	20
Maximum concentration allowable for prolonged exposure*	10
Maximum concentration allowable for short exposure, one-half to one hour*‡	50 to 100
Dangerous for even short exposure	400 to 500

† (U. S. Dept. of Interior, Bureau of Mines, 98, 1915)
* (FIELDNER, A., and KATZ, S.: *Eng. & Mining Jour.*, 107: 693, 1919)
‡ (LEHMANN: *Arch. f. Hyg.*, 18, 180, 1893)

erant in domestic and small commercial units. In this connection the escape of the gas serves as its own warning agent. From the Table XLV, giving the physiological response to various concentrations, it will be noticed that it is dangerous and irrespirable. Low concentrations are offensive and momentarily irritating. Simferopol[913] reported sulphur dioxide as an injurious impurity in the air of rooms in a fruit preserving factory.

Sulphur dioxide has been used for many years in the United States for the disinfection of ships.[914] Very few deaths have been reported from its use.

913. SIMFEROPOL, L.: *Gigiena truda i. tekhnika bezopnosti*, 5: 90, 1934.

914. WILLIAMS, C. L.: Pub. Health Reports, Reprint No. 1609, 49: 89, 1934.

On December 3 and 4, 1930, hundreds of people were taken ill and sixty-three persons died during a heavy fog.[915] The explanation of this occurrence was that the surrounding factories south of Luttich increased the concentration of sulphur dioxide and hydrofluoric acid in the air. There was very little air current on those days, and the concentrations of the gases were so markedly increased that they caused a long series of poisonings. Rostoski and Crecelius[916] report an explosion of a tank containing cellulose and sulphur dioxide. Eighteen persons were severely poisoned and several died. One patient died ten and a half months after the poisoning from a suppurative bronchitis, bronchiectasis, and emphysema. Schade[917] reported that the sulphur dioxide present in air in the city of Pittsburgh is too small to be a cause of concern from a hygienic standpoint. Meiter and Traubert[918] report that the average amount of sulphur dioxide content of the air at the Pittsburgh Experimental Station of the Bureau of Mines was 0.16 part per million. The maximum, 1.1 parts per million, was found on two days; less than the minimum detectable (0.1 part per million) on 141 days. They found that the concentrations tended to be higher on foggy or smoky days.

Sulphur dioxide is a fire hazard; the newspapers make frequent mention of cases. An example of this was a fire at Mission and 22nd streets in San Francisco, California. Captain Walter D. Griffin, of Company No. 21, responded to an alarm and when he arrived at the fire, a refrigerating plant located in the basement was emitting heavy fumes of sulphur dioxide. The following day Captain Griffin developed pneumonia from which he died, two months later.

Symptoms: Twenty parts per million parts of air cause an immediate irritation of the eyes. Amounts greater than this are apt to cause suffocation. The air-passages are highly irritated through the formation of sulphurous acid on their surface. Four hundred parts of sulphur dioxide in one million of air are dangerous to breathe for one hour; this amount

915. STORM VAN LEEUWEN, W.: *München. med. Wchnschr.*, 78:39, 1931.

916. ROSTOSKI and CRECELIUS: *Deutsches Arch f. klin. Med.*, 168: 121, 1930.

917. SCHADE, C.: *J. Indust. Hyg.*, 15:150, 1933.

918. MEITER, E. G., and TRAUBERT, C. E.: U. S. Bureau of Mines, R. I. 3005, June, 1930.

"elicits respiratory reflexes. Rarely causes death from edema of the larynx. Trachea and bronchi inflamed. Lung edema is rare."[919] Coughing and sneezing are readily induced. Both men and animals may be habituated to its inhalation. According to Tidy,[920] mice can be brought to tolerate twice the amount they could at first. Air containing from 0.03 to 0.04 gm. per thousand did not affect workmen more severely than amounts from 0.01 to 0.02 gm. affected those unaccustomed to breathing the gas.[921] I found that the majority of guinea pigs exposed for fifteen minutes to 1% sulphur dioxide were killed. Animals that recovered from this amount died within twenty-four hours. All of these animals had a severe conjunctivitis. The cornea becomes opaque, and there are dyspnea, cyanosis, and convulsions. Taken internally, there is catarrh of the stomach and chronic sulphuric acid poisoning. According to Kobert,[922] sulphur dioxide has been used for murder only once, and sulphurous acid only once with suicidal intent. The effects on vegetation are greater than on animals. Suits for damages against industrial plants emitting sulphur dioxide for the destruction of trees and other plants are frequent.[923]

Chronic catarrh has been noted following long exposure.[924] Pedley,[925] on the other hand, found no increased incidence of respiratory disease in Canadian paper mills using the sulphite process, and evidence from other industries, such as smelting, is negative. Kehoe and his associates[926] studied the effect of prolonged exposure to sulphur dioxide on 100 workmen exposed to this gas in the course of their employment. Forty-seven had from four to twelve years' exposure, the severity of which fluctuated through a wide range (seventy

919. HENDERSON and HAGGARD: Noxious Gases, Monograph Series.
920. TIDY: Forensic Medicine and Toxicology, 495, 1877.
921. LEHMANN, B. K.: Arch. f. Hyg., 18:180, 1893.
922. KOBERT: Kompendium der Toxikologie, 147, 1912.
923. SCHROEDER and REUSS: Die Beschädigung der Vegetation durch Rauch und die Huettenrauch-Schaden, 1883; also JUST and BLAINE: Landw. Versuchsst., part 2, 1889; WITHROW, J. R.: Atmospheric Pollution from Sulphuric and Plant Fumes, Chem. & Metall. Eng., 26:972, 1922; and PERROT, G.: Sulphur Dioxide as a Factor in the Smoke Problem of Salt Lake City, U. S. Bureau of Mines, Report of Investigations, No. 2128, 1920.
924. VON JAKSCH, R.: de Vergiftungen, 2nd ed., Vienna, 1910.
925. PEDLEY, F. G.: J. Indust. Hyg., 6:28, 1924.
926. KEHOE, R. A., MACHLE, W. F., KITZMILLER, K., and LE BLANC, T. J.: J. Indust. Hyg., 14:159, 1932.

parts per million by volume) but was still higher in the years before 1927. They found a significantly higher incidence of chronic, slight nasopharyngitis, and of alteration in sense of smell and taste. The men did not seem more susceptible to ordinary colds, but the average duration of colds was two to three times longer than the average for the control group. They also found a higher rate of abnormal urinary acidity, of dyspnea on exertion, of increased fatigue from work, and of sluggish or hyperactive reflexes, which indicated that sulphur dioxide did not have an effect on the human organism.[927]

Treatment: Workmen and firemen exposed to sulphur dioxide fumes should wear gas masks. When a person has been exposed to the gas, inhalations of oxygen should be given to lessen the respiratory effect, and alkaline drinks should be administered immediately.

Postmortem Appearances: The blood is very dark, and sometimes has an acid reaction. The hemoglobin is changed firsι through loss of oxygen, then by decomposition to hematin, as with mineral acids. The respiratory tract is inflamed and the lungs are edematous.

Tests: The characteristic odor of burning sulphur, its bleaching action, blue color with starch and iodic acid. This last test is sensitive one to 3,000. There is also an intensely suffocating odor. Take about 25 gm. of the sample in a 200-cc. Erlenmeyer flask, add several cc. of strong hydrochloric acid and sulphuric acid and free zinc and place a piece of lead acetate paper over the Erlenmeyer flask. In the presence of sulphur dioxide a darkening due to hydrogen sulphide will give the same reaction as the sulphide above. The official quantitative method is used. Distill 20 to 100 gm. of the sample (adding recently boiled water if necessary) in a current of carbon dioxide, after the addition of about 5 cc. of a 20% glacial phosphoric acid solution, until 150 cc. have passed over. Collect the distillate in about 100 cc. of nearly saturated bromine water, allowing the end of the condenser to dip below the surface. The method and apparatus may be simplified without material loss in accuracy by omitting the current of carbon dioxide, adding 10 cc. of the phosphoric acid instead of 5 cc. and dropping into the distillation flask, immediately before attaching the condenser, a piece of sodium bicarbonate weigh-

927. EVERS, A.: *Arch. f. Hyg.*, 106:255, 1931.

ing not more than 1 gm. The carbon dioxide liberated is not sufficient to expel entirely the air from the apparatus, but it will prevent oxidation to a large extent. When the distillation is finished, boil off the excess of bromine, dilute the solution to about 250 cc., add 5 cc. of dilute hydrochloric acid with 10% barium chloride solution. Boil for a few minutes longer; allow to stand over night in a warm place; filter through a weighed Gooch crucible, or through an ashless filter paper; wash with hot water; ignite at a dull red heat; and weigh as barium sulphate. Conduct a blank determination on the apparatus and reagents, and correct the result accordingly.

CARBON DIOXIDE (CO_2)
(Molecular Weight 44. Synonyms: Fixed-Air; Choke-Damp, Carbonic Acid, Carbonic Anhydride and Black-Damp)

THIS gas is not used at all in domestic refrigerants, but finds commercial application. It is little used for refrigeration purposes in small systems because of the necessity of high pressure, and thus heavy machinery. One thousand pounds per square inch is not an unusual pressure in apparatus for the liquefaction of carbon dioxide. It is one of the most common of all gases, being abundantly produced by a large number of natural and artificial processes, such as respiration, decay, alcoholic fermentation, combustion of coal and wood, lime-burning, etc. It is one of the gases found in mines as the result of the presence of material which, being oxidizable, takes up the oxygen from the air. "Black-Damp" consists of 87% nitrogen and 13% carbon dioxide.[928] If the air is deficient in oxygen due to the presence of this gas, a lighted candle will be extinguished. Not all gases have this property. Schultzik[929] found that this gas contained 26% carbon dioxide, 3% oxygen, and about 5% to 10% carbon monoxide. He also found that while most flames are extinguished by 10% carbon dioxide, acetylene does not go out until 26% to 31% is reached. It is present even in the purest air. Over the ocean, or on a mountain top, the atmosphere contains 0.03% by volume. It is a heavy gas, having a specific gravity of 1.52 compared with air, and on account of its weight is rather slowly diffusible. For these reasons it is not infrequently found in caves, old

928. HALDANE: *Brit. M. J.*, 2:16, 1930.
929. SCHULTZIK: *Zentralbl. f. Gewerbehyg.*, 5:76, 1928.

wells, cisterns, and other low and confined places, and has often been the cause of death of persons entering them.[930]   In cities, and especially around factories and in crowded halls, the amount may rise some hundreths of 1%. The discomfort and ill effects of bad ventilation are, therefore, not usually due to carbon dioxide itself or to the correspondingly slight decrease of oxygen, but to other factors, such as excessive moisture, high temperature, and lack of air motion.

Leaks of carbon dioxide gas would be difficult to locate because of the fact that it has no warning agent (see Tests, page 447), being colorless, odorless, and stable under ordinary conditions.

Numerous cases have been reported of the sloughing following the handling of dry ice. If a considerable quantity of dry ice were shipped in a baggage car the concentration of carbon dioxide might reach a dangerous point. The dry ice (carbon dioxide snow, solid carbon dioxide) which is used to preserve for short periods substances such as ice cream and ices, can cause injury to the skin. Mansens[931] has produced even skin cancers in animals by applying it. Linseed oil production in Holland, with evolution of carbon dioxide, has been the cause of many fatal poisonings. Green fodder in silos and residue in brewery vats have caused fatal poisoning in this country and in England. Making compressed yeast caused six cases in a German factory recently. In Grant Park, Chicago, two men cleaning out a cesspool were overcome by the gas and killed. An examination of the air several hours after the accident showed that it contained 26% carbon dioxide.[932]

Action on the Body: Carbon dioxide acts locally at the point of application, or remotely on the brain and spinal cord. Applied to the skin it produces a prickling or twitching, together with a feeling of warmth which, if the contact be continued, is followed by anesthesia. In olden times local anesthesia was brought about by rubbing the skin at the place to be operated upon with vinegar and powdered marble.[933] More

930. BRIAND and CHAUDE: Manuel Complet de Medecine Legale, 6th ed., 1858.

931. MANSENS, B.: *Nederl. tijdschr. v. geneesk.*, 75:1444, 1931.

932. See also BREZINA, E., and TELEKY, L.: Internationale Ubersicht über Gewerbekrankheiten nachden. Berichten der Kulturlander, 1914-18; 1920-26; 1927-29.

933. DEMARQUAY: *Compt. rend.*, 61:166, 1865.

profound symptoms arise when larger surfaces are affected. Bathing water charged with carbon dioxide causes a diminution of sensitiveness, reddening of the skin, warmth, prickling, and lowering of the pulse rate.

In the ordinary conditions and activities of life every movement of the body or limbs results in the production of an increased amount of carbon dioxide, and requires the absorption of an amount of oxygen corresponding to the energy expended. The carbon dioxide thus produced diffuses from the active muscles into the blood, by which it is carried to the so-called respiratory center controlling the activity of the muscles of the chest and diaphragm, and stimulates this center to increased activity. The increased respiration supplies the oxygen needed to make good the deficit, or "oxygen debt," due to the muscular work. Thus, as was first pointed out by Miescher, "carbon dioxide spreads its protecting wings over the oxygen supply of the body."

Carbon dioxide renders arterial blood venous more rapidly than other gases. It acts on diluted blood as other weak acids. The hemoglobin is converted into acid hematin. A slight increase in the number of erythrocytes was noted in rabbits exposed to 4% carbon dioxide for four days.[934] A solution of oxyhemoglobin treated with carbon dioxide yields a two-banded spectrum. On the evacuation of the carbon dioxide, the solution not coming in contact with the air, reduced hemoglobin is produced.[935] Muscular tissue loses irritability and becomes rigid in gaseous mixtures containing much carbon dioxide. Ciliary movements are also arrested.

The brain and spinal cord are first stimulated, causing increase of blood-pressure,[936] peristaltic movement, and reduction in pulse-rate, followed by more intense respiration and less psychic excitability, and finally paralysis. Absorption takes place through all mucous membranes, the lungs, the subcutaneous tissues, and also by the skin. Carbonates are changed to bi- or acid-carbonates in the blood or tissues. The elimination is quantitative, and occurs by the lungs, urine, skin secretions, and intestinal discharges. Death is ascribed to

934. DUFTON: Proc. Physiol. Soc., Lond., 51:5, 1917.
935. BUCKMASTER: Proc. Physiol. Soc., Lond., 51:105, 1917.
936. CATHCART: J. Physiol., 49:301, 1915; ITAMI, S.: J. Physiol., 45:338, 1912.

carbon dioxide poisoning, sufficient oxygen being supplied, to an excessive stimulation of the cerebrospinal system producing asphyxia, differing, however, from ordinary asphyxia, in which a loss of stimulation, especially of the heart, is due to the want of oxygen.[937]

Symptoms: High concentrations lead to sudden death from suffocation. When the amount of carbon dioxide does not cause insensibility, there is a tendency toward giddiness, somnolence, and loss of muscular power. Profuse perspiration and nausea are common. Drumming in the ears and quickened breathing follow. Sometimes mental excitement and cramps are noted. If oxygen deficiency is excluded by inhaling gas mixtures containing 20% oxygen, no effects occur until the concentration is 3%, when there is hyperpnea and discomfort; 8.5% produces in man in a few minutes distinct dyspnea, rise of blood pressure, and congestion which becomes unsupportable in twenty minutes, but disappears promptly in fresh air. The symptoms gradually increase in severity up to 15%. However, this it not dangerous to animals for an hour, and probably not to man. With 25% to 30% the stimulant phenomena pass into depression, with diminished respiration, fall of blood pressure, and coma, generally without convulsions. Workmen entering vats should be cautioned regarding this gas, and should not attempt to recover anyone rendered unconscious, until a supply of oxygen or air has replaced the high concentration of carbon dioxide.

Treatment: The body should be removed as speedily as possible to fresh air and given inhalations of oxygen. Resuscitation may take place after long insensibility, as has been shown by experiments on animals and experience with human beings.

Postmortem Appearances: Postmortem appearances are those of death from asphyxia. There is nothing very characteristic in the general appearance, and death may be ascribed to apoplexy or to some other cause.

Tests: When carbon dioxide is passed through lime water it causes a turbidity. Barium hydroxide is a better test than calcium hydroxide (lime water). The air is shaken with or

937. KOBERT, R.: Lehrbuch der Intoxikationen, Stuttgart, 2nd ed., 1121, 1906; HERMANN, L.: Lehrbuch der exper. Toxikologie, Berlin, 121, 1874.

drawn through a quantity of this solution of known strength, and the loss of alkalinity determined by titration with dilute acid. Fifty cc. of barium hydroxide solution are added to a bottle of five or six liters capacity, which has been filled with the air of the room by a flexible bellows pump. After thoroughly shaking the liquid with the air and after the lapse of half an hour, the turbid liquid is transferred to a stoppered separating funnel, the stem of which passes through a rubber stopper fitted to the neck of a bell-jar. One end of a piece of narrow flexible metallic tubing is inserted in the second perforation in the stopper, and the other end of the tube fits a small cork which closes the top of the tap-funnel provided with an asbestos plug, previously washed with baryta water. The bell-jar also contains sticks of moist potassium hydroxide, to free the air in the jar of carbon dioxide. The barium hydroxide liquid is thus filtered in an atmosphere free of carbon dioxide. An aliquot portion of the filtered liquid is titrated with nitric or hydrochloric acid, phenolphthalein being used to indicate the point of neutralization.[938] When the amount of carbon dioxide is large, its quantity may be determined by observaion with an eudiometer with the aid of potassium hydroxide solution. The dried air may also be drawn through a weighed vessel containing potassium hydroxide solution, when an increase in weight will show the amount of carbon dioxide in the volume of air submitted for analysis.[939]

When the air of a well, vat, or similar receptacle is to be tested, a sample for examination may be obtained by lowering into it a bottle containing fine sand and inverting by means of a cord attached to the bottom; when the sand running out is replaced by the air, the bottle is raised, mouth up. Using the Petterssen-Palmquist method, the carbon dioxide can be determined in air in a 25-cc. sample with an accuracy of one part in 10,000, and there is no necessity of making corrections for variations in pressure and temperature. This is accomplished by using a compensating tube filled with air and in communication with one side of a manometer tube; the buret containing the air to be measured is attached to the other side of the

938. WILLIAMS: Commemoration Volume, University College, Sheffield, 132, 1897.
939. See VAN SLYKE and CULLEN: J. Biol. Chem., 30:289, 1917; J. Biol. Chem., 30:347, 1917.

manometer tube; the compensating tube and buret are of nearly the same capacity and are in water. If the temperature of the water around the tubes changes during the experiment, the effect on the volume of air in each tube is the same. The carbon dioxide is absorbed in an Orsat gas pipet containing a solution of potassium hydroxide.[940]

AMMONIA (NH₃)
(Molecular Weight 17.032)

AMMONIA is used in both small and large refrigerating units. At ordinary temperatures it is a colorless gas with a specific gravity of 0.597. It is one of the products of the putrefaction of nitrogenous substances. It has the chemical formula of NH_3, or, in water, NH_4OH. Its synonyms are ammonium hydrate and ammonia-water. Ammonia in the form of ammonium hydroxide may act on the skin, and, if it penetrates deeply, might cause blistering. This also happens on ingestion or inhalation. It is an irritant and a corrosive agent, in the form of a gas or aqueous solution. At present ammonia is used more widely than any other refrigerant, commercially, despite its irritant and corrosive properties, because of the fact that its high latent heat of vaporization makes it exceptionally adaptable for refrigeration purposes. Furthermore, the operating pressures are considerably less than those for carbon dioxide, and ethane, thus reducing the cost of an installation. Ammonia does not ordinarily affect iron and steel. As it attacks copper and brass, brass valves and similar fittings are not used in ammonia systems. One-twentieth volume in 1,000 of air imparts a strong odor to the air; 0.3 to 0.35 volumes per 1,000 is the strongest concentration bearable for half an hour. It does not act as a real poison, however, but only as an irritant upon the mucous membrane, which can be borne much better by those accustomed to it. Mixtures of two volumes per 1,000 when inhaled for a long time, or five volumes per 1,000 for a short time, produce a severe and consequently dangerous irritation of the respiratory organs and the mucous membrane of the eye, but only locally, without causing injury to the other organs or their functions. One per cent is liable to be fatal.

It has one advantage shared by sulphur dioxide, that it,

940. DENNIS, L. M.: Gas Analysis, 382, 1913; TASHIRIA: Proc. Soc. Biol. Chem., 14:41, 1912.

itself, is a warning agent. Ammonia under high pressure may form an explosive mixture, especially in combination with oil vapor. It is combustible when admixed with air, the proportion being 16.1% by volume lower limit, 26.4% upper limit.

Many accidents have occurred from pipes breaking in cold-storage plants or cylinder heads blowing out, the concentration of the gas being so great as to cause death within a few minutes. Two very serious accidents, causing the death of a number of men, occurred in a large packing house in Chicago, in 1907. "The alterations in respiration and the action of the heart as the result of inhaling ammonia are produced reflexly from the irritation of the upper respiratory tract. This reaction consists in a general vasoconstriction and considerable increase of breathing; if the concentration is high respiration is stopped. The effects of inhaled ammonia are entirely upon surface tissues; none is absorbed."[941]

TABLE XLVI

PHYSIOLOGICAL RESPONSE TO VARIOUS CONCENTRATIONS OF AMMONIA

	Parts of Ammonia per million parts of air.
Least detectable odor*	53
Least amount causing immediate irritation to the eye*	698
Least amount causing immediate irritation to the throat*	408
Least amount causing coughing*	1,720
Maximum concentration allowable for prolonged exposure‡†	100
Maximum concentration allowable for short exposure (one-half to one hour)‡†	300 to 500
Dangerous for even short exposure (one-half hour)†	2,500 to 4,500
Rapidly fatal for short exposure	5,000 to 10,000

* (U. S. Dept. of Interior, Bureau of Mines, Technical Paper, 248, 1921.)
‡ (RONZANI, E.: *Arch. f. Hyg.*, 70:217, 1909.)
† (LEHMANN, K.: *Arch. f. Hyg.*, 5:1, 1886.)
(HENDERSON, Y., and HAGGARD, H. W.: Noxious Gases, Monograph Series No. 35, 1927.)

Tests: Characteristic odor, compare known amounts with color obtained with Nessler's Reagent, or weigh as ammonium platinic chloride.

941. HENDERSON and HAGGARD: Noxious Gases, Monograph Series, No. 35, 126, 1927.

DICHLORMETHANE (CH₂Cl₂)
(Molecular Weight 85)

DICHLORMETHANE has a density (air=1) of 3, and a boiling point of 105° C. It is a white water liquid at normal atmospheric temperature and pressure. It is very similar to dichlorethylene. It is, however, non-combustible, resembling trichlorethylene in this respect. With regard to combustibility, the Underwriters' Laboratories of Chicago, in their report on the fire hazard of dichlormethane as a refrigerant, draw the following conclusions: "The general fire hazard of dichlormethane is judged to be very much less than that of ammonia. At normal temperature mixtures of dichlormethane vapors with air in certain proportions are capable of weakly propagating flame when subjected to strong sources of ignition. At high temperature the vapors are moderately combustible."

The apparent ignition point of dichlormethane is relatively high, 662°C. (1223.6°F.) Mixtures of dichlormethane are not readily ignited by application of sparks or flame. The minimum fatal concentrations in five-hour test runs are: dichlormethane 5% by volume, dichlorethylene 2.7%, carbon tetrachloride 1.6%, trichlorethylene 1.5%.

DICHLORODIFLUOROMETHANE

TO OVERCOME some of the difficulties of the other refrigerants in domestic and refrigerating appliances, a new compound, dichlorodifluoromethane, known to the trade as F-12 was introduced. CF₂Cl₂, is a clear water white liquid, boiling at —21.6°F. (—29.8°C.).[942] For the thermodynamic properties of dichlorodifluoromethane the A. S. R. E. Circular No. 12, A. S. R. E. Data Book, 1931, should be consulted.[943]

Sayers, Yant, Chornyak and Shoaf[944] report that dogs, monkeys, and guinea pigs were exposed to air containing 20% by volume of dichlorodifluoromethane vapor for seven to eight hours daily on five days, and for four hours on the sixth day of each week during a twelve-week period. This exposure produces mild to moderate to marked generalized tremor in dogs and mild to moderate generalized tremor in monkeys.

942. TROUTAN, HILLDEBRAND: *J. Indust. & Eng. Chem.*, 4:23, 1931.
943. See Tech. Papers Nos. 1 to 12 of the Kinetic Chemicals, Inc., Wilmington, Delaware.
944. SAYERS, R. R., YANT, W. P., CHORNYAK, J., and SHOAF, H. W.: U. S. Bureau of Mines, Dept. of Commerce, R. I. 3013, May, 1930.

When they attempt to walk, they act very much like persons suffering from alcoholic ataxia. They react to light and stimuli, and do not become unconscious. The maximum severity of symptoms is reached in the first ten to twenty minutes of an exposure. A tolerance is developed with

TABLE XLVII

PHYSIOLOGICAL RESPONSE TO VARIOUS CONCENTRATIONS OF SOME COMMON GASES AND VAPORS IN AIR

Vapor or Gas	A Kills most animals in a very short time		B Dangerous in 30 to 60 minutes	
	Per cent by volume	Relative Order	Per cent by volume	Relative Order
Phosgene..........	0.02— 0.05	1	0.0025	1
Chlorine..........	.10	2	[1,2].004— .006	2
Bromine..........	.1	3	.004— .006	3
Hydrogen sulphide....	[2].06— .10 / [1].1 — .20 / [3].1 — .30	4	[1,2].05 — .07	6
Hydrocyanic acid.....	[2].048	5	[1,3].012— .015	4
Hydrogen chloride....	[1].1 — .2 / [2].5	6	.15 — .2	7
Sulphur dioxide......	[2].2	7	.04 — .05	5
Carbon monoxide.....	[2].5 — 1	8	.2 — .3 / .2	8
Ammonia...........	.5 — 1	9	.25 — .45	10
Benzene...........	1.9	10	No data	
Gasoline..........	2.4	11	1.1 — 2.2	11
Methyl bromide......	[5]2 — 4	12	[5].2 — .4	9
Chloroform.........	[1]6.8 — 8.2	[4]13	1.4	12
Carbon tetrachloride..	4.8 — 6.3	14	2.4 — 3.2	14
Ethyl bromide.......	[5]10 — 20	15	[5]1 — 2	13
Methyl chloride......	[5]15 — 30	16	[5]2 — 4	15
Ethyl chloride.......	[5]15 — 30	17	[5]6 —10	16
Carbon dioxide......	[2]30		[2]6 — 8	....

Vapor or Gas	C Maximum amount for 60 minutes without serious disturbances		D Slight symptoms after several hours or maximum amount for prolonged exposure	
	Per cent by volume	Relative Order	Per cent by volume	Relative Order
Phosgene..........	No data	0	0.0001	1
Chlorine..........	0.0004	2	.0001	1
Bromine..........	.02 — .03	7	[1].01 — .015	7
Hydrogen sulphide...	.02 — .03	7	[1].01 — .015 / [2].02	7
Hydrocyanic acid.....	.005— .006	4	.002— .004	3
Hydrogen chloride....	.005— .01	5	.001— .005	4
Sulphur dioxide......	[1].005— .02	6	[2].01 / [3].001	[4]2
Carbon monoxide....	[2].05 — .10 / [1].05	9	[1].05 / [2].04	9
Ammonia..........	[2].03	8	[1].01	6
Benzene...........	.31 — .47	11	[3].15 — .31	13
Gasoline...........	.43 — .71	14	No data	0
Methyl bromide......	[5].1	10	[5].005 — .017	5
Chloroform.........	.5 — .6	13	[2].2	8
Carbon tetrachloride..	.4 — .6	12	.16	11
Ethyl bromide.......	[5].6	15	[5].17 — .3	12
Methyl chloride......	[5].7	16	[5].05 — .10	10
Ethyl chloride	[5]4	17	[5]2	14
Carbon dioxide.......	[2]4 — 6	....	[2]2 — 3	....

1 Bureau of Mines Technical Paper 248, 1921.　　2 International Critical Tables, vol. II, 1927. 3 HENDERSON, YANDELL, and HAGGARD, H. W., Noxious Gases, A. C. S. Monograph No. 35, 1927.　　4 Depending on value taken.
5 Data from Figures 2, 3, 4, and 5, of Public Health Bulletin No. 185.
Where no reference number is given results are from references 1, 2, and 3.

(Table from U. S. Bureau of Mines, Report of Investigations, R.I. 3013, May, 1930.)

successive exposures, as manifested by decrease in severity of the symptoms. Guinea pigs exhibit no significant symptoms. The number of red blood cells and hemoglobin tended toward a slight increase during the first two or three weeks of the test, but thereafter was normal and similar to control animals; also, the number of white cells was the same as the controls. Differential white cell examinations showed a slight increase in the polymorphonuclear neutrophils and a slight decrease in lymphocytes in the blood of animals exposed to dichlorodifluoromethane. "No fatalities occurred among the dogs and monkeys. The fatality among the guinea pigs used for symptoms, weight, and fatality observations was two out of a group of sixteen exposed to gas, and one out of a group of sixteen controls during the twelve-week period, thus indicating no effect of exposure on fatality." Autopsies performed on all animals revealed no gross pathology attributable to the exposure to dichlorodifluoromethane. "In so far as the results of animal experimentation serve as a measure of hazards to persons, the investigation has shown that the possibilities of public health and accident hazards resulting from exposure to dichlorodifluoromethane when used as a refrigerant are remote."

ACROLEIN (C_2H_3CHO)

ACROLEIN occurs chiefly when fats are strongly heated by the oxidation of glycerine. Pure acrolein is a colorless liquid which boils at 52° C. It is soluble in two to three parts of water, ether, ethanol, or methyl chloride. It has a vapor pressure at 10°C. of 137 mm., and at 30°C. of 330 mm. On exposure to the air it slowly oxidizes to acrylic aldehyde.

Acrolein is liberated from the boiling of lubricating oil. It is often found in the exhaust gases from internal combustion engines. It is used as a tracer gas in the refrigerant methyl chloride. It is very irritating to the mucous membranes, acting upon the upper respiratory tract in relatively low concentrations when inhaled. Chemical Warfare Service reports that the lowest concentration at which 60% of the white mice used in an experiment died was 0.3 to 0.4 mg. per liter; the substance was inhaled for ten minutes. Irritation of the nose is produced at a concentration of 0.09 mg., irritation of the throat at 0.01 mg., and lacrimation is produced at 0.015 mg. It responds to tests for aldehydes.

ALKALOIDAL POISONS

M OST alkaloids are of vegetable origin, although certain ones, such as epinephrine, may be of animal or synthetic origin. They are physiologically active in very minute doses, acting rather specifically on the nervous system, i.e., they are specific nerve protoplasmic poisons. The physiologic effects observed depend upon the site of action and the species of animal. In general, the greater the nervous development of a species, the greater are the effects produced. For example, the fatal dose of morphine in frogs is approximately 750 mg. per kg., while in man the fatal dose is about 2 mg. per kg. The fatal dose of strychnine in a frog is about 100 mg. per kg. and in man about 0.75 mg. per. kg. Poisoning by alkaloids, accidental or intentional, is one of the more common forms of poisoning. It occurred even in ancient times. One of the most noted cases of poisoning in ancient times was the death of Socrates from drinking hemlock, of which the active principle is coniine.

Alkaloids may be defined as substances containing carbon, hydrogen, nitrogen, and, with two notable exceptions, oxygen. They are feebly basic substances, insoluble in water, but forming water soluble salts with inorganic acids. The nitrogen nearly always forms a link in a closed carbon chain. The more common nuclei about which the structures are built are pyridine, pyrrol (see page 455), quinoline, and isoquinoline. The salts formed are additive rather than substitutional products. Most of the alkaloids are optically active. Slight changes in the structural arrangement of alkaloids many times greatly modify their physiological action. For instance, the addition of a methyl group to the hydroxyl at 3 in morphine greatly reduces its toxicity and its addiction power; while having less effect in reducing, its properties are changed still further. Likewise the structural relationship between atropine and cocaine may be seen by studying their formulas. The physiological effects and therapeutic uses of these two drugs are quite different. The addition or substitution and the removal of such radicals as hydroxyl, methyl, ethyl, propyl, etc., acetyl, phenyl, etc., or their tautomeric rearrangement, may greatly modify or even destroy the physiological effects. The future offers great hope in the synthesis of new alkaloids which are more specific for certain actions and are

less toxic.   Chemists are attempting to increase the margin
of safety between the therapeutic and toxic doses.   In the
drug addiction laboratories of the Universities of Virginia and
Michigan, just such an attempt is being made to correlate
physiological activity with changes in chemical structure. The
following are the structural formulas for the common alkaloidal nuclei

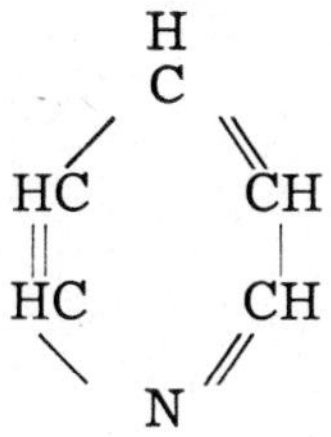

Pyridine

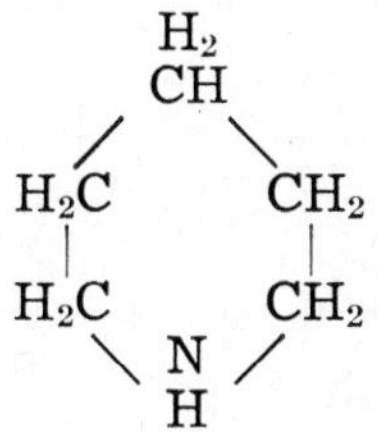

Piperidine

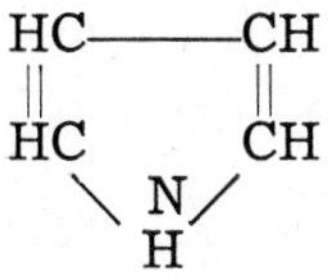

Pyrrol

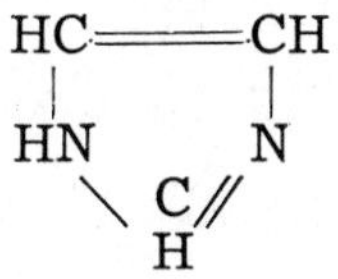

Glyoxalin

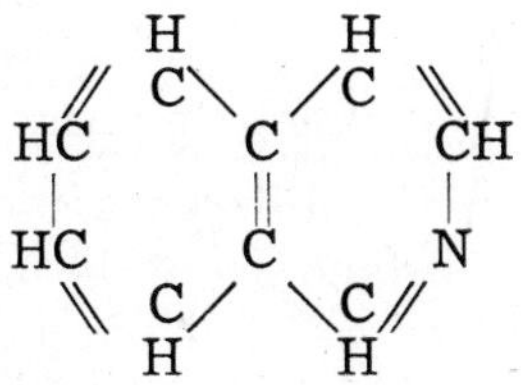

Isoquinoline

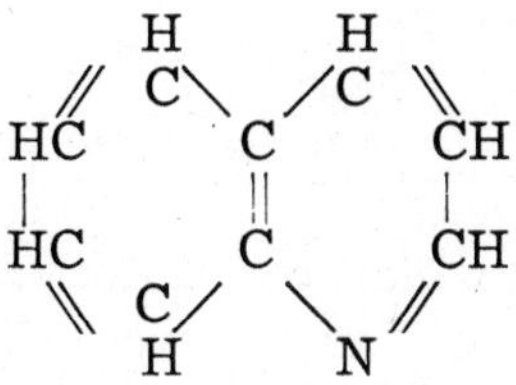

Quinoline

The nitrogen is in the form of either a secondary or
tertiary amine, usually the latter.

Identification of Akaloids: The identification ot alkaloids
is based upon their separation from animal tissues and their
recognition by characteristic tests.   Ptomaines are the chief
substances liable to be confused with alkaloids in analysis.

They are formed by bacterial decomposition of animal and vegetable proteins and are usually open carbon chains. Indol is an example of a closed chain, while cadaverine is an example of an open chain and incidentally a primary amine. Indol is a secondary amine. Although certain ptomaines resemble some of the vegetable alkaloids, they are never identical. Some of the alkaloids simulated by ptomaines are aconitine, coniine, codeine, colchicine, strychnine, and veratrine. Differentiation of these drugs from ptomaines may be found under their respective headings.

The identification of alkaloids may be made on extracted material, on the original sample which may be the free alkaloid, or on a salt of the crude drug made by studying their color reactions, precipitation reactions, melting points, optical rotation, biological activity, and pharmacognosy. While the alkaloids have rather definite solubilities in various liquids either as the free alkaloids or as salt, this property is used for separation rather than identification. In making analyses, it is also important to run suitable controls. In case of doubt, check the agents with known drugs. Most of the tests for alkaloids are rather delicate, particularly the color reactions, and amounts far less than therapeutic quantities can be identified. In extracting tissues there is an inevitable loss of the substance being recovered, and the tissue used is only a fraction of the entire body in which the drug may be more or less uniformly distributed. It is thus seen that delicate tests are rather essential.

(a) Color Reactions: Some substances not alkaloidal, especially closely related to alkaloids, give similar tests. However, in practically every case slight differences will be found which can differentiate the substances. It is usually necessary to run several tests to rule out all but one definite alkaloid. It is important in some color tests to note the sequence of shades and color changes. A final color may be entirely different from the initial color. In performing these color reactions it is rather obvious that there should be no impurities present. The presence of a ptomaine might obscure the picture, or the presence of more than one alkaloid may lead to error. It would be well to run side by side with the unknown substance, a known sample of the suspected alkaloid, or several samples if necessary, and identify the unknown by the direct simultaneous comparison of the color changes. These tests are usually best made by placing a particle of the solid residue on a porcelain titration plate, or white porcelain, and adding to this a drop of reagent with a small glass rod. The color reaction of alkaloids may be classified according to Henry[945] as:

It is produced by dehydrating agents such as concentrated sulphuric acid;

It is given by oxidizing agents, such as nitric acid, chlorine, sulphuric acid, potassium dichromate, manganese dioxide, lead oxide, cerosoceric oxide, etc.;

It is yielded by oxidizing agents which on their reduction, produce color productions, such as, iodic acid, chromic, molybdic, tungstic, and vanadic acids;

It is produced by special reagents such as ferric chloride.

1. Concentrated Sulphuric Acid: No color or only a faint straw color is given with aconitine, atropine, cocaine, codeine, scopolamine, gelsemine, morphine, nicotine, quinine, quinidine, and strychnine. Mere traces of impurities, either in the reagent or the alkaloid, may produce a color. Morphine may turn light red and gelsemine yellow to brown. Yellow, orange, or brown colorations are given by berberine, delphinine, gelsemine, and lobeline. Veratrine has an initial yellow coloration. Red, purple, or violet colors are given by impure aconitine, apomorphine, brucine, impure cocaine, coniine, impure gelsemine, nicotine, and physostigmine.

2. Concentrated Nitric Acid: No color with aconitine, atropine, cinchonine, coniine, gelsemine, morphine, nicotine, or veratrine. Red, purple, or violet colors are given by impure aconitine, apomorphine, berberine, brucine, and physostigmine. Impure morphine may be red.

3. Molybdic Sulphuric Acid (Froehde's Reagent): This reagent is prepared by dissolving one or two mg. of molybdic acid in 1 cc. of concentrated sulphuric acid. Older directions specify as high as 5 or 10 mg. of molybdic acid per cc., but higher concentrations lessen the sensitivity of the reagent. Sodium molybdate may be used in place of molybdic acid. This reagent is rather specific for morphine, although some other drugs give color reactions. This reagent should be freshly prepared. Morphine is at first violet-red, then changes

945. Allen's Commercial Organic Analysis, 4th ed. 6:198, 1912.

to a dirty green, yellow, and finally pink.   No other alkaloid gives these same color changes.   No color is given by atropine, cinchonine, hyoscyamine, nicotine, scopolamine, and strychnine.   Yellowish colorations are produced by aconitine and colchicine.   Red shades are noted with brucine and veratrine. Blue is given by codeine; green by apomorphine, berberine, and quinine.

4. Vanadic-Sulphuric Acid (Mandelin's Reagent): Dissolve 5 mg. of ammonium vanadate in concentrated sulphuric acid.   This reagent is most distinctive in its test for strychnine, the initial color being deep violet-blue, changing to deep purple and then to cherry-red, and on long standing, becoming yellow.

5. Formalin Sulphuric Acid (Marquis' Reagent):   This reagent is made by mixing one drop of formalin (40% formaldehyde solution) in 1 cc. of concentrated sulphuric acid. This reagent is of special value in the detection of morphine.

6. Selenious Sulphuric Acid (Mecke's Reagent):   Dissolve 5 mg. of selenious acid in 1 cc. of sulphuric acid.[946]

Mecke's Reagent: 0.5 gm. selenious acid dissolved in 100 cc. concentrated sulphuric acid.   The test is specific for substances containing the phenol group.   Nitro groups interfere completely with the reaction.   The test is not distinctive for morphine alkaloids; a negative test is conclusive but a positive is not.   Phenols, p. cresol, tyrosine, pyrocatechin, hydroquinine, adrenaline, are phenolic compounds of biologic occurrence and give a color reaction.

7. Arsenic Sulphuric Acid (Rosenthaler Reagent): Dissolve 10 mg. of potassium arsenate in 1 cc. of concentrated sulphuric acid.

8. Perhydrol-Sulphuric Acid (Schaer's Reagent): Dissolve 0.1 cc. of Merck's pure 30% perhydrol (30% hydrogen peroxide) in 1 cc. of concentrated sulphuric acid.   Always prepare fresh before using.   This reagent is of special value in the opium group and the atropine group.

9. Nitric Sulphuric Acid (Erdmann's Reagent): Mix one drop of 1% nitric acid in 2 cc. of sulphuric acid.   (See No. 2.)

(b) **Precipitation Reagents:**   To determine the presence of alkaloids in unpurified residues obtained in the extraction

946. LEVINE, V. E.:   *J. Lab. & Clin. Med.,* 11:809, 1926.

processes (see the section on General Considerations, page 30). General reagents, known as alkaloidal precipitants are employed. Many, if not all, of these reagents also precipitate protein material, so that the purification processes must be very carefully conducted before one is able to draw any conclusions from the results obtained. In performing the test for the presence of alkaloids by the use of these general precipitants, great care must be taken to conserve the material, as the residues are usually very small. The method used by Gadamer[947] is very efficient and reliable. A small portion of the dried residue obtained in the extraction process is treated with a single drop of 2% sulphuric acid and slightly warmed to bring it into solution. By means of a fine pointed glass tube transfer a portion of the solution to a small watch glass resting upon a black background and then add a small drop of reagent. If an alkaloid is present, a precipitate will be observed at the point of contact of the two liquids, or even throughout the mixture. The most serviceable and reliable of these three agents are the following:

1. Iodine Solution (Wagner's Reagent): Prepare the solution by dissolving 18 gm. of potassium iodide in about 90 cc. of distilled water and then dissolving 12.692 gm. of iodine crystals in the solution. Dilute this solution to 1000 cc. and a decinormal solution is obtained. For rough qualitative work, one part of iodine, two parts potassium iodide, and 100 parts of water may be used. The reagent must be used in acidulated solutions, not alcoholic, and added in excess. The precipitates of varying shades of dark brown to black are flocculent and amorphous, although they may become crystalline. Sodium thiosulphate dissolves the alkaloidal precipitate the periodide being reduced to a hydriodide. When the latter is made alkaline and treated with an immiscible solvent the pure alkaloid is recovered.

2. Potassium Mercuric Iodide Solution (Mayer's Reagent): For qualitative use, add to a solution of mercuric chloride a little more than enough of a solution of potassium iodide to dissolve the colored precipitate at first formed. (13.576 gm. of mercuric chloride and 49.8 gm. of potassium iodide dissolved in distilled water and diluted to one liter.) For quantitative

947. Lehrbuch der Chemischen Toxikologie, Göttingen, 482, 1909.

purposes, the solution should be N/20, containing 6.798 gm. of mercuric chloride and 25 gm. of potassium iodide dissolved in one liter of distilled water. This reagent should be applied in an acidulated solution in the absence of alcohol and acetic acid. The precipitates are yellowish white in color, and are crystalline or become so on standing. On treating the precipitate with stannous chloride, then adding caustic potash to alkalinize, and extracting with an immiscible solvent the free alkaloid is obtained. Van der Heyde[948] recommends this reagent as the most delicate and reliable for detecting atropine in small quantities of blood serum.

3. Potassium Cadmium Iodide Solution (Marme's Reagent): An excess of cadmium iodide is added to a boiling saturated solution of potassium iodide. When no more goes into solution an equal volume of cold saturated solution of potassium iodide is added. For qualitative work this reagent is made by dissolving 10 gm. of potassium iodide and 5 gm. of cadmium iodide in 100 cc. of water. The reagent is used in an acid solution in the absence of alcohol. The precipitates are flocculent and crystalline and are soluble in an excess of this reagent or in alcohol. On treating with alkali and extracting with the proper solvent, the free alkaloid is obtained.

4. Potassium Bismuth Iodide Solution (Dragendorff's Reagent): This reagent is prepared the same as the preceding, substituting bismuth iodide for cadmium iodide. Used in acidified aqueous solutions, it produces orange-red precipitates.

5. Phosphomolybdic Acid (DeVry's Reagent): Dissolve 150 gm. of ammonium molybdate in a liter of water and add this solution slowly to a liter of concentrated nitric acid. Add a warm solution of sodium phosphate until precipitation of ammonium-phosphomolybdate is complete. The yellow precipitate is filtered, washed with water, and dissolved in hot sodium carbonate. The solution is evaporated to dryness and ignited at low red heat until all ammonium salts are volatilized. The residue is moistened with nitric acid and again ignited. The sodium phosphomolybdate thus produced is then dissolved in ten times its weight of a mixture of one volume of concentrated nitric acid and nine volumes of distilled water, to obtain the final reagent. This reagent forms yellow amorphous precipitates with most alkaloids, some becoming crystalline on

948. Van der Heyde: *J. Lab. & Clin. Med.*, 7:280, 1922.

standing. Some alkaloids which possess a reducing action turn blue or dissolve with a blue color when ammonia is added. These are aconitine, atropine, berberine, codeine, colchicine, coniine, morphine, nicotine, and physostigmine.

6. Phospho-Tungstic Acid (Scheibler's Reagent): Dissolve 100 parts of sodium tungstate and 60 to 80 parts of sodium phosphate in 500 parts of water and add nitric acid until distinctly acid. Alkaloids may be recovered from their phospho-tungstate precipitates by mixing the moist precipitates with sodium carbonate and extracting rapidly with strong alcohol.

7. Bromine and Hydrobromic Acid (Wormley's Reagent): Hydrobromic acid is saturated with bromine. The precipitates are usually yellow and amorphous. This reagent is of value in micro-chemical work.

Freshly prepared solution of tannic acid precipitates alkaloids nearly quantitatively in neutral solution. They dissolve in acid solution.

9. Picric Acid (Hager's Reagent): This reagent gives yellow crystalline precipitates of many alkaloids. Nelson and Leonard[949] state that the most commonly occurring alkaloids may be identified with the microscope by their picrate crystals prepared under standard conditions.

10. Picrolonic Acid (Knorr's Reagent): This reagent precipitates alkaloids practically quantitatively. Picrolonic acid is 1 p-nitro-phenyl, 3 methyl, 4 nitro, 5 pyrazolon. Prepare 600 cc. of 90% nitric acid, keeping it ice-cold in a wide-mouthed bottle. Add 200 gm. of methyl-phenyl-pyrazolon, 1 gm. at a time keeping it stirred constantly, preferably with a mechanical stirrer and maintaining the temperature below fifteen degrees. The preparation should be carried out in a hood. When all of the methyl-phenyl-pyrazolon has been added stir the mixture for thirty minutes, filter by suction in a Buchner funnel covered with asbestos, and wash with dilute nitric acid and then with water. This crude production, which is trinitro-methyl-pheny-pyrazolon, is treated with 1,500 cc. of 33% acetic acid and stirred for twenty to forty minutes at not over 60° C. on a water-bath. The yellow crystals formed are placed in a Buchner funnel and washed with water. They are

949. NELSON and LEONARD: J. Am. Chem. Soc., 44:369, 1922.

ground in the water with 150 gm. of crystallized sodium pyrazolate and carbon dioxide. The salt is recrystallized from 75% alcohol. Small portions of the crystals are added to warm concentrated hydrochloric acid. Picrolonic acid separates as yellow meal powder. It is washed with water on an asbestos filter to remove the acid and sodium chloride. For use it is dissolved in alcohol in saturated solution. About 2.1 gm. are soluble in 100 cc. The precipitates formed by picrolonic acid are yellow or red, and decompose on heating. To recover the alkaloid from its picrolate, the latter is warmed with dilute sulphuric acid, with alkaloid passing into solution and picrolonic acid precipitating in pale yellow crystals. This mixture is extracted with acetic ether, the picrolonic acid passing into the ether and the alkaloid remaining in the aqueous solution. This reagent is of value in purifying strychnine, coniine, nicotine, brucine, morphine, codeine, atropine, quinine, and hydrastine. Aconitine, cocaine, and caffeine do not furnish definite compounds.

11. Platinum and Gold Chloride: These, as other heavy metals, form double salts with alkaloids. They are quite insoluble and crystalline. An estimation of the platinum or gold content gives a quantitative determination of the alkaloid.

The fact that a precipitate, or turbid solution is obtained with any of the above reagents, does not in itself signify the presence of an alkaloid. Leukomains, ptomaines, or even proteins, may still be present in the partially purified extracts. Careful purification with alcohol or other solvents should remove all traces of protein matter. Leukomains may be precipitated by potassium mercuric iodide, phosphomolybdic acid, or iodine. This is actually no more than a turbidity. Even a considerable precipitate is not proof that a poisonous alkaloid is present. This specific test should be run on the residue, such as the color tests or biologic tests already enumerated. Most alkaloids are better recognized by their color reactions, but certain ones are most conclusively proved by their biologic reaction. These are aconitine and atropine, while strychnine and cocaine biologic tests give very strong confirmation.

Stability of Alkaloids: Some alkaloids are quite stable in the presence of putrefying organic matter, notably strychnine, while others deteriorate rapidly. Morphine is detected with difficulty. Davoll took nine portions of putrefied material (reported as the organs of an animal buried forty-five days in a container, "a tight wooden box," in March and April) and extracted them first with alcohol acidified with acetic acid, later with hot amyl alcohol.[950] The final extracts prepared for qualitative reactions gave no indication of morphine. LeFort's test was made with iodic acid followed by ammonia. In all cases, however, the ordinary test of iodic acid and starch gave the blue color of liberated iodine.   To determine the trust-worthiness of (1) LeFort's and Froehde's test; (2) the method of extraction from tissue presented under the heading of Morphine (page 565); and (3) the liability of interference from production of tissue putrefaction when air is excluded, the following experiment was performed by Prescott:[951] About 2.5 kg. of finely chopped ox-liver were placed in a large bottle (a) securely stoppered with a perforated cork connected with a bent glass tube. The cork was sealed with paraffin and the outer end of the glass tube was allowed to dip into a cistern of mercury, thoroughly excluding all communication with the outside air. Putrefaction was now allowed to go on in a warm room for about fifty days. Gas was given out during the earlier part of the decomposition. Into another bottle (B) another 2.5 kg. of finely chopped ox-liver were placed with 0.52 gm. of morphine intermixed (about one part in 5,000) and this bottle sealed in a similar manner and set aside for thirty-five days. Contents of bottle (a) gave absolutely negative results with Froehde's reagent and LeFort's reagent and extracted by the process detailed under Morphine (page 565), or by Kippen-berger's proposed process. From bottle (B) the positive test for morphine, by the LeFort reagent, was obtained from a portion extracted by the method detailed under Morphine, while the portion extracted according to Kippenberger's method[952] yielded negative results.

To investigate the loss of alkaloid under conditions of actual animal poisoning, when the poison is physiologically distributed among the tissues with putrefactive changes in confinement from air after death, Smith and Prescott pro-

950. DAVOLL: *J. Am. Chem. Soc.*, 16:805, 1894.

951. PETERSON, HAINES, and WEBSTER: Legal Medicine and Toxi-cology, 434, 1923.

952. SMITH, H. T.: in work under Prescott's observation, University of Michigan, 1894.

ceeded as follows: 1.5 gm. of morphine were given by mouth to a 15-kg. dog. Two hours later the animal was killed by anesthesia and the body placed in a sheet iron box hermetically sealed on February 20. In the following month a 30-kg. dog was killed with anesthesia without the administration, and the body sealed up the same as the other. The two boxes were buried on March 20, in a wooden case three feet under the soil. On May 8, after seven weeks' burial and ten and a half weeks of enclosure of the body containing morphine, the two boxes were exhumed. The box containing the larger body, the one sealed up later, had burst from gas pressure within and its contents were in a state of decomposition more advanced than that of the small body. From each body the stomach, the intestines, and the liver were taken together for analysis by the method given under Morphine for separation from tissues, and also by the process proposed by Kippenberger. In the final results each of the putrefied extracts from the body of the animal poisoned by morphine gave distinct reactions for morphine by Froehde's test and LeFort's test, but gave no reactions for morphine with the ferric chloride, sulphuric and nitric test. The control animal, not poisoned, gave no reactions for morphine. With Kippenberger's process, the final residues failed to yield any reaction for morphine.

Quantitative Determination of Alkaloids: The quantitative estimation of an alkaloid in tissues examined can be only an approximate one. If the final residue is not sufficiently purified, a positive error arises; while the attempt to procure a perfectly pure alkaloid leads to more or less loss of substance, thus introducing a very decided minus error. The analyst must report his finding as so much alkaloid actually recovered and be content with this approximate result, never going so far as to state that the amount reported represents the exact quantity of alkaloid present in the tissues. It is not always possible to obtain quantitative values of the alkaloids, owing to the very small amount sometimes isolated, yet in every case of toxicological importance some statement regarding quantities isolated must be given.

A gravimetric method is the most satisfactory. This consists in weighing the amount of pure alkaloid isolated from a given quantity of tissue. The amount of tissue employed in the extraction should be an aliquot part of the total weight of the special tissue. Having determined the amount of the alkaloid in the tissue extracted, a simple calculation will yield the total quantity in the whole organ, assuming, of course, that the alkaloid is equally distributed throughout the organ.

As a check upon the gravimetric determination dissolve the residue after weighing, in 1 cc. of alcohol or ether. A volumetric estimation of the alkaloid present is made by adding a known volume of N/100 sulphuric acid and a little water to the dissolved alkaloidal residue. Warm slightly to insure complete solution of the alkaloid and titrate to excess of acid present, using N/100 sodium hydrate solution as the neutralizing agent, and cochineal, methyl-red, or iodeosin as an indicator. Subtraction of the amount of alkali solution added to produce a neutral reaction from the amount of N/100 acid originally employed yields that amount of acid combined with the alkaloid. Each cubic centimeter of N/100 acid thus combined represents 1/100,000 of the molecular weight of the alkaloid to be determined expressed in grams.

ACONITUM

A CONITE is the dried tuberous root of Aconitum napellus, commonly known as monkshood. The unground roots measure from 1 to 3.5 cm. in diameter by 4 to 10 cm. in length, and are of a fusiform shape. They are dark brown and marked with coarse whitish root scars longitudinally wrinkled, internally whitish and light brown and having a very slight odor. They have a sweetish taste, producing in a few minutes a tingling and numbness of the lips and tongue. The powder is grayish-brown, and the starch granules are .0.003 to 0.02 mm. in diameter. There are several alkaloids in the drug, but the chief one of toxicological importance is aconitine. Aconitine is acetyl-benzoyl-aconine $(C_{34}H_{47}NO_{11})$. The total alkaloidal content of the root varies from 0.75% to 1%. Commercial aconitine usually has some of the relatively inert alkaloids present and therefore must be standardized. Chemical analysis will not show the absolute percentage of aconitine present in the root, therefore physiological tests must be made. The small amount necessary to cause certain effects is not detectable by chemical means. Aconitine is crystallizable from alcohol, forming colorless, rhombic prisms or plates. The bitter taste of aconite is due to the less poisonous alkaloids present as impurities. Both aconitine and tincture of aconite are standardized by assay on guinea pigs. U.S.P. X specifies that aconite shall assay between .055 and .065 mg. per kg. body weight MLD. The tincture shall assay between 0.35 and 0.45 cc. per kg. MLD. In these tests guinea pigs shall weigh between 275 and 325 gm., and two of three guinea pigs shall be killed within six hours.

Aconitine forms white crystals which, when heated rapidly at 195° C. (383° F.), will melt. When heated slowly, decomposition takes place and it melts at 182° C. (359.6° F.), but when ignited it leaves no residue. The hydrochloride melts at 149° C., the hydrobromide at 163° C., and the nitrate at 198° C. Aconitine is soluble in 3,200 parts of water and 3,580 parts of benzine. It is soluble in alcohol in the ratio of one to twenty-eight, in ether at the ratio of one to sixty-five and in benzene at one to seven. It is very soluble in chloroform. The optical rotation for aconitine in ethyl alcohol in 3.73% solution is (a) 23°/D= 11.01. A 1.95% solution of aconitine hydrobromide in water has a specific rotation of (a) 20°/D=30.47.

Identification: Since aconitine is a fairly unstable alkaloid its recovery and identification are difficult. The alkaloid readily undergoes hydrolysis, breaking down even in boiling water and yielding acetic acid, benzoic acid, and aconine ($C_{25}H_{41}NO_9$). Aconine is easily soluble in water, and is more bitter than aconitine, but does not produce the same physiological effects. Its specific rotation in water is (a) D= —23, being dextrorotatory.

Chemical Tests:

1. PRECIPITATION: The general precipitating reagents give precipitates with aconitine. Gold chloride gives a yellow amorphous precipitate which can be crystallized from alcohol. This salt ($C_{34}H_{47}NO_{11}HCl\ AuCl_3$) melts at 145° C. and contains 20% gold. The hydrate with three molecules of water melts at 136° C. and contains 19% gold.

2. MOLYBDIC-SULPHURIC ACID REAGENT (Froehde's): This reagent when added to the salt residue obtained from extraction gives a blue color turning green.

3. SELENIOUS-SULPHURIC ACID (Mecke's): This gives no color in the cold, but on warming a dark brown to violet color is produced.

4. RESORCIN-SULPHURIC ACID: A portion of the solid

residue is warmed with a few drops of concentrated sulphuric acid and a small crystal of resorcin added. The color becomes orange to yellowish-red.

5. ALVAREZ'S REACTION: A portion of the solid residue is treated with five to ten drops of pure bromine. Heat on a water-bath and add 1 to 2 cc. of concentrated nitric acid and evaporate to dryness adding a little more bromine as the nitric acid loses its color in the process. Add 0.5 to 1 cc. of saturated alcoholic sodium hydroxide and again evaporate to dryness. The residue becomes red to brown depending on the amount of aconitine present. When cool add five to six drops of 10% copper sulphate solution, and a deep green color will be produced. This green color will be given by as little as 0.1 mg. of aconitine. None of the better known alkaloids was found by Alvarez to give this reaction.[953]

6. PHOSPHOMOLYBDIC ACID TEST (Palet):[954] Prepare the reagent by dissolving one gm. of sodium molybdate in 25 gm. of concentrated (85%) phosphoric acid. Add a few drops of this to a portion of the purified solid residue and heat directly over a small flame until vapors appear. A brilliant violet color indicates the presence of aconitine.

Biological Tests:

1. TINGLING OF THE LIPS: An aqueous solution of the free alkaloid or salt is bitter and produces numbness and tingling. A single drop of a solution containing one mg. in 100 cc. (one to 100,000) can be detected by this test. An extract of 6 mg. of the root in 4 cc. will produce a tingling and numbness which may last as long as one-half hour.

2. ANIMAL EXPERIMENTS: A solution injected hypodermically in a mouse or into the lymph-sac of a frog will cause the death of the animal within an hour when it contains as little as 1 mg. of aconitine in 100 cc., or 20 mg. of aconite root extracted into a 4-cc. solution. An electrocardiographic tracing of the heart action shows the muscles in tetany followed by a peculiar wave-like action with final arrest in diastole.

Pathology:

1. There are no characteristic changes seen at autopsy: The lung, liver, kidneys and brain are generally found somewhat congested. Effusions may be observed in the

953. *Chem. News*, 91:179, 1905.
954. *J. Pharm. Chem.*, 19:295, 1919; *Analyst*, 46:193, 1921.

pericardium and in the ventricles of the brain. The stomach is somewhat reddened. The blood is found abnormally fluid, and sometimes is a bright red color.

2. Separation of aconitine from the tissues:

Precautions must be taken to avoid hydrolysis of the alkaloid. The process directed for atropine may be used, extracting with alcohol at room temperature for a time and then at a temperature of not over 60° C. Then allow the extracts to stand in an icebox, remove the fat and evaporate the filtrate at a low temperature under a vacuum, using ether and chloroform as the immiscible solvents.

3. Deposition in the body:

Besides the stomach, the urine, kidneys, and liver are to be examined. Aconitine is excreted in the urine and saliva. Palet[955] has shown by experiment on white rats, injected subcutaneously with lethal doses of aconitine and buried in metallic boxes, that the alkaloid could be readily detected after a lapse of two months. He also showed[956] that there is a putrefactive product formed which may be confused with aconitine.

Poisoning—Dosage:

1. Lethal Dose: A lethal dose of aconitine or aconite produces a diminution in the force and frequency of the pulse, a cold and clammy skin, and a tingling and numbness of the mouth, face and throat. In somewhat larger doses there is also burning of the throat and stomach, increased salivation, nausea, retching and vomiting, grinding of the teeth, and extension of the numbness and tingling to other parts of the body, especially at the fingers. There is difficulty in swallowing and speaking, and pain in the eyes and head. There are usually cramps in the extremities, and muscle activity varying from tetany to convulsions. The pulse is slow, feeble, and irregular and there is a marked pallor. The respiration is shallow and rapid, but later becomes slower. Purging is usually not present, and the output of urine is diminished as a rule. There is a general picture of prostration, although delirium and stupor are absent.

2. Fatal Dose: The therapeutic dose of aconitine is 0.15 mg. or 0.00015 grams, and of the tincture 0.6 cc. As little as 2 mg. of aconitine may produce death, while a more certain fatal dose is 4 or 6 mg. Aconitine may be absorbed through the skin and produce poisoning.

955. *Semana med.*, 26:166, 1919.
956. *Semana med.*, 26:424, 1919.

3. FATAL PERIOD: The shortest fatal period on record is eight minutes. Death usually occurs in three or four hours in most cases of poisoning, and may be as long as four days.

4. TREATMENT: The stomach should be emptied and washed with tannic acid or powdered charcoal. Stimulants such as ammonia, alcoholic drinks, digitalis, strychnine, and caffeine should be administered. Warmth should be maintained.

Case Histories: Poisoning by aconite is usually accidental.

CASE 1: 0.4 of a mg. of aconitine nitrate in solution was taken by a feeble man sixty-one years of age. He immediately suffered from burning and constriction of the mouth and stomach, and his skin became cold. For two days he took repeated doses of that amount until 9.2 mg. had been taken. He suffered from violent symptoms of aconite poisoning, and it was believed he would die. Nevertheless he recovered. From the same solution of the alkaloid the physician who had prescribed it, took about 4 mg. of the aconitine nitrate. Symptoms of poisoning appeared in fifteen minutes. There was a burning in the mouth and abdomen, pallor, feebleness, shallow and irregular pulse, pupils at first constricted and then suddenly dilated. Vomiting was induced and ether given hypodermically. Later there were convulsions and dyspnea. The heart failed, and the patient died five hours after taking the poison.[957]

CASE 2: Four teaspoonfuls of tincture of aconite were taken by a man sixty years old. Tingling of the face, drawing of the facial muscles, intense coldness, weak pulse, dyspnea, and blindness followed. Under treatment with emetics,—tincture of digitalis, wine and brandy, and strychnine,—the patient recovered.[958]

CASE 3: A man died suddenly from poisoning by aconite or aconitine, administered presumingly by his wife and a farm hand. Suspicion being aroused, the body was exhumed 323 days after burial. The dose must have been enormous, because 4.8 mg. of aconitine were separated and weighed. The identification of the alkaloid seems to have been very conclusive, the following results being reported: bitter taste with tingling in the tongue, melting point of the alkaloid 168.8°C., and melting point of the crystalline chloraurate 136°C., and show-

957. BUSSCHER: *Berl. klin. Wchnschr.*, 17:337, 1880.
958. WARRINER: *Med. Rec.*, 39:521, 1891.

ing 19.86% gold. The benzoyl radical was demonstrated.[959]

CASE 4: A man, of age thirty-eight, was given a prescription calling for a grain of aconitine in twenty capsules, with directions to take one every three hours. One capsule was taken at 7:30 P.M. One hour later the patient complained of prickling sensations in the body and extremities, and of increasing weakness. At 10:30 a second capsule was given. Five hours later the patient complained of faintness and tingling sensation. The body was covered with a cold sweat. Pupils were dilated. There were no convulsions, vomiting, or diarrhea. The patient was very restless, became unconscious, and died five hours and twenty minutes after taking the second capsule (total dose: 6 mg., or 0.1 grain). Postmortem examination showed the lungs markedly edematous and engorged with blood. The heart showed general excessive hypertrophy and a marked arteriosclerosis. There was acute parenchymatous degeneration of the myocardium. There was passive congestion of the kidneys and liver, and marked parenchymatous degeneration. The gastro-intestinal tract showed no gross changes. Chemical examination of the stomach gave a non-crystalline alkaloid of bitter taste and producing a tingling sensation of the tongue. The alkaloid was precipitated from solution by Wagner's, Mayer's, and Sonnenschein's Reagents. Amorphous precipitate with gold chloride. Electrocardiographic tracings of the heart of a frog weighing 40 gm., poisoned with one-fortieth grain of the alkaloid, showed a quickening of the beat at first, later beats slow and irregular, with final arrest in diastole in one hour. The residue obtained from the kidney had a slightly bitter taste and produced a tingling sensation of the tongue.[960]

CASE 5: The subject ate freely of meat with "horse-radish" sauce made by mistake from aconite root. Fifteen minutes after dinner he experienced a tingling of the body and was giddy and restless. The skin was cold and clammy. The pupils were dilated. The heart was irregular, and pulse of 70. Respiration was shallow and barely perceptible. No vomiting. There was twitching of the left shoulder and facial muscles. He was treated with apomorphine, digitalin, strych-

959. CAREL: St. Paul M. J., 8:666, 1906.
960. McNALLY, W. D.: Legal Medicine and Toxicology, PETERSON, HAINES, and WEBSTER, 2:440, 1923.

nine, and recovered. Examination of the sauce revealed the presence of aconitine.[961]

CASE 6: A case of poisoning from aconitine, causing cardiac collapse,[962] is reported here to acquaint physicians with the possibility of its unsuspected occurrence. Aconite finds little usefulness nowadays, and therefore might be over-looked. Poisonings are rare in modern literature. In perusal of the literature, as far back as 1883, only three cases in man with specific mention of its effect on the heart are found. Also, this is apparently the only case in man in which electrocardiographic records were obtained.

The case: A merchant, of age thirty-one, weight 242 pounds, drank a small amount of whiskey at 4:00 P.M. The estimated quantity taken was probably less than three drams (11 cc.). At first he felt exhilarated and took a long walk, but a half-hour later he felt depressed. At night he went to a theatre. While there, at about 9:30, he became weak and dizzy, had difficulty in breathing, and felt quite faint as though dying, perspired profusely, and his skin was white, cold and clammy. He was given spirits of ammonia, but failed to be relieved. A positive collapse for two hours resulted, while he was taken home and put to bed. There was no vomiting or diarrhea, or tingling of the mouth, stomach, or skin. A moderate salivation was present. The chief complaint in the morning was weakness and faintness, and uneasiness over the precordium. Externally normal, except pale, and skin cold. Breathing normal. Heart enlarged slightly to left; sounds almost imperceptible; no murmurs or other abnormal observations. Pulse 40, weak and almost imperceptible. Blood pressure 75 systolic, and 40 diastolic. Electrocardiograms were taken at this time. Serological and chemical blood and urine examinations were negative. He was given stimulating treatment with digitalis, thyroid extract a half grain three times a day, and KI ten grains three times a day, atropine sulphate 1/100 grain two or three times a day, but these had no effect on pulse and made the patient worse. During the first week he complained of syncope. Pulse quite imperceptible, 40 to 48. Blood pressure remained 80 systolic, and 40-45 diastolic. The second week the pulse became more rapid, the blood pressure

961. LIVINGSTON: *Brit. M. J.,* 1:928, 1915.
962. HARTUNG, E. F.: *J.A.M.A.,* 95:1265, 1930.

began to rise and there were attacks of syncope. By the end of the fourth week the blood pressure was 125 systolic and 80 diastolic, pulse 60-80. The patient always complained of uneasiness over the precordial area. The whiskey he had taken was analyzed and found to contain aconitine. Examination of the electrocardiograms taken about eighteen hours after ingestion showed sinus bradycardia. Subsequent E.K.G.'s revealed an increase in the P-R interval to 28. He has now returned to normal health.

CASE 7:[963] One has occasionally met with a case of poisoning by aconite; for example, the liniment of aconite, belladonna, and chloroform, or the case of Dr. L. who murdered his brother-in-law with aconite. A chemist, thirty-four years of age, at 8:00 P.M. took a dose out of a bottle containing a proprietary influenza mixture, and soon afterward became ill and asked to be taken to a hospital. He was then vomiting; the vomitus was blood-stained. He stated that he could not see, and was "going in the legs." His pulse was regular at 80; pupils dilated but equal and regular. He was cyanotic and became unconscious, dying about 10:00 P.M. without convulsions. It is stated by Taylor that 1/2000 part of a grain may be recognized by the taste test, and will kill a mouse within a few minutes. Autopsy showed blood dark, with very few clots. The mucous membrane of the stomach and upper gut was reddened and covered with much mucus. The government analyst found that the influenza mixture (0.8 oz.) contained 1.5 grain aconitine, this only partly in solution. Aconitine was also isolated from the organs.

ATROPINE

THIS group includes hyoscyamine and scopolamine, as well as atropine. They are obtained from a number of plants of the order solanaceae. The more important ones are Atropa belladonna (deadly nightshade), Hyoscyamus niger (henbane), Datura stramonium (thorn-apple or jimson weed), Mandragora officinarum (European mandrake), Scopola japonica (Japanese belladonna), Scopola atropoides, Duboisia myoporoides. These alkaloids occur in different parts of the plants and in varying amounts in different species. Atropine is the racemic form of hyoscyamine and occurs in the root and

963. PALMER, A.: *M. J. Australia,* 1:29, 1933.

leaves of atropa belladonna. Hyoscyamine occurs as the principal alkaloidal constituent of other parts of fresh belladonna and later undergoes partial racemization. Stramonium and hyoscyamus contain only hyoscyamine. Scopolamine is the principal constituent of duboisia and scopola, being obtained commercially from the latter and occurs in traces in belladonna root. U. S. P. belladonna foila contains not less than 0.3% of mydriatic alkaloids, dose 0.06 gm. (one grain); and the root not less than 0.45%, dose 0.045 gm. (0.75 grain). Hyoscyamus U. S. P. contains not less than 0.040% alkaloids, dose 0.25 gm., (four grains). Stramonium U.S.P. contains not less than 0.30% alkaloids, dose 0.075 gm. (1.25 grains).

Properties: Atropine ($C_{17}H_{23}NO_3$—M. W. 289.19) forms shining needle-like crystals, or rhombic plates, which melt at 115.5° C. It is odorless, bitter and acrid in taste, alkaline to litmus, phenolphthalein, etc. The hydrochloride melts at 165° C., and the sulphate at 194° C. It is optically inactive. It dissolves in water to 0.16%, in ether to 2%, in glycerine and ether to about 4%, and is freely soluble in alcohol, benzene and amyl alcohol; chloroform dissolving 28.6%. The salts are freely soluble in water, but nearly insoluble in ether (one to 3,000).

Hyoscyamine ($C_{17}H_{23}NO_3$—M. W. 289.19) crystallizes from alcohol or benzene in needles which melt at 108.5° C. The hydrobromide melts at 152° C., and the sulphate at 206° C. It is levorotatory (a) 15°/D=—20.3. On heating at 110° C it becomes the optically inactive atropine. Hyoscyamine is nearly insoluble in water, but dissolves with ease in alcohol, ether, amyl alcohol, chloroform, and benzene. The salts are freely soluble in water. Dyoscyamine hydrobromide occurs as white prismatic, deliquescent crystals almost insoluble in ether (one to 2,260), but readily soluble in alcohol, chloroform, and water.

Scopolamine ($C_{17}H_{21}NO_4$—M. W. 303.17) is amorphous, but the hydrobromide forms rhombic crystals. The alkaloid melts at 55° C., and the hydrobromide at 194° C. The specific rotation for the alkaloid (a) 15°/D=—14.97, and for the hydrobromide (a) 18°/D=—26.0. A 2.65% solution of the alkaloid-alcohol gives (a) 15°/D=—13.7. In alcoholic solution it changes to optically inactive atroscine (analogue of atropine). It is somewhat more soluble in water than atropine, and is freely soluble in the organic solvents. The salts are freely soluble in water.

Homatropine ($C_{16}H_{21}NO_3$—M. W. 275.27) crystallizes from ether in prisms which are hygroscopic and melt at 97.5° C., and the hydrobromide at 212° C. with decomposition. The hydrochloride dissolves in water to 16%, in alcohol to 2.5%, in chloroform to about 0.23%, and is insoluble in ether.

Structural Formulas: The atropine group of alkaloids and cocaine are built around the tropine nucleus.

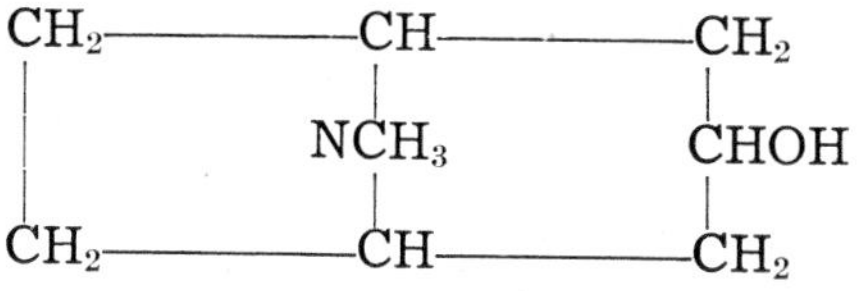

$$
\begin{array}{ccc}
CH_2\text{———}& CH\text{———} & CH_2 \\
| & | & | \\
& NCH_3 & CHOH \\
| & | & | \\
CH_2\text{———} & CH\text{———} & CH_2
\end{array}
$$

Tropine

It is to be noted that the pyridine ring structure exists in tropine. Atropine is the tropeic acid ester of tropine.

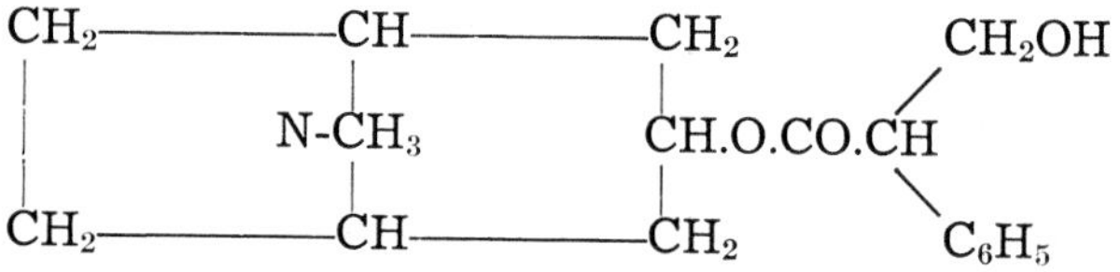

$$
\begin{array}{cccc}
CH_2\text{———}& CH\text{———} & CH_2 & CH_2OH \\
| & | & | & \nearrow \\
& N\text{-}CH_3 & CH.O.CO.CH \\
| & | & | & \searrow \\
CH_2\text{———} & CH\text{———} & CH_2 & C_6H_5
\end{array}
$$

Hyoscyamine is the stereoisomer.

In scopolamine the tropine nucleus has undergone a modification, the new nucleus being scopoline to which tropeic acid is attached to form scopolamine.

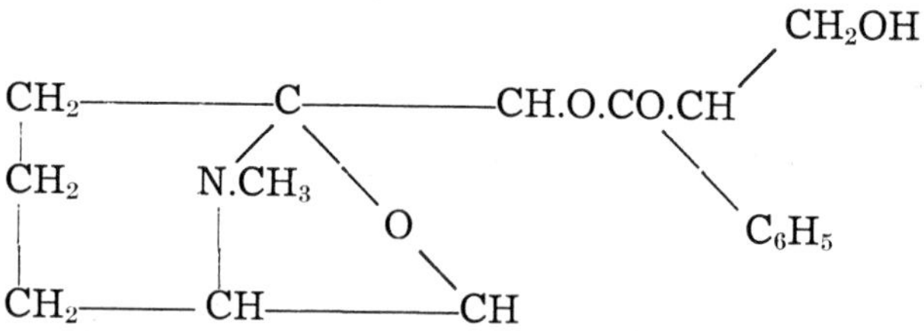

$$
\begin{array}{c}
CH_2OH \\
\nearrow \\
CH_2\text{———}C\text{———}CH.O.CO.CH \\
| \quad \diagup \diagdown \qquad \searrow \\
CH_2 \quad N.CH_3 \quad \diagdown \qquad C_6H_5 \\
| \qquad \quad | \qquad O \\
CH_2\text{——}CH\text{———}CH
\end{array}
$$

Scopolamine

The similarity of cocaine will be found under that heading.

Pharmacology: Atropine (1) paralyzes the parasympathetic nervous system by action of the myoneural junctions;

(2) increases the excitability of the motor areas of the brain including the medulla; and (3) in larger doses paralyzes the higher centers. It has a slight local analgesic action. By its action on the parasympathetic nervous system it produces, in small doses, certain cardinal effects. When administered internally, parenterally, or locally to the eyes, it will cause the pupils to dilate, this being due to the unopposed action of the sympathetic-innervated radial muscle fibers, following paralysis of the parasympathetic constrictor fibers. Although small doses may directly stimulate smooth muscle fibers, the usual effect is a relaxation of the muscle fiber through nerve paralysis. There is a marked diminution of the secretions of the sweat glands, with dryness of mouth, throat and skin. The bronchial musculature is relaxed. The intestines and uterus are relaxed. The effect on the heart rate is variable, since there is a combination of medullary stimulation and peripheral paralysis. The early stimulation of the vagus centrally is usually followed by the peripheral paralysis, i.e., a slowing up followed by acceleration. After the effect of the drug wears off, the rate may again be slowed up before becoming normal from a compensatory reaction. The respiration is stimulated by action on the medulla. After large doses death occurs from medullary paralysis.

The action of hyoscyamine is the same as atropine, differing only in degree. Hyoscyamine has the same effect on the central nervous system, but about twice the effect on the peripheral nerves. This is explained by the fact that hyoscyamine is purely levorotatory and about forty times as active as the dextrorotatory isomer which is present in atropine. In contrast to atropine, scopolamine causes an initial depression of the higher centers; in larger doses there is a delirium and excitement (it is this property which produces the "twilight sleep" when combined with morphine). The peripheral effects are similar to hyoscyamine, i.e., twice the potency of atropine. However, the duration is less.

Symptoms: Poisoning may occur from the ingestion of the berries of belladonna, particularly in children, and from eating thorn apples or henbane. Accidental overdoses of the drugs may produce symptoms of poisoning, or the drug may be taken with suicidal or homicidal intent. The margin of safety between the therapeutic doses and the fatal doses is extremely great compared with most other drugs. Large doses which produce severe symptoms may not endanger life. Certain individuals possess an idiosyncrasy to these alkaloids. This idiosyncrasy is manifested by reactions similar to other drug idiosyncrasies.

The first symptom of poisoning is that of dryness of the mouth and throat, with difficulty in swallowing, and a sensation of burning and thirst. Vision becomes impaired through dilatation and loss of accommodation, and the eyes present a rather prominent brilliant staring appearance. The voice is husky and the tongue is red. The skin, and particularly the face, becomes red. Cerebral stimulation is evidenced by delirium and delusions. With paralysis, the delirium gives way to drowsiness and stupor. The heart rate is quite high (170), and the respiration quickened. The delirium manifests itself in different ways, there being at times dizziness with headache, hallucinations, and maniacal demonstrations in which the individuals may run, dance, and perform various idiotic and raving movements; they may become hilarious, or bellicose, and mutter, laugh, cry, or talk. Chorea-like movements may occur, but convulsions are rare. In fatal cases there is a rapid and intermittent pulse, with coldness of the extremities and a deep coma. Hyoscyamine has similar central effects, but the peripheral effects are more powerful and of shorter duration. Scopolamine, on the other hand, produces more profound depression of the central nervous system, with an absence of the flushing of the skin, tachycardia, and excitement. Hallucinations may be present and the individual loses a certain amount of inhibitory control. It is this property which has given rise to the use of scopolamine as a so-called "truth serum." In many cases of poisoning, and even following therapeutic doses, there is a retention of urine from paralysis of the bladder, and catheterization is necessary.

Fatal Dose: As indicated, the fatal dose of these drugs is quite high; while 1 to 2 mg. may cause distinct symptoms, 100 mg. is probably the usual fatal adult dose. In children it may be considerably less. The smallest amount of atropine known to have caused death is 0.4 mg. instilled into the eye of a four year old child. A few cases are reported where death has occurred from 2 to 6 mg. of atropine sulphate.

While such small quantities have proved fatal, recovery has occurred after doses as high as 500 mg. have been taken. Leschke reports that five berries of the night-shade have caused death, while recovery has taken place after twenty berries have been eaten. The ingestion of these berries, and thorn apples, frequently leads to a nauseating irritation of the stomach, so that a large part of the ingested material may be vomited. The author[964] recovered 2.2 mg. (1/30 grain) of alkaloid from the stomach contents of a child dead from the effects of eating stramonium seeds. In this case, however, the amount isolated represents, of course, only a fraction of the amount taken, so that the fatal dose was undetermined. In one case, Duffin[965] reported a child two and one-half years of age dying from eating sixteen grains of the seeds, while in the case above cited the boy ate about 180 seeds. Concerning the lethal dose of hyoscyamus, hyoscyamine, homatropine, and scopolamine, little is known. No fatal cases of poisoning with homatropine have been reported.

Fatalities from scopolamine have occurred following anesthesia, but the blame cannot be placed entirely on the scopolamine. Death has occurred with as little as 0.6 mg. of scopolamine, and recovery has occurred from doses of 7 to 15 mg. There was reported a case of recovery following 500 mg. of scopolamine hydrobromide by mouth. Fowl and herbivorous animals show no toxic effects from ingesting plants containing these alkaloids. Solanine, an atropine-like alkaloid, occurs in potatoes under certain conditions, particularly in young and sprouting potatoes, which may contain this alkaloid in the peel. This accounts for potato poisoning which has occurred occasionally. Lickint[966] reported a non-fatal poisoning from 500 mg. of scopolamine. Shoemaker[967] cites three cases of death from only 0.25 mg., 1.0 mg., and 1.5 mg. scopolamine combined with 0.75 cg., 1.5 cg., and 2.5 cg. morphine respectively. Fowelin[968] reported a case of death from 0.6 mg. scopolamine, plus 0.4 cg. pantopon., plus 2 cg. morphine. Others have reported much higher amounts causing death: Zimmerman, 7 mg., Voss, 10 mg., and Kobert, 10 mg.

964. McNally, W. D.: *J.A.M.A.*, 65:1640, 1915.
965. Duffin: *London Med. Gaz.*, 15:194, 1834.
966. Lickint: *München. med. Wchnschr.*, 78:1991, 1931.
967. Shoemaker: *Deutsche med. Wchnschr.*, 1909.
968. Fowelin: *Zentralbl. f. Chir.*, 1911, 1927.

Gottlieb[969] states the toxic as well as lethal dose of scopola-mine is large in both man and dogs. In dogs an effect is seen with 1 mg., but they have endured 1,000 mg., while in man it depends upon the individual susceptibility, which varies greatly. A fifty-two year old druggist took about 50 cc. of 1% solution of scopolamine, equal to 500 mg. scopolamine hydrobromide. Shortly he noticed a salty taste in his mouth, a hum in his ears, and then dizziness, which became so intense that it was necessary for him to lie down. In a little while he was unconscious. Two hours later he was given 2 cc. of camphor oil, and 1 cc. caffeine, and after forty-five minutes was brought to a hospital. His face was red, and he had an exceptionally dry mouth, and a maximal mydriasis. The extremities were limp; reflexes normal; Babinski sign posi-tive in the right arm. The maximally dilated pupils did not react to light. Pulse was slow, breath fast and uneven, stopped occasionally for a few seconds. He was given 1 cc. cardiazol, lobeline, and pilocarpine, and his stomach was washed with 30 liters of warm water, containing tannin. Then 200 cc. of 15% magnesium sulphate were given. During the night convulsions occurred, so that 2.25 gm. of chloral hydrate were given. After sixteen hours he answered questions, and twenty hours after the intake of the scopolamine all the symptoms were gone.

Regenbogen [970] reported a case of a twenty-four year old man who took 350 mg. of scopolamine by mouth. After one-half hour, unrest occurred, then unconsciousness. The hospital report was: deep coma, tetanic stiffness of all body muscles, face scarlet red, pulse weak 160, extrasystole, Babinski, Oppenheim, Rossolimo, Mendel-Bechterew, and Gordon all positive. Patellar and Achilles tendon reflex increased. Abdominal reflex weak, positive. Sensitiveness greatly increased. After injection of ipral, pulse stronger, blood pressure increased, breathing deeper, slower, more regular. Next day he was conscious. After three days the patient was normal. He evidently had an individual suscepti-bility to scopolamine in that the poison was slowly absorbed and broken down in the liver. Perhaps the optical reaction plays a role. According to Hug, the levoscopolamine is two

969. GOTTLIEB, R.: Exper. Pharmacol, 1920.
970. REGENBOGEN, E.: *Deutsche med. Wchnschr.*, 59:1209, 1933.

to four times more poisonous than the optically inactive.

CASE 1: A boy, of age seven, ate some 180 stramonium seeds at 5:00 P.M. He ate supper at 6:00 P.M. He went to bed at 8:00 feeling well. At 12:15 A.M. he complained of being cold. One-half hour later he was delirious and tossed about in bed. One hour later he fell asleep, breathing heavily. He died at 6:00 P.M. No convulsions, vomiting, or diarrhea were present. A postmortem made twenty-four hours after death showed no evidence of skin rash, pupils were not dilated to any special degree, lungs were slightly distended and showed hypostatic congestion in the posterior portion. There were numerous small petechiae over the pericardium, with a slight passive hyperemia of the liver. A portion of the stomach contents, amounting to 130.5 gm., was submitted for analysis. This consisted of poorly masticated food, mostly vegetables and about twenty kidney-shaped seeds, 2 mm. long and 2.5 mm. wide, and of a brownish color. Two and two-tenths mg. of an alkaloid giving Vitali's test were extracted. This alkaloid produced mydriasis in animals.[971]

CASE 2: A man, twenty years of age, a senior pharmacy student, took 7.5 grains (500 mg.) of atropine sulphate at 9:30 A.M. At 11:00 A.M. the pulse was 170, respiration 44, temperature 104°. The pupils were dilated, skin flushed, lips parched, and delirium was present. The abdomen was silent. Moist rales in the lungs and cyanosis gradually developed. Gastric lavage was then employed, using large quantities of sodium bicarbonate solution. Fifty cc. of saturated magnesium sulphate were left in the stomach. Blood pressure was 180/60. Five hundred cc. of blood were withdrawn. The cyanosis and rales diminished. An indwelling catheter was inserted. Ten per cent CO_2 and 90% O_2 were given as needed. Before phlebotomy was done the hemoglobin was 115%. Continuous hypodermoclysis was started and cold sponges were administered. On recovery, he stated that he experienced dizziness, developed a blurring of vision and dryness of the mouth and throat, and then remembered nothing. The dose which he took was 1,000 times the therapeutic dose.[972]

CASE 3: A boy, six years of age, ate atropa belladonna berries. Dilated pupils, itching and dryness of the skin,

971. McNALLY, W. D.: J.A.M.A., 65:1640, 1915.
972. COMROE, B. I.: J.A.M.A., 101:446, 1933.

delirium and unconsciousness followed. The boy recovered.[973]

CASE 4: A woman applied a belladonna plaster to her breast; dimness of vision, thirst and a rash followed.[974]

CASE 5: A man, aged 57, wore a "strong belladonna plaster" over his loins. He developed dryness of the mouth and tongue, numbness of the hands and feet, dimness of vision, delirium, and coma. He was treated with physostigmine and recovered.[975]

CASE 6: A child, of three, ate stramonium seeds. The symptoms were dilated pupils, bright red, hot, dry skin, pulse full, and tetanic convulsions. Treatment consisted of gastric lavage, potassium bromide and chloral hydrate. The child recovered.[976]

CASE 7: Scott reported cases of poisoning in three boys, aged eight, ten, and twelve years, who ate berries found growing on an unfrequented ledge of rock. Examination showed flushed face, pupils widely dilated and fixed, voice weak and speech thick, showing a partial paralysis of the throat muscles. Mucous membrane of the mouth and throat was dry. Muttering delirium and periods of hyperexcitability alternated with periods of stupor, during which the respirations were slow and full. On attempting to walk, the gait was staggering and uncertain. The temperature at no time was over 100°, and the respiration 20 to 30.[977]

CASE 8: A paranoic, aged thirty-three, took 15 mg. of scopolamine hydrobromide. Three-quarters of an hour later the patient showed congestion of the face, slow strong pulse, pupils dilated, and not reacting to light, muscular contractions and clouded consciousness. Treatment by gastric lavage and camphor. The patient recovered.[978]

CASE 9: A woman, aged twenty-nine, had a pre-anesthetic injection of one-eighth grain of morphine and one-one-hundredth grain of scopolamine hydrobromide. About one-half hour later she fell asleep with stertorous breathing. She was slightly cyanotic; pupils were moderately dilated, but reacted to light; skin was dry and pale; superficial reflexes were

973. SCOFIELD: *Lancet,* 2:199, 1895.
974. GRIFFITH: *Brit. M. J.,* 1:1060, 1891.
975. HOWARTH: *Lancet,* 1:204, 1894.
976. PACE: *Med. & Surg. Reptr.,* 45:26, 1881.
977. SCOTT, Z. R.: *Atlantic M. J.,* 26:34, 1922.
978. STOLLE: *Allg. Ztschr. f. Psychiat.,* 57:151, 1900.

abolished. Pulse and respiration were normal; the latter becoming shallow and less frequent. The patient died two hours after receiving the injection.[979]

CASE 10: This case is the famous "Crippen Case," perhaps the most sensational poisoning case of this generation. Dr. Crippen was tried and convicted of poisoning his wife with hyoscine hydrobromide. The remains of a human adult, probably in early or middle life, consisting of heart, lungs, kidneys, stomach, intestines, and portions of skin and muscles, mixed with quick-lime, were found beneath the floor of the coal cellar of Crippen's house. In the viscera Dr. Willcox found an alkaloid which produced complete paralysis of the pupils in cats, for several days. By the Stas-Otto process he obtained a mydriatic alkaloid, which gave a purple color with Vitali's test. By purification he found that the alkaloid was gummy and not crystalline and with Wormley's reagent gave brown spheres. He, therefore, concluded that hyoscine was present. The quantities found in various organs amounted in all to two-fifths grain of hyoscine hydrobromide. The lungs contained only the merest trace, much less than the organs. Distribution pointed conclusively to administration by mouth and excluded the possibility of alkaloids being of putrefactive origin, as the best preserved organs yielded the largest percentage of alkaloid.[980] This case is of special interest as one of the first on record where the wireless aided in the capture of a murderer. The captain of a certain ship as it entered a Canadian port, received a wireless message from England which gave a description of Crippen and his secretary.

CASE 11: A physician in Chicago in 1935 prescribed a 10% solution of atropine sulphate to be applied by means of a dropper to the nose of a seven year old child. Three hours after the first application, the child died.

CASE 12: Comroe[981] reported a senior pharmacy student, aged twenty, who purposely took by mouth 7½ grains of atropine sulphate, dissolved in water. The patient recovered, although the stomach was not evacuated until one and one-half hours following ingestion of the drug. Acute pulmonary edema was one of the outstanding features of the case.

979. ELY: New York M. J. (etc), 84:799, 1906.
980. J.A.M.A., 55:1744, 1910.
981. COMROE, B. I.: J.A.M.A., 101:446, 1933.

CASE 13: Wolfe[982] reported the hypersensitivity, of a woman fifty-nine years of age, to atropine ointment which was applied after an iridectomy. She became restless at night. The lids of the operated eye were slightly red, but there was no swelling. This redness and swelling increased until the wheals had become an angry red papule. Skin tests confirmed that she was sensitive to atropine.

CASE 14: Jaeger[983] reports the case of a seventy-five year old woman who took 150 atropine tablets (100 tablets of atropine sulphate 0.0005 gm., and 50 tablets 0.00075 gm.) at one time. The symptoms were unconsciousness, dry mucous membrane, dry, hot, scarlet-red skin, especially in the face. Maximum mydriasis, loss of accommodation of the pupils, strong pulsation of the carotid, weak pulse (over 110). Breath uneven, and cramps in the muscle.

Fatal Period: Symptoms of poisoning begin to appear within a few minutes after absorption. The course of poisoning is not rapid, and the majority of fatalities occur within twenty-four hours.

Treatment: Gastric lavage, using plain water first, and then some precipitant, such as a solution of iodine, tannic acid and charcoal. If iodine is used, the amount should be roughly four times the weight of the atropine to be precipitated. The iodine solution should not be allowed to remain in the stomach. In moderate poisoning, morphine is of advantage if given hypodermically. In severe poisonings, where the depressant effect of atropine on the respiration has become manifest, morphine may further depress the respiration. If the respiration does become markedly depressed, caffeine and artificial respiration should be employed. Coramine may also be of value. Pilocarpine and physostigmine may be used, but these drugs do little more than merely alleviate the peripheral symptoms, and victims do not die from these peripheral symptoms. If there is extreme excitement or violent delirium, chloroform or ether may be employed.

Tests: Poe and Roe[984] report a number of reactions, the results of Vitali's test as applied to a number of substances other than atropine. With apomorphine, berberine, colchicine,

982. WOLFE, O. R.: *J.A.M.A.*, 97:460, 1931.
983. JAEGER, H.: *Med. Klin.*, 29:1377, 1933.
984. POE, C. F., and ROE, C.: *J. Lab. & Clin. Med.*, 18:743, 1935.

cryptopine, ergotine, homatropine, quinidine, and physostig-mine, grayish-brown to yellowish-brown colors were obtained. With cinchonine an orange color was obtained; codeine, a yellowish-red; daturine, deep reddish-violet; hydrastine, yellow; quinine, orange-red color, while scopolamine gives deep violet, and veratrine a light rose-violet. No color was obtained by aconitine, brucine, caffeine, cinchonidine, cocaine, catarnine hydrochloride, delphinine, dionine, emetine, beu-caine hydrochloride, gelseminine, heroin, morphine, nar-ceine, nicotine, papaverine, pelletierine, pilocarpine, piperine, pseudopelletierine, sanguinarine NO_3, sparteine, solamine, theobromine, theophylline.

A number of substances that cover up Vitali's test when present in equal amounts are: peralga, phenanthrene, phenol-phthalein, salvarsan, tetra bromphenolphthalein, tryptophane, vanillin. When the following substances were present five times as much as atropine, the characteristic Vitali's reaction did not appear: benzoin, brucine, codeine, emetine, hydrastine, morphine, narceine, physostigmine, skatole, thymol, and many others.

O'Kelly, Arlie, and Poe[985] used para-dimethyl-aminoben-zaldehyde, prepared by dissolving in concentrated sulphuric acid and 0.4 cc. of water. They used for their test solution 1 mg. atropine per cubic centimeter, which was evaporated to dry-ness and tested with two to three drops of the reagent and warmed on the water-bath for five minutes. Atropine, bella-donnine, brucine, hyoscyamine, scopolamine, solanine gave reddish-violet colors. Apomorphine, daturine, delphinine, emetine, heroin, morphine, narceine, narcotine, papaverine, quinidine, sanguinarine, and veratrine gave brown to brown-ish-violet colors. Berberine, cryptopine, piperine, gave greenish reactions. There was no color reaction with aconitine, caffeine, cinchonidine, cinchonine, cocaine, codeine, colchicine, cotarine hydrochloride, dionine, ergotine, beucaine hydrochloride, gel-semine, homatropine, hydrastine, nicotine, pelletierine, phena-caine, physostigmine, pilocarpine, pseudopelletierine, quinine, sparteine, strychnine, theobromine. The following substances when present in equal amounts with atropine completely obscured in reaction: aspirin, aminoazo-benzene, amyl alcohol,

985. O'KELLY, ARLIE A. and POE, C. F.: *J. Lab. & Clin. Med.*, 18: 1235, 1933.

antipyrine, benzidine, skatole, sparteine, strychnine, colocynthine, elaterine, guaiacol, morphine, isobutyl alcohol, narcotine, o-nitrobenzaldehyde. When present in five times the amount of atropine, 1, 2, and 4 dinitro aniline completely obscured the reaction in delphinine.

The separation of atropine, hyoscyamine, etc., from animal tissues follows the author's method as given on page 30. When poisoning has resulted from the swallowing of seeds of hyoscyamine, the contents of the stomach should be examined for the presence of seeds. The stramonium seeds are flattened, kidney-shaped, brownish-black to black, 2 mm. long by 2.5 mm. wide, and externally marked with a network of punctate depressions. Hyoscyamus seeds are 1 mm. long, kidney-shaped, rough, grayish-brown in color. Belladonna seeds are 3 mm. long, kidney-shaped, gray to brown, and smoother than the hyoscyamus seeds.

The alkaloidal solution is added to an excess of decinormal aqueous iodine solution in potassium iodide. The precipitates are stirred, drained, washed, dried, and weighed as atropine hydroiodide octa-iodide. This weight multiplied by 0.202 gives the quantity of atropine as free alkaloid. The reaction with this alkaloid as with other alkaloids is not 100%. Parallel analysis, using control samples, would demonstrate the loss by extraction. Most of the alkaloids would be found in the chloroform extract. The combined chloroform extract is shaken with water slightly acidified with acetic acid, the water extract is then separated and shaken with chloroform which has been made alkaline with ammonia and shaken successively with three portions of chloroform. After evaporation on a small watch glass, a small portion of this last chloroform extract shows the presence of material of tissues. The purification is repeated as before, beginning with the acidified solution until the purified extract is obtained. Keep in mind that with each purification, there is a loss of alkaloid.

Distribution in the Body: Cloetta[986] reported that atropine disappears from the blood stream. It is excreted in the urine, mostly, unchanged, chiefly within thirty-six hours. The excretion is not complete, as some of the atropine is dissolved in the body and becomes another base. Fickewirth and Heffter

986. CLOETTA: *Arch. f. exper. Path. u. Pharmakol.*, 119:125, 1908; 64:427, 1911.

state that atropine resists putrefaction, and can be found even months after burial.[987] A putrefactive alkaloid, as ptoma-tropine, has caused confusion in the tests for atropine, when the extracts have not been properly purified, as given under isolation.

Ipsen[988] isolated 0.2642 gm. (4.077 grains) of pure atro-pine sulphate from a cadaver, after more than three years' burial. The author extracted 2.2 mg. of alkaloid from the stomach contents of a child who had died from the effects of eating stramonium seeds. After its administration, Dragen-dorff detected atropine in the urine, in the liver, and in the kidneys of a cat, but none was found in the spleen. After 2.8 grains (0.1863 gm.) had been administered by mouth to a cat, weighing six pounds, twenty-four hours later it was found in the blood. Dragendorff also gave one grain (0.06 gm.) of atro-pine daily to a rabbit weighing three and a half pounds. Atro-pine was found in the urine each day.

Chemical Tests:

1. Vitali's Test: In a small porcelain dish place some of the residue obtained from the extraction process, or evaporate a portion of the chloroform extract, adding a few drops of fuming nitric acid and evaporate to dryness on a water-bath. Allow the colorless, or, at most, slightly yellow, residue to cool and add a few drops of fresh alcoholic potassium hydrate solution. A beautiful violet color is produced, which soon fades to a dark red, and then disappears. This color may be made to reappear by adding a few more drops of the alcohol potash solution. If the alkaloid is confined to a very small spot on the porcelain dish it is possible to detect as small amounts as 0.001 mg. of atropine. The same play of colors is noted with hyoscyamine and scopolamine, but not with homatropine. Arnold[989] has modified this test by adding to the dry residue, moistened with sulphuric acid, a fragment of sodium nitrite. To this slightly yellowish spot add a few drops of fresh alcohol potash, when there will be observed a violet color fading to violet-red, pale rose and finally disappearing entirely. A sufficient amount of the alcoholic potash must be added to neutralize the sulphuric acid which is used in the test.

987. FICKEWIRTH and HEFFTER: Biochem. Ztschr., 40:36, 1912.
988. IPSEN: Vrtljschr. f. gerichtl. Med., 31:308, 1906.
989. ARNOLD: Arch. de pharmacod., 20:561, 1882.

Flückiger[990] added sodium nitrate instead of nitrite. To the residue moistened with sulphuric acid, homatropine reacts the same as all members of this group.

2. Gerrard's Test: To a portion of the purified residue add a few drops of a 2% solution of mercuric chloride solution in 50% alcohol. When the residue is warmed gently, a yellow to brick-red color is produced, due to precipitation of the mercuric oxide. Homatropine reacts positively to this reagent, while scopolamine gives neither a yellow nor red precipitate. Gerrard reports white precipitates, which may become slightly yellow on heating with strychnine, brucine, morphine, codeine, veratrine, aconitine, coniine, gelsemine, caffeine, cinchonine, cinchonidine, quinine, and quinidine.

3. Gulielmo-Sohn Reaction: Take a small portion of the residue, heat in a test-tube with 1 cc. of sulphuric acid until the acid begins to color, and after cooling add 2 cc. of water drop by drop along the side of the tube; an odor suggestive of flowers will be obtained. If a small crystal of potassium permanganate be introduced before the water is added, the odor will be like that of bitter almonds.

4. Wormley's Bromine Test:[991] An aqueous solution of hydrobromic acid saturated with bromine produces with atropine or hyoscyamine and their salts, even in such dilute solutions as one to 10,000, a yellow amorphous precipitate which becomes crystalline in a short time. This is insoluble in acetic acid, and only very sparingly soluble in excess of mineral acids or fixed caustic alkalis. Wormley regards this reaction as being characteristic for atropine and hyoscyamine. While most alkaloids produce yellowish precipitates with this reagent, none becomes crystalline except those members of this group, and with meconine, which differs from that produced by atropine in its crystalline form. Opianyl (meconine) does not respond to the physiological test, or to Vitali's reaction for atropine. Veratrine produces a yellow precipitate; it does not assume a characteristic form such as hyoscyamine, which appears in brownish needles in leaf-like crystals like those from the leaf of a flower. Veratrine gives with para-dimethyl-amino-

990. FLÜCKIGER: *Pharm. J. & Trans.*, 16:601, 1888; *Chem. Centralbl.*, 504, 1886.

991. WORMLEY: Micro-Chemistry, 2nd ed., 642, 1885; *Am. J. Pharm.*, 66:513, 1894.

benzaldehdye a brownish-violet color instead of the reddish-violet color that atropine gives.

Carr[992] states that the crystals with scopolamine are tabular in form and are often arranged in leaf-like rosettes, even in dilutions of one to 2,000. He further indicates that homatropine and caffeine give crystalline precipitates with Wormley's reagent. For microscopic purposes this test may be made by adding a drop of the reagent to a drop or two of an aqueous solution of the salt of the supposed alkaloid on a glass slide. Allow to evaporate at room temperature. The characteristic crystals described above will be seen when examined under the microscope.

5. Physiological Test: Atropine dilates the pupils (mydriasis) and renders them insensible to light; it also paralyzes accommodation (cycloplegia), the lens being adjusted only for far vision. These actions are entirely peripheral and consist in paralysis of the oculomotor endings. The atropine effects may be removed by drugs which stimulate the oculomotor endings (pilocarpine, physostigmine, muscarine), and vice versa. Dissolve a small portion of the alkaloidal residue in four or five drops of a very dilute sulphuric acid solution and introduce a drop of this solution into the eyes of experimental animals. The mydriasis may last for several days.

BRUCINE ($C_{23}H_{26}N_2O_4$)

BRUCINE is an alkaloid of nux vomica and is related to strychnine in its chemical constitution, and in its physiological action. It is a monacid, tertiary base. It appears that brucine is the dimethoxyl derivative of strychnine. Brucine and strychnine can be separated by treating with cold absolute alcohol or acetone, which dissolves the brucine, leaving the strychnine, or from their oxalates in absolute alcohol, the strychnine oxalate being dissolved. It occurs as a white, odorless, crystalline powder, or colorless, transparent monoclinic prisms or shining leaflets. It is very bitter in taste. It is levorotatory. Brucine crystallizes from water with two to four molecules of water, and from alcohol with two molecules of water, melting in its water of crystallization at about 100° C. The anhydrous base dried at 150° C., melts at 178° C. It is soluble in chloroform and benzene, acetone, and ether, and

992. CARR: Allen's Commercial Organic Analysis, 4th ed., 6:308, 1912.

much more soluble in water than strychnine. It forms well defined salts; the hydrochloride, hydroiodide, nitrate and sulphate
are all soluble in water. It is precipitated by the general alkaloidal reagents.

Tests: (1) Brucine and strychnine do not give the same
reaction with sulphuric acid and oxidizing agents. Sulphuric
acid gives no color, but if a trace of nitric acid is added on the
point of a glass rod, a blood-red color develops with brucine,
which when gently warmed turns to yellowish-red, and finally
yellow. If to this residue a fresh solution of stannous chloride
(one to nine hydrochloric acid) or a colorless ammonium sul-·
phide be added, a purple color is produced. (Morphine gives
an orange color.) (2) Nitric acid gives a scarlet or blood-red
color, which on heating changes to yellowish-red and finally
yellow. (3) Potassium dichromate in aqueous solution of
brucine gives a yellow precipitate, soluble in nitric acid with
a red color. (4) Mercurous nitrate added to an aqueous solution gives no color in the cold, but on warming turns a carmine
color. Ammonia fumes applied to an evaporated solution in
nitric acid change the color to grass green, which changes to
violet when dissolved in hydrogen peroxide. (5) Blyth's
Test: [993] To an alcoholic solution of brucine, a small amount
of methyl iodide is added; circular rosettes of crystal groups
appear. Strychnine does not give a similar reaction, and does
not interfere with this test if present. (6) To test for strychnine
in the presence of brucine, dissolve in sulphuric acid and add a
trace of nitric acid, and after the red color has turned to yellow,
add a small crystal of potassium permanganate or potassium
dichromate. The fading purple test reaction shows strychnine,
and brucine, being decomposed by conversions into derivatives.

Isolation from Tissues: The procedure is similar to that
for strychnine with the exception that it must not be heated
with sulphuric acid on the water-bath, as directed, as it is
decomposed readily by oxidizing agents.

Symptoms of Poisoning by Brucine: The symptoms of
poisoning by brucine are essentially those of strychnine. However, the convulsive seizures noted with strychnine do not
always appear under the influence of brucine. Brucine is
much weaker and less toxic than strychnine.

993. BLYTH: Poisons, Their Effects and Detection, 4th ed., 351, 1906.

Fatal Amount: Andral[994] found brucine to have one-twelfth the strength of strychnine, while Magendie states this ratio to be one to twenty-four. Falck,[995] in his experiments on rabbits, injected subcutaneously brucine nitrate in varying doses, showed that the minimum lethal dose for rabbits was 23 mg. per kilo, while under the same experimental conditions, that of strychnine was 0.6 mg. per kilo. The ratio of the lethal dose of strychnine to brucine was thirty-eight and a half to one. From animal experimentation, the fatal dose of brucine for man would be twenty to twenty-five grains. Postmortem appearances are the same as under strychnine.

COCAINE ($C_{17}H_{21}NO_4$)

COCAINE is the chief alkaloid of the leaf of erythroxylon coca, constituting about 0.75% of the freshly drief leaf. Erythroxylon is indigenous in South America, but has been introduced into India, Ceylon, and Java. Besides cocaine, several other alkaloids are found in this leaf, such as hygrine, cinnamyl-cocaine, a-truxillin (cocamine), b-truxilline, benzoyl-ecgonine, and tropacocaine. One gm. of cocaine is soluble in 600 cc. of water, in 6.5 cc. of alcohol, in 0.7 cc. of chloroform, in 3.5 cc. of ether, in 12 cc. of olive oil, and in 30 to 50 cc. of liquid petrolatum, at 25° C. (U.S.P.,XI,123.) Cocaine melts between 96° and 98° C. A saturated aqueous solution of cocaine is alkaline to litmus paper, and is levorotatory. On saponification with water, cocaine splits into methyl alcohol and a base, benzoyl-ecgonine; while this base is further split into benzoic acid and ecgonine if the saponification be conducted with mineral acids or alkalis, as follows:

$$C_{17}H_{21}NO_4 + 2H_2O = C_9H_{15}NO_3 + C_6H_5COOH + CH_3OH$$

cocaine   ecgonine   benzoic acid   methyl alcohol

Like atropine, ecgonine belongs to the tropan-ring system and differs from tropin in the replacement of a hydrogen atom of the second atomic group. The group relations are shown by the similarity of the basic groups.

Symptoms: "Fatal cases run a very rapid course, with anxiety, sudden fainting, extreme pallor, dyspnea, sometimes brief convulsions, arrest of respiration, and death generally in

994. ANDRAL: cited by HUSEMAN: *Arch. f. exper. Path. u. Pharmakol.,* 9:429, 1878; MAGENDIE: *J. de physiol. et de path. gén.,* 3:267, (TAYLOR gives these figures as Andral 1/6, and Magendie 1/12.)

995. FALCK: *Vrtljschr. f. gerichtl. Med.,* 23:78, 1875.

a few minutes. With smaller doses or slower absorption there are confusion, laughter, vertigo, motor excitement; quickened pulse and palpitation; irregular dilated pupils and exophthalmos; nausea; vomiting and abdominal pain; great anxiety, disturbance of cutaneous sensation (worms under skin), finally delirium, dyspnea, and Cheyne-Stokes respiration, convulsions, unconsciousness; and death by collapse and asphyxia. However, if death has not occurred in a few minutes, the patient will almost always recover. Unconsciousness and Cheyne-Stokes respiration may persist for one or two hours. Recovery may be followed by more lasting psychic depression and melancholia."[996] Occasionally individuals are seen who have acquired the cocaine habit. During a period of the year 1909, a great many of these cases were seen, but in the last few years I have not seen any. The individual usually snuffs a small portion of the crystals, which are known to the habitué as "snow." In large centers such as Chicago, the police are called to pick up so-called "snow parties." The effect of snuffing the cocaine is such as to give the individual a sense of elation, and physical vigor. He has the sensation of being a millionaire. He wants to talk more than usual while under the influence of cocaine. With an increased dose, this snuff may develop increased mental condition, a period of delusion, and then mania. These conditions are succeeded by depression, and tremors, with a pale pasty face. The worst effect of this drug on the habitué is that he has a craving for more of it, similar to that of morphine, and he will pawn his furniture and his clothes to obtain it.

Fatal Dose: Mayer[997] states that a large proportion of anesthetic accidents are due to a mistake in the drug, its concentration and dosage. It is difficult to state the lethal dose or quantity, as it varies with individual susceptibility. Mannheim[998] considers one gram as the lethal dose, whether given by mouth or otherwise, but many cases are reported in which larger amounts have not caused death, and on the other hand, smaller doses have proved fatal. Thus 0.04 gm. has caused death when given subconjunctivally;[999] 0.648 gm. when taken

996. MAYER: from SOLLMAN: A Manual of Pharm., 3rd ed., 1927.
997. MAYER, E.: J.A.M.A., 77:1336, 1921.
998. MANNHEIM: Ztschr. f. klin. Med., 16:380, 1890.
999. ABADIE: Internat. klin. Rundschau, 2:1746, 1888.

by mouth,[1000] 1.5 gm. by rectum,[1001] and 0.03 gm. by urethra.[1002]

Fatal Period: In accidental poisoning from the administration of too strong a solution, or in an addict taking an overdose, death occurs in a few minutes. If a patient survives for half an hour, there is usually recovery.[1003]

Treatment: The stomach should be washed out immediately with water containing sodium bicarbonate, 60 grains to the pint. If a solution of permanganate is at hand, wash out the stomach with one small crystal to each eight ounces of water. Give inhalations of ammonia. Convulsions can be allayed either by ether, chloral, or chloroform. If there is any disturbance of breathing, artificial respiration should be practised at once, and cardiac massage applied after respiration fails. Inhalations of oxygen with 5% carbon dioxide should be given. Tatum, Collins and Atkinson[1004] report that the tolerance of animals is increased by sodium barbital and paraldehyde. Leschure[1005] has reported that sodium barbital in doses of 6 to 12 grains by mouth allays symptoms of cocaine if given one half hour before anesthesia. Weiss[1006] has shown that calcium injections do not increase the toxicity of cocaine.

In the treatment of chronic cocaine poisoning the individual must be treated the same as a morphine habitué, gradually withdrawing the drug from the patient. This is usually best conducted in a sanitarium, away from friends and relatives who might supply the drug.

Postmortem Appearances: The postmortem findings are not characteristic. The spleen, lungs, brain, liver, kidneys, and meninges are markedly congested, while the mucous membrane of the stomach may show slight hyperemia. Those who are addicted to snuffing of cocaine, may show perforation of the nasal septum.

Tests: Great difficulty is encountered in obtaining tests for cocaine from tissues on account of the ease with which this alkaloid leads to hydrolysis or saponification, giving, first, methyl alcohol, and then benzoic acid.

1000. CURGENVEN: *Quart. M. J.,* 4:152, 1895.
1001. SZUMAN: *Therap. Monatsch.,* 2:393, 1888.
1002. HAYNES: *Med. News,* 65:144, 1894.
1003. HAINES: in Hamilton's Legal Medicine, 1:428, 1894.
1004. TATUM, COLLINS, and ATKINSON: *J.A.M.A.,* 64:117, 1925.
1005. LESCHURE: *J.A.M.A., January* 15, 1927.
1006. WEISS, SOMMA: *J.A.M.A.,* 81:1282, 1923.

1. To a fragment of the residue from the alkaloidal extraction, or if the powder has been submitted for examination, take a minute fragment on a microscopic slide, add a drop of dilute hydrochloric acid and a drop of gold chloride test solution. Stellate crystals resembling fern-fronds will appear immediately, having a melting point of 198° C. (388.4°F.).

2. To a fragment or a crystal, or a few drops of an aqueous solution, add platinic chloride test solution. A yellow precipitate appears which, under the microscope, will be found to be feather-like or arranged in stellate form. In more dilute solutions, the crystals may appear as carpet tacks consisting of short, well formed prisms with a single branch from the center.

3. Giesel[1007] treated an aqueous solution of potassium permanganate, obtaining a purple violet precipitate of cocaine permanganate. Occasionally a brown hydrated manganese dioxide appears instead of the crystals. Seiter[1008] recommends the addition of one drop of a 25% solution of sulphuric acid to be added to the aqueous cocaine solution and then 1 cc. of a saturated permanganate solution. This can be conducted on a slide under a microscope with a drop quantity under a low magnification; the characteristic violet-red plates of cocaine will appear.

4. Metzger's Test: To an aqueous solution of cocaine hydrochloride add a 5% solution of chromium trioxide (chromic acid), or a 7.5% solution of potassium dichromate. A yellow precipitate is produced, which redissolves on shaking the mixture. On adding concentrated hydrochloric acid a permanent orange-colored crystalline precipitate of fine needles is formed, and the solution remains yellow for several days. This reaction is shown in solutions of one to 1,000 and is not duplicated, according to Metzger,[1009] by any of the other common alkaloids.

5. Guerbet's Test for Benzoic Acid: As stated before, cocaine is quite easily hydrolized or saponified in the above tests and, therefore, the analyst should test for the presence of benzoic acid which is characteristic for cocaine. To 0.1 mg. or

1007. GEISEL: Pharm. Ztg., Berl., 31:132, 1886; Chem. Centralbl., 1448, 1887.
1008. SEITER: Am. J. Pharm., 83:265, 1911; SEITER and ENGER: Am. J. Pharm., 83:195, 1911; and see HANKIN: Analyst, 36:2, 1911.
1009. METZGER: Pharm. Ztg., Berl., 34:697, 1889.

more of the alkaloidal residue, add three or four drops of fuming nitric acid and take up the mixed nitro compounds with
one drop of a 10% solution of stannous chloride, heat for two
or three minutes, cool and add two drops of a 1% solution of
sodium nitrite and two or four drops of a 1% solution of B-
naphthol in 10% ammonium hydroxide. A deep orange-red
precipitate is formed in the presence of benzoic acid. If this
precipitate be dried and dissolved in 1 cc. of concentrated sulphuric acid a violet-red solution is obtained which, on pouring
into water, changes to a brilliant orange-yellow color, still
visible with 0.01 mg. of benzoic acid.

6. Potassium Ferrocyanide Test: Potassium ferrocyanide
is a very useful reagent for the detection of cocaine. It forms
in a weakly acid solution of cocaine, large rosettes (up to 2
mm.). The rosettes are very similar to those formed from an
ammoniacal solution of zinc oxalate. Chromates form yellow
drops; picrates a fine granular yellow precipitate. The tartrate and oxalate are very easily soluble.

Separation from Animal Tissues: After the alcohol extracts have been obtained with very low heat, distill off the
alcohol with a high vacuum. After purification as given under
alkaloids (page 30), extract with petroleum ether. Then
remove fatty substances with benzene. I have failed a number
of times to find cocaine in cadaveric material where it was
alleged that cocaine had been taken. On the other hand I have
found it in the stomach and contents where death occurred
shortly after ingestion of the poison.

CODEINE

CODEINE is a morphine derivative, methyl morphine,
$C_{17}H_{18}(CH_3)NO_3$, the methyl group, being substituted for
the phenolic hydrogen, of the morphine molecule. It occurs
as white, prismatic, crystals. It crystallizes from water with
one molecule of the solvent, and melts under boiling water to
an oily liquid. It crystallizes from ether, carbon disulphide,
or benzene in anhydrous prisms melting at 155 C. Odorless,
and slightly efflorescent in warm air, levorotatory, and alkaline to litmus. Soluble in 120 parts water, two parts alcohol,
0.5 parts chloroform, eighteen parts ether and thirteen parts
benzene; insoluble in petrolic ether, and only slightly soluble
in fixed alkalis. It dissolves readily in acid-forming salts,

from which solution it is precipitated by sodium hydroxide but not by ammonium hydroxide. Heated with strong mineral acids, codeine is converted into apomorphine, therefore some of the tests for morphine will not differentiate the two alkaloids. Codeine is present in opium only to the amount of about one-twenty-fourth that of morphine (about 0.3%). The United States Pharmacopeia dose for the alkaloid and its two salts (phosphate and sulphate) is 0.03 gm., or 0.5 grain.

Codeine Phosphate, $C_{18}H_{21}NO_3.H_3PO_4.2H_2O$, contains not less than 70% anhydrous codeine. It occurs as fine, white crystals, or a white crystalline powder. It is odorless. Soluble in 2.3 parts water, 325 parts alcohol, 4,500 parts chloroform and 1,875 parts ether. It is efflorescent in the air, and faintly acid to litmus.

Codeine Sulphate, $(C_{18}H_{21}NO_3)_2H_2SO_4.5H_2O$, is found in long, glistening, colorless needle-shaped crystals, or a white crystalline powder. It is odorless, efflorescent in air. Soluble in thirty parts water, 1,280 parts alcohol. Insoluble in chloroform and ether. Neutral to litmus.

Symptoms: Codeine administered in moderate quantities resembles morphine in its action in man, but it is less narcotic, less constipating, and less apt to induce tolerance and habit. It is, therefore, especially valuable in conditions in which the sedative action must be continued for some time, and in patients who do not tolerate morphine. One grain of codeine induces sleep and relieves pain in about the same degree as one-fourth grain of morphine. The sleep is said to be not so deep and restful as that from morphine, as the patient is awakened by slight noises, is restless, and often is not re-freshed when he awakens. Larger quantities at times, instead of producing deeper sleep, increase the restlessness, and cause a considerable exaggeration in the reflex excitability. Its depressant action is not as great, or as enduring, as that of morphine, but the stimulation is more evident and involves not only the cord, but also the medulla and lower parts of the brain. The respiration is slowed, as with morphine, but the amount used must be at least four times that of morphine, larger doses failing to further influence the respiration. Codeine depresses the central nervous system, although in large doses it has some stimulating effects. In sleep the pupils are contracted; during the restless state they are dilated.

Codeine has a much milder action on the bowels and stomach, although doses sufficient to cause narcosis produce constipation. Lewin reports with doses of 0.8 gm., weakness, vertigo, myosis or mydriasis, loss of consciousness, delirium, contraction of the muscles, pulse increase, dyspnea and collapse. Doses of 0.1 to 0.012 gm. showed head pains, roaring ears, restlessness, slow pulse, abdominal pain, and vomiting. There is no tolerance acquired to codeine, regardless of the length of time used, but instead the patients become more susceptible, and doses which at first gave relief are nauseating after continued use. Codeine addiction, although of rare occurrence, has been reported by Gitterman,[1010] and Rogues de Fursac and Monestier.[1011] Codeine should not be used to replace the morphine of the habitue.

Fatal Dose: A dose of 0.3 gm. (4.5 grains) would most probably produce very unpleasant and very dangerous symptoms. Recovery has been reported from doses of eight grains in two cases.

Treatment: This would be the same as for morphine.

Tests: Codeine and morphine resemble each other in some of their color tests, but they can be distinguished from one another by their solubility in the ordinary organic solvents. Codeine is readily soluble in chloroform and ether, morphine is not. Codeine is precipitated by an excess of alkali hydroxides, but not by ammonia, while morphine is soluble in an excess of alkali hydroxides and is precipitated by ammonia. Codeine does not reduce iodic acid. Codein gives no blue color with neutral ferric chloride solution. Codeine gives no Prussian-blue color with ferric chloride and potassium ferricyanide. Sulphuric acid gives no color, but if a trace of arsenate, dilute nitric acid, or ferric chloride be added, a blue color is produced, which changes to red upon addition of a drop of nitric acid.

1. Nitric acid gives a yellow color, the crystals are orange-colored until dissolved.

2. Marquis' reagent gives a deep purple color, so closely resembling the shade produced by morphine that it is worthless as a distinguishing test.

1010. GITTERMAN: *Deutsche Med.-Ztg., Berl.,* 1891.

1011. ROGUES DE FURSAC, J., and MONESTIER, M.: *Ann. de méd. Legale, Par.,* 4:119, 1924; BONHAEFER and SCHWARTZ: *Deutsche med. Wchnschr.,* 56:1043, 1930; HEINMANN, W., and HATRY: *Med. Klin.,* 26: 9669, 1930; FOLEY: *Pennsylvania M. J.,* 36:44, 1932.

3. Froehde's reagent produces no color at first, but a blue color gradually appears.

4. Vanadium-sulphuric acid gives a green, changing gradually to blue.

5. Sulphuric acid with ammonium persulphate gives an orange color.

6. Sulphuric acid with ammonium selenite gives a green color.

7. When dissolved in sulphuric acid, and a drop of cane sugar (10%), a violet-red color appears which changes rapidly to deep red on heating, which is similar to morphine.

8. Codeine picrate prepared by precipitating from hydro-chloride acid solution and recrystallized from 10% acetic acid, melts at 195.5° C.

9. The micro-chemical method as devised by Tunmann[1012] is a means of differentiating morphine from codeine. The unknown is sublimed, covered with a watch glass, and a drop of hydriodic acid introduced at the edge. A granular precipitate forms which disappears on heating. The crystals of morphine tetraiodide form immediately upon cooling, but more rapidly in the presence of ethyl alcohol. The morphine tetraiodide crystals are always flat, rectangular plates 30μ to 50μ broad 80μ to 120μ long, are prismatic and of a brownish-red color. Most of the crystals are united to ladder and step-like aggregates 1 mm. or more long, which are combined to stars and crosses. Codeine triiodide crystals are paler, thicker, and smaller, about one-third those of morphine. Single crystals are rare, forming half-moon like triangles with a concave base and a blunted apex.

They are mostly twin crystals which always grow out on the convex side, giving butterfly and goblet-like forms.

Isolation from Tissue: Codeine is separated from the tissues by the same method as that described under Morphine. It is extracted from an alkaline solution by ether, amyl alcohol, chloroform, or benzene. Codeine is found in the stomach, intestines, blood, liver, and other organs, whether it was taken by mouth or hypodermically. It is excreted mainly in the urine and feces.

Ethyl Morphine, $C_{17}H_{18}(C_2H_5)NO_3$.—Dionine is the hydro-chloride of ethyl morphine closely related to codeine and

1012. TUNMANN: *Apoth. Ztg.*, 31:148, 1916.

resembles it in all its properties, but possesses no advantage over codeine. It is removed from alkaline solution by ether and chloroform, but is insoluble in petrolic ether. It decomposes at 110 to 115° C. without melting. It is a white crystalline powder, readily soluble in water and alcohol.

1. Froehde's reagent gives a green to deep green and eventually a blue color, differing somewhat from codeine.

2. Nitric acid gives a yellow color.

3. Ferric chloride containing a trace of potassium ferricyanide gives a blue-green color.

4. Marquis' reagent gives a purple color.

5. Mandelin's reagent gives a green color.

6. Codeine gives a precipitate on adding a few drops of ammonia water, soluble in excess, while dionine requires a greater excess of ammonia water to dissolve it, and it soon separates again on standing.

Benzyl Morphine, $C_{17}H_{18}NO_2C_6H_5CH_2$—Peronine is the hydrochloride of benzyl morphine. It is extracted from alkaline solutions by ether and petrolic ether.

1. Fröehde's reagent gives a brown, violet, brownish-green turning to slate color.

2. Marquis' reagent gives a purple shade.

3. Mandelin's reagent gives an olive brown color.

4. Nitric acid gives a yellow color.

Apomorphine, $C_{17}H_{17}O_2N$, is prepared by the action of some dehydrating substance upon morphine. Apomorphine is morphine less one molecule of water. The depressant action of morphine is greatly reduced on the central nervous system, but the stimulating action is the same. This stimulation is most developed in the vomiting center of the medulla oblongata.

Apomorphine in one-twelfth to one-sixth grain doses causes vomiting and nausea within ten to fifteen minutes. This subsides immediately after the evacuation of the stomach, but with larger doses continued nausea may persist, followed by depression and sleep, with salivation, tears and cold perspiration, muscular weakness, fast pulse. These effects are regarded as sequelae of the emetic action and not due directly to the drug. This depression and weakness in a few cases, passed into alarming collapse, but no actual fatalities are recorded due to apomorphine.

Apomorphine is the most powerful emetic known. Its action is on the vomiting center of the medulla, and is not a local one on the stomach. This is apparent from the fact that vomiting is produced more promptly and with a smaller dose if administered hypodermically than when given by mouth. No emesis is produced if apomorphine is placed in the stomach after the vessels supplying that organ have been ligated. Apomorphine is not excreted into the stomach, like morphine, and it is stated that it has been found in the mucous membranes of the air passages. It is possible that it may be decomposed in the tissues. Emesis may be indicated in poisoning, and here apomorphine is especially useful. But in a great majority of cases a better method of treatment is repeated washing of the stomach with a stomach tube, for in narcotic poisoning apomorphine sometimes does not act, owing to the depression of the vomiting center, and in corrosive poisoning a certain amount of danger attends its use, as the pressure on the walls of the stomach exerted by the contraction of the diaphragm and abdominal muscles may lead to a rupture of the weakened walls of the organ. In irritant poisoning, on the other hand, the reflex vomiting set up is generally sufficient to empty the stomach, and the indications are rather to allay the gastric irritation than to increase it by causing violent movement of the abdominal walls as produced by apomorphine.

Diacetyl Morphine, $C_{21}H_{23}NO_5$, (Heroin), is an artificial derivative of morphine with which it shares all the disadvantages and over which it has no important advantages. It was originally introduced with the claim that therapeutic doses not only lessen the cough reflex and slow the respiration, but also that the inspirations are deepened and more powerful, so that the alveolar air is more effectively ventilated. It has, however, been shown that there is no real difference from morphine in these respects. It is now generally conceded that heroin is as effective as morphine in cough, but not more so; that it is less effective against dyspnea; and that it is more liable to produce habit and toxic effects.

Heroin is prepared by the acetylization of morphine, the hydrogen atoms of the alcohol and phenol groups of morphine being replaced by the acetic radical. It occurs in white prisms or as white crystalline powder, odorless, having a bitter taste.

It melts between 171 and 173°C. It is soluble in 1,700 parts of water, thirty-one parts alcohol, 1.4 parts chloroform, 100 parts ether; very soluble in benzene. Heroin is precipitated by alkalis, but is soluble in excess. When heated in solution it decomposes to monoacetylmorphine. With potassium hydroxide it is saponified to morphine and acetic acid. These factors must be considered in quantitative work, where a smaller quantity than that declared is found; it must not be considered conclusive that the proper quantity was not originally present, but a further examination must be made for morphine. This deacetylization of heroin takes place to a great extent in the body, so that, in cases of poisoning, morphine is usually found present. (Heroin is no longer an official drug.)

Tests: 1. Heroin differs from morphine in being extracted from alkaline solution by chloroform.

2. Froehde's reagent gives a brilliant crimson purple color, soon fading.

3. Marquis' reagent gives a crimson color, soon fading.

4. Sulphuric acid with hexamethylene tetramine gives a golden-yellow color, changing to saffron and finally blue. (Morphine gives a purple color.)

5. Neutral solutions do not liberate iodine from iodic acid.

6. Ferric chloride gives no blue color.

7. The picrate recrystallized from alcohol (50%) melts at 200 to 205° C.

8. When heroin (0.1 gm.) is heated with alcohol (1 cc.) and sulphuric acid (1 cc.), ethyl acetate is formed, which is recognized by its odor. (Morphine and codeine do not give this test.)

9. Sulphuric acid with chloral hydrate gives a brownish-red color. (Morphine gives a violet, and codeine a bluish-green, (changing to red).

10. Platinic chloride gives rosette crystals, (McNally's test), which melt at 223° C.[1013] Morphine gives an amorphous precipitate.

Symptoms: Heroin resembles morphine in its general results, but acts more strongly on the respiration, and is therefore more poisonous. The advantages claimed for heroin by its advocates have not been confirmed. The depressant effects

1013. McNally, W. D.: *J. Lab. & Clin. Med.*, 2: 649, 1917.

on the cerebrum appear to be greater than those of codeine. Large doses have caused excitement and convulsions in animals and man. The more common symptoms are headache, disturbance of vision, slow small regular pulse, restlessness, cramps in the extremities, slight cyanosis, respiration slow and deep, death from respiratory paralysis.

Heroin is excreted unchanged in the urine, some also being found in the feces. It can be extracted from the saliva of race horses. In many states, the saliva of every winner is tested for alkaloids. When it is given for some time, the tissues learn to destroy it, and it no longer appears in the excretions. A certain tolerance is observed, the narcotic action becomes less marked and may entirely disappear, but the poisoning effect of large doses still remains.

Treatment: The treatment for heroin poisoning is the same as that given for morphine, with special attention given to the control of the respiratory paralysis.

Fatal Dose: The toxic dose of heroin is not certain, but a therapeutic dose which at times amounts to one-sixth grain must be regarded as very near the toxic dose. Poisonings have been reported from one-twelfth grain, while recovery has taken place after two grains.

McNally[1014] reported the following: W. K., of age twenty, a salesman, was admitted to a hospital in an unconscious condition and died seven hours later. The physical examination was comparatively negative save for coolness of the body, blue mottling of the abdomen, and a weak and irregular heart. The pupils were contracted. The pulmotor was used for intervals of three-fourths and one-half hour, respectively. The stomach was washed out with permanganate solution. Respirations were very slow, being thirteen per minute on admission to the hospital, and after the first use of the pulmotor, forty-two. They fell to sixteen when the pulmotor was used the second time. Just before death they were nineteen per minute. Postmortem examination showed the following: Pupils of the eyes were equal and dilated. External surfaces of the brain presented no change. Upon sectioning the pons, medulla, and cerebellar hemispheres, no gross alterations or evidences of disease were noted. An engorgement of the abdominal veins

1014. McNally, W. D.: *J. Lab. & Clin. Med.,* 2:570, 1917.

and marked passive hyperemia and edema of the lung were found; petechial hemorrhages in the epicardium and in the lining of the greater antrum of the stomach; dilation of the mitral ring; persistent lymphoid tissue in the thymic body; hyperplasia of the lymph nodes of the spleen, the lymph glands, the stomach, the small and large bowel, and of Peyer's patches; hyperplasia of the aorta; and slight chronic catarrhal prostatitis left obliterative fibrous pleuritis. The urine contained albumen and sugar in considerable quantity. In the toxicological examination of the viscera in this case, 0.3022 gm. of alkaloid was recovered. The portion extracted from the liver, kidney, spleen, the preservative in which the organs were held, the intestines and intestinal contents, all gave the reactions for morphine. The alkaloid extracted from the stomach and stomach content responded to the tests for heroin.

Isolation from Tissues: Owing to the hydrolysis of heroin to morphine, the usual method of extraction from the tissues fails to show its presence. The experiments of McNally indicate that the deacetylization of heroin does not take place in the stomach and stomach contents, while morphine is found in the other organs examined. McNally[1015] advances a method for its separation from tissue by successive portions of 50% alcohol acidified with a few drops of 10% tartaric acid. Keep the temperature of the sample close to 50°C. Allow the combined extract to remain in a cool place until the fat separates. The fat is separated in a separatory funnel, and washed with acidified water, and the washings are added to the main extract. If the sample is allowed to stand over night, considerable extraneous matter settles to the bottom of the flask and can be removed by filtration, washing the residue with 50% alcohol. Evaporate the alcoholic extract under diminished pressure, the water-bath being kept well under the boiling point. The pasty residue is taken up with a little cold acidified water, and the extraneous matter filtered off. The filtrate is allowed to filter into 95% alcohol, the protein substances and other impurities thus becoming granular on standing, and capable of easy filtration. The alcohol is evaporated off under diminished pressure, until the liquid in the distilling flask amounts to about 20 mils. This residue is taken

1015. McNally, W. D.: *J. Lab. & Clin. Med.*, 2: 649, 1917.

up with cold water, acidified with tartaric acid, and filtered. To the filtrate is added 1 gm. of "alcresta" (Lloyd's reagent), and the mixture well stirred. The alcresta, together with its adhering substances, is filtered off and the liquid tested for alkaloids. If any alkaloid remains in the filtrate, more alcresta is added and the mixture filtered. Transfer the alcresta containing the alkaloid to a glass separatory funnel and extract with successive portions of ammoniated chloroform. The chloroform is evaporated, leaving the free alkaloid as a residue. If any fat accompanies the alkaloid, dissolve the residue in a 0.5% hydrochloric acid solution, filter, and re-extract with ammoniated chloroform. The alkaloid is weighed and submitted to the tests above outlined for heroin. The purity of the residue may be shown by volumetric methods, the melting point, and crystalline appearance of the platinum salt. In most of McNally's extracts a brown residuous product was obtained, a crystalline residue appearing in only one instance.

Pseudomorphine, $(C_{17}H_{18}NO_3)_2$, may be considered as a condensation product of two molecules of morphine with a loss of two atoms of hydrogen. It is sometimes found present in opium or is prepared by the mild oxidation of morphine. Soluble in ammonia and alkalis, insoluble in water, acids, alcohol or ether. It crystallizes in leaflets, which decompose without melting. This product is of little importance in toxicology, because it is not poisonous; but it might enter into a case, as to whether it is present as a condensation product of morphine.

1. Sulphuric acid and sugar give a green color, changing to brown.

2. Sulphuric acid with a trace of iron gives a blue to green color.

Papaverine, $C_{20}H_{21}NO_4$, is an alkaloid obtained from opium, belonging to the benzyl isoquinoline group. It is not a morphine derivative. The papaverine group includes most of the other opium alkaloids not yet mentioned. Papaverine, narcotine, and narceine are the most important to the drug analyst. Papaverine appears as fine, white, rhombic prisms or needles, or sometimes in scales. It is odorless and tasteless. It is nearly insoluble in cold water, and slightly soluble in alcohol, ether, chloroform and benzene—somewhat more soluble in these liquids when hot, but deposited by them on cooling. It melts at 147° C. It is easily removed from an acidified solution by chloroform, and partially by ether. Narcotine is also removed by chloroform, but the alkaloids of this group may be separated by dissolving in oxalic acid, and concentrating the solution until papaverine oxalate crystallizes out. Papaverine also forms a very insoluble benzoate.

Tests: 1. Papaverine aqueous solution (one to ten) with a few drops of hydrochloric acid, and a few drops of potassium ferricyanide solution, gives a lemon-yellow precipitate. (Distinctive from other opium alkaloids.)

2. Marquis' reagent gives a colorless, at most, a faintly yellowish-green solution, gradually changing to deep rose and finally brown. (Morphine and its esters give purple or violet color.)

3. Sulphuric acid gives at most a very faint pinkish-brown or brown (limit of cryptopine, thebaine, or other organic impurities).

4. When a mixture of hydrochloric acid solution and a few drops of iodic acid solution is shaken with chloroform, the chloroform layer should not be colored violet (morphine).

5. Froehde's reagent gives a purple, gradually changing to blue.

6. Sulphuric acid and potassium dichromate give a purple, blue, green and finally deep blue.

7. Sulphuric acid with ammonium persulphate gives a yellow.

Warren[1016] reports the following specific reaction for papaverine (he states that only one other alkaloid, that from sanguinaria, gives this same test): Papaverine and potassium ferricyanide are mixed dry, then treated with Marquis' reagent, which gives a light blue, changing to violet and finally green fading to brownish-yellow. If selenious acid is added as the oxidizing reagent, the sanguinaria alkaloid gives a purple, while papaverine gives a greenish-blue to deep blue. The picrate melts at 179 to 181° C., the picrolonate at 220° C. When oxidized with potassium permanganate it forms a number of compounds, one of which is papaveraldine, $C_{20}H_{19}NO_5$, melting at 210° C. Papaveric acid, $C_{16}H_{13}NO_7$, is another oxidation product. It is dibasic, containing a ketone

1016. WARREN: *J. Am. Chem. Soc.*, 27:2402, 1915.

group, and when fused with alkalis is converted into protocatechuic acid.

Action: Papaverine is a comparatively weak poison. Its action on the central nervous system is about midway between morphine and codeine. Even large doses do not produce the amount of excitement caused by codeine or the soporific action of morphine. Small doses are followed by sleep and slow respiration, but these are not increased with larger doses. The heart beat is slower, but the blood pressure is scarcely affected. Papaverine is completely destroyed in the tissues. Single dose one-half grain to one and one-third grains, daily dose 7.5 grains. Single doses of fifteen grains are said to be non-toxic.

Preparations: Papaverine Hydrochloride, $C_{20}H_{21}O_4N.HCl$, contains not less than 88% of papaverine. It occurs in fine white crystalline powder, or in small monoclinic plates or prisms. It is odorless, with a bitter taste, and is permanent in air. It is sparingly soluble in water, soluble in alcohol and chloroform, insoluble in ether, and acid to litmus.

Papaverine Sulphate, $(C_{20}H_{21}O_4N)_2H_2SO_4$, contains not less than 85% papaverine. It occurs as white crystalline powder. It is odorless, with a bitter taste, slightly hygroscopic. It is soluble in water, alcohol, and chloroform; insoluble in ether. It is acid to litmus.

Papaveramine, $C_{21}H_{21}NO_5$, is found as an impurity with papaverine, which it resembles in its chemical properties. It is slightly soluble in water, ether, and benzene; soluble in alcohol, and in chloroform. Crystals melt at 128 to 129° C. This alkaloid present in papaverine will cause a violet-blue color with sulphuric acid.

Thebaine, $C_{19}H_{21}NO_3$, is soluble in alcohol, ether, chloroform and benzene, almost insoluble in water and alkalis, insoluble in petrolic ether. When heated to 130° C. it sublimes to caffeine-like crystals. (Papaverine, narceine, and narcotine do not sublime.) It crystallizes from alcohol in leaflets which melt at 193° C. Thebaine is very poisonous, producing symptoms resembling those of strychnine, but less active. It differs from morphine and codeine in its color reactions, giving with nitric acid a yellow color, and with sulphuric acid a reddish-brown. Froehde's reagent gives reddish brown. The picrate melts at 189 to 191° C.

Narcotine, $C_{22}H_{23}NO_7$, is present in opium to the amount of about 5%. It is extracted from opium with ether. Denarcotized opium is a well known commercial product. It resembles papaverine rather than morphine in action, but has even less depressant effects. It is a much less poisonous alkaloid than morphine or codeine, and very large quantities have been given with little or no narcosis. It is soluble in chloroform and benzol, slightly soluble in alcohol and ether, petrolic ether, hot water; insoluble in cold water and alkalis. It melts at 176° C.

1. It is precipitated by the general alkaloidal reagents.

2. Narcotine, treated with sulphuric acid, is decomposed into opianic acid and hydrocotarnine. The opianic acid is then tested for as follows:[1017] Dissolve in sulphuric acid (10%), heat gently after adding potassium permanganate solution (2%) until pink color is removed. Dilute with alcohol and test as follows: Mix one part of the alcoholic solution with two parts concentrated sulphuric acid and 0.1 part of phenolic solution; with a 5% alcoholic solution of gallic acid, get a blue color changing to greenish-brown. A 5% alcoholic solution of guaiacol gives a red, changing to a blue when heated on the water-bath; with a-naphthol, a gooseberry-red; and with b-naphthol, a wine-red. (Hydrastine gives the same colors under this treatment, as it is also decomposed to opianic acid.)

3. An alcoholic solution of narcotine (one to 100), plus concentrated sulphuric acid, plus solution of gallic acid (5%), and heated on the water-bath, gives an emerald-green color, changing to blue. (Hydrastine and hydrastinine also give these colors.)

4. Sulphuric acid gives a pale yellow solution, gradually turning to red.

5. Sulphuric acid, plus nitric acid, gives a red color.

6. Sulphuric acid, plus sodium hypochlorite, gives a red color.

7. Marquis' reagent gives a purple to slate color, fading.

8. Froehde's reagent gives a deep green.

9. Sulphuric acid and ammonium persulphate give an orange-red color.

10. The picrate melts at 141° C.

Narceine may be prepared from narcotine by digesting the

1017. LABAT: *Bull. Soc. Chem.*, 4:5, 1909.

latter with excess of methyl iodide for ten hours, heating on the water-bath to remove the excess iodide, dissolving in alcohol, and treating with chlorine in excess. Let stand a few hours to precipitate yellow crystals. The filtrate on evaporation gives a brownish gum, becoming crystalline narcotine methyl chloride, which gives narcine by neutralizing with sodium hydroxide and passing in a current of steam. Narceine occurs as colorless, prismatic needles, melting at 170 to 171° C. It is soluble in alcohol, alkalis, and hot water; slightly soluble in water and chloroform; insoluble in ether, benzol, and petrolic ether. It is extracted in the alkaline alcohol-chloroform fraction with morphine.

1. Mayer's reagent, mercuric chloride, or potassium ferrocyanide, give no precipitate. Gold and platinic chlorides, picric acid, tannin, and potassium bichromate give a precipitate on standing.

2. Iodine gives a brown precipitate; if excess iodine is removed by ammonia the precipitate is blue.

3. The picrate melts at 127 to 128.5° C. The platinochloride darkens at 190°, and melts at 198 to 199° C.

4. Sulphuric acid gives a brown color, changing to yellow-green and finally blue.

5. Froehde's reagent gives greenish-brown.

6. Marquis' reagent gives brown, green on edges.

7. Sulphuric acid with a trace of tannic acid gives a green color. (Narcotine and hydrastine give the same color.)

8. Sulphuric acid with a trace of resorcinol, when warmed, gives a crimson to cherry-red, changing to blood-red on cooling, and fading to orange.

9. Sulphuric acid, with ammonium persulphate, gives a violet, changing to blood-red to yellow.

10. Hydrochloric acid dilute with chlorine water, followed by an excess of ammonia water ,gives an orange-red color. (Thebaine gives a reddish-brown.) It has distinct acid properties.

Narceine has little or no action of any kind, being the weakest opium alkaloid in its effect. Its salts are broken up in aqueous solution, so that it is probably absorbed very slowly and imperfectly.

Laudanine, $C_{20}H_{25}NO_4$, crystallizes from alcohol or chloroform in prisms melting at 166° C. It is optically inactive. It is soluble in alcohol and ether.

1. Ferric chloride in a neutral solution gives a green color.

2. Sulphuric acid gives a pink tint, changing to violet on heating.

Laudanine, laudanidine, laudanosine, tritopine, and codamine are all closely related, being strong poisonous alkaloids.

Laudanidine melts at 177° C. and is levorotatory. It is separated from laudanine as a hydrochloride, which is very soluble in water.

Laudanosine melts at 89° C., and is soluble in alcohol, ether, chloroform, and benzene; insoluble in water and alkalis. It is dextrorotatory. Ferric chloride and sulphuric acid separately give no color.

Tritopine melts at 182° C. It is soluble in chloroform and slightly in ether; soluble in alkalis, but re-precipitates in an excess.

Codamine melts at 121 to 126° C.; is soluble in chloroform, ether, alcohol, and benzene, and somewhat soluble in water. Nitric acid gives a deep green color. Sulphuric acid with a trace of ferric chloride gives a greenish-blue color.

Dilaudid[1018] is obtained by the hydrogenation of morphine in a warm acid solution in the presence of a large excess of palladium, platinum, or their respective salts, used as a catalyst. It is a white crystalline powder, containing 88.66% of its alkaloid base. It is readily soluble in water (one to three) and in hot alcohol. But it is only sparingly soluble in cold alcohol, and is insoluble in ether. When dissolved in water, dilaudid gives a neutral solution which, when treated with ammonia or sodium carbonate, liberates the base, a white crystalline powder having a melting point of 259 to 260° C.

Zahler[1019] observed a slight decrease in the pulse rate and also in respiration. There was also a slight initial increase in blood pressure, followed by a drop, not exceeding 10 mm. The skin first became flushed, but soon returned to normal. Alvarez[1020] found that dilaudid has a less constipating action and less euphoria; the appetite is less disturbed, and its use causes less habituation. He gives two cases, in which 2.5 and 10 mg. a day were taken, with no difficulty in stopping. It does not

1018. KING, M. R., HIMMELSBACK, C. K., and SANDERS, B. S.: U. S. Pub. Health Service, Suppl. No. 113 to Pub. Health Reports, 1935.

1019. ZAHLER, HEINRICH: *Deutsche med. Wchnschr.*, 56:522, 1930.

1020. ALVAREZ, W. C.: *Proc. Staff Meet., Mayo Clin.*, 7:480, 1932.

have the calming effect of morphine. However, it does have
some advantages over codeine. Zahler found that the daily use
of the drug over a period of three months caused no discernible
decrease in its therapeutic value. He found that 5 mg. by mouth
was about as effective as 2 mg. subcutaneously. Hoesselin[1021]
found a similarity between dilaudid and morphine on respiration, pulse, and blood pressure. Intravenous injection of 4 mg.
of dilaudid, caused a drop of blood pressure from 130/65 to
120/60, a decrease in pulse rate from 70 to 66, and a decrease in
respiration from sixteen to thirteen within fifty minutes.
Basch[1022] found dilaudid five times more effective than morphine, and almost free from undesirable side-effects when used
as an analgesic in gall-stone colic, renal calculus, and other
painful disorders. Stroud[1023] reports the use of dilaudid in the
pains of cancer. He finds it an effective analgesic for constant
pain, and claims it is better than any other opiate. Stroud believes it is less habit forming, although his observations were
not conclusive; it caused less deterioration of character, and
morale, with less troublesome side actions. Eddy[1024] states that
it is a powerful analgesic and can depress respiration profoundly. Its efficiency is about equal to that of morphine, i.e., the ratio of their effective doses is equal to the ratio of their toxic
doses. King, Himmelsbach, and Sanders have arrived at the
following conclusions from substituting dilaudid for morphine:
"(1) Dilaudid is an effective substitute for morphine. (2) Dilaudid possesses definite addiction liability. (3) Definite mor-
phine-dilaudid cross-tolerance exists. (4) The potency of dilaudid is approximately four times that of morphine, but the
duration of its action appears to be considerably less than that
of morphine. (5) In the presence of a daily laxative, equally
effective doses of dilaudid are as constipative as morphine. (6)
In equally effective doses, dilaudid appears to affect sleep as
does morphine. (7) Dilaudid appears to possess no therapeutic
advantage over morphine."

Dilaudid is generally given in a dose about one-fifth that
of morphine; one-twentieth of a grain of dilaudid takes the
place of one-fourth of a grain of morphine. Its effect is usually

1021. HOESSELIN, H. VON: Klin. Wchnschr., 9:1382, 1930.
1022. BASCH: Fortschr. d. Med., 44:622, 1926.
1023. STROUD, C. M.: J.A.M.A., 103:1421, 1934.
1024. EDDY, NATHAN B.: J.A.M.A., 100:1032, 1933.

apparent within fifteen minutes, and continues for four to eight hours. The same type of depressive effects may result from overdoses, and it is not free from addictive properties.[1025]

COLCHICUM

THE meadow saffron, colchicum autumnale, contains two poisonous alkaloids of importance: colchicine and colchiceine. The root, or corm, and seeds are both used commercially. The corm, assayed by the U. S. P. process, should contain not less than 0.35% colchicine, and the seeds 0.45%. In the U. S. P. XI, the seed is official as colchici semen, and is practically inert.

The root is externally brownish and finely wrinkled, internally whitish, with numerous circular groups of fibrovascular bundles, giving the surfaces of the transverse sections a papillose appearance. The odor is slight; the taste sweetish, bitter, and somewhat acrid. The dose is four grains.

The seeds are subglobular, about 2 mm. in diameter, very slightly pointed at the hilum; externally reddish-brown, finely pitted. They are internally whitish, bony hard, nearly inodorous; their taste is bitter and somewhat acrid.

Tinctura Colchici is prepared from the seed, and yields from each 100 cc. not less than 0.036 gm., and not more than 0.044 gm. colchicine. The dose is 2.0 cc. (30 minims).

Colchicine, $C_{22}H_{25}O_6N$, occurs as pale yellow amorphous scales, or powder, turning darker on exposure to light. It is practically odorless. One gram is soluble in 22 cc. of water, in 220 cc. of ether, and in 100 cc. of benzene at 25°C. It is freely soluble in alcohol and chloroform, and is insoluble in petroleum benzin. Colchicine melts at between 142 and 146°C. Colchicine is the methyl ester of colchiceine or acetotrimethylcolchicinic acid, and, on heating with mineral acids, it is readily split up into methyl alcohol and colchicine. The latter, on heating with hydrochloric acid, loses an acetyl group as acetic acid, and then three methyl groups as methyl chloride, leaving colchicinic acid, $C_{15}H_{11}N(OH)_3(COOH)$.

Tests: Dilute acid solutions of colchicine are precipitated by most of the alkaloidal reagents, except platinic chloride and picric acid. Gold chloride slowly throws down colchicine from

---

1025. For an excellent bibliography, see Suppl. No. 113 cited in Ref. 1018.

its acidified solution in the form of a yellow amorphous precipitate which changes to a crystalline form.

Sulphuric Acid Test: Colchicine dissolves in concentrated sulphuric acid to a yellow solution. To this solution add a drop of nitric acid, the color changes to green, blue, violet, wine red, and finally green. The addition of concentrated sodium hydroxide in excess, gives an orange-red. It dissolves in nitric acid, giving a deep purple or bluish color. With ammonium vanadate it gives a yellowish-green color. Sulphuric acid and bichromate give a green color, soon fading. Marquis' reagent gives reddish crystals and a yellow liquid. Ferric chloride when added to an aqueous solution of pure colchicine produces no color, but, upon heating, a brownish-red color is produced, which changes to brownish-black. (Colchiceine will not give this reaction.) Ferric chloride added to an alcoholic solution of colchicine gives a garnet-red color immediately. Mandelin's reagent gives green to greenish-brown. Froehde's reagent gives brownish-orange. Mecke's reagent gives citron yellow to yellow-brown. Vitali's reagent gives dark brown.

Barillot's Test: Some of the ether or chloroform residue of the alkaloid is mixed with 1 cc. sulphuric acid and 0.2 gm. of oxalic acid. This golden-yellow mixture is sealed in a small glass tube and heated to 120°C. for one hour. The tube is then opened and the content, which is dark reddish-brown, is diluted with water. Add an excess of alcoholic sodium hydroxide, followed by an excess of acetic acid, which causes a yellow precipitate to form. Extract with chloroform and evaporate to dryness, leaving a yellow residue, which becomes a violet red on treatment with concentrated nitric acid, and raspberry red with concentrated sulphuric acid. (This test differentiates colchicine from morphine and codeine, both of which give a blue color, and from ptomaines which give no similar color.)[1026]

A non-poisonous substance giving many of the reactions for colchicine has been found among the normal constituents of beer, being apparently derived from hops. Putrefying cadavers yield substances which bear a close resemblance to colchicine, and might easily be mistaken for this alkaloid in toxicological work.

Biological Tests: Animals have shown great differences in

1026. *Bull. Soc. Chim.,* 3rd series, 11:514, 1894.

their sensitivity to colchicine, and the amount generally obtainable in toxicological cases is not sufficient for animal tests. Experiments have shown that a cat requires 0.5 to 1 mg. per kilo, a dog 1 to 5 mg. per kilo, a rabbit 7 mg. per kilo, and a frog 100 mg. to 1 gm. to produce death. White mice succumb to a dose of 0.05 to 0.2 mg. of colchicine; the symptoms progress slowly, but appear in about twenty-four hours. This slow progression of symptoms is typical for colchicine.

Extraction from Tissue: This alkaloid is separated from the tissue by the usual method outlined, with the following alterations and precautions. Colchicine is readily saponified by heating with acids or alkalis; therefore great care should be taken in the extraction process, not allowing the temperature to exceed 50°C. (122°F.). Colchicine is extracted from acid as well as alkaline solutions by amyl alcohol, chloroform, and benzol. To purify the colchicine extract, dissolve in warm water, filter, then extract with petroleum ether, which removes the fatty and resinous material, after which extract with chloroform. Another method is to precipitate the colchicine with tannic acid and filter, washing the residue on the filter paper with water. Mix this precipitate with freshly prepared lead hydroxide, dry, grind to a powder, and extract with chloroform. The extracts of the urine, kidneys, and intestines submitted from autopsy give the better yields of colchicine. Obolonski states that colchicine is stable for several months after death, having found it present after 258 days.[1027]

Poisoning by colchicum is found quite frequently in the literature: homicidal, suicidal, and accidental, proving fatal in many cases. In 132 cases reported as poisoned by colchicum, 118 were accidental, six suicidal, and eight homicidal.

Symptoms: No symptoms whatever are caused by small doses of colchicum. Large doses (4 to 5 mg.) cause diarrhea with griping in susceptible persons, and in the therapeutic use purging is often observed. This drug is slow in action, showing symptoms several hours after large as well as small doses.

In poisoning, whether injected or given by mouth, the symptoms arise from the alimentary tract; pain in the gastric region is followed by salivation, nausea, vomiting, and diarrhea. At first the evacuations are the ordinary contents of the stom-

1027. OBOLONSKI: *Vrtljschr. f. gerichtl. Med.*, 1888.

ach and intestines, but afterwards a quantity of sticky mucous fluid is ejected, often containing blood. Later, depression, apathy, and collapse follow. Movements are slow and difficult, especially in the posterior extremities, which eventually become completely motionless. The paralysis then increases upward until the fore limbs and respiratory muscles are involved, when death occurs from asphyxia. Consciousness remains until death, though there is some giddiness and precordial anxiety, and occasionally some confusion or even delirium preceding the collapse. In man at least, it would appear that the gastrointestinal irritation is not altogether an inflammatory action, since the intestines may appear quite normal after death, and there is seldom more than a simple catarrh of the duodenum. When ecchymoses, etc., have been found, they have been ascribed to the mechanical effects of the extremely energetic peristalsis.

The heart action and blood pressure in animals remain unaffected, while in man the pulse may become small, rapid, and thready; this no doubt is due to the collapse. The respiration is slow, though deep and full at first. Later it becomes shallow, and death is due to failure of respiration, the heart continuing to beat for some time later. The central nervous system is depressed, but this is thought to be due to the effect upon the abdominal organs, rather than directly on the nervous system. The leukocytes in the peripheral circulation are at first reduced, and later increased beyond the normal amount. The kidneys in some cases show complete anuria, in others increased urination. With small doses the urea and uric acid output is increased, but with larger doses the urea and uric acid are lessened. Bloody urine sometimes results.

Externally, colchicum is a local irritant, causing redness and smarting when applied to the skin. The dust when inhaled produces sneezing and conjunctival hyperemia, also a burning sensation in the mouth and throat.

Fatal Dose: Death from 0.05 of a grain has been reported occurring from twelve hours to ten days after ingestion. One-third of a grain (0.02 gm.) of the pure alkaloid, colchicine, is very liable to cause death. Kobert, from experimental work with dogs, calculated that one grain would be fatal for man; a violent diarrhea has resulted from the ingestion of one-twelfth of a grain (0.005 gm.).

Fatal Period: In the majority of fatal cases from a single dose, death has taken place in about twenty-four hours. Since this poison is excreted very slowly, repeated doses may be cumulative.

Treatment: In the treatment of colchicum poisoning give a cathartic and an emetic at once, also large quantities of water to act on the kidneys. Tannic acid forms an insoluble tannate and should be administered in large amounts; opium to check the vomiting and diarrhea, and to relieve the pain; with stimulants to counteract the depression.

Postmortem Appearances: The alimentary tract shows all the evidence of an acute gastro-enteritis, with numerous hemorrhagic areas especially in the upper part of the bowel, although mild cases may reveal nothing more than simple catarrhal inflammation of the duodenum.

CONIUM

CONIUM MACULATUM (spotted or common poison hemlock) grows wild in the United States and Europe. Conium contains six alkaloids, coniine, $C_8H_{17}N$, methyl-coniine, $C_9H_{19}NO$, and ethyl-piperidine. They are found in all parts of the plant, in the greatest amount in the unripe fruit which is used as the drug. Coniine predominates, the amount of the other alkaloids being proportionately very small. Conhydrine

| Pyridine | Piperidine | Coniine |

the next highest in quality is found in only about 0.05 the amount of coniine. This plant is of historical interest; Socrates was put to death by drinking its infusion. I have not seen one case in the examination of many thousands of bodies for poisons. An occasional case is found in the literature. Recently two cases have been reported.[1028] Comparative studies

1028. TERRELL, L. L.: *Kentucky M. J.*, 29:595, 1931; ERSKELUND: *Ugesk. f. laeger.*, 96:1257, 1934.

of the action of piperidine, coniine, and coniceine have been made by Kroger and Koll[1029] and Skezama.

Coniine is one of the simple derivatives of piperidine, obtained by reduction from pyridine. By substituting methyl, ethyl, propyl, and other alkyls for hydrogen, a series of alkaloids can be produced. Propyl-piperidine is coniine, being the first alkaloid synthetisized. The synthetic coniine has properties identical with the natural alkaloid, except that it is optically inactive. Coniine, $C_8H_{17}N$, when pure, is a colorless, oily liquid, with the odor of tobacco when concentrated, but, when diluted, has the characteristic mousy odor. Age and light darken the alkaloid. It is strongly alkaline in reaction. It melts at —2.50°C., and boils at about 166°C.

Volatile at ordinary temperatures, it distills readily with steam, or alcohol vapors. Its specific gravity is 0.8444 at 20°C. Rotation, (a) =16.4° at 19°C., the rotatory power being diminished upon dilution. Coniine solidifies to a crystalline mass in the cold, becoming fluid at —2°C. It is soluble in fifty parts of water, and readily soluble in alcohol, ether, petrolic ether, ethyl acetate, benzene and acetone. It forms a definite compound with carbon disulphide, which when evaporated leaves needle-like crystals. Coniine readily forms salts, which are colorless, odorless, and soluble in water, alcohol, and chloroform, but not in petrolic ether. On inverting a beaker moistened with hydrochloric acid over a drop of coniine white fumes are produced, forming the crystalline coniine hydrochloride. This reaction is similar to that given by nicotine, which gives an amorphous instead of a crystalline salt. The hydrochloride may also be formed by passing dry hydrogen chloride through an ether solution of coniine. The large rhombic crystals of coniine hydrochloride melt at 220°C. (428°F.). Nearly all the general alkaloidal reagents precipitate coniine if not too dilute. The platinic chloride salt, $(C_8H_{17}NHCl)_2 PtCl_4$, orange yellow crystals, melting at 175°C. (347°F.), crystallize from hot alcohol as deep red four-sided plates. Gold salt, $C_8H_{17}NHClAuCl_3$, crystals melt at 77°C. (170.6°F.). Gold and platinic chlorides give no precipitate in dilutions of one in 100. The hydroiodide melts at 165°C.; the hydrobromide at 211°C.; picrate, small yellow prisms, at 75°C.;

1029. KROGER and KOLL: *Arch. f. exper. Path. u. Pharmakol.*, 162: 375, 1931; and SKEZAMA: *Mitt. d. med. Gesellsch. zu Tokio*, 47:1291, 1933.

cadmio-iodide at 118°C.; picrolonate at 195.5°C. Coniine is prepared synthetically by reducing allyl-pyridine with sodium in alcohol.

Methyl-coniine is derived from coniine by replacing the hydrogen atom attached to N by a methyl. It is a colorless liquid; levorotatory; alkaline; of specific gravity 0.8318 at 24°C.; boiling at 173 to 174°C.; and with specific rotation (a)$D = 81.33°$.

Traces of coniceine are found in commercial coniine. It is also a colorless liquid, with an odor like coniine, of specific gravity 0.8825 at 22.5°C., boiling at 171 to 172°C., remaining liquid at —50°C., and optically inactive. It is slightly soluble in water, and has an alkaline reaction, and a sharp burning taste. It is easily reduced to inactive coniine by tin and hydrochloric acid, or sodium and alcohol. It is easily prepared from coniine by decomposing the bromo derivative with alkali. Stannic chloride produces a double salt melting at 215°C. The gold chloride melts at 69 to 70°C.; hydrochloride at 143°C.; hydrobromide at 139°C.; hydroiodide at 102°C.; picrate at 62°C. Is it said to be twelve to fifteen times more toxic than coniine.

Conhydrine is derived from coniine by replacing the H atom of the alpha propyl group by OH. It is crystallized from ether in colorless leaflets, dextrorotatory, melting at 118 to 121°C., boiling at 220 to 225°C. The odor is the same as coniine. It is soluble in alcohol and chloroform, less soluble in water and ether. It may be separated from coniine by cooling to 5°C., collecting the crystals on glass wool and washing with petrolic ether. Its gold chloride melts at 133 to 134°C. Its proportion to coniine in hemlock is about one to twenty. Conhydrine heated with phosphorous pentoxide in an atmosphere of hydrogen in a sealed tube is converted into b-coniceine.

Pseudoconhydrine is a stereo-isomer of conhydrine. It is dextrorotatory, (a)$D = 10.98°$; melts at 100 to 106°C.; boils at 230 to 236°C. It is alkaline, and is soluble in water and organic solvents. This alkaloid differs from conhydrine in that it is stable in the air, and is difficultly soluble in alcohol. The melting point of the crystals from petrolic ether is 52 to 69°C. The platinic chloride melts at 185 to 186°C.

Chemical Tests: 1. An aqueous solution is alkaline to litmus and phenolphthalein, reddening in alcoholic solution of the latter, which differentiates it from nicotine. Aqueous

solutions of both coniine and nicotine turn red with phenolphthalein, which color disappears with nicotine on shaking
with chloroform, but remains with coniine. Chlorine water
becomes turbid with coniine, but clear with nicotine. Bromine
water is clear with nicotine, but forms crystals with coniine.

2. Sodium nitroprusside produces no color at first, but
upon stirring, a red tint appears, finally yellow. This color is
changed to bright yellow with alkalis, and destroyed with
acids.

3. If 0.5 mil. of a strong alcoholic solution is boiled with
a few drops of carbon bisulphide and then an excess of water
added, a brown color will be obtained by copper sulphate and
ferric chloride, a green color by nickel chloride and cobalt
chloride. Uranium nitrate gives a red color. If shaken with
ether or toluene these colors will generally go into the solvent.
(Nicotine does not give these colors, but piperidine reacts
almost similarly. Lobeline and sparteine give a greenish or
no color with copper sulphate.)

4. Concentrated sulphuric and nitric acids give no color
with coniine, but give orange to green with coniceine. Alloxan
gives deep purplish red color with white needle-shaped
crystals. If potassium hydroxide is added a purple color and
a mousy odor are obtained; if warmed with dilute sulphuric
acid and potassium dichromate, butyric acid forms and is
recognized by its odor.

The separation of coniine from the tissues is carried out
in the same manner as outlined under Nicotine (page 549).
Many putrefactive substances, either exogenous or endogen-
ous, may be found in cadaveric material which closely resemble
coniine. The positive identification of coniine, therefore, is
very difficult, and often impossible in the presence of a large
quantity of decomposed animal tissues.[1030] Some of these
putrefactive bases, as cadaverin and putrescin, are derivatives
of piperidine, and are easily converted into piperidine. These
ptomaines do not give the biologic tests for coniine, but the
amounts necessary for such tests are not always available.
Therefore a positive statement must be carefully guarded.
The postmortem findings, symptomatology, and biologic test

1030. See SELMI, SULLE: *Ptomaine* 22, 1878; OTTO: Anleitung zur
Ausmittelung der Gifte, 6th ed., 1892; BOURDEL and BONTEMY: *Ann.
d'hyg.*, 3rd series, 55:352, 1880; KROGER: *Arch. f. exper. Path. u. Pharmakol.*, 162:342, 1831.

must all be indicative of coniine poisoning, using the chemical test as further proof.

Symptoms: Poisonous doses produce the general symptoms of weakness, languor, and drowsiness, but not actual sleep. Movements are weak, slow, and unsteady, and the gait is staggering. Generally there are nausea and vomiting, with profuse salivation. The intelligence usually remains clear. The pupils are ordinarily somewhat dilated, and ptosis also occurs, indicating that the dilation is due to oculomotor paralysis. In many instances imperfect vision results from paralysis of accommodation. The speech is thick, and the hearing is imperfect. There are tremors and fibrillary contractions of the muscles, with occasional convulsions. The breathing becomes weaker and slower, and death occurs from its arrest. Externally there is no action on the unbroken skin. On bruised surfaces, in large doses it is said to have a depressant effect on the sensory nerves. Anemia was reported by Turell.

Coniine does not cause any action of importance on the central nervous system. It is possible in fatal poisoning that the respiratory center may be depressed, but most observers believe that the terminal asphyxia is due to paralysis of the nerves of the respiratory muscles, and that the twitching and tremors arise from a partial paralysis of the peripheral nerves. The heart is affected through the stimulation and subsequent paralysis of the ganglia on the inhibitory fibers, which first causes slowing and then acceleration of the pulse. The blood pressure is at first increased from stimulation of the ganglia on the course of the vasoconstrictor nerves. The respiration is accelerated at first, but soon becomes slow and labored, then irregular and finally ceases.

Fatal Dose: Kobert states that about two grains of coniine is the lowest fatal dose, and that one-half to one grain is a poisonous quantity.

Treatment: Emetics should be administered and the stomach washed out; then tannic acid given freely, and the stomach again washed out. Strychnine is given as a respiratory stimulant, with other stimulants hypodermically. Warmth should be applied to the surface, and artificial respiration resorted to. Coniine is excreted rapidly by the urine, so that the effects pass off rapidly if death does not result. Low protein and salt-free diet protects the kidneys.

Postmortem Appearances: Postmortem findings are not characteristic. No distinctive lesions are found, but only the usual indications of death from asphyxia, such as engorgement of the organs, with dark venous blood, which becomes brighter red on exposure to air.

ERGOT

ERGOT is the dried sclerotium of claviceps purpurea, developed on rye plants. It is cylindraceous, obscurely three-angled, tapering toward both ends, obtuse, somewhat curved, from 1 to 4.5 cm. long and 3 to 5 mm. thick longitudinally furrowed. Externally it is dark purple or dark reddish-brown; internally it is white, tinged with purple or gray. Its odor is characteristic, but free from mustiness or rancidity; its taste is oily, somewhat acrid, and disagreeable. Powdered ergot is grayish to purple brown, containing purplish and whitish fragments of the outer tissue and the thin-walled cells. It deteriorates with age, and should not be kept longer than one year. The U. S. P. preparation of fluidextractum ergotae possesses a potency, per cubic centimeter, equivalent to not less than 0.5 mg. of ergotoxine ethanesulfonate. The powdered ergot is extracted with .petroleum benzin. The benzin is rejected, and after the drying of the drug, it is then extracted by ninety-eight volumes of diluted alcohol, and two volumes of hydrochloric acid. The dose is 2 cc. (thirty minims).

Ergot is of some importance in toxicology, as its preparations have caused poisoning, and epidemics have been widespread from consuming bread and grain which contained this drug. The chemistry of ergot has been investigated by many, and a number of alkaloids have been isolated, with amines of strong action. Many preparations are manufactured under copyrighted names, claiming to be pure products, free from irritating substances. Ergot contains a coloring substance which is a means of identification. It also contains 30% of oil and fat. Its alkaloidal content is 0.2% to 0.3%. Perlow and Blech reported a case of ergotamine tartrate poisoning with impending gangrene of the feet in which a complete cure was effected by papaverine hydrochloride.*

Ergot also contains a substance which Wengell called ergoxanthein or ergot yellow. Schmidt called this pigment schlererythrin. It is an amorphous red powder, soluble in alcohol

* *J.A.M.A.*, 109:27, 1937.

and glacial acetic acid, slightly soluble in ether, and insoluble in water and petrolic ether. Ammonia, alkali hydroxides, carbonates, and bicarbonates give a red to red-violet color. Ether solution plus sodium hydroxide is deep red. Calcium hydroxide, barium hydroxide, and lead acetate give blue-violet precipitates; iron chloride a deep green precipitate; chlorine and bromine, lemon-yellow. To separate, an alcoholic extract of the sample is acidified with tartaric acid and digested with alcohol, filtered, evaporated, and the residue extracted with ether. The ether is then filtered into a separatory funnel and shaken with a saturated sodium bicarbonate solution, which becomes a violet color. If the ether is shaken with ammonia, and the aqueous liquid separated and precipitated with basic lead acetate, the precipitate colors a saturated borax solution a red-violet color. In "New and Nonofficial Remedies" it has been shown that ergot contains alkaloids which are specific for ergot, and a number of amines. These amines, however, are decomposed products of proteins, and probably do not exist in fresh ergot. Ergotoxine, or hydroergotinine, an amorphous alkaloid, occurs in alcoholic extracts.

Ergotoxine, $C_{35}H_{41}O_6N_5$, was first isolated by Kraft, who called it hydro-ergotinine. It was later studied by Barger and Dale. Ergotoxine is a light white powder. It begins to soften at 155° C., and melts gradually at 162 to 164° C. It is soluble in alcohol, acetone, ethyl acetate, and chloroform; slightly soluble in ether, benzene and amyl alcohol; insoluble in petrolic ether. It is precipitated readily by all the alkaloidal reagents. When boiled with acetic anhydride, a molecule of water is split off and ergotinine is formed. Crystalline salts are easily formed with acids. Ergotoxine phosphate crystallizes in slender, colorless needles, melting at 186 to 187° C., soluble in 313 parts of alcohol. It causes the characteristic reaction of ergot on the cockscomb, and is concerned in the uterine and vascular effects. It is rather unstable, and by loss of water changes into an anhydride, crystalline ergotinine, $C_{35}H_{39}O_5N_5$, which, possibly because of its low solubility in physiological solutions, is quite weak in action. Both the alkaloids ergotinine and ergotoxine dissolve in dilute sodium hydroxide.

Ergotinine, $C_{35}H_{39}O_5N_5$, crystallizes in long needles. It is the anhydride of ergotoxine, containing one less molecule of water. Either alkaloid can be easily transformed into the other, which might explain some of the discrepancies in the literature regarding them. When heated rapidly it darkens first, then melts at 229° C. It is soluble in alcohol, acetone, ethyl acetate, and chloroform, moderately soluble in ether, benzene and amyl alcohol, nearly insoluble in petrolic ether. A solution of ergotinine in sulphuric acid, with ferric chloride, gives an orange-red color, becoming deep red, with a blue to bluish-green margin. A solution in glacial acetic acid, with ferric chloride to which sulphuric acid is added, gives a violet zone at the point of contact. Ergotinine and cornutine are probably synonymous with different authors. Solutions of ergotinine have a bluish-violet fluorescence, especially when acidified. It is strongly dextrorotatory. Ergotinine is readily converted into ergotoxine by the action of the alkalis and acids in aqueous solution; the reverse change is brought about by heating ergotoxine in methyl alcohol with acetic anhydride.[1031]

Tyramine, $C_8H_{11}NO$, para-hydroxyphenylethylamine, OH . C_6H_4 . $CH_2CH_2NH_2$, crystallized from alcohol, forms hexagonal leaflets, melting at 161° C. Because of its solubility in water, this base is difficult to isolate. It is extracted from a concentrated solution rendered alkaline by sodium carbonate, with amyl alcohol. It is not toxic, but probably is responsible for the pressor action of ergot.

Acute Poisoning: Acute poisoning by ergot is very rare, and is caused accidentally except in some cases where it has been employed to produce abortion. The symptoms are vomiting, burning pains in the abdomen, tingling of the extremities, great thirst, diarrhea, collapse with weak rapid pulse, cold skin, hemorrhage from the uterus, abortion, and often icterus. There is ecchymosis in many organs and in the subcutaneous tissues, suppression of urine, prostration, coma, and death from respiratory and cardiac failure. Death may occur in a few hours, or be delayed a few days. In cases of recovery, abnormal symptoms persist for a few days. Sometimes a cataract forms in the eyes. Therapeutic doses of ergot generally cause no ill effects except in pregnancy, when it causes a contraction of the uterus and abortion. In some fatal poisonings abortion occurred.

Chronic poisoning is very rarely caused by the medicinal

1031. See BARGER: Allen's Commercial Organic Analysis, 7:17, 1913.

use of ergot. Some epidemics have occurred from eating bread made with grain containing ergot. In 1926-1927, there occurred a severe epidemic of 11,319 cases of poisoning in Russia, in the district between Kasan and the Ural Mountains. Of these, 1,618 were admitted to the hospital and ninety-three died.

The clinical picture of ergotism appears in two forms, the convulsive and the gangrenous. The convulsive form occurs when ergotine has been taken in small amounts, corresponding to an ergot content of bread of 10 to 20% at most, usually less than 10%. The gangrenous form, on the other hand, is more common in those cases in which the ergot content of the bread has been 30 to 50%.

The symptoms are of two types, those causing a nervous disorder, and those causing gangrene. In some cases both types have been found, but, as a rule, one prevails. The gangrenous type generally develops in the fingers and toes. Sometimes the entire leg or arm becomes cold and numb, dark, dry, hard and shrunken, and falls off with little or no pain, and no hemorrhage. Gangrene also occurs in the internal organs. Cataracts are common. The symptoms of spasmodic ergotism are drowsiness, depression, weakness, giddiness, headache, and cramps in the limbs, with itching. In severe cases, convulsions, generally clonic and often epileptiform, occur. There is mental weakness and sometimes complete dementia. In animals, restlessness, salivation, vomiting and purging, depression, ataxia, clonic convulsions, and death by paralysis of the respiratory center occur. Gangrene is common in the pig, in which the ears, the extremities, and pieces of skin of the trunk become hard and dry and finally fall off.

Speck[1032] reports the danger of ergotism from the use of ergotamine tartrate which was marketed under the name of "gynergen." (This gynergen is equal to 50% ergotamine tartrate.) During the course of nine days he gave 11 cc. gynergen, equivalent to 5 cc. ergotamine tartrate. There were cramp-like pains and a dry gangrene on the toes. Panter reports a case with central disturbances which recovered. Nielsen reports a suicide after the taking of fifteen tablets of gynergen. Labbi reports cramps in the coronary vessels. Fomina reported the passage of active substances of ergot

1032. Speck, W.: *Med. Klin.*, 26:1521, 1930.

into the milk of nursing mothers.[1033] Therefore, caution should be used in the administration of ergot after delivery.

Fatal Dose and Period: The fatal dose of ergot and its preparations cannot be stated definitely, because of the variation in strength. Thirty grains (1.95 gm.) have caused severe poisoning,[1034] but recovery has followed 150 grains (9.72 gm.). Gangrene and death have been said to follow ten grains. Death is more likely to follow the long continued use of small medicinal doses than after one large dose.[1035] According to Barger, 0.3 gm. of ergotoxine per day must be something like the upper limit of the amount required to produce serious gangrene.[1036]

Treatment: Wash out the stomach with water containing eighty to 100 grains of sodium bicarbonate. Give 0.5 to 1.0 gm. sodium tetrathionate dissolved in 10 cc. of sterile distilled water intravenously daily. Empty the bowels by soapsuds enemas, and purgatives, such as calomel and castor-oil. Treat symptomatically. Give stimulants, such as strychnine and coffee. If gangrene sets in, the parts should be bathed with warm water and wrapped in a soothing ointment.

Postmortem Appearances: Hyperemia may be noted throughout the kidney, uterus, liver and lungs. Hyperemic and ecchymotic areas may appear in the stomach and bowels.

Chemical Tests: The detection of ergot in flour is best done by the method of Gruber:[1037] A few mg. of flour are distributed in a drop of water on a slide, and covered with a cover slip. The slide is then heated slowly until the starch grains burst. Besides the burst grains of rye starch and the fragments of the husk, one sees the ergot particles, sometimes recognizable by their reddish-brown edge, otherwise a colorless mass of irregular polygonal cells with oil drops accumulated around the particles. With an ergot content of 0.1%, one or two particles will be found in each preparation, but with only 0.05%, one should no longer find a particle in every preparation.

The detection of ergot in bread is carried out by the method

1033. Fomina, P. I.:   *Arch. f. Gynäk.,* 157:275, 1934.
1034. Meadows: *Med. Times & Gaz.,* 2:397, 1879.
1035. Davidson: *Lancet,* 2:256, 1884.
1036. Barger: *Pharm. J.,* 110:470, 1920.
1037. Gruber, Thieme: "Uber Mutterkorn in Getreide, Miehl, und Brot," *Veröffentl.* a. d. Geb. d. Med., 1930.

of Hartwich as follows: "The bread is soaked for twenty-four hours in water, and then boiled for a long time with 1.5% hydrochloric acid, the acid being frequently poured off and renewed. The sediment is then examined microscopically."[1038]

At the present time the tests for ergotinine and ergotoxine are impossible to differentiate. There are certain color reactions that may be regarded as characteristic of the alkaloids of ergot without reference to the specific alkaloid involved.

GELSEMIUM

THE dried rhizome and roots of gelsemium sempervirens are cylindrical, usually in cut pieces of variable length, externally light yellowish-brown, with purple-brown longitudinal lines. The bark is about 1 mm. thick, the wood is pale yellow, porous but tough, with numerous distinct medullary rays. The odor is pronounced and characteristic; the taste aromatic and bitter. The dose is 65 mg. (one grain). This drug is no longer official in the U. S. P. preparations. Of fluidextractum gelsemii the dose is 0.05 cc. (one minim). Of tinctura gelsemii, 10% alcoholic extract, the dose is 0.5 cc. (eight minims).

The alkaloids contained in gelsemium are gelsemine, gelseminine, sempervirine, gelsemidine, gelsemoidine, and gelsemicine.

Gelsemine, $C_{20}H_{22}N_2O_2$, occurs as white glistening prisms, which melt at 178° C. It is soluble in chloroform, ether, and alcohol, and sparingly soluble in water.

Toxicity: M.L.D. - 180 mg. per kilo weight in experimentation with white rabbits. Seven mg. of gelsemine HC1 caused a fall in blood pressure in cats, and a total dose of 12 mg. caused death. Concentration of one to 10,000 and one to 20,000 diminished the contractions in the intestines of rabbits.[1039] Local application to the eye of 0.1% gelsemine HCl solution into the conjunctival sac produced mydriasis. With gelsemine HC1 a maximal dilation of the pupil to 3 mm. occurred at the end of three hours and disappeared twenty-four hours later. On the other hand, the homatropine mydriasis reached its maximum of 3.25 mm. within fifty minutes, but lasted for only eight hours.

Tests: The pure alkaloid when dissolved in concentrated sulphuric acid gives no color, but upon the addition of an oxi-

1038. HARTWICH: "Die menschlichen Genusmittel," Leipzig, 1911.
1039. CHOU: *Chinese J. Physiol.*, 5:131, 1931.

dizing agent, an intense red or purplish color develops, changing to blue or bluish-green and finally to blue or green. Gelsemine generally is contaminated with gelseminine: if sulphuric acid be added, a reddish or brown tint appears, gradually turning pink, and, upon heating, purple and chocolate tints develop. Upon adding oxidizing agents to an impure gelsemine dissolved in sulphuric acid, a red to purple tint develops, with purplish-red streaks following the course of the oxidizing agent. This finally turns blue-green. Nitric acid upon warming becomes red, turning to dark green.

Pure gelsemine has very slight toxic action; the effects of the commercial preparation are thought to be due to the gelseminine present.

Persons are reported to have been poisoned by eating honey gathered by bees from gelsemium flowers.[1040] Boutelle[1041] reports a case of a young man who died four hours after he had taken two tablespoonfuls of the liquid fluid extract. Symptoms usually seen are: double vision, dilatation of the pupils with loss of accommodation, dropping of the lower jaw, general slow pulse which appears to be dependent on respiration, low temperature, and death caused by respiratory failure. The effects usually appear after about one-half hour, but sometimes immediately. The principal alkaloid, gelsemine, was isolated in a pure state by Gerrard.[1042] Thompson[1043] isolated, besides gelsemine, another amorphous alkaloid which was named gelseminine. Cushny[1044] found this substance to be much more powerful than gelsemine; a dosage of 0.35 mg. per kilo of the former being fatal to rabbits. His colleagues found later that Thompson's gelsemine was a mixture of three substances which they termed sempervirine, gelsemidine, gelsemoidine; but each of these substances was not as toxic as the original substances.[1045]

By subcutaneous injections the MLD for albino rats is

1040. WOOD, H. C., JR., and LA WALL, C. H.: U. S. Dispensatory, Philadelphia, 1900.

1041. BOUTELLE, J. T.: Boston M. & S. J., 91:321, 1875.

1042. GERRARD, A. W.: Am. J. Pharm., 55:256, 1883.

1043. THOMPSON, J.: Pharm. J., 17:805, 1887.

1044. CUSHNY, A. R.: Arch. exper. Path. u. Pharmakol., 31:39, 1893.

1045. CHILLINGWORTH, E. P.: J. Am. Pharm. Ass., 4:315, 1914; SAYRE, L. E., and WATSON, G. N.: J. Am. Pharm. Ass., 8:708, 1919; SAYRE, L. E.: J. Am. Pharm. Ass., 1:458, 1912; 3:314, 1914; STEVENSON, A. E., and SAYRE, L. E.: J. Am. Pharm. Ass., 4:60, 1915.

0.00010 to 0.00012 per gm. of body weight. The same results are obtained with intraperitoneal injection. By intravenous injections the MLD in milligrams per kilo weight for rabbits is 0.05 to 0.06 and for dogs is 0.5 to 1.0 mg. The main symptoms of toxicity in mammals were depressed respiration, tremors, incoordination of movement, paralysis of extremities, convulsions, urination, retching, and salivation. Death results from respiratory failure. Artificial respiration alone may save the animal from a small lethal dose. The author studied subsequently the pharmacological action of gelsemicine on the respiration, and found that in dogs and rabbits gelsemicine hydrochloride in minute doses produces a stimulation of the respiration. In larger doses a depression preceded by a transient stimution, and in toxic doses a progressive depression resulted. Anesthetized and morphinized animals are more susceptible to the drug. From his experimental work he concluded that the respiratory action of gelsemicine is chiefly due to the action on the respiration center.

Gelseminine: Gelseminine occurs as an amorphous basic substance, which has not been crystallized. It is probably a mixture of two or more alkaloids. Sayre showed gelseminine was a mixture of sempervirine, gelsemidine, and gelsemoidine. This mixture is more potent than any of the alkaloids of gelsemium. It is precipitated by the usual alkaloidal reagents, and gives color reactions the same as gelsemine. It also produces mydriasis. When administered intravenously into rabbits, it produced a quieting down of the animal, followed by excitement, weakness of extremities, shallow and low respiration, convulsions, urination, and salivation, and finally death from respiratory failure. The MLD for the rabbit was found to be 0.08 mg. per kilogram of body weight.

Sempervirine: Sempervirine crystallizes from chloroform in reddish-brown needles, which are soluble in chloroform and alcohol, slightly soluble in water, and almost insoluble in ether, benzene and petrolic ether, with a melting point of 223° C. From alcohol it crystallizes as red ortho-rhombic crystals, melting at 254° C. The nitrate, crystallizes from either alcohol or chloroform and melts at 283° C., with decomposition. The hydrochloride is readily soluble in water and alcohol. A yellow precipitate is formed with platinic chloride, potassium chromate, and sodium nitrate. It is precipitated by the usual alkaloidal

reagents. The MLD is 5 mg. per kilogram of rabbit, 100 mg.
per kilogram of frog. It causes no dilatation of pupils, but otherwise its poisoning effects are the same as those of gelsemicine.

Scopoletine: Scopoletine, $C_9H_5O_3OCH_3$, crystallizes from
alcohol in long colorless needles. It sublimes at 140-170° C.,
and melts at 204° C. This product has also been called gelse-
minic acid. It is readily soluble in chloroform from acid solutions.

Tests: Upon shaking the chloroform solution with dilute
ammonia, the ammonia solution shows a distinct blue fluorescence. This reaction is very useful in analytical work for
showing the presence of gelsemium.

Gelsemidine: Gelsemidine is amorphous. It is soluble in
chloroform and alcohol, but insoluble in ether. Its hydrochloride is very soluble in water and alcohol, but is insoluble in ether
and chloroform. It is found in minute amounts in gelsemium.

Gelsemoidine: Gelsemoidine is amorphous. It is soluble in
water, alcohol, and chloroform, but insoluble in ether. It does
not form crystalline salts, and is hygroscopic. Its hydrochloride is soluble in the same solvents as the alkaloid. This also
exists in very small quantities in gelsemium.

Gelsemicine: Gelsemicine has a molecular formula of
$C_{20}H_{25}O_4N_2$; its specific rotation in alcohol 140°. It is recrystallized from acetone in ortho-rhombic prisms, which melt at 171°
C. It forms a monohydrochloride very soluble in water. Gelsemicine is highly potent, producing the usual toxic effects of
gelsemium in mammals. Gelsemicine was found to be very
toxic to mammals, and death resulted a short time after the injection of the drug. The MLD for frogs by injection into the
anterior lymph sac is 0.020 to 0.030 mg. per gram of body
weight. Death follows as slow depression without convulsions.
The time for this to occur varies from several hours to several
days.

Tests: Chemical: 1. Sulphuric acid dissolves the gelsemium
alkaloids with a yellowish or brownish color. If a piece of solid
potassium dichromate, manganese dioxide, or cerosoceric acid
be drawn through the solution, a reddish-purple or cherry-red
color is shown along the path of the crystal. This color changes
to a blue green. (The pure separated alkaloids do not give this
reaction. Gelsemine gives a crimson color, changing to green
and finally yellow. Sempervirine is at first green, changing to

yellowish-green. Gelsemoidine is at first purple changing to green.)

2. Nitric acid gives no color with the pure isolated alkaloids. With the combined gelsemium alkaloids, nitric acid gives a yellowish or brownish-green color, changing to deep green.

The presence of gelsemium is not difficult to establish. Scopoletine is easily identified, and then the identification of the other alkaloids makes it complete. The pure alkaloids are easily identified; the only substances for which they might be mistaken are strychnine and yohimbine, and they can be differentiated from these bases because a residue evaporated with nitric acid does not give a purple color with alcoholic potash.

To test for scopoletine and the other alkaloids, extract with alcohol, filter and evaporate the alcohol, dissolve the residue in dilute hydrochloric acid, and filter into a separatory funnel. This solution is then shaken with chloroform. The chloroform is separated and shaken with water made alkaline with ammonia. If scopoletine is present, the aqueous layer will show a blue fluorescence. If a further identification of scopoletine is desired, the chloroform solution is extracted with water, filtered and evaporated, and the residue crystallized out of alcohol. These crystals are subject to sublimation at 150° C., and the melting point determined. The acid solution, after the removal of scopoletine, is rendered alkaline, extracted with ether, then chloroform, and tested for its individual color reactions.

Symptoms: External: Gelsemium or its alkaloids applied to the skin have no effect, but, if dropped into the eye, cause momentary smarting and hyperemia of the conjunctiva and rapid dilatation of the pupil, with paralysis of accommodation. The symptoms of gelsemium poisoning so closely resemble those of conium that it is very difficult to make a diagnosis. Gelsemium is more depressant to the central nervous system than conium.

Treatment: Wash the stomach thoroughly with warm water. Give internal and external stimulation to increase the warmth of the body and blood circulation; respiratory stimulation; digitalis hypodermically for the heart, morphine and atropine for the respiration.

Postmortem Appearances: These appearances are all normal, except for a superficial venous injection and congestion of some of the organs.

HYDRASTIS

COMMONLY called "goldenseal," hydrastis consists of the dried rhizome and roots of hydrastis canadensis. The therapeutically important alkaloids contained in Hydrastis canadensis are hydrastine, found in amounts varying from 0.5% to 3%, with greatly lesser amounts of berberine and canadine.

Hydrastine, $C_{21}H_{21}NO_6(CH_2O_2C_9H_7NCH_3C_{10}H_9O_4)$, is readily decomposed into hydrastinine, $(CH_2O_2C_9H_7NCH_3)$, and opianic acid. It is related chemically to narcotine, which differs only in possessing one more methoxyl group. Narcotine when decomposed also forms opianic acid. Hydrastine is white to creamy white glistening prisms, sometimes of large size. It is odorless; bitter in taste; permanent in the air; soluble in 135 parts of alcohol, 124 parts of ether, two parts of chloroform, and almost insoluble in water; levogyrate; melts at 131° C.; contains no water of crystallization; alkaline to litmus paper. The dose is 0.2 grain.

Hydrastinine Hydrochloride, $C_{11}H_{11}NO_2HCl$, is the hydrochloride of an artificial alkaloid derived from hydrastine. It occurs as light yellowish needles, or a yellowish-white, crystalline powder, odorless, and of bitter taste. It is very soluble in water and alcohol, and in 286 parts chloroform and 1,300 parts ether. It melts at 212° C., and is neutral to litmus. Its aqueous solution, when highly diluted, shows a blue fluorescence.

Tests: 1. Sulphuric acid gives a yellow color; on heating this changes to purple.

2. Sulphuric acid containing a trace of molybdic acid gives a green color, changing to olive green and then to brown.

3. Nitric acid gives a reddish-yellow color.

4. Sulphuric acid containing a trace of selenous acid gives a yellowish-red color, changing to brown.

5. If a crystal of hydrastine is dissolved in dilute sulphuric acid and a solution of potassium permanganate (one to ten) is added, a blue fluorescence is developed (distinction from hydrastinine).

6. Hydrastine with Froehde's reagent gives no reaction at first, but on standing a deep green.

7. Bromine solution produces a yellow precipitate, soluble in ammonia water, forming an almost colorless solution.

8. Potassium dichromate produces a precipitate, which re-

dissolves if gently heated, but on cooling it separates in glistening crystalline needles. Sulphuric or nitric acid produces a deep yellow color.

9. Sulphuric acid with a crystal of ammonium vanadate gives a light brown, changing to dark brown.

Hydrastinine hydrochloride has a very limited use in medicine. Hydrastinine is an oxidation product of hydrastine. The hydrochloride is formed by passing dry hydrogen chloride through a chloroform solution of hydrastinine. Hydrastinine melts at 116 to 117° C. It is soluble in ether, chloroform, petrolic ether, benzene, alcohol, and slightly soluble in water. Its water and alcohol solutions are fluorescent.

Tests: 1. Froehde's reagent and ammonium vanadate give the same colors as hydrastine.

2. Nessler's reagent gives a black precipitate. (Morphine, apomorphine and picrotoxine are the only substances giving this same reaction.)

3. Mandelin's reagent gives a pink, changing to bright red, then to brick red.

4. Marquis' reagent gives no color.

Opianic acid is detected as follows: The acid solution of hydrastine is oxidized with permanganate, and alcohol is added to obtain a concentration of 1% opianic acid. One part of this alcoholic solution is treated with two parts sulphuric acid and tested. Gallic acid gives a blue color which, upon warming, changes to brown. Guaiacol produces red changing to blue, (a) naphthol a gooseberry red; (b) naphthol a red wine. Codeine a violet to blue. Methylnaphthol violet, soon fading. (Narcotine and laudanosine give the same colors.)

Berberine, $C_{20}H_{17}NO_4$, occurs as yellow prismatic crystals. It is odorless, and has a very bitter taste. It is somewhat soluble in cold water, chloroform and benzol, but is insoluble in ether and petrolic ether. Most of its salts are less soluble than the free alkaloid. It is best removed from solutions by a mixture of alcohol and chloroform.

Tests: 1. Berberine is precipitated by the general alkaloidal reagents.

2. Froehde's reagent gives a greenish-brown to dark brown or violet color.

3. Nitric acid gives a reddish-brown liquid, which, when diluted with water, gives a yellow precipitate partially soluble

in ammonia water. To another portion add strong alcoholic potash; note odor and color.

4. Sulphuric acid gives an orange-yellow solution, changing on warming to olive green, which changes to a violet or a brownish-green upon adding potassium bichromate.

5. Sulphuric acid with a crystal of sodium nitrate gives a violet streak.

6. Sulphuric acid added to a solution of berberine, and treated with chlorine water added, so that it rests on the surface, causes a bright red zone to be formed at the junction of the two liquids.

Isolation from Tissues: The tissue is treated according to the general method for alkaloidal extraction. The acidified residue is rendered alkaline with ammonia water and extracted with ether four times. This ether extract is shaken out with dilute hydrochloric acid, which is separated and made alkaline with ammonia, and shaken out with four portions of ether. Then this ether extract is washed with water, filtered into a tared dish, the ether evaporated, and the residue weighed and tested for hydrastine. Berberine in mixtures with hydrastine is separated by precipitating the acid solution with potassium iodide, which precipitates the berberine, leaving hydrastine in solution.

Symptoms: In frogs hydrastine causes increased reflex irritability, with tetanus resembling that of strychnine, also terminating in paralysis. In man toxic doses cause general feebleness, tremor, dyspnoea, incoordination of movements, clonic and then tonic convulsions, and tetanus. Berberine in large doses lowers the temperature, increases peristalsis, and causes death by central paralysis.

IPECACUANHA (IPECAC)

IPECAC consists of the dried rhizome and roots of cephaëlis ipecacuanha, known in commerce as Rio, or Brazillian, ipecac, or of cephaëlis acuminata Karsten, known in commerce as Cartagena, Nicaragua, or Panama ipecac.

Ipecac yields not less than 2% of the ether-soluble alkaloids of ipecac, and contains not more than 5% of its overground stems, and not more than 2% of other foreign matter. The roots are in cylindrical pieces, mostly curved and sharply flexuous, occasionally branched, from 3 to 15 cm. long and 1 to 4 mm. thick. They are reddish-brown to dark brown, either smooth or closely annulated, with thickened, incomplete rings, and usually exhibiting transverse fissures with vertical sides. The bark is smooth and thin, easily separated from the tough, fibrous wood. The odor is distinctive, the dust sternutatory. The taste is bitter, nauseous, and acid. The rhizomes are cylindrical, about 10 cm. long and 2 mm. thick. They are longitudinally wrinkled, with few elliptical scars and a distinct pith about one-sixth of the entire diameter. The outer layer is dark brown, the cortex grayish white. The wood is light yellow.

Powdered ipecac is light brown in color. Elements of identification are the cork cells; the starch grains single and up to five to seven compound, the single grains up to 0.015 mm. in diameter (Rio) and up to 0.02 mm. in diameter (Cartagena); raphides of calcium oxalate up to 0.05 mm. in length, and fragments of the porous tracheids. The dose as expectorant is 0.06 gms. (one grain); as emetic, 1 gm. (fifteen grains).

The U. S. P., XI, preparations are: fluidextractum ipecacuanhae, pulvix ipecacuanhae et opii, syrupus ipecacuanhae (from fluidextract).

Fluidextractum Ipecacuanhae: Fluidextract of ipecac yields from each 100 cc., not less than 1.8 gm. and not more than 2.2 gm. of the ether-soluble alkaloids of ipecac. The dose as expectorant is 0.06 cc. (one minim); as emetic 1 cc. (15 minims).

Syrupus Ipecacuanhae is prepared from the fluid extract: Fluidextract of ipecac, 70 cc.; glycerin, 100 cc., and a sufficient quantity of syrup to make 1000 cc. The dose as expectorant is 0.75 cc. (12 minims); as emetic, 15.00 cc. (four fluidrachms).

Pulvis Ipecacuanhae et Opii (Dover's powder) consists of ipecac, in very fine powder, 10 gm.; powdered opium, 10 gm.; lactose, coarsely powdered, 80 gm., to make 100 gm. It is grayish-white or very light brown; exhibiting coarse, angular, frequently more or less cone-shaped, colorless fragments from 0.03 to 0.40 mm. in length. It is very slowly soluble in water and in chloral hydrate test solution, and has the quality of strongly polarizing light with a strong display of color (fragments of lactose). Other elements of identification are the tissues of ipecac described above.

Ipecac is used for its emetic and expectorant properties, and in the treatment of amebiasis. Alkaloidal principles are: Emetine, $C_{25}H_{27}(OCH_3)_4 (NH)N$; cephaeline, $C_{25}H_{27}(OCH_3)_3(OH)$

(NH)N; psychotrine, $C_{25}H_{26}(OCH_3)_3(OH)N_2$. Emetine is methyl-cephaeline, and cephaeline is obtained from psychotrine by reduction. All three are derived from isoquinoline. Emetine and cephaeline resemble each other in their action, while psychotrine is almost inert.

Hesse[1047] reports in addition to these, hydroipecamine, isomeric with cephaeline, and ipecamine, isomeric with psychotrine.

Emetine when pure is amorphous and nearly colorless, becoming darker on exposure to light. It is strongly alkaline, completely neutralizing acids; is optically inactive, and melts at 70°C. It is readily soluble in alcohol, ether, chloroform, and benzene, but only slightly in water and petrolic ether. Emetine forms well-defined salts. The hydrochloride is a white or slightly yellowish crystalline powder, without odor, soluble in water, and alcohol, and gradually darkening on exposure to light. The sulphate, acetate, and oxalate are amorphous, and very soluble in water. The hydrobromide and hydroiodide are sparingly soluble, and separate on adding a soluble bromide or iodide to a solution of emetine hydrochloride. The nitrate is also sparingly soluble, and may be obtained as a resinous mass on adding potassium nitrate to a solution of the hydrochloride.

Emetine, $C_{30}H_{44}N_2O_4$, was first prepared by Glenard,[1048] and later studied by Paul and Cownley.[1049] As described by these workers, emetine is a nearly colorless base, which is apparently uncrystallizable. It melts at about 68°C. (15.4° F.), rapidly acquiring a yellowish color on exposure to light. It is only slightly soluble in water, but dissolves readily in alcohol, ether, chloroform, and benzene, though only very sparingly in petroleum ether even when hot. On evaporation of any of these solutions, emetine is left as a transparent varnish-like residue, which is strongly alkaline to litmus and neutralizes acids completely. When precipitated from the solutions of one of its salts by alkali hydroxides, emetine is soluble in excess of the reagents. Emetine is probably a quinolin derivative, being a diacid-tertiary diamin containing four methoxyl groups.

1047. HESSE: Annalen, 405, 1914.

1048. GLENARD: Am. de chim. et phys., 8:233, 5 s., 1876.

1049. PAUL and COWNLEY: Pharm. J., 24:61, 3 s., 1893; 25:111, 373, and 690, 3 s., 1894; see also CRIPPS: Pharm. J., 1:160, 4 s, 1895; FRERICHS and TAPIS: Arch. d. Pharm., 260: 390, 1902; KARRER: Gesellsch., 49: 2057, 1916.

Emetine Hydrochloride, $C_{30}H_{44}N_2O_4 2HCl$, contains variable amounts of water of crystallization. It occurs as a white or very slightly yellowish crystalline powder, without odor. On exposure to light it gradually darkens. It is freely soluble in water and alcohol, its aqueous solution being slightly acid to litmus. Its aqueous solutions yield precipitates with iodine in potassium iodide, with mercuric-potassium iodide, and with platinic chloride. A 5% solution of this salt, mixed with potassium bromide or iodide, yields a dense precipitate, which dissolves on the addition of alcohol, this solution giving, when slowly evaporated, tufts of silky needles of the hydrobromide or hydroiodide.

Cephaeline when freshly precipitated is colorless, but soon turns yellow when exposed to light. It melts at 102° C. An alcohol or ether solution, when evaporated, leaves a transparent varnish, but if evaporated in a closed tube, silky needles are deposited. It is much more soluble in petrolic ether than emetine, and differs from that alkaloid by dissolving readily in alkali hydroxides. The hydrochloride forms transparent rhombic crystals.

Psychotrine is found only in small quantity, (0.04% to 0.06%). When pure, the yellow prisms melt at 138° C. It is soluble in alcohol, chloroform, and alkalis, but sparingly soluble in ether, differentiating from emetine and cephaeline. Ammonia solution gives a blue fluorescence.

Tests: The alkaloids of ipecac are so closely associated with each other, that their chemical reactions will be given for them in combination. They are precipitated from acid solution by the usual alkaloidal reagents.

1. Sulphuric acid gives pale yellow, changing to brown on warming.

2. Ferric chloride gives a blue color, later becoming green.

3. Calcium hypochlorite followed by a drop of acetic acid gives an orange or lemon-yellow color.

4. Froehde's reagent with the combined alkaloids gives a yellowish-pink color, changing to green, which on adding hydrochloric acid changes to greenish-blue and then to rose with green edges. Froehde's reagent with pure emetine gives a bright grass green; with cephaeline, no color.

5. Potassium ferricyanide and ferric chloride added to a hydrochloric acid solution give a Prussian-blue color.

6. The alkaloids of ipecac can be distinguished from those of opium by Froehde's reagent and hydrochloric acid.

Emetine gives, with Froehde's reagent, a dirty green, which turns grass green on addition of hydrochloric acid. Cephaeline turns purple-red with hydrochloric acid and immediately changes to Prussian-blue. Psychotrine with Froehde's gives a dull purple color, turned dull green by hydrochloric acid. A mixture of the alkaloids with Froehde's reagent turns purple-bluish to violet, which after addition of hydrochloric acid turns an intense blue. Opium alkaloids with Froehde's reagent give a characteristic purple, which disappears with hydrochloric acid.

7. Millon's reagent in a one-to-fifty solution of emetine is colorless in the cold, but upon heating turns yellowish. Cephaeline is violet in the cold, on heating it becomes dark brown.

8. Mercuric acetate in a one to fifty solution of emetine is unchanged in the cold, but upon heating becomes turbid and yellowish. Cephaeline is colorless in the cold, but becomes violet and later dark gray on heating.

9. The microscopical examination of psychotrine crystals furnishes valuable information in the detection of ipecac alkaloids. A chloroform solution is shaken with a small amount of dilute acid, and evaporated on a watch glass. Another watch glass is moistened on the inside with ammonia and placed over the acid solution. The ammonia vapor liberates the alkaloid as very minute octahedral crystals.

When these alkaloids are found in only small amounts, a definite conclusive identification cannot be made, as it is not always easy to detect them if other alkaloids are present.

To separate emetine and cephaeline, the hydrochloric acid solution of the alkaloids is made alkaline with ammonium hydroxide and shaken with ether. The ether solution is then shaken with dilute ammonium hydroxide, which, after washing with ether, is added to the original aqueous solution, which should contain all of the cephaeline. The emetine is obtained by evaporation of the ether. The alkaline aqueous solution is made acid with hydrochloric acid, then alkaline with ammonium hydroxide and extracted with ether-chloroform (one to six) which removes the cephaeline.

Estimation in Tissues: These alkaloids are extracted from the tissues by the general method already outlined. They are easily extracted from alkaline aqueous solutions by ether.

Symptoms: Ipecacuanha powder is a powerful local irritant to the skin, causing redness, vesication, sometimes pustulation and ulceration. Some individuals are so susceptible to
its irritant action that a very small quantity causes swelling
and injection of the conjunctival and nasal mucous membranes,
with irritation of the eyes, salivation, coughing, sneezing, and
bronchial catarrh. It possesses some antiseptic properties, destroying the bacilli of anthrax, but not affecting the spores.

Whether given by mouth, subcutaneously, or intravenously, the symptoms are the same, occurring in a very short time.
When taken internally emetine has a bitter acrid taste, causing
salivation, nausea, and vomiting. If the vomiting is profuse,
no further effects are produced. In doses too small to provoke
vomiting, there is a prolonged nausea, with increased salivation
and perspiration. The emetic action of ipecac is due to its irritating effects on the mucous membrane of the stomach. If
this action were due to the absorption of the drug, a smaller
dose injected hypodermically, or a smaller dose injected intravenously, should have the same effect. But it has been found,
that an amount sufficient to cause vomiting when swallowed,
does not have the same effect when injected.

Toxic doses cause nausea, vomiting, purging, abdominal
pains, frequently bloody stools, vertigo, lethargy, muscular
weakness, convulsive movements, low blood pressure, collapse,
and death from cardiac failure (diastolic arrest). In cases where
death follows shortly after administration, no pathological lesions are found after death. If death has been prolonged for
about a day, the stomach and intestines have the appearance
of acute gastro-enteritis. The mucous membrane is swollen,
congested, covered with mucous secretions, with occasional
ulceration. The heart is stopped in diastole. The blood clots
slowly. Other organs show no pathology.

NICOTINE

DEATH by nicotine is very infrequent, which is all the more
remarkable when we consider the large amount of nicotine consumed each day. However, since 1920, when the author
reported five cases,[1050] there has been an increase in reports of
fatal cases of nicotine poisoning. Nicotine is the only alkaloid

1050. MCNALLY, W. D.: *J. Lab. & Clin. Med.*, 4:4, January, 1920.

of tobacco (nicotiana tabacum) which possesses any toxicological interest, although at least three other alkaloids (nicotinine, nicoteine, and nicotelline) have been isolated from tobacco by Pictet and Rotschy.[1051] Nicotine, next to caffeine, is the most popular and most widely used alkaloid. The every day uses of both alkaloids are mere habits, not addictions as with the opiates, and the use of either can be discontinued without serious consequence. The effects of smoking are due in a large measure to the absorption in the body of the alkaloid nicotine; as it is an alkaline substance, its continual contact with the delicate cells of the lungs during the inhalation of the smoke must cause irritation. Some of the nicotine in tobacco is present as a free alkaloid, readily volatile, and easily extracted with petrolic ether; the remainder is combined as salts with organic acids.[1052] During smoking these salts are dissociated, a portion of the nicotine is burned, and a part passes into the smoke. Moist tobacco gives off more nicotine during combustion than the drier tobacco. In the smoke there will be found a large number of substances other than nicotine. During the process of smoking there is virtually a chemical factory in operation. The smoke contains over twenty products of decomposition and combustion, chief of which are nicotine, pyridin, picoline, ammonia, oxides, nitrogen, carbon monoxide, carbon dioxide, cyanides, arsenic, hydrogen sulphide, methyl alcohol, fatty acids, formaldehyde, lutidin, collidine, and phenolic bodies.[1053] The nicotine content of tobacco varies; that of pipe tobacco from 1.25 to 2.8%; of cigars from 0.91 to 1.9%; of cigarettes from 0.43 to 3.34%.[1054] Asherson[1055] asserts that 6 to 8 mg. of nicotine reach the mouth from a cigarette smoked in the usual way. Winterstein and Aronson[1056] state that 13 to 15% of the nicotine content of cigars and cigarettes is absorbed by the organism. The continued use of tobacco apparently creates a tolerance for nicotine and the

1051. PICTET and ROTSCHY: Ber. d. deutsch chem. Gesellsch., 34: 696, 1901.

1052. GARNER: U. S. Dept. of Agriculture, Bureau of Plant Industries, Bull. 102, 1908.

1053. McNALLY, W. D.: Am. J. Cancer, 85:6, 1932.

1054. THURSTON: Bull. Agricultural Comm., Bureau of Drugs, Ohio, 1914; BAILEY: Conn. Agricultural Exper. Sta., Bull. 295, 1927; 307, 1928.

1055. ASHERSON: Chem. News., 120:150, 1919.

1056. WINTERSTEIN, A., and ARONSON, E.: Ztschr. f. Hyg. u. Infektionskr., 108:530, 1928.

products of combustion; otherwise cases of poisoning would not be limited to the beginner.

Pure nicotine is a colorless, and almost odorless oil, which, after standing exposed to the air, turns brown and assumes the peculiar smell of tobacco. It has a sharp, burning taste. It boils without decomposition at 246.1° C. under 730.5 mm. pressure, or at 246.7° S. under a pressure of 745 mm. Its specific gravity is 1.0092 at 20° C. (68° F.). It is strongly levorotatory, its specific rotatory power, according to Jephcott,[1057] is—168.40 to —168.66 at 20° C. Its refractive index is 1.53 at 20° C., that of the commercial nicotine used as an insecticide (95%) being 1.525, according to Fryer and Fryer.[1058] It is capable of distillation, without decomposition, with steam or in a vacuum. It is soluble in water (5% of nicotine is soluble at any temperature in water and 15% of water in nicotine), alcohol, amyl alcohol, ether, petroleum ether, benzene, chloroform, and oils. The solubility curve shows the formation of a definite hydrate which separates out from the excess of either water or nicotine between the temperatures of 60° and 210° C. This was reported by Hudson.[1059] The aqueous solution of nicotine is strongly alkaline in reaction. In the absence of other basic substances, it may be easily determined by titration with standard acid, using methyl red, methyl orange, cochineal, iodeosin, as indicators,[1060] one cc. of N/50 sulphuric acid being equal to 0.003246 gm. of nicotine.

Symptoms: Small doses of nicotine, such as obtained from smoking the first cigar, cigarette or pipe, produce giddiness, headache, nausea, and vomiting. Larger doses will produce cold, clammy sweats, disturbance of vision, profuse salivation, vomiting, diarrhea, and collapse. These symptoms may also be seen after the first attempt at smoking. When nicotine is taken in poisonous doses the patient complains of a hot burning sensation in the mouth, esophagus, and stomach. In several cases seen by the author this burning was so intense that the patients tore open their collars. Where large doses have been taken, death may occur within three minutes and the above symp-

1057. JEPHCOTT: *J. Chem. Soc.*, 115:104, 1919.
1058. FRYER and FRYER: *Analyst*, 44:104, 1919.
1059. HUDSON: *Ztschr. f. phys. Chemie*, 47:113, 1904.
1060. SCHICK and HATES: *Ztschr. f. Untersuch. d. Nahrungs u. Genusmittel.*, 28:269, 1914.

toms be absent, except the burning in the mouth, esophagus, and stomach. Where death does not occur rapidly, there is vertigo, mental confusion, great muscular weakness, restlessness, and abdominal pain. The pulse may be feeble, soft, and rapid, or irregular because of the extrasystoles, while respiration is quick, deep, and labored. There is usually a fall in the blood pressure. Clonic convulsions appear, later accompanied by fibrillary twitching of various muscles, and tetanic spasms have been reported.[1061] There may be disturbances of vision with scotoma, narrowing of the field of vision, and diminution of the sharpness of the sight in the center of the field. Workers in tobacco factories complain of disorders of vision. Among sixty-five cases of tobacco amblyopia, there were eleven cases of neuritis with a picture of pseudotabes, with absence of the knee-jerks, lancinating pains, and uncertainty of movements. The frequency of sterility among female tobacco workers and heavy smokers is very noticeable. Nicotine temporarily has a stimulating effect, due to an excitation of the sympathetic nervous system with increased outpouring of adrenalin from the suprarenals—hence the raised blood pressure and blood sugar, the increased capacity for work and the relief from hunger, thirst, or fatigue.

Emanuel[1062] reported that the smoking of seven or more cigarettes caused the appearance of nicotine in the milk of wet nurses examined. He found that more nicotine was excreted in the urine than in the milk, the greater quantity being eliminated four to five hours after smoking. If fifteen or more cigarettes are consumed daily, or even larger quantities, nicotine is absorbed, and under these conditions untoward effects may be expected in the baby. Faulkner[1063] reported cases of nicotine poisoning by absorption through the skin. A man sat down in a chair on which 40% nicotine solution had been spilled. Fifteen minutes later he began to feel nauseated and lost consciousness. In the hospital he was semi-comatose, and was writhing, moaning, and having rapid, irregular, gasping respirations. Heart beat was 86, temperature 95.6° F., respiration 40; pupils pin-point; blood pressure 110 systolic and 45 diastolic;

1061. See OKUSHIMA: *Acta scholae med. univ. imp. in Kioto*, 3:151, 1919; *Chem. Abst.*, 15:271, 1921.

1062. EMANUEL, W.: *Ztschr. f. Kinderh.*, 52:41, 1931.

1063. FAULKNER, J. M.: *J.A.M.A.*, 100:1664, 1933.

pulse feeble, extremities cold. There were no tendon reflexes, no local skin reactions. Two per cent sugar and acetone were found in the urine. He was given caffeine with sodium benzoate, and recovered in four days. Three weeks after leaving the hospital he still had weakness, sweating, vertigo, insomnia, nervousness, and substernal pressure. Lockhart[1064] reported the case of a girl who spilled 7.5 cc. of 95% free nicotine on the sleeve of her overalls. She immediately removed the overalls and washed her arm with hot water, wiped off the sleeve, put the overalls on again and went back to work. Twenty minutes later she collapsed. For half an hour she was on the verge of death, but recovered. Vomitus three hours later contained nicotine. Fretwurst and Hertz[1065] report the case of a man spraying 18 liters of a nicotine solution which he had prepared from a 96% solution by diluting it one to four. Sometimes the wind was blowing against him, so that a small portion of the material was falling on him in the form of a fine fog. He completed his work in three-quarters of an hour and appeared to be normal. Soon after this he began to vomit some greenish-yellow material which had a strong odor of nicotine. The symptoms were the same as described above. Five hundred cc. of urine were examined and found to contain 26 mg. of nicotine. In this case the hemoglobin was 104%; R.B.C. 5,680,000; W.B.C. 23,000. The blood sugar was increased to 1.75%. The elevation of the blood sugar may be explained on the basis of an increased production of adrenalin caused by the nicotine. The nicotine in this case could have entered either by skin absorption or inhalation.

Fatal Period: Most of the cases that I have seen died within a few minutes after taking preparations that were being used as insecticides. Large doses of pure nicotine may prove fatal within a few seconds. Death has been reported in the cases of suicides in a few seconds. Sonnenschein[1066] reported the cases of two suicides who died in three and five minutes, respectively, after swallowing one or two ounces of tobacco. Weidanz reported the death of one child, and the serious illness of two others from the use of tobacco powder sprinkled on the skin for favus. Husemann [1067] cites a case, seen by Hellwig, of two broth-

1064. LOCKHART, L. P.: *Brit. M. J.*, 1:246, 1933.
1065. FRETWURST, F., HERTZ, A.: *Ztschr. f. klin. Med.*, 122:641, 1932.
1066. Cited by WEIDANZ: Heilkunde, 333, 1907.
1067. HUSEMANN: Handbuch der Toxicologie, 481, 1862.

ers who died after continuous smoking of seventeen and eighteen German pipefuls of tobacco. Merriam[1068] alludes to an instance of death in a child from the incautious employment of a strong decoction of tobacco, as a lotion for ringworm of the scalp. A man[1069] died three hours after using a tobacco decoction for the cure of an eruptive disease. Grahl,[1070] of Hamburg, relates a case where an ounce of tobacco was boiled in water fifteen minutes and the infusion was administered on the advice of a female quack. The individual was seized in two minutes with vomiting, violent convulsions, and stertorous breathing, and died in three quarters of an hour. Travagot[1071] records a case where two ounces and one dram were used in place of a dram and a half for an injection in a man affected with ascarides. Death occurred in eighteen minutes. In another case[1072] a man died in one hour after an enema of two drams of tobacco in eight ounces of boiling water. Feil[1073] reports a case of a woman, fifty-two years of age who took an insecticide containing 12% nicotine in mistake for cascara, dying in twenty minutes. I found a record of one case of the French poet, Santeul,[1074] where death did not occur for two days after the drinking of wine in which Spanish snuff had been placed by a practical joker. Another instance where death did not occur for several days is that of a child, aged three, who used an old pipe for blowing soap bubbles for one hour. Symptoms of poisoning developed, and the child died on the third day.[1075]

Fatal Quantity: From one case where a liquid was drunk containing 42.4% of nicotine, I recovered one-half grain of nicotine.[1076] Kobert states the smallest fatal dose for an adult is one grain.[1077] As most of the cases that have been fatal have taken large doses, it is a difficult matter to state just how much is necessary to produce death. I reported two individuals who drank about 30 cc. of an insecticide containing 39.84% of nico-

1068. MERRIAM: *London Med. Gaz.*, 40:1, 561, 1839 .
1069. *J. de chim. med.*, 329, 1830.
1070. GRAHL: *Hufel Ard's J. d. Prak. Heilk.*, 121:4, 100.
1071. TRAVAGOT, M.: *Gaz. med.*, Paris, November 28, 1840; *Edinburgh M. & S. J.*, 105:558, 1841.
1072. *Edinburgh M. & S. J.*, 110:159, 1813.
1073. FEIL: *Cleveland M. J.*, 15:174, 1916.
1074. FONTANELLE, JULIA: *J. de chim. med.*, 2:652, 1836.
1075. *Pharm. J.*, 377, 1877.
1076. McNALLY, W. D.: *J.A.M.A.*, 127:377, 1921.
1077. KOBERT: Lehrbuch der Intoxikationen, 2:1064, 1906.

tine and died within five minutes. Macht and Davis[1078] reported the toxic dose for cats using 4 1-b nicotine as 1.3 mg. per kilogram. Franke and Thomas[1079] reported the effects of nicotine administered by mouth, vein, and subcutaneously or intramuscularly. The dose had little effect upon the time of death. Death occurred in two minutes by intravenous injection, and in three or four minutes when administered by mouth or intramuscularly. In his work on experimental dogs he reported 10 mg. per mouth as killing 57% of them. Three mg. administered by the veins killed all the dogs; 15%, however, survived 5 mg. Muscular injection of 7.7 mg. killed one animal, and another animal survived 23 mg. given subcutaneously.

Treatment: The stomach should be washed out immediately with water containing activated carbon, which absorbs the alkaloid. In the absence of this or finely pulverized charcoal, give the patient strong tea or tannic acid in the lavage water to precipitate the alkaloid. Intravenous injection of one-thirtieth grain of strychnine sulphate should be given, followed by friction rubs, warmth, promotion of respiration, and the inhalation of oxygen. Recovery is possible if seen early and the above treatment instituted.

Statistics: Case 1. The historic case of the trial of the Count of Bocarme in 1850 for the murder of his brother-in-law, Gustav Fougnies, is of interest because Stas made an analysis determining nicotine in the case, and it was from this that the Stas method was developed.[1080]

Case 2. Taylor, in 1858, reported a man drinking an unknown quantity of nicotine. He collapsed immediately and died in three to five minutes.[1081]

Case 3. In 1859 an army officer was found dead. Near the body was found a bottle which contained the nicotine.[1082]

Cases 4 and 5. Kruger reports two children becoming ser-

1078. MACHT, D. I., and DAVIS, MARY E.: *J. Pharmacol. & Exper. Therap.*, 50:93, 1934.

1079. FRANKE, F. E., and THOMAS, J. E.: *Proc. Soc. Exper. Biol. & Med.*, 29:1177, 1932.

1080. ORFILA: Toxikologie, *Wharton & Stilles' Med. Jurisprudence*, 2:603, 1884; see also: Proces de comte et de la comtesse de Bocarme devant la cour d'assises de Hainault, Mons, 1851; STAS: *Bull. Acad. roy de méd. de Belgique*, 52:9, 202, 1851.

1081. TAYLOR: Die Gift in Gerichtl. Med. Berichung, 1863.

1082. FONSAGRIVES and BESNOU: Cited by MASHKA, Handbuch d. Gerichtl. Med., 2, 1882.

iously ill because they had an infection and their scalp was sprayed with tobacco powder.[1083]

Case 6. A man applied to himself a decoction of tobacco for the cure of an eruptive disease. Death took place in three hours, with the usual symptoms of tobacco poisoning.[1084]

Case 7. Fretwurst and Hertz reported a twenty-nine year old gardner who was spraying fruit trees with nicotine which he had prepared himself from a 96% solution in dilution, one to four. He sprayed about eighteen liters of this solution in three-quarters of an hour. Five minutes after the work was finished symptoms set in.[1085]

Case 8. Regenbogen reports the case of a gardener's assistant, fifteen years old, as working with "vomasol" which contains nicotine. It was used as a fumigator against insects.[1086]

Case 9. Schmidt reported a thirty-three year old man as taking 4 gm. of pure nicotine with suicidal intent. He presented severe intoxication with cramps, but, since he vomited, death did not occur.[1087]

Case 10. Auche reported a case of a man suffering from pediculi pubis. He rubbed his entire body with a decoction which he had made by boiling 3,000 grains of tobacco in two liters of water. He was seized with vertigo, nausea, heaviness of the head, disturbance of vision, cold sweats, extreme pallor, trembling, and weakness of the limbs. The pupils were slightly dilated but retained the power of accommodation; they reacted to light. There was difficulty of respiration and of speech. The symptoms gradually subsided after three hours.[1088]

Case 11. Mashka, in 1855, reported a sailor with a mental disturbance, as swallowing one-half to one ounce of tobacco. In the hospital, he suddenly collapsed while bathing. Thirty minutes later there were cramps, diarrhea, vomiting. Death occurred after seven hours.[1089]

Case 12. An eighteen year old girl received a tobacco enema and fainted after thirty minutes.[1090] She collapsed after one

1083. WEILL, DUFOURT, and DELAUSE:　Gerichtl. Med., 4:395, 1924.
1084. NOMIAS:　Am. J. M. Sc., 75:268, 1865.
1085. FRETWURST and HERTZ:　Ztschr. f. klin. Med., 122:641, 1932.
1086. REGENBOGEN:　Samml. Vergift. Falle, 3, A:123, 1932.
1087. SCHMIDT, M.:　Ztschr. Gerichtl. Med., 14:559, 1930.
1088. AUCHE:　Am. J. Pharm., 63:463,1891.
1089. Handbuch d. Gerichtl. Med., 2, 1882.
1090. Cited by MASHKA.

hour. Death occurred an hour and a half after the enema.

Case 13. Reynolds reported the death of an infant five months old who was given milk into which tobacco had been put by mistake. After two feedings of the milk the child became cyanotic and collapsed. There was profuse sweating of the head. Extremities were cold and clammy, with twitching of the muscles of the face. Both pupils were widely dilated. Pulse was weak and irregular. Respiration was slow and labored. Treatment with atropine, strychnine, brandy, epinephrine, coffee, enemas, etc., was of no avail. The infant died.[1091]

Case 14. Riedel reported a man as dying suddenly while eating after drinking a glass of wine in which another guest had poured some "snuffing tobacco" for a joke.[1092]

Case 15. Classen reports a farmer as dying from a drink that his friend had made from the residue of several pipes.[1093]

Cases 16 and 17. Sonnenschein reported two suicides by ingestion of tobacco. Death occurred within three and five minutes, respectively.[1094]

Cases 18 and 19. Husemann cites a case seen by Hellwig of two brothers who died after continuous smoking of seventeen and eighteen German pipefuls of tobacco.[1095]

Case 20. Morgan reports the death of a child from drinking water taken from a well in which there had lain a package containing tobacco.[1096]

Case 21. A man drank an unknown quantity of liquid containing 44.84% nicotine. The concentrated solution of the insecticide was kept in a cognac bottle, a small portion of which was diluted in a large volume of water for spraying lettuce and radishes. A similar bottle containing liquor was kept on the shelf alongside the insecticide. The man took one swallow of the liquid containing the nicotine, realized immediately his mistake, ran seventy-five feet to the house, and raised a bottle of milk to his lips, but dropped dead before he was able to take a drink of the milk.[1097]

Case 22. Under the influence of liquor, a man went to the

1091. REYNOLDS: *J.A.M.A.*, 62:1723, 1914.
1092. RIEDEL: WEIDANZ: *Ztschr. f. d. ges. gerichtl. Med.*, 33:52, 1907.
1093. CLASSEN: Cited by WEIDANZ: see Ref. 1092.
1094. Cited by WEIDANZ: see Ref. 1092.
1095. HUSEMANN: Handbuch der Toxicologie, 481, 1862.
1096. Cited by WEIDANZ: see Ref. 1092.
1097. MCNALLY, W. D.: *J. Lab. & Clin. Med.*, 5:4, 1920.

kitchen of his home and drank from a whiskey flask, an unknown quantity of insecticide containing 43.24% nicotine, causing death in a few minutes.

Case 23. The circumstances are very similar to the last case, although the man was not intoxicated. The insecticide was not analyzed, but from the minutes of the coroner's inquest it was learned that the insecticide contained nicotine and was used for spraying plants.[1098]

Cases 24 and 25. These occurred on November 7, 1918, at Morton Grove, Illinois. Two men, celebrating the first report of the Armistice, visited the home of a mutual friend, who was asked to give them a drink of liquor. Three bottles of beer were opened, and the host then recalled having a bottle of whiskey in the pantry, which he produced and poured out three whiskey glasses full. The capacity of the glasses was 90 cc. and they were said to have been two-thirds filled with the fluid from the whiskey flask. The two visitors drank about half of the portion given them, one making the remark "what funny tasting booze." Both men had a sensation of choking, dropped to the floor gasping for air, became cyanotic, dying within five minutes. Neither of them vomited. One had a frothy mucus coming from his mouth and nose, and had urinated and defecated. The host claimed he drank some of his liquor and immediately produced emesis by drinking a large quantity of water with salt. A postmortem examination upon the bodies, made three hours after death, showed an intense hyperemia of all the organs. The stomachs were highly congested, having the odor of alcohol. Upon opening the thoracic and abdominal cavities, no distinct odor of nicotine was noted. The heads were not posted. The stomachs were removed for chemical examination. The stomach and content of E. N. weighed 345 gm. A volatile distillate of 200 gm. of stomach and content showed the presence of .4465 gm. of nicotine, making a total of .7702 gm. in the organ. The stomach and content of F. P. weighed 659 gm. From 115 gm. I recovered .8673 gm. of nicotine, making a total of 4.9609 gm.[1099]

Case 26. J A., on November 6, 1919, took half an ounce of an insecticide which, upon analysis, contained 40.86% nicotine. After taking the poison he walked up a flight of stairs from the basement of his home to the kitchen, where he vomited; he

1098. McNally, W. D.   1099. McNally, W. D.

then walked about twenty feet to his bedroom and dropped
dead. The time estimated by his family was less than five minutes after he started to walk from the basement until death
occurred. There was no autopsy. The Coroner's verdict was
"took nicotine with suicidal intent while temporarily insane.[1100]

Case 27. The case of E. H. P. occurred September 22,
1919.[1101] A camouflaged breakfast and robbery had been staged
to give the appearance of murder. The deceased was found
gagged and bound in a large armchair in the kitchen of his
home. Upon the handkerchief gag and upon his shirt were
brown stains; on the floor was a broken tumbler. The ropes
binding the arms were not securely tied on the left arm, and
the right arm had nine and a half inches of slack, which was
sufficient to permit a person to slip down in the chair and drink
from a glass tumbler. The postmortem examination of the
body demonstrated a hyperemia of all the organs; otherwise
nothing grossly was observed except a peculiar odor in the
stomach. A chemical examination of the organs revealed the
presence of nicotine. Nicotine was found on the gag and on the
bosom of the shirt. In the coffee and milk on the table tests
failed to show the presence of nicotine. The brain contained
none, the kidneys and liver gave only traces.

Case 28. D. D. male, on March 11, 1920 after drinking
heavily took one ounce of an insecticide containing nicotine. No autopsy was held. The verdict of the Coroner's
jury was "suicide while despondent and temporarily insane."
An ounce bottle which had contained nicotine was submitted.[1102]

Case 29. G. S., on May 7, 1920, is said to have taken nicotine
by mistake for cascara, and was found dead in bed with no
glass or bottle nearby. The postmortem demonstrated a hyperemia of all the organs. A chemical examination of the organs
revealed that death was due to nicotine poisoning. The result
of the chemical examination can be seen in Table XLVIII.[1103]

Case 30. M. M., a housemaid, on July 19, 1920, took an
unknown quantity from a bottle labeled "Nikoteen" containing
28.60% nicotine. She had been drinking heavily and when
told her services were no longer required, took the poison and

1100. McNALLY, W. D.

1101. The newspaper publicity given this case may have been
responsible for other poisonings by nicotine, as was previously noted in
connection with deaths by mercuric chloride; McNALLY, W. D.: *Med.
Rec.*, February, 1, 1919. 1102, 1103: See Refs. 1104, 1105.

was found dead the next morning. A postmorten was made and the organs submitted for chemical examination. The verdict was "suicide while temporarily insane." Investigation revealed that she had been confined in an asylum for four months the year prior to her death.

Case 31. F. R. D., a boy seven years of age, on September 12, 1919, was given one-half of a dram of an insecticide in mistake for a cough mixture. The bottles were practically of the same design, both containing a dark brown liquid. The child walked eighteen feet after taking the liquid, and died within five minutes. There were no organs submitted. A chemical examination of the insecticide gave 31.55% nicotine.[1104]

	Bowel	Stomach	Stomach Content
E. P. H. Undetermined	(A) In 807 gm. 782.7 mg. (B) 97.0 mg.	(A) In 138 gm. 990.5 mg. (B) 717.6 mg.	
G. S. Accident		(A) In 224 gm. 441.79 mg. (B) 200.7 mg.	(A) In 310 cc. 3184.2 mg. (B) 1271.7 mg.

TABLE XLVIII

NICOTINE IN MILLIGRAMS

(A)—In total weight material received.

(B)—In 100 gm.

	Stomach and Content	Liver	Kidney	Urine
M. M. Suicide	(A) In 276 gm. 9.6 mg. (B) 3.5 mg.	(Nicotine liquid 20.06%)	(A) In 282 gm. 1610.2 mg. (B) 571 mg.	(A) In 173 gm. 9.1 mg. (B) 5.3 mg.	(A) In 135 gm. 14.4 mg. (B) 10.7 mg.	(A) In 280 cc. 1.1 mg. (B) 0.4 mg.
M. V.	(A) In 478 gm. 65.1 mg. (B) 13.6 mg.	(A) In 161 gm. 18.5 mg. (B) 11.4 mg.		(A) In 1255 gm. 37 mg. (B) 2.9 mg.	(A) In 372 gm. 16.1 mg. (B) 4.6 mg.	

Case 32. M. V., of Los Angeles, was found dead the morning of April 5, 1921, and her body was shipped to Chicago. The mysterious circumstances surrounding this death caused exhumation of the girl's body, April 10, 1921. The death certificate gave the cause of death as "diphtheria," evidence of which could not be seen by the Cook County pathologist at the autopsy. The postmortem showed that an abortion had been recently performed. A chemical examination of the organs revealed that death was due to nicotine poisoning.[1105]

Case 33. Kuhn and Esser reported a case of a man drinking an unknown amount of an insecticide, which contained 36.2% of pure nicotine. The organs, including the stomach

1104, 1105. MCNALLY, W. D.:   J. Lab. & Clin. Med., 2:8, 1922.

contents, were also examined chemically, and in 680 gm. of organs and blood, 0.2320 gm. of nicotine were found.[1106]

Postmortem Appearances: Lami made a postmortem examination of a three year old girl who died one hour after drinking a nicotine-containing insecticide. He found hyperemia of the meninges and of the brain, as well as of the esophagus and stomach.[1107]

In most of the cases that I have observed, death occurred rapidly and the autopsy revealed more or less intense gastroenteritis. The blood is dark and fluid. Congestion of the brain and internal viscera is usually found. Kuhn and Esser in their cases reported the intestinal mucosa to be very hyperemic and also the meningeal vessels as being strongly injected. The brain sections disclosed punctate hemorrhages.

Chemical Tests for Nicotine: During the process of making the alkaline distillate, the odor of nicotine may be apparent to the chemist. The general alkaloidal reagents will precipitate nicotine from quite dilute solutions, a point of distinction from coniine. Potassium chloro-platinate solutions and epichlorhydrin were found to be useful. P-dimethylaminobenzaldehyde is a very sensitive reagent. The free nicotine is dehydrated to nicotyrine by means of a silver nitrate. Since pyrrole and pyrrolidine also give a violet coloration with dimethylaminobenzaldehyde, high dilution and a second treatment with silver acetate may be necessary to insure an exclusive test for nicotine. One part in 50,000 may be detected in this way. Furfural reacts both with pyrrole and with nicotyrine in phosphoric acid solution, giving rise to a deep yellow color, which persists on heating, in the presence of silver acetate, provided only nicotine was originally present. Often many of the reactions described for nicotine do not take place, and in some instances the tests are found not to be typical for nicotine.

Nicotine when freshly distilled in water is white, but soon turns brown upon standing. It has a boiling point of 246.7° C. (476.06° F.) at 745 mm. pressure. Tincture of iodine gives a yellow precipitate which soon becomes purplish or reddish-brown; phosphomolybdic and phosphotungstic acids give precipitates even at dilution of one to 40,000; gold chloride pro-

1106. KUHN, A.,and ESSER, A.: *Deutsche Ztschr. f. d. ges. gerichtl. Med.*, 21:305, 1933.
1107. Cited by LESCHKE: Clinical Toxicology, 1934.

duces a yellow or brown amorphous precipitate, especially in neutral solutions of nicotine, which precipitate is readily soluble in excess of nicotine and in caustic alkalis, but insoluble, or nearly so, in acetic and hydrochloric acids, a distinct cloudiness being observed at dilutions of one to 10,000; platinum chloride gives a yellow amorphous precipitate, which soon becomes crystalline, at a dilution of one to 5,000 of nicotine; mercuric chloride produces a white, curdy precipitate, which becomes crystalline on standing in dilutions of one to 3,000, which precipitate is soluble in acetic and hydrochloric acids and also in ammonium chloride, but from this latter solvent the nicotine separates to some extent on standing for a time; picric acid gives an amorphous precipitate which soon changes into crystalline tufts, the reaction indicating nicotine in a dilution of one to 25,000; potassium mercuric iodide, likewise, gives a crystalline precipitate at a dilution of one to 25,000. With coniine the concentration of the alkaloid must be considerably greater than that mentioned above before reactions occur. Silicotungstic acid, or potassium silico-tungstate, when added to a solution of nicotine containing an excess of free hydrochloric acid, yields an immediate precipitate at dilutions of one to 300,000, while at a dilution of one part of nicotine per million, a crystalline precipitate appears on allowing the mixture to stand for twenty-four to forty-eight hours. Coniine, with this reagent, yields precipitates only at dilutions of one to 5,000 or stronger.

Roussin's Test: If an ethereal solution of iodine is added to an ethereal solution of nicotine, a brownish-red amorphous precipitate is produced which, after standing for some hours, is converted into a crystalline mass of long, ruby-red needles. This reaction occurs at a dilution of about one to 100, while with more dilute solutions the amorphous phase of the reaction may be absent. These crystals are known as "Roussin's crystals," and are not formed with coniine. If the nicotine be resinous these crystals are formed with difficulty.

Melzer's Test: If a drop of nicotine or 0.5 to 1 cc. of a dilute solution of nicotine be heated to boiling with 2 or 3 cc. of epichlorhydrin, the mixture becomes distinctly red. Coniine gives no reaction with this reagent.[1108]

1108. MELZER: *Ztschr. f. anal. Chem.*, 37:357, 1908.

Crystallization Test: If a few drops of nicotine be placed on a watch glass and a few drops of concentrated hydrochloric acid on another watch glass, one of these glasses being inverted over the other, a white cloud is produced, which is not as dense as in the case of coniine. In the case of nicotine no crystals will be observed on the glasses, while with coniine a prompt appearance of crystals of coniine hydrochloride will be noted. If this test be made by evaporating a few drops of concentrated hydrochloric acid with a few drops of nicotine, a varnish-like residue will appear, which is amorphous, but which will change to a distinctly crystalline deposit on allowing it to stand in a desiccator over sulphuric acid for some time. With coniine, the formation of crystals is almost immediate.

Schindelmeiser's Test: If nicotine that is not resinous is treated with a drop of formaldehyde solution (which should not contain any formic acid), and then with a drop of concentrated sulphuric or nitric acid, the mixture assumes an intense rose-red color. If the nicotine and formaldehyde be allowed to stand for several hours, a solid compound is formed which gives a more pronounced color on the addition of nitric acid. If this latter technique is employed the formaldehyde must not be in excess, otherwise the solution becomes green after a time and rapidly decomposes. This test is not given by coniine, trimethylamine, piperidine, pyridine, or aniline, nor by the ptomains resembling nicotine.[1109]

Tunmann's Test: Dissolve a few crystals of para-dimethyl-aminobenzaldehyde on a watch glass in a drop of fuming hydrochloric acid, adding thereto from the side a drop of the aqueous solution of nicotine. A rose color develops immediately at the surface of contact, then a violet-red zone results, and finally the entire liquid becomes violet-red. The color increases in intensity and persists for ten to twenty-four hours. On like treatment coniine and pyridine give no color. Aniline yields, in not too dilute solutions, a red color, but immediately precipitates a dyestuff in the form of red needles. By this test nicotine may be readily detected in cigar smoke.[1110]

If proper precautions are taken, p-dimethylaminobenzaldehyde becomes a sensitive reagent. The free nicotine is de-

1109. SCHINDELMEISER: *Pharm. Centralhalle*, 40:703, 1899.
1110. TUNMANN: *Apoth.-Ztg.*, 33:485, 1918; *Chem. Zentralbl.*, 2: 227, 1919.

hydrated to nicotyrine through the use of silver nitrate.

Separation from the Tissues: Nicotine may be separated by the Stas-Otto process. Dangelmayer[1111] has shown that trichlorethylene extracts nicotine quantitatively from alkaline solutions, and that the nicotine may be recovered by shaking this extract with dilute sulphuric acid. However, if nicotine is suspected, it can be separated easier in the alkaline volatile distillate and precipitated as the silicotungstate. It has been shown by Bertrand and Javillier[1112] that the precipitation of nicotine in the presence of an excess of hydrochloric acid proceeds quantitatively when silicotungstic acid or potassium silicotungstate is added to a hydrochloric acid solution of nicotine. This property enables us to make a quantitative determination of the amount in the tissues, without the same possibilities of error inherent in the other methods. In the process recommended, advantage is taken of the fact that nicotine is volatile with steam from alkaline solutions. A definite amount of the finely divided organ, or a definite volume of the stomach contents or other fluid, is placed in a distilling flask and a sufficient amount of water and sodium hydrate solution added to make the mixture of the consistency of thin gruel and strongly alkaline in reaction. A few pieces of glass or pumice may be placed in the flask to prevent bumping. Distillation is then carried out with a rapid current of steam in the usual manner, the distillate being collected in a large flask with 15 or 20 cc. of 10% hydrochloric acid. Continue the distillation until a portion of the distillate shows no opalescence when treated with a few drops of the 10% solution of silicotungstic acid followed by a few drops of hydrochloric acid (if nicotine be present in a solution of one in 300,000, an opalescence will appear almost immediately). After the distillation is complete, make the distillate up to a definite volume and filter through a dry filter, testing a portion of the filtrate with methyl orange or methyl red to be certain that the reaction is still acid. With a buret measure an aliquot portion of the filtered

1111. DANGELMAYER: *Chem. Ztg.*, 42:290, 1918; *Chem. Abst.*, 13: 2958, 1919.

1112. *Bull d. sc. pharmacol.*, Par., 16:7, 1909. *Bull. Acad. roy. de méd. de Belgique*, 1042, 1909; *Bull. Soc. Chem.*, 10:241, 1909; and see also GUGLIALMELLI and HARDH: *Ann. soc. quin. Argentina*, 7:121, 1919; MCNALLY, W. D.: *J. Lab. & Clin. Med.*, 5:213, 1920; TAIGNER: *Ztschr. f. anal. Chem.*, 63:346, 1919; HEIDUSCHKA and WOLF: *Schweiz. Apoth. Ztg.*, 58:213 and 229, 1920.

distillate, allowing it to flow into a beaker or small flask. Add a few cubic centimeters of the 10% hydrochloric acid (3 or 4 cc. for each 100 cc. of liquid taken), and follow this with a few cc. of 10% solution silicotungstic acid (the author recommends 1 cc. for every 0.01 gm. of nicotine suspected); mix thoroughly and allow to stand for eighteen to twenty-four hours. At the end of that time filter the crystalline precipitate through a quantitative known ash filter, and wash with water containing a little hydrochloric acid. The original filtrate should be tested with a few drops of the nicotine distillate in order to insure an excess of the reagent in the original mixture, and likewise the washing should be continued until all of the excess silicotungstic acid is removed from the precipitate. After the washing is complete, transfer the filter and precipitate to a weighed platinum crucible, dry carefully, and incinerate first over the ordinary Bunsen lamp and then over the blast lamp for a few minutes. Cool in a desiccator to constant weight. If the weight of the incinerated residue be multiplied by 0.114 the product yields the amount of nicotine in the aliquot portion of the distillate taken for the determination, as the composition of the precipitate given by silicotungstic acid with nicotine is $12WO_3 . 2H_2O . 2C_{10}H_{14}N_2\text{-}5H_2O$. Proper calculation gives the total nicotine in the complete distillate, and likewise in the total original organ from which the portion was taken for determination.

During the extraction of decomposed organs, certain decomposed products in a concentrated form yield reactions from the alkaline ether extract that resemble nicotine. However, at greater dilutions and after purification, the residue from the alkaline extractions fails to give tests for nicotine.

Rorsch, Fassbender, Schwanert, Liebermann, and Selmi have found nicotine-like substances in decomposing animal tissues when there was no possibility of true nicotine being present.

OPIUM

OPIUM is the air-dried, milky exudation obtained by incising the unripe capsules of papaver somniferum, or its variety, album de Candolle. It may be described as rounded, somewhat flattened, masses, usually 8 to 15 cm. in diameter; externally dark brown, covered with fragments of poppy leaves; more or less plastic when fresh, becoming hard and brittle or tough on keeping; internally dark brown, somewhat lustrous. It has a characteristic odor, and its taste is very bitter. The dose is 0.06 gm. (one grain). Opium in its normal moist condition yields not less than 9.5% of anhydrous morphine.

Opium Granulatum is opium dried at a temperature not exceeding 70° C. and reduced to a coarse powder. Granulated opium yields not less than 10% nor more than 10.5% anhydrous morphine. Its description is the same as that of powdered opium.

Opium Pulveratum is opium dried at a temperature not exceeding 70° C. and reduced to a very fine powder yielding not less than 10% and not more than 10.5% anhydrous morphine. In description it is light brown, or yellowish-brown to brownish-red, more or less irregular and granular fragments. Its dose is 0.06 gm. (one grain).

Pulvis Ipecacuanhae et Opii contains 10% opium, 10% ipecac, 80% lactose. It is a grayish-white or very light brown powder, very slowly soluble in water, and strongly polarizing light with a strong display of color. Other elements of identification are the tissues of ipecac and the capsules of opium poppy. The dose is 0.3 gm. (five grains).

Tinctura Opii contains 10% extract of granulated opium. The dose is 0.6 cc. (ten minims).

Tinctura Opii Camphorata contains 0.4% extract of powdered opium plus 0.4% benzoic acid, 0.4% camphor, and 0.4% oil of anise. The dose is 4 cc. (one fluid dram). Tincture of opium yields from each 100 cc. not less than 0.95 gm. and not more than 1.05 gm. of anhydrous morphine.

Morphinae Hydrochloridum, $C_{17}H_{19}O_3N \cdot HCl \cdot 3H_2O$, consists of white, silky, glistening needles, cubical masses, or a white glistening powder. It is odorless, and stable in air; soluble in 17.5 parts of water, fifty-two parts of alcohol, 0.5 parts of boiling water; and soluble in glycerin, but insoluble in chloroform and ether. The dose is 0.008 gm. (one-eighth grain).

Morphinae Sulphas, $(C_{17}H_{19}O_3N)_2H_2SO_4 \cdot 5H_2O$, consists of white, feathery, silky crystals, cubical masses, or white crystalline powder; odorless and stable in the air; soluble in 15.5 parts water, 565 parts alcohol, insoluble in chloroform and ether. The dose is 0.008 gm. (one-eighth grain).

Codeina, $C_{17}H_{18}(CH_3)O_3N.H_2O$, codeine, methylmorphine, is obtained from opium or prepared from morphine by methylation. It is colorless, and slightly efflorescent in warm air, and is soluble in 120 parts of water, two parts of alcohol, 0.5 parts of chloroform, eighteen parts of ether and thirteen parts of benzene. The dose is 0.03 gm. (one and on-half grains).

Codeinae Phosphas, $C_{17}H_{18}$ (CH_3) $O_3.H_3PO_4$. $1\frac{1}{2}H_2O$, contains not less than 67% of anhydrous codeine. It consists of fine, white needle-shaped crystals, or a white crystalline powder. It is odorless, and is soluble in 2.3 parts of water, 325 parts of alcohol, 4,500 parts chloroform, and 1875 parts of ether. The dose is 0.03 gm. (one and one-half grains).

Codeinae Sulphas, $(C_{17}H_{18}(CH_3(O_3N)_2H_2SO_4 . 5H_2O$, consists of long, glistening, white, needle-shaped crystals, rhombic prisms, or a crystalline powder; odorless and efflorescent in the air; soluble in thirty parts of water, 1280 parts of alcohol; insoluble in chloroform and ether. The dose is .03 gm. (one and one-half grains).

Apomorphinae Hydrochloridum, $C_{17}H_{17}O_2NHCl_{1/2}H_2O$, is the hydrochloride of an alkaloid prepared from morphine by the abstraction of one molecule of water. It consists of white or grayish-white glistening crystals, acquiring a greenish tint upon exposure to light and air. It is odorless, and is soluble in fifty parts of water, fifty parts of alcohol, and very slightly soluble in chloroform and ether. The dose as expectorant is 0.001 gm. (one-sixtieth grain); as emetic hypodermically, 0.005 gm. (one-twelfth grain). Apomorphine hydrochloride must be rejected if it at once imparts an emerald-green color to 100 parts of distilled water when shaken with it.

Opium owes its therapeutic activity to about twenty alkaloids of which morphine, codeine, papaverine, narcotine, and thebaine are the most important. The total amount of alkaloids in opium varies from 5% to 25%, different varieties containing very different quantities of each alkaloid. For example, the morphine content of some samples of opium may vary from 3% to 23%. These alkaloids are found in opium in combination with meconic, lactic, and sulphuric acid.

Kerbosch investigated the distribution of the alkaloids in various parts of the plant.[1113] In the seeds he found traces of narcotine and an amorphous alkaloid, which, after germina-

1113. *Arch Pharm.,* 248:336, 1910.

tion, contained considerable quantities of narcotine, codeine, morphine, papaverine, and thebaine. The flowering plant, up to ripening time, contains narcotine, papaverine, codeine, and morphine in all parts except the hair. The latex varies in its alkaloidal content in different parts of the plant. The alkaloids contained in opium in their relative proportional amounts are as follows:

Morphine, $C_{17}H_{19}NO_3$		9%
Narcotine, $C_{22}H_{23}NO_7$		5%
Papaverine, $C_{20}H_{21}NO_4$		0.8%
Thebaine, $C_{19}H_{21}NO_3$		0.4%
Codeine, $C_{18}H_{21}NO_3$		0.3%
Narceine, $C_{23}H_{27}NO_8$		0.2%
Cryptopine, $C_{21}H_{23}NO_5$		0.08%
Pseudomorphine, $(C_{17}H_{18}NO_3)_2$		0.02%
Laudanine, $C_{20}H_{25}NO_4$		0.01%
Lanthopine, $C_{23}H_{25}NO_4$		0.006%
Protopine, $C_{20}H_{19}NO_5$		0.003%
Codamine, $C_{20}H_{25}NO_4$		0.002%
Tritopine, $(C_{12}H_{27}NO_3)_2$		0.0015%
Laudanosine, $C_{21}H_{27}NO_4$		0.0008%

Morphine, codeine, meconidine, codamine, laudanine, laudanidine, laudanosine, protopine, and cryptopine have a narcotic or tetanic action; the others are practically inactive from a toxicological viewpoint. The analysis of opium would not necessitate the identification of all the alkaloids but would be sufficient if the more familiar ones such as morphine, codeine, thebaine, narcotine narceine, and papaverine, were identified, with the presence of meconic acid.

Opium, and its alkaloids and derivatives, are used in many medicinal preparations, such as cough syrups and lozenges, soothing syrups, diarrhea mixtures, neuralgia remedies, anodynes, cholera mixtures, coryza mixtures, consumption remedies, habit cures, asthmatic remedies, suppositories, and many foreign, especially Chinese, remedies.

Morphine, $C_{17}H_{19}NO_3$, is a complex derivative of phenanthrene. It contains two OH groups (one phenolic, the other alcoholic) in which substitutions can be made by either alkyl or acid radicals. The more important alkyl esters are the monomethyl (codeine) and the dimethyl (thebaine):

$$C_{15}H_{14}ON \begin{cases} \text{-OH} \\ \text{-CHOH} \\ \text{-CH}_2 \end{cases} \qquad C_{15}H_{14}ON \begin{cases} \text{-OCH}_3 \\ \text{-CHOH} \\ \text{-CH}_2 \end{cases} \qquad C_{15}H_{14}ON \begin{cases} \text{-OCH}_3 \\ \text{-COCH}_3H \\ \text{-CH} \end{cases}$$

Morphine	Codeine	Thebaine

The nature of these radicals, whether acid or alcoholic, aromatic or aliphatic, modifies the actions quantitatively but only in degree. Replacement of one hydroxyl group (codeine) diminishes the narcotic action and increases the respiratory and tetanic action. When both OH groups are replaced by acids (diacetyl morphine), the narcotic effects are stronger than with codeine, and the tetanic action is weaker than with morphine.

The different behavior of opium alkaloids to solvents affords a valuable means of distinguishing and separating them. They are precipitated from concentrated solutions of their salts by alkali hydroxides and alkali carbonates, some of the precipitates dissolving in excess of the reagent. Most of the opium alkaloids (except papaverine and laudanosine) have a levorotatory action on polarized light, but the specific rotatory power varies greatly with the solvent and the concentration of the solution, and because of this fact has a very limited practical value. The alkaloids give characteristic color reactions with certain chemical reagents, which, combined with their melting point, crystalline form, and solubility provides a means of identification. The salts of papaverine and narcotine, especially with organic acids as acetic and benzoic, are very unstable, being decomposed even by cold water. Hence, when the acid salts are treated with a neutral solution of sodium acetate, or even with a slight acid solution, the free alkaloid is precipitated. This reaction will distinguish these from the others. Morphine, codeine, and thebaine are titrated accurately by standard mineral acids, using litmus or methyl orange as indicators, but they have no action on phenolphthalein.

Papaverine, narcoteine, and narceine have no effect upon litmus, and their salts may be titrated with standard alkali and litmus just as if the acids were uncombined, the first two of these showing their feeble basic characteristics by the fact that they are extracted by chloroform from acid solutions.

Morphine, an alkaloid, found most abundantly in opium,

is the constituent responsible for most of the poisonous effects of opium. Morphine occurs as colorless, or white, shining rhombic prisms, fine needles, or as crystalline powder. It crystallizes from alcohol as prisms, containing one molecule of water. It is odorless and permanent in the air. It is soluble in 3,340 parts of water, 210 parts of alcohol, 1,220 parts of chloroform, 6,250 parts of ether, 125 parts of amyl alcohol; it is insoluble in benzene. It is levorotatory. The water of hydration is given off at 100° C., the alkaloid melting at 254° C. when heated rapidly. When heated slowly it begins to melt at 247° C. with decomposition. Morphine with its water of hydration melts at about 230° C. It is a strong tertiary base and also a monatomic phenol, dissolving in alkalis to form salts with one atom of the metal which is decomposed by carbon dioxide or ammonia. This reaction of forming salts with alkalis is used to good advantage in separating morphine from other alkaloids. It forms diacetyl and dibenzol derivatives. Acids, alkalis, and zinc chloride remove a molecule of water, converting it into apomorphine; soluble in ether and chloroform. Morphine is readily oxidized; weak oxidizing agents, such as gold, silver, and iodic acid, convert it into pseudomorphine, $C_{17}H_{19}NO_3 + O = (C_{17}H_{19}NO_3)_2 + H_2O$. Morphine is found in the alkaline ether and chloroform extracts when looking for alkaloids.

Symptoms: Poisoning by morphine or opium is chiefly due to the action of morphine, which makes up about half of the opium alkaloids. If taken by mouth the effects begin to appear in twenty to forty minutes; if taken hypodermically the symptoms appear much earlier, and narcotism is more likely to follow the early symptoms. The individual susceptibility to opiates varies greatly. Children are more susceptible than adults. The same high degree of susceptibility is shown by some patients with circulatory disorders, especially those with arteriosclerosis. Doses as low as one-fourth grain and even less have caused deep and prolonged unconsciousness, and death. The usual symptoms seen from an overdose of morphine are, first, a sense of mental exhilaration and physical ease, with a quickening and strengthening of the pulse, and then a depression of the brain, with special reference to its higher functions. Smaller doses, insufficient to cause this depression, cause a diminished sensibility to lasting impressions, such as pain, cough, hunger, and discomfort. Following this there may be dizziness and heaviness of the head, nausea, languor, and drowsiness, the pulse being reduced in frequency sometime before it is reduced in force. Where it is used in postoperative cases, doses as small as one-fourth grain may cause nausea. Some people, especially those with great susceptibility, may complain of itching of the skin and even erythema. As the action of the morphine continues, it produces sleep. There is a gradual loss of muscular power and a diminished sense of feeling. The pupils become contracted. The sensitiveness of the conjunctiva is contracted, and the pupils fail to respond to light. The respirations become less and less frequent, finally being reduced in some cases to four or five a minute, with stertorous breathing.

Tests: Morphine is precipitated by all the usual alkaloidal reagents, and gives distinct color reactions with a number of reagents.

1. Ferric chloride gives a deep blue color, changing to green with an excess of the reagent, and disappearing on heating or upon addition of acids or alcohol. (Pseudomorphine gives a blue color and codamine a dark green.) The material is best taken in the solid form. A stirring rod is rubbed through the residue obtained in the alkaline ether or chloroform extracts, and moistened with a neutral ferric chloride solution, one-to-fifteen dilution. There should be no free acid in the reagent, and it should not be alkaline enough to be at all turbid. The blue color produced by morphine with ferric chloride changes to an orange, which fades to yellow upon adding nitric acid. This test is not very satisfactory for morphine, as a large number of aromatic compounds with phenolic hydroxl in their structure give with ferric salts a blue, or a partly blue color. Prescott states that extracts from putrefactive tissues did not give the ferric chloride test, except in analysis where morphine was established by other reactions.[1114]

2. An aqueous solution reduces iodic acid with liberation of iodine, which when extracted with chloroform or carbon disulphide gives a violet color. There are two iodic acid tests for morphine: (1) LeFort's test which is iodic acid with ammonia and gives a mahogany color; (2) iodic acid and starch, which turns blue from the liberated iodine acting on the starch.

1114. PRESCOTT's Organic Analysis, 399.

LeFort's test is distinctive of morphine and is proof of the presence of morphine. The test without ammonia is not distinctive of morphine, but is given by any strong reducing agent. LeFort's test is a positive test, while the other is a negative test. The iodic acid in both tests acts as an oxidizing agent on the morphine, the ammonia used in the LeFort's test decolorizes the iodine and develops the color of the morphine oxidized product. LeFort's test is carried out as follows: To a small quantity of the unknown on a white porcelain plate, add a drop of iodic acid solution and let stand ten minutes. If any free iodine appears, which is noted by the color, it is carefully washed off by floating over it a few drops of chloroform. This is repeated until the residue is colorless. Let dry and add a few drops of ammonia water (10%) until a mahogany color develops showing morphine present. The decanted chloroform is evaporated and a small amount of starch paste is added, which will turn blue in the presence of free iodine.

A more convenient way would be to first apply the starch test thus: To the unknown on a white porcelain plate, add a small quantity of the starch paste, evaporate to dryness, and with a glass rod add a small quantity of iodic acid solution. Whether the blue color develops or not, add a few drops of ammonia water, which gives a mahogany color, showing the presence of morphine. This method avoids the loss of material by washing with chloroform.

LeFort recommends the following method for making the test: Narrow strips of filter paper are moistened with the unknown, and then the strips are dried and wetted again several times. This dry strip is moistened with iodic acid solution, partly dried, and then an excess of ammonia water applied. The mahogany color, will extend as far up the paper as the unknown was applied.

LeFort's test is distinctive of morphine. The delicacy is 1/6400 grain of pure morphine, but in the presence of foreign matter present in tissue extracts it is reduced to 1/1280 grain (0.00005 gm.).

3.   Concentrated nitric acid gives a deep red or orange-red color, the crystals dissolving to an orange-red solution, gradually fading on standing. Adding a drop of stannous chloride to the red solution causes no change (brucine turns purple).

4. Sulphuric acid gives a faint pink color when pure, the color soon fading.

5. Husemann's test: Concentrated sulphuric acid is added and then warmed to 100° C., then concentrated nitric acid, a chlorate, chlorine water, or sodium hypochlorite, is added, giving a blue or purplish color, changing to deep red and gradually fading.

6. Froehde's reagent, (1 to 2 mg. molybdic acid in 1 cc. concentrated sulphuric, freshly made), when added to the dry unknown on a white porcelain plate gives a deep purple color, fading to violet and becoming green. If allowed to stand this green color slowly changes to yellow, and finally to faint pink. If the amount of morphine is great the violet color remains for a long time, but the smaller the amount the quicker the change in color takes place. This test is distinctive for pure morphine, but with extracts from tissue which contain foreign matter one should be guarded in his deductions from this test alone. Poe and Stehley[1115] made a study of Froehde's test for morphine, to determine which group of chemical substances gave a morphine test, and upon mixing what substance interfered with the test. Procedure: 1 gm. sodium molybdate dissolved in 100 cc. C.P. concentrated sulphuric acid was the reagent used. The standard morphine was an alcoholic solution containing 1 mg. of morphine per cc. The compounds studied contained 1 mg. per cc., and such solvents were used as would readily dissolve the substance and readily evaporate. Insoluble substances were finely ground and suitably suspended in volatile liquids. Tests made:

(1) One cc. of the solution was evaporated and tested with three to four drops of Froehde's reagent.

(2) One c. of the solution plus 1 cc. of morphine solution was tested with three to four drops of Froehde's reagent.

(3) Five cc. of solution plus 1 cc. of morphine solution were tested with three to four drops of Froehde's reagent. The alkaloids and their salts gave the following color test:

Aconite	blue to green
Apomorphine	green to blue, trace of violet
Belladonnine	brown
Berberine	dirty brown

1115. POE, CHARLES F., and STEHLEY, PEARL SURBRUGG: *J. Lab. & Clin. Med.*, 18:375, 1933.

Brucine	reddish-violet to blue
Codeine	green to blue
Colchicine	brownish-orange
Cotarnine hydrochloride	brick red
Cryptopine	violet to green
Delphinine	brown, purple streaks
Dionine	greenish-yellow
Emetine	brown, trace of violet
Heroin	reddish-violet
Hydrastine	green to brown
Morphine	reddish-violet to green
Narceine	brown to green
Papaverine	light violet to green
Phenacaine	light green
Piperine	reddish-orange to brown
Quinine	pale green
Sanguinarine nitrate	brown to purple
Solanine	yellow
Veratrine	yellow to orange

No color was given by, atropine, caffeine, cinchonidine, cinchonine, cocaine, daturine, ergotine, betaeucaine hydrochloride, gelseminine, homatropine, hyoscyamine, nicotine, pelletierine, physostigmine, pilocarpine, pseudopelletierine, quinidine, scopolamine, sparteine, strychnine, theobromine, theophylline.

The amino acids gave the following:

Tyrosine	blue
Tryptophane	dirty green
Phenylglycine	brown
Aspartic acid	tan

No color with, alpha alanine, arginine, asparagine, betaine hydrochloride, phenylalanine, creatine, creatinine, glycine, hippuric acid, leucine.

Of twenty aliphatic acids tested only one, palmitic acid, gave a dirty brown, the others gave no color.

The sugars gave:

Levulose	light yellow
Xylose	gray

No color with galactose, lactose, glucose, sucrose, maltose, and a few others.

No color was given with urea and uric acid derivatives such as amytal, barbital, barbituric acid, biuret, guanine, ipral, luminal, peralga, urea, urethan, uric acid.

The following glucosides were tested:

Colocynthin	reddish-brown to purple
Convallamarin	brown
Digitalin	magenta, streaks of purple
Elaterin	olive green
Phlorizin	navy blue
Picrotoxin	yellowish-orange
Salicin	violet-blue to rose
Saponin	greenish-blue to streaks of violet
Arbutin	violet
Santonin	no color

Using equal amounts of the following substances and morphine, the test was completely obscured: azoxybenzene, para-aminoazobenzene, adrenalin, benzolacetophenone, nicotinic acid nitrate.

Using five times the amount of the following as of morphine, the test was obscured: amino-phenol, benzhydrol, b-napthalamine hydrochloride, piperine, phenolphthalein, sanguanine nitrate.

Rosenbloom and Mills[1116] show that putrefactive substances do not interfere with this test, as they did not obtain a morphine color test with decomposed material, whether of aerobic or anaerobic origin. Froehde's reagent will detect 1/6400 grain (0.00001 gm.) with a very distinctive reaction.

Sulphuric acid with other oxidizing agents gives color reactions as follows: with titanic acid, a pink violet to brown-red color; with selenous acid or ammonium-selenite[1117] dissolved in 100 gm. C.P. concentrated sulphuric acid, a blue to green, changing to olive-green when cold, and, on heating, to a brown color.

Mecke's reagent gives the following reactions:

1116. J. Biol. Chem., 15:327, 1913.
1117. LEVINE, V. E.: Mecke's reagent, 0.5 gm., J. Lab. & Clin. Med., 11:809, 1926.

Alkaloid	Cold	On Heating
Aconite	no color	dark brown violet
Apomorphine	dark blue violet	turns a dark brown
Atropine	no color	no color
Brucine*	yellow red	citron green
Caffeine	no color	no color
Cocaine	no color	rose yellow
Codeine	blue or emerald green	steel blue to olive
Colchicine*	citron yellow	yellow brown
Coniine	no color	no color
Delphinine*	deep brown	brown
Narceine	faint greenish-yellow	dark violet
Narcotine	greenish, steel blue to cherry red	
Nicotine	yellowish	yellowish
Papaverine	greenish, steel blue to deep violet	intense dark methyl-violet
Physostigmine	brownish-yellow	weak brown
Picrotoxin	almost colorless	yellowish-brown
Quinine	colorless	dark brown
Solamine	gray brown	gray brown
Strychnine	no color	no color
Thebaine	deep orange, fading	dark brown
Veratrine*	citron yellow, olive green	brownish-violet
Dionine	evanescent blue, emerald green	
Heroin	emerald green	
* Due to sulphuric acid alone.		

7. Pellagri's test: Dissolve the unknown in fuming hydrochloric acid, then add concentrated sulphuric acid and evaporate. Morphine is shown by a purple color at the edges, which changes to red after all the hydrochloric acid is evaporated. If this is dissolved in hydrochloric acid and then neutralized with sodium bicarbonate, it becomes violet. If hydriodic acid or dilute alcoholic iodine is added, the color changes to green, which, if shaken out with ether, turns purple.

8. Cane sugar is mixed with morphine, moistened with a few drops of water, and made into a paste. A few drops of sulphuric acid are allowed to flow alongside the mixture, and an intense purple color develops at the point of contact, changing to violet and green, to yellow (oxydimorphine is

colored green and codeine reacts similarly to morphine).

9. Marquis' reagent (3 cc. concentrated sulphuric acid plus two drops 40% formaldehyde) added to the dry residue on a white porcelain plate, gives an intense purple-red color, changing to violet, then blue. This reaction is quite distinctive, and is delicate to 0.02 mg. With this reagent codeine and apomorphine give a violet changing to blue, but not the initial purple-red color. Oxydimorphine shows a green color, changing to flame red. Dionine shows a dark blue violet. Heroin gives colors similar to morphine.

10. Denige's test: To 10 cc. of a dilute solution of morphine (over 0.3%) add 1 cc. hydrogen peroxide and 1 cc. ammonium solution and then one drop of copper sulphate solution (4%). Shake well, and a rose red to a deep red color appears, depending upon the concentration of the alkaloid present. (Codeine, thebaine, papaverine, narceine, and narcotine do not give the same colors, but oxydimorphine, apomorphine, heroin, and dionine give somewhat similar colors.)

11. Potassium dichromate and sulphuric acid give a green color. Vanadium-sulphuric acid gives a yellow, changing to violet brown, then to slate color.

12. Lautenschlaeger's test: This reagent is a solution of diazotized sulphanilic acid prepared as follows: Dissolve 0.2 gm. sulphanilic acid in 80 cc. distilled water, cooling with ice if necessary. Add 10 cc. N/10 hydrochloric acid and 10 cc. N/10 sodium nitrate solution. In making test, the unknown is dissolved in a small amount of sulphuric acid and made alkaline with sodium carbonate. To this is added an equal portion of the above reagent. Upon adding an acid it gives a red color, changing to orange. This reaction is sensitive in a dilution of one to 10,000. In a dilution of one to 1,000,000 the color is distinctly yellow, while with a dilution of one to 2,000 it is dark red. No other opium alkaloids give the same colors. Emetine gives red, sparteine gives yellow, physostigmine red, coniine bright yellow, nicotine brightly yellow. This color is stable only with morphine in an acid solution.

13. Crystals: Solutions of morphine give characteristic crystals with reagents such as iodine, palladous chloride, picrolonic acid, etc., and a microscopical examination of the forms of these compounds, is one of the most valuable means

of identifying the alkaloid and differentiating it from the others.

14. In conducting a biological test for morphine one injects under the back skin of a white mouse neutral hydrochloric acid solution of morphine.[1118] After a few minutes an "S"-forming curve of the tail will be noted, which will last for twenty hours with a dose of 5 mg. With a dose of 0.05 mg. it will last for forty-five minutes. The delicacy and reaction is placed at 1/100 of a mg. With smaller doses of morphine a certain number of white mice will show tetanic convulsions, as if strychnine had been administered. (Straub's test.)

Morphine is crystallized from a 95% alcohol solution. In rapid crystallization, such as occurs in cooling a warm alcohol solution, needles are obtained which are not distinctive. The crystallization should be slow enough to give columns whose end surfaces will clearly show their boundary lines. To retard or even prevent altogether the evaporation of the alcohol solution, it may be dropped upon a watch glass, which is then covered with another watch glass. It serves better still to place the solution on a watch glass or a glass slide, under a small bell jar, and place underneath a small roll of filter paper wet with alcohol. To obtain crystals from a minute amount, such as that extracted from the tissues, a final residue of such extractions is treated with warm alcohol in repeated portions of only a drop or two, and the solution, concentrated if need be, is drained into a cavity 4 or 5 mm. wide on a glass surface. A suitable receptacle is made by a section of glass tubing cemented upon a glass slide with a little paraffin. From time to time the result may be observed under a power of fifty diameters, which is suitable for the full examination of crystals.

Morphine crystallizes in columns, single and grouped, of the orthorhombic system, with the hexagonal end surfaces. The crystals begin to lose their water of crystallization at 75°C. The crystals blacken before melting, and melt at about 230°C.

These crystalline forms must also respond to the chemical tests for morphine before the chemist can make a positive report. These chemical tests may be applied to a minute crystal under a good hand magnifier.

1118. STRAUB, HERMAN: *Biochem. Ztschr.*, 39:216, 1912.

The Extraction and Isolation of Morphine: The material to be examined is divided as finely as possible, and a weighed aliquot portion is put into a flask connected with a reflux condenser. The material in the flask is covered with 50% alcohol, acidulated with tartaric or acetic acid, and the contents digested on a hot plate at about 70°C. for one hour. It is then cooled and strained. The residue is treated in the same manner a second and a third time. The alcoholic filtrate is evaporated, by means of suction, on a water-bath, to a syrupy liquid. To this is added 95% alcohol, and it is then allowed to stand until precipitation of the proteid matter is complete. This is washed a few times with alcohol. The alcohol is distilled off with suction, in a water-bath, and the residue brought to a syrupy consistency. This residue is treated with alcohol (95%), filtered and evaporated as before, and the purification continued until there is no precipitation caused by 95% alcohol. To the filtered liquid, lead acetate solution is added in slight excess. The precipitate, if obtained, is to be examined for the presence of meconic acid. The filtrate and washings are treated with hydrogen sulphide to precipitate all the lead, which, after standing for one hour or longer, is filtered out. The last filtrate, with washings, is evaporated to remove all the hydrogen sulphide, and extracted. The precipitate to be examined for meconic acid is now suspended in lead water and treated with hydrogen sulphide gas and filtered to remove all the lead. The filtrate from the lead sulphide is evaporated. The filtrate is to be kept clear, for meconic acid with ferric chloride gives a deep red or purplish-red color. This color is not readily destroyed either by boiling, by the addition of hydrochloric acid, or by mercuric chloride. (Difference from thiocyanic acid.) This color, however, is destroyed by the addition of stannous chloride, but it returns on addition of nitrous acid. Lead acetate gives a yellowish-white precipitate of lead meconate, which changes to red when touched with ferric chloride. Meconic acid will be extracted in the acid ether extract. The residue, if it contains meconic acid, will become pale yellow, gradually turning pale violet when treated with two drops of concentrated sulphuric acid. Ammonium vanadate reagent gives a purple to deep blue color. which gradually fades. Froehde's test gives a pale yellow to pale green color. Meconine with ammonium vanadate gives a pale yellow ammoniacal solution. The solution turns pale green-yellow, and gradually pale red. Extract morphine by use of chloroform in alkaline solution.

Kabasawa[1119] decomposes the proteins by means of papain digestion for twenty to eighty minutes, and extracts the morphine with hydrochloric acid, removing the ether soluble substances from the hydrochloric acid solution. The cleavage of the residual lipoids is obtained by heating on the water-bath for six hours. The extraction is made in a Soxhlet's apparatus, using a chloroform ethyl alcohol mixture. A re-extraction with hydrochloric acid is made, having the purified morphine extract in a volume of 25 cc. of N/200 hydrochloric acid. The quantitative iodometric procedure as given by Wada is recommended.

These chemical tests for meconic acid are distinctive and delicate. When applied to the contents of the stomach, if opium or laudanum is retained in this organ the tests for meconic acid offer a reasonable probability of its detection.

In the examination of the stomach contents for opium, it should always be carefully inspected for fragments of the mass of opium. Filtered and washed portions of the content are to be searched with hand magnifier and microscope, comparing with residues of opium similarly treated. Upon first opening the stomach, attention should be given to the odor, as to whether that of opium or laudanum can be distinguished.

Deposition in the Body: Kobert found only small and varying amounts of morphine in the urine.[1120] Wormley found it present in the urine of six patients who had taken morphine; in four of these not more than a trace, while in two a considerable amount.[1121]. Notta and Lugan found it constantly in the urine of persons taking morphine habitually, and it may be found when 0.1 gm. or more is taken daily.[1122] Borntrager could find no morphine in the urine of a person who took large doses daily by mouth, but found it in the feces.[1123] Subcutaneous injection in one person showed traces in the urine even when given in very small doses. In another person who was given much larger doses none appeared. Morphine is

1119. Kabasawa, W.: Jap. J. M. Sc. Tr., IV-Pharmacol., 8:97, 1934.
1120. Kobert: Lehrbuch der Intoxikationen, 971, 1906.
1121. Wormley: Univ. M. Mag., Phila., 2:399, 1890.
1122. Notta and Lugan: Arch. d. Pharm., 3 s., 23:512, 1885.
1123. Borntrager: Chem. Centralbl., 17:119, 1880.

eliminated largely through the mucous membrane of the stomach and intestines, either unchanged or slightly changed. As a result from a hypodermic injection, it appears in the alimentary canal. That morphine is, to a certain extent, eliminated by oxidation of the blood can hardly be doubted, as the alkalinity of the blood is conducive to the change. Morphine has been found in the liver, gall-bladder, kidneys, brain, spleen, blood, and stomach, intestines, urine, and feces. In a doubtful diagnosis of morphine poisoning, the urine and feces should be examined, but failure to find its presence should not be conclusive evidence against its presence in the system.

Mouneyrat reports a case of a man, victim of the morphine habit, who formerly took sixty-two grains daily, and recently thirty grains daily, but received no morphine for fourteen days before he died. Morphine was found mostly in the liver, also in the kidneys, and brain.

Homburger and Munch, using Autenrieth's modification of the Stas-Otto process with a five-hour extraction of the organs and three extractions with ether in both acid and alkaline solutions, followed by a final extraction with hot amyl alcohol, showed that 97.5% of the morphine injected into cats and rabbits can be recovered if the analysis be started soon after death.[1124] The yield in these tests indicated the following order of accumulation of morphine in the system of the cat: urine, liver, kidney, spleen, and stomach. With the rabbit the amounts found were stored in the following order: kidney, liver, urine, spleen, and stomach. They believe that loss of morphine in the cadaver is due to a preliminary drop due to splitting up of free morphine, and then a period during which the morphine is fairly constant, followed by a secondary drop due to the splitting up of the combined morphine. Morphine is a fairly stable alkaloid, but not as stable as strychnine.

Symptoms of Acute Poisoning: The action of morphine varies considerably in different animals. It acts chiefly on the central nervous system, but it also has an effect on some peripheral organs such as the intestines. Small quantities of morphine (one-eighth grain) decrease the voluntary movements and produce a drowsiness which soon passes into sleep, unless the patient is disturbed. If the patient is kept awake, his actions and movements show nothing abnormal, but his

1124. HOMBURGER and MUNCH: *J. Am. Chem. Soc.*, **38**:1873, 1916.

thoughts are not connected, and a desire to sleep predominates. If not disturbed for a few minutes he sinks into sleep, which is rather light, and there is no difficulty in arousing him. At this stage the imagination is not depressed to the same extent as the reason. The self control and judgment are lessened, and although the stream of thought may seem more rapid and the images more vivid than usual, the logical sequence of the ideas of time and space is lost. The patient enters a stage of dreams, during which pain is diminished, respiration slowed, and the pupils contracted.

In larger quantities (one-fourth to one-half grain) morphine produces a deep dreamless sleep from which one may still be easily aroused, but which returns immediately if undisturbed. With an increased dose the sleep deepens, and he sinks into a coma from which he cannot be awakened. At this stage the pulse is regular and full, the face is purple and congested, the pupils are contracted to a small point, the throat is dry, the skin feels warm, the respiration is weak and slow, and the temperature may be low. The patient generally awakens refreshed, feeling normal, except for a dryness of the throat, and perhaps a slight nausea.

The effects of morphine taken by mouth appear in from twenty to forty minutes. If taken hypodermically, they appear sooner. With toxic doses, as the poisoning advances, the body is covered with perspiration, the pulse becoming so weak it is almost imperceptible. The respiration grows slower and more stertorous and irregular. The limbs are relaxed, and death, due to respiratory failure, may be preceded by asphyxial convulsions. Death may occur in from two to ten hours. Recovery is possible even after coma and convulsions have developed, in which case the coma passes into a condition of slumber which may endure for twenty-four to thirty-six hours. If the patient survives forty-eight hours, the prognosis is favorable. The period when fatal depends little, if at all, upon the quantity of poison taken.

Postmortem: The appearances are simply those characteristic of asphyxia. The condition of the pupils varies. The pin-point pupil seen during life in a morphine poisoning usually disappears and a normal undilated pupil is seen. The gastric mucous membrane is sometimes reddened. The odor of the drug may be detected if opium has been taken.

Treatment in Acute Poisoning: The stomach is washed out repeatedly at short intervals, whether the poison was taken by mouth or by injection, as it is excreted into the stomach. Emetics should be given, especially apomorphine hydrochloride hypodermically. If narcosis has already set in, the effect of the emetic may be interfered with. A dilute solution of potassium permanganate in the form of a lavage 0.5 gm. per liter has been used successfully, as it has a chemical action on the drug. Atropine sulphate (0.05 grain) is given hypodermically. Tincture belladonna (2 cc.) by mouth may be repeated every fifteen minutes, but caution must be exercised in using this antidote, for cases of recovery from opium poisoning have been followed by death from the belladonna used as an antidote. Some advise the immediate use of 0.10 grain atropine in a single dose and not repeated. To decrease the solubility of the morphine, tannic acid, coffee, tea, and finally powdered charcoal in water, and an iodine solution may be given. Every effort should be made to arouse the patient and keep him awake, especially by walking him around, pinching the skin, slapping him, and by giving ammonia inhalations and artificial respiration if necessary. The patient under all conditions should be kept warm.

Tovell reports the following treatment of acute morphine poisoning:[1125] Empty the stomach, then give a lavage with sodium permanganate, 0.5 gm. per liter. Magnesium sulphate is administered and left in the stomach for a purgative. Keep awake and moving if possible, giving common cardio-vascular stimulants. A case is reported of a physician, sixty years of age, with cancer of the jaw, who administered to himself at the Mayo Clinic twenty-four one-fourth grain tablets hypodermically, in the thigh. Respirations were two to four per minute. Artificial respiration was given. A Magill catheter was put in the trachea with the aid of a laryngoscope. He was given a continuous flow of oxygen, with 10% of carbon dioxide added. The cyanosis disappeared, and respiration jumped to six per minute. The temperature was 102°F. A Lindy vest was also used. (This is a pneumatic vest containing two rubber bags which can be inflated and deflated causing alternate pressure and relaxation of the chest.)

Chronic Poisoning: Chronic poisoning is very common, the drug being taken either by mouth or hypodermically. To

1125. TOVELL, R. M.: *Proc. Staff Meet., Mayo Clin.*, V, 8:646, 1933.

the public chronic poisoning means addiction. However, other substances can form a habit, such as cocaine, Indian hemp, mariahuana, chloroform, chloral hydrate, alcohol, ether, and trichlorethylene. The effects of the prolonged use of these drugs is noted in the complete breakdown of moral, mental, and physical character of the addict. With opium, as previously noted, there are two distinct groups of alkaloids. The first of these, known as the phenanthrene group, possesses analgesic, narcotic, and addiction properties, of which morphine is the more important. The second, or isoquinoline, group is without narcotic effects and does not enter technically into the addiction situation. The gravity of addiction is not clearly understood or appreciated by the public. Some cases are very pitiful. The families are without proper food, clothing, and shelter. An addict will steal anything from strangers, friends or relatives to obtain money with which to purchase morphine. In one recent case a young man, twenty-five years of age, sold his mother's phonograph five different times, so that he might obtain funds to purchase the narcotic. Each time the phonograph was returned he promised not to take it again. Relatives may tolerate such treatment from an habitué, but he is soon deserted by all his friends.

The conventional idea of an opium addict is one who is pale, hollow-eyed, and cadaverous in appearance. This conception results partly from the more or less characteristic symptoms seen in chronic poisoning when the drug is withdrawn. It is then that the individual, because of suffering, makes himself known as an addict.

Many addicts appear physically normal when able to maintain an adequate balance in drug supply. Early withdrawal symptoms or lack of drug balance invariably give rise to more or less loss of weight, anemia, and disturbances of the digestion, with loss of appetite. Constipation is the rule, but it might alternate with diarrhea. The addict is subject to intercurrent diseases, both surgical and medical. Pulmonary tuberculosis occurs in about the proportion of one in every twenty, whereas irritation of the nose and throat is common. Skin abscesses occur in 5%, while scars from former abscesses are found in about two-thirds of all addicts. Syphilis occurs in about 18% of the individuals, whereas oral sepsis, pyorrhea, and carious teeth are common among them. The skin and mouth are dry;

the pupils are contracted; the heart is irregular; the gait is unsteady; there is nervousness and a lack of energy and will power. All sense of honor is lost, and statements are untrustworthy. A common result is sexual impotency, with melancholia and dementia. When deprived of the drug, the patient suffers agony. Marks of needles will be found on the arms and legs if the drug has been used hypodermically.

Treatment: The symptoms associated with the withdrawal of the drug, as seen in opium or opium alkaloid addiction, are striking phenomena. The five most common abstinence symptoms are fear, insomnia, restlessness, yawning, and chilly sensations lasting a few to several hours, and sometimes followed by sleep from ten to twelve hours. On awakening the symptoms are intensified; profuse perspiration, tremors, muscular twitching, sneezing, photophobia, vomiting, diarrhea, palpitation, and cramps being the most common. There are no specific cures for chronic opium poisoning. The general principle underlying the treatment of the addict is practically the same, but each case must be considered as a separate problem. It is absolutely impossible to treat addicts at home, or in an office. They must be placed in an institution, where they can be watched and treated as symptoms develop. Friends and relatives must be kept away. Even when imprisoned they obtain a supply through some underhand source. All food, tobacco, and supplies of any kind from friends or relatives should be prohibited in every penal institution. A universal rule should be established preventing gifts of any description from entering penal institutions. This would lessen the number of drugs, saws, knives, and guns introduced to prisoners. I have seen heroin introduced in plug tobacco, in which the outside leaf had been pulled away and a neat little pocket cut in the plug in which the drug was concealed. I have seen drugs introduced in fruit. Shoes have been submitted to me in the soles and heels of which pockets had been cut. The clothing may contain secret pockets so that after the addicts enter the institution, they are supplied from the amount they had with them. When these addicts enter, their clothing should be taken away from them.

If the facts have been disclosed showing the exact daily dosage of the narcotic usually taken, this dosage may be continued for several days, until the individual becomes ac-

customed to his surroundings and acquires a confidence in his
physician, for this is absolutely necessary. The drug is then
cut down to half the amount, and a purgative is given with a
motor stimulant. The Pettey treatment is very satisfactory
for routine procedure. Dr. Pettey uses the following prescription: Hydrargyri chloridi mite, 0.65 gm.; extracti cascarae
sagradae, 0.65 gm.; ipecacuanhae, 0.65 gm.; strychninae nitratis,
0.0162 gm.; atropinae sulphatis, 0.0013 gm. Mix and make
four capsules. One of these capsules should be given at 4:00,
and one at 6:00, 8:00 and 10:00 P.M., after the evening meal.
At 6:00 A.M. one-thirtieth of a grain of morphine is to be given
by hypodermic injection, and a bottle of magnesium citrate per
mouth. The above should be repeated at 8:00 and 10:00 A.M.
if good results have not been obtained. After this purgation,
one half of the usual dosage of the narcotic may then be given.
The next step in the treatment of the addict is to give an
infusion into the vein of one quart of sterile normal saline
solution. High blood pressure and arteriosclerosis are contra-
indications. It is best given at 3:00 P.M., and the patient
should be put to bed for a few hours after the infusion. The
following day at 4:00 P.M. a purgative capsule is again given,
and at 6:00, 8:00 and 10:00 P.M. the above treatment is repeated.
The drug can now be cut down to one-fourth the amount
formerly given, and it is decreased each day until an almost
infinitesimal dose is given, after which the saline solutions and
hypodermic injections should be stopped. In some patients
who are particularly intolerant to pain and discomfort, hyoscine may be used. Barbituric acid drugs fail to have a quieting
effect upon these individuals.

All classes of people are involved in chronic opium poisoning (which includes derivatives of opium). Eighty per cent are
of the underworld. Ninety thousand to one hundred thousand
addicts are in the United States. Drug addicts are found in
all races, all religions, and in all classes of society. There are
four males to one female addict in the white race. More negro
women are addicts than men. Addicts are more prevalent in
large cities. The youngest addict I have seen was eighteen
years of age, but they have been reported from fifteen years up.

Most of the cases of addiction I have seen did not come
from medical treatment, but rather from association with an
individual who was an addict and who wanted another person

to see "the soothing effect of an experiment," which was in reality the beginning of an addiction. Frequently, druggists and physicians become addicts because of the ease of access to the drug. The nervous, unstable person is more liable to contract the habit. The greatest aid in the prevention of this habit is to restrict the sales. Attempts along this line have been made, and an international agreement has been reached for limiting the world manufacture of narcotic drugs. Thirty-five countries have signed, thereby restricting the amount required for medicinal and scientific purposes. Institutions such as have been erected by the government at Lexington, Kentucky, and Fort Worth, Texas, represent a step in the right direction for the treatment of addiction.

Research should be encouraged to find drugs with a narcotic action, but non-habit forming. Through the activities of the National Research Council, Bureau of Social Hygiene, in cooperation with the Bureau of Narcotics, new chemical compounds are being prepared in the Cobb Chemical Laboratories, with the purpose of finding a combination with the phenanthrene ring which would give narcotic properties without addiction. Ninety such drugs have been studied at the University of Michigan, by Edmunds and Eddy.

Fatal Dose: The slight tolerance which develops in the addict, can be overstepped. I have seen addicts, accustomed to taking four grains at one dose, kill themselves by taking six grains. With the withdrawal of opium and its derivatives a toxine is said to be responsible for the symptoms. This, however, has not been proved. Two grains of morphine may be stated as the fatal dose for some people. I have seen several fatal cases of morphine poisoning in addicts, who had overstepped their dosage. Death may be caused by one grain or less in individuals who have an unusual susceptibility. Children are very susceptible to morphine poisoning, due to a lack or resistance in the respiratory nerve centers. Kobert states that morphine injected hypodermically exerts one to three times the amount of strength and rapidity as when taken by mouth.[1126] To lessen the tendency to nausea, small doses of atropine are combined with the morphine when given hypodermically. This, however, does not counteract the depression of respiration, which is a contra-indication for use of morphine.

1126. KOBERT: Lehrbuch der Intoxikationen, 970, 1906.

PHYSOSTIGMINE

THE ripe seed of physostigma venenosum (Calabar bean) yields not less than 0.12% of alkaloids. Common names for it are Calabar bean, chap nut, Eser's nut, and ordeal bean. The seeds occur oblong, somewhat reniform, 15 to 30 mm. long, 10 to 15 mm. thick. Externally they are reddish or chocolate brown, smooth, and somewhat roughened near the brownish black groove, which extends almost the entire length of the convex edge. The embryo is whitish. There is a bean-like odor. The taste at first is starchy, afterwards becoming acrid. The dose is 0.101 gm. (one and one-half grains).

Physostigmine Sulphas, $(C_{15}H_{21}N_3O_2)_2H_2SO_4$, occurs as a white, or yellowish-white, micro crystalline powder. It is odorless, and has a bitter taste. It is deliquescent, and turns reddish upon exposure to air and light. Physostigmine Sulphas has been deleted from the U. S. P., XI.

Physostigminae Salicylas, $C_{15}H_{21}O_2N_3.HC_7H_5O_3$, is the salicylate of an alkaloid obtained from the dried ripe seed of Physostigma venenosum Balfour. It is colorless, or faintly yellow, shining, odorless crystals. It acquires a red tint when long exposed to light and air. The dose is 0.002 gm. (one-thirtieth grain). One gm. is soluble in 75 cc. of water, in 16 cc. of alcohol in 6 cc. of chloroform, and in 250 cc. of ether, at 25° C. It is also called eserine salicylate.

Tests: 1. Neutral or only faintly acid to litmus paper. Physostigmine salicylate evaporated with a few drops of ammonia water gives a blue residue which, when dissolved in alcohol, gives a red fluorescent solution upon adding acetic acid. 2. Ferric chloride produces a deep violet color to an aqueous solution. 3. Chlorinated lime produces a red color to an aqueous solution. 4. Potassium hydroxide produces a cherry red color to an aqueous solution. 5. Platinic chloride produces no precipitate. (Distinction from the sulphate.)

6. Nitric acid produces the same colors as for sulphate.

Physostigmine, also known as eserine, is the poisonous alkaloid contained in Calabar bean. The drug is rarely used in medicine, but the sulphate and salicylate of the alkaloid are employed. Physostigmine crystallizes from a mixture of benzol and petrolic ether in prisms melting at 86 to 87°C. It is dimorphous, the modification melting at 105 to 106°C. Both modifications are levorotatory to the same degree, —75.8.

It is slightly soluble in water and petrolic ether, readily soluble in other organic solvents. Franco states that physostigmine or eserine poisoning is rare.[1127] It sometimes occurs as the result of a mistake, or by over-dosage, or from a hypersensitivity on the part of the patient. In a review of the literature he found only three reports of autopsies, and one of these had ingested Calabar beans, from which this poison is extracted. No report exists in the literature in which physostigmine is said to have been used for criminal purposes. However we possess a very rich literature concerning animal experiments with this substance. Franco reports two deaths: a man sixty-one years old and a woman thirty-two who died from taking a small quantity of physostigmine sulphate. Kubli reported a patient suffering from glaucoma who was given eight drops of eserine solution, which was followed by the symptoms of the poisoning, stertorous breathing, and cyanosis, lasting for about three-quarters of an hour.[1128]

Dullop reported a case of a woman who had a cataract in the left eye, and a considerable conjunctival irritation. She was given eserine. After the use of this substance she had an abundant lacrimation for about a quarter of an hour, with chronic spasms of the eyelids. After another quarter of an hour there was a spasmodic rigidity of the lips, and after some time she began also to show disturbance of memory. She made an uneventful recovery.[1129] Lodderstaedt reported a case of chorea.[1130] Leibholz reported two cases of physostigmine poisoning.[1131] Folli reported one case of eserine poisoning.[1132] Other cases have been observed by Speer.[1133] Kratter reported a fatal case of poisoning.[1134] Olsen in 1923,

1127. FRANCO, E. E.: Arch. d'anthrop. crim., 50:850, 1930.

1128. KUBLI: Zur Lehre von Glaukom-Monat. Bl. f. Ahkde, 8:421, 1880.

1129. DULLOP: Lancet, 26:621, 1887.

1130. LODDERSTAEDT: Berl. klin. Wchnschr., 17:336, 1888.

1131. LEIBHOLZ: Vrtljschr. f. gerichtl. Med., Berl., April, 1892; Bd. III, T. 2 S., 284.

1132. FOLLI, F.: Imola. Tip. Galenti, 6, 1896.

1133. SPEER, G. G.: Therap. Gaz., 27 and 20:443, 1904. And see HEUBNER, W.: Pharmakologische und chemisches ueber das Physostigmin, Arch. f. exper. Path. u. Pharmakol., 53:313, 1905.

1134. KRATTER: Eine Todliche Physostigminsvergiftung, Vrtljschr. f. gerichtl. Med. 3s. Suppl. Bd., 43:272, 1912. See also NEUREITER, E.: Eine Todische Physostigminevergiftung, Deutsche Ztschr. f. d. ges. gerichtl. Med., 518, 1922.

reported a case of physostigmine poisoning.[1135] Gernhardt, in 1927, observed four cases of this poisoning.[1136]

Symptoms: The condition of the pupil of the eye is of no significance in physostigmine poisoning.[1137] The physiological effects manifested themselves in five to twenty-five minutes after the injection, and there was a marked cutaneous hyperesthesia, vomiting, convulsions, and diarrhea, paralysis of the diaphragm, spasm of the glottis with transient dyspnea, increased salivation, sweating, slowing of the respiration, and lowering of the temperature. Death usually occurs by respiratory paralysis.[1138] Physostigmine has a central and peripheral action.[1139] Harnack, Witkowski, Schweder, Magnus, and Kress have proved that the central action is shown in the paralysis of the brain and cord, after stimulation; while the peripheral action is indicated in the stimulation of the striped musculature and the glands leading to over-secretion, excessive mucous secretion, and stimulation of peristalsis .

Fatal Quantity: Death has been reported after eating six of the beans. Although a number of cases of intoxication have been reported, the exact amount of the dose taken is not ascertained. Leibholz reported the death of two women who in an attempt to commit suicide, took one ampoule containing 0.1 gm. of Merck's physostigmine sulphate.[1140] On the basis of self-experimentation, Christison reports quite marked toxic effects from taking six grains of the seed followed on the next morning by a further dose of twelve grains.[1141]

Postmortem Appearances: The most frequently encountered morbid changes found in individuals dead from eserine poisoning are congestion—the blood is fluid, and always dark in color—glandular hypersecretion, hemorrhage, excitory action on gastro-intestinal tract, and pulmonary edema. The mucous membrane of tongue and the pharyngeal walls is

1135. OLSEN: *Ugesk. f. laeger.*, 19:85, 1923.

1136. GERNHARDT, A.: *Klin. Wchnschr.*, 30:320, July, 1927, S. 1433.

1137. FRANCO: see Ref. 1127.

1138. STRUBELL: *Wein. klin. Wchnschr.*, 1105, 1906.

1139. HARNACK and WITKOWSKI: *Arch. f. exper. Path. u. Pharmakol.*, 5:401, 1876. And see SCHWEDER: Dissert., Dorpat., 1889; MAGNUS: *Pflüger's Arch. f. d. ges. Physiol.*, 18:1, 1905; and KRESS: *Pflüger's Arch. f. d. ges. Physiol.*, 109:608, 1905.

1140. LEIBHOLZ: *Vrtljschr. f. gerichtl. Med.* (III) 3:284, 1892.

1141. CHRISTISON: *Pharm. J.*, 474, 1855; see also FRASER: *Edinburgh M. J.*: 9:36, 1864.

strongly swollen and dusky colored; the epithelium is desquamated in the upper portion of the trachea; lower down the tracheal epithelium is swollen. The stomach is strongly distended, with the mucous membrane markedly reddened and swollen and covered with a tenacious mucus feeling almost soap-like. There is subpleural ecchymosis, and marked narrowing of the large intestine.

Chemical Tests: The chemical detection is facilitated by the rapid passage of the substance into the body fluids—blood, urine, saliva and bile.

1. Most of the common alkaloidal reagents precipitate it, some only in concentrated solutions.

2. Gold chloride gives a purple brown precipitate, which turns brown and finally, after some time, turns red. This gold salt melts at 163 to 165° C.

3. Ammonia or alkalis give a pink color, due to the formation of the oxidation product rubreserine.

4. Another oxidation product is eserine blue. This is formed when an alcoholic solution is treated with barium hydroxide solution and shaken with about one-fourth the volume of air. The red color first obtained changes to green and then blue, becoming deeper as more air is added. This product is soluble in chloroform and is extracted from the chloroform with dilute hydrochloride acid.

5. Sulphuric acid gives a yellow color, turning to orange.

6. Nitric acid gives a blood red color, turning to green upon evaporation.

7. The addition of alcoholic potash produces a brownish-green solution which turns green upon adding acetic acid.

8. Hydrochloric acid gives a pink or reddish color.

9. Froehde's reagent gives a violet color, turning brown.

10. Hot ammonia gives a yellow-red, on evaporation a blue or blue-green residue, soluble in alcohol, which turns violet red and fluorescent with acetic acid. Bromine water, not in excess, gives an intense red color.

Biological Test: Myosis is produced in a cat's eye with as little as 0.005 to 0.01 gm.[1142] If the biological test on the cat's eye is found to be negative, physostigmine cannot be detected chemically. Or if the test on the cat's eye is negative owing to an extremely small quantity of alkaloid present, its

1142. FUHNER, H.: Berlin, Springer Bd., 92, H., 5-6 Bez. S. 346, 1918.

presence can be detected with a method which is based on the synergic action of physostigmine with acetyl choline. By means of this test quantities even as small as 0.0001 mg. can be detected by the contraction of muscles of leeches. The iris shows different reactions in each individual. There are in man and animals various degrees of hypersensitivity toward this drug.

Isolation from Tissue: This alkaloid is separated from the tissues by the general method of isolation. (See page 30.) It is extracted from the alkaline extract by ether or chloroform. If the alkaloid is present, the acid extract has a reddish-brown color, which in the alkaline solution becomes red. Physostigmine is distributed fairly well throughout all the organs; it is separated unchanged in the urine. Putrefactive products of organs developed after several months have little effect upon the extraction and identification of this alkaloid.

PILOCARPUS

THE leaflets of pilocarpus jaborandi Holmes or of pilocarpus microphyllus Stapf yield not less than 0.5% .of alkaloids. Pilocarpine nitrate is an official preparation of the U. S. P., XI.

Pilocarpinae Hydrochloridum, $C_{11}H_{16}O_2N_2.HCl$, occurs colorless, odorless, faintly bitter in taste, hygroscopic. It is soluble in 0.3 parts of water, 0.3 parts of alcohol, 366 parts of chloroform; insoluble in ether. It melts between 195 and 198° C. It is slightly acid to litmus paper.

Pilocarpina Nitras, $C_{11}H_{16}O_2N_2HNO_3$, occurs as shining, colorless crystals. It is stable in the air. One gram of pilocarpine nitrate is soluble in 4 cc. of water and in 75 cc. of alcohol, at 25° C. One gram is soluble in 21 cc. of alcohol at 60° C. It is insoluble in chloroform or in ether. The average dose is 0.005 gm., or one-twelfth grain.

Tests: 1. Sulphuric acid plus a crystal of potassium dichromate gives a bright grass green color.

2. Dissolve 0.02 gm. of the hydrochloride in 2 cc. of water, add 2 cc. of a faintly acid hydrogen dioxide solution, and cover with about 1 cc. of benzene. Add three or four drops of a solution of potassium dichromate (one to 300) and shake gently. The benzene layer becomes a violet color, while the aqueous remains yellow. This test is distinctive, no other

alkaloid giving the same colors. Do not use more than 0.02 gm. of the salt or the color will not be characteristic, instead it will turn to the blue. The dose is 0.005 gm., or one-twelfth grain. The alkaloids occurring in the various species of pilocarpus are pilocarpine, $C_{11}H_{16}N_2O_2$, isopilocarpine, $C_{11}H_{16}N_2O_2$, a stereoisomer, pilocarpidine, $C_{10}H_{14}N_2O_2$, jaborine, $C_{11}H_{16}N_2O_2$.

Pilocarpine is the only alkaloid of pilocarpus used medicinally. When pure it is crystalline, but it is usually seen as an oily syrup, as it is very hygroscopic. It is soluble in water, caustic alkalis, alcohol, chloroform, benzene, but less so in ether. Its solution is dextrorotatory (a) $D = 100.5°$.

3. Mayer's reagent and iodine cause a precipitate. The reagents used for color reactions with other alkaloids give no specific colors with pilocarpine.

4. Helch's test is applied to an aqueous solution of the hydrochloride as follows, and is specific: To the aqueous solution, add 2 cc. of an acid solution of hydrogen peroxide, 2 cc. of benzene, and a few drops of potassium dichromate (0.3%). If pilocarpine is present, the benzene layer upon shaking becomes purple to blue. Pyridine and quinoline give a violet color, which soon fades. Apomorphine gives a violet, changing to green on separating the benzene, and upon adding dilute stannous chloride. Antipyrin gives a blue color, distinguished from that of pilocarpine by shaking the benzene layer with water containing a trace of hydrochloric acid, and treating this acid layer as before with peroxide, dichromate, and benzene, when the color will return, which is not the case with pilocarpine.

5. Bromine at high temperatures forms bromcarpinic acid, $C_{10}H_{15}N_2O_4$, melting at 209° C.

Isolation from Tissues: Pilocarpine is separated by the general methods for alkaloids (see page 30) from weak ammoniacal solutions with chloroform, but not from caustic alkali solutions.

Symptoms: Poisoning causes a marked secretion of saliva, excessive perspiration and tears, nausea, retching, and vomiting, pain in the abdomen, violent movement of the intestines, with profuse watery evacuation. The pulse is sometimes quickened, sometimes slow and irregular. The pupils are contracted. The respiration is quick and dyspnoeic, with rales over the bronchi. There are giddiness and confusion, with sometimes tremors and feeble convulsions. Eventually slower respiration and weakness occur, but consciousness remains until breathing ceases. The action of pilocarpine on the sweat glands renders it the most powerful sudorific in the pharmacopeia. It is used to remove excess fluid accumulations in the body.

Death very rarely results from the use of pilocarpine. When it does occur, it is by paralysis of the heart or edema of the lungs.

Treatment: In addition to the general treatment for alkaloidal poisoning, is the physiological antidote atropine.

QUININE

QUININE, $(C_{20}H_{24}O_2N_2.3H_2O$, has a molecular weight of 378.25 (U. S. P., XI). It is an alkaloid obtained from cinchona. A white, micro-crystalline powder, quinine is odorless, and has a bitter taste, which is intense and persistent. It is efflorescent in dry air. One gram of quinine is soluble in 1560 cc. of water, in 0.8 cc. of alcohol, in 1.1 cc. of chloroform, in 1 cc. of ether, and in 1890 cc. of ammonia water, at 25° C. A solution of quinine in dilute sulphuric acid shows a vivid blue fluorescence. Add two or three drops of bromine test solution to 5 cc. of a saturated, aqueous solution of quinine, and follow with 1 cc. of ammonia test solution. The liquid acquires an emerald-green color, due to the formation of thalleioquin.

Quinine is used extensively in large doses as a routine in the treatment of malaria, as a general protoplasmic poison. It is toxic to all cells, and even to unorganized ferments; but it has an especially high toxicity for ameboid cells, and is relatively non-toxic for higher organisms. It exerts a very selective action on the malarial parasites and is, therefore, a specific against malarial disease, provided sufficiently large doses are administered.

I have never seen a death due to this alkaloid, although cases of poisoning have been reported. Dawson and Garbade[1143] report cases of idiosyncrasy due to quinine, cinchonidine, ethyl hydrocupreine, and others of the cinchona series. These authors say many people have taken quinine for some time, later developing a sensitiveness to it. Hemoglobinuria may be produced with quinine in idiosyncrasy, and also with cinchonine.

1143. DAWSON, W. T., and GARBADE, F. A.: *J. Pharmacol. & Exper. Therap.*, 39:417, 1930.

Willimot reported a fatal case of quinine poisoning.[1144] Raven reported a fatal case of poisoning after taking forty-eight five-grain doses (total 240 grains) of quinine sulphate.[1145] Husemann reported two grains fatal to a typhus convalescent patient. Starkenstein considers the average fatal dose to be 10 to 12 gm., but cases taking 12, 15, and 20 gm. have recovered.[1146] Willimot reported a two and one-half year old girl taking 130 gr., dying in three and one-half hours. He reported another child five years old taking 25 gm., recovering in four hours. Both had pain in the stomach, and nausea. The elder child recovered after an emetic. The younger child began vomiting and purging, and later had convulsions. The child, when seen by a physician in the hospital, was in a state of asphyxia. The skin was cyanotic, and there was frothing at the mouth and nostrils, and hypothermia, with pulse and respiration almost imperceptible. At autopsy, there was marked lividity, the eyes were prominent, tongue protruding, viscera congested, blood nearly black. There were petechiae in the heart, suprarenals, kidneys, and stomach. Quinine was found in the stomach contents. There were traces in the liver, but in no other organs was any found.

Burgess and Usher reported ten cases where quinine idiosyncrasy was present from the use of alcoholic tonsorial lotions.[1147] These lotions contained quinine. Beer reported the case of a woman thirty years of age, who drank one-half glass of quinine solution (about 15 gm. of quinine).[1148] Within a short time she became unconscious, and for twenty-four hours she lost the ability to speak and was not able to move. After twenty-four hours, consciousness returned and she noticed that she was blind. Twenty-four hours later she was able to distinguish her fingers before her eyes. Four days later an examination showed widely dilated pupils which did not react to light and accommodation, or at least sluggishly so, nystagmus, ptosis, and clonic spasms of the eyelids. When examined with the ophthalmoscope the papilla of the optic nerve was pale and atrophic. The arteries were thready, and the veins more or less narrow, rarely dilated. The retina usually shows thready

1144. WILLIMOT, S. G.: *Lancet*, 2:1133, 1931.
1145. RAVEN: *Brit. M. J.*, 2:59, 1927.
1146. STARKENSTEIN: ROST-POLIL: Toxikologie, Berlin, 433, 1929.
1147. BURGESS, J. F., and USHER, B.: *Canad. M. A. J.*, 23:45, 1930.
1148. BEER, LEON: *Ztschr. f. Augenh., Berl.*, 74:50, 1931.

arteries and narrow veins. As a whole the retina is ischemic. Vision usually returns in these cases in from twenty-four to forty-eight hours and gradually improves, but it must be remembered that the condition may last for months before any improvement can be noticed. Since quinine is used extensively in hair tonics the ophthalmologist would do well to question some of his male patients regarding the use of such tonics. The manner in which quinine acts on the eye is not clear. Chorades is of the opinion that quinine causes a constriction of the end arteries.[1149] As the result of the constriction of these arteries degenerative changes of the retina are apt to occur, with a resulting atrophy of the optic nerve. As time goes on, central vision is restored.

Quinine stimulates contraction and increases the tone of the uterus. It is used by the obstetrician in doses from 15 to 20 grains in labor to intensify weak contractions. In larger doses it has been used as an abortifacient.

Suicides with quinine in Bulgaria have been reported to be on the increase.[1150] In the last four years they constitute one-third of all other cases of suicide. Out of 166 cases of poisoning observed by the above author in the clinic during the last ten years, there are eighty-six cases of quinine poisoning, eighty-two of these occurring within the last seven years, against fifty-one suicides with other poisons. Lavier reported five patients receiving 16 gm. of quinine by mistake.[1151] Reactions were all identical. They collapsed, the pulse was small, and the cardiac action became weaker. One of the patients died after about ten minutes. Two other patients had a period of chronic spasms followed by tonic convulsions, with opisthotonos. Two other patients also collapsed, but they vomited quite profusely and evacuated in this manner a good portion of the ingested poison. For about ten minutes they had clonic spasms, which were followed by a tonic stage. They remained in a comatose state for about forty hours, with a temperature of about 36° C., with a small pulse and a weak heart action. Treatment consisted in administration of caffeine and camphorated oil. As these two

1149. CHORADES: Zur Frage des Chininamblyopie, *Dnepro-Petrowskij med. zur.*, *Jg.* 5 Mr. 7-8, 1926 (Ref. in *Zentralbl. f. d. ges. Ophth., Berl.*).

1150. *Arch. f. Schiffs-u. Tropen-Hyg.*, 38:288, 1934; MINKO DOBREFF: Statistics on Premedicated Quinine; Self-Poisonings in Bulgaria.

1151. LAVIER, PAR. G.: *Bull. Sac. path. exot.*, 24:184, 1931.

patients improved, they both complained of extreme weakness, which disappeared in eight days. One of the patients had an attack of quinine amblyopia, which subsided completely after about one month. The fifth patient recovered relatively quickly. At autopsy on the one who died in ten minutes, there was marked congestion of the lungs and hyperemia of both kidneys.

Leschke[1152] described a case of quinine poisoning reported by Goldmann: "A man, twenty, took 19 gm. of quinine sulphate in solution as a means of committing suicide. The symptoms consisted in loss of consciousness and damage to the kidneys. The blood sugar was 56 mg. per cent. The axillary temperature was 36.4° C. The consciousness returned as a result of camphor and strychnine injections. The power of hearing was restored, although there were still severe drumming noises in the ears. There was, however, complete blindness. Later the sight was regained, except that a concentric limitation of the field of vision was still present some months later.

Quininae Dihydrochloridum, $C_{20}H_{24}N_2O_2.2HCl$, is a white powder, odorless, very bitter tasting alkaloid. One gram is soluble in 0.6 cc. of water and in 12 cc. of alcohol, at 25° C. It is slightly soluble in chloroform, and very slightly soluble in ether. An aqueous solution is strongly acid to litmus paper, and has a blue fluorescence.

Quininae Hydrochloridum, $C_{20}H_{24}O_2N_2HCl.2H_2O$, has been deleted from the eleventh revision of the U. S. P.

Quininae et Urae Hydrochloridum, $C_{20}H_{24}O_2N_2.HCl.CO-(NH_2)_2.HCl.5H_2O$, occurs as colorless, translucent prisms, white granules, or a white powder. It is odorless, and has a very bitter taste. One gram is soluble in 0.9 cc. of water, and in 2.4 cc. of alcohol, at 25°C. The dose, hypodermic, is 1 gm. (fifteen grains).

Quininae Aethylcarbonas, $C_{23}H_{28}O_4N_2$, occurs as white, fine, soft needles, usually matted together in fleecy masses. It is odorless, and practically tasteless. It darkens on exposure to light. It is slightly soluble in water, 1 gm. is soluble in 2 cc. of alcohol, in 1 cc. of chloroform, and in about 10 cc. of ether, at 25° C. It is readily soluble in dilute acids. It melts at 89° to 91°C.

Quinina Sulphas, $(C_{20}H_{24}O_2N_2)_2.H_2SO_4.2H_2O$, is the sulphate of an alkaloid obtained from cinchona. Quinina sulphas

1152. LESCHKE, ERICH: Clinical Toxicology, 191, 1934.

occurs as fine, needlelike, white crystals, frequently cohering in masses. The salt is odorless, has a very bitter taste, and darkens on exposure to light. One gram is soluble in about 90 cc. of water, and in 10 cc. of alcohol, at 25° C. One gram is soluble in about 15 cc. of boiling water. It is soluble in chloroform, but almost insoluble in ether. Dose, 1 gm. (fifteen grains).

Quininae Bisulphas, $C_{20}H_{24}O_2N_2.H_2SO_4.7H_2O$, occurs as white or colorless crystals, usually needle-like, or a white crystalline powder. It is odorless, and has a very bitter taste. It effloresces on exposure to dry air, and turns yellow on exposure to light. One gram of quinine bisulphas is soluble in 9 cc. of water, in 23 cc. of alcohol, in 15 cc. of glycerine, in 625 cc. of chloroform, and in 2500 cc. of ether at 25° C.

Quininae Hydrobromidum, $C_{20}H_{24}O_2N_2HBr.H_2O$, and Quininae Tannas, have been deleted from the eleventh revision of the U. S. P.

Quinidine Sulfate of the U. S. P., XI, is the sulfate of an alkaloid obtained from cinchona. It occurs as fine, needle-like white crystals, frequently cohering in masses. The salt is odorless, has a very bitter taste, and darkens on exposure to light. One gm. of quinidine sulfate is soluble in about 90 cc. of water, and in 10 cc. of alcohol, at 25°C. One gm. is soluble in about 15 cc. of boiling water. It is soluble in chloroform, but almost insoluble in ether. The dose is 0.2 gm. (three grains).

CINCHONA

CINCHONA (Peruvian bark) is the dried bark of cinchona succiruba Pavon et Klotzsch, or its hybrids, known in commerce as red cinchona, or of cinchona ledgeriana Moens et Trimen, cinchona calisaya Weddell, or hybrids of these, with other species of cinchona, known in commerce as calisaya bark or as yellow cinchona, yielding not less than 5% of alkaloids. It occurs in quills or chips, curved, or in broken fragments. The bark from 2 to 9 mm. in thickness, externally brown or reddish brown. The outer bark may be absent, the color externally is then cinnamon brown. The odor is slightly aromatic, the taste is bitter and somewhat astringent.

The various species of cinchona contain over thirty alkaloids. The better known of these, and those used for therapeutic purposes, are quinine, quinidine, cinchonine, and cupreine. The others are said to resemble these in their effects on the system, although very little is known regarding them. These alkaloids are derivatives of quinoline. Quinine and quinidine are isomeric, $C_{20}H_{24}N_2O_2$. Cinchonine and cinchonidine are isomeric, $C_{19}H_{22}N_2O$. Quinine and cinchonidine are levorotatory; quinidine and cinchonine are dextrorotatory. Cinchona bark contains several acids, as tannic, quinic, caffeic, and oxalic, and other neutral bodies, as quinovine, quinovic red, cinchol, cholesterol, etc. Cinchona and its alkaloids probably enter into more combinations and have a wider field of application, than any other drugs used in medicine. They are prepared as pills, tablets, extracts, elixirs, wines, syrups, capsules, and bitters.

Tests: 1. Dissolved in sulphuric, tartaric or acetic acids cinchona gives a blue fluorescence. Cinchona alkaloids also give this color.

2. Thalleioquin test: If to 1 cc. of an aqueous solution of quinine (one to 100) containing just sufficient sulphuric acid to effect a complete solution, there be added 2 cc. of bromine test solution, followed by 1 cc. of ammonia water, the liquid should acquire an emerald green color. LaWall modified the thalleioquin test; with his modification he claims to detect one in 200,-000 of quinine.[1153] To 100 cc. of quinine sulphate solution (one to 200,000) in a Nessler tube, are added five drops of potassium bromate solution (0.5 gm. potassium bromate, 10 cc. hydrobromic acid, 10%, and 90 cc. water) well mixed; and this, treated with ten drops of stronger ammonia water, produces a green tint, with the cinchona alkaloids responding to the thalleioquin test. This can also be modified as a confirmatory test, by following the bromine water with a few drops of potassium ferro or ferricyanide solution and then ammonia water, which gives a red color, instead of green. This color can then be extracted with chloroform. This test is extremely delicate, and characteristic for cinchona alkaloids, but must be very carefully applied if only small amounts are available. The thalleioquin test is also given by quinidine, cupreine, hydroquinine, hydroquinidine, and diquinicine, but not by cinchonine, cinchonidine, or quinamine. Morphine, caffeine, or antipyrine, in certain proportions, interfere with this test, but cocaine, codeine, atropine, and strychnine do not. The quinine extract should be as pure as possible before the test is applied.

1153. LaWall: *Am. J. Pharm.*, 84:484. 1912.

3. Dissolve in a mixture of acetic acid and alcohol (fifteen to six), add 0.5 cc. sulphuric acid and heat to boiling, then add 7 cc. of a saturated solution of iodine in alcohol slowly. Bronze or olive green crystals of quinine iodo-sulphate will separate on cooling. These crystals are insoluble in cold water.

4. Dissolve in 1 cc. of dilute sulphuric acid and dilute with water to 20 cc., neutralize with ammonia water, add one drop hydrogen dioxide and one drop of copper sulphate solution, and boil. An intense red color develops, which slowly changes to blue and finally green. (Quinidine also gives this test.)

5. One gram of quinine should dissolve completely in a slightly warmed mixture of absolute alcohol and ether (six to three), and the solution should remain clear on cooling (absence of cinchonine and cinchonidine).

6. Potassium iodide does not give a precipitate with quinine. This distinguishes quinine from quinidine and cinchonidine, but not from cinchonine. Potassium ferrocyanide gives a reddish-brown color, but no precipitate. (With quinidine a white flocculent precipitate, with cinchonine and cinchonidine, a white precipitate, soluble in excess.)

7. Mercuric chloride gives no precipitate with dilute quinine solutions, but gives an immediate precipitate with cinchonine, cinchonidine, and quinidine. All the general alkaloidal reagents precipitate quinine. Phosphotungstic acid gives a pink fluorescence. The picrate, which melts at 125 to 126° C., should always be prepared in the identification of quinine.

Symptoms: Cinchona owes its effect on the body almost entirely to its quinine content. The bark, however, is more of a gastric irritant than quinine, and is also a decided astringent. Large doses have caused febrile paroxysms, beginning with a chill, and terminating with slight perspiration.

Externally quinine has no influence upon sound skin, but it is distinctly irritant to mucous membranes and raw surfaces. Internally, in doses of ten grains or more, quinine causes a sense of fullness in the head, tinnitus aurium, slight deafness, disorders of vision, and sometimes blindness. The physiological effects differ greatly in different individuals, and various idiosyncrasies regarding its influence have frequently been noted. Workers in cinchona bark have developed a peculiar rash. Occasionally it is the cause of cutaneous eruptions, such as erythema, urticaria, herpes, purpura, and even gangrenous affections. The effects upon the eye have been described.

The tincture and fluid extractum are no longer official in the U. S. P. The tincture cinchonae compositas is made from the percolation and extraction of 100 gm. of cinchona powder, 20 gm. of serpentaria, and 80 gm. of orange peel per 1000 cc.

SCOPARIUS

SCOPARIUS is found in the dried tops of cytisus scoparius (broom plants). It occurs as thin, flexible, branched twigs, 2 to 3 mm.thick, externally dark green, with five wings and numerous reddish-brown cork patches. Internally it is yellowish. It has a peculiar odor and a bitter taste. The dose is 1 gm. (fifteen grains). This drug contains a resinous substance called scoparin, and the alkaloid sparteine, $C_{15}H_{26}N_2$.

Sparteine Sulphas, $C_{15}H_{26}N_2H_2SO_4.5H_2O$, occurs as colorless, rhombohedral crystals, or as a crystalline powder. It is odorless, slightly saline and somewhat bitter in taste. It is acid to litmus paper and hygroscopic. It is soluble in 1.1 parts of water, and in 2.4 parts of alcohol; insoluble in chloroform and ether.

Sparteine, $C_{15}H_{26}N_2$, has been used to slow the pulse in cardiac disturbances, but its reactions are uncertain, and the drug has fallen largely into disuse. It weakens the heart and cannot take the place of digitalis. Sparteine is not official in the U. S. P., XI. Pure sparteine is a colorless, oily liquid, heavier than water, and forms crystalline salts resembling aniline. It has a very bitter taste. Sparteine darkens and thickens upon exposure to air. It is soluble in alcohol, ether, chloroform, petrolic ether, slightly soluble in water, and insoluble in benzol. When pure it boils at about 320° C.

Tests: 1. Mineral acids give no color. Sparteine is volatile with steam. It is precipitated by the general alkaloidal reagents (see page 30). The platinochloride melts at 244° to 257° C., with decomposition; the gold chloride at 175° to 180° C., with decomposition; and the picrate at 178° to 180° C.

2. Ferric chloride and potassium thiocyanate, when dried, give a violet to reddish color.

3. An ether solution of sparteine gives a black periodide precipitate. This precipitate, if dissolved in boiling alcohol, on cooling separates out in green needles.

4. Ammonium sulphydrate gives an orange-red color.

5. Dry sulphur added to an ether solution of sparteine gives a bright red precipitate when hydrogen sulphide is added. (Coniine gives an orange turbidity.)

Isolation from Tissue: Sparteine is separated from tissue by steam distillation into an acid solution. It is shaken out of the ammoniacal solution with petrolic ether. For quantitative determination the ether extract is evaporated, and the residue dissolved in dilute hydrochloric acid and precipitated by 10% silicotungstic acid or its potassium salt. The precipitate is dried and weighed. Its composition is $SiO_2.12WO_3.2H_2O.2C_{15}H_{26}N_2 7H_2O$.

Symptoms: The general effects of sparteine are almost identical with those of coniine, but it is much less poisonous. It causes death by paralysis of the terminations of the phrenic nerves in the diaphragm. Poisonous doses cause trembling, incoordination, increase of the reflexes, clonic and tonic convulsions, followed by enfeeblement of all the functions, paralysis, and death from asphyxia.

STRYCHNINE AND NUX VOMICA

NUX VOMICA is the dried ripe seed of strychnos nux-vomica Linne, and yields not less than 2.5% of alkaloids, of which shall be not less than 1.15% of strychnine. The seed is orbicular, nearly flat, occasionally somewhat bent, from 10 to 30 mm. in diameter, and from 3 to 5 mm. in thickness; externally grayish or greenish-gray, covered with appressed hairs, giving it a silky luster; very hard when dry. Internally it shows a thin and hairy seed coat and a large grayish white endosperm at one end on which is embedded a small embryo with two broadly ovate, five- to seven-nerved cotyledons. It is inodorous, and its taste is intensely and persistently bitter. The preparations recognized by the U. S. P., XI, are the extract and the tincture. Powdered nux vomica is light gray in color, and very bitter in taste. The dose is 0.1 gm. (one and a half grains).

The powdered extract yields not less than 7 gm. and not more than 7.75 gm. of strychnine. The dose is 0.015 gm. (one-quarter grain).

The tincture for each 100 cc. yields not less than 0.018 gm. and not more than 0.120 gm. of strychnine. The dose is 1 cc. (fifteen minims).

Strychninae Nitras, $C_{21}H_{22}O_2N_2.HNO_3$, is the nitrate of an alkaloid obtained chiefly from nux vomica. It occurs as colorless, glistening needles, or a white, crystalline powder. It is odorless and stable in the air. One gram of strychnine nitrate is soluble in 45 cc. of water, in 150 cc. of alcohol, in 50 cc. of glycerine, and in 105 cc. of chloroform, at 25°C. It is insoluble in ether. It is levorotatory. The dose is 0.002 gm. (one-thirtieth grain).

Strychninae Sulphas, $(C_{21}H_{22}O_2N_2).H_2SO_4.5H_9O$, is the sulphate of an alkaloid obtained chiefly from nux vomica. It occurs as colorless or white crystals, or a white, crystalline powder. It is odorless, and is efflorescent in dry air. One gram of strychnine sulphate is soluble in 35 cc. of water, in 81 cc. of alcohol, and in 220 cc. of chloroform, at 25° C. It is freely soluble in glycerine, but insoluble in ether. The dose is 0.002 gm. (one-thirtieth grain).

There have been separated from nux vomica about nine alkaloids—strychnine, brucine, strychnicine, curine, curarine, tubocurarine, protocurine, protocuridine, and protocurarine—but the only two of therapeutic and toxicological value are strychnine and brucine.

Strychnine is the most important of the alkaloids of the strychnos group, both therapeutically and toxicologically. It was discovered by Pelletier and Caventou in 1818.[1154] In seventy-eight cases of strychnine poisoning investigated by me from 1912 to 1936, thirty-three were accidental, four were homicides, and forty-one were suicides. In 1936 only two suicides by strychnine were reported by the Coroner of Cook County. Strychnine is a monacid, tertiary base combining with one equivalent of acid to form salts. Its chemical formula is $C_{21}H_{22}N_2O_2$. It is distinguished as an alkaloid of very stable composition, resisting various ordinary decomposing influences further than most organic compounds, while still capable of very decisive chemical reactions. It is the only alkaloid that we can subject to strong sulphuric acid during the process of purification and still obtain characteristic reactions. It occurs in colorless, transparent, prismatic crystals (of the rhombic system), or as a white crystalline powder; odorless, permanent in the air. Samples kept in bark-stoppered bottles do not

1154. PELLETIER and CAVENTOU: *Am. de chim. et phys., Par.*, 2 s., 26: 44, 1924.

undergo a change in weight after twenty years. It is very intensely and persistently bitter in taste, the bitterness being manifest in extremely dilute solutions. However, some persons are unable to distinguish dilute solutions of one to 10,000. I have two or three students in my Materia Medica class every year who are unable to distinguish dilute solutions of both strychnine and quinine. One gram of strychnine dissolves in 6420 cc. of water, 136 cc. of alcohol, 5 cc. of chloroform, and in 180 cc. of benzene at 25° C. (77° F.); also in 3100 cc. of boiling water ,and in 34 cc. of boiling alcohol; it is very slightly soluble in ether. It crystallizes from benzene in octahedral crystals. Well formed crystals may be obtained by the gradual addition of water to the alcoholic solution, a fact of importance in the identification of this alkaloid in toxicological examinations. Its saturated solutions are alkaline to litmus and are levorotatory. Its melting point when heated in small amounts is 268° C. (514.4° F.) according to Lobisch and Schoop and confirmed later by Vanderkleed,[1155] although Stoehr and, later, Beckurts state this to be 265 to 266° C. (509 to 510° F.). It is precipitated from solutions of its salts by the general alkaloidal reagents (page 30), picrolonic acid being especially valuable as a purifying reagent. It is precipitated by the fixed alkali hydroxides and carbonates, and is not readily soluble in excess of these reagents, although ammonia undoubtedly dissolves the precipitate when in excess to a more or less extent.

Tests: 1. A solution of strychnine salt is precipitated by the general alkaloidal reagents and by fixed alkali hydroxides and carbonates, in which it is readily soluble in excess, although ammonia dissolves it to a less extent when in excess.

2. The bitter taste of strychnine is more intense than that of any other known substance. It can be detected in a solution of one to 600,000 to 700,000.

3. Sulphuric acid gives no color.

4. Froehde's reagent gives no color.

5. Erdmann's reagent gives no color.

6. Nitric acid gives a yellow color.

7. The Fading Purple test is very sensitive and characteristic, and important as a means of identifying strychnine. The

---

1155. Lobisch and Schoop: *Monatschr. f. Chem.*, 9:858, 1888; Vanderkleed: Allen's Commercial Organic Analysis, 6:442, 1912.

alkaloid is dissolved in sulphuric acid and treated in the cold with an oxidizing agent, which gives an evanescent play of various bright colors. The test in detail is carried out as follows: The crystals, or the residue evaporated from the chloroform extract on a white porcelain plate, is dissolved in a few drops of sulphuric acid. A small crystal of potassium dichromate is slowly drawn through this liquid with a thin glass rod. The changes in colors are a momentary deep blue, changing to deep violet, then to purplish-red, cherry red, and finally to orange or yellow. These colors are more or less fleeting, depending upon the amount of alkaloid present. In the presence of small amounts this play of colors may be so rapid that the bluish tint disappears immediately while with large amounts it may persist for quite some time before fading. Other oxidizing agents have been employed, such as manganese dioxide, cerosoceric oxide, ammonium vanadate, and potassium ferricyanide, but potassium dichromate is used to a greater extent, and gives very satisfactory results. A distinctive reaction can be obtained with 1/27027 grain (0.0000025 gm.) of strychnine. When the quantity is very small it is advisable to dissolve the oxidizing agent in the acid before adding to the unknown, as in Mandelin's reagent the ammonium vanadate (1%) is dissolved in concentrated sulphuric acid. This reaction, while very characteristic of strychnine, is also given by other drugs which are extracted from alkaline solutions under the same conditions. Yet there might be differences in the reactions to show that the product is not strychnine. There would always be a doubt, unless substantiated by other tests.

Poe and O'Day[1156] recommend that the reagent be prepared by dissolving one part of finely ground ammonium vanadate in 200 parts cold C. P. concentrated sulphuric acid. This reagent gives a violet-blue to orange-red color, finally changing to yellow. These authors tested over 500 different alkaloids in this manner. Brucine gave an orange-yellow color, codeine a yellow to caramel, apomorphine a gray-black to brown-black color, morphine gave the same as apomorphine. Gelsemium, hydrastis, opium, sanguinaria, and yohimbine give a purple color with sulphuric acid and dichromate. The similarity of the color reactions of strychnine and yohimbine is to be noted, as

1156. POE, CHARLES F., and O'DAY, DAVID W.: *J. Am. Pharm. Ass.*, 19:1292, 1930.

both drugs are used for the same purposes. Some glucosides and other principals produce colors, but they are removed by the acid immiscible solvents. Substances completely covering up the strychnine test when present in equal amounts are: aspirin, salicylic acid, b-naphthol, and pyrogallic acid. Substances completely covering up strychnine tests when present in five times the amount of strychnine are apomorphine, colchicine, tryptophane, aspirin, salicylic acid, and tannic acid.

The fading purple test is interfered with by the presence of much morphine or brucine. To remove brucine, dissolve in about 2 cc. dilute sulphuric acid, add 2 cc. nitric acid, and let stand a few hours. Make alkaline with excess of sodium hydroxide solution and extract with ether. The ether extracts the brucine and leaves the strychnine in the solution, which can then be extracted with chloroform. Another procedure is to dissolve the residue in sulphuric acid and add a trace of nitric acid. Brucine gives a red color changing to yellow. Then add a crystal of potassium dichromate, which when stirred in will turn blue or reddish-violet in the presence of strychnine. Gelsemine gives a reddish-purple to cherry red, without the initial blue or blue-violet. Geissospermine shows a reaction with this test similar to that of strychnine, but it is colored purple with nitric acid, strychnine showing no color. Cod-liver oil when pure produces a display of colors from purple to crimson to brown. Colocynth resin gives a very similar color test, but can be removed by acid ether.

8. Evaporated with nitric acid, strychnine gives a yellow color to the residue, which turns purple upon the addition of alcoholic potash. (Similar to atropine, colchicum, yohimbine.)

9. Deniges' test: To prepare the zinc amalgam used in this test, treat granular zinc with some concentrated hydrochloric acid to clear the surface. Pour off the acid and cover the zinc with tartar emetic solution (1%), shaking for one hour, when 1 cc. of a saturated solution of mercuric chloride is added for each gram of zinc. Add a few drops of hydrochloric acid. Let stand one-half hour and pour off the liquid. The zinc is washed and dried. To make the test add about one gram of this zinc amalgam to the dry alkaloid, or its solution, followed by 0.5 cc. hydrochloric acid. Stand for about twenty minutes and pour off the liquid, to which add a few drops of potassium ferrocyanide solution (0.02%), when a pink rose

red color is produced. The test is useless if the residue is impure.

10. Malaquin's test: One cc. of a solution of the strychnine salt (one to 1000) is mixed with 2 cc. of hydrochloric acid and one gram of granulated zinc. After a few minutes it is heated quickly to boiling, cooled, and carefully poured over 2 cc. of sulphuric acid so as to form a separate layer in the test tube. A rose-red ring will form at the junction of the two layers if strychnine is present, and upon standing the entire solution becomes red. On heating the color is not changed, but it is rendered colorless by potassium sulphocyanate, ammonia, or sodium hydrogen sulphate in excess. According to Malaquin the only other known alkaloid which gives this reaction is veratrine, but this is differentiated by the fact that when the mixture of sulphuric acid and the treated alkaloids are boiled this is changed to a dirty yellow with veratrine. This test is very characteristic and will detect one part in 1,000,000.

11. Crystal test: A few drops of the chloroform extract are evaporated on a glass slide, and dissolved in a drop of dilute acetic acid, and the excess acid evaporated. To this add a drop of potassium dichromate solution, and then stir with a narrow glass rod, and allow to crystallize. The crystals under the microscope are found to be octahedral and dendroidal in form. The octahedral crystals are distinctive, as the dichromate itself will form dendroidal crystals.

12. Nitric acid and potassium chlorate, after warming, give an intense scarlet color. Upon adding ammonia this turns brown, and, upon evaporation to dryness, a dark green, which turns orange brown with potassium hydroxide, and green again with nitric acid.

13. Moisten the dry substance with a solution of zinc chloride (one to thirty) and evaporate to dryness. A scarlet color is produced. (Veratrine also gives red and delphinine a red brown. Brucine prevents the formation of the scarlet color, and a dirty yellow develops.)

The Biologic Test: A very slightly acidulated aqueous solution of the purified extract is given to a small frog, either hypodermically into the lymph sac immediately beneath the skin of the back at the root of the hind leg, or by blowing into the stomach through a small tube. The time is noted and the frog is observed. A period of uneasiness with accelerated respiration precedes the tetanic spasms. The paroxysms at first have remissions, and their return is hastened by agitation or vibration, as by striking upon the table. Wormley obtained with frogs weighing 15 to 50 grains distinct symptoms in from ten to thirty minutes with 1/5000 grain of strychnine; with 1/500 grain in three to four minutes, and death in from fifteen to thirty minutes. Kobert mentions one-thirtieth grain as a fatal dose for frogs. Very small doses of morphine with young white mice frequently cause convulsions similar to the action of strychnine.

Symptoms: The time of appearance of the symptoms will depend upon the manner of introduction and upon the individual differences. If taken by mouth, the time of action will be controlled by the condition of the stomach, whether empty or full, and the nature of the food present. If administered by subcutaneous injection, the place of administration will affect the promptness of its action. Strychnine will act more quickly than preparations of nux vomica. The symptoms never appear sooner than fifteen minutes and are not generally delayed beyond a half hour. The first symptoms are a feeling of uneasiness with a heightened reflex irritability, followed by muscular twitching in some parts of the body. With larger doses this is followed by a sense of impending suffocation, and convulsive movements begin which have the effect of mechanically causing the patient to cry out or to shriek. Then follow the characteristic spasms, which set in with great violence. These are at first clonic, and then tonic. Opisthotonos results from the extensor muscles overcoming the flexors, the feet being curved inwards. The spasms again become clonic, with intermissions and repetitions. With each successive attack the symptoms become more violent, the patient resting on his head and feet, the remainder of his body arched above the bed. The eyes are staring, the face livid, the chest and abdomen stiff as board. The pulse is very rapid, and the sense of touch, sight, and hearing are abnormally acute. The respiration at first is labored and dyspnoeic, and then is temporarily arrested by the spasmodic contraction of the diaphragm. The patient is entirely conscious and usually suffers excruciating pain. Foaming at the mouth may occur from the interference with respiration, and the asphyxia resulting from the latter induces cyanosis, dilatation of the pupils, and eventually coma. The patient lies exhausted and covered with a cold sweat. The slightest noise or disturbance will bring another convulsive seizure. The number of seizures varies, but three or four are usually fatal. Death is then due to asphyxia and exhaustion.

Fatal Dose: One-half grain of strychnine has proved fatal in several instances. In one case a woman twenty-two years of age died after five hours from the effects of half a grain of strychnine administered through mistake by a hospital nurse.[1157]

Fatal Period: Death usually occurs within one hour, and is rarely delayed beyond three hours. I have a record of one case dying within fifteen minutes from the time the strychnine was given. If a patient having taken strychnine survives four hours the chances for recovery are good. Several deaths have been reported from about three-fourths of a grain,[1158] and also from one grain.[1159] The average fatal dose for man is usually placed from half a grain to one and three-fourths grains. There certainly would be more recoveries from the effects of half a grain than from the effects of one and three-fourths grains, irrespective of treatment. However, recovery has been reported following the taking of 9, 15, 19, 20, 27, 32, and 40 grains.[1160] In these cases it is to be remembered, however, that emetics had been given. The result of any poisonous dose is governed by a considerable number of factors, of which the dose is but one. Some cases have been reported which indicate that a cumulative action follows repeated doses of strychnine.[1161]

Treatment: Haggard and Greenberg[1162] report three cases

1157. *Lancet,* 2:291, 1856.
1158. WATSON: *Lancet,* 1:73, 1846; OGSTON: *Lancet,* 1:428, 1856; SOCQUET, OGIER, and BALTHAZARD: *Ann. d'hyg.,* 4 s., 7:523, 1907.
1159. DILL: *Lancet,* 2:533, 1873; DECOURCILLON: *Med. Arch.,* 3:31, 1869.
1160. In this connection see LEE: *Med. Bull.,* 5:82, 1883; PARKER: *Med. Leg. J.,* 2:375, 1884; BERRY: *Phila. Med. Reg.,* 1:566, 1887; CONNER: *Ohio Med. Rec.,* 4:12, 1879; GRAY: *Brit. M. J.,* 1:486, 1880; DAVIS: *Cincin. M. & Dent. J.,* 2:65, 1886-7; NIEDNER: *Charité-Ann., Berl.,* 29:26, 1905; WILSON: *Am. J. M. Sc.,* n. s., 48:70, 1864.
1161. BOOTH: *M. Times & Gaz.,* 13:35, 1856; PEREIRA: Mat. Med., 656, 1872; DUTGER: *Med. & Surg., Rep.,* 13:2, 1865; HUNTER: *M. Times & Gaz.,* 2:5, 1867; GREENWOOD: *Lancet,* 1:654, 1856; MEIER: *Berl. klin. Wchnschr.,* 62:1225, 1905; CLARK: *Chicago M. Times,* 43:109, 1910.
1162. HAGGARD, H. W., and GREENBERG, L. A.: *J.A.M.A.,* 98:1133, 1932.

of Dr. James S. Martin, of Waterbury, Connecticut, in which apomorphine apparently saved life following ingestion of fatal doses of strychnine. One-tenth and one-fifth grain doses of apomorphine were used, the smaller dose in a child. They reported that rats were saved from the two times fatal dose, but not the three times lethal dose of strychnine. One-third of the lethal dose of phenobarbital in rats will protect them against the three times lethal dose for strychnine. Barlow[1163] reports that pentobarbital, in small repeated doses by vein, antidotes up to thirty-five times the minimum lethal dose of strychnine for rabbits. One hundred per cent of all animals receiving fifteen lethal doses of strychnine or less, recovered. He suggests for man one-tenth grain of pentobarbital per pound of body weight. Barlow suggests fractional intravenous injections of pentobarbital, the initial dose being one-tenth of a grain of sodium pentobarbital per pound of body weight and one-twentieth grain per pound of body weight when convulsions reappear. Caution should be exercised when more than four injections have been given during the first two or three hours. Barbiturates are not as specific as the early claims indicated. Apomorphine can be given, one-tenth of a grain for adults, for its emetic action causes evacuation of the unabsorbed strychnine from the stomach. The stomach should be washed out with potassium permanganate solution, diluted to the color of port wine. Give chloral hydrate per rectum to control convulsions when barbiturates do not act readily. One gram of Mercks "Carbo Medicinalis" will bind 580 mg. of strychnine. When this is available the stomach should be washed out with it immediately.[1164] Swanson administered intravenously single equivalent effective doses of sodium amytal and pentobarbital sodium in rabbits poisoned by strychnine.[1165] Dawson, Taft and Barlow reported the injection of small effective doses of barbituric acid derivatives repeated at intervals as judged by the non-recurrence of strychnine convulsions. Gold and Gold[1166] give the results in a larger series of experiments, and show that there is no

1163. BARLOW, O. W.: J.A.M.A., 98:1980, 1932.
1164. DAWSON and TAFT: Proc. Soc. Exper. Biol. & Med., 28:917, 1931. And see J. Lab. & Clin. Med., 17:325, 1932; Gaz. méd de France, 389, 1933; Arch. internat. de pharmacodyn. et de thérap., 46:137, 1933.
1165. SWANSON, E. E.: J. Lab. & Clin. Med., 17:325, 1932.
1166. GOLD, D. A., and GOLD, H.: J.A.M.A., 100:1589, 1933.

appreciable antagonism between apomorphine and strychnine in dogs, that the reflex hyperexcitability from non-fatal doses of strychnine is not diminished, and that death from doses fatal to untreated animals is not prevented by the administration of apomorphine. Patients recover after administration of apomorphine even if twice the lethal dose of strychnine has been taken. Flanden and Bernard report a fatal phenobarbital poisoning from massive doses in a case of strychnine intoxication.[1167]

Stalberg and Davidson report an unusual delay in the appearance of the actual convulsions, forty-nine hours after the ingestion of the poison.[1168] The convulsions occurred during a period of five and one-half days. The authors gave intravenous injections of sodium amytal, which, they claim, saved the life in this particular case. Tribrom-ethanol anesthesia, which was supplemental to the sodium amytal, was given. They report a case of a woman thirty years of age, weighing 150 pounds, accidentally swallowing, after a light breakfast, one and three-fourths grains of strychnine in the form of sugar-coated pills. Hosse says strychnine poisoning is rarely seen in adults.[1169] In 467,500 admissions to the Bellevue Hospital during the past eleven years, only six cases were observed. There was only one case in children in the past five years out of 13,500 patients. Nitzescu reports the suppression of the experimental epileptic attack and of strychnine convulsions by intravenous injections of paraldehyde.[1170] In the experiments with paraldehyde, the writer used 1.2 and 1.3 mg. per kilogram of body weight of the rabbit. The convulsions appeared after fifteen, seventeen, ten, fourteen, and thirteen minutes. Injection of 5 cc. and of 10 cc. of the paraldehyde solution, as soon as the first convulsions appeared, intercepted the attack immediately and completely. Nitzescu believes that, in the treatment of tetanus by general anesthesia, the chloroform might be replaced by paraldehyde, and the injection renewed several times if necessary. Kempf, McCallum, and Zerfas report the successful treatment of eleven cases of strychnine poisoning. In ten of these cases the authors used

1167. FLANDEN and BERNARD: *Bull. et mém Soc. méd d. hôp. de Paris*, 49:1550, 1933.
1168. STALBERG, S., and DAVIDSON, H.: *J.A.M.A.*, 44:1781, 1915.
1169. HOSSE, L.: *Arch. Pediat.*, 40:264, 1923.
1170. NITZESCU, I. I.: *Compt. rend. Soc. de biol.*, 110:1220, 1932.

sodium amytal, and in one they used sodium pentobarbital.[1171] The authors report Cases 1 and 2 which follow:

CASE No. 1: V. H., a white woman, aged nineteen, well developed and well nourished, was brought into the Indianapolis City Hospital at 5:15 P.M., October 26, 1928. She had taken 100 one-thirtieth grain (0.002 gm.) each strychnine sulphate tablets at 1:00 P.M. after a heavy meal. She had been given morphine one-half grain (0.03 gm.) hypodermically, about fifteen minutes before admission. She was having mild convulsive twitchings at this time, and an attempt at gastric lavage was made. She immediately had a severe generalized convulsion with opisthotonos, trismus, risus sardonicus, complete extension of the extremities, and cyanosis. Attempts to induce ether anesthesia increased the convulsions. She had five such convulsions in fifteen minutes, and, during the fifth, she was given eight and a half grains (0.55 gm.) of sodium amytal intravenously. The convulsion stopped and the patient relaxed completely and went to sleep. At 7:30 the patient awakened, drank a glass of water, and dropped back to sleep. She roused slightly at 10 o'clock and, at this time, appeared to be slightly hypersensitive, but she soon fell asleep again and had no further convulsions. She was transferred to the ward, where for two days she suffered from a rather severe gastritis, which caused her to vomit frequently. On the third day she was normal and was released from the hospital. This was the first case of strychnine poisoning treated with sodium amytal.

CASE No. 2: W. T., a white man, aged forty-eight, took one and one-fourth grains (0.08 gm.) of strychnine in the form of one-fourth grain tablet triturates at 2:00 A.M., November 24, 1930. He was hyperexcitable, but did not have a complete convulsion. He was given 7.5 grains of pentobarbital sodium intravenously and slept until 5:30. There were no further symptoms and the patient was released after twenty-four hours. This was the first case of strychnine poisoning to be treated with pentobarbital sodium. The authors conclude: "A drug that can be given in quantity just sufficient to stop convulsions and in such a manner that a definite result may be obtained at once is almost necessary to save life. A soluble barbiturate, such as sodium amytal, sodium pentobarbital, or phenobarbital sodium, is the only available drug that can, on present evidence, be

1171. KEMPF, McCALLUM, and ZERFAS: J.A.M.A., 100:548, 1933.

safely administered in this manner to human beings."

CASE No. 3: Rose[1172] reports a case of strychnine poisoning in a young woman swallowing one ounce of liquor strychnine hydrochloridae, i.e., approximately 0.24 gm. (four grains) of strychnine hydrochloride. Half on hour later convulsions commenced, and these continued for another half hour before she was attended by a private practitioner, who administered 0.015 gm. (one-fourth grain) of morphine hypodermically, and 7.0 cc. (two drachms) of liquor morphinae hydrochloridae by mouth, with ether anesthesia. She was sent to a hospital still anesthetized, and a gastric lavage was performed with four pints of weak potassium permanganate solution two hours after she had taken the drug. She was given 7.2 gm. (120 grain) of potassium bromide and convulsions recommenced. Under chloroform anesthesia, 0.42 gm. (seven grains) of "sodium luminal" in 5% solution was injected intravenously; this kept her deeply unconscious for three hours, after which she had another convulsion. She was again anesthetized with chloroform and 1 gm. of "sodium evipan" in 10.5 cc. of distilled water was injected intravenously. This rendered her unconscious for a further three hours, after which she did not have any more convulsions, except for a slight spasm of both hands, which was easily controlled by 7.2 gm. (120 grains) of potassium bromide given by mouth. The patient left the hospital five days later apparently none the worse for her experience.

CASE No. 4: B. D., of Lincoln, Illinois, gave a young woman strychnine in a ham sandwich. Convulsions did not occur for one hour after. The patient died within an hour and a half from the time of the administration of the poison. B. D. was tried for murder, but was acquitted.

Separation of Strychnine from Tissues: Take at least 100 gm. of the finely comminuted organs and proceed as under separation of alkaloids (see page 30), using 50% alcohol. This procedure should be followed, as the mere extraction with acidulated water might not take out other substances that would aid in the preparation of the particular medication taken or given the individual. If it is certain that no other drug was used, then the tissue can be strongly acidulated with sulphuric acid and digested on the water-bath for about two hours. The

1172. ROSE, THOMAS: *M. J. Australia*, 1:213, 1935.

mixture is strained through a cloth and evaporated on the water-bath to about one-third of its volume. Add to this five or six times the volume of 94% alcohol. The organic matter is filtered off and washed with alcohol of the same strength as that of the filtrate. The filtrate can be evaporated under a vacuum to a syrupy liquid, and then transferred to a Squibb's separatory funnel with an equal volume of chloroform. Before extracting with chloroform, the liquid is made slightly alkaline by the addition of ammonium hydroxide solution. By using this method more emulsions are obtained than by the longer method previously described. Extract several times with chloroform, evaporating the chloroform extracts in a small beaker. The residue will have considerable extraneous organic matter in addition to the alkaloid. This residue can be purified by adding dilute sulphuric acid, filtering through a small filter paper, and extracting with chloroform after making it alkaline with ammonium. The residue will still contain impurities which can be removed by treatment with hot concentrated sulphuric acid. Heat on the water-bath for an hour and a half or in a dry oven fifteen to twenty minutes, the temperature not to exceed 120°C. The residue is now black from the action of the sulphuric acid. Stir with 1 or 2 cc. of water, and filter through a small cone of filter paper. The filtrate is washed with distilled water. The filtrate is made alkaline with ammonium and extracted as before with chloroform, keeping in mind that with each purification, a certain amount of the alkaloid is lost. If the residue, after this purification with sulphuric acid, still contains extraneous matter, it can be subjected to another treatment with sulphuric acid as before. The purified material is weighed in a beaker and saved for chemical and biological tests. The treatment with sulphuric acid would rule out certain putrefactive products obtained during the extraction process, which might confuse the analyst. If the preparation contained decomposed products giving a chemical test similar to that of strychnine, these same substances would fail to give the biological test, which should always supplement the chemical test.

Deposition of Strychnine in the Body: When a person dies suddenly from strychnine, the greatest amount will be found in the stomach and contents. It is almost always found in the liver and kidneys. Under certain conditions strychnine may be found in all the organs of the body. It has been found in the brain and blood. It is eliminated in the perspiration, and the saliva, and much more by the urine,[1173] and not at all by the feces. If the poison had been found in extremely small amounts minus the typical symptoms of strychnine poisoning, the toxicologist should endeavor to determine whether the strychnine had been administered for therapeutic purposes.

Detection in the Body after Prolonged Periods or Burning: Strychnine resists decomposition in the body. I have found it in the organs of a body exhumed two years after burial. Lesser[1174] detected strychnine in the completely mummified body of a woman 337 days after death, while Kratter[1175] discovered it in the body of a man, which had been buried five years and eight months and had been externally converted into adipocere. In the case of Mrs. Richard Budde, Eagle River, Wisconsin, where an attempt had been made to burn the body, I found 0.146 grain in the stomach and kidney. The liver failed to show the presence of strychnine. The lungs, which were carbonized, also failed to show the presence of strychnine. In this body the arms, legs and head had been burned off, nothing but the trunk remaining. Budde was tried for murder but was acquitted. Within two hours of his release from jail he was found dead from strychnine poisoning.

Failure to Detect: When the analyst extracts a large sample of tissue, if death were due to strychnine I believe it would always be found. However, my preceptor, Haines, states that he examined the stomachs of two children who died suddenly with all the symptoms of strychnine poisoning, but that he could not obtain any indication of the poison in the analysis of either case. Aikman[1176] reported a child two years old, taking an unknown number of A, B and S tablets which were sugar coated. He died in about five hours. Another child, four years of age, took ninety sugar-coated Hinkle pills. The patient died eight hours later. Barbiturates were not used in treating these cases. Every year there are cases of children dying of strychnine poisoning from the eating of brightly colored cathartic and tonic pills. Laws should be enacted prohibiting

1173. KOBERT: Lehrbuch der intoxikationen, 1161, 1906.
1174. LESSER: *Vrtljschr. f. gerichtl. Med., Berl.*, 3 F., 15:270, 1898.
1175. KRATTER: *Vrtljschr. f. gerichtl. Med., Berl.*, 3 F., 33:131, 1907.
1176. AIKMAN, J.: *J.A.M.A.*, 95:1161, 1930.

the promiscuous sale of these preparations by druggists. They should be sold only as prescribed by the physician. The patient should be cautioned regarding the dangerous strychnine contained in these brightly colored tablets.

VERATRUM

VERATRUM VIRIDE (green hellebore, American hellebore) consists of the dried roots and rhizome of veratrum viride Aiton. The rhizomes are more or less conical, varying from 2 to 7 cm. long and 1.5 to 3 cm. in diameter. They are externally light to dark brown or brownish-black, rough and wrinkled, and inodorous, with a bitter and acrid taste. The roots are numerous, nearly cylindrical, from 3 to 8 cm. long and 1 to 4 mm. in diameter, and whitish. The powder is grayish-brown to dark brown in color and strongly sternutatory. The dose is 0.1 gm. (one and one-half grains). The tincture is a 10% extract in alcohol; its dose is 1 cc. (fifteen minims).

Veratrine is a mixture of alkaloids obtained from the seed of Asagroea officinalis. It is a white or grayish-white amorphous powder, odorless, but causing intense irritation or sneezing when even a minute quantity reaches the nasal mucous membrane. It has an acrid taste, causing tingling and numbness of the tongue. It is soluble in 1,750 parts of water, 2.2 parts of alcohol, three parts of ether; insoluble in petroleum benzene. It melts at 152°C. It is alkaline to litmus. The dose is 0.002 gm. (one-thirtieth grain).

Tests: 1. Sulphuric acid when heated gives a cherry red color, which is a very characteristic test.

2. Mecke's reagent produces a brownish-green color.

3. Sulphuric acid with sugar gives a green color, changing to blue, then fading.

4. Sulphuric acid in the cold gives a yellow color, changing to orange with strong greenish fluorescence in reflected light. On standing the color changes to red, then to a deep carmine red.

5. Froehde's, Mandelin's and Erdmann's reagents give the same colors as sulphuric acid.

6. Bromine water added to the sulphuric acid solution gives a purple color.

The other alkaloids of veratrum give the following colors when treated with sulphuric acid: jervine—yellow, brownish-yellow and then bright green; rubijervine—yellow-orange, then dark red; veratralbine—the same as veratrine; pseudo-jervine—yellow, then bright green; protoveratrine—greenish-blue, then violet; protoveratridine—violet, then cherry-red.

7. Hydrochloric acid dissolves veratrine without color, but upon boiling gives a bright red color, which is stable for weeks. This test is characteristic but not very delicate.

8. Nitric acid gives a yellow color. Cevadine gives the same color; sabadine, and sabadilline are colorless; veratralbine gives a rose color, changing to pale yellow.

9. Vitali's test: dissolve in fuming nitric acid and evaporate to dryness, leaving a yellow residue. Cool and then add a few drops of alcoholic potassium hydroxide solution. A reddish-violet color is obtained. (Strychnine and atropine also give this same reaction.)

10. Weppen's test: one part of veratrine is mixed with six parts of powdered cane sugar and treated with sulphuric acid. A yellow color is obtained, changing to a grass-green, then blue, finally colorless. (This test is characteristic of the veratrum alkaloids.)

Biological Test: If a small quantity of a slightly acid solution of veratrine is injected into the lymph sac of a frog, there occur movements as if the animal were going to vomit, the heart action is slowed, and the movements are awkward and clumsy, which shows spasmodic contractions of the muscles and the inability to relax. The power of coordination is lost.

Isolation from Tissues: As this poison is eliminated by the kidneys, the urine and kidneys should be subjected to analysis. The procedure for isolating veratrine from the tissues is carried out the same as for atropine. The best solvent is chloroform in alkaline solution.

Symptoms: Fatal results from veratrum are of rare occurrence, notwithstanding the severity of the symptoms caused by its use. This is probably due to the emetic action, produced by large doses. Symptoms of poisoning caused by veratrum appear within a short time and may be delayed an hour or more. They begin with prickling and burning in the mouth followed by an intense burning pain in the stomach. There is great thirst, with difficulty in swallowing, then salivation, nausea, and persistent vomiting, and violent purging with severe abdominal colic. The prickling sensation spreads to the skin, which becomes reddened with intense itching, followed by profuse perspiration. Sneezing, lacrimation, and coryza may occur. There is restlessness, cold extremities, and vertigo, with dilated pupils and almost complete lack of vision. The pulse is at first slow, but later becomes feeble, thready and rapid, owing to paralysis of the vagus. Respiration is gasping, shallow and superficial, sometimes with dyspneic attacks. Death is usually due to respiratory failure, but may be due to cardiac weakness or collapse from prolonged vomiting and consequent prostration.

Fatal Dose: The fatal quantity cannot be definitely stated. Harris[1177] reported recovery from 3.7 cc. of the tincture. A woman, fifty years of age took 4.3 cc. of a fluid extract in two doses. Vomiting occurred in two hours and continued for four weeks, when the patient died.[1178]

Treatment: The stomach is thoroughly washed with warm water. The patient should be kept flat on his back, with the head lower than the feet. Vomiting should be restrained. Warm applications should be made to the extremities, and external stimulants employed. A dose of tincture of opium per rectum, undiluted spirits per mouth, and ammonia at discretion should be given; with strychnine and digitalis for respiratory failure.

Postmortem Appearances: The appearances are not distinctive. There is congestion of the lining of the stomach and bowels, and sometimes hyperemia of the brain.

YOHIMBINE

YOHIMBINE represents the pharmacologic therapeutically effective principal of a rubiaceae of West Africa called coryanthe yohimbe.[1179] According to Raymond-Hamet this substance is supposed to be chemically and biologically identical with the base quebrachine.[1180] Cases of poisoning have occurred from its use as an aphrodisiac. The lack of agreement concerning substances of the same name explains not only differences of opinion found in the literature[1181] but explains also a

1177. HARRIS, J. C.: *Boston M. & S. J.*: 72:249, 1865.
1178. JOHNSON, T. M.: *Buffalo M. & S. J.*, 45:133, 1866.
1179. HESSE, E., LANGER, J.: *Med. Klin.*, 27:1536, 1931.
1180. RAYMOND-HAMET: *Compt. rend. Acad. d. sc.*, 187:142, 1928.
1181. FURBRINGER: *Deutsche med. Wchnschr.*, 1364, 1925.

series of intoxications which have been observed in the last four years.

Biologically the yohimbine preparations are characteristic, having the following effects: When applied locally on the mucosa this substance produces anesthesia, as can be seen from the fact that rabbit's cornea which has been treated with a 1% solution of this substance becomes anesthetized for about a half hour. The toxic symptoms arising from the absorption of this substance manifest themselves in the form of salivation, increased respiration, and repeated defecation. In suitable animals, such as dogs, one can observe strong erections and coitus movements. With reference to the circulatory system we find a fall in blood pressure, and sometimes myocardial damage, the damage involving particularly the conduction system of the heart with the result that the efficiency of the heart is decreased. Hesse noted the effects consist of a slowing of the pulse, a decrease of the pulse amplitude, disturbances in the conduction mechanisms in the heart, and finally stoppage of the heart in diastole. Raymond-Hamet[1182] have shown that animals which have been treated with yohimbine did not respond to adrenalin with a rise in blood pressure but rather with a fall in blood pressure, and it has been therefore concluded that the fibers of the sympathetic nerve may be classified with excitatory and inhibitory ones. The rise in the blood sugar level which is observed after the administration of adrenalin is offset by yohimbine.

TREMETOL

THE names "trembles" and "milk sickness" have been applied to illness following the drinking of milk from cows which have eaten richweed or snake root. The only constituent responsible for this poisoning is tremetol. This illness is found chiefly in the States bordering the Ohio River and in the Midwestern section of this country. In 1928 I saw three cases, with one death, in Streator, Illinois.

The symptoms include lassitude, pains in the legs, loss of appetite, obstinate constipation, and vomiting, and the breath has a peculiar odor. The disease has been transmitted to calves, lambs, and young rabbits[1183] by the mothers of these

1182. RAYMOND-HAMET: *Compt. rend. Acad. d. sc.*, 180:2074, 1925.
1183. U. S. Dept. of Agriculture, Farmers' Bull. No. 1593.

animals. Cats have been poisoned by milk from affected cows, and there are many more or less well authenticated reports of the poisoning of other animals in the same manner. Even the meat of poisoned animals may poison other animals eating the same. Many accidents occur from the consuming of milk or butter of cows affected with trembles.

White Snake Root, or Richweed: Eupatorium uticoefolium is a slender, erect perennial herb, belonging to the family compositae. Its leaves, which are three to five inches long, are opposite, broadly ovate, pointed, sharply toothed and thin, and have rather long petioles. It is most commonly known as white snake root. Other names which have been applied to it are white sanicle, Indian sanicle, deerwort, boneset, poolwort, poolroot, richweed, squaw-weed, whitetip, and steria. Milk, meat, and butter produced from cows affected with trembles should always be avoided.

Tremetol is a cumulative poison, as was demonstrated in the experimental feedings which were made in several successive doses given in one day.[1184] Acetonuria is, however, a serious complication of the disease and likely to be fatal.

The disease should be treated symptomatically to overcome the acidosis. Give intravenously calcium gluconate and sodium bicarbonate by mouth until the urine is alkaline. Hypodermatoclysis into the breast of one liter of normal saline and 5% glucose should be given to overcome the vomiting. Enemas of 3% sodium bicarbonate and 5% glucose may also be given.

Cattle should be kept away from fields where this plant is known to grow.

SULPHANILAMIDE
(Para-Aminobenzene Sulphonamide)

DOMAGK,[1184-A] who was working with azo dyes, noticed that the presence of a sulphonamide group lessened the efficiency of the dye as an antiseptic and caused it to protect infected mice. Levaditi and Vaisman[1184-B] confirmed the re-

1184. Couch, J. F.: Reprint from *J. Am. Veterinary Med. Assoc.*, 73:26, N. S., No. 5, 603, 1928; *J. Agricultural Research*, 35:6, 547, 1927.

1184-A. Domagk, Gerhard: *Ang. Chem.*, 48:657, 1935; *Deutsche med. Wchnschr.*, 61:250, 1935.

1184-B. Levaditi, C., and Vaisman, A.: *Compt. rend. Soc. de Biol.*, 119:946, 1935.

sults of Domagk. Horlein,[1184-C] Nitti and Bovet,[1184-D] Cole-brook,[1184-E] and Long[1184-F] noticed that mice were not protected against strains of low virulence. Goissedet, Despois, Gailliot, and Mayer[1184-G] confirmed the work of Tréfouel, Nitti, and Bovet that azo-linkage was not necessary for action on streptococci and found that benzylideneaminosulphonamides were active, also sodium p - aminobenzenesulphonamidemethylenebisul-phite.

Since it has been used upon human beings, toxic ef-fects of the drug have been noted: depression of the liver function and hemolytic anemia. Not all patients react the same to this drug. Every physician should have repeated examinations made of the patient's blood. In one case in which I gave eleven tablets, in twenty-four hours, for a sinus infection, a drop of 700,000 cells in the red count occurred. The patient became depressed, nauseated, and was unable to eat. His condition improved in another thirty-six hours after stoppage of medication. Harvey and Janeway[1184-H] reported three cases of severe hemolytic anemia during the treatment of a streptococcic sore throat and a meningococcic meningitis, with sulphanilamide. In one of these, on the fifth day, there was a drop from 4,900,000 to 1,570,000 cells in the red count. The hemoglobin dropped from 101% to 30%. There was a marked leukocytosis, with 87,000 white blood cells, of which 1% were myeloblasts, 20% juvenile neutrophils, 53% poly-morphonuclear neutrophils, 2% eosinophils, 14% lymphocytes, and 7% monocytes. The drug was discontinued and the pa-tient was given three transfusions of citrated blood of 500 cc. each during the next forty-eight hours. A rapid improvement in his condition was noted. All three patients recovered after medication was stopped and transfusions of blood were given.

Toxicities of prontosil and p-aminobenzenesulphonamide base and hydrochloride were compared, giving the drugs in suspension of gum acacia, by mouth, to mice weighing 19 gm.

1184-C. HORLEIN, H.: Proc. Roy. Soc. Med., 29:313, 1936.
1184-D. NITTI, F., and BOVET, D.: Compt. rend. Soc. de Biol., 119: 1277, 1935.
1184-E. COLEBROOK, L., and KENNY, M.: Lancet, 1:1279, 1936.
1184-F. LONG, P. H., and BLISS, ELEANOR: J.A.M.A., 108:32, 1937.
1184-G. GOISSEDET, P., DESPOIS, R., GAILLIOT, P., and MAYER, R.: Compt. rend. Soc. de Biol., 121:1082, 1936.
1184-H. HARVEY, A. M., and JANEWAY, C. A.: J.A.M.A., 109:12, 1937.

to 22 gm.[1184-I] Twelve mg. of prontosil proved to be innocuous, 25 mg. killed four out of six mice, 50 mg. five out of six, and 100 mg. six out of six. Sulphonamide is produced in the body from prontosil by reduction of the dye. Therefore, it would seem plausible that the bactericidal effect of the prontosil upon hemolytic streptococci was due to the presence of sulphonamide that is formed.[1184-J]

The drug may be given six to ten tablets daily, by mouth, in divided doses, or by hypodermoclysis using 100 to 400 cc. of an 0.8% solution in normal saline. Total dosage should not exceed 5 gm. in twenty-four hours. Cecil[1184-K] stated that daily doses of seventy-five to eighty grains may be given by mouth without untoward effects.

Branham and Rosenthal[1184-L] reported that, dosage being equal, subcutaneous administration was more effective than oral in meningococcus and pneumonococcus in mice. Borat,[1184-M] reported a death from agranulocytosis after treatment with prontosil flavum.[1184-N]

Cyanosis is an indication for the immediate withdrawal of the drug and for oxygen therapy. A red blood cell count and hemoglobin examination should be made every twenty-four hours. A drop in either is an indication for discontinuance of the medication. Renal insufficiency is a contraindication to the use of this drug. Caution should be used in the administration of this drug to a patient already anemic. Kohn[1184-O] reported a case of acute hemolytic anemia during treatment with sulphanilamide. Bucy[1184-P] reported a toxic optic neuritis in a girl aged sixteen, as the result of the administration of sulphanilamide. Skin eruptions have been reported by Menville and Archinard, Goodman and Levy, and Frank.[1184-Q]

1184-I. BUTTLE, G. A., GRAY, W. H., and STEPHENSON, D.: *Lancet*, 230:1286, 1936.

1184-J. COLEBROOK, L., BUTTLE, G. A., and O'MEARA, R. A. Q.: *Lancet*, 231:1323, 1936.

1184-K. CECIL, R. L.: Paper read before the staff of New York Polyclinic Medical School and Hospital, January 13, 1937.

1184-L. U. S. Pub. Health Reports, 52:685, 1937.

1184-M. J. GG. Univ. Amsterdam, Internal Hospital Department.

1184-N. *Lancet*, 1:1519, 1937.

1184-O. KOHN, S. L.: *J.A.M.A.*, 109:1005, 1937.

1184-P. BUCY, P. C.: *J.A.M.A.*, 109:1007, 1937.

1184-Q. MENVILLE, J. G., and ARCHINARD, J. J.: *J.A.M.A.*, 109:1008, 1937; GOODMAN, M. H., and LEVY, S. C.: *J.A.M.A.*, 109:1009, 1937; FRANK, L. J.: *J.A.M.A.*, 109:1011, 1937.

Other references:

SCHREUS, PH.: *Deutsche. med. Wchnschr.*, 61:255, 1935.
LEVADITI, C. and VAISMAN, A.: *Presse med.*, 43: 2097, 1935.
KLEE, PH., and ROMER, H.: *Deutsche med. Wchnschr.*, 61:253, 1935.
TREFOUEL, J., MME. TREFOUEL, NITTI, F., and BOVET, D.: *C. R. Soc. Biol.* 120:756, 1935.
HUBER, H. G.: *München. med. Wchnschr.*, 83:2014, 1936.
JAEGER, K. H.: *Deutsche. med. Wchnschr.*, 62:1831, 1936.
HORLEIN, H.: *Proc. Roy. Soc. Med.* 29:313, February, 1936.
GOISSEDET, P., DESPOIS, R., JOILLOT, P. and MAYER, R.: *C. R. Soc. Biol.* 121:1082, 1936.
PROOM, H.: *Lancet,* 1:16, 1937.
LYTH, H.: *Brit. M. J.,* 1:584, 1937.
DISCOMBE, G.: *Lancet,* 1:626, 1937.
PALMER, W. H.: *Brit. M. J.,* 1:472, 1937.
PLUMER, H. E.: *New England J. Med.,* 216:77, 1937.
FOULIS, M. A., and BARR, J. B.: *Brit. M. J.,* 1:445, 1937.
SOUTHWORTH, H.: *Proc. Soc. Exper. Biol. & Med.,* 36:58, 1937.
GROSS, P., COOPER, F. B. and MELLON, R. R.: *J. Bact.* 33:72, 1937.
ROSENTHAL, S. M.: Public Health Rep., 52:48, 1937; 52:192, 1937.
FRANK, L. J.: "Dermatitis from Sulfanilamide," *J.A.M.A.,* 109:13, 1937.
SCHWENTKER, F. F., GELMAN, S. and LONG, P. H.: *J.A.M.A.,* 108:1407, 1937.
BUTTLE, G. A. H., PARISH, H. J., McLEOD, M. and STEPHENSON, D.: *Lancet,* 1:681, 1937.
COOPER, F. B., GROSS, P. and MELLON, R. R.: *Proc. Soc. Exper. Biol. & Med.* 36:148, 1937.
KOHN, S. E.: "Anemia During Treatment with Sulfanilamide," *J.A.M.A.,* 109:13, 1937.
BUCY, PAUL C.: "Toxic Optic Neuritis Resulting from Sulfanilamide," *J.A.M.A.,* 109:13, 1937.
SCHONBERG, I. L.: "Purpuric and Scarlatinaform Eruption Following Sulfanilamide," *J.A.M.A.,* 109:13, 1937.
NEWMAN, BEN A., and SHARLIT, HERMAN: "Sulfanilamide: A Photosensitizing Agent of the Skin," *J.A.M.A.,* 109:13, 1937.
GOODMAN, M. H., and LEVY, CHARLES S.: "Eruption During Administration of Sulfanilamide," *J.A.M.A.,* 109:13, 1937.
SCHWENTKER, F. F., CLASON, F. P., MORGAN, W. A., LINDSAY, J. and LONG, P. H.: *Bull. Johns Hopkins Hosp.,* 60:297, 1937.
MENVILLE, JOHN G., and ARCHINARD, JOHN J.: "Skin Eruptions in Patients Receiving Sulfanilamide," *J.A.M.A.,* 109:13, 1937.
BALLENGER, EDGAR G., ELDER, OMAR F., and McDONALD, HAROLD P.: "Sulfanilamide and Thermotherapy," *J.A.M.A.,* 109:13, 1937.

VOLATILES, DISTILLATES, AND SOLVENTS

PETROLEUM DISTILLATES

PPROPERTIES: The petroleum distillates having a boiling point between 30°C. and 90°C. are used for motor fuels and are known as gasoline. The paraffin hydrocarbon mixtures with a boiling point below 150°C. are known as benzine, gasoline, petroleum, naphtha, etc. They consist of pentane, heptane, and hexane. Those substances with a boiling point between 70°C. and 150°C. are used chiefly as solvents. From 150°C. to 270°C. are the boiling points of kerosene, and over 270°C. will be found the various lubricating oils, such as vaseline and paraffin.

Petroleum naphtha[1185] is a generic term applied to refined, partly refined, and unrefined petroleum products of which not less than 10% distills below 347°F. (175°C.), and not less than 95% of which distills below 464° F. (240° C.).

Petroleum spirits is a refined petroleum distillate with a minimum flash point of 70° F. (21° C.).[1185]

Hayhurst reports a case of a man aged forty-eight who worked with "mineral spirits" as a degreasing agent. This substance was composed of hydrocarbons similar to gasoline, 95% by volume distilling below 203° C., the residue being heavy mineral oil. This patient developed a number of symptoms, the chief ones being smarting and running eyes, burning sensation in nose and throat, headache, dizziness, anorexia, nausea, sometimes vomiting, "naphtha jags", nervousness, prostration, muscular twitchings, loss of strength, and gradual loss of weight from 138 to 121 pounds. In 1923 this patient was examined and found to have a persistent cough; he raised a good deal of morning sputum, complained more or less of headache, tinnitus, especially at night; his weight was 104, and there was corresponding weakness and loss of strength; his sleep was disturbed, and unrefreshing. He was able to work about the house and yard but unable to use the street cars alone; his vision was 20/30 each eye, and there was senile puffiness of both lower lids. Hearing in the right ear was nearly gone, and was impaired in the left ear. Tongue reflexes were normal.[1185]

The man who took this patient's place in 1919 had quit,

1185. HAYHURST, E. R.: *Indust. Med.*, 5:53, 1936.

so the patient said, because of stomach trouble and later died. Another employee in the same work died with pneumonia two days after ceasing work. Another large and well developed man had a downward course also.

Symptoms: Hayhurst reports three series of chronic poisonings from petroleum distillates, each representing two or more cases, as well as a group of six significant individual cases from as many different sources.[1185] The period of exposure was from five weeks to three or four years before employment disability began.

The typical picture associated with the disability came on with the complaint of loss of weight, worry, and a feeling of "slipping" in physical and mental well being. The author groups the objective findings as follows: (1) loss of weight from 10% to 60% over months of time, with periods of partial recovery almost to normal; (2) pulse rate increased, sometimes notably; (3) blood picture showed severe secondary anemia—60-90% hemoglobin, red cells decreased 20-35% color index less than 1, slight leukocytosis of 10,000 to 14,000; (4) skin irritation; (5) mouth infection; (6) diarrhea; (7) mental depression, and even slowed mentality.

Nunn and Martin report seven cases of gasoline poisoning and sixty-five cases of kerosene poisoning in children ranging in age from ten months to four years. In the kerosene poisoning cases the mortality was 9.2%, and in the gasoline cases 28%.[1186]

Price reports four cases of poisoning in children who drank kerosene.[1187] One experienced no untoward effects; one went into immediate collapse from which there was rapid recovery; one had considerable respiratory difficulty for eighteen hours, with subsequent recovery; and one died. The ages of these children ranged from eleven months to two years. The pulse was rapid but strong, respiration slightly labored, and there was a mild degree of cyanosis. The stomachs of these children were washed out and they were given caffeine, atropine, and dextrose intravenously. In these four cases there was no constant picture accompanying the drinking of kerosene. This can be explained by the fact that the ingested kerosene may have been of different fractions, as the toxicity will vary

1186. Nunn, J. A., and Martin, F. M.: *J.A.M.A.*, 103:472, 1934.
1187. Price, J. P.: *J.A.M.A.*, 99:214, 1932.

in direct proportion to the content of its volatile products. There is no known antidote for kerosene. Stomachs should be washed out at once and a mild laxative administered; treat the patient symptomatically.

Tucker[1188] demonstrated the oxidation products of petroleum oils exposed to the air at temperatures below 150°C. to be a complicated series of compounds with acidic properties.[1189] The lubricating fractions of petroleum are not toxic to foliage until they are oxidized to asphaltogenic acids. Using apricot leaves as a testing medium, it was found that the toxic threshold is reached when approximately 0.5% of asphaltogenic acids are formed.

Schneider caused acute poisoning in children by the ingestion of 8 to 10 gm. of benzine; an adult recovered after drinking 0.25 liter.[1190] The toxic dose is 7.5 gm. per kilogram of body weight. Benzine enters the body in two ways, by inhalation and by drinking which occurs through error. It is a cerebrospinal poison, with narcotic action similar to ether and chloroform. The symptoms of poisoning by benzine are drunkenness, later unconsciousness with cyanosis, cramps, reflex disturbances, paralysis, followed by death. In case of recovery there is a disturbance for months of the central nervous system, a retrobulbar neuritis, and epilepsy. If taken internally, it causes vomiting, stomach pains, difficulty in swallowing, fever, bronchial symptoms, kidney disturbances, and disturbances of the digestive tract.

The fatal dose of kerosene has never been determined. As much as a liter has been taken without causing death, but children have died after taking small but unknown amounts. In several newspaper accounts a dose as small as four ounces was reported as having caused the death of a three-year-old infant.

Gasoline escaping from the tanks at filling stations may impart an odor to spring water for as much as 100 feet away from the station, and it has been known to pollute the water in a flowing spring to such an extent that it was unfit for drinking purposes.[1191]

1188. TUCKER, R. P.: *Indust. & Eng. Chem.*, 28:458, 1936.
1189. STAEGER, H. C.: *Indust. & Eng. Chem.*, 17:1272, 1925; HASLAM, R. T., and FROLICH, P. K.: *Indust. & Eng. Chem.*, 19:292, 1927.
1190. SCHNEIDER, H.: *Med. Klin.*, 29:1168, 1933.
1191. VER STEEG, KARL: *Science,* 76:235, 1932.

METHYL ALCOHOL

METHYL ALCOHOL is variously known as methanol, carbonol, wood alcohol, pyroxylic spirit, wood spirit, wood naphtha, Columbian spirit, Colonial spirit, methyl hydroxide, Manhattan spirits, standard wood spirits, green wood spirits. When purified it is used under the name "Columbian spirits" and "Eagle spirits." It is obtained by the destructive distillation of wood. Its chemical formula is CH_3OH. It occurs in commerce in varying degrees of purity.

Properties:

Purity, 99.8% to 100% methyl alcohol.

Specific gravity, 0.792 to 0.793 at 20°C.

Acidity: no more than 0.01%, calculated as formic acid.

Color, water-white.

Distillation range: below 64°C., none; above 66°C., none.

Acetone: less than 0.03%, by weight.

Non-volatile matter: not more than 0.0025%.

Odor: free from odor foreign to pure methanol.

Flash point: 14°C. (57.2°F.).

Weight per U. S. gallon: 6.64 pounds at 60°F.

Melting point—97.8°C.

Critical pressure: 78.7 atmospheres.

Critical temperature: 240°C.

Heat of combustion: 5,334 calories per gm.

Refractive index: 1.329 at 20°C.

Specific heat: 0.645 from 23°C. to 43°C.

Latent heat of vaporization: 262.8 calories per gm. at 64.5°C.

Dielectric constant: 31.2 at 20°C.

Vapor pressure: 0°C., 29.6 mm. of mercury; 20°C., 96.0 mm. of mercury; 40°C., 260.5 mm. of mercury; 60° C., 625.0 mm. of mercury.

The crude wood alcohol contains much acetone, some ethyl-methyl-ketone, methyl and dimethyl acetate, furfural, allyl alcohol, and other bodies that give it an extremely disagreeable odor and taste. It found extensive use during prohibition as a denaturing agent for alcohol. The purified alcohol is colorless and has an odor and taste similar to that of ethyl or grain alcohol. When it burns, however, the odor of formaldehyde is easily detected. On oxidation it yields formaldehyde and formic acid. It finds extensive use as a solvent, especially in varnishes and as an anti-freeze for automobiles. It has been taken as a beverage, causing hundreds of cases of death and blindness.

It is used in a large number of occupations, such as by aniline dye makers, anti-freeze makers, art glass workers, artificial flower makers, artificial silk makers, automobile painters, bookbinders, bronzers, cementers (rubber shoes), driers (felt hats), dry cleaners, dye makers, explosive workers, feather workers, felt hat makers, furniture polishers, hardeners (felt hats), lacquerers, lacquer makers, linoleum makers, methyl alcohol workers, methyl compound workers, millinery workers, painters, paint makers, patent leather makers, perfume makers, photo-engravers, photographers, wood polishers, polish makers, rubber workers, shellackers, shellac makers, soap makers, stiffeners (felt hats), varnishers, varnish makers, vulcanizers, wood alcohol distillers, woodworkers.

Throughout the prohibition period deaths occurred from its use as an adulterant of whiskey and other beverages. In one instance a bartender diluted, and colored with caramel, five gallons of wood alcohol and dispensed it to five of his customers. Four of them died, from the effects of wood alcohol poisoning, and the fifth one became blind. This man took only two one-ounce glasses of the diluted beverage; he stated that the other men had taken from four to six glasses of it.

In New York there were seventy-four wood alcohol deaths from January 1, 1930, to March 31, 1931. From newspaper records, over 400 fatalities occurred in the United States from October 10, 1930, to April 22, 1931. A number of these deaths came from drinking radiator alcohol, some of which had been colored blue. Many of the deaths in Pennsylvania were definitely ascertained to have been caused by this "blue methanol," particularly those cases at Titusville and Uniontown. Seven deaths occurred in Raton, Colfax County, New Mexico, on March 23, 1931, from drinking radiator alcohol. Anti-freeze mixtures should all contain some substance which causes vomiting, with the addition of something with a disagreeable odor which will inform the ignorant that they are dealing with a non-beverage substance. Every barrel should be labelled in large red letters, "POISON—WOOD ALCOHOL." The laity, not being well informed, do not know that methyl alcohol is wood alcohol. The words *wood alcohol* should be preserved and used on all commercial packages. This is one way that will safeguard the lives of people and keep them absolutely protected against the illegal use of this substance for beverage purposes.

In 1904 Buller and Wood[1192] collected 275 cases of serious poisoning by methyl alcohol; in 153 blindness, and in 122 death, occurred. Many cases of wholesale poisoning have occurred both in the United States and abroad.[1193] In Berlin[1194] about 130 men drank "brandy" composed of two-thirds methyl alcohol and one-third ethyl alcohol; fifty or more died, forty-two became blind or had impairment of vision, and thirty-two recovered.

Baskerville[1195] collected 725 published cases of poisoning resulting from the drinking of wood alcohol; there were 390 deaths, ninety cases of total blindness, and eighty-five of impaired vision; in about 100 cases the results were not specifically stated. Baskerville also collected sixty-four cases of poisoning by the inhalation of methyl alcohol.[1196] Blindness has resulted from the external use of methyl alcohol.[1197]

Methyl alcohol is more volatile than ethyl alcohol, and the inhalation of its vapors by painters and by other workmen has frequently caused death or blindness. Repeated application to the skin may also cause blindness. I have caused the death of rabbits in from ten to twelve days by the daily application of wood alcohol to a shaved area (2 in. x 2 in.) on their backs. It matters little whether it is synthetic methanol or wood alcohol prepared by distillation, it is still a poison. The constant exposure to small doses produces cumulative effects in the internal organs.

Action: The first toxic effect of wood alcohol was reported by McFarlan in 1855. Since its introduction at the close of the Civil War in 1865, methyl alcohol has been increasingly used as an article of commercial application and its use has increased

1192. Buller and Wood: *J.A.M.A.*, 43:972, 1904.
1193. Cf. Strohmberg: *Petersb. med. Wchnschr.*, 31:55, 1904 (55 deaths).
1194. Cf. Stadelmann and Magnus-Levy: *Berl. klin. Wchnschr.*, 49:193, 1912.
1195. Baskerville: 2nd Rep., Factory Investigation Comm., New York, 2:921, 1913.
1196. Cf. also Wood: *J.A.M.A.*, 59:1962, 1912 (Case 2).
1197. Cf. Wood: *J.A.M.A.*, 60:1762, 1913.

markedly since it has been synthetized from carbon monoxide, water gas, and carbon dioxide. It soon found use as a substitute in medicine, bay rum and toilet waters.

Some time ago the medical fraternity found that people were becoming blind in a mysterious manner, and before long it was recognized that methyl alcohol was the element causing the trouble. Casey Wood and Buller brought clearly to our attention that blindness and eye disturbances followed the use of wood alcohol.

This substance is a poison when taken internally in beverages, or if inhaled, or absorbed through the skin. The effects of a small dose of methyl alcohol upon animals do not differ markedly from those of ethyl alcohol. The toxicity of methyl alcohol is increased by its impurities, consequently the toxic dose and symptoms will vary according to the impurity. The symptoms, may, however, appear more slowly and the duration of the intoxication be more prolonged; the condition of coma caused by methyl alcohol may continue for two, or three, or even for more than six, hours. In numerous experiments, however, it never continued for twenty-four hours. Methyl alcohol is less inebriating than ethyl alcohol, or grain alcohol. In acute fatal intoxications of the lower animals, methyl alcohol is found to be slightly less toxic than ethyl alcohol.[1198]

Methyl alcohol in the lower animals, affects most powerfully the more highly differentiated nervous structures, as is shown by the prolonged coma, and it is a well recognized fact in pharmacology that poisons which affect the highly differentiated nerve structures very powerfully are proportionately more dangerous the higher developed is the nervous system of the animal. Methyl alcohol remains in the body five to ten times as long as grain alcohol, because it is oxidized comparatively slowly. The body has great difficulty in disposing of methyl alcohol; some is slowly excreted in the urine, and in the expired air.[1199] Asser recovered after seven days, 55.8% of 25 cc. given to a dog.[1200] Some is excreted into the stomach[1201] and is doubtless reabsorbed from this organ or from the intestines.

1198. HUNT: Loc. cit.: NICLOUX and PLACET: *J. de physiol. et de path. gén.*, 14:916, 1912.

1199. VOLTZ and DIETRICH: *Biochem. Ztschr., Berl.*, 40:15, 1912.

1200. ASSER: *Ztschr. f. exper. Path. u. Therap., Berl.*, 15:322, 1914.

1201. BONGERS: *Arch. exper. Path. u. Pharmakol.*, 35:415, 1895.

The body oxidizes methyl alcohol slowly and incompletely with the formation of formic acid.[1202] In one of Pohl's experiments 60 cc. of methyl alcohol were given to a dog and the maximum amount of formic acid did not appear in the urine until the fourth day, and there was an abnormal amount present three days later. There is a profound disturbance of metabolism; a condition of acidosis develops,[1203] and there is also a marked increase in the excretion of lactic and other organic acids. Nine people out of ninety-four poisoned died in a methyl alcohol poisoning epidemic at Odessa in 1932. These poisonings occurred in men unloading wood alcohol, which they consumed. Poisoning symptoms occurred about eight or twelve hours after consumption of the methyl alcohol, and were in all probability due to the products of oxidation, formaldehyde, and formic acid.

Symptoms: The condition of stimulation such as is seen in grain alcohol seems to have been rarely reported in methyl alcohol poisoning. The symptoms are hyperemia, and cyanosis of the face and mucous membrane of the mouth, as well as excitement. There are depression, weakness, headache, nausea, pains in the epigastric and temporal regions, dyspnea and cyanosis, delirium or a maniacal condition, or stupor, the patient being aroused by pain and vomiting, cold sweats and subnormal temperature, and dilated pupils not reacting to light. There may be long continued coma, and death from failure of the respiration. But in other cases consciousness has been preserved almost until death. Convulsions may precede the death. A condition of coma may continue for three or four days, and recovery, except for blindness, occur.[1204] I have seen fatal cases in which the symptoms did not appear for thirty-six hours, the victims working the following day after the consumption of the poisonous beverage. The symptom[1205] which has aroused most

1202. POHL: *Arch. f. exper. Path. u. Pharmakol.*, 31:281, 1892; RABINOVITCH: *Arch. Int. Med.*, 29:821, 1922.

1203. KROL: *Arch. Int. Med.*, 72:444, 1913; HARROP and BENEDICT: *J.A.M.A.*, 74:25, 1920; VAN SLYKE and PALMER: *J. Biol. Chem.*, 41:567, 1920.

1204. MOULTON: *J.A.M.A.*, 37:1447, 1901; SWADENER: *J.A.M.A.*, 60:1479, 1913.

1205. THOMPSON: *Med. & Surg. Rep.*, 77:97, 1897; WOODS: Loc. cit.; HARLAN: *Ophth. Rec.*, 10:81, 1901; WURDEMANN: *Am. Med.*, 2:995, 1901; MOULTON: *Therap. Gaz.*, 8:335, 1899; BURNETT: *Therap. Gaz.*, 10:801, 1901; BULLER and WOOD: Loc. cit.; FRIEDENWALD: *Ophth. Rec.*, 10:429, 1901; WOOD: *New York M. J.*, 81:5, 1905; and many others.

interest is blindness, as has been reported by a number of American ophthalmologists.

Blindness has occurred in a large percentage of severe cases of poisoning; it is bilateral, and may set in within a few hours or it may be delayed for several days. There will be first a feeling of pain about the eyes, and tenderness on pressure over the lids, discomfort on looking around, slight photophobia, and dilatation of the pupils. The patient may go along for twenty-four to forty-eight hours and then complain of disturbances of vision or become totally blind. Sight may be restored in a few days only to be lost again within two or three weeks. The blindness is due to atrophy of the optic nerve.[1206]

Central scotoma was observed, and in some cases peripheral vision was preserved, but the field was always narrowed. Sometimes the color sense was chiefly affected.[1207]

Gifford has reported a case in which the only symptom of the poisoning was blindness, in which a man became temporarily blind in three days from drinking cologne spirits made with methyl alcohol.[1208] The other symptoms were so slight that the patient failed to remember he drank the cologne. This is unusual, as nearly all the cases that I have seen have complained of pain in the abdomen. In other cases in which a large quantity of the poison had been taken, the patients were comatose for two or three days and then awoke almost blind.[1209]

Eight gm. of methyl alcohol were found to affect the eyes seriously.[1210]

The diagnosis is based on the symptoms and the presence of abnormally large amounts of methyl alcohol in the urine.

Birch-Hirschfeld describe experiments upon three monkeys; pure methyl alcohol, diluted with several times its volume of water, was given in doses of from three to six or seven ccm. every day or two. When it became evident that the animals were at the point of death, they were killed in order that the eyes and optic nerves could be obtained in good condition

1206. See FRIEDENWALD: *Ophth. Rec.*, 10:429, 1901; BIRCH-HIRSCH-FELD: *Arch. f. Ophth. (von Grafe's)*, 54:68, 1902; and UHTHOFF: Graefe-Saemisch Handbuch, 2nd ed., 5:11, 1907.

1207. BURNETT: *Ophth. Rec.*, 11:309, 1902.

1208. GIFFORD: *Ophth. Rec.*, 10:342, 1901.

1209. HARLAN: *Ophth. Rec.*, 10:81, 1901.

1210. *Pharm. Centralhalle*, 52:335, 1911; 51:64, 792, 1910; *Chem. Abst.*, 5:2278, 1911.

for microscopical study. The first monkey received 28 ccm. of methyl alcohol in this way, and was in a dying condition on the eighth day. The second animal was moribund on the fifteenth day after receiving 79 ccm. of the alcohol, while the third animal was in a dying condition on the eleventh day after having been given 56 ccm. of the alcohol.[1211]

Birch-Hirschfeld describe experiments with seven rabbits and three hens, where the feeding of 70 ccm. of methyl alcohol in fourteen days produced sight disturbances noticeable on the second day. The hens lost sight rapidly and died within a few days. A longer period was required to produce blindness in the rabbits.[1212]

The following cases show the effects of inhalation:[1213]

Case 1: A worker died on the fourth day after varnishing beer vats. He suffered from headaches, delirium, blindness, stupor, and convulsions. The diagnosis was wood alcohol poisoning.

Cases 2 and 3: Both cases died from inhalation while varnishing beer vats. The varnish contained wood alcohol.

Cases 4, 5 and 6: Varnishing beer vats, worked two days, and one became ill with nausea and dizziness, and finally lost his sight.

Cases 10 and 11: Misses E. W. and L. K. worked at pencil varnishing. They suffered from headache, dizziness, and nausea followed by blurred vision, all of which occurred twice daily while at work. Both claimed that in the open air the symptoms vanished. The constant attacks caused a gradual impairment of vision.

Case 12: Was blinded by use of wood alcohol during the process of work at copper refining.

Loewy and Von der Heide state that if the air that is breathed contains 0.2% of methyl alcohol, it has a toxic effect upon animals when inhaled for a sufficiently long period.[1214] There has been found 0.05% to 0.6% in workrooms. It is recommended that the concentration be kept below one part per million. Eisenberg exposed animals to one ounce of methyl alcohol soaked up by cotton suspended in the ceiling of the ani-

1211. BIRCH-HIRSCHFELD: *Arch. f. Ophth.*, 54:68, 1902.
1212. BIRCH-HIRSCHFELD: *Klin. Monatsbl. f. Augenh.*, 38:682, 1900.
1213. Bull. State of New York Dept. of Labor, No. 86.
1214. LOEWY and VON DER HEIDE: *Bull. No.* 15, 1930.

mal cages for periods varying from fifteen to sixty minutes three times daily.[1215] Three animals died under these conditions within ten days. The quantity of exposure was then reduced to one-half the amount. No other animals died, but apparently they were sacrificed and the tissues of all were examined. Koller reports a case of complete blindness with recovery of vision, following the drinking of whiskey containing 34% methyl alcohol.[1216] The actual amount of methyl alcohol ingested was about 20 cc. Langgaard believes that small repeated doses of methyl alcohol are more toxic than ethyl alcohol.[1217] Lewin demonstrated the toxicity of methyl alcohol both by inhalation and ingestion through the stomach.[1218]

Schweinitz states that blindness and atrophy of the disc have followed the ingestion of two to five drams (7.8 to 19.4 gm.) while recovery after drinking one-half pint (236 cc.) of this liquor has been observed.[1219] Tyson and Schoenberg demonstrated experimentally the toxic influence of methyl alcohol by inhalation.[1220] They also state that during 1912 the literature showed 100 cases of amblyopia and death from inhalation of methyl alcohol, which is only a small per cent of the actual cases. Tyson refers to thirteen cases of blindness from inhalation and reports three new cases in varnishers.[1221]

Toxicity: Sklianskaya, Urieva, and Mashbitz[1222] found that acetone depresses the cardiac activity more powerfully than methyl alcohol in the entrance phase. The recovery of cardiac function occurs much better after acetone than after methyl alcohol. So far as the setting in of narcosis is concerned, the toxicity of acetone is greater than that of methyl alcohol. With the increase of low concentrations the toxicity of acetone and methyl alcohol increases quickly and sharply; with

1215. EISENBERG, A. L.: *Am. J. Pub. Health,* 7:765, 1917.

1216. KOLLER, C.: *Med. Rec.,* 68:10, 1905.

1217. LANGGAARD, A.: *Berl. klin. Wchnschr.,* 49:1704, 1913.

1218. LEWIN, L.: *Chem. Centr.-Bl.,* 1:672, 1911; *Apoth.-Ztg.,* 26: 545, 1911.

1219. SCHWEINITZ, G. E.: Diseases of the Eye, 10th ed., 1580, 1924; *Ophth. Rec.,* 10:289, 1901.

1220. TYSON, H. H., and SCHOENBERG, M. J.: *J.A.M.A.,* 63:915, 1914; *Chem. Abst.,* 9:2942, 1915.

1221. TYSON, H. H.: *Zentralbl. f. Biochem. u. Biophys.,* 15:205, 1912.

1222. SKLIANSKAYA, R. M., URIEVA, F. E., and MASHBITZ, L. M.: *J. Indust. Hyg.,* 18:106, 117, 1936.

higher concentrations the toxicity remains about uniform. According to the mortality of white mice, methyl alcohol is considerably more toxic than acetone or its mixtures, the toxicity of the latter being approximately that of acetone. The comparative toxicity of these solvents is different, depending upon whether the criterion accepted is setting in of narcosis or mortality of mice. With a mortality of white mice as a criterion, methyl alcohol is more toxic than acetone. In the combined action of mixtures of acetone and methyl alcohol, the action of acetone predominates in high concentrations, and that of methyl alcohol in low concentrations

Macht states: "The toxicity of the normal alcohols, methyl alcohol, ethyl alcohol, butyl alcohol, and amyl alcohol, increases with their place in the aliphatic series, as indicated by the lethal dosage for cats, and by their effects on isolated frog's heart and plain muscle preparations. The secondary propyl, butyl and amyl alcohols were found to be less toxic than the corresponding primary alcohols. In discussing the toxicity of alcohols a distinction should be made between the acute or immediate, and the secondary or remote effects of the drugs, as it is well illustrated in the studies on methyl alcohol and $PhCH_2OH$.[1223]

Methyl alcohol is distinctly toxic when ingested by rabbits, and possesses a toxicity greater than that of ethyl alcohol in equal doses.[1224]

In 1926 the first synthetic methanol came from Germany. In the summer of that year, several drums of this material found their way to Buffalo, causing over twenty-five deaths. Methanol caused thirty-four deaths in New York City in October, 1928. Previously, in that year, pure methanol was used in whiskey supplied by a Baltimore druggist, causing five or six deaths.

There were thirty deaths in Illinois in 1929, traced to a methanol beverage. In April and the first half of May, 1930, autopsies in New York City showed that of thirty-seven deaths from acute alcoholism, thirty were due to methanol alone.[1225]

It has been shown from experiments on rats and dogs that the total amount of methanol absorbed through the respiratory

1223. MACHT, D. I.: Chem. Abst., 15:122, 1921.
1224. BERTARELLI, E.: Ann. d'hyg., 42:665, October, 1932.
1225. Chicago's Health, 33:24, August 19, 1930.

tract varied from 0.32 to 0.35 gm. per kilogram of body weight.

Fatal Dose: One to two ounces has proved fatal in a number of cases.[1226] The author has seen a number of cases of death occurring from three to four ounces. Ring[1227] reported death from three to five ounces. Recovery has taken place from as much as six to eight ounces, when the substance had been taken within a short time. Moulton[1228] reported a drinking bout in which five men drank about a half pint of wood alcohol each. Two died within twenty-four hours, two recovered entirely, while the fifth recovered with complete atrophy of the optic nerve of the right eye and great contraction of the field of vision of the left eye. Blindness or serious impairment of vision has been reported from 15 cc.,[1229] 20 to 23 cc.,[1230] and 60 cc. Much larger amounts have been taken without either temporary or permanent injury to the eyes. Buller and Wood concluded that if ten persons drank four ounces of methyl alcohol within three hours all would have marked abdominal distress, four would die, two of them becoming blind before death, and six would eventually recover, of whom two would be permanently blind.

Fatal Period: Two Polish women died within eighteen hours after drinking an unknown amount of wood alcohol. The wood alcohol had been cooked with coffee, with the mistaken idea that the coffee would detoxify the alcohol. Wood alcohol was found in the liver, kidneys, bowel, and urine. Death has been reported as early as one hour. The majority of the cases, however, do not die until after twenty-four hours. Death may be delayed for three or four days. I have seen several cases where the men were very sick but made a complete recovery after four days.

Treatment: The stomach should be washed out with water containing 5 gm. of sodium bicarbonate to the pint of water. Haskell, Hileman and Gardner[1231] attempted to prevent death by alkaline treatment; their results however, have not been

1226. SWADENER: *J.A.M.A.*, 60:1479, 1913; PIERCE: *Boston M. & S. J.*, 160:232, 1909.

1227. RING: *Tr. Am. Ophth. Soc.*, 9:529, 1902.

1228. MOULTON: *Ophth. Rec.*, 8:335, 1899.

1229. RAUB: *Ophth. Rec.*, 8:169, 1899; BURNETT: Loc. cit.; BULLER and WOOD: *J.A.M.A.*, 43:972, 1904 (also pp. 1058, 1117, 1213, and 1289).

1230. BULLER: *Montreal M. J.*, 33:29, 1904 (two cases); KOLLER: *Med. Rec.*, 49:10, 1905.

1231. HASKELL, HILEMAN, and GARDNER: *Arch. Int. Med.*, 27:71, 1921.

very encouraging. Morphine may be given to relieve pain. Stimulants, such as camphor, caffeine, and strychnine, may be given.

Postmortem Appearances: Grossly there is nothing characteristic about the organs after death by wood alcohol poisoning. There is hyperemia of the mucous membrane of the stomach and duodenum, and usually small hemorrhages; the lungs are hyperemic and edematous; edema and congestion of the brain and meninges with increase in the cerebrospinal fluid are reported; the mucosa of the bladder was found hyperemic in a few cases.

Burhans described the postmortems of eleven cases.[1232] External examination revealed two types of bodies, the flaccid of which there were nine, and the spastic of which there were two. The cyanosis was marked, the color being almost indigo blue. The bodies were hyperextended, the arms flexed at the elbows, the thighs flexed on the abdomen and the legs on the thighs. The bladder and rectum had emptied. The skin was pink. Only the brain showed any gross pathological change. There was an increased amount of cerebrospinal fluid and a mild degree of edema of the brain. The optic nerves all showed edema, and those of the individual who had been sick for four days had undergone cloudy swelling and marked degeneration. Gross examination found the heart and lungs characterized in the spastic cases by a contraction of the heart until it was half the normal size. The lungs were completely filled with air, the individual dying at the end of an inspiratory breath. In the flaccid cases the heart, particularly the right side, was dilated. The lungs were congested and edematous, the dependent portions being full of fluid. The mucosa of the esophagus and stomach showed varying degrees of pathology. The mucosa of the stomach of the individual who died twelve hours after drinking the methyl alcohol, was only mildly congested. In one individual who had been sick three days the esophageal mucosa and mucosa of the stomach at the esophageal opening and in the prepyloric area was ulcerated and eroded. There was congestion of the liver in every case. Microscopically there was degeneration of the liver cells. In an individual who lived four days there was an acute yellow atrophy. The pancreas showed the un-

1232. BURHANS, E. C.: *Illinois M. J.*, 58:260, 1930.

usual feature of hemorrhagic pancreatitis. The kidneys of all evidenced degeneration to a greater or lesser degree.

MacDonald reports the pathology of methyl alcohol amblyopia.[1233] The epithelium was missing over a considerable portion of the cornea. The iris showed cystic degeneration of the pigmented epithelial layer. The ciliary body showed moderate round-cell infiltration. The vessels were congested. In one case examined by MacDonald the ganglion cells were decreased in number and degenerated, and cystic spaces were seen throughout the layer. The nerve fiber layer showed considerable distortion; particularly in the region of the disc. The pigmented epithelium of the retina showed migration of the pigment granules. The vessels of the choroid were markedly congested. He believes that the changes which occur later, and which result in optic atrophy, are due to ascending degeneration of the nerve fiber following upon the damage to the ganglion cell.

Isolation: Methyl alcohol will be found in the acid distillation, previously described.

Detection: Deniges' Test:[1234] To 1 cc. of the distillate add 5 cc. of 1% permanganate and 0.2 cc. of concentrated sulphuric acid. Mix and after two or three minutes decolorize by the addition of 1 cc. of 8% solution of oxalic acid. Allow to stand and add 1 cc. more of sulphuric acid. Shake until completely decolorized. Upon addition of 5 cc. of a colorless fuchsine solution, after standing one minute, a characteristic violet color will appear (0.1% will give the color).

Trillat Method:[1235] To 50 cc. of the sample add 50 cc. of water and 8 gm. of lime, and fractionate by the aid of Glinsky bulb tubes. Dilute the first 15 cc. of the distillate to 150 cc., mix with 15 gm. of potassium dichromate and 70 cc. of dilute sulphuric acid (one to five), and allow to stand for an hour with occasional shaking. Distill, reject the first 25 cc., and collect 100 cc. Mix 50 cc. of the distillate with 1 cc. of redistilled dimethylaniline, transfer to a stout tightly stoppered flask, and keep on a bath at 70° to 80° C. for three hours, with occasional shaking. Make distinctly alkaline with sodium hydroxide solution and distill off the excess of dimethylaniline,

1233. MacDonald, A. E.: 13th Meet. Ophth., Amsterdam, 1929.
1234. Deniges: *Chem. Centralbl.,* 1:1992, 1910.
1235. Abst. *Analyst.,* 24:13, 211, 1899.

stopping the distillation when 25 cc. have passed over. Acidify the residue in the flask with acetic acid, shake, and test a few cc. by adding four or five drops of a 1% suspension of lead dioxide. If methyl alcohol is present, there occurs a blue coloration which is increased by boiling. Ethyl alcohol thus treated yields a blue coloration which changes immediately to green, later to yellow, and becomes colorless when boiled.

Riche and Bardy Method: This method depends on the formation of methylaniline violet. It is conducted as follows: "Place 10 cc. of the sample previously redistilled over potassium carbonate if necessary, in a small flask with 15 gm. of iodine and 2 gm. of red phosphorus. Keep in ice water for ten to fifteen minutes or until action has ceased. Distill, on a water-bath, into about 30 cc. of water (methyl and ethyl iodides formed). Wash with dilute alkali to eliminate free iodine. Separate the heavy oily liquid that settles, and transfer to a flask containing 5 cc. of aniline. If the action is too violent, place the flask in cold water; if too slow, stimulate by gently warming the flask. After an hour boil the product with water, cool, and add about 20 cc. of 15% sodium hydroxide solution; when the bases rise to the top as an oily layer, fill the flask to the neck with water and draw them off with a pipet. Oxidize 1 cc. of the oily liquid by adding 10 gm. of a mixture of 100 parts of clean sand, two of common salt, and three of cupric nitrate; mix thoroughly; transfer to a glass tube; and heat to 90° C. for eight to ten hours. Exhaust the product with warm alcohol, filter, and dilute to 100 cc. with alcohol. If the sample is free from methyl alcohol the liquid has a red tint, but in the presence of 1% of methyl alcohol it has a distinct violet shade; with 2.5% the shade is very distinct and still more so with 5%. To detect more minute quantities of methyl alcohol, dilute 5 cc. of the colored liquid to 100 cc. with water and dilute 5 cc. of this again to 400 cc. Heat the liquid thus obtained in a porcelain dish and immerse in it a fragment of white merino wool (free from sulphur) for thirty minutes. If the alcohol is pure the wool will remain white, but if methyl alcohol is present the fiber will become violet, the depth of tint giving a fairly approximate indication of the proportion of methyl alcohol." In the presence of ethyl alcohol the solution becomes slightly red.

Immersion Refractometer Method: "Determine by the

immersion refractometer at 20° C. the refraction of the distillate obtained in the determination of alcohol. If the refraction shows the percentage of alcohol agreeing with that obtained from the specific gravity, it may be assumed that no methyl alcohol is present. If, however, there is an appreciable quantity of methyl alcohol, the low refractometer reading will at once indicate the fact. If the absence from the solution of refractive substances other than water and the alcohols is assured, this difference in refraction is conclusive of the presence of methyl alcohol. The addition of methyl alcohol to ethyl alcohol decreases the refraction in direct proportion to the quantity present; hence the quantitative calculation is made readily by interpolation of the figures for pure ethyl and methyl alcohol of the same alcoholic strength as the sample being used."[1236]

Example: "The distillate has a specific gravity of 0.97080, corresponding to 18.38% alcohol by weight, and has a refraction of 35.8 at 20° C. by the immersion refractometer; in interpolation in the refractometer table readings of ethyl and methyl alcohol corresponding to 18.38% alcohol are 47.3 and 25.4, respectively, the difference being 21.9; 47.3 — 35.8 = 11.5; (11.5 ÷ 21.9) 100 = 52.5, showing that 52.5% of the total alcohol present is methyl alcohol."

Quantitative Determination: In a personal communication Harger has submitted a modified Wright-Elvove test, which in turn is based upon that of Deniges' test, which is a short cut for determining the presence of methyl alcohol in urine, spinal fluid, and protein-free filtrate without distillation. (I prefer to make all tests upon the distillates.) Harger recommends this procedure: Place 2 cc. of urine in a test-tube. Add to this one drop of 95% ethyl alcohol followed by 1 cc. of a permanganate solution. Dissolve 3 gm. of potassium permanganate in 100 cc. of water containing 15 cc. of phosphoric acid (ortho, syrupy). Mix and allow to stand for ten minutes. At the end of this time, decolorize the excess of permanganate by adding 1 cc. of the oxalic acid solution. (Oxalic acid: Slowly pour 50 cc. of concentrated sulphuric acid into 62 cc. of water. Cool and dissolve in the solution 5 gm. of oxalic acid.) After about one minute, the solution should be perfectly clear. Now

1236. *J. Am. Chem. Soc.*, 27:964, 1905; also Methods of Analysis, Association of Official Agricultural Chemists, 4th ed., **578, 1935.**

add 2 cc. of Schiff's reagent and mix well. (Schiff's reagent can be used in the Deniges' method as above described.) Dissolve 0.2 gm. of rosaniline (fuchsin) in 120 cc. of hot water, cool, and add this to a solution of 2 gm. of sodium bisulphite in 20 cc. of water. Now add 2 cc. of concentrated hydrochloric acid and dilute to 200 cc. This reagent becomes colorless or light brown in about an hour. If placed in a glass-stoppered bottle containing very little air, it will keep for several months. (However, it becomes less sensitive with age, and to obtain best results one should use a solution not more than a month old.) If methyl alcohol is present, the fluid will assume a violet or pink color within an hour. If much methyl alcohol is present, the solution may become a violet or pink within ten minutes. If no color develops within two hours, toxic quantities of methyl alcohol are not present.

For the quantitative determination prepare a series of standards in 2 cc. of water containing 0.2 to 1.0 mg. of methanol. Run these simultaneously with the unknown according to the method above outlined and compare with a colorimeter. If the unknown gives a color much stronger than that of the highest standard, it should be diluted until it gives a color within the range of the standards used. With protein-free filtrates or distillates from urine, blood, or tissues, the error by this method should not exceed 5%. To determine whether all of the alcohol present is methanol, a portion of the distillate may be run by the dichromate method.[1237] For the simultaneous determination of methanol and ethanol in biological material see Russell and Thienes.[1237] This method has been modified and used in Harger's laboratory, as follows: Prepare a volatile distillate in the usual manner using 100 gm. of tissue, distilling until 100 cc. of distillate have been obtained.

Removal of Formaldehyde: Weigh out 1 gm. of pyrogallol and place this in a small funnel which is supported in the neck of a 100-cc. glass-stoppered bottle. Measure out 20 cc. of the tissue distillate and introduce this into the bottle through the funnel so that it washes the pyrogallol into the bottle. Wash into the bottle any liquid adhering to the funnel by means of 2 cc. of water. Now add 5 cc. of concentrated sulphuric acid to the contents of the bottle. Stopper, and

1237. HARGER, R. N.: *J. Lab. & Clin. Med.,* 20:746, 1935. RUSSELL and THIENES: *Proc. Soc. Exper. Biol. & Med.,* 30:23, 1932.

shake the bottle vigorously, and allow it to stand for ten minutes. At the end of this time, transfer the contents of the bottle to a small distilling flask and rinse out the bottle with two 2-cc. portions of water, adding the rinsing to the distilling flask. Distill until about 12 cc. of distillate have collected. Disconnect the distilling flask and wash out the condenser, catching the washings in the receiving flask. Make the distillate up to a convenient volume and use an aliquot of this for the determination of methanol and ethanol.

Simultaneous Determination of Methanol and Ethanol: The apparatus consists of a reaction tube connected to a train of tubes containing in turn concentrated sulphuric acid, dehydrite, ascarite, and dehydrite. The reaction tube is made of pyrex with inside dimensions approximately ten and a half inches by one and five-eighths inches, which is closed by a two-hole rubber stopper carrying a bubbler tube which reaches almost to the bottom of the pyrex tube, the upper end of the bubbler tube expanding to a diameter of about one-third inch, which serves as a funnel for introducing fluids into the tube. The other hole of the rubber stopper carries an outlet tube. If desired, this part of the apparatus may be made entirely of glass, thus avoiding the possibility of reagents coming in contact with the rubber stopper. However, we have run numerous analyses with the tube closed by means of a rubber stopper and have not observed any errors due to this arrangement. The outlet tube is connected in turn with an all-glass gas washing tube which contains concentrated sulphuric acid, then with a tube containing dehydrite, which in turn is connected with an ascarite tube which is followed by a second dehydrite tube. Ascarite, as purchased, soon becomes too dry to efficiently absorb carbon dioxide. This ascarite should be subjected to a preliminary moistening process by drawing air through it which is partially charged with water vapor by being passed through the sulphuric acid of specific gravity about 1.5. Water should not be used, as this tends to clog the ascarite at the end of the tube.

Place in the reaction tube exactly 15 cc. of 2% potassium bichromate solution, followed by 30 cc. of concentrated sulphuric acid. Mix the two fluids and place the tube in a beaker of ice water. During this preliminary aeration, the ascarite tube and dehydrite tube following it should not be placed in the train. The intake of the bubbler tube should be connected to a guard tube containing ordinary soda lime or ascarite. After three or four minutes of aeration, the ascarite tube and the dehydrite tube following it should be connected and a measured portion of the solution to be analyzed introduced through the bubbler tube into the reaction tube, followed by enough water to make a total of 15 cc. The bichromate used will easily oxidize 50 mg. of ethanol or 25 mg. of methanol or a corresponding mixture of the two alcohols, leaving a sufficient excess of the bichromate to insure completion of the reaction. Reconnect the guard tube to the bubbler inlet, mix the contents by gently shaking and forcing the liquid to the bottom of the bubbler tube by blowing into the guard tube. Immerse the reaction tube in vigorously boiling water for a period of ten minutes. At the end of this time remove the boiling water-bath and substitute an ice water-bath. Cool for five minutes. During this fifteen-minute period, the air current should be discontinued, leaving the outlet open to take care of fluctuation in volume. Now draw a current of air through the apparatus for ten minutes. The air current should be slow for the first two minutes, after which it may be increased to the limit of the capacity of the sulphuric acid gas washing tube. The increase in weight in the ascarite tube and the dehydrite tube following it represents the carbon dioxide formed from the methanol. From this figure one should subtract a blank which varies as follows with the ethanol oxidized:

No ethanol, subtract 0.3 mg.

1 to 10 mg. of ethanol, subtract 0.6 mg.

10 to 20 mg. of ethanol, subtract 0.8 mg.

20 to 40 mg. of ethanol, subtract 1.2 mg.

This blank is due to a slight amount of carbon dioxide in the sample analyzed, which, together with the wash water, measures 15 cc., and also to the fact that about 1% of the ethanol is oxidized to carbon dioxide. To calculate the methanol, multiply the corrected weight of carbon dioxide by 0.727.

Transfer the contents of the reaction tube to a 250-cc. volumetric flask and add distilled water to make up the mark. Transfer the contents of this flask to a 700-cc. flask which is connected to a condenser by means of a Kjeldahl connecting bulb. Distill until exactly 100 cc. of distillate have been collected. Titrate the distillate with N/20 NaOH, using phenol-

phthalein as the indicator.   The distillate contains 47% of the
acetic acid formed.   From the titration figure subtract a blank
of 0.15 cc., this blank not being affected by the presence of
methanol in the sample.   To calculate for ethanol, multiply the
corrected volume of N/20 NaOH by 0.489 (100/47 x 2/3) which
gives the mg. of ethanol in the sample used.   Table **XLIX**
shows typical results with the method, using a mixture of
ethanol and methanol the composition of which was unknown
to the analyst.

TABLE XLIX

SIMULTANEOUS DETERMINATION OF METHANOL
AND ETHANOL

Sample	ETHANOL Mg. per cc.		METHANOL Mg. per cc.	
Number	Used	Found	Used	Found
1.	2.08	2.17	0.79	0.78
1.	2.08	2.20	0.79	0.71
2.	1.46	1.51	1.63	1.56
2.	1.46	1.61	1.63	1.63
3.	2.01	2.15	1.35	1.24
3.	2.01	2.27	1.35	1.26
4.	4.68	4.73	0.00	0.11
4.	4.68	4.71	0.00	0.03
5.	2.93	3.00	0.24	0.45
5.	2.93	3.04	0.24	0.34
6.	1.65	1.56	0.74	0.79
7.	0.00	0.08	2.36	2.34
7.	0.00	0.03	2.36	2.25
7.	0.00	0.02	2.36	2.28
8.	0.87	0.94	1.38	1.29
8.	0.87	0.94	1.38	1.29
9.	1.96	2.05	1.38	1.34
9.	1.96	spilled	1.38	1.31
10.	2.30	2.31	0.93	0.91

To check the results calculated from the carbon dioxide
and acetic acid formed, one may determine the excess of
bichromate by a suitable method to see if the bichromate
consumed corresponds to the alcohols found.   One mg. of
ethanol should consume 4.24 mg. of bichromate, and one mg.
of methanol 9.14 mg. of bichromate.   In the foregoing table
there was an agreement between the bichromate consumed
and the alcohol present.

In order to determine the volume of solution to place in the reaction tube, one may make a preliminary test upon the reducing power of this solution by placing in a test-tube 1 cc. of the 2% bichromate solution and 4 cc. of water, followed by 5 cc. of concentrated sulphuric acid. Mix well and to the resulting hot solution slowly add, with stirring, the solution to be tested until the yellow bichromate is replaced by green. About ten times this volume of solution is the proper sample to take, provided its volume does not exceed 15 cc.

Micro-Method:[1238] Compare with standard tubes containing not over 1 cc. of standard methanol. It is best to use only 2 cc. of the sample solution, adding 0.5 cc. of 4% ethyl alcohol and sufficient water to make 4 cc. Approximate readings may be made in thirty minutes, precise ones after one hour, but best under two hours for the color fades later. Do not make any readings after this time. The limit of detection is 0.2 cc. of the standard 0.04% methanol.

Atkinson found allyl alcohol to the extent of 0.5% in one sample of chemically pure methyl alcohol. The toxicity of it is 150 times that of methyl alcohol.[1239]

Formic acid is a normal and fairly constant constituent of human urine. Its detection on a qualitative basis in urine is not proof of methyl alcohol poisoning. Quantitative tests are requisite, 1 gm. or more per day being essential.[1240]

Fellenberg states that methyl alcohol in urine is determined by a modification of Deniges' method.[1240] On a pectin-free diet very small amounts of methyl alcohol occur in the urine (about 0.4 to 1.0 mg. per 750 grains), and on a fast it is reduced to one-half. A diet rich in pectin whether raw, containing pectase, or cooked and pectase-free, makes little difference in the methyl alcohol secretion.

Levy reports that methyl alcohol may be found in the urine, blood, and cadavers after six months' burial.[1241]

1238. CHAPIN, R. M.: *J. Indust. & Eng. Chem.*, 13:943, June, 1921.
1239. ATKINSON, H. V.: *J. Pharm.*, 25:144, 1925; *Chem. Abst.*, 19: 3126, 1925.
1240. AUTHENRIETH, W.: *J. Am. Chem. Soc.*, 118:909, 1920. See also JANSCH, H.: *Vrtljschr. f. gerichtl. Med., Berl., Sanitatswesen.*, 62:3, 1921. And FELLENBERG, V. T.: *Mitt. a. d. Geb. d. Lebensmittelunt. u. Hyg.*, 6:24, 1915; *Chem. Abst.*, 9:2262, 1915.
1241. LEVY, L.: *Berl. klin. Wchnschr.;* abst. *J.A.M.A.*, 3:2, 1912. See GETTLER, A. O.: *J. Biol. Chem.*, 42:311, 1920, for an excellent and extensive study of methods for detection of methyl alcohol.

ETHYL ALCOHOL*

F ROM the earliest records of the development of human society we find reports of the physiological effects of fermented beverages. Until comparatively recent times, these were preparations of moderate alcohol content produced by the natural fermentation of mixtures containing starches and sugars. Inasmuch as the fermenting activity of most yeasts is inhibited in solutions containing 10% to 12% of alcohol, the alcoholic strength of these beverages was necessarily low. With the discovery of distillation methods, it was soon learned from these fermented mixtures of comparatively weak intoxicating power could be distilled a fluid of very great potency. As a result we are now confronted with toxicological problems arising from these two classes of beverages: **fermented** and **distilled.** The average alcohol content of the common alcoholic beverages is as follows:

Fermented Liquors
Beers ....4 to 6% by volume.
Ales ....5 to 8%.
Wines (natural) ....5 to 16%. (These may be "fortified" to an alcoholic content of 16 to 20% by the addition of alcohol.)

Distilled Liquors
Gin ....35 to 45%.
Whiskeys and
Brandies ....40 to 55%.

In medical practice, the U. S. Pharmacopeia recognizes the following:

Alcohol dehydratum—Not less than 99% by weight.

Alcohol—Not less than 92.3% by weight (or 94.9% by volume).

Alcohol dilutum—41.5% by weight (49% by volume).

Spiritus frumenti (whiskey)—47% by volume.

Spiritus vini vitis (brandy)—48 to 54% by volume.

In addition to these, there is easy access to many other preparations which contain sufficient concentrations of ethyl alcohol to be toxicologically significant. Among these are patent medicines (many of which owe their chief pharmacological activity to their appreciable alcohol content), flavoring

* By CLARENCE W. MUEHLBERGER, PH.D., Chicago.

extracts,[1242] hair tonics, toilet waters, and "canned heat" (denatured alcohol solidified to a gel by means of a small amount of cellulose nitrate).

Denatured alcohol is the ordinary 95% alcohol of commerce which has been rendered unpalatable by the addition of various substances of unpleasant taste or odor. Alcohol so denatured is exempt from the taxes which are imposed upon alcohol used for beverage purposes. Except for special purposes, denatured alcohol is so treated as to render its solutions exceedingly unpleasant and even nauseating if used for beverage purposes. This is designated as **completely denatured** alcohol. Formerly this denaturing was accomplished by the addition of 5% crude wood distillation spirit (methyl alcohol) to 95% of commercial ethyl alcohol. During the Prohibition era, a large number of deaths following the drinking of denatured alcohol solutions were attributed to this 5% of methyl alcohol, and it was subsequently replaced by various oxidized petroleum derivatives which were exceedingly unpleasant in both odor and taste. It seems highly improbable that the small amount (5%) of methyl alcohol in the earlier "denatured" formula was of any material toxicological significance.[1243]

The illicit "bootleg" distilled liquors of the Prohibition era were also reputed to be exceedingly dangerous, and numerous deaths were reported, particularly from the Atlantic Coast, as a result of "poison moonshine." While it is true that these crude liquors did contain greater amounts of fusel oils, esters, and aldehydes than are ordinarily found in properly rectified liquors, careful investigations[1244] have indicated that the really toxic agent of these preparations was simply ethyl alcohol. MacNider[1245] observed extensive albuminuria in animals fol-

1242. For cases of epidemic poisoning from Jamaica ("Jake") ginger during the latter part of the prohibition era, see SMITH, M. I., ELVOVE, W. H., and FRAZIER, W. H.: "The Pharmacological Action of Certain Phenol Esters with Special Reference to the Etiology of so-called Ginger Paralysis," U. S. Pub. Health Reports, 45:2509, 1930.

1243. Unpublished work by LOEVENHART and KEHR: University of Wisconsin, 1926, and personal communication of W. P. YANT, U. S. Bureau of Mines, Exper. Sta., Pittsburgh, 1935.

1244. MCNALLY, W. D.: J.A.M.A., 83:1680, 1924; GERTY: Am. J. Pub. Health, 14:603, 1924; BIGELOW, LYTHGOE, and HUNT: New England J. Med., 198:227, 1928; HOWARD: New England J. Med., 200:933, 1929.

1245. MACNIDER: J. Pharmacol. & Exper. Therap., 26:97, 1925.

lowing the administration of so-called "moonshine" liquors. He attributed this to their high content of aldehydes.

It should be noted that some alcoholic liquors owe at least a part of their toxic action to substances other than alcohol. Thus the hallucinations and epileptiform attacks so frequently observed in the chronic drinkers of absinthe are probably referable to the oil of wormwood which it contains.

Some idea of the extent of fatal alcoholism may be obtained from McNally's report[1246] of the number of cases investigated by the Coroner of Cook County (Illinois) in which the diagnosis was made either upon the history of alcoholism or by chemical analysis of the vital organs. A more recent report by Leary[1247] gives similar figures for the Southern Medical Examiner's District of Suffolk County, Massachusetts.

TABLE L
DEATHS DUE TO ALCOHOL

Year	Alcoholism Cook County, Illinois. (Total population about 4 million)	Suffolk County, Massachusetts (Total population about 600,000)
1910	215	......
1911	76	......
1912	108	......
1913	66	123
1914	91	117
1915	110	112
1916	87	152
1917	88	146
1918	46	55
1919	55	82
1920	41	25
1921	97	57
1922	158	85
1923	180	171
1924		198
1925		220
1926		171
1927		200
1928		191
1929		188
1930		148
1931		182
1932		168
1933		182
1934		279
1935*		300

(Note: the years 1920–1932 are bracketed in the margin with the word "PROHIBITION".)

* LEARY, private communication.

1246. McNALLY, W. D.:   *J.A.M.A.*, 83:1680, 1924.
1247. LEARY: *New England J. Med.*, 214:15, 1935.

Leary points out the general downward trend of temperance, especially during the war period (1917-1920) when it was quite unfashionable and unpatriotic to become drunk; the increase in alcoholism during the early part of the Prohibition era, followed by an additional sharp rise after the repeal of the 18th Amendment. In all probability, these sharp rises are largely due to the increase in the consumption of stronger (distilled) alcoholic liquors.

With the extremely widespread use of alcoholic beverages throughout the world, it is not surprising to find that ethyl alcohol looms as one of our very important toxic substances. Deaths attributed to alcoholism, both acute and chronic, reach a very high figure, although the reliability of such statistics is problematical. It is exceedingly difficult to fairly differentiate cases of alcoholism from other pathological conditions which may be concomitant factors materially contributing to the death of the individual. Obviously such pathological conditions can only be discovered by a complete necropsy; in the absence of a necropsy they are largely conjectural. This is particularly true in deaths attributed to chronic alcoholism. In **acute** alcoholism, it is probable that very few fatal cases result from ethyl alcohol poisoning uncomplicated by other pathologic factors. Unless a person is drinking very strong alcoholic liquor in large quantities and at a very rapid rate (as in drinking a quart of whiskey on a wager) the body furnishes its own protective mechanism. With any drinking at a reasonably slow rate, the individual passes into a stuporous condition in which he is physically unable to imbibe further. This condition of stupor or mild coma leaves a considerable margin of safety below a fatal alcoholic depression. So unless there is some other complicating pathological factor (such as serious cardio-circulatory disease) cessation of alcohol intake is followed by gradual recovery.

Physical Properties: Pure ethyl alcohol is a clear, colorless, mobile fluid having a specific gravity of 0.7939 (at 60° F. or 15.6° C.), a boiling point of 78.3° C., and a freezing point of —130°C. It has a characteristic odor and a sharp burning taste. It is very hygroscopic and readily withdraws water from tissues. When its aqueous solutions are distilled, the alcohol is concentrated in the low-boiling distillate and may be so concentrated up to about 95% strength. At this concentration a constant-boiling mixture (boiling point=78.1° C.) is formed. This constant boiling mixture has a specific gravity of .8141 at 15.6° C. Alcohol solutions of high concentration have very excellent solvent properties which are not only utilized in the manufacture of pharmaceutical preparations, but also in the arts and in chemical industries. Strong alcohol solutions are readily flammable and burn with a faint bluish flame. This combustion involves the oxidation of the alcohol to carbon dioxide and water. Chemical oxidizing agents oxidize alcohol readily, first to acetaldehyde and then progressively to acetic acid. Very powerful oxidizing agents oxidize alcohol partially to carbon dioxide. Dehydration, either by very active chemical dehydrating agents or by catalytic means, decomposes alcohol into ethylene and water.

Pharmacologic Action: (Space will only permit a casual discussion of the pharmacologic aspects of alcohol action. For a more complete discussion, the reader is referred to "Alcohol and Man," an excellent symposium on various phases of alcohol action, edited by Haven Emerson and published in New York by MacMillan (451 pages) in 1932.)

Alcohol is definitely poisonous to all forms of life. It acts as a protein precipitant in higher concentrations. Alcohol solutions are toxic to bacteria, the maximum bactericidal action occurring at approximately 70% alcohol concentration. Concentrations either higher or lower than 70% are definitely lower in antiseptic value. The mild local irritant action of alcohol is probably due to its dehydrating effect and its ability to precipitate proteins. Concentrations of greater than 50% alcohol are very painful if injected subcutaneously or intramuscularly. If injection is made near a nerve, strong alcohol solutions produce paralysis and sometimes destroy the nerves. Alcohol may be considered to be a food in the sense that it furnishes a readily available energy supply. However, there are so many other less objectionable sources of energy available that its use as a food is rarely indicated.

Alcohol is rapidly absorbed from the gastro-intestinal tract, from all mucous surface, and from the lungs. It is doubtful if any absorption takes place through the intact skin. When taken by mouth, alcohol is absorbed into the blood stream at a very rapid rate. The rate of this absorption depends, of course, upon the concentration of alcohol consumed as well as upon the quantity and nature of the material already in the stomach.[1248] Harger's experiments on fasting dogs[1248] have shown that at the end of the first half hour 58% of the ingested alcohol was absorbed from the gastro-intestinal tract; at the end of the first hour 88% and at the end of one and a half hours 93% had been absorbed. The absorbed alcohol is carried by the blood to all parts of the body and in the post-absorptive period (after the first hour following ingestion) is fairly equally distributed in the watery tissues of the body **approximately** in the same ratio as their water content. Thus one finds that the alcohol content of materials rich in water such as urine, saliva, or blood is very high, whereas the alcohol content of muscle is comparatively low. As one might expect from their water content, blood corpuscles have a lower alcohol concentration than blood plasma. The alcohol content of blood plasma is 10% to 20% higher than that of whole blood and in the post-absorptive period approaches height of the urine alcohol.[1249] The secreted cerebrospinal fluid has approximately the same alcohol content as the circulating blood; however, because of its very slow downward movement, there is a considerable lag in the change of lumbar fluid alcohol as compared with blood alcohol.[1250]

Following absorption alcohol is detoxified, largely by oxidation to carbon dioxide and water,[1251] but to a minor extent

1248. SOUTHGATE, H. W.: "The Effect of Alcohol, Under Varying Conditions of Diet, on Man and Animals, with Some Observations on the Fate of Alcohol in the Body," *Biochem. J.*, 19:737, 1925. HARGER, R. N., and HULPIEU, H. R.: "Extent of Absorption of Alcohol at Various Intervals After Oral Administration," *Proc. Soc. Exper. Biol. & Med.*, 32:1247, 1935.

1249. MILES, W. R.: "The Comparative Concentrations of Alcohol in the Human Blood and Urine After Intervals of Digestion," *J. Pharmacol. & Exper. Therap.*, 20:265, 1922; WIDMARK, E. M. P.: "Die theoretischen Grundlagen und die Praktische Verwendbarkeit der gerichtlichmedizinischen Alkoholbestimmung," Berlin, 1932, p. 20.

1250. ABRAMSON, L., and LINDE, P.: "Zum Ubergang des Athylalkohols in die Spinalflüssigkeit beim Menschen," *Arch. internat. de pharmacodyn. et de theráp.*, 39:325, 1930; GETTLER, A. O., and FREIREICH, A. W.: "Determination of Alcoholic Intoxication During Life by Spinal Fluid Analysis," *J. Biol. Chem.*, 92:199, 1921; NEWMAN, H. W., and MERTENS, H. G.: "Reliability of Spinal Fluid Analysis in the Diagnosis of Drunkenness," *Proc. Soc. Exper. Biol. & Med.*, 30:727, 1932-33; also *Arch. Neurol. & Psychiat.*, 30:1092, 1933.

1251. ATWATER, W. O., and BENEDICT, F. G.: "An Experimental Inquiry Regarding the Nutritive Value of Alcohol," *Mem. Nat. Acad. Sc.*, 8:231, 1902.

by excretion in the expired air and by way of kidneys. Perspiration and feces contain only traces of alcohol. As might be expected, there is a fairly constant relationship between the alcohol content of the blood and that of the expired air.[1252] Because of admixture with varying amounts of unbreathed air, the determination of the true alcohol content of exhaled air presents difficulties which have caused some workers[1253] to discard the alcohol content of exhaled air as an indication of the intensity of the pharmacological response to alcohol. Harger avoids this by determining the alcohol: CO_2 ratio in expired air and calculating the volume of the air sample from the quantity of CO_2 which it contained. By this procedure, a very satisfactory correlation between the alcohol content of blood and expired air may be obtained.

During the period of absorption of alcohol from the gastrointestinal tract, the alcohol content of the urine rises much more slowly than that of blood. However, as the absorption becomes more complete (following forty-five to sixty minutes after ingestion) the alcohol content of the urine reaches and then exceeds that of blood. In the post-absorptive period, the urine approaches blood plasma in its alcohol content which suggests that the alcohol passes through the kidneys by diffusion from the blood. During this period, the urine is definitely higher than whole blood in its alcohol content, although the ratio of the two is fairly constant.[1254] Urine contains about one-third more alcohol than the blood. The analysis of the urine contained in the bladder affords an approximate average of the alcohol concentration of the urinary output since the previous voiding. For this reason the urine alcohol does not reflect the pharmacologic intensity of alcohol action as accurately as does the blood alcohol.

In the blood there is a slight loss of alcohol as it passes from the arterial to the venous circulation. This loss is par-

1252. LILJESTRAND, G., and LINDE, P.: "Uber die Ausscheidung des Alkohols mit der Expirationsluft," Skandinav. Arch. f. Physiol., 60:273, 1930; HAGGARD, H. W., and GREENBERG, L. A.: "Studies in the Absorption, Distribution and Elimination of Ethyl Alcohol," J. Pharmacol. & Exper. Therap., 52:137, 1934; HARGER, R. N.: Unpublished material presented at A.M.A. meeting at Cleveland, Ohio, in June, 1934.

1253. SMITH, S., and STEWART, C. P.: "Diagnosis of Drunkenness from the Excretion of Alcohol," Brit. M. J., 1:87, 1932.

1254. SOUTHGATE, H. W., and CARTER, G.: "Excretion of Alcohol in the Urine as a Guide to Alcoholic Intoxication," Brit. M. J., 1:463, 1926.

ticularly great during the rapidly changing conditions of the absorptive stage.[1255]

Alcohol is oxidized in the body, particularly in the liver, but to some extent in all the tissues.[1256] Widmark[1256] attempted to express this detoxification during the post-absorptive period in a mathematical equation, as follows:

Where C_t=the alcohol concentration calculated as mg. alcohol per cc. of the blood at time$=_t$.

β=the rate of disappearance of alcohol from the bloodstream in per cent per minute (independent of concentration or quantity taken) . . . A constant for each individual and averaging 0.0025% to 0.0026% per minute.

r=saturation factor representing the ratio of the average concentration of alcohol in the entire body to concentration in the blood. A constant for each individual, averaging 0.68 for men and 0.55 for women. This is in agreement with the value of 0.62 given by Haggard and Greenberg.

p=the body weight of individual in kilograms.

A=total alcohol consumed in gm.

t=time in minutes following ingestion of alcohol.

C_0=concentration (theoretical) of alcohol in the blood stream at time of ingestion assuming absorption to be instantaneous.

Then $C_0 = \dfrac{A}{pr}$

$C_t =_0 -\beta t$ and $A = pr (C_t + \beta t)$

While these formulas enable one to **estimate** the concentration of alcohol in the blood at any particular time following ingestion of alcohol, and also to estimate the quantity of alcohol consumed, these estimates are frequently in error due to the fairly wide variability of the constants β (0.0016 to 0.0040)

1255. CARLSON, A. J., and co-workers: "Studies on the Possible Intoxicating Action of 3.2% Beer," Univ. of Chicago Press, 1934; SOUTHGATE, H. W., and CARTER, G.: see Ref. 1254; HAGGARD and GREENBERG: see Ref. 1252.

1256. PRINGSHEIM, J.: "Chemische Unterschungen über das Wesen der Alkoholtoterenz," Biochem. Ztschr., 12:143, 1908. WIDMARK, E. M. P.: "Les lois cardinales de la distribution et du metabolisme de l'alcohol ethylique dans l'organisme humaine," 1930, Lund, Sweden.

and r (0.46 to 0.90). If one has already measured these constants for an individual, the calculation may be made quite accurately. For men a slight and not entirely certain negative correlation was found between the factor r and the body weight p, but for women this value was more negative.

There is some question as to whether or not the rate of alcohol metabolism is constant and independent of the amount of alcohol taken. Mellanby's[1257] observations on humans indicate that alcohol is oxidized at a rate of about .15 gm. per kilogram body weight per hour. Haggard and Greenberg[1252] have shown that this rate of oxidation is not a constant, but that during each hour the body is capable of oxidizing about one-sixth of the absorbed alcohol remaining in it.

It is certain that the rate of detoxification is so great that after twenty-four hours, only traces of alcohol may be found in the blood and tissues, even following an acute alcoholic debauch. One may still find a fairly high concentration of alcohol in the lumbar fluid after twenty-four hours, and if the urine has not been voided for a long period of time (which is rare), it may contain considerable alcohol after twenty to twenty-four hours.

Tolerance: It is common knowledge that among humans there is not only a wide range of natural susceptibility to alcohol but also an acquired tolerance in those who have imbibed freely and frequently over a period of time. The nature of the tolerance has been the subject of considerable experimentation and much speculation, but its exact nature is still somewhat obscure. It appears that in alcohol habitues, the rate of alcohol metabolism is somewhat more rapid than in abstainers.[1258] Gettler's experiments on dogs tend to bear out his contention, although his selection of control animals was unfortunate. Likewise a single experiment by Turner[1258] also supports this view. Newman and Cutting, experimenting on three dogs, were unable to discover any significant change in alcohol metabolism

1257. MELLANBY, E.: Med. Research Com., Special Rp. No. 31, London, 1919.

1258. BOGEN, E.: *California & West. Med.,* 44:262, 1926; PRINGSHEIM, J.: see Ref. 1256 (on animals); SCHWEIZHEIMER, W.: "Der Alkohlogehalt des Blutes unter Vereschiedenen Bedingungen," (in humans), *Deutsches Arch. f. klin. Med.,* 109:271, 1913. GETTLER, A. O., and FREIREICH, A. W.: "The Nature of Alcohol Tolerance," *Am. J. Surg.,* 27: 328, 1935. TURNER, R. G.: "Blood Alcohol and Its Relation to Intoxication," *J. Pharmacol. & Exper. Therap.,* 44:305, 1932.

when these animals were habituated to alcohol.[1259] It is possible that their negative results were due to the comparatively short period of habituation of their animals.

As to whether habitual drunkards absorb alcohol more rapidly or more slowly than abstainers, there is very little agreement. The differences, if any, appear to be slight. Apart from differences in rates of absorption and detoxification, the only apparent explanation of the tolerance is due to an acquired resistance of the body tissues in withstanding the effects of alcohol. There is no direct evidence of this whatsoever. As a matter of fact, within the limits of normal biologic variation which one observes with any drug (particularly those drugs which have their chief effect on the nervous system), drunkards and abstainers show approximately the same intensity of intoxication when they have the same alcohol concentration in their blood. This observation suggests that if tissue tolerance does exist, it probably is not very extensive in effect.

"Normal Alcohol": If the tissues of persons who have not partaken of any alcohol be analyzed, they will be found to contain very slight amounts of volatile reducing substances.[1260] These are equivalent to about 0.005% alcohol or less and are of no toxicological significance. Although Gettler, Niederl and Benedetti-Pichler[1261] have actually isolated alcohol from normal human tissues and identified it by means of boiling point and conversion to ethyl benzoate, ethyl iodide, etc., Harger and Goss[1262] point out that a large proportion of the volatile reducing substances as well as alcohol which previous workers were able to isolate by distilling normal tissues, were not preformed alcohol but alcohol resulting from decomposition during storage and distillation. It appears that alcohol, if it does exist as a normal constituent of the body, occurs only in exceedingly minute amounts which are of no toxicological significance.

1259. NEWMAN, H. W., and CUTTING, W. G.: "Alcohol Injected Intravenously: Effect of Habituation on Rate of Metabolism," *J. Pharmacol. & Exper. Therap.*, 55:82, 1935.

1260. See McNALLY, W. D., EMBREE, H. C., and RUST, C. A.: "Alcoholic Content of Normal Placental Tissues," *J. Biol. Chem.*, 74:219, 1927; GETTLER, A. O., and TIBER, A.: "The Alcoholic Content of the Human Brain," *Arch. Path.*, 3:218, 1927.

1261. GETTLER, A. O., NIEDERL, J. B., and BENEDETTI-PICHLER, A. A.: "The Isolation of Pure Anhydrous Ethyl Alcohol from Non-Alcoholic Human and Animal Tissues," *J. Am. Chem. Soc.*, 54:1476, 1932.

1262. HARGER, R. N., and Goss, A. L.: "The So-Called Normal Alcohol of the Body," *Am. J. Physiol.*, 112:374, 1935.

Symptoms of Acute Poisoning: In acute alcoholism, the symptoms arising from the action on higher nerve function vary over a considerable range. The other symptoms are fairly constant. Following ingestion there is a general feeling of warmth and light-headedness usually associated with a slight flushing of the skin, especially of the face. In this early stage of intoxication, the changes in behavior may vary, although the subject usually becomes much more talkative, bolder, (due to release from ordinary inhibitions), and self-confident. He is much more candid than usual and more likely to say exactly what he thinks regardless of circumstances. This is exemplified by the old saying, "In vino veritas." Even in this early stage, psycho-physiological tests[1263] show an interference with the accurate performance of tasks involving concentration, rapid response to stimuli and correct judgment.

As the intoxication progresses, personality changes become more evident, and it is here that the greatest variation is observed.[1264] Many persons become hilarious, sing, shout, dance, and show their good feeling in other ways. Some individuals become very quiet, even sullen and morose; others become irritable and combative; others have fits of weeping, remorse and despair. This emotional instability is accompanied by an increase in muscular incoordination and a slowing of response to stimuli.

Further absorption of alcohol produces even more marked incoordination which gives rise to a slurring of the speech (particularly with the enunciation of "s" sounds), a staggering gait and a dulling of all sensation and ability to make judgments or remember what has taken place. This confusion develops into a stupor and finally, if sufficient alcohol has been taken, into a coma. During these latter stages both respiration and pulse rate are decreased and the body temperature falls. The skin is cold and cyanotic. Death from uncomplicated alcoholism usually results from respiratory failure.

Symptoms of Chronic Poisoning: Chronic alcoholism is more properly a problem of neurology and psychiatry than of toxicology. Chronic use of alcohol is frequently adopted by an individual who is incapable of making the necessary environ-

1263. MILES, W. R.: "Alcohol and Human Efficiency," Carnegie Inst., Washington, Pub. No. 333, 1924.
1264. FLEMING, R.: *Am. J. Psychiat.*, 92:89, 1935.

mental adjustment, in order to escape from his unpleasant circumstances. It may take the form of steady drinking, periodic drinking, or comparatively infrequent debauches (dipsomania). Steady drinkers and periodic drinkers who consume rather large amounts of alcohol frequently suffer from skin disorders, gastritis, particularly following a period of heavy drinking, cirrhosis of the liver, and fatty changes in the heart muscle and other tissues. Neurological disturbances, in cases of heavy drinking, take the form of delirium tremens, a condition characterized by vivid hallucinations of hearing and sight, acute mania frequently followed by exhaustion and collapse. More moderate chronic use of alcohol results in Korsakoff's psychosis, typified by loss of memory and complete disorientation, along with polyneuritis, with tremors of the extremities, lips and eyelids, and with either numbness or tingling sensations or shooting pains in the hands and feet. The dipsomaniac remains entirely normal and sober for long periods of time, but succumbs to rare attacks of an irresistible desire for liquor. Such debauches of intense drinking may last for one or two days or for over a week, usually terminated by acute gastritis and complete nervous breakdown of the victim. The patient may have little or no recollection of what happened during the drinking period.

Practically all cases of chronic alcoholism show some mental abnormality and should, therefore, be investigated as psychiatric problems.

Treatment: In acute alcoholic poisoning, treatment consists of:

1. Prevention of further absorption—by producing emesis by means of apomorphine injections, or by resorting to gastric lavage.

2. Combating the effects of the absorbed alcohol by giving inhalations of a mixture of 93% oxygen and 7% carbon dioxide.[1265]

3. Giving the patient supportive treatment as symptoms indicate, such as wrapping in blankets or applying hot water bottles to maintain body temperature, or the administration of cardiac stimulants or artificial respiration.

Fatal Dose: Owing to the wide range of susceptibility to

1265. HUNTER, T. F., and MUDD, S. G.: *Boston M. & S. J.*, 190:971, 1924. ROBINSON, L. F., and SELESNICK, S.: *J.A.M.A.*, 105:1734, 1935.

alcohol, it is difficult to establish any particular quantity as a fatal dose. Death frequently occurs when the alcohol concentration of the tissues amounts to 0.5% or more. Usually 150 to 450 cc. of alcohol taken during a very short period of time are necessary to produce fatal concentrations in the tissues.

Fatal Period: Death from acute alcoholism usually takes place within twelve hours following drinking. Coma of more than twelve hours' duration almost always results fatally.

Postmortem Appearance: There is little to be observed at postmortem which is diagnostic of alcoholism. Upon opening the thoracic and abdominal cavities, and particularly when opening the skull and removing the brain coverings, the odor of alcohol may be noted. In acute poisoning the irritant effects of strong alcohol solutions may be noted in the hyperemia of the esophagus, stomach, and duodenum. If coma has been of several hours' duration, considerable edema is to be expected, particularly of the brain and to some extent of the lungs. There may be some fatty degeneration and cirrhosis of the liver as well as minor changes in the kidneys, but these are usually the result of chronic use rather than of a single fatal debauch.

Chemical Tests: Alcohol, along with other so-called "volatile" poisons, is removed from tissues and biological fluids by distillation from a faintly acid solution and tests subsequently made on the distillate. Because of the great frothing tendencies of such materials, the distillation is ordinarily made by steam rather than by direct distillation. Frequently, it is found advisable to utilize protein precipitants in the distillation to minimize this frothing tendency. In fresh tissues the isolation of alcohol in reasonably pure state by such steam distillation is quite simple. However, where putrefaction has been extensive, or where foreign chemicals such as embalming fluids have been introduced into the specimen, not only is the chemical analysis rendered more difficult, but the results also are much less reliable and significant from the toxicological viewpoint. For this reason, it is important that the material be obtained as fresh as possible, kept in a refrigerator, and analyzed with the least possible delay. Preservatives should be avoided except for the possible use of small amounts of sodium oxalate or sodium fluoride as an anti-coagulant for blood specimens.

If qualitative tests show the presence of such impurities as aldehydes or hydrogen sulphide, in the distillate, these may be removed by treatment, first with silver acetate solution and subsequent distillation from a solution rendered slightly alkaline with sodium hydroxide. If acetone is present (as in the urine of diabetics) it may be removed by treatment with Scott-Wilson's alkaline mercuric cyanide reagent. (Scott-Wilson's reagent is made by dissolving 1 gm. of mercuric cyanide in 60 cc. of water, then adding 18 gm. of sodium hydroxide which has been dissolved in 60 cc. of water, and finally adding 0.29 gm. of silver nitrate dissolved in 40 cc. of water. If turbid, allow to settle and decant the clear fluid. Distillation of the specimen from a mixture containing one-fourth its volume of the reagent will eliminate acetone, volatile acids, aldehydes, and sulphides.) The purified distillate may then be used for alcohol analysis.

Qualitative Tests: These are only of value in identifying the material in the distillate as being ethyl alcohol. The important question of how much ethyl alcohol is present must be answered by means of a quantitative determination.

1. **Chromic Acid Reduction Test:** Mix 5 cc. of distillate in a small Erlenmeyer flask with 3 cc. of concentrated sulphuric acid, and at once add a solution of potassium dichromate containing 17.042 gm. per liter from a graduated pipet. If alcohol is present, the first few drops of the orange colored dichromate solution will quickly turn to a bluish-green. If the addition of the dichromate be continued until the reaction mixture becomes a yellowish-green rather than a bluish-green, a rough estimate of the amount of alcohol present may be made. One cc. of the dichromate solution oxidizes 4 mg. of alcohol to acetic acid with the resultant reduction of hexavalent chromium (orange color) to the bluish-green trivalent state.

2. **Iodoform Reaction:** About 10 cc. of distillate are treated with a solution of iodine in potassium iodide sufficient to color the mixture a deep brown. Then 5% sodium hydroxide solution is added drop by drop until the brown color changes to a yellow. On warming this mixture in a steam-bath, the characteristic odor of iodoform indicates the presence of ethyl alcohol. On cooling the mixture (in a refrigerator over night, if necessary) the characteristic small hexagonal crystals of iodoform will separate out and may be recognized with low power

magnification on a microscope slide. Substances such as acetaldehyde, acetone, lactic acid, etc., give this reaction, so these must be eliminated from the distillate before making the test.

3. **Acetaldehyde Test:** Ten cc. of distillate are placed in a test-tube and a spiral of copper wire heated to redness is quickly plunged into the contents of the tube. The tube is kept cool in a beaker of cracked ice, and the oxidation by means of the heated copper spiral is repeated about ten times. The content of the tube is then treated with 2 cc. of colorless reduced (with SO_2) fuchsin solution. (Schiff-Elvove reagent: 0.1 gm. basic fuchsin dissolved in 60 cc. hot distilled water, cool, and add solution of 1 gm. anhydrous sodium sulphide C. P. in 10 cc. of distilled water. Cool nearly to room temperature, stir, and add 2 cc. of concentrated hydrochloric acid. Dilute to 100 cc. and allow to stand for several hours before using. This solution will retain its sensitivity for about a week if kept in a glass-stoppered bottle in a refrigerator.) The mixture is then allowed to stand for about ten minutes. If alcohol is present a red color is produced by the acetaldehyde which is formed in the oxidation of alcohol. The intensity of the red may be used to approximate the quantity of alcohol present.[1266]

4. **Ethyl Benzoate Test:** Treatment of 10 cc. of distillate with a few drops of pure benzoyl chloride, shaken well and followed by 5 cc. of 5% sodium hydroxide solution (or sufficient to make the reaction permanently alkaline after the excess of benzoyl chloride has been hydrolyzed), and heated in a steam-bath, will give the odor characteristic of ethyl benzoate if alcohol is present. If the odor is not noticeable, the excess sodium hydroxide may be neutralized so that the mixture is barely alkaline, then cooled and extracted in a separatory funnel with pure ether. On evaporating the ether solution on a steam-bath the warm residue will have the odor of ethyl benzoate even if the amount of alcohol present is slight.

If the alcohol is present in sufficient quantity and concentration, a similar procedure may be employed, replacing the few drops of benzoyl chloride with 100 mg. of powdered (three to five) dinitrobenzoyl chloride. The ethyl ester isolated by evaporation of the ether extract,[1267] will permit the identifica-

1266. GETTLER, A. O.: *New England J. Med.*, 201:724, 1929.
1267. MALONE, G. B., and REID, E. E.: *J. Am. Chem. Soc.*, 51:3423, 1929.

tion to be made by means of its melting point. The ethyl ester melts at 91°C.

5. Identification of Pure Alcohol: If present in sufficient quantity the alcohol may be actually isolated and identified by means of its physical properties and by means of its derivatives. The details of this micro-chemical procedure are given by Gettler and his associates.[1268]

Quantitative Determination: Space will not permit a complete discussion of the myriad techniques which have been employed by various investigators for the determination of ethyl alcohol. For discussions of the literature of these various procedures, the reader is referred to papers by Gettler, Harger and Haggard.[1269]

All of the methods for determining alcohol consist of two steps: (1) the separation of the alcohol from body tissue and fluids either by means of areation or by distillation, and (2) the determination of the isolated alcohol either by physical or chemical means. Ordinarily urine or protein-free filtrates from blood may be distilled directly. Isolation from other tissues is almost invariably made either by aeration or steam distillation. For determining the quantity of alcohol which has been separated from tissues, most workers have discarded the physical methods such as measurement of specific gravity or refractive index of the distillates.[1270] Bock[1271] has more recently reported satisfactory results using the interferometer for the measurement of refractive index. However, the difficulties involved in the application of such physical methods and the uncertainty as to just what substance is responsible for the increase in refractive index renders this procedure of doubtful value in medicolegal work.

Of the chemical methods, practically all of the satisfactory procedures are based upon the oxidation of alcohol. The oxidation to acetaldehyde is difficult to control and methods based upon the reaction give only approximate results. The oxidation to acetic acid is easily controlled and is quantitative. The most common oxidizing agent for this purpose is chromic acid, and in most methods the determination is based upon the

1268. In *J. Am. Chem. Soc.*, 54:1476, 1932.

1269. GETTLER, A. O., and TIBER, A.: *Arch. Path.*, 3:75, 1927; HARGER, R. N.: *J. Lab. & Clin. Med.*, 20:746, 1935; HAGGARD and GREENBERG: see Ref. 1252.

1270. GETTLER and TIBER: see Ref. 1269.

1271. BOCK, J. C.: *J. Biol. Chem.*, 93:645, 1931.

amount of chromic acid which is reduced by the alcohol. It is possible to determine the acetic acid by distillation and titration, utilizing the Duclaux principle.[1272] This latter procedure is employed by Gettler and Tiber.[1273] By the use of more powerful oxidizing agents, such as iodine pentoxide or potassium permanganate,[1274] alcohol may be oxidized beyond the acetic acid stage, at least a portion of the alcohol finally being changed to carbon dioxide and water. These oxidations do not proceed quantitatively to the carbon dioxide end-product, and for that reason are probably not as precise as those involving the easy and definite oxidation to acetic acid.

The chromic acid oxidation methods are practically all modifications of the original Nicloux procedure.[1275] Almost every worker who has employed this principle in determining alcohol has made his own modification of the original method, so that variations are legion.

A method which during the past four years has given very satisfactory and reliable results in the Cook County (Illinois) Coroner's Laboratory is based on the procedure employed in the Carlson Research. The reagents and solutions required are:

.3472 N Potassium Dichromate Solution—Made by dissolving 17.042 gm. of pure dry potassium dichromate (reagent grade) in sufficient distilled water to give a total volume of 1000 cc. Each cc. of this solution is capable of oxidizing exactly 4 mg. of ethyl alcohol to acetic acid.

Approximately (N/20) Sodium Thiosulphate Solution — Made by dissolving 12.5 gm. of pure sodium thiosulphate crystals in sufficient boiled (to eliminate dissolved CO_2) distilled water to give a total volume of 1000 cc. This solution must be standardized against the potassium dichromate solution.

Starch Indicator Solution—About 0.5 gm. "soluble starch" is placed in a beaker and mixed with sufficient cold distilled water to make a thin paste; 250 cc. of boiled distilled water are then added quickly and the mixture stirred. The resulting solution should be nearly clear. When cool it is ready for use. If kept in a refrigerator it retains its sensitivity to free iodine

1272. UPSON, F., PLUM, H. M., and SCHOTT, J. E.:   J. Am. Chem. Soc., 39:731, 1917.
1273. See Ref. 1269.
1274. FRIEDMANN, T. E., and RITCHIE, E. B.:   Proc. Soc. Exper. Biol. & Med., 30:451, 1933.
1275. NICLOUX, M.:   Compt. rend. Soc. de biol., 48:841, 1896.

for several days, but for accurate work it is best to prepare a fresh solution each day.

Saturated Picric Acid Solution—Picric acid is twice recrystallized from hot distilled water, and a saturated aqueous solution (about 14 gm. per liter) made from crystallized products.

Potassium Iodide—Pure reagent quality crystals are used. These must be free from iodate or other substances which liberate iodine in **dilute** sulphuric acid solution.

Sulphuric Acid—Chemically pure concentrated (95%) acid is used. The distilled water used must be particularly free from grease or other organic reducing substances.

Apparatus—The apparatus consists of a steam generator (A), distilling flask (B), condenser (C), and receiver (D).

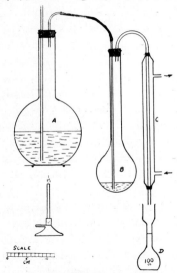

SCALE

FIG. 20
Apparatus for Alcohol
Determination

The steam generator is composed of a three-liter Florence flask fitted with a rubber stopper, delivery and safety tubes. It is heated by a large Bunsen burner and is connected to the distilling flask by a short length of heavy-wall rubber tubing. The distilling flask, which contains the specimen, is an 800-cc. long-neck Kjeldahl flask. It is not necessary to heat the distilling flask except by means of the steam from the steam generator. The condenser jacket is removable and the condenser tube is made of a long length of 9-mm. tubing bent as indicated. This avoids one extra connection at the condenser. Needless to say, the rubber stopper and connections at the neck of the distilling flask must be absolutely tight. For small specimens (less than 50 gm.) a 300-cc. Kjeldahl flask is used instead of the 800-cc. size, and the distillate received in a smaller Kohlrausch sugar flask. A rapid current of cooling water is sufficient to condense the alcohol without loss. It is not necessary to pack the receiver in ice.

For analysis, weighed specimens of hashed tissue or measured volumes of blood or urine are employed. If an ample supply of material is available, samples of 50 gm. or 50 cc. are used. These are slowly distilled in a current of steam and the distillate received in a 100-cc. Kohlrausch sugar flask. Blood specimens froth badly, especially during the first part of the distillation, and for this reason a volume of saturated picric acid solution equal to the blood sample is added to the blood in the distillation flask. Even with this precaution, the analysis of blood is difficult and the distillation must be **very slow** at first to avoid frothing. Needless to say, if the coagulated blood froths up in the flask near the condenser connection, the determination must be discarded. Tissue specimens or urine do not froth badly, and the use of picric acid is unnecessary. Distillate is collected equivalent to twice the weight of the sample (100 cc. distillate for a 50-gm. sample). This is tested for aldehydes, acetone, and sulphides, and if present, these are removed as indicated in the qualitative tests.

Methanol is tested for, using the U.S.P., XI, test. Either 5-cc. or 10-cc. portions* of distillate (representing 2.5 to 5.0 gm. of specimen) are accurately pipetted into large test-tubes (20 to 25 mm. diam.); 5 cc. portions of standard (.3472 N) potassium dichromate sufficient to oxidize exactly 20 mg. of alcohol, are accurately pipetted into each tube and mixed thoroughly by shaking. About 5 cc. of concentrated sulphuric acid are also pipetted into the tube while the contents are being shaken. This results in the evolution of some heat. The tube containing the mixture is then placed in a bath of boiling water for fifteen minutes to complete the oxidation of the alcohol to acetic acid. The amount of oxidizing agent remaining after all the alcohol has been oxidized to acetic acid is then determined iodometrically. The tube and contents are cooled and the contents poured into a 500-cc. Erlenmeyer flask containing 250 cc. of cold distilled water. After shaking, about 3 gm. of pure potassium iodide crystals are added, and after standing about five minutes the liberated iodine (yellowish-brown color) is titrated with the standard sodium thiosulphate solution. Upon addition of the sodium thiosulphate, the yellowish-brown color of the solution becomes progressively lighter. When it has become a pale yellow, 2 cc. of starch solu-

* For specimens of unusually high alcohol content, such as stomach contents, it may be necessary to use smaller amounts of the distillate (0.5 cc. to 2.0 cc.).

tion are added. This reacts with the remaining free iodine to produce a deep blue color. The addition of sodium thiosulphate solution is continued until the deep blue of the starch-iodine color just fades out to the **very pale** bluish-green color of chromium sulphate. With very little practice this end-point can be read very accurately.

Needless to say, all apparatus must be scrupulously clean, since grease or other organic matter acts as a reducing agent similar to alcohol. Glassware and volumetric apparatus should be cleaned with hot potassium dichromate-sulphuric acid cleaning solution and then thoroughly washed with distilled water.

A blank determination should be made, using everything in the analysis except the specimen of tissue, blood, or urine. The titration in such a blank should be the same as that obtained when one uses distilled water instead of tissue distillate. For forensic purposes it may be desirable to standardize the procedure by analyzing an alcohol solution of known content. However, experience has shown that if the potassium dichromate solution is prepared as indicated, each cc. will oxidize exactly 4 mg. of ethyl alcohol.

Sample Calculation:
50 gm. of hashed liver used for analysis and 100 cc. of distillate collected.
5 cc. of this treated with 5 cc. of .3472 N $K_2Cr_2O_7$ and 5 cc. of H_2SO_4 required 18.5 cc. of $Na_2S_2O_3$ to reduce the liberated iodine.
5 cc. of water $+$ 5 cc. of .3472 N $K_2Cr_2O_7$ $+$ 5 cc. of H_2SO_4 required 34.5 cc. of $Na_2S_2O_3$.
The amount of oxidant used up by the alcohol in the sample is therefore equivalent to the difference in these titrations or 34.5 cc. $-$ 18.5 cc. $=$ 16.0 cc.

1 cc. of $Na_2S_2O_3 = \dfrac{20}{34.5}$ or .580 mg. of alcohol.

Alcohol in 5 cc. of distillate $=$ 16.0 $\times$ .580 $=$ 9.28 mg.
Alcohol in entire 50 gm. of liver specimen was 20 times this or 185.6 mg.

% alcohol in liver $= \dfrac{.1856 \times 100}{50} = 0.37\%$

Harger Micro-Method:[1275-A] Where the amount of material available for analysis is very limited, one of the micro-methods is indicated. Of these, the procedure of Harger appears to offer the least difficulty. In principle, it employs the Nicloux

1275-A. HARGER, R. N.: "A Simple Micro-method for the Determination of Alcohol in Biologic Material," *J. Lab. & Clin. Med.*, 20:746-751, 1935.

method of oxidizing the alcohol to acetic acid by means of an excess of chromic acid but differs in the ingenious manner by which the excess of oxidant is determined. Instead of employing the standard iodometric procedure, Harger uses a reducing agent composed of ferrous sulphate which has been strongly colored by methyl orange. In using this reducing agent, the excess of oxidizing agent is detected by its bleaching-out effect on the azo dye (methyl orange). The first drop of excess reducing agent produces a red color. Thus the use of expensive potassium iodide is avoided, and also the nuisance of making fresh starch indicator is obviated.

The following solutions are utilized in the procedure:

.0434 N Potassium Dichromate Solution—Prepared by dissolving 2.129 gm. of pure dry powdered crystals of reagent quality $K_2Cr_2O_7$ in sufficient distilled water to make exactly 1,000 cc. One cc. of this solution will oxidize exactly 0.5 mg. of ethyl alcohol or 0.232 mg. of methyl alcohol.

20% Ferrous Sulphate Solution: 50 gm. of $FeSO_4.7H_2O$ dissolved in 150 cc. of water, 30 cc. of concentrated sulphuric acid added, and finally diluted with water to a volume of 250 cc. In a glass-stoppered flask, this solution undergoes very little oxidation over a period of a year.

Methyl Orange (0.1%): Dissolve 1 gm. of methyl orange in one liter of water in which 1 gm. of sodium hydroxide has been dissolved. Filter off any insoluble residue. This solution will keep indefinitely.

62% Sulphuric Acid: Pour one volume of concentrated C.P. sulphuric acid (95% strength) into an equal volume of distilled water and allow to cool to room temperature before use.

Red Reducing Fluid: Into a clean 100-cc. Erlenmeyer flask, place 35 cc. of 62% sulphuric acid and 5 cc. of 0.1% methyl orange solution. Pipet 1 cc. of the 20% ferrous sulphate solution into the flask, mix and cool to room temperature before use. About 2.5 cc. of this solution are required to reduce 1 cc. of the standard potassium dichromate solution. This solution deteriorates slowly, especially in warm weather, but may be used for three or four days.

Isolation of Alcohol: Tissues or urine are rendered slightly acid by the addition of tartaric acid and steam distilled, collecting an amount of distillate equal to the weight of the sample. Ordinarily this distillate is diluted to exactly fifty times its original volume, and 5 cc. portions (representing 0.1 gm. of original specimen) used for subsequent analysis. If the alcohol content of the tissue is particularly high or low, this dilution is altered suitably.

To avoid the troublesome foaming which results when blood specimens are steam distilled, a protein-free filtrate is obtained by the Folin-Wu[1275-B] method. Five cc. of this filtrate (representing 0.5 cc. of blood) are diluted with 20 cc. of water in a 125-cc. Pyrex distilling flask, a few glass beads added and the mixture slowly distilled until about 12 cc. of distillate have been collected. This is diluted to 25 cc. volume, and 5 cc. (equivalent to 0.1 cc. of blood) used for analysis.

Analysis of Distillates: Into a test-tube (about 17 mm. x 150 mm.) are measured 5 cc. of distillate (containing less than 0.5 mg. of alcohol) and 1 cc. of standard potassium dichromate solution. After shaking, 5 cc. of concentrated sulphuric acid are added and mixed thoroughly by means of a clean glass stirring rod. The warm mixture is allowed to stand for ten minutes, then cooled in a water-bath to room temperature and titrated with standard red reducing fluid (using a 5-cc. micro-burette) until a permanent pink color results. During the titration, Harger uses an ingenious scheme for air-stirring, employing a vacuum pump. Into another tube are placed 5 cc. of distilled water instead of 5 cc. of diluted distillate. Because the sulphuric acid used often contains a trace of reducing material, a second cc. of dichromate solution is added to one of the completed titrations and again titrated.

Calculation:

U = Titration figure for unknown

W = Titration figure for distilled water

B = Titration figure for extra cc. of bichromate

Q = Quantity of blood, urine, or tissue represented by the aliquot analyzed.

Then $\dfrac{W-U}{B \times Q}$ x 0.5 = mg. ethyl alcohol per cc. or gm. of sample.

The micro-method of Widmark[1275-C] is widely used for blood and urine analysis in Europe. It is not so readily adapt-

1275-B. FOLIN, O., and WU, H.: "A System of Blood Analysis," *J. Biol. Chem.*, 38:82, 1919.

1275-C. WIDMARK, E.: "Eine Mikromethode zur Bestimmung von Athylalkohol in Blut," *Biochem. Ztschr.*, 131:473-484, 1922.

able to tissue analysis and requires apparatus specially made by a glass-blower.

Gettler's Method:[1275-D] This method which is employed for **precise** determinations of alcohol in tissue in the laboratories of the New York Medical Examiner's office is based upon the oxidation of alcohol to acetic acid with the subsequent distillation and titration of that acid.*

The tissue is first chilled, then ground up and a 500 gm. portion placed in a two-liter flask. To this are added 600 cc. of distilled water, 5 cc. of saturated tartaric acid solution, and 1 cc. of white mineral oil. The mixture is then distilled with steam until 800 cc. of distillate have been collected. Twenty gm. of potassium dichromate and 40 cc. of concentrated sulphuric acid are placed in a 500-cc. flask, and 300 cc. of the distillate (representing 187.5 gm. of tissue) are added. The flask is connected to a well cooled condenser by means of a Hopkins distilling head and distilled slowly. The rate of distillation is controlled so that forty-five to fifty minutes are required to collect exactly 250 cc. of distillate. This is then mixed and 50 cc. (representing 37.5 gm. of tissue) is titrated using N/20 sodium hydroxide solution and phenolphthalein indicator. Each cc. of N/20 sodium hydroxide solution neutralizes acetic acid equivalent to 2.3 mg. of ethyl alcohol. Subtracting from this titration the acidity resulting from the distillation non-alcoholic tissue (1.32 cc. for brain), Gettler found that he could account for 83.6% to 86.3% of the alcohol added to brain tissue. His results obtained by titration were therefore multiplied by 1.167 to correct for this loss. Because of the manipulation involved, the high "blank", and the uncertainty of the amount of loss inherent in the method (13.7% to 16.4%), it is much less accurate than the other methods given.

Interpretation of Results: The making of qualitative and quantitative tests for ethyl alcohol in tissues or body fluids is simply a matter of ordinary chemical analytical procedure and can be performed by any skilled analyst. The results are fairly accurate, and errors of more than 1% of the total alcohol present are inexcusable. On the other hand, experience has shown that while a high degree of precision may be obtained with

---

1275-D. GETTLER, A. O., and TIBER, A.: "The Quantitative Determination of Ethyl Alcohol in Human Tissues," *Arch. Path.*, 3:75-83, 1927.
* For routine work the method given in Ref. 1260, page 641, is used and results reported as "1 plus," "2 plus," "3 plus," or "4 plus."

homogeneous and easily measured substances such as blood, urine, spinal fluid, and saliva, this degree of accuracy cannot be expected with tissues such as liver, kidney, brain or stomach. In other words, if one takes hashed liver tissues and weighs out two separate samples which are carried through the usual analytical process of distillation, etc., the results of these two duplicate analyses cannot be reasonably expected to agree closer than within 1% of the total alcohol present. Our experience has been that tissue analyses in which alcohol values are given to the third significant figure, are misleading. Furthermore, such accuracy is not only impractical from the analytical viewpoint, but also of no toxicological significance. There is no difference in the conclusion to be drawn if the brain, liver or kidney contains either 0.25% or 0.26% of alcohol.

Non-fatal Cases—Drunkenness: In determining whether or not an individual is "drunk" we must first establish just what we mean by that term. The terms "intoxication" and "drunkenness" are frequently used as synonyms. However, common usage of the term "drunk" by the laity has come to imply a stage of intoxication where the symptoms are obvious. In the medical literature one finds a wide variety in the interpretation of the term. Some[1275-E] hold that "any demonstrable alteration in behavior resulting from the ingestion of alcohol constitutes some degree of drunkenness." Others imply that the degree of physical or mental impairment must be quite extreme before the individual may be said to be drunk.*

A somewhat modified form of this view is taken in certain European countries[1275-F] where it is held that alcoholic intoxication must be so extreme as to produce obvious alteration of physical behavior and control before the individual may be

1275-E. See Ref. 1250.

* This attitude is exemplified by the old bar-room quatrain, utilized by bartenders as a criterion of the point beyond which a customer should not be sold further drinks:

> "He is *not* drunk who, from the floor,
> Can rise again and drink once more.
> But he *is* drunk who prostrate lies,
> And can neither drink nor rise."

Cited by HALL, W. W.: "Drunkenness, Naval Medicolegal Aspects of the Diagnosis," *U. S. Naval Med. Bull.*, 34:149-163, 1936.

1275-F. Alcohol Investigation Committee of British Medical Research Council Report—"Alcohol: It s Action on the Human Organism," 2nd ed., London, 1923, 170 pp.

said to be "drunk." This view is supported by Turner.[1275-G] A fair attitude appears to lie between these two extremes.

It seems reasonable to define "drunkenness" as the state where the alcohol effect interferes with normal function.[1275-H] Whether or not a person is to be considered "drunk" depends upon the nature of the activity in which he is engaged. Thus a person may have taken several "highballs" and seated himself in his home to listen to the radio. For such activity, he might be considered to be quite sober. But if this same man were to undertake a task involving quick and accurate response to stimuli, and sound judgment, such as driving a high-powered motor car through crowded city streets, he might be considered to be definitely "drunk."

That there are various grades of alcoholic intoxication has been known for centuries.* Probably the best classification, based upon clinical observation is that of Bogen who recognizes five stages: (1) sub-clinical; (2) excitement; (3) confusion; (4) stupor; and (5) coma.

Inasmuch as the "drunk" implies not only an observation, but a judgment as well, it is probably wise to avoid using it in medicolegal cases. If one gives an opinion as to the stage or grade of alcoholic intoxication of an individual, the jury may then draw their own conclusion as to whether or not he was "drunk" within the legal sense of the term. In this way the toxicologist may avoid the criticism that he is invading the province of the jury.

Until quite recent years, the sole criterion of alcoholic intoxication was a clinical examination of the subject. Observations were made as to the odor of alcohol on the breath, flushings of the face, dilation of pupils, ability to stand steadily in an erect position with eyes closed (Romberg test), the ability to coordinate muscular activities as typified by walking a straight line, climbing steps, inserting a key in a keyhole, pick-

---

1275-G. TURNER, R. G.: "Blood Alcohol and Its Relation to Intoxication in Man," *Proc. Soc. Exper. Biol. & Med.,* 32:1548-1552, 1935.

1275-H. WILSON, G.: "The Definition of Drunkenness," *Police Journal,* (London), 1:594-604, 1928.

* Shakespeare recognized three stages, as evidenced by the following conversation in TWELFTH NIGHT (Act 1, Scene 5, lines 122-128):

Lady Olivia: "What's a drunken man like, fool?"

Clown: "Like a drowned man, a fool and a madman. One draught above heat makes him a fool. The second mads him and a third drowns him."

ing up pins or bits of paper, etc., alterations in speech—particularly in the enunciation of "s" sounds, and general orientation as revealed by conversation. While such tests are valuable in recording the condition of an individual, they are certainly far from quantitative, and depend largely upon the judgment of the observer for whatever accuracy they may afford. Unfortunately alcohol usage is one subject upon which many individuals have very strong personal opinions and prejudices which interfere with reasoned judgment of the observer. Furthermore, there are other conditions, such as nervous diseases, diabetes, traumatic injuries to the brain or other nerve centers, uremia, shock, etc., which might give rise to conditions which could easily be mistaken for alcoholic intoxication. The odor of alcohol on the breath merely indicates that the individual had been drinking—and even this odor may be simulated by other beverages or by the acetone-breath of diabetics.[1275-I]

As a very important adjunct to such clinical tests, Europeans have developed chemical methods which are certainly at least as reliable and probably of greater quantitative significance than ordinary clinical observations. These have been based upon analyses of blood, urine, breath, saliva, or spinal fluid. Although they have long been accepted by European courts, such tests have not yet been adopted extensively in this country largely because of our presumption of the innocence of the accused and our guarantee that he shall not be required to give self-incriminatory evidence. One cannot demand that a suspect give a specimen of his blood, urine, saliva, or spinal fluid for test. In all probability one could legally analyze the expired air by the method of Harger without violating the constitutional rights of the subject. Likewise if a suspect is placed in a cell fitted with a urinal which is connected to a dry bottle instead of a sewer, a sample of urine may often be obtained without asking for it. However, the best chemical criterion of the degree of alcohol intoxication is furnished by the analysis of a blood specimen[1275-J] taken at the time, although analyses of saliva, breath and urine may furnish very valuable information. The alcohol concentration of the saliva and breath paral-

1275-I. Bogen, E.: "Alcohol and Man," edited by Haven Emerson. New York, 1932, Chap. 6, pp. 126-152. See also *J.A.M.A.*, 89:1508, 1927 and *Am. J. M. Sc.*, 176:153, 1928.

1275-J. Kozelka, F. L.: "Medicolegal Aspects of Alcoholism," *Wisconsin M. J.*, 34:816-821, 1935.

lels that of blood.[1275-K] The secreted urine also represents an approximate average of the alcohol content of the secreted urine during the period since the last voiding. Its analysis, therefore, does not give such a reliable index of the condition of the subject **at the time,** as does the blood. The probable condition of the subject for a short time prior to the taking of the

TABLE LI

RELATION BETWEEN CLINICAL INDICATIONS OF ALCOHOLIC INTOXICATION AND CONCENTRATION OF ALCOHOL OF THE BLOOD AND URINE

Stage	Blood Alcohol	Urine Alcohol	Clinical Observations
Sub-clinical	0-.11	0-.15 .1 to .15%* (inebriation)	Normal by ordinary observation, slight changes detectable by special tests.
Emotional Instability	.09-.21	.13-.29 .20 (characteristic state of drunkenness)*	Decreased inhibitions; emotional instability; slight muscular incoordination; slowing of responses to stimuli.
Confusion	.18-.33	.26-.45	Disturbance of sensation; decreased pain sense; staggering gait; slurred speech.
Stupor	.27-.43	.36-.58	Marked decrease in response to stimuli. Muscular incoordination approaching paralysis.
Coma	.36-.56	.48-.72	Complete unconsciousness; depressed reflexes; subnormal temperature, anesthesia; impairment of circulation; possible death.
Death (Uncomplicated)	over .44	over .60	

* VELIO, PAND, VAN TENNSCHE, M.: *Arm. Hyg. publ. Ind. Sociale,* 15:1, 1936.

specimen may be approximated if it can be established that no alcohol had been ingested in the interim. As has been pointed out previously, lumbar spinal fluid does not reflect the alcohol content of the circulating blood and its alcohol content is practically useless as an index of alcoholic intoxication. Cisternal fluid closely approximates blood in its alcohol content,

1275-K. ABELS, J. C.: "Determination of Ethyl Alcohol in Saliva," *Proc. Soc. Exper. Biol. & Med.,* 34:504-505, 1936.

but because of the difficulty and danger of withdrawing a specimen, it should never be done in a living individual. This is particularly true when one can obtain more reliable material (blood) much more easily and safely. It is, of course, understood that the alcohol contained in the stomach represents **unabsorbed** alcohol and does not give any index as to the stage of intoxication of an individual. Alcohol in the stomach merely indicates that the individual had been drinking some alcoholic material.

The relationship between the alcohol content of the blood (and, to a lesser degree of certainty, that of the urine) and alcoholic intoxication is given by the modification of Bogen's table in Table LI.

These stages have been cleverly illustrated by Dr. Esther Bogen Tietz, particularly with reference to the alcohol content of the urine.

It will be noted that these stages overlap. There is no sharp line of demarcation where one stage leaves off and another commences. They shade into each other.

The value of chemical tests in determining the degree of alcoholic intoxication is largely in detecting the earlier stages. One hardly needs a chemical analysis of blood to demonstrate a condition of alcoholic stupor or coma; such conditions are self-evident. However, in the earlier stages the chemical tests may be exceedingly valuable in arriving at a correct conclusion.[1275-L] It may be generally stated that within the bounds of biologic variation (which amounts to about plus or minus 10% to 15% in the human) all persons, regardless of their previous experience in drinking alcoholic beverages, are equally intoxicated when the concentration of alcohol in their blood stream is equal. Different persons manifest their intoxication in different ways, especially in the period of emotional instability. Some sing hilariously, some are jovial, some are silent or morose or melancholy, some are pugnacious, some are seized with fits of weeping—but apart from their personality differences, they are in the same **stage** of intoxication.

In many instances, chemical tests are of value in excluding alcoholism as a causative factor in cases of stupor or coma. It should be noted that the amounts of acetone encountered in

1275-L. Schmidt, M.: "Alcohol Studies: II—Concentration of Alcohol in the Blood," *J. Indust. Hyg.*, 16:355-365, 1934.

body fluids in cases of diabetes do not interfere materially with the correct interpretation of chemical tests.

It is important to note that while the chemical tests are of chief diagnostic value in the earlier stages of intoxication, these are the stages of greatest medicolegal interest. It is in the early stages of intoxication that drivers of motor cars are particularly dangerous and when pedestrians are unusually careless or reckless. The toll of dead and injured as a result of motor car accidents is unquestionably higher because of intoxication of drivers. In fact, in a survey of the causes of motor car accidents in England, a committee appointed by the British Medical Association estimated that 25% of road accidents of motor cars were referable to low grade alcoholic intoxication of the drivers.[1275-M] Heise,[1275-N] in his observations of motor car accidents on the National Highway at Uniontown, Pennsylvania, found that two thirds of the drivers who had accidents, had been drinking.

Fatal Cases: As has been previously pointed out, a large number of fatalities attributed to acute alcoholic intoxication are undoubtedly complicated by other pathological conditions. It is unusual to find a case where an otherwise entirely normal individual dies as a result of uncomplicated acute alcoholism. Only where strong alcoholic beverages are taken quickly and in large quantity, are such fatalities observed. Such cases result when persons drink on a wager or engage in drinking bouts to see whose resistance is greatest. With drinking of even strong liquor at a comparatively slow rate, alcohol automatically acts as its own protective agent. When a person arrives at the stupor stage, he is not in a condition to continue drinking and fatality is avoided.

The distribution of alcohol in the various tissues is of considerable importance in the correct interpretation of the alcoholic condition of the deceased. If there is a high alcohol content of the stomach (over 0.7%) it indicates that the deceased had been drinking during the two or three hours prior to his death. On the other hand, if there is still an appreciable amount of material in the stomach, and its alcohol content fairly closely

1275-M. "The Sub-intoxicated Driver," *J.A.M.A.*, 106:1580-1581, 1936.

1275-N. HEISE, H. A.: "Alcohol and Automobile Accidents," *J.A.M.A.*, 103:739-741, September 8, 1934.

approximates that of other body tissues (liver, kidney, or brain), it suggests that the deceased had not been drinking during his last hours.

Apart from the gastro-intestinal tract, the other organs contain alcohol which reaches them by way of the blood stream. Hence their alcohol content is a measure of **absorbed** alcohol. If one takes the alcohol concentration of the blood as 1.00, the alcohol concentration of the kidney will be about .90 to .95 and that of the liver and brain about .80 to .90. Thus one can make a fair **estimation** of the alcohol content of one tissue from that of another.

Two questions often arise in fatal cases where alcoholism is suspected of playing some role in causing death:

1. Did death result from acute alcoholic poisoning?
2. In what stage of alcoholic intoxication was the deceased at the time of death?

The answer to the first question depends upon the alcoholic content of the tissues and the other pathological changes disclosed by the necropsy. If there is no serious pathology and the blood contains more than 0.43% alcohol, the kidney more than 0.39% alcohol or the liver or the brain more than 0.35% to 0.39% alcohol, one may fairly assume that death resulted from acute alcoholism. If, on the other hand, one finds serious pathology such as extensive cardio-circulatory disease or liver or kidney lesions, it would be fair to assume that in the presence of lesser concentrations of alcohol (0.25% to 0.35%) death was due to a combination of the pathologic lesions found, and acute alcoholism. Death from chronic alcoholism is difficult to diagnose from postmortem information, and must be based largely upon the history of the case.

The answer to the second question is based upon the distribution of alcohol in the body tissues. As has been pointed out previously, one can draw quite accurate conclusions regarding the stage of alcoholic intoxication from the blood analysis. Also one can make farily accurate inferences of the blood alcohol from the alcohol content of other tissues such as liver, kidney, or brain. It should be noted that, for the purpose of medicolegal interpretation of the extent of alcoholic intoxication, the analysis of the brain is of no greater significance than that of the liver, kidney, or blood.

The state of preservation of the tissues is of considerable

importance. There is some postmortem fermentation of the tissues and particularly of the stomach contents where putrefaction has progressed for several days in a warm environment. The extent of alcohol production by such fermentation does not exceed 0.02% to 0.10% of alcohol in the tissues and rarely introduces a serious error into the toxicologic interpretation of the chemical results. On the other hand, Nicloux[1275-O] has shown that tissues containing appreciable amounts of alcohol, actually lose alcohol as putrefaction advances. Where the body has been embalmed, the toxicologist is confronted with a more complex problem. Embalming fluids almost invariably contain formaldehyde and methyl alcohol as well as small but toxicologically significant amounts of ethyl alcohol. These interfere with the ordinary determination of ethyl alcohol using the Nicloux principle. However, upon oxidation with chromic acid, both formaldehyde and methyl alcohol are oxidized to carbon dioxide and water. If ethyl alcohol is present it is oxidized to acetic acid which may be distilled off and titrated.[1275-P] If ethyl alcohol is present in the embalming fluid used, it is impossible to give any opinion as to alcoholism in the deceased. Koopmain and Kempski[1275-Q] believe that without simultaneous determination of the alcohol content of the urine and of the blood there can be no definite conclusions regarding the degree of drunkenness.

BUTYL ALCOHOL

BUTYL ALCOHOL, $CH_3(CH_2)_2CH_2OH$, has a specific gravity of 0.810 to 0.815 at 20°C. It boils between 112° and 118° C., and its flash point is 35°C.

Smyth[1276] has shown that animals have survived 164 exposures to this substance. In spite of the very low concentration in which this was used, the tested animals showed a definite change in the blood picture; there was decrease in the red cells and a relative absolute leukocytosis. The period of exposure was four hours each day for six days. Similarly,

1275-O. NICLOUX, M.: *Compt. rend. Soc. de biol.*, 120:1301, 1935.

1275-P. ABERNETHY, R. J., RUSSELL, E. R., and THIENES, C. H.: "The Estimation of Ethyl Alcohol in Brain," *J. Lab. & Clin. Med.*, 19:1014-1018, 1934. WREDE, KARL, and SCUBA, H.: "Estimation of Alcohol in the Blood: Heiduschka and Steulmaim Method," *Zentralbl.*, 78:267, 1937.

1275-Q. KOOPMAIN, H., and KEMPSKI: *München. med. Wchnschr.*, 84:780, 1937.

1276. SMYTH, H. F.: *J. Indust. Hyg.*, 10:73, 1928.

turpentine was used on four animals, and all but one, which died from infection, made an excellent recovery, gained in weight and showed no skin or blood changes. At autopsy there was a slight fatty degeneration in the kidney.

Amyl alcohol, $C_5H_{11}OH$, has a boiling point of 137°C. Its specific gravity is about 0.81 at 25° C. It is slightly soluble in water. Jacobi and Speer describe a fatal case of amyl aclohol poisoning in an epileptic aged twenty-two.[1277] Through a mistake the nurse had given the patient 35 cc. in place of 6 gm. prescribed as an enema, as bromides had no effect upon his seizures. After twenty-four hours, edema of the lungs and cardiac insufficiency were present. At the end of forty-two hours severe gastric hemorrhage occurred, consisting of about one liter of coffee ground substance. There was complete loss of reflexes but, shortly after, this returned, beginning with the plantar. The patient died a few hours later. No autopsy was obtained. The author states that Anker in 1892 reported a woman's attempt at suicide by taking 27 gm. of amyl alcohol, approximately the same amount that his patient received.

Amyl acetate, known as banana oil, has been used as a solvent for many years. It causes irritation of the eyes, throat and nose. Workmen complain of headache, tightness of the chest and a dry cough. St. George* reported a death from inhalation of amyl acetate and another from inhalation of ethyl acetate. In the case of the amyl acetate the autopsy revealed an edema of the glottis and a diffuse irritation of the respiratory and gastrointestinal tracts and a tracheo-bronchitis and pleuritis. In animal experiments, edema and a pneumonic infiltration of the lung and a fatty infiltration of the liver are noted. A workman inhaling ethyl acetate for three hours complained of a "stomatitis," bleeding gums, and blood stained tissues. In St. George's case the autopsy showed a marked congestion of the eyes and viscera, fluid blood in the vessels, petechial-like hemorrhages throughout the serous cavities and mucous membranes.

Diacetone alcohol has a specific gravity of 0.95 to 0.92 at 20° C. It is miscible with distilled water in all proportions. It distills between 60° and 75° C. Its molecular weight is 7.65 at 68° F. It is also miscible with all common solvents. In industry it is used as a solvent for oils and resins.

1277. JACOBI and SPEER: *Therap. Halbmonatsch.*. 34:445, 1920.
* ST.GEORGE, A. V.: *Am. J. Clin. Path.*, 7:69, 1937.

The solvents methyl, ethyl, butyl and amyl acetates are very important constituents of cellulose acetate coatings and nitro-cellulose and cellulose lacquers. Most of these are used in spray guns which have largely replaced the brushing and dipping. The danger in the use of these substances arises when the solvents contain alcohol, ether, or benzol, or when the pigment which is contained in the lacquers is inhaled. I have seen cases of spray gun workers who had, according to the x-ray pictures, a mottling in the lungs very similar to that seen in first degree silicosis. Workers in amyl acetate frequently complain of headaches and irritation of the eyes.

Butyl Acetate, $CH_3CO_2C_4H_9$, has a specific gravity of 0.872 to 0.880 at 20° C. Its molecular weight is 116.1. It has a melting point of —76.8° C., and a boiling point of 116.3° C. Butyl acetate is used for dehydrating purposes, and as a solvent for nitrocellulose and mineral and vegetable oils, natural resins and many synthetic resins. It is used extensively in the manufacture of nitrocellulose lacquers, and in the making of artificial silk, photograph films polishes, and safety glass. Although this substance is used extensively in industry, poisoning has not been reported from its use.

Acetone, $CH_3.CO.OH_3$, is used as a solvent for cellulose acetate and nitrocellulose and in making celluloid, artificial silk, and smokeless powder. The Bureau of Mines, experimenting on animals, reports an acute narcotic effect stronger than that of chloroform and death from 110 mg. per liter of air. Flury and Zernik,[1278] however, have administered as much as 125 and 178 mg. per liter without killing the animal. I have not seen a case of acetone poisoning.

Furfural, as reported by McGuigan,[1279] is locally corrosive and anesthetic in action, is about one-half as toxic as phenol and one-third as toxic as formaldehyde for goldfish, and is similar to chloral in its action on frogs. I tried to use furfural in embalming fluid and found that the fluid turned dark and discolored the skin. I also found that furfural is irritating to the eyes.

Dioxan is diethylene dioxide, and it has been reported[1280]

1278. FLURY, F., and ZERNIK, F.: *Schadliche Gase,* Berlin, 1931.
1279. McGUIGAN, H.: *J. Pharmacol. & Exper. Therap.,* 21:65, 1923.
1280. YANT, W. P., SCHRENK, H. H., WAITE, C. P., and PATLY, F. A.: U. S. Pub. Health Rep. 45:2023, 1930.

by Yant and his associates that this substance causes acute poisoning from the vapors, the symptoms consisting of irritation of the eyes, nose, throat, air passages and lungs, with narcosis if the concentration is high.

Barber reported five men who died as the result of working in a process in which dioxan (diethylene dioxide) was used.[1281] "The morbid anatomy was proved to be hemorrhagic nephritis in four cases submitted to autopsy, associated with central necrosis of the liver, which was proved by histological examination in three cases. There is evidence that a few intense exposures to the chemical dioxan are much more serious than repeated slight exposures. There is little evidence of disease from chronic poisoning, but those exposed to the chemical showed a definite degree of increase of leucocytes, particularly the neutrophils."

Triortho-Cresyl Phosphate, the phosphoric ester of cresol, was substituted during prohibition days for Jamaica ginger, and caused thousands of cases of "Jake paralysis." During 1930 and 1931 poisoning from the substance occurred on a large scale in Oklahoma and Southern California, due to drinking of Jamaica ginger. About 15,000 persons were affected in ten days. The poisoning was followed by general weakness and a feeling of tingling and burning of the hands and feet, and in about a thousand of the cases there was paralysis of the extremities. Clinically, the condition resembles lead poisoning, owing to degeneration of the peripheral nerves and anterior horn cells, of the cord particularly in the cervical and lumbar regions. Triortho-cresyl phosphate is used in lacquers, and may at some future time again be of interest as a poison, although it is not very volatile.

Test for Amyl Alcohol Vapors in Air:[1282] Collect the air in a dry flask of known capacity and quickly add 20 cc. of 96% alcohol previously diluted with an equal volume of water; stopper, and shake vigorously. Agitate for two or three hours, then filter if necessary. To 1 cc. add 0.1 cc. of a 1% solution of furfural, and carefully run in 5 cc. of concentrated sulphuric acid (s.g. 1084) along the side of the test-tube, mixing slowly while cooling with a water jet. Prepare color standards from amyl alcohol in the same manner. Place all the tubes in boiling water

1281. BARBER, H.: *Guy's Hosp. Rep.*, 84:267, 1934.
1282. KOREMAN, I. M.: *Arch. f. Hyg.*, 109:108, 1932.

for three minutes. Cool thoroughly and compare colors. The value multiplied by 20 gives the quantity of amyl alcohol or amyl acetate vapor in the volume of air examined. For very weak vapor concentrations a series of flasks may be used with 96% alcohol which is afterward diluted with an equal volume of water before colorimetrization. Grease must not be used on stopcocks.

To get a synthetic vapor concentration to test the method, laboratory air was passed through soda lime and calcium chloride, then over a surface of amyl alcohol in a U-tube until a desired weight had been removed. Against concentrations of 0.17 to 0.57 mg. of the alcohol per liter of air, the findings averaged within 5% of the expected value, with a minimum variation of 10%. Results with the acetate were practically the same.

Vapors of methyl or ethyl alcohol, ethyl ether, acetone, or amylene-free benzene are detrimental to the determination, but with vapors of benzene containing unsaturated hydrocarbons the results show the sum of the latter plus the amyl alcohol or acetate. Oil of turpentine interferes by producing colors with the furfural and acid.[1282]

FORMALDEHYDE (HCHO)

FORMALDEHYDE is a colorless gas, with a characteristic pungent odor, prepared by the oxidation of methyl alcohol. It condenses at —20° C. (—4° F.) and solidifies at —90° C. (—130°F.). It is freely soluble in water. On heating with dilute caustic alkali it separates into methyl alcohol and formic acid: $2CH_2O + KOH = CH_4O + HCOOH$. On standing with ammonia it yields hexamethylentetramin: $6CH_2O + 4NH_3 = (CH_2)_6N_4 + 6H_2O$. The United States Pharmacopeia (U. S. P., XI) states that it is an "aqueous solution containing not less than 37% of CH_2O, with variable amounts of methanol to prevent polymerization". This is sold under the name of formalin. Prior to June 21, 1906, it was used extensively as a preservative for milk and other articles of food. It is used as a preservative in the chemical industry in the preparation of substitutes for ivory—celluloid and horn—made by the action of formaldehyde on casein. It is also used in making bakelite, an artificial resin from condensing formaldehyde with phenol.

The vapors of formaldehyde are very irritating to the mucous membranes, and the workmen engaged in the manufacture and handling of it often suffer from severe coryza, conjunctivitis, and bronchitis.

Formaldehyde, when applied to unbroken skin, hardens the epidermis and produces an anesthesia. A stronger solution causes superficial necrosis of the nails and skin, often causing a persistent eczema. It is very painful when applied to the abraded skin. An aqueous solution containing one part of formaldehyde in 2,000 is very irritating to the skin. Long continued application of strong solutions leads to ulcerations and gangrene; weak solutions lead to eczema. Some embalmers develop severe dermatitis and have to discontinue their work for months before they resume embalming of bodies with solutions containing formaldehyde.

The fatal dose for mammals intravenously is about 0.07 to 0.09 gm. per kilogram of body weight.

In cases of formaldehyde poisoning, the patient's stomach should be washed out with a very dilute ammonia solution. It should be repeatedly washed out with water containing one teaspoonful of sodium bicarbonate to the pint of water. McGuigan[1283] says that formaldehyde is absorbed from all parts of the alimentary tract and lungs. It may oxidize in the tissues, especially the liver, to formic acid. A part of the formic acid may appear in the urine, but small quantities are also completely destroyed. A person who has taken methenamine or hexamethylentetramin liberates formaldehyde which may be found in the urine, depending upon the acidity, the concentration, and the time of standing. Smith[1284] found 0.05 gm. always gave formaldehyde in acid urines, while 0.03 gm. was inconstant.

Formaldehyde will be found in the acid distillate of all embalmed bodies. I have had three cases of poisoning by formaldehyde which were accidental, the men believing that they were drinking alcohol contained in bottles which had previously held Bourbon whiskey. One case drank six ounces with suicidal intent. The symptoms are burning sensation in the mouth, esophagus, and stomach, similar to that produced by carbolic acid and bichloride of mercury. Death may occur in twenty-four to forty-eight hours. Autopsy showed severe gastritis with erosions (in two of the cases mentioned above). Autopsy in the accidental case showed a puckering of the eso-

1283. McGuigan, H.: J.A.M.A., 62:984, 1914.
1284. Smith, G. G.: Boston M. J., May 15, 1913.

phagus and stomach, with marked hyperemia of all the organs. In non-fatal cases the urine is suppressed for twelve to twenty-four hours and then generally contains albumin, blood, and casts. Following the taking of formaldehyde there is diarrhea, tenesmus, sore mouth, and dysphagia. The largest quantity from which recovery has been reported is 60 cc.

Formaldehyde has a corrosive effect on the eyes if the concentration reaches 4,900 parts per million of air for three hours. Iwanoff[1285] says that damage to the lungs, which will not pass off for several days, can be produced by exposure to 0.8 mg. per liter of air for four hours. If it lasts as long as eight hours, pneumonia may follow. The danger limit for cats is not much over 200 parts per million. The physiological action has been attributed to the decomposition of formaldehyde into formic acid and methyl alcohol. McCord found formaldehyde rash developing in women who applied celluloid and viscose caps on medicine bottles, the material containing free formaldehyde.[1286]

Tests: Formaldehyde gives all general aldehyde reactions.

1. With Nessler's reagent it gives a yellow to reddish-yellow color, and upon heating a black precipitate forms.

2. Upon standing with ammonium silver nitrate solution it will be reduced, with the formation of a silver mirror.

3. To 2 cc. of the distillate add 1 cc. of concentrated sulphuric acid; cool, and add 5 cc. of reduced fuchsin solution. Mix and allow to stand. The presence of formaldehyde is indicated by the violet-red color which gradually develops.[1287] The fuchsin solution is prepared by dissolving 0.02 gm. powdered fuchsin in 120 cc. of hot water; cool to room temperature. Then 2 gm. of anhydrous sodium sulphite are dissolved in 20 cc. of water and added to the fuchsin solution. Add to this 2 cc. of hydrochloric acid (specific gravity 1.19) and dilute to 200 cc. with water. In about an hour this is ready as a reagent.

4. To 5 cc. of concentrated sulphuric acid add a few drops of distillate, from two drops to 2 cc., depending upon the concentration of formaldehyde present. Allow to cool and add a few milligrams of morphine. A violet-red color develops if formaldehyde is present (Marquis test).[1288]

1285. IWANOFF, N.: *Arch. f. Hyg.*, 73:307, 1911.

1286. McCORD, CAREY P.: Indust. Rep., Retail Credit Assn., 3:4, 1928.

1287. See ELVOVE: *J. Indust. & Eng. Chem.*, 9:295, 1917; also WIELAND and SCHEWING: Ber. 54, 25:27, 1921.

1288. See GETTLER, A. O.: *J. Biol. Chem.*, 42:311, 1920, for complete list of references on tests.

5. To 15 cc. of milk in a casserole add 2 cc. of distillate, and then a drop or two of dilute ferric chloride and 5 cc. of concentrated hydrochloric acid. The mixture is gently heated. A violet color develops if formaldehyde is present in the original material examined. The violet color may appear on the edge of the liquid where it comes in contact with the formaldehyde. Where very much is present the color will appear throughout the top of the liquid (Hehner test). To 1 cc. of distillate add one drop of 1% carbolic acid solution, underlaying this with pure sulphuric acid; a caramel red ring will be obtained in dilutions as great as one to 200,000.

6. If the amount of the formaldehyde is not too small, a very characteristic and useful test is to obtain crystals of hexamethylentetramin, $6CH_2O + 4NH_3 = (CH_2)_6N_4 + 6H_2O$, after treating the formaldehyde with ammonia and evaporating slowly. If some of the residue from this reaction is dissolved in water and treated with bichloride of mercury, phosphoric and molybdic acids, (Mayer's or Wagner's reagent), a crystalline double salt is obtained similar to that found with alkaloids. This reaction is very useful for the microscopic determination of formaldehyde.

7. To 2 cc. of distillate add eight drops of 5% solution of phenylhydrazine hydrochloride and one drop of 0.5% sodium nitroprusside solution and five drops of 10% sodium hydroxide solution. If formaldehyde is present a blue color is developed, which changes to green and then to yellowish-red. Acetaldehyde produces a red color.

8. To 3 cc. of distillate add 0.05 gm. of resorcin and one drop of 50% sodium hydroxide solution. Heat, and in the presence of formaldehyde a beautiful red color will appear.[1289]

9. To 5 cc. of distillate add 0.5 cc. of sulphuric acid and a few drops of dimethylanilin, and heat to 40° C. (104° F.) for an hour in a sealed tube. Alkalinize the product with sodium carbonate and evaporate the excess of dimethylanilin. Acidify with acetic acid and add a trace of lead dioxide. The presence of formic aldehyde will be shown by the production of an intense blue color.[1290]

Estimation: Formaldehyde may be determined by its reaction with neutral ammonium salts whereby hexamethyl-

1289. LEBBIN: *Chem. Centralbl.*, 1:641, 1899.
1290. TRILLAT: *Chem. Centralbl.*, 2:585, 1898.

entetramin is formed, as indicated in the following equation: $6CH_2O + 4NH_4OH = (CH_2)_6N_4 + 10H_2O$. We use a definite amount of the distillate with an excess of ammonia. Cork the flask, and shake frequently for a period of two or three days to convert the formaldehyde into hexamethylentetramin. Transfer this to a platinum dish and evaporate nearly to dryness on the top of a closed water-bath. The dish is then transferred to a desiccator, and the drying is continued over sulphuric acid to a constant weight. The percentage of formaldehyde is calculated from the weight of hexamethylentetramin, making a correction for the residue left by the formaldehyde itself by direct evaporation.

Formaldehyde may be assayed as follows:

1. Transfer about 3 cc. of solution of formaldehyde to a tared flask containing 10 cc. of distilled water, stopper the flask tightly, and determine the exact weight of the solution taken. Add 50 cc. of normal sodium hydroxide, and follow this immediately but slowly through a small funnel with 50 cc. of hydrogen peroxide T.S. that has been previously neutralized to bromthymol blue T.S. with normal sodium hydroxide. Heat the mixture cautiously on a water-bath for five minutes, shaking occasionally. Allow the mixture to cool, rinse the funnel and inner walls of the flask with distilled water, and, after allowing it to stand for thirty minutes, add two to five drops of bromthymol blue T.S., and titrate the excess of alkali with normal sulphuric acid. Each cubic centimeter of normal sodium hydroxide is equivalent to 0.03002 gm. of formaldehyde.

2. To 100 cc. of the distillate add 10 cc. of N/10 silver nitrate with a few drops of 50% nitric acid, in a 200 cc. flask. Add 10 cc. of solution of potassium cyanide containing 3.1 gm. of potassium cyanide, and make up with water to the 150 cc. mark Shake, filter, and titrate 100 cc. of filtrate with tenth-normal ammonium sulphocyanate, using ferric chloride as indicator. Acidify another portion of 10 cc. N/10 silver nitrate with nitric acid; add 10 cc. of potassium cyanide solution to which 100 cc. of formaldehyde distillate obtained above have been added. Make the whole up to 150 cc., filter, and titrate as before 100 cc. of the filtrate with 10 cc. ammonium sulphocyanate for excess of silver. The amount of potassium cyanide used up by the formaldehyde in terms of N/10 ammonium sulphocyanate is found by multiplying by 2 the difference between the two

results, and the total formaldehyde is calculated by multiplying by 3 the amount found in the 100 cc. of distillate.

3. Iodometric method:[1291] Mix 10 cc. of the aldehyde solution, which should not exceed 3% formaldehyde, with 25 cc. tenth-normal iodine solution. Add drop by drop a solution of sodium hydroxide until the liquid is clear yellow. The solution is set aside for ten minutes, after which hydrochloric acid is added to set free the uncombined iodine; the latter is titrated back with N/10 thiosulphate. Two atoms of iodine are equivalent to one molecule of formaldehyde. The amount of iodine taken up multiplied by 0.1183 gives the amount of formaldehyde.

PARALDEHYDE ($CH_3.CHO$)$_3$

PARALDEHYDE is a polymer of acetaldehyde. It has a molecular weight of 132.09, and is a clear transparent liquid which has a strong, characteristic, not unpleasant odor but a disagreeable taste. The specific gravity is about 0.99 at 25°C. It distills between 120° and 125°C., and boils at 124°C. When heated with a small amount of dilute sulphuric acid it is converted into acetaldehyde, recognized by its odor. Poisoning by paraldehyde is very rare.

Symptoms: The patient may fall asleep ten to fifteen minutes after taking 2 cc. of paraldehyde. However, I have seen one case in which a half-ounce of the substance had no ill effect whatever. The man was in the habit of taking one-fourth to one-half ounce daily to allay nervousness. If he exceeded this amount, it caused him to have nausea, headache, and dizziness. The usual effects of amounts exceeding 2 cc. are deep stupor and complete relaxation of the muscles; the face is flushed, and the pupils are somewhat contracted. Habitual use of paraldehyde is known in India, but it is uncommon.[1292] The symptoms in chronic paraldehyde poisoning vary. There are usually disturbances of the digestion, thirst, emaciation, general muscular weakness, and mental failure, with tremors of the hands and tongue. Skin eruptions similar to those caused by chloral hydrate have been reported. Individuals develop a paraldehyde habit, just as they develop the morphine habit.

Fatal Dose: Death has been reported in four hours from

1291. *Zetts. anal. Chem.*, 36:18, 1897; abst. *Analyst*, 22, 221.
1292. CHOPRA, R. N., and CHOPRA, G. S.: *Indian M. Gaz.*, 67:481, 1932.

22.5 cc.[1293] However, three and a half ounces caused a severe but not fatal poisoning. Those accustomed to the use of paraldehyde can take very large doses, as in the case of the patient mentioned above. Doses of one ounce have been taken for months without causing any symptoms. On the other hand, two ounces a day have led to severe reaction.[1294]

Treatment: The treatment is to wash out the stomach, and give barbiturates or morphine to quiet the nerves.

Postmortem Appearances: The postmortem appearances are not characteristic. Schneider[1295] found that the changes due to paraldehyde poisoning are mainly loosening and swelling of the mucous lining of the stomach, with gradual sloughing of the surface tissues. The author noted injury to the liver cells. He cites instances from the literature in which 75 gm. were taken by a patient but did not lead to fatal poisoning, while in another patient 50 gm. caused death.

ACETALDEHYDE (CH₃.CHO)

ACETALDEHYDE is a colorless, irritating liquid, having a peculiar odor, and boiling at 20°C. (69.8°F.). It is used in the chemical industry, in the quick vinegar process, in the manufacture of mirrors, and by dye makers, explosive workers, pyroxylin plastic workers, synthetic resin makers, and varnish makers.

Symptoms: Acetaldehyde causes irritation of the mucous membranes of the mouth, the eyes, and the respiratory tract; it also causes dyspnea, cough, acceleration of the pulse rate, and profuse night sweats.

Acetaldehyde will be found in the acid distillate, and responds to the general tests for aldehydes as given under Formaldehyde (see page 668).

Estimation: 1. Prepare aldehyde-free alcohol by first redistilling the ordinary 95% alcohol over caustic soda or potash, then add from 2 to 3 gm. per liter of m-phenylenediamine hydrochloride, digest at ordinary temperature for several days (or reflux on the steam-bath for several hours), and then distill slowly, rejecting the first 100 cc. and the last 200 cc.

2. Fuchsin solution: Dissolve 0.05 gm. of pure fuchsin in

1293. *Lancet*, 2:423, 1890.
1294. REINHOLD: *Therap. Monatsh., Berl.*, 2:300, 1897.
1295. SCHNEIDER, P.: *Wien. klin. Wchnschr.*, 42:357, 1929.

500 cc. of water, add 5 gm. of SO_2 dissolved in water; make up to a liter, and allow to stand until colorless. Prepare this solution in small quantities, as it retains its strength for only a very few days.

3. Prepare the standard aldehyde solution according to the directions of Vasey as follows: Grind aldehyde ammonia in a mortar with ether and decant the ether. Repeat this operation several times, then dry the purified salt in a current of air and finally in a vacuum over sulphuric acid. Dissolve 1.386 gm. of this purified ammonium aldehyde in 50 cc. of 95% alcohol; to this add 22.7 cc. of normal alcoholic sulphuric acid; then make up to 100 cc., and add 0.8 cc. to compensate for the volume of the ammonium sulphate precipitate. Allow this to stand over night and filter. This solution contains 1 gm. of acetic aldehyde in 100 cc., and will retain its strength.

The standard found most convenient for use is 2 cc. of this strong aldehyde solution diluted to 100 cc. with 50% alcohol by volume. One cc. of this solution is equal to 0.0002 gm. of acetic aiaehyde. This solution should be made up fresh every day or so, as it loses its strength.

Determine the aldehyde in the distillate. Dilute from 5 to 10 cc. of the distillate to 50 cc. with aldehyde-free alcohol (50% by volume), add 25 cc. of the fuchsin solution and allow to stand for fifteen minutes at 15°C. The solutions and reagent should be at 15°C. (59°F.) before they are mixed. Simultaneously prepare standards of known strength in the same way. Compare the red color developed in the unknown with that in the standard. From this the amount is calculated.

A method originally proposed by Reiter[1296] has been modified by Roques with good results: A sodium sulphite solution is made by dissolving 12.6 gm. of anhydrous sodium sulphide in 400 cc. of water, adding 100 cc. of normal sulphuric acid, diluting to 1000 cc. with alcohol of 96% and filtering after twenty-four hours. A convenient quantity of the alcoholic solution of aldehyde to be examined is placed in a 100-cc. stoppered flask, mixed with 50 cc. of the sulphite solution and made up to 100 cc. with 50% of alcohol. A second quantity of 50 cc. of the sulphite solution is placed in a similar flask and made up to 100 cc. with the same alcohol. After heating to 50°C. at least four hours, 50 cc. are withdrawn from each flask, and the sulphurous acid

---

1296. REITER: *J. Soc. Chem. Indust.*, abst., 16: 606, 1897.

determined by means of tenth-normal iodine solution; the difference is the quantity of sulphurous acid that is in combination with the aldehyde:

1 cc. of N/10 iodine=0.0022 gm. of aldehyde.

If the liquid to be examined contains less than 1% of aldehyde, the sulphite solution must be diluted; for 0.5% of it should be diluted with an equal volume of alcohol of 50%, and N/20 iodine should be used; for 0.1% the sulphite should be diluted with alcohol of 50% to ten times its ordinary volume, and centinormal iodine solution should be used.

CHLORAL HYDRATE (CCl₃.CH(OH)₂)

$$\text{CHLORAL HYDRATE (CCl}_3.\text{CH(OH)}_2)$$

CHLORAL HYDRATE is a colorless, transparent, crystalline substance, having an aromatic, penetrating and slightly acrid odor and a slightly bitter, caustic taste. Its molecular weight is 165.39. It slowly volatilizes when exposed to the air. One gram of chloral hydrate is soluble in 0.25 cc. of water, in 1.3 cc. of alcohol, in 2 cc. of chloroform, and in 1.5 cc. of ether at 25°C. It is decomposed by alkali into chloroform and formates and water at ordinary temperature. If the acid distillate is not exhausted, it will be found in the alkaline distillate as chloroform or as a formate.

Chloral hydrate has been used as "knockout drops" for the purpose of producing sleep, for robbery, and for other crimes. In a number of instances, where it was given in an alcoholic beverage, death was caused when only its hypnotic effect was desired. In one instance Dr. W. H. Burmeister, Coroner's Physician, submitted organs of a man found in the Chicago river, and expressed the opinion that the man had not drowned. A chemical examination of the organs revealed that the man had been poisoned by chloral hydrate. Investigation revealed that he had been "jack rolled" on Madison street, Chicago. Chloral hydrate passes into the fetus and may cause its death without killing the mother.[1297]

Chopra[1298] states that addiction to chloral hydrate is of recent origin. The addicts are mostly between the ages of twenty-one and forty years, and in the majority of cases they

1297. *Pharm. J.*, 27:629, 1908.
1298. CHOPRA, R. N., and CHOPRA, G. S.: *Indian M. Gaz.*, 67:481, 1932.

are also addicted to alcohol or opium. Addiction was found mostly among the liquor drinkers who want its intoxicating effect. The authors describe forty cases, and state that the habit is harmful and dangerous, and more liable to produce pathological changes in the organs and immediately fatal results than any other drug of addiction used in India.

Symptoms: When 1 to 2 gm. of chloral hydrate are given per mouth, drowsiness is produced in ten to fifteen minutes, and quiet, sound sleep within an hour. The sleep may last for several hours, but the patient can be easily and completely awakened, and is refreshed, without any depressing after-effect. However, in cases where there is a weakened heart action, as in delirium tremens, or the insomnia of continued fever, death may result very rapidly from failure of the heart, in some cases occurring even before drowsiness is noticed. Occasionally chloral hydrate may produce excitement and delirium. Nausea and vomiting may be the result of the local action of the drug upon the stomach. It has been found impossible to arouse a man from sleep if he has been given an overdose of the drug together with alcohol; the respiration is irregular and shallow and the pulse is scarcely perceptible; the pupils are moderately contracted, making one think that the patient had taken morphine; the pupils are rarely dilated; the face is cyanotic, or, in the early stages, flushed. On account of the dilatation of the vessels, the extremities are cold, and the blood pressure and temperature are slightly lower, but little more than in natural sleep. In respiratory and circulatory diseases these depressant effects may be more pronounced and may lead to some cyanosis. If the dose of 2 to 3 gm. is exceeded, the patient passes into stupor and coma with complete muscular relaxation. The action is very similar to that of chloroform. Large doses always cause a marked fall in temperature on account of the cutaneous vasodilatation coupled with the production of heat from the muscular relaxation.

According to Sollmann and Hatcher, the temperature regulation in deep coma resembles that of cold-blooded animals.[1299]

Death is ordinarily caused by paralysis of the respiratory center. It is possible that cardiac paralysis in an already weakened heart may cause death, as in the case of chloroform. Sudden death is common among habitual chloral hydrate

1299. SOLLMANN and HATCHER: *J.A.M.A.*, 51:487, 1908.

takers, and may occur after doses slightly larger than those which the patient has been taking.

In chronic chloral hydrate poisoning, a scarlatina-like rash or vesicles, or superficial ulceration of the roots of the nails, may be seen. There is frequently a disturbance of digestion, with diarrhea and loss of weight.

Fatal Dose: Death has been reported from doses as small as 1 to 3 gm., and recovery has taken place from 10 to 28 gm. The average fatal dose is placed at about 10 gm. Caution must be used in giving over the therapeutic dose.

Fatal Period: The fatal period is dependent upon the size of the dose and the condition of the individual who has taken the drug. Thirty grains caused death in thirty-five hours. Doses of seventy-five grains have caused death in fifteen minutes to one hour. Death has taken place within ten minutes after taking twenty to thirty grains. Where death has occurred rapidly from such small doses, there must have been some cardiac involvement before taking the chloral hydrate. The number of cases of chloral hydrate poisoning are not as numerous as formerly, because of the introduction of the barbiturates.

Treatment: The same general measures should be used as described on pages 11-14. Wash out the stomach. Administer hypodermically strychnine, caffeine, and caffeine with sodium benzoate. The temperature of the patient should be maintained by the use of electric pads, hot water bottles, and blankets.

Postmortem Appearances: The gross appearance of the organs in a case of chloral hydrate poisoning offers nothing characteristic. The contents of the stomach may have the odor of chloral hydrate. However, this odor is frequently masked by alcoholic beverages taken by the individual. Fatty degeneration of the heart, liver, and kidneys is seen in chronic cases of chloral hydrate poisoning.

Isolation: Chloral hydrate is isolated in the acid distillate of a steam distillation. It is decomposed by alkalis, giving rise to chloroform and formates, and if not all removed by the acid distillate it is found in the alkaline distillate as chloroform, or as a formate.

Tests: 1. Boil a few cc. of the acid distillate with 0.2 gm. of solid sodium thiosulphate. This gives a turbid liquid of blue-red color. After the addition of a few drops of potassium hydroxide solution the turbidity disappears and the color of the liquid becomes brownish-red. A portion of the distillate may be heated under a reflux condenser with magnesium oxide on a water-bath, which causes magnesium formate and chloroform to be produced

$$2CCl_3CHO.H_2O + MgO = 2CHCl_3 + (HCO_2)_2Mg + H_2O$$

A few cc. of the solution in the flask, after the decomposition of the chloral hydrate, will give tests for chloroform (see under Chloroform page 687). The balance of the liquid is filtered from the insoluble material, the liquid is acidified with tartaric acid, and the formic acid is distilled off and identified by the following test:

Upon boiling a solution of formic acid with acidified potassium permanganate, the latter is reduced and the color of the solution disappears.

When a few drops of mercuric chloride are added to a solution of formic acid, a white precipitate of mercurous chloride will be formed. Silver nitrate solutions are reduced by formic acid, with the production of a black precipitate of metallic silver

$$2HgCl_2 + H.CO_2H = 2HgCl + 2HCl + CO_2$$

2. When phloroglucin and sodium carbonate and chloral hydrate are allowed to stand at room temperature for about one-half hour, a lilac to orange to blood-orange to deep red color develops. As small as 0.01 mg. of chloral hydrate in 1 cc. may be detected by this method. Chloroform does not give this reaction. Formaldehyde and acetaldehyde interfere in that they give a reddish color. If the distillate contains considerable chloral hydrate, 1 cc. may be used for the test. However, it is better to use 5 cc. to which are added four drops of saturated solution of phloroglucin and 2 cc. of 20% sodium carbonate. Upon standing a lilac to orange to blood-orange to deep red color develops.[1300]

3. In the absence of acetaldehyde, chloral hydrate gives with phenylhydrazine a light crystalline condensation product which is characteristic for both substances. Upon the addition of phenylhydrazine to chloral hydrate and sodium acetate, a white clouding will develop with the formation of long, colorless needles thrown out of solution. These crystals are first

1300. GETTLER, A. O.: Proc. Soc. Exper. Biol. & Med., 16:110–116, 1919.

yellow and then, after an hour's standing, become dark brown in color. This reaction is also given by naphthol hydrazine and diphenylhydrazine. Benzol phenylhydrazine gives no crystalline condensation product with chloral hydrate.

4. When yellow ammonium sulphide is added to a dilute solution of chloral hydrate, there is formed a white, later rose-red clouding. The substance formed is soluble in a drop of alcohol.

5. To 2 cc. of distillate are added six drops of saturated resorcin solution and 1 cc. of saturated sodium carbonate. Let stand for one hour. Dilute by adding 10 cc. water, and a beautiful green fluorescence will appear if chloral hydrate is present. Chloroform will not give this reaction. Caution should be used in this reaction as resorcin itself may give a fluorescence. Schwarz[1301] claims that there is a red color in addition to a green fluorescence. Gettler says that with chloroform, a green fluorescence never appears and that with chloral hydrate, even in minute amounts, fluorescence always occurs, and, although the red color does not appear in very dilute solutions, the green fluorescence is always present, especially if the produced reaction is diluted with 10 cc. of water. The test is sensitive for 0.1 mg. in 1 cc., and substances of an aldehyde character do not give this reaction.

Estimation: Chloral hydrate can be converted into chloroform and the amount of this determined, or it can be converted into formic acid and added to an excess of mercuric chloride solution, weighing the precipitated mercurous chloride.[1302] Chloral hydrate may be estimated in the aqueous solution by neutralization to remove any free acid. Titrate with normal sodium hydroxide. The amount of chloral hydrate can be determined from the amount of normal alkali used.

Chloral hydrate is separated in the urine partly as urochloral acid, $C_8H_{11}.Cl_3O_7$. Urochloral acid is crystalline, and soluble in water, alcohol, and ether. It reduces copper from Fehling's solution. Urochloral acid, on boiling with either dilute sulphuric acid or hydrochloric acid, forms trichlorethyl alcohol and glycuronic acid. To separate urochloral acid, evaporate the urine to a syrupy consistency at the heat of the water-bath. Acidulate with sulphuric acid and extract in a

1301. SCHWARZ: *Ztschr. f. anal. Chem.,* 27:668, 1888.
1302. *Arch. f. exper. Path. u. Pharmakol.,* 46:347, 1901.

Squibb's separatory funnel with a mixture of three volumes of ether and one of alcohol; the ethyl alcohol is separated and distilled, leaving an acid residue. Neutralize with potassium hydroxide or potassium carbonate, and evaporate. The residue is extracted with 90% alcohol and filtered. To the filtrate add ether, which forms a precipitate which is washed with ether and absolute alcohol. The precipitate is boiled with absolute alcohol and filtered hot. On cooling, the potassium salt of urochloral acid separates in tufts and silky needles. The crystals are dried over sulphuric acid and repurified by washing with alcohol and ether. The melting point of urochloral acid is 142°C.

During the acid distillation of chloral hydrate, chloroform is liberated to the extent of 2.36%. In the average case of chloral hydrate poisoning chloroform is always found, even if the stomach content is acid. During the usual procedure of adding magnesium oxide to the stomach content it was found that only 20.8% of the chloral hydrate was recovered as chloroform. The slight alkalinity due to sodium bicarbonate, calcium carbonate, and magnesium oxide found in antacid medication, is found to liberate from 2% to 21% of chloroform from chloral hydrate if added to the stomach content. In the examination of the stomach content for the presence of chloral hydrate the quantitative results never show the correct amount of chloral hydrate, as decomposition of this substance takes place in the steam distillation with the presence of free alkali. The alkalis that may be present are magnesium oxide, sodium bicarbonate, or calcium carbonate which have been used for the treatment of hyperacidity. In persons who have taken or been given chloral hydrate, the stomach content will show very much less chloral hydrate than was originally taken or given, because of the decomposition of the chloral hydrate by these substances.

CHLOROFORM ($CHCl_3$)
(Molecular Weight 119.38)

CHLOROFORM has been largely supplanted by ether, ethylene, and nitrous oxide. Statistics show that deaths from chloroform anesthesia have varied from one in 1,000 to one in 5,900. Occasional deaths have been reported when chloroform was used for criminal purposes, it having figured in several sensational murders in Cook County. A doctor was sentenced to Joliet (Illinois) for murdering his wife by chloroform. In the celebrated Wynekoop case, chloroform was administered in quantities which could have accounted for death, although the hemorrhage resulting from a bullet wound which coursed through the body also could have been responsible. In this case 750 gm. of brain yielded 358.7 mg. chloroform (5.52 grains); 220 gm. liver yielded 19.6 mg. (0.30 grains) of chloroform; 205 gm. stomach and content yielded 59.04 mg. (9.2 grains); 100 gm. kidney yielded 17.32 mg. (0.27 grains) of chloroform. Gettler and Blume gave the following table for the chloroform content of the brain in cases in which death involved the administration of chloroform:[1303]

TABLE LII
CHLOROFORM CONTENT OF BRAIN

Case	History	Mg. Chloroform in 1,000 gm. Brain
1	Suicide by inhalation	432
2	Suicide by inhalation	480
3	Suicide by inhalation	410
4	Suicide by inhalation	390
5	Homicide by inhalation	372
6	Homicide by inhalation	384
7	Homicide by inhalation	374
8	Anesthesia for abortion, shock	162
9	Anesthesia for abortion, hemorrhage	60*
10	Anesthesia for operation on tonsils, shock	136
11	Anesthesia for minor operations, shock	135
12	Anesthesia for minor operation, shock	145
13	Anesthesia for minor operation, shock	120
14	Anesthesia for minor operation, shock	122
15	Anesthesia for abortion, shock	182
16	Anesthesia for minor operation, shock	70†

* Patient came out of anesthesia; died of hemorrhage.
† Patient died from shock during administration of chloroform; was not fully anesthetized.

Table LIII shows the rate of disappearance of chloroform from the dog's brain during recovery from anesthesia.

It is highly improbable that an adult could be put to sleep by chloroform without consent. Children, however, might be anesthetized.

Properties: Chloroform is a clear, colorless, mobile liquid having a characteristic ethereal odor and a burning, sweet taste. It is not inflammable, but the heated vapor burns with a green flame. It is soluble in 210 volumes of water, and

1303. GETTLER, A. O., and BLUME, H.: *Arch. Path.*, 2:841, 1931.

miscible with alcohol, ether, benzene, petroleum, benzine, and with fixed or volatile oils. Chloroform boils at 61.0°C. but is volatile at lower temperatures. Its specific gravity is 1.474 to 1.478 at 25°C. The chloroform used for anesthesia is free from hydrochloric acid and phosgene. When chloroform is decomposed by flame, phosgene (carbonyl chloride, $COCl_2$), chlorine, and hydrochloric acid are liberated. Fatal poisoning has been reported from the action of these products.[1304] The addition of alcohol, with storage in the dark, prevents such decomposition. On heating with alcoholic potash, it is decomposed into potassium chloride and a formate, while on heating with alcoholic potash and ammonia it yields potassium cyanide.

TABLE LIII
AMOUNT OF CHLOROFORM IN DOGS' BRAINS

Dog	Body Weight Kg.	Weight of Brain Gm.	Time in Minutes			Mg. of Chloroform in Brain at Death	
			To Anesthetize	Until First Signs of Recovery	Until Placed on Floor	In Entire Brain	Calculated to 1,000 Gm.* of Brain
1	8.5	80	15	6	8	4.10	51.3
2	5.7	75	15	5	17	2.50	33.3
3	6.3	69	15	4	6	2.25	32.6
4	6.9	70	15	6	10	1.65	23.6
5	9.4	82	12	5	10	0.87	10.6
6	5.2	52	15	5	6	0.27	5.2
7	11.3	60	15	4	8	0.01	0.16
8	7.6	60	15	..	....	16.20	270.0
9	6.3	65	15	..	....	18.50	284.6
10	7.6	68	7			37.50	551.5

* Chloroform content of human brain is best reported on 1,000 gm. basis; in order to facilitate comparison, the chloroform in the dogs' brains was also calculated to 1,000 gm. portions.

Physiological Action: Chloroform is more irritant than ether in equal concentrations, and can be employed as a rubefacient. Accidents have happened where individuals have poured chloroform upon a bandage, causing marked blistering. Irritation is due largely to coagulation of the protoplasm. The first effect of the evaporation of chloroform is a cooling sensa-

1304. GERLINGER: Arch. f. exper. Path. u. Pharmakol., 47:428, 1902; BETACH: Brit. M. J., 1:63, 1905; ARMAND and BERTIER: Rev. de chir., Paris, 32:37, 1905; ACHARD, LEBLANC, and BINET: Arch. de méd. expér. et d'anat. path., Par., 28:628, 1920; WIKI: Rev. méd. de la Suisse Rom., 41:38, 1921; LAQUEUR and MAGNUS: Ztschr. f. d. ges. exper. Med., 13:31, 1921; HERTZMANN: Ztschr. f. d. ges. exper. Med., 13:180, 1921.

tion to the skin, which is later followed by a burning sensation
and redness. When chloroform was used as an anesthetic, it
was necessary to put vaseline upon the skin to prevent burning
during the production of anesthesia. Its irritant action on
mucous membranes is even more evident.

Symptoms: It is customary to recognize three stages in
the symptoms produced by chloroform. The first stage is that
of excitement. There is a feeling of warmth—first of the face,
then of the entire body—followed by a tingling sensation of the
skin. There are ringing and roaring sounds in the ears, and
vision becomes distorted. Consciousness is soon lost, and the
patient may struggle violently and indulge in profane or abusive language. The second stage is that of surgical anesthesia;
the muscles are relaxed, the patient lies perfectly still with
regular but rather slow and shallow respiration, and is entirely
insensible to pain. This stage may be maintained for hours. If
the inhalation of chloroform is discontinued at this stage, the
patient usually awakens within twenty to forty minutes, but
he may not awaken for several hours. Vomiting, which may
occur at almost any stage, may persist for some time. There is
usually some confusion of ideas also. The third stage is that
of paralysis, and it is characterized by a fall of blood pressure
and the failure of the respiration and heart. The skin becomes
dark and cyanotic, and the pupils dilate widely. There has
been a discussion in progress for many years as to the cause of
death in chloroform inhalation; some maintain that it is due to
failure of the heart, others to failure of the respiration. It
seems probable that in most cases in which death occurs late in
the anesthesia the respiration ceases first; in many cases life
may be maintained for some time by means of artificial respiration, the heart continuing to beat fairly well. In other cases the
heart is so deeply poisoned that it is unable to beat long after
the respiration has ceased, although artificial respiration is
maintained; this occurs most frequently when the chloroform
vapor is inhaled in concentrated form.

Very many of the deaths from chloroform have occurred
early in the anesthesia—at the very beginning of the operation
or even before the operation was commenced—or when the
patient had been allowed partially to come out and chloroform
was again administered. In most of these cases of sudden death
the heart stopped suddenly and before the respiration. This

form of death has been attributed to a sudden overloading of the heart with concentrated chloroform vapor. Pohl[1305] found that dogs could be killed in this way, and that the blood in the left side of the heart might contain ten times as much chloroform as that in the right side. A lethal amount of chloroform may be absorbed from a few deep inhalations. Embley[1306] has adduced a number of experiments and arguments to show that over-acidity of the vagus nerves leading to permanent stoppage of the poisoned heart may be responsible for this form of death, and states that in dogs it may be prevented by section of the vagi or by their paralysis with atropine. Levy,[1307] on the other hand, believes that in these cases there is a condition of very light anesthesia during which the heart is easily thrown into ventricular fibrillation with immediate death. He states that this form of death does not occur during deep anesthesia. The fibrillation is especially likely to occur from sensory nerve stimulation; reflexes through the accelerator nerves or an increased secretion of the adrenal glands may be a factor, for it was found that the injection of epinephrine into animals in light chloroform anesthesia would cause ventricular fibrillation. Whatever the explanation of this form of death, it is recognized that it is dangerous to operate under imperfect chloroform anesthesia. The condition of the patient is also frequently a factor in the fatal case. It is dangerous to administer chloroform to the very old, to those suffering from fatty heart, atheromatous arteries, diabetes, chronic diseases of the kidneys, or in status lymphaticus. Many fatalities occur among drunkards; it has been stated that the mortality among these has been as high as from 10 to 13%. Death occasionally results from suffocation due to the drawing into the air passages of vomited matter. Death occasionally occurs under chloroform when every precaution is taken; as such cases occurred in operations before the introduction of anesthetics, it seems very probable that sometimes death is not due to the anesthetic at all.

Death in deep anesthesia usually is due to paralysis of respiration with more or less involvement of circulation. With chloroform there is a progressive fall of blood pressure and finally cessation of the heart beat, but the pulse has generally

1305. POHL: *Arch. f. exper. Path. u. Pharmakol.*, 28:239, 1891.
1306. EMBLEY: *Brit. M. J.*, 1:817, 885, 951, 975, 1902.
1307. LEVY: *Heart*, 4:319, 1913; 5:299, 1914.

become imperceptible before the respiration finally stops.

Delayed chloroform poisoning may develop within twenty-four to forty-eight hours, and has been known to occur as late as one week after the anesthetic was given. The patient becomes restless, and vomits repeatedly; jaundice, tenderness over the liver, delirium, and coma appear. There may also be cutaneous hemorrhages.

Symptoms following the ingestion of chloroform are due to the local irritant action and also to the effects after absorption. Vomiting usually results, and there is sometimes involuntary evacuation of the bowels. However, in the Ursula Lang case in Milwaukee, Wisconsin, the patient did not vomit after two ounces of chloroform were given per mouth in a suicidal pact. It was thought at first that the girl was given the drug by inhalation, but from the finding of considerable chloroform in the bowel, I came to the conclusion that the chloroform had been taken by mouth. If the chloroform is absorbed, the symptoms may resemble those caused by inhalation of the drug. I have seen several cases of habitues who inhale chloroform for its stimulating effect. When taken by mouth, a period of excitement appears, and the patient staggers like a drunkard. Some are unconscious within ten minutes. The skin becomes cyanotic, cool; respiration is irregular and stertorous, and the breath smells of chloroform; the pulse is weak and irregular. The pupils may be dilated or contracted. Coma may continue for many hours and recovery may still take place, but abdominal pain, bloody diarrhea, swelling of the liver, jaundice, and painful micturition may continue for several days. Death may occur from pulmonary edema or failure of the heart, but more frequently from gastritis. In a series of fifty-seven cases collected by Eliot fifteen died, while of seventeen cases reported by Hirsch seven died.[1308]

Fatal Dose: When constant, 1.5% concentration of chloroform causes death in animals in one hour, and Geppert[1309] has shown that it requires the same concentration of chloroform vapor to anesthetize the lower animals as man. This would soon be fatal to man; hence, the rule is laid down that patients should not receive air containing more than 3.5% of chloroform

1308. ELIOT: *Med. Rec.*, 27:29, 1885; HIRSCH: *Ztschr. f. klin. med.*, 24:190, 1894.
1309. GEPPERT: *Deutsche med. Wchnschr.*, 25:447, 1899.

vapor. Fifteen drops of chloroform have caused death, while on the other hand twenty-two and a half ounces have been inhaled and the patient recovered. The fatal dose when taken per mouth is difficult to determine. In the Ursula Lang case two ounces caused death, while other cases have recovered from administrations as large as six ounces; 40 mm. (3.7 gm.) have caused severe but not fatal poisoning.[1310]

Fatal Period: Death has occurred before anesthesia was fully produced—within ten to fifteen minutes after the beginning of the administration of the anesthetic. Death may occur at any stage of chloroform inhalation.

Treatment: In case of the failure of respiration during the inhalation of chloroform the administration of the anesthetic should be immediately stopped, and the head should be lowered and the feet raised so as to drive the blood to the brain. Artificial respiration should be commenced, and the patient given inhalation of 10% carbon dioxide in oxygen. Injection of epinephrine into the pericardial sac has apparently saved life in cases in which the heart has failed as the result of a long continued anesthesia.

Postmortem Appearance: If the drug has been taken per mouth, there is marked hyperemia of the buccal mucosa, esophagus, and stomach. Congestion of the lungs, bronchi, and kidneys has been reported. If death occurs in a short time, chloroform will be found in the stomach content, in the liver, kidneys, blood, and brain. If death has been delayed for several days, jaundice and fatty degeneration of the heart, liver, and other organs may be found.

Gettler reports the case of a girl found dead in a doctor's office, whose brain showed 150 mg. of chloroform.[1311] The doctor claimed that the girl came into his office and died during a conversation. The quantitative chemical examination proved conclusively that she could not have walked into the physician's office. Autopsy disclosed that an incomplete abortion had been performed. Flagg states that a previous condition of suffering or anxiety renders a subject, otherwise able to resist large doses, liable to collapse from even a small dosage. In the stage of induction, chloroform death occurs as follows: There is a spasm of the respiratory tract due to a large amount of chloroform

1310. MARSHALL: *Med. News,* 73:654, 1898.
1311. GETTLER: *Med. Times,* 58:246, 1930.

accumulating in the mask; following relaxation of the spasm, spontaneously or otherwise, the patient breathes deeply; a lethal dose of chloroform is carried to the heart muscle which, weakened by the previous spasm, suddenly and permanently dilates. This is the usual cause of death of the large and alcoholic and athletic type of individual. Secondly, there is a vagus inhibition causing paralysis of the heart muscle which sometimes occurs in high strung, neurotic individuals. Embley and Martin have found that the action of chloroform in the blood in such quantities as may occur in inhalation of 1% to 3% vapor in air paralyzes the neuro-muscular mechanism of the blood vessels.[1312]

Tissot reported more than 70 mg. chloroform per 100 cc. of arterial blood often causes death.[1313] Chloroform in the brain is in equilibrium with that in the blood. If a fatal dose ensues at the moment of the heart's arrest, the amount in the venous blood is more than in the brain, but later the amount in the brain is often higher than in the venous blood. The amount in the venous blood is always less than in the arterial blood.

Meyer and Gottlieb direct attention to the narrow margin between the therapeutic and the lethal dose of chloroform.[1314] They found in deep narcosis with a compensating heart that the blood contained 0.35%, whereas in a dog anesthetized to the point of cardiac failure the chloroform content of the blood is 0.058%. The left ventricle, which is the principal factor in heart failure, contained 0.22%, whereas the right heart contained only 0.02% of chloroform. While respiration ceases first, the heart is primarily affected. Abel has found in the stage of complete anesthesia that the brain contains three times more chloroform than an equal weight of blood.[1315] The blood contained 0.015% and the brain 0.0418%. Most of the chloroform is in the red corpuscles, the serum containing very little.

Isolation: Chloroform will be found in the acid distillate. If the stomach content is alkaline, an examination must be made for the presence of formic acid, as the expert would be unable to say whether the chloroform found was administered as such or as chloral hydrate, as the latter is decomposed by alkali to the formation of chloroform, as previously mentioned.

1312. EMBLEY and MARTIN: J. Physiol., 32:147, 1905.
1313. TISSOT: Compt. rend. Acad. d. sc., 142:234, 1906.
1314. MEYER and GOTTLIEB: Experimentelle Pharmakologie, 1926.
1315. ABEL: Bull. Johns Hopkins Hosp., January, 1925.

Tests: 1. To 25 cc. of volatile distillate add one drop of anilin and 1 cc. of alcoholic potassium hydroxide; warm; the offensive odor of isobenzonitrile is produced. This will detect the presence of one part of chloroform in 5,000 parts of water.

$$CHCl_3 + C_6H_5NH_2 + 3KOH = C_6H_5NC + 3KCL + 3H_2O$$

This reaction is also given by chloral, bromoform, iodoform and trichloracetic acid.

2. Boil 20 cc. of the distillate with 0.3 gm. of resorcin and 0.5 cc. of 10% sodium hydroxide. The fluid becomes yellowish-red and shows a greenish-yellow fluorescence. The red color is due to sodium roseolate and the fluorescence to fluorescein.

3. When the distillate is boiled with Fehling's solution, a precipitate of red cuprous oxide forms. This becomes the basis for the quantitative determination. Cuprous oxide may be weighed or the amount of unchanged copper may be determined with a standard solution of dextrose. Two equivalents of copper (2Cu) correspond to one equivalent of chloroform ($CHCl_3$):

$$CHCl_3 + 5KOH + 2CuO = Cu_2O + 3KCl + K_2CO_3 + 3H_2$$

4. When chloroform is warmed with a solution of alpha- or beta-naphthol in strong caustic potash, a blue color is formed which throws down a bright red precipitate upon addition of acid. Exposure to the air causes the blue color to become green, and finally brown.[1316]

5. Chloroform yields triethyl ether of orthoformic acid when boiled with alcoholic potassium hydroxide:

$$3C_2H_5OH + 3KOH + CHCl_3 = 3KCl + CH(OC_2H_5)_3 + 3H_2O$$

After diluting with water and evaporating the alcohol, the material is acidified with tartaric acid and the formic acid distilled off and tested as given under Chloral Hydrate (page 676).

6. Ragsky described a process in which chloroform was decomposed by heat into perchlorbenzene, chlorine and hydrochloric acid.[1317] The distillate is introduced into a flask provided with a doubly perforated cork. Through one of the perforations passes a funnel tube, and through the other a delivery tube, bent at right angles. The flask is placed on a water-bath

1316. LUSTGARTEN: *Ztschr. f. anal. Chem.*, 22:97, 1892; *Monatsh. f. Chem.*, 3:722, 1892.

1317. RAGSKY: *J. f. prakt. Chem., Leipz.*, 46:170; see also BASSET· *Jahrb. d. Chem.*, 608, 1867; and RAMSAY: *Jahrb. d. Chem.*, 628, 1886.

and connected with a piece of hard glass tubing eighteen inches long, which is heated for about four inches by a broad Bunsen burner. About four inches in front of the heated portion the tube passes through a Liebig condenser having a length of six inches, and beyond the condenser a piece of filter paper, moistened with a mixture of starch paste and potassium iodide. The end of the tube is connected with a set of Liebig bulbs containing a solution of silver nitrate, and these are in turn connected with an aspirator. After the tube has been heated to bright redness the mixture in the flask is distilled at a gentle heat, while a current of air is slowly drawn through the system by the aspirator. Any chloroform vapor that may be present is decomposed for the most part according to the equation: $6CHCl_3 = C_6Cl_6 + 6HCl + 6Cl$. With 150 cc. of blood taken from the carotid of a dog anesthetized with chloroform the writers were able to show all three products with the greatest ease. The perchlorbenzene forms beautiful needles just in front of the flame; the chlorine decomposes the potassium iodide, liberating iodine, which turns the starch blue, and hydrochloric acid, passing into the bulbs, precipitates silver chloride which may be identified by appropriate tests.

Estimation: 1. Ludwig's apparatus is used in the estimation. Flask A contains a little pure water, enough to serve as a valve for the two glass tubes running to the bottom of the flask. Tube B contains glass beads. U-shaped tube C contains silver nitrate solution. To start the determination, the tube and beads within it are heated to a faint glow. The chlorine-free air is drawn through the apparatus from left to right. All the air going through the apparatus must pass through silver nitrate solution. If after a few minutes no turbidity is noticed in the silver nitrate solution, the air passing through and the water in the flask are chlorine free. The next step is to add a measured amount of the distillate containing the chloroform, through the thistle tube, into flask A. It is then put in a warm water-bath at 60°C. (140°F.). The stream of air passing through gradually forces all the chloroform through the red-hot tube. Here the $CHCl_3$ is burned; converting all the chlorine into HCl. This passes on and is collected in the U-tube in the form of AgCl. When all the chloroform has been burned up, the AgCl is collected, washed, and weighed. From this weight the amount of chloroform is calculated.

2. Nicloux method:[1318] To 20 cc. of blood, or other aqueous liquid, 95 cc. of alcohol and 5 cc. of a 5% alcoholic solution of tartaric acid are added. The mixture is placed in a Kjeldahl flask fitted with a cork through which passes one tube of a Reitmair bulb—upon whose other tube a continuation has been fused, which is bent downward and passes to the bottom of a graduated cylinder in such manner that its point is below the level of 10 cc. of alcohol placed therein—and 40 cc. are distilled over. All of the chloroform present passes into the distillate, which is then transferred to a flask, along with 10 cc. of alcohol used to wash the cylinder. To the 60 cc. now in the flask 10 cc. of a 10% alcoholic solution of caustic potash (free from chloride) are added, the flask is fitted with an Allihn, or other effective, reflux condenser, and the content is boiled moderately for an hour. After cooling, the content of the flask is transferred to a beaker and 15 cc. of water, used in two portions to wash the flask, are added. The content of the beaker is accurately neutralized with sulphuric acid, using phenolphthalein as indicator, 0.5 cc. of a 5% solution of neutral potassium chromate is added, and the liquid titrated with a standard solution of silver nitrate containing 8.535 gm. to the liter, 1 cc. of which represents 2 mg. of chloroform. The process is affected with a minus error of 2%, which is constant. Tissues are hashed and mixed with 95 cc. of alcohol, and 5 cc. of 5% alcoholic tartaric acid solution to 20 gm. of tissue, and the process carried on as above.

This method consumes less time than that of Ragsky's method previously described.

Fujiwara[1319] describes the pyridine color reaction with chloroform and related substances which is sensitive to one part in one million. In 1926 Cole[1320] described a chromatophylic method for the quantitative determination of chloroform, using the method of Fujiwara. In 1931 Gettler and Blume[1321] modified this method: Take 5 cc. of acid distillate for the chromatophylic determination and compare the color obtained with colored glass discs of the Helliga-Klett type. All material to be used for the isolation of volatile solvents should be thoroughly

1318. NICLOUX: Compt. rend. Soc. de biol., 60:88, 1906.
1319. FUJIWARA: Sitzungsb. u. Ablandl. naturfors. Gesellsch., Rastock, 6:1, 1914.
1320. COLE: J. Biol. Chem., 71:173, 1926.
1321. GETTLER, A. O., and BLUME, H.: Arch. Path., 11:555, 1931.

chilled in the refrigerator before the sample is comminuted. The acid distillate can be prepared as given previously.

By this method it was found that compounds such as bromoform, chloral, and iodoform also give a Fujiwara color reaction. Chemically pure, colorless pyridine must be used in the test. For the preparation of the standard 1 gm. pure chloroform is weighed in a glass-stoppered weighing bottle, and dissolved in 900 cc. of water in a liter volumetric flask; 5 cc. of hydrochloric acid are added and enough water to make one liter. The whole is then thoroughly mixed. The solution contains 1 mg. of chloroform in 1 cc. A series of standards can be prepared containing 0.5 mg., 0.1 mg., 0.01 mg., 0.005 mg., and 0.0025 mg. respectively in 1 cc. These standards must be prepared each week even if refrigerated.

Gettler recommends a series of glass discs varying in depth from orange-pink color to blood red color, simulating the various depths of color obtained with chloroform when subjected to the pyridine test. Small discs are cut and fitted into the wheels of a Helliga-Klett colorimeter. These color discs are standardized by chloroform solutions of known concentrations. In the absence of these discs the color can be compared in other types of colorimeters. The standards are prepared as follows: In five clean dry 50-cc. test-tubes 5 cc. of five standards are measured. In a similar tube 5 cc. of distillate is pipetted. To each are added 5 cc. of chemically pure, colorless pyridine and 10 cc. of sodium hydroxide. The content of the tubes is mixed thoroughly. The tubes are corked loosely to avoid evaporation. The tubes are placed in a boiling water-bath for exactly one minute and then cooled quickly with tap water; 20 cc. of water are added to each tube and mixed. The color of the unknown is compared to the colors of the five standards. If 100 gm. of tissue were used and 250 cc. of distillate obtained, the amount of chloroform in the 100 gm. would be calculated as follows:

The standard divided by unknown times value of standard used in mg. of chloroform times 25 divided by 5 times 1.087 equals the mg. of chloroform in 100 gm. of tissue. As it is possible to recover only 92% of the chloroform, a correction factor of 1.087 is used. The use of pyridine and sodium hydroxide solution makes an excellent qualitative test to use routinely for the presence of chloroform. Using this method, Gettler found that nine patients who died after chloroform anesthesia in the preparation for surgical operation gave the following amounts of chloroform: from the brain 120 to 182 mg.; from the lungs 92 to 145 mg.; from the liver 65 to 88 mg., in 1,000 gm. of tissue.

BROMOFORM (CHBr₃)
(Molecular Weight 250.99)

B ROMOFORM is a colorless, heavy liquid, boiling at 148° to 150° C. (298.4° F.). It has a sweetish taste, and an odor similar to chloroform. Its specific gravity is 2.808 at 25° C. It is very slightly soluble in water, but is soluble in alcohol, ether, benzene, and in fixed volatile oils, and is slightly volatile at ordinary temperatures. It is not inflammable, but when vaporized its vapor burns. It has been administered in liquid form in the treatment of convulsive affections, especially whooping cough.[1322]

The symptoms are very similar to those caused by chloroform taken internally. There is intoxication, sometimes excitement, then a tendency to sleep, anesthesia, feeble respiration, contracted pupils, and coma.

Three drops are said to have caused serious symptoms in a child of four. One dram caused the death of a child two years of age in five hours.[1323] However, recovery has taken place from as high as 9 gm.

The treatment is the same as under Chloroform (page 685).

Bromoform reacts chemically the same as chloroform, giving the isonitrile reaction, the pyridine reaction, naphthol, resorcine, and Ragsky tests. To differentiate from chloroform, test for the presence of bromine in the silver precipitate in the Ragsky test, as follows: The silver precipitate is dried and then fused with a sodium and potassium carbonate mixture. This is extracted with water. The silver halide is now in the form of an alkaline salt. Bromine can be separated by means of chlorine, the bromine being detected by shaking with carbon disulphide which assumes a reddish-yellow color. Ether or chloroform may be used instead of the carbon disulphide, but the solution is pale yellow. Starch gives a reaction, but is less delicate than with carbon disulphide.

For the estimation of bromine the liberated bromine is

1322. BORGER: *München. med. Wchnschr.*, 43:469, 1896; CHENEY: *Arch. Pediat.*, 14:112, 1887.
1323. MULLER: *München. med. Wchnschr.*, 55:1211, 1908.

made to act upon potassium iodide, and iodine which is liberated is estimated by standard solutions of sodium thiosulphate.

METHYL BROMIDE (CH_3Br)

METHYL BROMIDE is used in the manufacture of antipyrine and certain dyes. Attention was called to its toxic effects when it was used as a refrigerant, causing several deaths in Connecticut. Sayers, Yant, Thomas, and Berger[1324] reported that an atmosphere containing 5% to 9.6% by volume of methyl bromide vapors caused uneasiness in guinea pigs immediately after being placed in the test chamber, and after one or two minutes they were helpless. Death occurred as quickly with 5% as with 9.6%. Concentrations of 2.2% caused coughing in seven minutes which was followed by a retching-like action, unsteadiness in eight to fifteen minutes, and marked weakness at the end of thirty minutes. Exposure to 0.54% for ten minutes caused no apparent symptoms. Exposure to 0.05% to 0.06% caused no symptoms other than slight salivation and nasal discharge after four and a half hours. Increasing weakness, roughened fur, and physical signs of pneumonia and lung irritation were observed in the animals that died after the test.

Postmortem on the animals that died showed moderate degeneration of the heart muscles; the lungs were congested, hemorrhagic, and frequently edematous; the liver was congested, degenerated and occasionally slate gray in color; there were a few cases with a congested pancreas; the spleen occasionally was congested, edematous, and degenerated; there were a few cases with congested suprarenals; kidneys were congested and edematous; intestines were congested, frequently containing bile-tinged or blood-tinged fluid; and the brain occasionally was congested. The degree of these changes varied with exposure, but in general the changes were the most severe in animals that died immediately after, or within twenty-four hours following, long exposure to comparatively low concentrations.

DIMETHYL SULPHATE ($(CH_3)_2SO_4$)

MOHLAU[1325] reported two cases of poisoning by this substance. Exposure caused irritation of the throat and eyes. As time progressed the irritation of the throat and eyes

1324. Sayers, R. R., Yant, W. P., Thomas, B. G. H., and Berger, L. B.: U. S. Pub. Health Bull. 185, March, 1929.
1325. Mohlau: J. Indust. Hyg., 2:239, 1920; see also Weber: Chem. Centralbl., 1:364, 1902.

and bronchial inflammation increased. The symptoms were followed by acute congestion of the lungs and edema of the throat and larynx. Recovery was slow.

CARBON TETRACHLORIDE (CCl₄)
(Molecular Weight 153.83)

CARBON TETRACHLORIDE is a clear, colorless, mobile liquid. It has a characteristic ethereal odor, resembling that of chloroform. It is soluble in about 200 times its volume of water. It is miscible with alcohol, chloroform, ether, benzene, and with petroleum benzene, and dissolves most of the fixed and volatile oils. It has a specific gravity between 1.558 to 1.590 at 20°C. It distills between 76° and 78° C.

Carbon tetrachloride finds extensive use as a non-inflammable rubber solvent, as a fire extinguisher, as a delousing agent, and in medicine, as an anthelmintic. It is found in some occupations such as those of airplane dope workers, rubber cementers, rubber cement mixers, degreasers in textiles, degreasing plants, dry cleaners, electroplaters, fire-extinguisher makers, lacquerers, lacquer makers, metal-polish makers, paraffin workers, perfume makers, refrigerator makers, mechanical parts degreasing, rubber workers, vulcanizers, and also in x-ray apparatus. Carbon tetrachloride has come into extensive use as a fire extinguisher, and also as a non-inflammable cleaning agent. The tetrachloride appearing on the market is often disguised by the addition of odorous substances or mixed with small amounts of chloroform or petroleum oils. It is sold under various trade names, such as "carbona" and "pyrene." In the experiments conducted by the United States Bureau of Mines[1326] carbon tetrachloride was sprayed on heated iron or an excelsior fire in a gas-tight room of 1,000 cubic feet capacity. The use of 0.3 to 1.0 liter of the tetrachloride resulted in the contamination of the air in the chamber with phosgene to the extent of fifteen to 168 parts per million parts of air. This is equivalent to a production of 0.4 to 4.5 liters of phosgene. A number of fatalities from phosgene poisoning have resulted from the use of carbon tetrachloride fire extinguishers in confined places such as ships, mines and buildings. The phosgene coming in contact with moisture liberates hydrochloric acid. When carbon tetrachloride was

1326. U. S. Dept. of Interior, Bureau of Mines, Tech. Paper 248, 1921.

first used as an anthelmintic a number of accidents occurred because it was given to chronic alcoholics and people suffering from heart and kidney diseases. The organs most commonly involved are the liver and the gastro-intestinal tract. It has been shown by a number of research workers that it causes a calcium deficiency, and the use of alcohol renders one more susceptible to its effects.

Toxicity: Rabbits succumb to 4 cc. per kilogram, while dogs are apparently not affected by 25 cc. per kilogram by mouth. The difference depends on absorption, for both animals are about equally susceptible to inhalation. Monkeys are uninjured by 1 to 5 cc. by mouth, every two or three days for twelve to sixteen doses. Fats and alcohol increase the toxicity.[1327]

A healthy young man about thirty-six years of age, on July 2, 1934, cleaned a rug with one gallon of carbon tetrachloride, taking about three hours for the work. Within twenty-four hours he began to vomit, and, on three occasions, he vomited blood. He complained of headache and weakness. He developed an icteric tinge of the sclera, tenderness over the right lower liver border, albuminuria, hematuria, and slight swelling of the ankles. The blood pressure at this examination was 158/120, and the temperature was 101.6.° He had occasional coughing spells, and rales posteriorly at both lung bases. He developed a hiccough lasting for seven days. The reflexes were normal. On the ninth day the patient was very dyspneic, somewhat cyanotic, and his bronchitis was worse. There was a subicteric tinge to his skin. His pupils reacted to light and accommodation. On the tenth day his pulse was 104.° Rales on both sides of the chest were increased. He was given 50 cc. of 50% glucose intravenously. On the eleventh day his lungs were quite edematous. He felt drowsy and somewhat irrational, and slept most of the time. He was given 5 cc. calcium gluconate intravenously, also 1000 cc. of 5% glucose subcutaneously. The following day there was a marked diuresis. Then he began to improve. The non-protein nitrogen on admission was 130 mg. per 100 cc., creatinine, 12.4 mg. per 100 cc. On leaving the hospital, July 12, 1934, his non-protein nitrogen had dropped to 40 mg. per 100 cc. the creatinine being 2.7 mg. per 100 cc.

1327. HALL: *J.A.M.A.*, 77:1641, 1921. HALL and SCHLLINGER: *J. Agric. Research*, 29:319, 1925; 23:165, 1923.

This young man developed a nephritis, myocarditis, and from the symptoms had fatty degeneration of the liver. He was very nervous and continued to have trouble with his heart, and a year and a half after the accident he committed suicide. An autopsy was not possible as he lived in another city.

McGuire reported seven cases of poisoning among the employees of a felt manufacturing plant.[1328] The patients were all Italians, and were wine drinkers. The symptoms were nausea and vomiting, which lasted from one to three days. Three vomited small amounts of blood; six had diarrhea, five complained of headache; four complained of burning or smarting about the eyes and mouth; two had liver enlargement with jaundice; four had kidney irritation, one of which was an acute nephritis. This man also had bronchopneumonia.

Minot and Cutler experimenting with dogs, found at autopsy that the liver appeared yellowish and was soft and friable.[1329] The gastro-intestinal tract usually contained old blood, with hemorrhagic areas in the pyloric end of the stomach and in the upper third of the small intestine. They found that dogs poisoned by carbon tetrachloride could be successfully treated by intravenous injections of calcium chloride. Calcium lactate was given by mouth, when vomiting was not persistent. Ammonium chloride and hydrochloric acid were also effective, as well as parathyroid extract.

Tomb and Helmy report that in experiments with carbon tetrachloride there is an accumulation of guanidine in the blood and a severe subsequent hypoglycemia.[1330] Calcium salts prevent this intoxication, but do not protect the liver or prevent the accumulation of guanidine in the blood.[1330]

Lehmann[1331] concludes that the industrial use of carbon tetrachloride is of very little, if any, toxicological significance, unless it is subjected to a high degree of heat. A case similar to the one I have mentioned above, was reported by Lacornu and Pecker in 1932.[1332] They mention the case of a man who worked for two hours in a confined space with carbon tetra-

1328. McGuire, L. W.: *J.A.M.A.*, 99:988, 1932.
1329. Minot, A. S., and Cutler, J. T.: *J. Clin. Investigation*, 6:359, 1928.
1330. Tomb, J. W., and Helmy, M.: *J. Trop. Med.*, 36:265, 1933. And see *J. Pharmacol. & Exper. Therap.*, October, 1931.
1331. Lehmann: *Zentralbl. f. Gewerbehyg.*, 7:123, 1930.
1332. *Presse méd.*, 40:386, 1932.

chloride. This man became jaundiced, his liver was enlarged, the urine contained albumin, and he finally developed anuria, and died on the eighth day. If carbon tetrachloride is used with a good draft or in an open space, there is little danger from its inhalation.

Wilcox and Dudley[1333] report a number of cases of toxic jaundice caused by carbon tetrachloride, and state that even when death does not occur, the liver might be damaged. Three cases, subjected to the vapor of carbon tetrachloride in extinguishing fires, showed impairment of renal function, and in one case there was complete suppression of the urine for ten days. One case began with vomiting and gastric disturbances, and a few days later developed a mild jaundice. At the end of ten days the patient suddenly had an epileptiform convulsion, with blood pressure of 220 mm., hemoglobin and blood urea of 300 mg. per 100 cc. Edema of the lungs developed and in one case there was complete suppression of urine but the man eventually recovered.[1333] Leoncini described a fatal case of carbon tetrachloride poisoning, including an autopsy, arising from the use of a fire extinguisher containing carbon tetrachloride.[1334]

Most of the carbon tetrachloride produced today does not contain carbon bisulphide, since new processes remove every trace of this impurity. Carbon tetrachloride for medicinal use contains no sulphur compounds, or other foreign impurities. The product is 99.99% pure. In the late 1860's carbon tetrachloride was tried out as an anesthetic in England, but was soon found to have a much narrower therapeutic range than chloroform. Carbon tetrachloride was used very little until 1921, when it was introduced into medicine as an anthelmintic. Hall demonstrated this on dogs in 1921, and it was confirmed on man by Nicholls and Hampton in 1922, and especially by Lambert in 1922. When dogs were exposed to the fumes of carbon tetrachloride in air mixtures of known proportion, all the stages of narcotic effects were observed; 40 mg. per liter caused the animal to become restless and uneasy; 51 mg. per liter caused marked muscular restlessness and hypertonia,

1333. WILCOX, W., and DUDLEY, S. F.: *Brit. M. J.*, 105, January, 1934. And see DUVOIR, M., GUIBER, and DESOILLE, H.: *Chem. Abst.*, 28: 2412, 1934.

1334. LEONCINI, F.: *Rassegna di med. appl. lavoro indust.*, 5:6, 1934.

and increased salivation, and the animal became unsteady; 57 mg. per liter caused coarse intermittent tremor of the head, with fibrillary muscle twitchings; 73 mg. per liter caused the animal to lose the power of coordination and balance, so that it was unable to keep on its feet, and there was also a very marked tremor of the head; 133 mg. induced a quiet sleep, with cessation of all voluntary and involuntary muscular movements. On inhalation of this mixture, it takes between nine and thirteen minutes before the narcosis is complete. Animals inhale this mixture for one hour without dying. The amount of carbon tetrachloride likely to be absorbed through the skin is uncertain. Experimental investigations have demonstrated a slight degree of absorption through the skin of the rabbit's ear. It produces a somewhat stronger local irritation of the skin than chloroform.

The greatest danger of intoxication from carbon tetrachloride is the inhalation of the fumes of the volatile fluid. A good down draft ventilation is necessary to remove it completely from air. In 1907 Colman reported a case of intoxication, and he strongly deprecated the use of carbon tetrachloride in the dry shampoo.[1335]

Dingley reported a case of carbon tetrachloride poisoning from the bursting of a patent fire extinguisher. A man inhaled the carbon tetrachloride from the fire extinguisher and died within forty-five minutes.[1336] Wirtschafter describes five cases of carbon tetrachloride intoxication in men employed in dry cleaning and exposed to fumes eight to ten hours daily for one to six months.[1337] All complained of headache, dizziness, nausea, vomiting—which was severe in two, diarrhea with abdominal pain in two, weakness and loss of weight, insomnia in one, irritability in another, and lethargy in a third. One man had polyuria. Wirtschafter thinks that, as a result of the low blood sugar caused by carbon tetrachloride intoxication, the retina is deprived of an adequate supply of glucose for normal metabolism and function. Inasmuch as there is also a deranged fat metabolism in such intoxication, there is according to Adler[1338] some substance present in the liver and in

1335. COLMAN, H.: *Lancet,* 1:1709, 1907.
1336. DINGLEY, L. A.: *Lancet,* 1:1037, 1926.
1337. WIRTSCHAFTER, A. T.: *Am. J. Pub. Health,* 23:1035, 1933.
1338. ADLER, F. H.: MacMillan, 1933.

certain fats which is concerned with the rod-visual purple function of the retina.

Hausemann and Helly reported the case of a disinfector, aged forty-six years, who, while using carbon tetrachloride for the examination of insects, inhaled the fumes of the fluid. He had attacks of vomiting, and died on the twelfth day after the intoxication. Death was hastened by a pre-existing condition of nephritis.[1339]

Pagniez, Plichet, and Koang reported the case of a painter inhaling air laden with fumes of carbon tetrachloride. He suffered severe attacks of gastro-intestinal disorder, and a week later nephritis occurred with severe anasarca, pronounced oliguria, moderate hypertension, and a marked increase in the non-protein nitrogen content of the blood. The symptoms subsided in four weeks.[1340]

Butch reported a case of a man, aged fifty-four, who was cleaning old telephones, for which he used a solution containing 60% carbon tetrachloride and 40% gasoline, in a room with poor ventilation. After working for six months it was necessary to hospitalize the patient. On admission there were signs of cirrhosis of the liver. After four months' treatment he was able to return to work.[1341]

Brandt reported a case in a shoe repair shop where carbon tetrachloride was used as a solvent for rubber soles.[1342] Richet and Conder reported a case of nephritis following the use of carbon tetrachloride.[1343] The patient had the typical symptoms of carbon tetrachloride, in addition to a bloody diarrhea, which disappeared on the third day. Physical examination on the third day revealed an enlarged liver. The patient made an uneventful recovery. Scheurlen and Witsky report a leather dresser working in a room without sufficient artificial ventilation. Death was caused by damage to the liver.[1344]

Poindexter and Greene report a fatal case of an Italian, aged

1339. HAUSEMANN and HELLY: Rev. suisse d. accid. du travail (etc.), Genève, 23:50, 1929.
1340. PAGNIEZ, P., PLICHET, A., and KOANG, N. K.: *Presse méd.*, 40:1146, 1932.
1341. BUTCH, W.: *J.A.M.A.*, 99:728, 1932.
1342. BRANDT, A.: *Gewerbepath. u. Gewerbehyg.*, 3:335, 1932.
1343. RICHET, C., and CONDER, R.: *Bull. et mém.*, 35:1247, 1932.
1344. VON SCHEURLEN and WITSKY, H.: *Zentralbl. f. Gewerbehyg.*, 22:60, 1935.

forty-six, who for the past eleven years had been a cleaner of clothes. His work consisted of washing clothes in an open receptacle in a poorly ventilated room. The cleaning fluid consisted of a mixture of 55% carbon tetrachloride and 5% naphtha and benzine. Autopsy revealed an advanced toxic cirrhosis of the liver, hemorrhages, and old infarcts of the right kidney with compensatory hypertrophy of the left kidney.[1345]

Tietze's first case reported, complained of dizziness and buzzing in the ears, tremors of the right hand, and spells of unconsciousness. When brought to the hospital the patient was stuporous. The urine contained albumen and a sediment containing white cells, a few red cells, and hyaline and granular casts. The blood pressure was 145. During the night he had two epileptiform seizures characterized by tonic and clonic spasms. He made an uneventful recovery. A second case from the same factory, developed tremors of the right hand, extreme flexion of the right arm, torsion of the head, pain in both arms, and an inarticular speech. This patient suffered from nervousness more than the first patient, but he also made an uneventful recovery.[1346]

Henggeler reports the case of a fifty-four year old janitor who was working in a school house, waxing the floors of the different rooms, with wax containing carbon tetrachloride.[1347] On the third day of this work it was storming and raining, so he worked with the windows closed. There were six individuals who participated in this work. At the end of this stormy day two of them complained of malaise, headache, and nausea. The following day two more complained of nausea, headache, and fever. One was taken to a hospital where he was almost completely anuric, and had a violent headache, hiccough (this is the first case that I have found where hiccoughs were reported in addition to my case above), and extreme nausea. The stools were bloody, the reflexes were decreased, and the general condition was poor. The pulse was normal in rate and intensity. During the second week there developed a weakening of the visual acuity and a deafness which lasted for a few

1345. POINDEXTER, M. D., and GREENE, C. H.: *J.A.M.A.*, 102:2015, 1934.

1346. TIETZE, A.: *Arch. f. Gewerbepath. u. Gewerbehyg.*, 4:732, 1933.

1347. HENGGELER, A.: *Schweiz. med. Wchnschr.*, 12:223, 1931.

days. Vomiting and hiccoughs continued until the twenty-second day, when the patient received injections of cardiazol, which caused the nausea and vomiting to disappear. One and a half months later the patient was fully recovered. Glaser reports the case of a workman who died during the filling of fire extinguishers.[1348] Other cases similar to this have been reported.[1348]

When used as an anthelmintic, the adult dose is 2 to 3 cc.

Horrocks reported the death of a Filipino child, following the treatment of ascariasis with carbon tetrachloride.[1349] The child was given a mixture which contained 0.041 gm. of santonin, 0.185 cc. oil of chenopodium, and 0.431 cc. of carbon tetrachloride with castor oil to make up the total volume of 3 cc. This was followed in one hour by 20 cc. of castor oil. The child died on the twenty-third day. Autopsy revealed that the liver was small and flabby, and showed irregular yellow mottling. The intestine showed an area of injection.

Haigler reported several cases of poisoning by carbon tetrachloride aboard the U. S. S. Lexington, in December, 1929.[1350] A considerable quantity of the chemical in tin containers was received on board this ship, but none was found to be leaking, although some were rusted. In connection with this case it was found that some of the containers had rusted through and there had occurred consequently some leakage. Therefore six men were ordered to remove the defective cans, emptying them into a gasoline drum. During the work some of the bottoms came off and about two or three quarts were spilled, liberating dense vapors. Within a period of approximately five minutes, two members of the party collapsed and became anesthetized. The remaining tried to rescue their friends, but were overcome by the fumes and also became unconscious. When removed from the source of contamination and into fresh air they revived, and all made uneventful recoveries. The fatality rate for the average dose of 3 cc. has been one death in 50,000 persons.

Becher reports a case of a woman seventy-six years old,

1348. GLASER: Deutsche Ztschr. f. d. ges. gerichtl. Med., 471, 1928. For other cases see CADE and MAZEL: Bull. et mém. Soc. méd. d. hôp. de Paris, 1923; FLORET: Zentralbl. f. Gewerbehyg., 8:28, 1920; JAQUET: Deutsches Arch. f. klin. Med., 71:370, 1901.

1349. HORROCKS, CAPT. G. E.: Mil. Surgeon, 74:246, 1934.

1350. HAIGLER, F. H.: U. S. Nav. M. Bull., 30:137, 1932.

who drank one-fourth liter of a cleaning fluid containing carbon tetrachloride.[1351] For six hours she was unconscious. When revived she vomited, and complained of pain in the stomach and back. The urine contained a moderate number of leukocytes, a few red cells and albumen, with oliguria. The urine also showed the presence of hyaline and granular casts. After two weeks it was negative for albumen, and the oliguria subsided. On the twenty-fourth day blood chemistry revealed a decrease in the blood urea, and at this time it was present to the extent of twice its normal value. The most outstanding symptoms in this case were a relative bradycardia, and rise in blood pressure associated with renal disease. The hypertension probably was the result of the renal insufficiency.

Smyth reviewed the literature and found twenty-seven fatal cases of acute poisoning. Of these fourteen followed its internal administration as an anthelmintic. Of the other thirteen cases only six occurred in the United States—one a baby, who died after having adhesive strips removed with the help of carbon tetrachloride. He found ninety-six cases of acute, subacute and non-fatal poisonings, but eighteen were not industrial. Of the industrial cases, thirty-three occurred in this country, but not all are typical since thirteen were in persons using mixed solvents.[1352]

Dudley refers to Moller who has published a comprehensive review of the toxicology of carbon tetrachloride poisoning in which he examined forty-three reports and papers on the subject.[1353] Seven Italians, who were exposed to carbon tetrachloride vapor while cleaning felt hats, acquired headache, nausea, vomiting, smarting eyes and mouth, jaundice, enlargement of the liver, and definite signs of kidney irritation. In one of this series acute nephritis and bronchopneumonia developed. In another accident three men were exposed to carbon tetrachloride vapor. One had trivial symptoms only, but the other two, eight days after an attack of acute gastro-intestinal disturbances, developed "oliguria, moderate hypertension, and generalized edema." One of the men died; the other after his blood urea had risen to 375 mg. per 100 cc. recovered within a month. Mention is made of another accidental case

1351. BECHER, E.: München. med. Wchnschr., 77:891, 1930.
1352. SMYTH, H. F.: Indust. Med., 4:12, 1935.
1353. DUDLEY, S. F.: J. Indust. Hyg., 17:93, 1935.

followed by a single case having symptoms identical with the foregoing, who recovered after the blood urea figure had reached 480.

Gonzales reports the case of a housemaid, aged forty, who, using a gallon container of "Quick as a Wink" cleaning fluid, poured almost the entire content in a basin and dipped some garments in the liquid.[1354] She was found dead beside the basin. At autopsy the body was negative except for a moderate grade of chronic diffuse nephritis, pial edema, and injection of the laryngeal and bronchial mucosa. A chemical examination of the organs revealed the presence of carbon tetrachloride and dichloropropane. The analysis showed 18 mg. in 500 gm. of brain, 26.5 mg. in 500 gm. of lung, and 1.45 mg. in 500 gm. of liver, of chlorinated hydrocarbons of low boiling point. Analysis of the cleaning fluid indicated that 60% of it was carbon tetrachloride and 40% dichloropropane.

Robbins found in experiments with dogs, that bone marrow contained the most carbon tetrachloride, with the liver content next highest. Small quantities were found in blood, brain, kidney, lungs, etc. Practically all the carbon tetrachloride was excreted in the lungs and scarcely any in the urine.[1355]

Davis conducted experiments in a room 20 x 20 x 10 feet, having a capacity of 4,000 cubic feet, and containing 113,347.5 liters of air.[1356] He exposed four different individuals for thirty minutes to an atmosphere containing 1 mg. per liter of air, and found that three out of the four had no effects whatsoever, and that one was slightly nauseated and nervous: pulse 120, respiration 28, blood pressure 145. Urinalysis gave negative results in all cases.

In a second experiment Davis exposed four persons to 0.5 mg. per liter for two and one-half hours. The persons ranged in age from thirty-five to forty-eight years. There were no symptoms. The blood pressure ranged from 115 to 130. The blood pressure and other physical conditions were not given before entering the gas chamber. In a sixth experiment he exposed three subjects to 0.25 gm. per liter from three to seven minutes. The subject exposed for seven minutes had nausea,

1354. GONZALES, T. A.: *J.A.M.A.*, 106:286, 1936.
1355. ROBBINS, B. H.: Abst. *J. Pharmacol. & Exper. Therap.*, 37: 203, 1929.
1356. DAVIS, PAUL A.: *J.A.M.A.*, 103:962, 1934.

vomiting, and felt dizzy and sleepy. The blood pressure of two of the subjects was 150. Pulse ranged from 110 to 130, respiration from 22 to 28. Urinalysis disclosed no albumin, no sugar, no casts, no sediment, increased phosphates and acidity. Examination two weeks later showed that no ill effects were caused by the exposure. The author refers to a case in which a toxic amblyopia was present, and states that the examination of the visual fields may be a valuable procedure for the early detection of carbon tetrachloride intoxication.

Moller reports six cases, three of which were from having the hair shampooed with cleaning fluid containing carbon tetrachloride, and two from cleaning dresses with carbon tetrachloride.[1357] The sixth is that of a workman who was repairing a container using carbon tetrachloride. He felt ill and before he left for home had vomited several times. He had a diarrhea, and felt tired but returned to his work. He became jaundiced, and four days later was so weak he was unable to return to work. He was cyanotic and dyspneic, with a pulse rate of 112. He had nose bleeding, and small subconjunctival hemorrhages. The lungs showed a moderate amount of dullness, and there were many moist rales. The liver was enlarged and somewhat tender on palpation. The urine contained some albumen and casts, and the white blood count was 15,000. This patient made an uneventful recovery.

Lamson[1358] and others have subjected dogs to the fumes of carbon tetrachloride of various concentrations. In a concentration of 0.58 volumes per cent the animal becomes restless and uneasy. There is an increase of salivation. In a concentration of 0.74 volumes per cent there occurs marked muscular restlessness and hypertonia. The animal is unsteady and the salivation is increased. Concentration of 0.83 volumes per cent caused coarse intermittent tremor of the head and fibrillary muscle twitchings. In a concentration of 1.06 volumes per cent the animal loses the power of coordination and balance. It is unable to keep on its feet. There is a very marked tremor of the head. Concentration of 1.94 volume per cent induces a quiet sleep, with cessation of all voluntary and involuntary movements. It takes from nine to thirty minutes of inhalation of this mixture before the narcosis becomes complete, and the

1357. MOLLER, KNUD: J. Indust. Hyg., 15:418, 1933.
1358. LAMSON, P. D.: J. Pharmacol. & Exper. Therap., 29:191, 1926.

animals may inhale this mixture for one hour without dying.

Treatment: The treatment begins with removal of the individual from the source of the vapor. Alkalinization with a calcium salt, and preferably intravenous injection of calcium gluconate, or ingestion of glucose, is recommended. Hospital cases should be given intravenous injections of physiological salt or normal salt and glucose by hypodermoclysis. Digitalis should be given to strengthen the heart. Special attention should be paid to keeping the kidneys and bowels working.

McConnell* reports that in cases of acute poisoning stimulants such as epinephrine are dangerous as first aid measures in resuscitating persons overcome by these vapors.

Every precaution should be taken to prevent the inhalation of this gas, concentration should be kept below 0.01%. The use of a down draft should prevent cases of poisoning in industrial plants. Carbon tetrachloride should never be sold in quantities larger than one pint to the laity, thus preventing many accidental deaths. The plant physician should be very careful in the selection of people working with all chlorinated hydrocarbons. Those having nephritis, diabetes, myocardial degeneration, high blood pressure, and those using alcohol, should not be permitted to work with carbon tetrachloride.

Lehmann[1359] gives an extensive study of the hazards of carbon tetrachloride. Schibler[1360] reports a case of acute yellow atrophy of the liver caused by acetylene tetrachloride. These cases resemble those of carbon tetrachloride very much.

Symptoms: Robbins found that dogs given carbon tetrachloride through the gastro-intestinal route excreted almost all of it through the lungs. None was found in the urine. Bollman and Mann,[1361] experimenting with dogs showed it to be capable of setting up lesions in the liver with symptoms characteristic of portal obstruction, although death usually was caused by intestinal hemorrhage, or rupture of a duodenal ulcer. Having this in mind, plant physicians should under no circumstances employ an individual having symptoms of gastric or duodenal ulcers. Lamson and his associates,[1362] giving

* McCONNELL, W. J.: *J.A.M.A.*, 109: 763, 1937.

1359. LEHMANN, K. B.: *Zentralbl. f. Gewerbehyg.*, 7: 123, 1930.

1360. SCHIBLER: *Schweiz. med. Wchnschr.*, 10: 1079, 1929.

1361. BOLLMAN, J. L., and MANN, F. G.: *Ann. Int. Med.*, 5: 699, 1931.

1362. LAMSON, P. D., ROBBINS, B. H., and WARD, C. B.: *Am. J. Hyg.*, 9: 430, 1929.

carbon tetrachloride inhalations, produced necroses in the liver with bilirubinuria, the effect being increased by a digestible fatty food. This condition was also accelerated by the administration of alcohol, given before the dose of the solvent (carbon tetrachloride). This effect of alcohol has been noted by a number of observers, on human beings. Takahashi, working with rabbits, found renal injury with a decreased output of ethereal sulphates and increased output of nitrogen, but the most striking lesions were in the liver.

Headache, hiccough, nausea, vomiting, diarrhea, pain and tenderness in the liver region, and jaundiced sclerae characterize the early stages; oliguria, urine containing albumen and casts follow next; then symptoms of uremia, increasing in severity as the suppression of urine becomes complete. Death is preceded by uremic convulsions.

Minot[1363] found that when the toxic action could be traced to alcohol, the reason for the toxicity was lack of calcium in the diet, for a negative calcium balance causes over-susceptibility to carbon tetrachloride. Holland, Kehrer and Oudendahl[1364] report a death from central necrosis and fatty degeneration of the liver and kidneys, resulting from carbon tetrachloride poisoning. MacMahon and Weiss[1365] describe an unusual case in which the blood in the right side of the heart and the large pulmonary arteries contained an extremely high percentage of fat (60%). The probable source of this fat was the liver, which was severely damaged, large, and full of fat. The patient was an alcoholic, and his sensitiveness to carbon tetrachloride was increased not only by the action of alcohol in aiding the absorption of carbon tetrachloride, but also by the synergistic action of the two in causing liver damage. Rosenthal and Lillie[1366] reported the production of lipemia in a dog by feeding it carbon tetrachloride. Sartorius and Boedicker[1367] report an accident similar to that reported by Henggeler (page 699) where a fluid was used to clean the floors in

1363. MINOT, A. S.: *Proc. Soc. Exper. Biol. & Med.*, 24:617, 1927.

1364. KEHRER, J. K. W., and OUDENDAHL, A. J. F.: *Nederl. tijdschr. v. geneesk.*, 70:746, 1927.

1365. MACMAHON, H. E., and WEISS, S.: *Am. J. Path.*, 5:623, 1929.

1366. ROSENTHAL, S. M., and LILLIE, R. D.: *Am. J. Physiol.*, 97:131, 1931.

1367. SARTORIUS, F., and BOEDICKER, W.: *Zentralbl. f. Gewerbehyg.*, 8:103, 1931.

a schoolhouse. The mixture was found to contain carbon tetrachloride and chloroform. Koelsch[1368] reported that some men become accustomed to these vapors, while others find them unendurable. Gerbis[1369] found that some workmen developed a mild addiction to this narcotic. This would not seem unusual, as I have seen a number of women who were addicted to inhaling chloroform.

Veley[1370] reoprted one death and serious illness from its use as a dry shampoo. Levassort[1371] reported one case with unconsciousness, convulsive movements, nausea, and a long continued condition of malaise. The carbon tetrachloride used was contaminated with carbon disulphide.

Kobert[1372] gives the deadly concentration per liter for man as 300 to 400 mg. Men are able to stand one-half to one hour in a concentration of 70 mg.; from one-half to one hour without very serious effects in 25 to 40 mg. per liter. Ten mg. over a long period of time would cause only the slightest symptoms.

Tests: When a copper cone is heated over an alcohol lamp, or a Bunsen burner, a greenish color will be imparted to the flame in the presence of a halogen. In the presence of chlorine there will be obtained a green color, while with bromine and iodine more of a blue flame will appear. When the flame remains colorless, is it the proof of absence of a halogen. Carbon tetrachloride is isolated from the organs by distillation. Carbon tetrachloride gives the isonitrile reaction. It does not give the naphthol and resorcine reaction. By converting it into phosgene and passing it into a cold saturated solution of aniline in water, a precipitate of diphenylurea will be obtained which is weighed or determined in terms of its nitrogen by the Kjeldahl method:

$$COCl_2 + 4C_6H_5NH_2 = CO(NHC_6H_5)_2 + 2C_6H_5NH_2HCl$$

Hydrogen chloride and chlorine must be removed before passing the phosgene into the aniline water. The phosgene is extracted by passing the gas through a 2% solution of sodium iodide in acetone; and titrating the free iodine with thiosulphate or arsenite. Chlorine is removed by solid antimony

1368. Koelsch, F.: *Handb. d. soz. Hyg.*, 2:352, 1926.
1369. Gerbis, H.: *Zentralbl. f. Gewerbehyg.*, N. S. 4:330, 1927.
1370. Veley: *Lancet*, 2:1162, 1909.
1371. Levassort: *J.A.M.A.*, 60:1719, 1913.
1372. Kobert, R.: *Kompendium der Toxikologie*, 5th ed., 1912.

sulphide or mercury sulphide. If hydrochloric acid is present, antimony sulphide cannot be used, as it liberates hydrogen sulphide which reacts with the sodium iodide. The hydrochloric acid is removed by passing the gas through zinc dust. The reagents used to remove these gases must be free of moisture, as water decomposes phosgene.

Egidio[1373] reports that carbon tetrachloride is detected by a method similar to that used by Vitali for the detection of chloroform and chloral. Experiments in which guinea pigs ingested carbon tetrachloride showed that its presence could be proved by this method in the viscera twelve days after death. This test is sensitive to 0.00055 gm. carbon tetrachloride in 30 cc. alcohol, and can be used for its detection by condensing the production of hydrogen combustion, passing it into NH_4OH, acidifying with HNO_3, and titrating with $AgNO_3$.

Ethylsilicate when introduced into small animals intraperitoneally, intravenously, orally, or upon the skin shows an unusual toxicity. McCord* found that, when even so small a quantity as 0.02 cc. of ethylsilicate per 100 gm. of animal weight, is introduced intravenously the animal dies within five minutes. The point of action is limited to the capillaries of the lung tissue, with slight involvement of the capillaries of the heart. Within five minutes there is hemorrhage into the lung sacs, and rupture of the capillaries of the lungs occurs, and death apparently is due, in the case of rabbits, to air aspirated through the ruptured air sacs, leading to air emboli.

TETRACHLORETHANE ($CHCl_2$—$CHCl_2$)

TETRACHLORETHANE, prepared industrially by the action of chlorine upon acetylene, is a heavy, colorless, oily liquid with a boiling point of 147° C. (296.6° F.) and a specific gravity of 1.614. The vapor is about six times heavier than air, a very important factor in connection with the dangers from its industrial use. It is non-inflammable, and has a sickening sweet odor suggestive of chloroform. It is an excellent solvent for certain types of cellulose esters, resins, etc., and was used extensively during the war as an ingredient in some

---

1373. EGIDIO, CIARAVINO: *Boll. chim. farm., Milano,* 74:741, 1935; Chem. Abst. 30:2, 409, 1936.

* McCORD, CAREY P.: *J.A.M.A.,* 109:767, 1937.

of the airplane "dopes," or varnishes, with which the wings and other parts of airplanes were painted. It is also used in the manufacture of non-inflammable films, lacquered goods, and artificial silk.

Zangger saw seven cases of poisoning among the workers in a chemical industry. In spite of differences in age, all the workmen had the same symptoms.

Lehmann and his associates[1374] showed, in animal experiments, that the vapors of tetrachlorethane have a narcotic action similar to that of chloroform, but about four times as toxic. Jungfer and Willcox[1375] reported cases of poisoning from the use of "dope" in airplane factories. The outstanding symptom was jaundice. This "dope" contains, as one of its constituents, tetrachlorethane. The German preparation contains more than 60%, the English about 12%, together with a number of other solvents.

Grimm reported eighteen cases of poisoning in Germany, and in England at least seventy cases of jaundice, with twelve deaths.[1376]

Symptoms: The early symptoms begin with abnormal fatigue, discontent, general nervousness, and loss of appetite, which are followed by nausea, vomiting and dizziness. The blood at this stage of poisoning is striking, and is of aid in diagnosis. There is a progressive increase of large mononuclear cells, often reaching 40%; there are many immature large mononuclears, a slight elevation in the white cells, and a progressive but slight anemia. Willcox and Grimm[1377] describe several cases as having the symptoms of general malaise, drowsiness, vomiting, constipation, and headache, followed after a period of days or even weeks by intense jaundice, with pale stools and bile-stained urine; vomiting becoming worse, confusion, stupor, delirium, and coma, usually followed by death. A purpuric rash, hemorrhages, hematemesis, also convulsions and suppression of the urine occurred. If the patient was removed from the exposure when the jaundice was slight, complete recovery occurred, but slowly. If the jaundice is severe, the patient will not recover.

1374. LEHMANN: *Arch. f. Hyg.*, 74:1, 1911.
1375. JUNGFER: *Zentralbl. f. Gewerbehyg.*, 2:222, 1914; WILLCOX: *Lancet*, 2:1489, 1914.
1376. GRIMM: *Vrtljschr. f. gerichtl. Med.*, 48: II Suppl. 192, 1914.
1377. WILLCOX: *Lancet*, 1:544, 1915.

Postmortem Appearances: Schibler reported acute yellow atrophy of the liver. There is marked fatty degeneration in the kidneys and liver cells.[1378]

Treatment: Give glucose or calcium gluconate intravenously, and calcium gluconate wafers by mouth. The patient should not be returned to this type of work.

Dichlorethylene has caused death. The autopsies showed an excess of fat in the blood suggesting embolism rather than asphyxiation. The lethal dose for cats in thirty minutes was 44,000 parts per million.

Tetrachlorethylene is less narcotic, although the toxicity for cats is very closely that of dichlorethylene, 37,000 parts per million being lethal for cats in thirty minutes.

Cyclohexanol acetate, $(CH_2)_5.CO.OC.CH_3$, is a hydrogenated phenol used in pyroxylin lacquers. It is not very volatile and evaporates more easily than other solvents. From animal experiments it is thought to paralyze the central nervous system, and to be more toxic than benzene but not as much of a hazard as the latter because of its lesser volatility.

Waite, Patty and Yant* reported that ethylene glycol ("cellosolve") caused death of guinea pigs, the autopsy showing congestion and edema of the lungs. When the animals died three days after exposure, a bronchopneumonia was found.

1378. SCHIBLER, W.: *Schweiz. med. Wchnschr.*, 59:1079, 1929; abst. in *J.A.M.A.*, 94:66, 1930.

* WAITE, C. P., PATTY, F. A., and YANT, W. P.: Public Health Report, 45:1459, 1930.

DRUGS AND MISCELLANEOUS

IODOFORM (CHl_3)
(Molecular Weight 393.77)

IODOFORM occurs as a fine, lemon-yellow powder, or lustrous crystals. It has a peculiar, very penetrating odor. It is insoluble in water, to which, however, it imparts its odor and taste.

One gram of iodoform, U. S. P., XI, is soluble in 66 cc. of alcohol, in 80 cc. of glycerine, in 10 cc. of chloroform, in 7.5 cc. of ether, in 2.8 cc. of carbon disulphide, and in 34 cc. of olive oil, at 25° C. Most of the cases of poisoning from iodoform have been medicinal, resulting from the use of the drug as a surgical dressing, or from its long continued use on wounds.

Symptoms of acute iodoform poisoning are very complex and variable, sometimes one and sometimes another predominating. There is general malaise for a few hours or a day, the patient may become restless and sleepless and may suffer from nausea, headache, giddiness, and mental confusion, and then pass into a condition of great depression resembling melancholia; hallucinations and delusions of persecution and suicidal impulses may follow. The period of depression may be followed by mania and violent delirium, with other symptoms resembling meningitis.

Very few cases of poisoning occur, as iodoform has been largely replaced by non-odorous antiseptics.

The amount of iodoform necessary to cause death when taken internally is not known. Individuals seem to differ greatly in their susceptibility to the drug. Thirty grains and sometimes even twenty have caused death, while recovery has followed the taking of 120 grains.

The treatment consists in removing the dressing containing this drug. The barbiturates may be given to check the mania and delirium.

Postmortem appearances are fatty degeneration of the heart, liver, and kidneys. Edema of the pia mater and of the lungs and acute nephritis have been found in some cases.

Detection: The tissues or other material under examination are made alkaline with caustic potash, and subjected to steam distillation. The distillate is treated with a few drops of caustic potash, and any iodoform present is shaken out with ether in a separatory funnel. After the ether evaporates, the iodoform remains as hexagonal stars or other hexagonal forms which may be recognized under the microscope. Iodoform always yields the odor of isobenzonitrile when warmed with aniline and alcoholic potassium hydroxide. A red color is given when iodoform is present, with pyridine and sodium hydroxide.

A similar color is given when phenol and resorcine and sodium hydroxide are added to a few drops of a solution of the suspected substance in alcohol and the mixture warmed over a small flame. This precipitate is soluble in alcohol with a carmine-red color. The red color is discharged by mineral acids and restored by alkalis. This red substance has all the properties of rosolic acid, and is produced by chloroform as well as iodoform.

SULPHONMETHANE

SULPHONMETHANE (sulphonal, sulphonmethanum, U. S. P.) is diethyl-sulphone-dimethyl-methane, $(CH_3)_2C(SO_2\text{-}C_2H_5)_2$. It occurs in colorless, prismatic crystals that are without odor and nearly tasteless, melting at 125° C. (257° F.). Sulphonmethane is sparingly soluble in cold water readily soluble in hot water, and soluble in alcohol and ether.

Symptoms: The medicinal dose: seven to fifteen grains (0.5 to 1 gm.) of sulphonmethane usually produces sleep, but sometimes nausea, headache, dizziness, and irregular gait result.

After large doses the symptoms are exceedingly variable. Among those noted are the following: mental confusion, motor disturbances, as shown by an irregular gait or paralysis, stupor, insensibility, more rarely excitment and convulsions. In very severe cases the respiration is stertorous and irregular, the pulse scarcely perceptible, and there is marked cyanosis. Death usually results from failure of respiration, even though artificial respiration is given. Sometimes the secretion of urine is suppressed, and death results from anuria. Coma has continued for six days with recovery.

Fatal Dose: Death has frequently followed doses of seventy-five grains to one ounce. Thirty grains caused death in a neurasthenic woman.

Fatal Period: Death may occur in a few hours or in a few days.

Treatment: The stomach should be washed out, and diuretics, purgatives, strychnine and other stimulants administered.

Isolation: Sulphonal will be found in the evaporation of the acid ether extract, and is best identified by its melting point.

If sufficient material is obtained, a portion of it is melted with potassium cyanide which develops a mercaptan odor, and forms potassium sulphocyanate. This is dissolved in water, the addition of ferric chloride giving a blood red color. When heated in a test-tube with powdered charcoal, sulphonal forms mercaptan, acetic acid, formic acid, and sulphur dioxide. If 0.1 gm. of sulphonal be heated in a test-tube with 0.1 gm. of sodium salicylate, an odor of mercaptan develops; if this mixture be treated with five drops of sulphuric acid, a turbid red solution is obtained having the odor of methyl salicylate. If some of the tablets or powder taken by the patient are submitted, the charcoal test may be applied. Heat some of the powder with powdered charcoal in a test-tube. The odor of mercaptan may be noted, and the vapors will change blue litmus paper red.

Sulphur dioxide may be shown by its bleaching action on a piece of filter paper moistened with blue starch iodide suspended in the mouth of the tube.

TRIONAL AND TETRONAL

TRIONAL and tetronal are very similar in both chemical and physiological properties to sulphonmethane. Trional melts at 76° C., and tetronal at 89° C. Both will be found in the acid ether extract; as they all give the same chemical tests, the melting point must be relied upon to distinguish these three.

BARBITAL

BARBITAL was introduced by Fisher and Mering in 1905 under the name of "veronal." It is, chemically, diethyl-barbituric acid (diethyl malonyl urea, malo-urea); $CO(NHCO)_2C(C_2H_5)_2$; it is derived from diethylmalonic acid and urea. Its molecular weight is 184.11. It is a white, crystalline powder, melting at 188° to 189° C. (370.4° to 372.2° F.); odorless and faintly bitter. It is stable in the air. One gm. is soluble in 150 cc. of water, 14 cc. of alcohol, 75 cc. of chloroform, 35 cc. of ether at 25° C., and in 13 cc. of boiling water (U.S.P., XI).

In 1905 Kress[1379] published a long list of cases in which untoward results had followed its use. Since that time a large number of cases of poisoning have been reported. A number of these have been accidental. Most of the cases I have seen were suicides or attempts at suicide. I have seen a number of cases of addiction to barbital and barbital compounds. Lambert[1380] has said that the habitual use of barbital produces distinct psychosis, with hallucinations and delusions of persecution, requiring at best several weeks for recovery. The laity is using a great deal more of this drug than is generally realized. This drug should only be sold on prescription and the physician is responsible largely for its misuse. In Colorado a state law prevents the sale of this class of compounds unless prescribed by a duly licensed physician.

Barbital is excreted slowly, so that continued doses may produce serious cumulative effects. The margin between the ordinary therapeutic dose (0.5 gm.) and the toxic dose (usually 8 to 10 gm.) is somewhat wide, so that the ordinary dose taken by an individual has little effect upon the blood pressure and respiration. Fatal collapse has been reported in several cases from relatively small doses (ten to fifteen grains or 0.65 to 1 gm.).[1381] I have seen more than twelve individuals recover from a dose as large as 10 gm.

Barbital and its derivatives have largely supplanted sulphanol, trianol, tetranol, and chloral hydrate in nervous insomnia. Some persons, however, are very sensitive to the barbiturates, becoming delirious after a dose as small as one-half grain. Barbital has caused conditions resembling alcoholic intoxication, disturbance of speech, delusion, tremor, ataxia, loss of memory. Repeated doses of one and a half grains have caused loss of weight, anemia, hematoporphyrinuria, and oliguria. Postoperative cases given barbiturates developed

1379. KRESS: *Therap. Monatsh., Berl.*, 19:467, 1905; see also SEIFERT: *Die Nebenwirkungen d. moder. Arzneimittel*, 99, 1915.

1380. LAMBERT, A.: *J.A.M.A.*, 96:286, 1931.

1381. *J.A.M.A.*, 53:1833, 1909.

dullness, drowsiness, nausea, vertigo, asthenia, and skin rashes. Others have a marked depressing effect from one and a half grains which causes them to feel markedly depressed twenty-four hours after taking the drug.

Dreyfus recommends this drug in treatment of delirium tremens, using 0.5 gm. three times a day. Wolfram employs it against vomiting, seasickness, migraine, and for combination anesthesias.[1382] If more rapid action is desired the soluble barbital may be used, 1 gm. of which is soluble in 5 cc. of water at 25° C. and in 2.5 cc. of boiling water.

Barbital produces sleep in about one-half hour. Respiration and circulation are little affected by a therapeutic dose of 5 grains. The minimum fatal dose of barbital by mouth for rabbits was found by Maloney and Tatum to be 0.2 to 0.275 gm. Eddy found the minimum fatal dose for dogs varied from 0.4 to 0.6 gm. per kilogram of body weight.[1383]

Roemer found that the fatal dose by subcutaneous injection was 1.5 gm. per kilogram for frogs, 0.35 gm. for cats. Impens states that the fatal dose whether administered by mouth or subcutaneously was practically the same. Sollmann gives the fatal dose of barbital for rats as 0.31 gm. per kilogram when administered hypodermically. Barbital caused, in addition to its effect upon the central nervous system, profound fall of blood pressure due to a peripheral paralysis of the blood vessels comparable to that caused by arsenic.[1384] There is also a fall of temperature.

Barbital is largely excreted unchanged in the urine. It is excreted slowly, sometimes not reaching a maximum until the second day, and continuing on the third and even up to the sixth day.[1385]

Symptoms: The patient, when first seen by the physician, is usually in coma with reflexes and pupillary reaction retained and even exaggerated. Chang and Tainter reported an unusual case where 18 gm. (278 grains) of sodium barbital had

1382. WOLFRAM: Merck's Reporter, 20:259, 1906.
1383. MALONEY and TATUM: J. Pharmacol. & Exper. Therap., 44: 337, 1932. EDDY: J. Pharm., 33:43, 1928. SEEVERS: J. Pharm., 42:217, 1931.
1384. ROEMER: Arch. f. exper. Path. u. Pharmakol., 66:24, 1911. IMPENS: Deutsche med. Wchnschr., 38:945, 1912. SOLLMANN: Manual of Pharmacology, 4th ed., 4:771, 1932. JACOBJ: Arch. f. exper. Path. u. Pharmakol., 66:24, 1911.
1385. KOPPANI: J. Pharmacol. & Exper. Therap., 52:121, 1934.

been taken with suicidal intent.[1386] This case was characterized by deep coma of six days' duration, rapid pulse and respiration and high temperature, in contrast to the usual picture of severe depression of temperature and respiration. Respiration was regular with a rate of about 42 per minute; pulse 164, rectal temperature 102.8° F. During the next two days the temperature progressively rose to 107.2° with a pulse rate of 200 and respiratory rate of 54 per minute. Temperature, pulse and respirations gradually decreased until the ninth day, when the temperature had reached 100°, pulse 95, respirations 24. During this period the lungs were clear. No septic process was detectable to explain the high fever. The urine was heavily loaded with red cells and albumen.

Constricted pupils may confuse the physician with opium poisoning. However, in several cases that I have seen the pupils were widely dilated. Disturbances of vision may be present for a number of days. In addition to stupor, excitement or restlessness, restless sleep, trismus, delirium, and rise of temperature, the symptoms have suggested uremic coma, in other cases pneumonia.[1387] From the administration of one and a half grains I have seen mild erythema resembling a scarlet fever rash. In two individuals who were accustomed to taking six grains a day, acneform rash developed which disappeared on stopping the drug.

Coste and Bolgert[1388] report that they also found four cases of an ulcerous condition following poisoning by barbituric acid preparations. The location of the lesions was in the sacral region, the internal surface of the thighs, the buttocks and plantar region. They found ulcerations as large as the palm of the hand in the left popliteal region superimposed upon profoundly indurated areas similar to that described by Maillard, Levy and Fiehrer. In a second case large symmetrical blisters in both plantar regions were seen.

Treatment: Dawson and Taft, Barlow, Haggard and Greenberg, and Zerfas and McCallum[1389] have called attention

1386. CHANG, D. K., and TAINTER, M.D.: *J.A.M.A.*, 106:1386, 1936.
1387. WILLCOX: *Lancet*, 2:734, 1913.
1388. COSTE, F., and BOLGERT, M.: *Internat. M. Digest*, 23:270, 1933.
1389. DAWSON and TAFT: *Proc. Soc. Exper. Biol. & Med.*, 28:917, 1931. BARLOW, O. W.: *J.A.M.A.*, 98:1980, 1932. HAGGARD, H. W., and GREENBERG, L. A.: *J.A.M.A.*, 98:1133, 1932. ZERFAS, L. C., and McCALLUM, J. T. C.: *Anesth. & Analg.*, 8:349, 1929.

to the specificity of the barbiturates in strychnine poisoning because of their anticonvulsant efficiency. The reverse can be used for the treatment of barbiturate poisoning.[1390] A case report is given of a woman, aged forty-seven years, who had taken 15 gm. of a barbiturate and recovered following a dose of 0.06 gm. strychnine given within twenty-four hours. Ramond and Delay report a case in which a person, poisoned by barbital, died in spite of the enormous amount of strychnine (0.62 gm.) administered within three days. Flandin and Bernard[1390] report a temperature of 107.6° two hours after death.

Injections of strychnine to combat the toxic effects of barbituric acid derivatives according to the Idd method[1391] are accepted today in France as the only remedy offering any chance of success. Carriere[1391] states that one may use strychnine since no remedy should be neglected in the presence of the danger of death, but it should not be relied upon as the sole remedy; other remedies should be tried. He had excellent results with intravenous injections of coramine and a 30% solution of alcohol.

The stomach should be washed out, high colonic flushings and diuretics given. Injections of camphor, caffeine with sodium benzoate and other cardiac and vascular stimulants should be given. If the patient is unable to swallow, intravenous injections of glucose and normal salt should be used.

Sanderson[1392] reported a man twenty-six years of age who had taken 200 grains of barbital four hours previously. He was given 800 cc. of 20% glucose intravenously twenty-four hours after admission to the hospital. An hour later the patient had a chill, became restless and moved for the first time. At 6:00 o'clock the next morning he could swallow and talk incoherently. On the third day he was semiconscious. Five days after admission he was quite rational.

Buzzo and Bertani reported intravenous injection of coramine.[1393]

1390. Foreign letters, *J.A.M.A.*, 102:306, 1934.
1391. Foreign letters, *J.A.M.A.*, 103:270, 1934.
1392. SANDERSON, G. H.: *California & West. Med.*, 33:887, 1930.
1393. BUZZO, A., and BERTANI, O. C.: *Rev. asoc. méd. argent.*, 47: 398, 1933. CROHN: *Med. Klin.*, 28:1200, 1932; GLASSER, G.: *Berl. Med. Klin.*, 28:514, 1932; BARILARI, MARGULIS, and MARENZI: *Prensa méd argent.*, February 20, 1932; BARILARI and MARTINEZ: *Pub. en el Dia Med.*, July 24, 1933.

Lickint[1394] reported a case of dial poisoning. **Severe intoxi-cations with dial** (diallyl barbituric acid) are very rare, and few such cases have been reported. Thomel,[1395] and Wein-berg[1395] found a sense of depression of the head and marked tremor of the hands, and a slight ataxia the following day after taking this drug. Christoffel[1396] has described a staggering gait, a tremulous and stammering speech, and sensory decep-tions with 0.3 and 0.4 gm. of dial. Schmidt[1397] has observed tremor in the hands so severe that the patient was unable to hold a spoon following a dose of 0.1 gm. dial given twice a day over a long period of time. Müller[1398] gave 0.4 to 0.8 gm. of dial intravenously and subcutaneously for ten days. In thirty-three cases observed there were two with collapse, eight with fever above 38° C.; one-third of the cases showed albuminuria, and five cases showed urobilinogen. The author describes the case of a war veteran who had consumed 2.4 gm. of dial which he swallowed with the aid of an elixir. Twenty hours later he was brought into the clinic unconscious. The skin of the face was dark red. He had loud breathing; the pupils were con-tracted and reacted only sluggishly to light; he had a marked dermographia. The abdominal, cremasteric and patellar re-flexes were absent; there was no patellar or ankle clonus. Temperature was normal, pulse regular at a rate of 104 per min-ute. There was some urobilinogen and indican. The patient made an uneventful recovery.

Fatal dose: Death has followed the taking of less than 1 gm. Recovery has occurred, as in Chang and Tainter's case quoted previously, in which the patient took 18 gm. I have seen recovery in a number of cases where 10 gm. had been taken. In the case reported by Chang and Tainter, recovery occurred after the patient had been in a comatose condition for six days. Littell reports recovery after the taking of 120 grains on each of twelve successive days.[1399] Recovery, on the strength of Chang's and Tainter's case, may occur after any dose from 1 to 18 gm.

1394. LICKINT, F.: *Deutsche med. Wchnschr.*, 56:2001, 1930.
1395. THOMEL: *Deutsche med. Wchnschr.*, 49:1214, 1923. WEINBERG: *Deutsche med. Wchnschr.*, 40:1377, 1924.
1396. CHRISTOFFEL: *Schweiz. med. Wchnschr.*, 50:1123, 1920.
1397. SCHMIDT, C.: *Med. Klin.*, 40:1568, 1924.
1398. MÜLLER: *Ztschr. f. Neurol.*, 107:523, 1927.
1399. LITTELL, J.: *J.A.M.A.*, 77:1333, 1921.

Fatal Period: Death may occur in a short time from a fatal collapse by peripheral paralysis of the blood vessels. Usually life is prolonged for several days. Death seldom occurs under twenty-four hours. Embden[1400] reported that death did not occur in thirty-six hours after taking 20 gm. Germann[1401] reported death in seventy-nine hours after taking 200 to 250 grains. Recovery is possible after six days of coma.

Toxic Effect: Solis-Cohen and Githens[1402] state that more fatal accidents are now recorded in England from barbital than from any other drug. It can now be sold only on prescription in England and Wales. Two deaths were reported following doses of 0.7 gm., one was a healthy child of three years. Death may follow the use of 3 gm. even in a healthy adult.

Schroder[1403] reported a case in which death did not occur until eight days after taking the drug. This individual showed a deep coma with loss of reflexes of the extremities. Later, signs of circulatory failure developed, due to vasomotor paralysis of the peripheral vessels.

Ruhberg[1404] speaks of the non-narcotic addicts. The most striking of this group are caused by barbital and paraldehyde. Dannemann[1405] thinks a few of the cases of death were in individuals having an idiosyncrasy, making them susceptible to small or moderate doses of barbital.

Postmortem Appearances: In an acute case of barbital poisoning, there may be nothing characteristic seen grossly. Where life has been prolonged for a number of days, pulmonary edema, hyperemia, and edema of the meninges, and hyperemia of the liver and kidneys have been described. The heart usually shows marked dilatation. Bronchopneumonia has developed in a number of cases of barbital poisoning. One case has been reported which showed, in the ganglion cells, a peculiar type of albuminoid degeneration of the cell protein with collections of metachromatic particles. The metachromatic degenerative changes were most marked in the pons and in the medulla.

1400. *München. med. Wchnschr.*, 55:1050, 1908.

1401. *J.A.M.A.*, 46:1999, 1906.

1402. Pharmacotherapeutics and Materia Medica and Drug Action; New York, D. Appleton & Co., 1928, p. 195.

1403. *Deutsche Ztschr. f. d. ges. gerichtl. Med.*, 13:353, 1929.

1404. RUHBERG, G. N.: *Minnesota Med.*, 12:75, 1929.

1405. DANNEMANN, A. C.: *J. Nerv. & Ment. Dis.*, 69:33, 1929.

Isolation: The tissue is prepared as previously described for an alkaloidal extraction. The barbiturates will be found in the ether extract. On evaporating the ether the barbital remains in the residue as needle-like crystals. Only about 90% recovery is made using ether. Fischer and Hoppe[1406] claim that barbital can be found excreted unchanged in the urine, and in fatal cases in which the patient usually lived for twenty-four hours or longer a very considerable amount may be found in the urine. Van Itallie and Steenhauer[1407] recommend the extraction with ethyl acetate. With urine take 100 cc.; add 100 cc. neutral or basic lead acetate and filter. The filtrate is evaporated on the water-bath to 25 cc. and acidified with acetic acid. The warm solution is transferred to a separatory funnel and shaken twice with ethyl acetate. The latter is filtered through a dry filter paper, evaporated and the residue dissolved in 10 cc. of boiling water with 5 cc. of dilute sulphuric acid added. This is heated to a boil, and 10/N potassium permanganate added until the supernatant fluid is colorless. The excess is destroyed with a few drops of H_2O_2. The colorless solution is shaken twice with ethyl acetate, the latter filtered through a dry filter, evaporated, and the residue dried at 100° C., and weighed. This residue can be used for the various tests for barbital.

2. Identify barbital in the dry residue by first obtaining its melting point, which is 187° to 190° C. Millon's reagent: To an aqueous solution of the residue add an equal quantity of Millon's reagent. A gelatinous yellow precipitate forms, soluble in excess of the reagent.[1408]

3. Equal parts of alkaline residue and caustic potash are fused and dissolved, and the cool mass dissolved in a little water and divided into two parts. One portion is tested for the presence of hydrocyanic acid. The other portion is acidified with sulphuric acid, extracted with ether, and evaporated. The residue is diethylacetate, which is oily and has a rancid odor. A little of this added to a dilute solution of ferric chloride gives a red color.

4. A solution of chloro-iodide of zinc added to barbital

1406. FISCHER and HOPPE: *München. med. Wchnschr.*, **56**:1429, 1909.

1407. VAN ITALLIE and STEENHAUER: *Pharm. Weekblad*, **58**, 1921.

1408. See MOLLE and KLEIST: *Arch. d. Pharm.*, **242**:401, 1904.

gives a precipitate of small flat tabular crystals, gray to black-ish-red in color.

5. Hydriodic acid dissolves barbital sublimates, and often deposits large flat red crystals.

6. Potassium bromide solution of bromine gives flesh-colored needles and leaflets.

7. Sublimate dissolved in ammoniacal copper solution and allowed to evaporate, gives violet and pink monoclinic plates.

8. In the presence of phenobarbital, test No. 3 gives a pleasant odor of locust honey, while barbital yields a sour, rancid odor, and proponol has a spicy odor which soon changes to a pungent one.

9. Phenobarbital can be distinguished from barbital and proponal by dissolving 0.01 to 0.02 gm. of material in 5 to 10 cc. formaldehyde plus 4 cc. concentrated sulphuric acid. Upon standing a while, phenobarbital gives a brilliant rose-red then cyclamen-red to wine-red color. The other two become slight∙ly yellow.

10. Strzyzowski[1409] recommends the decolorizing of the extracted material with a few centigrams of charcoal before extraction with ether or ethyl acetate. The residue from the ether is sublimed in vacuum. On sublimation, crystals are formed which belong to the monoclinic variety. Microcrystal∙lographic inspection follows. This shows the treatment of bar-bital with silver nitrate whereby prismatic crystals are obtained which are very characteristic, and quantities smaller than 0.0005 gm. may be detected in this way.

Linegar, Dille and Koppanyi[1410] add 5 cc. of 10% copper sulphate solution to 25 cc. of urine and make alkaline with 10 cc. of 10% sodium tungstate solution; mix, filter, and add 4 cc. of 5% sulphuric acid to 30 cc. of filtrate with chloroform as usual.

1409. STRZYZOWSKI, C.: *Ann. de méd. lég.*, 13: 49, 1933.
1410. LINEGAR, C. R., DILLE, J. M., and KOPPANYI, T. J.: *J. Am. Pharm. Ass.*, 24: 847, 1935.

PHENOBARBITAL ($C_{12}H_{12}O_3N_2$)

PHENOBARBITAL (phenylethylbarbituric acid) has a molecular weight of 232.11. It occurs as small glistening crystals, or a white crystalline powder. It is odorless, and is stable in the air. Soluble phenobarbital, $C_{12}H_{11}O_3N_2Na$, has a molecular weight of 254.10 and occurs as flaky crystals, white crystalline granules, or a white powder; it is colorless, hygroscopic, and has a bitter taste. It is soluble in water and alcohol but practically insoluble in ether or chloroform. Phenobarbital melts between 173° and 177° C. A saturated aqueous solution of phenobarbital is acid to litmus paper. One gram of phenobarbital is soluble in about 1000 cc. of water, 8 cc. of alcohol, 40 cc. of chloroform, 13 cc. of ether, and about 700 cc. of benzene at 25°C. The dose for this drug is half a grain (0.03 gm.). The dose is the same for the soluble phenobarbital. It was formerly marketed under the name of "luminal." It differs from barbital in that one ethyl group (C_2H_5) has been replaced by a phenol group (C_6H_5).

Toxic affections occur more frequently from phenobarbital than from barbital. Gruber and Baskett[1411] have found that large doses of phenobarbital have a marked depressant action on the circulation and cause a fall in blood pressure from 10% to 80%. Phillips[1412] has collected references to sixteen cases of poisoning. Eight doses of one and a half grains were taken daily for eight days, producing a violent eruption accompanied by high fever and some irritation of the kidneys.

Wilcox[1413] reported that phenobarbital in the dose of 0.3 gm. has, in a number of instances, caused active poisoning. Wright[1414] reported a case of fatal poisoning from phenobarbital. The patient, a woman, had taken phenobarbital with suicidal intent. The drug was isolated from the brain, 90 mg. per 100 gm., and from the stomach and liver in much smaller amounts, 3 to 5 mg. per 100 gm. of tissue.

Rash is more apt to develop from phenobarbital than from barbital. I have seen a number of cases resembling scarlet

1411. U. S. Dispensatory, ed. 21, Philadelphia, J. B. Lippincott Co., 213 and 828, 1926.

1412. J.A.M.A., 78:1199, 1922.

1413. WILCOX, R. W.: Materia Medica and Therapeutics, 12th ed., Philadelphia, P. Blakiston's Son Co., 1929, p. 607.

1414. WRIGHT: Arch. Int. Med., 43:85, 1929.

fever, measles, and acne. I have given phenobarbital to three epileptic patients over a period of ten years in doses of from one and a half to four and a half grains a day and have not observed any untoward effect except erythema on two or three occasions.

Severe symptoms—dizziness, nausea, vomiting, double vision—resulted from a dose of 0.3 gm.[1415] Disturbances of speech, ataxia with inability to stand, and diminished reflexes followed the taking of 0.6 gm. in twenty-four hours, and in another case 0.9 gm. (with 0.2 gm. barbital) in four hours.[1416] Death has been reported from 15 gm. of soluble phenobarbital taken over a period of three weeks.[1417] Eschback[1418] reported a case of a forty-three year old woman who was depressed and worried. She ingested twenty tablets of phenobarbital, an equivalent of 2 gm. She became unconscious and could not be aroused even after the injection of caffeine and intramuscular injections of lobeline. The author then gave three injections of 2 mg. of strychnine at intervals of fifteen minutes, also without results. On account of the seriousness of the case and because death was expected, it was decided to give 1 cg. of strychnine. Five minutes later the patient came out of the coma, began to talk incoherently but rapidly, and eventually recovered.

Dial: Leschke[1419] found eight cases of severe but not fatal poisoning and nine fatal cases due to diallyl barbituric acid. The chief symptoms are coma, cyanosis, loss of reflexes, muscular relaxation, and sometimes incontinence of urine and feces. Death is due to respiratory or circulatory paralysis. Achard reported two fatal cases of diallyl barbituric acid poisoning and two with recovery.[1420] Kohn-Abrest reported a case of a patient who had taken 4.9 gm. of dial; he was in deep coma with reflexes abolished, and died the next day, after developing dyspnea with Cheyne-Stokes respiration and cyanosis.[1421]

1415. STEIN: *Therap. Halb Monatsch.*, 34:387, 1920.
1416. FARNELL: *J.A.M.A.*, 61:192, 1913.
1417. HUEBER: *München. med. Wchnschr.*, 66:1090, 1919.
1418. ESCHBACK, J. H.: *Bull. et mém. Soc. méd. d. hôp. de Paris*, 57:1183, 1933.
1419. *Med. Klin.*, 29:59, 1933.
1420. ACHARD, C.: *J. de méd et chir. prat.*, 100:277, 1929.
1421. KOHN-ABREST, L.: *Bull. et mém. Soc. méd. d. hôp. de Paris*, 54:261, 1930.

The postmortem findings in a case of diallyl barbituric acid poisoning are serious lesions of the liver, chiefly fatty degeneration. The cells present an abnormal clearness, with nuclear fragmentation and invasion of the protoplasm by transparent granulations.[1422]

Van der Horst and Van Hasselt report poisonings from iso-methyl-ethyl barbituric acid, cyclobarbital and diethyl-allyl-barbiturate in diethylamine.[1423] These authors reported a fatal case due to poisoning with diethyl-allyl-barbiturate in diethylamine, of a woman to whom injections were given for the control of an acute psychosis. On the day following the last injection the patient suddenly collapsed. The pulse was not perceptible and she finally died. Flandin[1424] reports the case of a woman of twenty-eight who had taken 3.6 gm. barbital with 3.6 gm. diallyl barbituric acid. The pulse became imperceptible, the respiration slow and irregular. The patient died from respiratory paralysis with terminal pulmonary edema.

Shinkle[1425] reports two cases of poisoning by allyl-iso-propyl barbituric acid combined with amidopyrine. The patient was given this barbital compound for withdrawal pains and sleeplessness in a cure for morphine addiction. She suddenly developed urinary incontinence and other symptoms suggestive of tabes. While in the hospital she passed into an acute psychosis with delirium.

Orford reported the case of a woman, aged thirty-nine, who took twelve dial tablets (eighteen grains). When seen two and a half hours afterward, she was cyanosed, respirations 6 to 8, eyes fixed, pupils dilated, reflexes gone, skin cold and clammy. She was given 3 cc. of coramine intramuscularly. In a few minutes her pulse, color, and respiration improved.[1426]

Glasser reports a patient who took thirty luminal tablets, 120 drops somnifen, five or six 2-cc. luminal ampoules, six pernocton ampoules intramuscularly, and possibly other hypnotics. Three intravenous doses at 5 cc. of coramine brought about recovery.[1427]

1422. Paris correspondent, *J.A.M.A.*, 92:662, 1929.
1423. VAN DER HORST, L., and VAN HASSELT, J. A.: *Psychiat. en neurol. bl.*, 37:158, 1933.
1424. FLANDIN, C.: *Bull. et mém. Soc. méd. d. hôp de Paris*, 49:561, 1933.
1425. SHINKLE, C. E.: *J. Med.*, 9:479, 1928.
1426. ORFORD, T. J.: *Canad. M.A.J.*, 30:65, 1934.
1427. *Med. Klin.*, 15, 1932.

Cohen and Gildea reported a patient who took as high as 2 gm. of phenobarbital daily.[1428]

Purves-Stewart and Willcox reported three cases of poisoning by barbiturates, one of whom had taken veronal 125 grains (twenty-five tablets); allonal 125 grains (twenty-five tablets); quadranox seventy-five grains (ten tablets), and ipral 150 grains (twenty tablets). She came out of coma in three and a half days, and finally completely recovered.[1429]

CINCHOPHEN AND NEOCINCHOPHEN

CINCHOPHEN (phenylquinoline, carboxylic acid, atophan, phenylcinchoninicum), $C_6H_5 . C_9H_5N . COOH$ consists of small, colorless, needle-like crystals, or a white to yellowish-white powder. It is odorless, and almost insoluble in cold water. One gram is soluble in about 400 cc. of chloroform, 100 cc. of ether, and in 120 cc. of alcohol at 25°C. It melts at 210°C., with partial decomposition. It is no longer official.

Cinchophen was introduced as a therapeutic agent for gout by Nicolaier and Dohrn in 1908.[1430] Phillips in 1913[1431] reported cutaneous manifestations, such as pruritus, angioneurotic edema, urticaria, and macular and papular rashes following its use, and Herrick, also in 1913,[1432] reported a case of urticaria and scarlet-fever-like rash. Its toxic effects were first published by Schroeder,[1433] who reported nine cases of his own and eight others reported to him by other physicians. In his experience the drug induced irritation of the alimentary tract as well as constitutional symptoms, such as itching and edema of the skin, fever and headache. Hanzlik and Scott[1434] reported a comparative study of the efficiency and toxicity of cinchophen, neocinchophen, and salicylic acid. Barron[1435] was probably the first to report a case of cinchophen poisoning. He attributed it to a case of severe allergic reaction, and then he sounded a

1428. COHEN, L. H., and GILDEA, E. F.:   *Arch. Neurol. & Psychiat.*, 31:1283, 1934.

1429. PURVES-STEWART, J., and WILLCOX, W. H.:   *Lancet*, 226 (1):6, 1934.

1430. NICOLAIER and DOHRN: *Deutsches Arch. f. klin. Med.*, 93:331, 1908.

1431. PHILLIPS, J.:   *J.A.M.A.*, 61:1040, 1913.

1432. HERRICK, W. W.:   *J.A.M.A.*, 61:1376, 1913.

1433. SCHROEDER: *Ugesk. f. laeger.*, 84:114, 1922.

1434. *J.A.M.A.*, 77:1230, 1921.

1435. BARRON, MOSES: *J.A.M.A.*, 12:2010, 1924.

note of warning against the indiscriminate use of both cinchophen and neocinchophen. Boros* reported ascites due to cinchophen poisoning. Also in 1924, Boot and Miller[1436] reported the results of treatment of twenty cases of acute rheumatic fever. They found that 75% of the cases treated showed toxic effects of some sort. Barron's case was a man of forty-four who had taken five to six tablets daily of seven-and-one-half grains dosage. His rheumatism was relieved and he had no further attacks for several months, when he again took the tablets. After taking two tablets he felt a peculiar sensation all over the body; itching and prickling were followed by numbness and a feeling of complete paralysis; he saw black before the eyes, but did not lose consciousness; and he had cold clammy perspiration, and pressure sense across chest in the region of the heart causing difficulty in breathing.

Worster-Drought[1437] reported liver damage. After this date the literature abounds with reports of liver damage due to cinchophen. The gross pathology was first demonstrated by Cabot.[1438] In the early part of 1926 Sir Langdon Brown[1439] reported two fatal cases of jaundice following the administration of atoquinol, and stated that he knew of two other cases. Evans[1440] reported three cases of toxic jaundice following the use of cinchophen, in one of which there were two separate attacks, one following the taking of thirty seven-and-a-half-grain tablets. Glover[1441] reported a case following the use of atoquinol, with indigestion and jaundice. Willcox[1442] reports that a man, aged sixty-nine, who had taken three five-grain tablets daily for a week, began to show jaundice, and after twenty-eight days died. Wells[1443] reports the case of a thirty-three year old woman who took twenty tablets averaging seven and a half grains over a period of four and a half to five months. She complained of pain and tenderness over the gall-bladder; she had a normal temperature; urine showed a trace of albumin.

* Boros, Edwin: *J.A.M.A.*, 109:113, 1937.
1436. *J.A.M.A.*, 82:1028, 1924.
1437. Worster-Drought, C.: *Brit. M. J.*, 1:148, 1923.
1438. Cabot, R. C., Cabot, H.: *Boston M. & S. J.*, 192:1122, 1925.
1439. *Brit. M. J.*, 2:37, 1926.
1440. Evans, G.: *Brit. M. J.*, 2:93, 1926.
1441. Glover, L. G.: *Brit. M. J.*, 2:136, 1926.
1442. Willcox, W. H.: *Brit. M. J.*, 2:273, 1926.
1443. Wells, C. J. L.: *Brit. M. J.*, 2:759, 1936.

The jaundice lasted three days, followed by death. The necropsy showed an acute yellow atrophy of the liver.

Loewenthal, Mackay, and Lowe[1444] reported two cases of acute yellow atrophy of the liver and suggested that albuminuria and nephritis should be considered as a contra-indication for the use of this drug. Rake[1445] calls attention to the benzene ring in the quinoline nucleus. From this the benzene ring can be obtained, and the toxic properties are accounted for. Sutton[1446] reported a case in detail, with autopsy by Simonds. Garzell[1447] reported three cases of poisoning with angioneurotic edema, urticaria, macular and papular rashes. Scully[1448] in 1924 reported idosyncrasy to cinchophen.

Rabinowitz[1449] reported seven cases from one hospital, and listed forty-three collected from the literature of atrophy of the liver due to cinchophen medication.

Neocinchophen, $C_{19}H_{17}O_2N$, has a molecular weight of 291.14. It is the ethyl ester of 6-methyl-2-phenylquinolin-4-carboxylic acid. It is a pale yellow, crystalline powder, odorless and tasteless, and is permanent in the air. Neocinchophen is nearly insoluble in water, is soluble in hot alcohol, and is very soluble in ether and in chloroform. The melting point is not below 74°C.

The early symptoms of intoxication by cinchophen and neocinchophen are malaise, anorexia, nausea, vomiting, diarrhea, urticaria, vasomotor disturbances, rashes, jaundice. Beaver and Robertson[1450] have reported the relatively rapid necrosis and autolysis of the hepatic parenchyma resulting in atrophy of the liver.

Treatment includes a large water intake, light, easily assimilable carbohydrate diet, glucose by mouth or intravenously, injections of calcium gluconate.

Of more than 100 cases reported the mortality rate was over 50%. Carroll and Elliott[1451] claim that the number of

1444. LOEWENTHAL, MACKAY and LOWE: *Brit. M. J.*, 1:592, 1928.
1445. RAKE, G. W.: *Guys' Hosp. Rep.*, 77:229, 1927.
1446. SUTTON, D. C.: *J.A.M.A.*, 91:310, 1928.
1447. GARZELL, S. L.: *New England J. Med.*, 206:183, 1932.
1448. SCULLY: *J.A.M.A.*, 83:623, 1924.
1449. RABINOWITZ, M. A.: *J.A.M.A.*, 96:1220, 1930.
1450. BEAVER, D. C., and ROBERTSON, H. E.: *Am. J. Path.*, 17:237, 1931.
1451. CARROLL, H. C., and ELLIOTT, C. A.: *M. Clin. North America*, 17:473, 1933.

unreported cases is very large. In some instances large doses of cinchophen are tolerated. In one case 2.5 to 6 gm. daily for a period of eighteen years for the relief of arthritis has been reported. On the other hand, two to three tablets have caused serious illness in people who had previously taken the drug.

Lerd[1452] reported a case where 6 gm. were taken over a period of a few days, which resulted in poisoning, jaundice, and death. Several factors enter into the tolerance to cinchophen. Probably there is a lowered glycogen content, hyperthyroidism, and hypersusceptibility.

Schwarz[1453] reported a case of poisoning from di-idoatophan (biloptin) in a woman thirty years of age who had been given 5 gm. of the drug in milk preparatory to the x-raying of the gall-bladder.

ORGANIC ACIDS OF THE FATTY ACID SERIES
ACETIC ACID

ACETIC ACID (acidum aceticum, CH_3COOH, molecular weight, 60.03) is official in the U. S. P., XI, as glacial acetic acid, (acidum aceticum glaciale), containing not less than 90% of $HC_2H_3O_2$. It is a clear, colorless liquid, having a pungent, characteristic odor, and, when well diluted with water, an acid taste. Glacial acetic acid is miscible with water, with alcohol, and with glycerine. Its specific gravity is from 1.047 to 1.050 at 25°C. It boils at about 118°C., and congeals at 14.75°C. Acetic acid is an aqueous solution containing not less than 36% and not more than 37% of $HC_2H_3O_2$. It is a clear colorless liquid, having a strong characteristic odor, and a sharply acid taste. The specific gravity is about 1.045, at 25°C. Dilute acetic acid (acidum aceticum dilutum) is an aqueous solution containing not less than 5.7 gm. and not more than 6.3 gm. of $HC_2H_3O_2$, in each 100 cc. The substitution by mistake of acetic acid for the dilute acid has caused serious illness. A clerk in a well-known chain drug store dispensed acetic acid in a prescription in place of the dilute acetic acid, the final product containing 24.18% of acetic acid. A severe pain of the mouth, throat, and stomach, was noted after the patient took several doses of this medicine before her physician

1452. LERD, S. C.: *Ohio State M. J.*, 28:28, 1932.
1453. *Ges. d. Artze. Wien. Seitz., g. v.*, 11:11, 1927.

was notified. A number of deaths have been caused from its accidental use. In 1909 Franz[1454] collected 256 cases of acetic acid poisoning in Germany; 46.2% of these occurred in children, with a mortality of 71.1%. Very few cases of poisoning with acetic acid are seen in America. (The few seen are usually found industrially.) In St. Petersburg in 1908, 34% of all the cases of suicide were due to this acid.

Acetic acid is the acid found in household vinegar, its strength ranging between 4% and 6%. Stoenesco[1455] reported that in the city of Bucharest, in the years 1891-1893, acetic acid caused more deaths than any other poison, eighteen out of eighty-five.

Symptoms: There is a burning taste in the mouth and esophagus, followed by pain in the stomach and radiating over the whole abdomen. Vomiting occurs, with labored noisy breathing, a short irritable cough, then collapse, and death within forty-eight hours. The symptoms sometimes simulate a ruptured gastric ulcer. The pain and distress may last for several weeks, depending upon the concentration of the acid taken. Glacial acetic acid produced blisters on the skin. Sklodowski cites eleven cases of acetic acid poisoning in which hemoglobinuria was a common feature. He considered this a help in a differential diagnosis from other poisons.[1456]

Treatment: The stomach should be washed out with water containing sodium bicarbonate, one teaspoonful to the pint. Treat as under corrosive poisons.

Postmortem appearances are similar to those of the corrosive acids. The mucous membrane of the mouth, throat, and stomach has a white scalded appearance, and there may be patches of corrosion and areas of acute inflammation.

Fatal Dose: Death has followed the swallowing of two tablespoonfuls[1457] by an adult, and a few drops have been fatal to children. Stumpf[1458] reported a fatal case of poisoning from a tablespoonful of the "essence of vinegar;" the patient, a man thirty-two years of age, suffered from severe diarrhea and a

1454. FRANZ: *Friedreich's Bl. f. gerichtl. Med.*, Nürnb., 60:401, 1909. Cf. BLEIBTREU: *München. med. Wchnschr.*, 55:1987, 1908.
1455. STOENESCO: *Ann. d'hyg.*, 4s., 1:525, 1904.
1456. SKLODOWSKI: *Presse méd.*, November, 1925.
1457. BLEIBTREU: *München. med. Wchnschr.*, 55:1987, 1908.
1458. STUMPF: *München. med. Wchnschr.*, 45:690, 1898.

weak heart. In Birkett's case,[1459] two to three ounces of a 33% acid immediately caused acute laryngitis in a drunken man of forty years, who was rescued by tracheotomy and artificial respiration. David[1460] reported the case of a woman who suffered severely from the effects of a quart of common vinegar swallowed with suicidal intent. In chronic poisoning from the drinking of acetic acid there follows a catarrhal condition of the stomach, a furred tongue, paleness of the skin, and anemia, loss of weight, emaciation, and a weakened pulse.

Isolation and Detection: Acetic acid is found in the acid distillate, after distillation with steam. An aliquot part of the distillate can be titrated with N/10 sodium hydroxide; 1 cc. of N/10 is equal to 0.006 gm. of acetic acid. If a portion of the acetic acid is neutralized with sodium hydroxide and evaporated to dryness, and the residue acidified with sulphuric acid, the odor of acetic acid develops. If to another portion, 1 cc. of alcohol is added, plus sulphuric acid, the pleasing odor of ethyl acetate is noted. A portion of the dried residue can be heated with arsenous acid in a dry hard glass tube, when the disagreeable odor of cacodyl develops.

FORMIC ACID (HCOOH)
(Molecular Weight 46.016)

FORMIC ACID is a colorless, irritating liquid, causing blisters when applied to the skin. It solidifies at 1°C. (33.8°F.), melts at 9°C. (48.2°F.), and boils at 99°C. (210.2°F.). It mixes with water and alcohol and has a reducing action, as it is readily oxidized to carbon dioxide, and therefore precipitates silver solutions. When taken internally it causes erosions similar to those caused by the mineral acids. The vapors are very irritating. According to Rubner and Hefter, solutions of 2% are distinctly harmful while 0.25% and 0.125% will cause distinct irritation. The salts of formic acids are poisonous in large doses, causing a drop in body temperature, acceleration of the pulse, and heart failure.

Isolation and Detection: Formic acid is found in the acid distillate. If death occurs early, or where life is prolonged, it is found in the urine as a formate. The urine is acidified with sulphuric acid and distilled with steam. For the determination

1459. BIRKETT: *Lancet*, 2:98, 1867.
1460. DAVID: *Brit. Am. J. Sc.,* September, 1847.

of formic acid Jones[1461] has worked out a method: The solution containing the formic acid is made alkaline with Na_2CO_3, warmed, and an excess of standard permanganate added. All the formic acid is oxidized, and a precipitate of manganese hydroxide thrown down. The solution is acidified with sulphuric acid, and a measured volume of oxalic acid added until all the precipitate has dissolved and the permanganate disappears. The excess of oxalic acid is then titrated with standard permanganate. A volume of oxalic acid equal to that taken is also titrated with the permanganate solution, and the difference between the result and the total permanganate required to oxidize the formic acid. The method is not reliable in the presence of much chloride.[1462]

Tests: 1. After neutralization with sodium carbonate both acetic and formic acid give, with iron chloride, a blue-red color. Upon warming the solution, the color becomes darker, and a reddish-brown precipitate is formed.

2. Bichloride of mercury, by heating with formic acid, is reduced to the insoluble mercurous chloride.

3. Silver nitrate is reduced by formic acid to metallic silver.

TARTARIC ACID ($C_4H_6O_6$)
(Molecular Weight 150.05)

TARTARIC ACID (acidum tartaricum) occurs as colorless translucent crystals, or a white, fine to granular crystalline powder. It is odorless, has an acid taste, and is stable in the air. One gm. of tartaric acid is soluble in 0.75 cc. of water, and in 3 cc. of alcohol at 25°C. It is tetravalent and bibasic, and forms large monoclinic prisms which melt at 170°C. (338°F.). Wholesale poisonings have occurred when it was used too strong as an ingredient in circus lemonade. A druggist was tried for manslaughter for having caused the death of a man, twenty-four, by giving him one ounce (31 gm.) of tartaric acid in mistake for aperient salts. The man died in nine days.[1463]

The symptoms are the same as for acetic acid.

Fatal cases of poisoning by citric acid have been reported by Kionka and Kornfeld.[1464]

1461. JONES, H. C.: *Am. Chem. J.*, 17:539, 1895.
1462. SUTTON: Volumetric Analysis, 11th ed., 115, 1924.
1463. GILL: *Lancet*, 1:18, 1845; *Ph. J. & Tr.*, 4:370, 1844 and 1845.
1464. KIONKA: *Aerztl. Sachverst.-Ztg.*, *Berl.*, 9:4, 1903. KORNFELD: Friedreich's Bl. f. gerichtl. Med. Nürnb., 53:359, 1902.

ETHER (C₄H₁₀O)
(Molecular Weight 74.08)

STATISTICS vary as to the number of deaths from ether when used as an anesthetic. From figures, one death in 2,500 to one in more than 50,000 anesthetizations have been reported.

Ether has been employed as a means of suicide, and death has resulted from its use as an intoxicant. Great precaution must be taken in the opening of cans or bottles of ether, as the vapor may catch fire from free flames or sparks many feet away. $C_2H_5 . O . C_2H_5$ is a transparent, colorless, mobile liquid, having a characteristic odor and a burning, sweetish taste. It is highly volatile and inflammable. Its vapor when mixed with air and ignited may explode violently. Ether is soluble in about twelve times its volume of water at 25°C. It is miscible with alcohol, benzene, chloroform, petroleum benzine, and with fixed and volatile oils. Its specific gravity is 0.713 to 0.716 at 25°C.; its boiling point is 35°C. The drinking of spirits of ether (Hofmann's anodyne), which is a mixture of one part of ether with three parts of alcohol, caused several deaths during the prohibition era.

Symptoms: The vapor is irritating to the larynx and gives rise to a feeling of suffocation, the respiration and heart are slowed reflexly and rendered irregular. The secretion of mucus and saliva is much increased. Sensation and consciousness are soon lost, and if too much ether is given death results, usually from failure of respiration. When ether is swallowed or taken internally there is an intense burning sensation in the throat and stomach, and a rapid, intense intoxication, similar to, but of a shorter duration than, that caused by alcohol. Individuals develop the habit of smelling and taking ether, similar to chloroform. The after-effects of the chronic indulgence of ether are trembling of hands, muscular weakness, cramps of the muscles, headache, etc.

The anesthetic stage is that which is aimed to be maintained. It is characterized by complete paralysis of the brain and of the motor reflex centers of the cord, and usually some depression of the medullary centers.

In the early stages, the pulse rate and blood pressure are increased by the reflexes, excitement, and incipient asphyxia.

During anesthesia, the effects are similar to those of alcohol, stimulant rather than depressant; the cutaneous and cerebral vessels are dilated, the pulse rate is increased 80 to 110, and the blood pressure is practically unchanged, or somewhat normal in man.[1465]

Fatal Dose: The fatal dose of ether when inhaled varies within wide limits. Cardiac patients die from small doses. It is necessary to maintain a concentration of about 6.7% by volume of ether vapor in the inspired air in order to maintain surgical anesthesia. A concentration of 9% has a distinctly depressing effects upon the medullary centers, and 11.2% causes respiratory paralysis in a few minutes in animals. The fatal dose when taken internally is not known; an individual recovered from seven drams (26 cc.). It is thought, however, that one fluid ounce (30 cc.) would be fatal to most adults.

Fatal Period: Death may occur at any stage, or before narcosis has been produced. Schram, van Leeuwen, and van der Made[1466] showed that with normal cats, concentrations of 0.13% to 0.14% of ether in the blood lowered the blood pressure considerably by action on the vasomotor and vagus centers, but the heart muscle is not affected by this concentration. Even with the fatal concentration, 0.17%, the heart is scarcely damaged, although the circulation is depressed before death. If artificial respiration is performed, cardiac arrest occurs with 0.25% of ether in the blood.

In the analysis of a case of death from ether,[1467] the brain contained 0.50, the liver 0.30, and the lung 0.34 cc. When the anesthetic had been stopped for eighty-five minutes, or when death occurred eighty-five minutes to twenty-five hours after anethesia, there was no ether found in the brain. This seems unusual, as ether can be detected on the breath of some patients after several hours.

Treatment: In cases of arrest of breathing during ether anesthesia artificial respiration should be promptly practised. Inhalations of oxygen and carbon dioxide should be given. Hypodermic injection of strychnine, ammonia, and camphor may be given as stimulants.

1465. SOLLMANN, T.:   Manual of Pharmacology, 3rd ed., 711, 1926.
1466. SCHRAM, P., VAN LEEUWEN, and VAN DER MADE: *Arch. f. d. ges. Physiol.*, 165, 123, 1916.
1467. GETTLER, A., and SIEGEL, H.:   *Arch. Path.*, 17:510, 1934.

Spirits of ammonia have been of material assistance in reviving some cases.

Postmortem Appearances: There is usually hyperemia of the mucous membranes, and if the autopsy be made soon after death, the organs have an odor of ether.

Detection: The pathologist, in submitting organs for the detection of volatile solvents, should have containers for the same that can be refrigerated before submitting to the chemist for examination. While toxicologist for the Cook County Coroner, I used large desiccators for the preservation of brain and other material, with a pyrex cover and ground-in pyrex stopcock. The ether that volatilized from the tissue was aspirated from the desiccator by being drawn out by means of a stopcock on the side of the desiccator. The material was then refrigerated again, finely comminuted, and distilled.

Gettler, Niderl and Benedetti-Pichler[1468] devised a specially constructed rectification flask, for the isolation of ether from tissue distillates. This rectification flask was modified by Gettler and Siegel so that the entire original distillate could be used for the isolation of ether. The bulb of the flask is of larger capacity (300 cc.). A glass tube running to the bottom of the flask is fused into the side of the flask for the introduction of the material from which the ether is to be isolated, and serves as a safety tube during the distillation, making it easier to empty and clean the flask. The uppermost S-shaped part is straightened out and points downward at an angle of 45° to the main tube of the flask. This was done so that all the ether could be collected in one portion rather than in a series of drops. In grinding up the tissue, the grinder should be cooled by applying ice. The material is weighed, mixed with 200 cc. of ice-cold water, and placed in a two-liter flask. An additional 300 cc. of water and 1 cc. of liquid petrolatum are added. The mixture is distilled with steam, a long, well cooled condenser, the tip of which has been bent to resemble an adapter, being used. The adapter should dip into 25 cc. of ice water contained in the receiving flask, which is covered with cracked ice. Two hundred cc. of the distillate are collected. The distillate is now poured through the safety tube into the rectification flask, described by Gettler.

1468. GETTLER, NIDERL, and BENEDETTI-PICHLER: *Mikrochemie,* 11:173, 1932; *J. Am. Chem. Soc.,* 54:1479, 1932.

AMYL NITRITE ($C_5H_{11}NO_2$)

AMYL NITRATE (amylis nitris, U.S.P., XI) has a molecular weight of 117.09. It contains not less than 80% $C_5H_{11}ONO$, and is a clear, yellowish liquid having a peculiar ethereal fruity odor and a pungent, aromatic taste. It is volatile even at low temperatures. The specific gravity is 0.865 to 0.875 at 25° C., and its boiling point is 97° to 99° C.

It is carried in thin glass capsules or "pearls," one of which is crushed in a handkerchief as needed and given for inhalations. It causes flushing of the face and the upper part of the body. Doses larger than 0.2 cc. may cause vomiting, unconsciousness, and collapse, with shallow respiration and possibly cyanosis. Disturbances of vision may follow. The symptoms following the internal administration are similar to those caused by inhalation of the drug. After doses of one teaspoon or more the symptoms are great weakness, cyanosis, a very feeble, thin, slow intermittent pulse, and gastric irritation. Recovery follows under appropriate treatment of emetics, strychnine, and digitalis. Cadwallader[1469] reported a fatal case of one-half ounce of amyl nitrite.

Isolation: Amyl nitrite will be found in the acid distillate which should be redistilled, using the Gettler micro-distillation apparatus as described under Ether (page 733).

Detection: The distillate may be tested for the presence of nitrite and amyl alcohol after heating with sodium hydroxide in a flask with a well-cooled reflux condenser. For the determination of amyl nitrite, take 3 mils of the purified substance which has been shaken with 0.5 gm. of potassium bicarbonate and carefully decanted into a tared 100-mil measuring flask containing about 20 mils of alcohol, and weigh accurately.[1470] Add sufficient alcohol to bring the volume to exactly 100 mils, and mix thoroughly. Introduce into a nitrometer exactly 10 mils of the alcoholic solution, followed by 10 mils of potassium iodide and 5 mils of dilute sulphuric acid. When the volume of gas has become constant, within thirty to sixty minutes, note the amount collected, multiply this volume in mils by 4.8, and divide the product by the original weight in grams of the amyl nitrite. At standard

1469. CADWALLADER: *Med. Rec.*, 50:816, 1896.
1470. FULLER, H. C.: Chemistry and Analysis of Drugs and Medicine, 1920, p. 734.

temperature and pressure the quotient represents the percentage of amyl nitrite in the liquid.

ETHYL BROMIDE

ETHYL BROMIDE is a heavy colorless, very volatile liquid with a chloroform-like odor. When inhaled it produces anesthesia or, rather, analgesia, with great rapidity. Consciousness returns within two or three minutes after the administration is discontinued.

Ethyl bromide has a boiling point of 38° to 40° C.

In a series of 60,000 cases there were sixteen deaths, i.e., one death in 3750. In another series there was one death in 5220 cases. Death may occur at any period of the administration, as within thirty seconds after the beginning, or hours and days afterwards,[1471] similar to the action of chloroform.

In order to isolate ethyl bromide from the tissues, the same precautions must be used as under Ether (page 733). Ethylene bromide decomposes quantitatively when heated with zinc and a little water, producing zinc bromide and ethylene gas:

$$C_2H_4Br_2 + Zn = ZnBr_2 + C_2H_4$$

This substance is more poisonous than ethyl bromide, and has been largely replaced by other anesthetics.

ETHYL CHLORIDE

ETHYL CHLORIDE (aethylis chloridum, U.S.P., XI) is extensively used as a local anesthetic. Glaister[1472] states that from twenty to thirty deaths have been reported from its use as a general anesthetic. It is usually dispensed in metal or glass containers with a small, constricted glass opening through which the ethyl chloride vapor is applied to the skin. It is a colorless, mobile, very volatile liquid with a characteristic ethereal odor and a burning taste. It is slightly soluble in water, freely soluble in alcohol and in ether. Its specific gravity at 0° C. (32° F.) is 0.921, and its boiling point is 12° to 13° C. It burns with a smoky green flame with the production of hydrochloric acid which may be detected in the usual manner. It causes a green tinge to a heated copper cone.

1471. Simon's Case, *Phila. M. J.*, 4:367, 1899; Sims: *Med. Rec.*, 17:361, 1880.

1472. Glaister: Medical Jurisprudence and Toxicology, 1915, p. 722.

ETHYLENE DICHLORIDE

ETHYLENE DICHLORIDE, $C_2H_4Cl_2$, has an extremely narrow boiling range of 82.5 to 84.0°C., and the lowest specific gravity of all commercial chlorinated solvents. It weighs only 10.4 pounds per gallon. It was first prepared more than a century and a half ago, and remained a costly reagent until 1927.

It is used for the extraction of gums, resins, and insecticides, the dewaxing of oils, and the degreasing of metals.

In combination with alcohol it is a solvent for nitrocellulose and for cellulose acetate.

Manifestations of intoxication by this substance are eye and nose irritation, vertigo, static and motor ataxia, retching movements, semiconsciousness, and unconsciousness accompanied by uncoordinated movements of the extremities. Death is likely if exposure is continued. (Experiments with guinea pigs with 6% vapors brought on symptoms within ten minutes —death within thirty minutes.)

Dimethyl acetonyl carbonyl is in principal use as a solvent for cellulose bodies. Action on animals is akin to that of acetone. It is more toxic than acetone; soporific in action. It lowers blood pressure.

Dimethyl-paraphenylendiamine is the most toxic of the phenylendiamines.

Ethylene chlorhydrin is taken into the body through skin absorption or through inhalation of vapors. It is narcotic in action. Death is due to respiratory failure.

Ethylene glycol (Prestone) is used as an anti-freeze. It is closely related to ethyl alcohol.

Sulphur monochloride is utilized in the rubber industry. Exposure produces symptoms similar to myelitis, jaundice, loss of weight, etc.

Toluylendiamine is a frequent constituent of hair and fur dyes. Has an action similar to phenylendiamine.

Trinitrotoluene causes skin affections, nephritis, cystitis, liver degeneration with jaundice, destruction of the blood cells, and methemoglobinemia.

During its manufacture poisoning may occur from the nitric acid fumes and toluene.*

* McCord, Carey P.: Industrial Hygiene for Engineers and Managers, 1st ed., 1931.

NITROGLYCERINE ($C_3H_5(NO_3)_3$)

NITROGLYCERINE (glyceryl trinitrate, or glonoin) is used in medicine as a remedy in angina pectoris. It is a pale, yellowish, odorless, oily liquid, nearly insoluble in the water, and soluble in absolute alcohol, ether and chloroform. When heated above 250°C. it explodes. It will also explode violently upon concussion. A 1% solution is used in medicine under the name of Spiritus glycerylis nitratis; also as tablets of glycerol trinitrate which contain 0.01 grain of nitroglycerine.

Many cases of nitroglycerine poisoning are caused in industry in men making dynamite and other high explosives. The men in industry suffer from the acute effects of this vasodepressant with headaches, flushed face, intense throbbing in the head, palpitation of the heart, and sometimes nausea and vomiting. Most workers acquire an immunity to the effects of nitroglycerine, but this immunity is only temporary, as it will be lost over a week-end or holiday. This does not serve to protect them from severe exposure. Laws[1473] states that headache following increased use of nitroglycerine may be preceded by complete loss of vision, and the patient may reach a maniacal state. Ebright described a case of a patient who became wild, irrational, and finally ran around shouting and hitting his head against trees, walls and other objects so that he had to be forcibly restrained. Laws found that all those working with nitroglycerine have large families and that sooner or later these men are troubled with a tachycardia on exertion. New men working in nitroglycerine are very susceptible.

The type of headache caused by nitroglycerine is throbbing, starting in the forehead and moving towards the occiput, where it remains for hours to several days. The patient often feels restless and tosses in bed. He may be nauseated and have diarrhea.

Alcohol increases the toxic symptoms by relaxing the blood vessels. Thus a man exposed to nitroglycerine the whole day may bring on a headache by simply drinking a cocktail.

Fatal Dose and Period: A few drops may prove fatal. One-fiftieth of a drop has produced most severe headache. Death may occur within two hours, or be delayed six hours or more.

Treatment: Elimination of the poison should be hastened

1473. LAWS: *J.A.M.A.*, 31:793, 1898.

by washing out the stomach and by administration of cathartics. Normal saline should be injected intravenously. The drinking of black coffee has been of service in relieving the headaches. Give injections of methylene blue.

Postmortem Appearances: The postmortem appearances are hyperemia of the brain and its membranes, and of the stomach and intestines.

Isolation: The same precautions as given under Ether (page 733) should be used in the isolation of the nitroglycerine. Werber's experiments[1474] on poisoned animals show that the poison is rapidly decomposed in the body, and is not likely to be found in the urine, blood, or liver. Werber's method consists of extracting the nitroglycerine from the organic material by treatment with chloroform or ether. Upon evaporation the organic solvent will remain as a viscous oil. Difficulty will be found in separating the fat which will accompany the ether or chloroform extract from organic material.

Tests: 1. The fraction of a drop heated in a capillary tube explodes.

2. For the presence of nitrites or nitrates, see tests under those subjects.

3. When a strong aqueous solution of yellow ammonium sulphide is added, glycerine and ammonium nitrite are formed:

$$C_3H_5(NO_3)_3 + 3(NH_4)_2S = C_3H_5(OH)_3 + 3NH_4NO_2 + 3S$$

4. The residue upon evaporation is extracted with alcohol, which upon evaporation leaves glycerine. This is identified by burning, which gives the penetrating odor of acrolein, and can be further identified by Schiff's reagent.

5. Another portion of the suspected substance is treated with yellow ammonium sulphide, an excess of lead carbonate, and a trace of lead acetate. After filtration the liquid is tested for a nitrite with metaphenylenediamin and sulphuric acid. Test for nitrites with Griess reagent (alpha naphthylamine and sulphanilic acid in acetic acid).

CARBON DISULPHIDE
(Carbon Bisulphide)

EXPOSURE to this chemical is found among ammonium salt makers, artificial silk makers, asphalt testers, carbon disulphide makers, celluloid makers, cementers (rubber shoes),

1474. *Ztschr. f. anal. Chem.*, 7:158, 1866.

cement mixers (rubber), dry cleaners, dryers (rubber), enamelers, glue workers, insecticide makers, match factory workers, oil extractors, paint makers, paraffin workers, putty makers, reclaimers (rubber), smokeless powder makers, sulphur extractors, tallow refiners, and vulcanizers.[1474-A] Pazen[1474-B] was the first to call attention to it as an occupational poison, although the poison was known in 1796. It boils at 46.5° C. It has a specific gravity of 1.262. It burns with a bluish flame, yielding carbon dioxide and sulphur dioxide. When passed through a red hot tube it yields carbon tetrachloride and sulphur monochloride. It dissolves in its own weight of sulphur at 38° C.

Poisoning by carbon disulphide occurs through breathing or getting the fluid on the skin. Oliver[1474-C] found that carbon disulphide was a very deadly poison to animals. Two types of poisoning are recognized, namely, the acute and the chronic. The symptoms of acute poisoning are characterized by circulatory disturbances, pallor, headaches, throbbing of temples, palpitation, fainting, and drowsiness. Digestive disturbances follow the above symptoms. There is nausea, vomiting, loss of appetite, occasionally diarrhea, sometimes colic and constipation. Carbon disulphide dissolves the lipoids of the blood and acts upon the central nervous system and the parenchymatous organs. There is weakness of the legs, incoordination, signs of great fatigue, unsteady gait, and a mania with homicidal and suicidal tendencies has been reported. Summerfield and Fischer[1474-D] reported that chronic symptoms may appear within a few weeks or months or after several years of work. Following the excitement stage, faintness, giddiness, drowsiness, exhaustion, and headache, there is a drunken gait, and exaggerated reflexes. A positive Romberg is usually found. Peripheral neuritis and digestive disturbances as seen in acute stage are present. Disturbances of taste, smell, and sight are common. In the stage of depression, there is pallor, and weakness. Organic nervous symptoms are common and consist of partial and complete paralyses, especially of the extensor group of muscles leading to wrist drop, steppage gait, and later contrac-

1474-A. McCord, Carey P.: Industrial Hygiene for Engineers and Managers, 112, 1931.

1474-B. Pazen: Chemie Industrielle, 1851.

1474-C. Sir Thomas Oliver, in Allbutt and Rolleston's System, 2:1, 102, 1909.

1474-D. Summerfield and Fischer: U. S. Labor Bull., 100, 1912.

tures. Skin pigmentation may be present. The patient cannot read because of disturbances of vision, disturbances of color fields, and retrobulbar neuritis. When removed from exposure, recovery may be slow, extending over a period as long as seventeen months. Substitution of other rubber solvents has made poisoning by this agent rare. Treatment consists of removal from exposure; artificial respiration may be necessary. Treat symptomatically. Wiley, Hueper and von Oettingen[1474-E] reported manifestations of the toxic effects of low concentrations of carbon disulphide in mice and rats which were exposed to CS_2-air mixtures of 1.09 mg. and 0.114 mg. per liter for eight hours a day over a period of twenty weeks. Several animals died during the experimental period. Operators should not be exposed to concentrations of carbon disulphide greater than 0.1 mg. per liter.

CYANIDES

SODIUM CYANIDE is used in industry in the case hardening of steel, and in the manufacture of cutlery, tools, springs, files, automobile and bicycle parts. Some machine shops temper their metal by dipping it in molten sodium cyanide. The material to be treated is suspended in the molten cyanide bath by means of wires, jigs, or baskets, and allowed to remain until the depth of the case required is obtained. It is then removed and immediately quenched in water, oil, or brine as the steel may require. This will produce a case of 10,000ths to 12,000ths of an inch. The cyanide bath may vary between 50% and 25% sodium cyanide. The average analysis of a typical cyanide bath would show sodium cyanide of 25% to 35%. The operating temperature for cyanide hardening will vary from 1400°F. (800°C.) to 1625°F. (885°C.), according to the composition of the steel being treated. The time of treatment varies from a few minutes to an hour. Small pieces are generally treated by placing a number in a strong mesh basket and immersing the whole for the desired length of time. The author had occasion to visit the R and H factory at Niagara Falls where cyanide eggs (cyanegg) were being made. The factory was a large, spacious building. The odor of cyanide was very apparent. The molten cyanide was poured out into molds forming the eggs. The men employed in this department worked there

1474-E. WILEY, F. H., HUEPER, W. C., and VON OETTINGEN, W. F.: *J. Indust. Hyg. & Tox.*, 18:733-40, 1936.

for many years and, according to the technical superintendent, never had any illness. The cyanide eggs contain 96% to 98% sodium cyanide and weigh approximately one ounce. This cyanide is also sold in granular form. The crystalline salt has a melting point of 556°C. (1040°F.).

Sodium cyanide is very deliquescent and is gradually decomposed by moisture and carbon dioxide if left in an open container. Fifty-eight and three-tenths grams are soluble in 100 cc. of water at 20°C. An aqueous, dilute solution of this substance, 0.25%, is used for the extraction of gold and silver from ores.

In some factories no hoods or other means of ventilation are provided over the cyanide baths, and in one shop I found 0.00048 gm. of hydrocyanic acid in 187 cubic feet of air. A test taken near the water-bath in which the metal was quenched gave 0.0006 gm. of hydrocyanic acid in twenty-four cubic feet of air. In one factory in which this test was made the men knew that the amount of gas given off was dangerous and they would run for an open door when quenching the metal.

In some electroplating works the cyanide baths are not protected by hoods, and cases of poisoning have occurred from inhalation of these fumes. F.G., an electroplater, testing out the strength of his cyanide solution, made an error and added acid instead of silver nitrate; a poisonous amount of cyanide was evolved. The man walked about eighteen or twenty feet away and dropped dead.

Burning celluloid gives off the fumes of hydrogen cyanide. I found the presence of cyanide in the blood of one of the victims of the Cleveland disaster. Kockel[1475] burned dinitrocellulose containing 40 to 50% camphor and found 0.05 gm. hydrocyanic acid. This is the amount of dinitrocellulose found in a small comb, and would be sufficient to poison a human being. The extraction of gold and silver from ores by the use of sodium cyanide causes the evolution of hydrocyanic acid gas.

Chronic poisoning is not seen in electroplating works, in tempering, or in the extraction of gold and silver by the use of the cyanides. However, Reed[1476] reported fourteen cases of chronic industrial poisoning from cyanogen chloride. The symptoms reported after exposure each day for eight months

1475. KOCKEL: *Vrtljschr. f. gerichtl. Med., Berl.*, 26:1, 1903.
1476. REED: *J. Indust. Hyg.*, 2:140, 1920.

were dizziness, nausea, profuse lacrimation, coughing, staggering, and prostration that lasted for several hours; there was also muscular weakness, congestion of the lungs, irritation of the skin, hoarseness, edema of the eyelids, conjunctivitis, and burning on urination. There were also periods when the pulse was irregular, but this bore no relation to the exposure. The weight of one man fell from 170 to 150 pounds. At the end of five weeks after changing occupations he had gained ten pounds.

Cyanide rash has been reported by factory inspectors, especially in Germany, consisting of itching, papules, and vesicles which may become infected. This rash has been attributed to the caustic action of quick lime more than to the cyanides. Braddock and Tingle[1477] reported that dermatitis in mill plants where the cyanide process of gold extraction is used is due to irritation by strong caustic and not to poisoning by cyanide, and that the immediate exciting agent is probably lime, whether as the oxide in the dust flying around the slaking barrel, or as a strong solution of the hydroxide in the mud of the mud press. Gasmaske[1478] reported two cases of chronic hydrogen cyanide poisoning due to long continued breathing of hydrogen cyanide. In one patient the dermatitis appeared on the hands. Both patients recovered when proper precautions were observed.

The report of the Cook County Coroner's Office for 1935 shows eight deaths due to cyanides, seven caused by potassium cyanide. This is an error, because potassium cyanide is rarely used. In my experience I found only two cases of potassium cyanide poisoning in about twenty years. Most of the deaths are due to sodium cyanide. Deputy Coroners are very prone to say "potassium cyanide," as the term is more familiar to them; this is especially true where chemical examination has not been made. In 1936 there were twelve deaths reported. Most of the cases of cyanide poisoning do not occur in industry; they are usually suicides.

Kobert[1479] reported two cases of chronic poisoning from the use of cyanides in gilding. Merzbach[1479] described a case of

1477. Braddock, W. H., and Tingle, G. R.: *J. Indust. Hyg.*, 12:259, 1930.
1478. *Gasmaske*: Chem. Abst., 28:2410, 1934.
1479. Kobert: Lehrbuch der Intoxikationen, Stuttgart, 836, 1902. And Merzbach, G.: *Hyg. Rundschau, Berl.*, 9:45, 1899.

chronic poisoning in a man forty-four years of age who had worked for thirteen years in an art printing establishment. His duty was to place copper plates in a solution of the double cyanide of silver and potassium, the galvanizing current splitting off the silver which was deposited on the copper, also releasing CN which in part joined the hydrogen given off by the same current from water. As the covers on these galvanizing tubs were imperfect the fumes of hydrogen cyanide escaped, and were inhaled by the workman. His illness began at about the end of the first year, and increased in severity until his death about six months after he was forced to stop work. It was characterized by severe gastro-intestinal disturbance, vomiting, abdominal cramps, obstinate constipation, and by general functional disturbance of the whole nervous system with involvement of the intellect.

Death occurred in a number of instances where the gas was used to kill vermin in ships, workshops, and dwellings. In 1924 the author reported[1480] six deaths following fumigation with hydrogen cyanide. The materials used in the fumigating process and their proportions were those recommended in a Farmer's Bulletin of the Department of Agriculture.[1481] The building to be fumigated was a restaurant, above which were two flats. The people in these flats were warned in a perfunctory manner by the fumigator that he was going to fumigate the restaurant below, and he suggested that they leave their windows open. The spaces around the water and steam pipes entering the ceiling were sealed with paper, but a shaft two feet by six inches leading to the flats above was not properly sealed. For each 100 cubic feet of space to be fumigated earthen ware jars or crocks having a capacity of about two gallons were used as generators. The water was added to the jars and the required amount of acid afterward to avoid spattering, which would occur in the reverse order. After the required number of jars were prepared, paper bags containing the cyanide were dropped into the dilute acid. The fumigator sealed the front door of the restaurant and placed a sign on the door warning the public not to enter. Six people living above the restaurant returned home and were overcome by the gas.

1480. McNally, W. D.: *Med. J. & Rec.*, February 6, 1924.
1481. U. S. Dept. of Agriculture, Farmers Bull., No. 699.

Because the shaft mentioned above was not properly sealed, the gas had entered the first and second apartments and caused the death of six people.

The U. S. Public Health Service has shown that an experienced man may be allowed to enter a room that has been fumigated if the air contains not more than 0.1 part in 1,000 of hydrogen cyanide; 0.5 parts per 1,000 can be breathed by a man for one minute without injury; 0.375 parts per 1,000 can be breathed for one and one-half minutes, and 0.25 parts per 1,000 for two minutes. Lehmann and Flury have established 0.1 mg. per liter of air as the utmost limit that should be permitted for continual exposure.

Hydrogen cyanide can be absorbed through the skin.[1482] Fairley, Linton, and Wild[1482] report that an atmosphere saturated with hydrocyanic acid is readily absorbed by a skin surface amounting to one-sixtieth of the body area of the guinea pig and will produce death if exposure is prolonged. Hydrocyanic acid passed through the skin of the rabbit, which, with its respiratory system protected or excluded, can tolerate a concentration which averages one in 210 for ninety minutes. Williams says that this absorption through the skin accounts for cases of poisoning where gas masks have been used, as the gas will penetrate clothing. It also accounts for cases of poisoning in persons who had put on clothing which had been recently fumigated. Miss C. S. entered her room the morning following fumigation and put on clothing which had been there during the process. She was immediately taken sick, became unconscious, and was removed to a hospital. An examination of the blood failed to show the presence of a cyanide. I gave her fifteen grains of sodium thiosulphate intravenously. She immediately come out of her semi-comatose condition. Part of the cyanide she had inhaled could have come from the clothing. The residual cyanide left in the plaster for days after fumigation releases small amounts of hydrogen cyanide. Cevidalli[1483] has attempted to show that wool absorbs hydrogen cyanide, and that this material gives off the poison gradually. Messerli reported a case of a man found dead in an apartment

1482. SCHUTZE: *Arch. f. Hyg.*, 98:70, 1927; DRINKER, P.: *J. Indust. Hyg.*, 14:1, 1932; WALTON, D. C., and WITHERSPOON, M.: *J. Pharmacol. & Exper. Therap.*, 26:315, 1925-26. FAIRLEY, A., LINTON, E. C., and WILD, F. E.: *J. Hyg.*, 34:283, 1934.
1483. CEVIDALLI: *Atti di Soc. med. chir., Padova, 1923.*

which had been disinfected for bedbugs the day before with hydrogen cyanide gas.[1484]

Lubenau[1485] has shown that it took eighteen days to rid a room completely of the gas after fumigation with hydrogen cyanide. It was found that at a low temperature and a high humidity the gas has a tendency to settle on the surface of common objects. Eighteen days afterward traces of hydrogen cyanide could still be found in the air, so it was necessary to institute thorough ventilation. After forty-one days the room was completely free of the gas, but adjacent rooms had also been fumigated and there was a considerable quantity of gas still present which had penetrated through the office material.

In addition to the uses already mentioned, cyanide is employed for the extermination of all animal and insect life in citrus groves, grain houses, shops, ships and dwellings; it is also used in photographing, silver plating, the gilding of metals, the cleaning of gold and silver, and in the manufacture of certain dyes. And it may be produced by bacteria in the body under the influence of bacillus pyocyaneus. Gettler and St. George[1486] report that in the city of New York 410 cases of death from cyanide occurred from January 1, 1918, to December 31, 1933; 329 of these were suicides, four were homicides, twenty-five accidental ingestion, and fifty-two from fumigation.

Of all the poisoning cases of recent years there has been no case that had attracted more attention than the Orpet-Lambert case. Motive paralleled motive; action paralleled action and opportunity paralleled opportunity. The case had many points in favor of suicide and many points in favor of murder. Each had access to the cyanide, but the evidence indicated that Orpet had access only to sodium cyanide. Samples of cyanide taken from the Orpet greenhouse showed it to be sodium cyanide. Several months after the finding of the body of the Lambert girl in the woods, a coat was submitted to me for examination. It was found to contain three spots about one-half inch in diameter and one-quarter of an inch apart in a straight line—the fact that they were in an abso-

1484. MESSERLI: *Schweiz. med. Wchnschr.*, 62:880, 1932.
1485. LUBENAU: *Ztschr. f. Med.*, 45:249, 1932.
1486. GETTLER, A. O., and ST. GEORGE, A. V.: *Am. J. Clin. Path.*, 4:447, 1934.

lutely straight line was important. In the examination of hundreds of blood stains and other spots found on clothing, I had never observed a parallel case in which spots were found in a straight line. The stains had a pronounced odor of cyanide, yet my test showed that sodium or potassium cyanides exposed to air for so long a period would not retain their odor. It was obviously a clever "plant" by someone desiring to strengthen the murder theory, and I testified to that effect. The chemist for the prosecution, the late Dr. Ralph Webster, stated that the spots were made by potassium cyanide. The experts for the State testified they were made by sodium cyanide. After the acquittal of Orpet the stains were examined by the late Professor Walter S. Haines and Mr. Carl Miner who found they were made by sodium cyanide, an entirely different substance from that found in the stomach. (See page 44.)

HYDROCYANIC ACID

HYDROCYANIC ACID (hydrogen cyanide or prussic acid, HCN) is a colorless, transparent liquid of a penetrating characteristic odor resembling that of peach kernels. Its specific gravity is 0.758 at 7°C. It boils at 26.5°C. (80°F.), and solidifies at —15°C. (5°F.); it is more or less easily decomposed by exposure to light. Even at temperatures below the boiling point it volatilizes so rapidly that if a drop falls on a glass plate a portion of it freezes. The pure acid is very unstable and is rarely seen, even in the chemical laboratory. A 2% solution was formerly a U. S. P. preparation. This preparation was colorless, with a characteristic odor and taste, and was not stable. It was found in preparations of wild cherry bark (prunus virginiana) and in the oleum amygdalae amarae, being derived from amygdalin. Hydrocyanic acid is also found as amygdalin in the kernels of various fruits. The peach stone contains 0.17%, the plum 0.56%, cherry 0.3%, apple 0.035%; the oil of bitter almonds contains 2% to 14%, and the substance is also found in tobacco smoke. Compounds containing the CN radical are toxic only as they liberate HCN. Ferro-, ferri- and subphocyanide are stable and, therefore, do not show these effects.

Potassium cyanide (KCN) is a white, deliquescent salt, odorless when perfectly dry, but emitting the odor of hydrocyanic acid when moist. It is soluble in two parts of water. The solution has an alkaline reaction, and decomposes slowly in the cold and rapidly upon heating. The sodium salt, being so much cheaper than the potassium salt, is used much more extensively. The sodium salt is used extensively in photographing, and silver plating, and in the cleaning of gold and silver and the manufacture of certain dyes. As previously mentioned, hydrocyanic acid vapors are emitted in some of these processes, and may give rise to poisoning. One part of hydrocyanic acid is contained in 2.5 parts of potassium cyanide; when the salt is taken into the stomach, hydrocyanic acid is slowly set free by the action of the acid of the gastric juice, so that the effects of potassium cyanide are practically the same as those of an equivalent amount of hydrocyanic acid. The salt, however, causes some corrosion at the point of application.

Physiological Action: Solutions of hydrocyanic acid, when applied to the skin, are absorbed, causing numbness and a partial loss of sensation. Upon the central nervous system this substance acts as a stimulant, causing excitement and then convulsions. The stage of stimulation is very brief, and is followed by paralysis of all parts of the central nervous system. Respiration is first stimulated, and then paralyzed. Circulation is similarly affected. The cyanogen ion is toxic to all forms of life except to certain fungi. Geppert showed that its effect upon protoplasm was due largely to its retarding process of oxidation; as a consequence, the tissue was no longer capable of absorbing oxygen, and in the higher animals the blood, not giving up its oxygen to the tissues, retains its bright arterial color in the veins.[1487]

When hydrocyanic acid is added to drawn blood, the latter loses its property or power to decompose hydrogen peroxide; the blood also retains its red color much longer than does normal blood. The color of hydrocyanic acid blood has been confused with the color of carbon monoxide blood. The chemical examination readily differentiates these two conditions. In cases of fatal poisoning, the dependent parts of the body are often of a bright red color similar to that of carbon monoxide poisoning.

Hydrocyanic acid is rapidly changed in the body to form sulphocyanides, and is eliminated in this form.[1488] Both the acid

1487. GEPPERT: *Ztschr. f. klin. Med.*, 15:208 and 307, 1888.

1488. McKELWAY, J. I.: *Am. J. M. Sc.*, 129:684, 1905; see also SCHWENKENBECKER: *Arch. f. Anat. u. Physiol., ph. Abt.*, 134, 1904.

and the alkaline salts in solution are rapidly absorbed from all surfaces, even from the uninjured skin.

Symptoms: After swallowing, hydrocyanic acid has been described as having an acid, harsh taste and causing a constriction in the throat. Other symptoms may not begin for several seconds, or even minutes and the patient may perform a number of conscious acts, such as walking across the room, rinsing the glass from which the poison was taken, or concealing the bottle or throwing it out of the window. For instance, a man in a downtown hotel in Chicago took a drink of sodium cyanide, walked to a window, and threw the bottle out the window. In another instance, a chemist soldered a .38 caliber revolver to a tin funnel, placed it over his heart, and, after drinking a quantity of sodium cyanide, shot himself. The amount of cyanide found in his stomach was sufficient to have killed him without his resorting to the firearm. I have seen several instances of this same method in suicide, the person fearing that the cyanide may not work. However, as a rule when a fatal dose has been taken, no voluntary acts of any importance are performed. In the case of Miss L. Z., a boy friend gave her a capsule containing sodium cyanide just as she was leaving the breakfast table. She walked one block to a street car and dropped dead. The boy friend was tried for murder, convicted, and sentenced.

Most of the cases of cyanide poisoning are found dead. It is seldom that one witnesses a death by this agency. Where life has been prolonged the description has been given of a constriction in the throat followed by salivation, nausea, and occasionally vomiting; these are followed by anxiety, confusion, vertigo, and headache. There is palpitation of the heart, a feeling of constriction in the chest, and the respirations become first rapid, then slow and irregular. The inspirations are very short, the expirations greatly prolonged. The patient becomes unconscious, and falls suddenly to the ground in convulsions not unlike those of epilepsy. The skin is covered with a cold sweat; the pupils are dilated and insensible to light. The eyes are glassy, staring, and very prominent, as in other cases of asphyxia. The mouth is covered with foam, which is sometimes blood-stained. The breath smells strongly of hydrocyanic acid. The convulsions may be general and lead to opisthotonos, or they may be confined to certain groups of muscles. The hands are usually clenched. Involuntary evacuations of the feces and urine may occur. The convulsive stage is followed by depression and paralysis. The patient remains unconscious and then becomes comatose. There is a complete abolition of the reflexes. In less severe cases, in which the patient recovers, the early symptoms are those described; the patient falls to the ground insensible, convulsions follow, succeeded by the stage of paralysis in which the respiration becomes slow and shallow. After a little while the respiration begins to improve and the patient awakens. Vomiting frequently occurs. The feeling of constriction in the chest and weakness, causing an unsteady gait, headache, difficulty in speech and drowsiness may continue for a few days. In the majority of the less severe cases recovery occurs within forty-eight hours. The mortality in cases of cyanide poisoning is over eighty per cent.

Hydrogen cyanide poisoning may result from inhalation of vapors of hydrocyanic acid, as illustrated in the six cases of death following fumigation. Hydrocyanic acid is fatal to animals in thirty minutes to an hour when present to the extent of 0.3 to 0.12 mg. per liter of air. Twenty to forty parts of hydrocyanic acid per one million parts of air cause slight symptoms after several hours' exposure. The maximum amount which can be inhaled for one hour without disturbance is fifty to sixty parts per million of air.[1489]

Diagnosis: The diagnosis of acute cyanide poisoning is easy. The characteristic peach kernel odor upon the breath is often sufficient. However, material should be submitted to the toxicologist for examination.

Fatal Dose: One-half dram of a 2% solution of cyanide is known to have caused death.[1490] A healthy woman, aged twenty-two, died in fifteen to twenty minutes after taking 0.9 grain (0.058 gm.) contained in a lotion. In another case a man took a similar dose and was insensible for four hours. One grain (0.064 gm.) of hydrocyanic acid would most certainly prove fatal. In like manner, 2.4 grains (0.15 gm.) of potassium cyanide would be a fatal dose. As with other poisons, recovery has taken place from larger doses. Recovery has been reported from the taking of what was estimated to be twenty, forty, and even fifty to sixty grains of potassium cyanide.

Fatal Period: Inasmuch as most cases of cyanide poisoning

1489. KOBERT: Kompend. der prak. Toxicol., Stuttgart, 1912.
1490. GARSTANG: *Lancet,* 2:15, 1888.

are found dead, the exact time of death is unknown. The fatal period depends upon circumstances attending the administration of the cyanide. Miss Z. took cyanide in capsules and walked a block before dying. In other instances I have histories where death occurred immediately upon taking the sodium cyanide in solution. A person may perform a number of acts after taking a fatal quantity of the poison. A white man, L. K., drank one-half glass of prussic acid which he had made by acidifying a solution of potassium cyanide. After drinking the solution he put the glass on the dresser and lay down on the bed, dying within a few minutes. In another case a woman, drank, with suicidal intent, two ounces of shoe cleaner containing sodium cyanide and died within five minutes. Some cases have been reported where life was prolonged nearly half an hour. After ingestion of three drams (11.1 cc.) of hydrocyanic acid, death occurred in twenty minutes. After one-half dram (1.87 cc.) death occurred in twenty minutes. In one instance a suicide lived for three and one-half hours after swallowing an unknown quantity of hydrocyanic acid.[1491] In the majority of cases recovery is the rule if the patient lives for an hour. This applies to sodium and potassium cyanide as well as to hydrocyanic acid.

Howard reported a case of a jeweler, aged forty-two, who was found in collapse by an assistant who had been absent only about ten minutes.[1492] The man was removed to a hospital, and died thirty minutes after admission. The stomach and content contained 11.8 grains of cyanide, the liver one-third grain, the kidneys one-tenth grain, and there were distinct traces in the blood from the thoracic cavity, and in the brain. A man died one hour and twenty minutes after ingesting an unknown quantity of hydrocyanic acid.[1493]

Treatment: In most instances of cyanide poisoning death occurs before the physician arrives. By telephone the physician can advise the administration of hydrogen peroxide or potassium permanganate in water, the water in the latter case to have a color corresponding to that of Burgundy red. These are given to the patient with the purpose of converting the hydrocyanic acid into the harmless oxamid. Vomiting should be induced by irritation of the pharynx or by household

1491. Brit. M. J., 1:131, 1883.
1492. HOWARD, C. D.: Boston M. & S. J., 196:58, 1927.
1493. Brit. M. J., 56, 1925.

emetics. Methylene blue[1494] has been demonstrated by Sah- lin,[1495] Eddy,[1495] Brooks,[1495] Hug,[1496] Hanzlik[1496] and others to antagonize the action of cyanide in animals. Hug[1497] has demonstrated that sodium nitrite is by far the better antidote than methylene blue for dogs. Wendel,[1497] also found that the principal action of methylene blue in counteracting the toxic effects of cyanide appears to depend on methemoglobin formation.[1497]

Chen, Rose, and Clowes[1498] have found that inhalation of amyl nitrite is much more efficient than methylene blue. They found that no animal was protected by methylene blue against three minimal lethal doses of cyanide. By the inhalation of amyl nitrite, dogs can tolerate four minimal lethal doses of sodium cyanide. One or two of their animals received four and a half minimal lethal doses and recovered completely. Even animals which are given larger doses survive longer when treated with amyl nitrite. This drug, in addition to being twice as effective as methylene blue, has the advantage of being readily administered by the respiratory route. The frequency of amyl nitrite inhalation should be reduced to once every thirty minutes, and finally every two to five hours as the pulse and respiratory rates approach normal.

In addition to the first-aid advice given by telephone, the stomach should be washed out by the physician while an attendant is giving inhalations of amyl nitrite. Artificial respiration should also be administered.

Trautman,[1499] from experiments made on rabbits, white rats and guinea pigs, found that injections of 1% methylene blue solution were of no value in the treatment of hydrocyanic acid gas poisoning if the animals had absorbed, by breathing,

1494. Methylthionine chloride, U.S.P., XI.

1495. SAHLIN, B.: *Skandinav. Arch. f. Physiol.*, 47:284, 1926. EDDY, N. B.: *J. Pharmacol. & Exper. Therap.*, 41:449, 1931. BROOKS, M. M.: *Proc. Soc. Exper. Biol. & Med.*, 29:1228, 1932; *Am. J. Physiol.*, 102:145, 1932; *J.A.M.A.*, 100:59, 1933.

1496. HUG, E.: *Compt. rend. Soc. de biol.*, 3:519, 1932. HANZLIK, P. J.: *J.A.M.A.*, 100:357, 1933.

1497. HUG, E.: *Compt. rend. Acad. d. sc., Par.*, 115:458, 1934. WENDEL, W. B.: *J. Pharmacol. & Exper. Therap.*, 54:283, 1935. HUG, E.: *Compt. rend. Soc. de biol.*, 112:511, 1933; WENDEL, W. D.: *J.A.M.A.*, 100:1054, 1933; *J. Biol. Chem.*, 100, 1933.

1498. CHEN, K., ROSE, C., and CLOWES, G.: *J.A.M.A.*, 100:1920, 1933.

1499. TRAUTMAN, J. A.: U. S. Public Health Reports, 48:1443, 1933.

lethal or near lethal doses of gas in a short period of time. My experience with humans indicates that amyl nitrite should be given in preference to methylene blue.

Draize[1500] advised intravenous injections of 2 or 3 cc. of 2% sodium tetrathionate per kilogram of body weight. This was effective in saving rabbits which had received orally three times the minimal lethal dose of hydrocyanic acid. He states: "Methylene blue administered intravenously in the form of a 1% aqueous solution does not afford as much protection. The intravenous injection of quantities in excess of 2 cc. of a 1% solution of methylene blue was injurious to the rabbit."

Christoni and Foresti[1501] found that sodium tetrathionate is very effective in converting the sodium cyanide into sulphocyanate ion. According to the reaction:

$$Na_2S_4O_6 + NaCN + 2NaOH = Na_2SO_4 + Na_2S_2O_3 + H_2O$$

The use of colloidal sulphur has been tried by a number of investigators.[1502] Pentathionate and hexathionate have also been suggested.

Lethal Dose: Hug has found that the lethal dose in dogs, if given intravenously at a velocity of 0.2 mg. per kilogram per minute, is 0.8 mg. per kilogram weight of animal.[1497] A very slow intravenous injection of 0.5 mg. of hydrocyanic acid per kilogram per hour is tolerated by the dog for ten hours. On the basis of his experiments Hug concludes that the fundamental factor which conditions the toxicity of hydrocyanic acid and the cyanides is the velocity of absorption.

The lethal dose for guinea pigs is 0.9 mg. per kilogram of animal, the poison being given subcutaneously.

Postmortem Appearances: Upon opening the body, the odor of hydrocyanic acid usually is detected. If it is not detected in the thoracic cavity the odor may be noticed when the skull cap is removed. The blood is generally of a red color, is uncoagulated, and engorges the veins and the right heart. A similar odor is noticed after nitrobenzene. The latter, however, persists for a long time if exposed to the air. The body usually

1500. DRAIZE, J. H.: *J.A.M.A.*, 101:1759, 1933.

1501. CHRISTONI, A., and FORESTI, B.: *Arch. internat. de pharmacodyn. et de thérap.*, 42:140, 1930.

1502. MILANESE: *Arch. internat. de pharmacodyn. et de thérap.*, 32:156, 1926; RAFFO: *Kolloid-Ztschr., Dresd. & Leipz.*, 2:358, 1908; FORST: *Arch. f. exper. Path. u. Pharmakol.*, 128:1, 1928.

has the appearance of a person in natural sleep. The dependent parts often show bright red or violet patches. The lungs, liver, kidneys, and spleen are usually highly congested. The stomach is usually edematous. The mucous membranes may be swollen and show punctate hemorrhages. Death occurs so rapidly in many of the cases that there is little time for changes to occur. Where life has been prolonged for several minutes to an hour the liver may show fatty degeneration, and extravasations of blood are found in the pia, brain substance, and cord. In some cases the mucous membranes of the esophagus and stomach are swollen and stained red or brownish-red by cyanhematin. Sometimes there will be found acute passive congestion of the liver, spleen, and kidneys; there is hyperemia and edema of the brain, and edema of the lungs.

In the case of W. H., 290 gm. of stomach and contents yielded 0.0337. gm. (0.52 grain) of hydrocyanic acid, equivalent to 0.95 grain sodium cyanide or 1.25 grains potassium cyanide; 725 gm. liver yielded 0.0157 gm. (0.24 grain) of hydrocyanic acid, equivalent to 0.44 grain sodium cyanide or 0.58 grains potassium cyanide; 160 gm. kidney yielded 0.0035 gm. (0.05 grain) of hydrocyanic acid, equivalent to 0.09 grain sodium cyanide, or 0.12 grain potassium cyanide. This man went to mail a letter and dropped dead on the way from the mail box.

B. G., on February 12, 1919, died a few minutes after taking unknown quantities of sodium cyanide; 220 gm. of stomach and content contained 0.0067 gm. of hydrocyanic acid, calculated to 0.0122 gm. sodium cyanide; 388 gm. of bowel gave 0.0067 gm. hydrocyanic acid, calculated to 0.0117 gm. of sodium cyanide; 913 gm. of liver gave 0.0460 gm. hydrocyanic acid, calculated as sodium cyanide; 142 gm. kidneys gave 0.0091 gm. hydrocyanic acid, calculated to 0.0165 gm. sodium cyanide.

Tests: The finely comminuted tissue is introduced into a distilling flask, acidified with sulphuric acid, and subjected to steam distillation. A portion of the distillate is reserved for quantitative examination The other portion is divided into separate parts and submitted to the following tests:

1. Smell cautiously of the distillate. The odor of the free acid may be noted.

2. Five cc. of the distillate are made alkaline. A few drops of yellow ammonium sulphide are added, and the mixture is evaporated to dryness. The residue is taken up with a small

quantity of HCL. The sulphur is filtered off, and to the filtrate add a drop of ferric chloride. The red ferric sulphocyanide is formed, and serves for detection of hydrocyanic acid in a dilution of one to 4,000,000.[1503]

3. To 10 or 25 cc. of the distillate made alkaline with a few drops of sodium hydroxide solution, 0.5 cc. of ferrous sulphate and 0.5 cc. of ferric chloride solutions are added. The solution is warmed and acidified with hydrochloric acid. A Prussian-blue is immediately precipitated. In some instances where the amount of cyanide is very small it is best to run this test in a porcelain casserole and allow to stand for several hours, when a fine precipitate of Prussian-blue may be noticed when it would have failed of detection otherwise. This reaction will show the presence of hydrocyanic acid one part in 50,000.

4. The Schonbein test:[1504] This test may be applied to the material before distillation. The material under examination is placed in a small flask and acidified with tartaric acid. The mouth of the flask is closed by a tightly fitting cork whose lower surface is provided with a slit into which is inserted a piece of filter paper that has been moistened in turn with a 5% tincture of guaiacum and 0.1% copper sulphate solution. In the presence of hydrocyanic acid the filter paper assumes a deep blue color. This test may be applied by the introduction of filter paper at the end of the adaptor while the distillation is being conducted. Möckel says this test is delicate to one part in 3,000,000. The blue color, however, is produced by many other substances, as chlorine, bromine, nitric fumes, ozone, and ammonia.

5. A purple precipitate will be formed when 1 cc. of the following reagent is added to a solution containing cyanide: 10 mg. ferrous ammonium sulphate and 10 cg. ammonium acetate dissolved in 50 cc. of water.

6. When a solution of the alkaline-reduced phenolphthalein and a little copper sulphate solution are added to the distillate a red color develops if cyanide is present.[1505] Oxidizing agents, as ferric chloride, nitrous oxide, hydrogen peroxide, will not react in this manner. This is sensitive one to 500,000.

7. Solutions of silver nitrate precipitate, from solutions of cyanides or hydrocyanic acid, silver cyanide. This is a white

1503. LINK and MOCKEL: Ztschr. f. anal. Chem., Wiesb., 17:455.
1504. Neues Repert. der Pharm. Bd., 18:356, 1868.
1505. WEEHUIZEN, F.: Chem. Centralbl., 1191, 1905.

anhydrous precipitate, soluble either in ammonia or in a solution of potassium cyanide.

8. Upon the addition of a few drops of sodium picrate to the cyanide solution, a red color develops. In a 1% solution the color develops rapidly. In more dilute solutions the reaction requires a longer time. If a strip of paper be moistened in sodium picrate solution and allowed to be suspended in a jar in which there are organs containing cyanide, after several hours a red color will develop.

9. Kobert's examination of the blood using the spectroscope: Two small bottles are filled with normal and suspected blood diluted one to 100. Both of these exhibit the absorption bands of oxyhemoglobin. The two bottles are corked and placed in a warm dark place for twenty-four hours. During this period the normal blood has become darker in color, and will show absorption bands of reduced hemoglobin. If the suspected blood also darkens and gives absorption bands of reduced hemoglobin, no cyanide was originally present, but if the suspected blood remains bright red and still gives the absorption bands of oxyhemoglobin, then cyanide was originally present.

10. If a piece of starch paper, which has been made slightly blue with a trace of iodine, is placed in the suspected solution, it will be decolorized at once if even a trace of cyanide is present. Delicate to one part in 1,000,000. Although this test is extremely delicate, the reaction is obtained by hydrogen sulphide, sulphur dioxide, uric acid, albumin, and alkalis.

11. To 5 cc. of distillate add a few drops of potassium nitrate solution, then two to four drops of ferric chloride and a few drops of sulphuric acid to get a bright yellow color. Heat to boiling. Add sufficient sodium hydroxide solution to remove the excess of iron and filter. To the filtrate add two drops of dilute ammonium sulphide solution. If the solution contained hydrocyanic acid, a violet color will appear and pass through blue, green, and yellow. This test is delicate to one part in 312,-000.[1506]

If the body has been previously embalmed, difficulty will be encountered in obtaining the above test because formaldehyde with cyanide forms an oxynitrile. If the autopsy is not made shortly after death, the presence of hydrocyanic acid may

1506. VORTMANN: *Monatschr. f. Chem.*, 7:416, 1886.

disappear. Traces of this substance are produced during the first few days of putrefaction.

12. When material contains non-poisonous potassium ferrocyanide, hydrocyanic acid will appear in the distillate from a solution acidified with tartaric acid. When an aqueous solution of mercuric cyanide is distilled with tartaric acid, the distillate will contain hydrocyanic acid only when a large quantity of mercuric cyanide is present. If the Reinsch test shows the presence of mercury, a soluble sulphide or hydrogen sulphide should be added to the suspected material, and the distillation resumed. Mercuric cyanide will be completely decomposed and the distillate will contain hydrocyanic acid.

13. Hydrocyanic acid may be detected by benzidine acetate. On a small filter paper disc which has been moistened with a drop of reagent, one drop of the unknown is mixed with a drop of dilute sulphuric acid. The test is best carried out on a porcelain dial with a watch glass placed over the filter paper to prevent evaporation. In the presence of hydrocyanic acid there will be formed an intense blue ring. The limit of detection is 0.25 gamma of cyanide, and the limit of dilution will be one to 200,000.[1507]

14. The brown spot on a filter paper or dial, due to freshly prepared cupric sulphide, will promptly disappear if one drop of cyanide solution is added. This is due to the formation of complex potassium cuprocyanide. The test is sensitive to 2.5 gamma of hydrocyanic acid, and the limit of dilution is one in 20,000.

15. Hydrocyanic acid can be detected by converting it into alloxan, and then, by ammonia, into oxaluramid and dialluric acid.

Estimation: When a solution of silver nitrate is added to an alkaline solution containing cyanogen, no permanent precipitate of silver cyanide appears until all the cyanogen has combined with the alkali and the silver to form a double salt (for example, KCy.AgCy). If the slightest excess of silver, over and above the quantity required to form this combination, is added, a permanent precipitate of silver cyanide is produced, the double compound being destroyed. If, therefore, the silver solution be of known strength, the quantity of cyanogen present

1507. MOIR, J.: *Chem. News*, 102:17, 1910; *Chem. Zentralbl.*, 2:688, 1910; PERTUSSI, C., and GASTALDI, E.: *Chem. Ztg.*, 37:609, 1913; SIEVERT, A., and HERMSDORFF, A.: *Ztschr. f. ang. Chemie, Berl.*, 34:3, 1921.

is easily found; one part of silver in this case being equal to two parts cyanogen.

1. To 50 cc. of distillate add 5 cc. of strong ammonia and 2 cc. of a 5% solution of potassium iodide. Add slowly from a buret N/10 silver nitrate with continual stirring. At the appearance of a permanent cloud in the liquid the addition of silver nitrate is discontinued. The titration is best conducted over a black background. One cc. of N/10 normal silver nitrate corresponds to 0.005396 gm. of hydrocyanic acid:

$$AgNO_3 + KCN = AgCN + KNO_3$$

2. The cyanide may be estimated in the distillate in which the material has been distilled over borax to remove traces of chlorine, and the distillate is treated with an excess of a dilute solution of silver nitrate containing a trace of nitric acid. The precipitated silver cyanide is collected on a weighed filter, thoroughly washed, dried at 100°C. (212°F.), and weighed.

BITTER ALMONDS

A LARGE number of plants contain, in small amounts, amygdalin and other glucosides yielding hydrogen cyanide.[1508]

The defense in certain cases will raise the point that the small amount of cyanide found by the chemist was derived from a certain specific food that contained amygdalin which, on hydrolyzing, gives hydrocyanic acid. In the case of H. A. the defense attorney raised the point that the wife of H. A. had eaten peanuts and bitter almonds shortly before death. A chemical examination, however, demonstrated the presence of sodium cyanide and free hydrocyanic acid; there were no remnants of peanuts or bitter almonds in the stomach or the stomach content. The police also found that H. A. had purchased sodium cyanide from a jeweler for the purpose of killing a dog. But, instead of killing a dog he used it on his wife.

Lange found amygdalin in some of the common seeds in amounts as follows: Peach 2% to 3% (0.11% to 0.16% hydrocyanic acid); plum and apricot 1% (0.05% hydrocyanic acid); apple 0.6% (0.03% hydrocyanic acid); cherry 0.8% (0.04% hydrocyanic acid).[1509]

The hydrolysis of amygdalin introduced into the body by

1508. CZAPEK: Biochemie der Pflangzen; DUNSTAN, H., and AULD: Proc. Roy Soc., London, 79B:315, 1907; ARMSTRONG: Proc. Roy. Soc., London, 79B:360, 1907; COMPTONS Chem. News, 106:163, 1912.

1509. LANGE: Kais ges. Amt., 25:478, 1907.

itself is usually harmless, although mild symptoms have been reported from it. However, it is frequently accompanied in nature by emulsion or other ferments which decompose it with the production of hydrocyanic acid.

$$C_{20}H_{27}NO_{11} + 2H_2O = 2C_6H_{12}O_6 + C_6H_5CHO + HCN$$

Amygdalin + Water = Dextrose + Benzaldehyde + Hydrocyanic acid

Jacobi reported the case of a woman who died after eating an unknown amount of bitter almonds.[1510] It was estimated, from the amount left in the box which the woman had purchased that morning, that about 100 gm. (175 pieces), corresponding roughly to about 3 gm. of amygdalin, or 0.18 gm. of hydrocyanic acid, had been taken.

Fifty to sixty bitter almonds are sufficient to produce death in an adult; children may die after the ingestion of four to six. Bitter almonds yield about 3% of amygdalin. Since amygdalin yields 5.9% of hydrocyanic acid, somewhat more than one ounce would be required to yield one grain, or 0.64 gm., of anhydrous hydrocyanic acid. In the case reported by Jacobi, the woman had taken almost four times the lethal dose.

Maschka reported a case in which two and a half ounces were taken with suicidal intent. The symptoms began in a few minutes. The woman died within an hour and a half from the first symptoms.[1511]

Haberda reported six fatal cases, one of which refers to a child, the five being suicides.[1512]

Baker reported a case in which a man said he had eaten two handfuls of bitter almonds; recovery followed.[1513] In another case of suicide, death resulted in two hours from a handful of bitter almonds. In Jacobi's case, death did not occur until three hours after ingestion of the poison.

Cases of poisoning have been reported from the eating of kernels of peach, cherry, apple. The symptoms are dizziness, accelerated pulse, cherry-red color of the face, and spasm of the esophagus and pylorus due to hydrocyanic acid. A girl of five lived seventy-two hours after eating an unknown quantity of cherry kernels. A woman was severely poisoned but recovered after consuming twenty kernels of apricot seeds.

1510. JACOBI: *Deutsche Ztschr. f. d. ges. gerichtl. Med.*, 21:15, 1933.
1511. MASCHKA: *Ztschr. f. anal. Chem. Wiesb.*, 12:4, 1873.
1512. HOFMANN-HABERDA: Lehrbuch d. gerichtl. med., 1927.
1513. BAKER: *Brit. M. J.*, 2:12, 1881.

Pester says that the bark and leaves of many plants of the plum family contain hydrocyanic acid in combination.[1514]

Cases of cyanide poisoning have been reported from eating certain varieties of the phaseolus lunatus. These beans contain a glucoside from which hydrocyanic acid is liberated in the intestines. From 8 to 56 mg. hydrocyanic acid may be obtained from 100 gm. of beans.[1515] The symptoms develop slowly, and are the same as following the consumption of kernels of the peach.

OIL OF BITTER ALMONDS

OIL of bitter almonds (oleum amygdalae amarae, U.S.P.) is a volatile oil obtained by distillation with water, from bitter almonds, and from other seeds containing amygdalin. The oil contains 85% benzaldehyde, and not less than 2% to 4% hydrocyanic acid. Part of the benzaldehyde is in loose chemical combination with hydrocyanic acid, forming benzaldehydcyanhydrine, but in the body the molecule is quickly and completely dissociated so that the toxicity of benzaldehydcyanhydrine corresponds closely to that of an equivalent amount of hydrocyanic acid.

The oil of bitter almonds is an ethereal oil which, on hydrolysis, yields hydrocyanic acid, benzaldehyde, and glucose. On distillation, both the cyanide and benzaldehyde must be determined. The cyanide comes in the first part of the distillate, the benzaldehyde a little later, yielding a milky distillate.

A number of cases of poisoning occurred from the use of this oil as a flavoring agent in confectionery. Witthaus reported that out of 492 cases of cyanic poisoning, sixty-five were due to the oil of bitter almonds. Some of these were suicides, and others were accidental. The symptoms following the ingestion of the oil of bitter almonds are the same as for hydrocyanic acid. Death may occur within ten minutes.

The fatal dose is ten drops. Taylor reports a case in which death occurred in one-half hour from seventeen drops. Recoveries have been reported with prompt treatment from doses of half an ounce.

1514. PESTER, S. D.: *Presse méd.*, 42:1006, 1903.

1515. SUNDENDORF and GEHRTZ: *Ztschr. f. Untersuch. d. Nahrungs.- u. Genussmittel, Berl.*, 38:350, 1920; DIENEMANN: *Deutsche. med. Wchnschr.*, 46:1364, 1920.

Oil of bitter almonds may be easily distinguished from nitrobenzene by heating on the water-bath for a little time with manganese dioxide and sulphuric acid; bitter almond oil treated in this way loses its odor; nitrobenzene is unaltered.

CYANAMIDE

CYANAMIDE, which is used as a fertilizer, has caused poisoning in laborers working with the chemical. The symptoms are a transitory redness of the face, headache, marked congestive hyperemia of the face and upper third of the body. Respiration is accelerated and deepened, and there is an irregular heart with lowered blood pressure, and a feeling of giddiness.

The severity and duration of the poisoning vary with the amount of cyanamide dust that may have been absorbed. Attacks usually last from one-half hour to two hours. Occasionally deep-rooted ulcers may appear on the skin, and on the mucous membranes there may be irritation such as conjunctivitis, laryngitis, bronchitis, tonsillitis, and rhinitis.

The double cyanides, such as potassium ferrocyanide, Prussian-blue, Turnbull's blue, are usually considered non-poisonous.

Cyanic acid, the cyanates and sulphocyanates, are nearly harmless. However, poisoning has occurred from thiocyanates used in the reduction of blood pressure.

Cyanogen, cyanogen iodide, cyanogen chloride, and nitroprussiate of soda are all very poisonous.

BENZENE (BENZOL) BENZINE

PURE benzene or benzol, C_6H_6, is a colorless, limpid liquid with a characteristic odor which is rather pleasant. It boils at 80.2° C. Its specific gravity is 0.879. It is soluble, 0.07 gm. in 100 cc. of water.

The commercial varieties contain some toluene, xylene, olefins, paraffins, and carbon disulphide. It is somewhat soluble in alcohol, and is an excellent solvent for rubber, gums, resins, celluloid, and fats of all kinds. It is used extensively in the rubber industry, in varnish and paint removing, in gilding and bronzing, in spray gun paints, coal tar paints, and to a small extent as motor car fuel. Pure benzene is not used in industry.

Winslow reports that occasional instances of acute benzol poisoning may be found in the medical literature extending back to 1862.[1516] He has found a record of over 100 cases of acute benzol poisoning, of which about one-half were fatal.

De Balsac and Agasse-Lafont report the occurrence of eight deaths and thirty-six cases of illness among 120 persons employed in the workshop in two months due to the use of benzene distilling about 80° C., where benzene had been used as a rubber solvent in an adhesive instead of an industrial benzene which contains only xylene, toluene, and cymene.[1517]

Benzol poisoning may result from absorption of the benzene by the respiratory tract, or the alimentary tract, or through the skin. In the majority of cases the poison enters the body by way of the respiratory tract, skin absorption being very slow, especially in those cases in which the hands are immersed in benzol. However, both skin and respiratory avenues may be involved simultaneously as in the case of a man whose overalls were soaked in benzol from a leak in a tank and who endeavored to wash the benzol down the sewer, during which process he inhaled a large amount of benzol fumes. Where the amount of benzol is considerable, or in a confined space, it may act as an asphyxiation agent.*

Symptoms: Inhalation of the fumes causes symptoms referable to effects upon the central nervous system. There are muscular tremors, salivation, violent twitchings, exhaustion, paralysis, quick respiration at first, then slow, then a rapid pulse, lowering of the temperature, and, in fatal cases, narcosis, convulsions, and death from paralysis of the respiratory center. Lehmann[1518] found no characteristic changes in the organs or in the blood, but Chassevent and Garnier[1519] found

1516. WINSLOW, C. E. A.: *J. Indust. Hyg.*, 9: 61, 1927.
1517. DE BALSAC, F. H., and AGASSE-LAFONT: *Bull. Acad. de Méd.*, July 4, p. 31, 1933.
* For a review of the literature dealing with health hazards in spray painting, Bull No. 15, Nat. Research Council of Canada, Ottawa, p. 44, 1930, contains a valuable bibliography. See also ENGELHARDT: Benzol vergiftung; SAMMELBERICHT: Sammlung von vergiftungsfallen, 2, 1931; KEESER, FROBOESE, TURNAU, GROSSE, KUSS, WILKE: *Schrift. a. d. Gesamtgeb. d. Gewerbehyg.*, No. 29, Berlin, 1930; LOEWENBERG: *Fortschr. d. Med.*, 10-12, 1932; MITNIK and GENKIN: *Arch. f. Gewerbepath. u. Gewerbehyg.*, 2: 457, 1931; and SCHWARTZ: *Deutsche med. Wchnschr.*, 449, 1932.
1518. LEHMANN, K. B.: *Arch. f. Hyg.*, 75: 1, 1912.
1519. CHASSEVENT and GARNIER: *Arch. internat. de pharmacodyn. et de thérap.*, 14: 93, 1905.

congestion of the abdominal organs and peritoneum, ecchymoses and ulcers along the upper border of the stomach in the mucous coat. Rambousek tested benzene on dogs and rabbits, finding the former the more susceptible. After-effects were noticed in those that survived; however, where death occurred, only a moderate hyperemia of the brain, lungs, and mesenteric vessels was found. Santesson,[1520] experimenting with crude and with pure benzene, was able to produce hemorrhages in the mucous membrane of the stomach and the intestines and in the lungs. He concludes that benzene dissolves the body fat, and that emboli of fat lodge in the smaller vessels, causing first stasis and then rupture of the vessel wall. Selling[1521] found blood changes in rabbits as a result of poisoning with pure and with commercial benzene, the most striking feature being a leucopenia which progressed till the white corpuscles numbered 400 in a cubic millimeter of blood. Selling made extensive animal experiments, and he was the first to assert that the essential characteristic of benzol poisoning is not the purpura hemorrhagica, but an extreme leucopenia caused by aplasia of the bone marrow, affecting especially the granular leucocytes, and to a slight degree the mononuclears. Ferguson and Hamilton[1522] state that the actions of benzene and toluene are very similar, but that benzene is the more powerful. The action of both of these substances is on the young blood cells. Like many poisons and many drugs which are used in medicine, the first effects of these substances are stimulating. Leucocytosis, erythrocytosis, and possibly thrombocytosis appear early, with histological evidence of hyperplasia. The ultimate result in clinical terms is an agranulocytic anemia, accompanied by purpura hemorrhagica and, as the pathological manifestation, an aplastic bone marrow. Rambousek finds that vapors of benzol mixed with air are very poisonous. He published a large number of serious and fatal cases, collected from the literature and from personal information. Selling's work led to the advocacy by Koranyi, of Hungary, of the therapeutic use of this leucocytic agent in the treatment of

1520. SANTESSON: *Arch. f. Hyg.*, 21:336, 1897.
1521. SELLING, L.: *Johns Hopkins Hosp. Rep.*, 17:183, 1916; also *Beitr. z. path. Anat. u. z. allg. Path.*, 51:576, 1911.
1522. FERGUSON, F., and HAMILTON, T. D.: *J. Indust. Hyg.*, 33:547, 1933.

leucemia. Duke[1523] reported variations in the blood count. Hurwitz and Drinker[1523] reported the factors of aplastic anemia, a decrease of defensive substances, precipitins, agglutinins, and opsonins. Hektoen[1523] reported the effect of benzene on the production of anti-bodies. Rusk[1523] reported lowered resistance to infections. This was also reported by Simonds and Jones,[1523] Smith,[1523] and Winternitz and Hirschfelder[1523] as resulting from the loss of these substances, as well as from the disappearance of phagocytic leucocytes. Many cases of benzene poisoning have happened while men were exposed to heavy fumes in cleaning out vats or painting in confined spaces. In these cases death occurred suddenly. However, many cases of benzene poisoning have been reported where death did not occur suddenly, when the people worked for hours, days, or weeks in connection with the use of coal tar paint, or when a sealing mixture of rubber dissolved in benzene was used.[1524] This form is characterized by profound blood changes of the aplastic type, and by lesions in the vessel walls which lead to multiple hemorrhages into the skin, and subcutaneous tissues, and from the gums, nose, throat, stomach, bowel, and uterus. Human beings and animals do not show the same effect upon the blood. Animals show the leukocytic toxic effect of benzol, while in human beings the outstanding feature is the destruction of the red blood cells; in one instance the red count ran down to 1,000,000. Hamilton[1525] reports the history of a case of benzol poisoning with a blood count of 6,800 white cells, but only 1,500,000 red cells; another with 7,000 white cells but only 1,900,000 red cells. Of seventy-seven blood counts collected from the literature, there were seventeen with a blood picture such as is seen in animals poisoned with benzol. Leucopenia was far in excess of anemia. However, there were twenty-two with the reverse, an excessive anemia with a moderate leucopenia. The clinical picture is one of progressive anemia with

1523. Duke, W. W.: *Arch. Int. Med.*, 11:100, 1913. Hurwitz, S. H., and Drinker, C. K.: *J. Exper. Med.*, 21:401, 1915. Hektoen, L.: *J. Infect. Dis.*, 19:69, 1916. Rusk, G. Y.: *Univ. California Publ. Path.*, 2:139, 1914. Simonds, J. P., and Jones, H. M.: *J. Med. Research*, 33:197, 1915. Smith, A. R.: *J. Indust. Hyg.*, 10:73, 1928. Winternitz, M. C., and Hirschfelder, A. D.: *J. Exper. Med.*, 17:657, 1913.

1524. Selling, L.: *Bull. Johns Hopkins Hosp.*, 21:33, 1910; and McClure, R. D.: *J.A.M.A.*, 67:693, 1916.

1525. Hamilton, Alice: Industrial Toxicology, 158, 1934.

a sense of malaise, fatigue, and weakness, then bleeding from the gums and nose, followed by rapid decline, petechiae, hemorrhage from the stomach, intestines, uterus and mouth, retinal hemorrhage, fever more or less intense, sometimes chills and delirium, and death from anoxemia and heart failure with pulmonary edema. Typically, the leucopenia should be a granulopenia, and in some cases the polynuclears do fall as low as 10% of the leucocytes. If there is a simultaneous infection there may be enough active marrow tissue left to produce a response in the form of increased polynuclears[1526] which would cloud the diagnosis of benzol poisoning, as only a leucopenia was considered. The red cells usually do not present any abnormality; however, stippling and even nucleated red cells may be found.[1527] The color index cannot be depended upon, as a review of seventy-five published cases showed that while the index was low in seventeen, in twenty-two it was high, and in thirty-six it was normal.

Bamesreiter exposed animals to concentrations from 14.5 to 120 mg. per liter with light benzine and heavier concentrations from 46 to 197 mg. per liter. The animals remained in these chambers until deep narcosis occurred, or until a period of six hours had elapsed, without the picture changing in the last half hour.[1528]

In some cases of benzol poisoning hemorrhages are absent, for even in cases with a marked loss of platelets, clinical purpura may fail to appear. Hogan and Schrader have reported an increase in the menstrual flow, or if pregnant, in the uterine flow.

In chronic poisoning the symptoms may not appear until sometime later. Rohner, of Iowa University, reported a case of a man who quit work because the fumes irritated his eyes. It was not until a month after his benzol exposure that he developed a fatal aplastic anemia. Four of Santesson's patients developed serious symptoms only after they had left the factory. Ordway and Gorham have reported that the marrow

1526. PAUL, W. D.: *J. Indust. Hyg.*, 193, 1927. MEDA, G.: *Il benzolismo professionale, Lavoro*, 13:264, 297, 326, 363, 1922.
1527. HUNTER, HANFLIG, and RONCHETTI, V.: *Atti. d. Soc. lomb. di sc. med. e biol., Milano*, 11:322, 1922; OETTINGER, W.: *These de Paris*, 1919, 1920.
1528. BAMESREITER, OTTO: *Arch. f. Hlg.*, 108:120, 1932.

is not always aplastic; it may show hyperplasia, but with a failure to deliver the new cells into the circulation.[1529] This same condition has been found in some cases of agranulocytic angina.

A diagnosis between benzol poisoning and pernicious anemia must be differentiated. In pernicious anemia there is hyperplasia of the marrow and great regenerative activity, especially in the production of the red cells, as shown by examination of the blood smear. The leucopenia in pernicious anemia is not usually marked. In benzol poisoning, however, leucopenia is marked, the hemorrhage being an outstanding feature. There is a high color index, with an involvement of the central nervous system. Martland reports that one cannot depend on the changes in the blood-forming organs alone for a diagnosis of benzol poisoning. In one instance he saw a marrow typical of pernicious anemia, and he has also seen a blood picture characteristic of myeloid leucemia. A woman who had been sealing with a thin benzol rubber cement in a canning factory gave a history of bleeding from the gums and nose for four days, with disturbances of vision and increasing weakness. A double retinal hemorrhage was found, and purpuric spots over the limbs. The red blood count was 5,000,000, the hemoglobin was 100%, the white cells 7,000, with 61% polynuclears. An abnormal feature of the blood was the absence of platelets. After admission to a hospital an anemia and leucopenia developed, and she died within four weeks, in spite of eight blood transfusions.

Lazarew came to the conclusion, after 1,200 experiments with white mice poisoned with different hydrocarbons, that the toxicity of benzine, with reference to acute poisoning, depends upon its content of paraffins, cycloparaffins, and aromatic hydrocarbons.[1530] With a small percentage content of benzol and its homologues, the toxicity of benzol vapor, at the same boiling point, is the greater the higher the cycloparaffine content and the less the paraffin content.

Brullowa and his associates conducted experiments with 100 rabbits, seventy guinea pigs, and thirty white mice by exposing them to vapors of various kinds of benzene. They found

1529. ORDWAY, T., and GORHAM, L. W.: *Oxford Univ. Press.*, 9:219, 1918.

1530. LAZAREW, N .W.: *Arch. f. Hyg.*, 102:227, 1929.

that in a single acute intoxication there often occurs a decrease in the quantity of erythrocytes and a fall in the hemoglobin.[1531]

Tschermkoff, Gadaskin, and Kowschar, after considering a number of laboratory experiments, came to the conclusion that the most important changes which occur after the inhalation of benzene may be referred to the central nervous system; the clonic spasms which follow benzol inhalation intoxication are caused by benzol and not the phenol which is the oxidation product of benzol present in the blood.[1532]

Lazarew, Brussilowskaja, Lawrom, and Lifschitz exposed mice and rabbits to the fumes of benzine and benzene and found that these substances, in the liquid state, can penetrate through the skin of the rabbit into the organism.[1533] Rabbits exposed to benzene fumes yielded a urine which gave a positive reaction for phenol. It was also shown that benzene was present in the expired air seven to nine minutes after immersion of the animal's paw in the fluid. The maximum concentration of benzine in the expired air was found to occur in about one-half hour (0.8 to 1 mg. per liter of air). Similar experiments made with benzene showed this substance in the expired air three to four minutes after immersion of the paw, the maximum concentration being found at 1.2 to 1.5 mg. per liter of air. Therefore, the authors conclude that benzene penetrates faster and in greater quantities through the skin and into the organism than does benzine.

Lewin has also conducted experiments along this line.[1534] His experiments were made in a closed space which was filled with benzene vapors at a concentration of 50 to 60 mg. per liter of air.

He summarizes his results as follows: In acute benzene intoxication there were (1) reaction of the reticulo-endothelial system; (2) hyperemia; (3) degeneration, and (4) siderosis. The hyperemia was particularly marked in the lungs and spleen, and in severe cases there was hypertrophy of the cells

1531. BRULLOWA, L. P., BRUSSILOWSKAJA, A. S., LAZAREW, N. W., LUBIMOWA, M. P., and STALSKAJA, D. I.: *Arch. f. Hyg.*, 104:226, 1930.

1532. TSCHERMKOFF, GADASKIN, and KOWSCHAR: *Arch. f. exper. Path. u. Pharmakol.*, 161:214, 1931.

1533. LAZAREW, BRUSSILOWSKAJA, LAWROM, and LIFSCHITZ: *Arch. f. Hyg.*, 106:112, 1931.

1534. LEWIN, I. E.: *Arch. f. Gewerbepath. u. Gewerbehyg.*, 3:340, 1932.

belonging to the reticulo-endothelial system. In such cases the spleen was invariably enlarged, owing to swelling of the endothelial cells lining the capsule of the spleen. Underneath the capsule were found myeloid metaplastic foci, and macrophages were present in the follicles. In the stratum fascicularis of the suprarenal bodies the author also saw swelling of the capillary endothelium and severe mitosis of the endothelial cells. In severe cases there was fatty degeneration of the liver and kidneys, this degeneration consisting essentially of neutral fats and lipoids. The degenerative changes were rather pronounced in the kidneys, which showed a typical picture of nephrosis. The bone-marrow also showed a considerable degenerative change. Here the author shows distinct increase in the number of megakaryocytes with pyknotic nuclei.

Frumina and Fainstein said that rubber factory workers who were exposed to about 3 mg. of benzine per liter of air showed vertigo, excitability, and loss of sleep.[1535] The objective symptoms were decreased hemoglobin and erythrocytic count, subnormal color index, punctate erythrocytes, and frequently a moderate leukocytosis.

Lestschinskaja[1536] poisoned some 751 white mice with different kinds of benzine, and found that the mortality of the mice appears to be a better and more reliable criterion for the toxicity of the poison than the side position and the disappearance of reflexes as suggested by Fuhner.[1536]

Vigdortschik, studying the chronic effect of benzine on workers, in 1929 and 1930 compared the pathological changes most frequently encountered in 451 female workers in the rubber industry (benzine), 412 weavers, and 384 cigarette girls. The components of all three groups were women of about the same age and working more or less under the same conditions. Among the rubber workers there was a high incidence of functional neuroses (neurasthenia, hysteria, etc.); this high incidence was found to be so great that it could hardly be considered accidental. Furthermore, the author found that these workers showed the highest incidence of bronchitis. These same workers had the highest anisonormocytosis and a certain

1535. FRUMINA, L. M., and FAINSTEIN, S. S.: *Zentralbl. f. Gewerbehyg.*, 21:161, 1934.

1536. LESTSCHINSKAJA: *Arch. f. Gewerbepath. u. Gewerghyg.*, 4:508, 1933. FUHNER, H.: *Biochem. Ztschr.*, 115, 1921.

degree of anemia. Conjunctivitis and skin diseases were also found very frequently among them.[1537]

Emile-Weil observed a case of a sixty year old rubber worker whose leukemia following benzol intoxication was gradual.[1528] The onset was characteristic by jaundice, which apparently developed without cause. Examination of the blood revealed a severe aplastic anemia, red blood cells, 1,800,000, hemoglobin 30%, no anisocytosis, polychromatophilia, poikilocytosis; 30,000 hematoblasts; white cell count 25,900, with a differential count of polymorphonuclear leukocytes 60%, lymphocytes 34%, large mononuclears 2%, and neutrophils 4%.

In another report on this condition the author[1539] states that he believes the hemorrhagic tendency which often accompanies the light anemias of benzene intoxication to be a prodromal sign of a syndrome of a grave anemia with purpura hemorrhagica, which is best called aleukemia hemorrhagic.

Peronnet states that the benzene content of the blood of guinea pigs subjected to inhalations of the vapor at concentrations of 20 mg. and 50 mg. per liter of air, respectively, is a linear function of the time of exposure to the vapor up to twenty minutes.[1540] At the time of certain acute symptoms of poisoning, the blood contains 2.60 mg. to 2.80 mg. benzene per 100 gm. The benzene rapidly disappears from the blood, largely through the lungs, without chemical change. It is also eliminated in the urine in the form of conjugated phenols.

Baker reported the case of a man forty-seven years of age, employed as an operative in an asbestos factory, who, two weeks prior to his admission to a hospital (April 26, 1928), had been in good health.[1541] At this time he began to have shortness of breath, pain beneath the sternum, with severe bleeding from the nose and mouth; a severe nosebleed lasting two days was one of the initial symptoms. About the same time he noticed hemorrhagic spots over the arms and legs. There were hemorrhages in the mouth from the gums, and there was a dis-

1537. Vigdortschik, N. A.: Zentralbl. f. Gewerbehyg., 10:219, 1933.
1538. Emile-Weil: Bull. méd., 46:750, 1932.
1539. Emile-Weil: Paris méd., 2:112, 1933.
1540. Peronnet, M.: J. de pharm. et chim., Par., 21:503, 1935; Chem. Abst., 29:7500, 1935.
1541. Baker, Frederick H.: Tr. Mass. Med.-Leg. Soc., 6:131, 1929.

tinct blurring of vision and dizziness upon bending over. For a few days before admission to the hospital, in addition to his hemorrhages, dizziness, and blurred vision, there was severe headache, both frontal and occipital, with a severe pain under the sternum. There was no edema and no cough. His blood pressure was 120 systolic and 70 diastolic. The examination on April 30, 1928, showed the hemoglobin to be 50%; red blood cells 1,000,000, white blood cells 1,700. Differential count showed polymorphonuclears 24%, lymphocytes 68%, mononuclears 8%, with a slight anisocytosis, and poikilocytosis. Platelets were markedly diminished. On May 4, 1928, the hemoglobin was 25%, red blood cells 1,070,000; white blood cells 11,000, polymorphonuclears 36%, lymphocytes 50%, mononuclears 12%, with marked achromia. On May 1, 1928, he was given one blood transfusion. On May 5, 1928, twenty-four hours before death, he had convulsions and anuria. Urine examinations showed blood in the sediment.

Von Hans Jost noted increased elimination of paired sulphuric acid and glycuronic acids, phenols, and hippuric acids, in the urine of printers.[1542] The increase of hippuric acid in the urine is explained as the result of the intake of toluene in the inspired air. The oxidation products of xylol are known for the dog, and one should take into consideration the normal urinary products, such as cresol and hippuric acid.

Nikulina and Titowa found thrombopenia very frequently among benzol workers (seventy-three out of seventy-six workers) while anemia and leukopenia occurred in scarcely half the cases.[1543] Anderson reports hyperplasia of bone-marrow, with benzol poisoning.[1544]

The conclusion that Ferguson, Harvey, and Hamilton have drawn is that benzene and toluene act in a similar way, but benzene is more powerful because it is more volatile.[1545] Both substances act on the red blood cells. The first effects are stimulating, followed by leukopenia, anemia, and thrombo-

1542. VON HANS JOST: Arch. f. Gewerbepath. u. Gewerbehyg., 3:491, 1932.
1543. NIKULINA, C., and TITOWA, A.: Arch. f. Gewerbepath. u. Gewerbehyg., 5:201, 1934.
1544. ANDERSON, D. H.: Am. J. Path., 10:101, 1934.
1545. FERGUSON, T., HARVEY, W. F., and HAMILTON, T. D.: J. Hyg., 33:547, 1933.

penia.   Both are powerful solvents of fat, and so act on the
nerve cells, capillary endothelium, and the parenchyma of organs, whence follow nervous symptoms and hemorrhages.

Sartorius and Sudhues report that it is possible to expose
rabbits several hours daily over a period of one and a half years
to benzol-air mixtures of 13.6 to 27.2 mg. per liter of air without noteworthy changes.   All animals, however, did not
show the same tolerance.[1546]

The nervous symptoms are muscular tremor, tonic and
clonic spasms, euphoria, insomnia, hallucinations, delirium,
inebriation, narcosis, convulsions, and the Parkinsonian syndrome.[1547]   As previously mentioned, leucopenia may exist as
one of the most important diagnostic symptoms, yet it may
exist as a physiologic state in the absence of any abnormal condition, and a true benzene poisoning may exist without any
leucopenia, as also mentioned before.   A low red count and
several other symptoms of the poisoning, such as local irritation, anemia, or nervous symptoms, can be found in workers
not exposed to benzene.

Torday,[1548] in an examination of sixty-one persons, found
the lowest of the white cells to be 6,700.   Galambos[1549] determined the normal variation in healthy persons as ranging
from a minimum of 3,500 to a maximum of 12,000, with 7,613 as
the mean.   Therefore, caution should be used in making a
diagnosis of benzol poisoning upon the blood count alone,
where the count is below 5,000. Some confusion may arise from
agranulocytosis. It is in the blood counts, the hemorrhage and
the gingivitis, that the greatest similarity is to be found between agranulocytosis and benzene poisoning.   Here again we
must rely on the fact of the exposure, and in benzene poisoning the spongy, inflamed gums seldom reach the gangrenous,
ulcerated, sloughing stage frequently encountered in agranulocytosis, which sloughing may embrace the pharyngeal tissues.
However, agranulocytosis may exist without this serious buccal involvement.   In benzene poisoning, high fevers are terminal, unless there is a simultaneous infection, while in agranulocytosis the fever is persistent and early.

1546. SARTORIUS, F., and SUDHUES, M.: Arch. f. Hyg., 110:245, 1933.
1547. McCORD, CAREY P.: J.A.M.A., 93:280, 1929.
1548. TORDAY, A.: Bull. Johns Hopkins Hosp., 37:14, 1935.
1549. GALAMBOS, A.: Folia haemat., 13:153, 1912.

Lewin,[1550] Lehmann,[1550] and Schwenke[1550] have reported that purified benzene is less toxic than the crude varieties. The impurities which are usually present in benzene when poisoning occurs do not cause the symptoms or the pathological picture, and hence it is my opinion that it is the benzene itself that causes the damage.

Starr described an outbreak of benzene poisoning in a millinery establishment in which twenty-two out of twenty-seven girls exposed, presented manifestations of benzene poisoning.[1551] Exposure was limited to the use of a rubber-benzene cement (with carbon disulphide and carbon tetrachloride as adjuvants). Certain groups of girls seemed to be more susceptible than others working with benzol. Batchelor,[1552] the National Safety Council investigation,[1553] and Rambousek[1553] advocate the substitution of the homologues of benzene, toluene and xylene. Toluene is more toxic than benzene as a producer of acute narcotic action.

Schwarz described a case of a man who drank refined benzene over a period of five or six weeks and developed a severe polyneuritis, which incapacitated him from walking, and in which there was abolition of all the tendon reflexes and reaction of degeneration of the affected muscles.[1554] He stopped taking the benzene, and after seven months was able to walk and resume work in an office, though the peroneal and tibial muscles on either side were still weak.

Pulford reports a case of a painter in whom the hemoglobin was 21%, the red blood count 1,200,000, and the white blood count 1,940.[1555]

Lignac experimented with 26 mice, giving them 0.003 cc. of benzol three times weekly.[1556] At first there occurred a pronounced proliferation of the lymphoid tissue, especially in the

1550. LEWIN, L.: München. med. Wchnschr., 54:2377, 1907. LEHMANN, K. B., et al.: Arch. f. Hyg., 71-72:307, 1909, 1910; and SCHWENKE, H.: J. Gasbel., 63:142, 1920.

1551. STARR, E. B.: J. Indust. Hyg., 4:203, 1922.

1552. BATCHELOR, J. J.: Am. J. Hyg., 7:276, 1927.

1553. Nat. Safety Council Investigation: Final Report of the Committee on Benzol (Chemical and Rubber Sections, Nat. Safety Council), May, 1926; and RAMBOUSEK, J.: Gewerbliche Vergiftungen, Leipzig, 431, 1911.

1554. SCHWARZ, H. G.: Deutsche med. Wchnschr., 58:449, 1932.

1555. PULFORD, D. SCHUYLER: California & West. Med., 35:361, 1931.

1556. LIGNAC, G. O.: Frankfurt. Fortschr., 9:403, 1931.

spleen, while the myeloid tissue was somewhat decreased. He found that if the benzol administration was continued, the mortality, especially of the female animals, increased considerably, death occurring under symptoms of hemorrhagic diathesis, general emaciation and atrophy, which was pronounced in the spleen. The considerable deposit of hemoglobinogenic pigments, namely, hemosiderin and hematin, and the increased destruction of the red blood cells in the spleen, point to an abnormal hemoglobin decomposition; it cannot be stated with certainty whether this is produced directly or indirectly by the benzol. In a study of twenty-eight cases, "leukemia" never revealed pictures suggesting those previously mentioned. The author concludes his work by the statement that "not every case of leukemia is produced by benzol", but that "arsenic, thorium, and also roentgen rays, given in certain amounts for a considerable length of time, may lead to the production of leukemia." Also the possibility of "spontaneous leukemia" cannot be excluded.

Kuntzen's experiments suggest that chronic intoxications with minute amounts of auto-gases (from benzol) may possibly contribute to the increases in general predisposition to thrombosis, and may partly be responsible for the increased frequency of thrombosis.[1557]

Smith reported a chronic case of benzol poisoning in a worker in an artificial leather shop, where he was applying a benzene-rubber compound to the material to be coated.[1558] Shortly after beginning this work he lost his appetite and felt nauseated at times while in the shop, vomiting about once a week. After working three months he noticed itching of the skin of the extremities and at the same time he began to bleed freely from the gums. His blood pressure was 125/80. The patient was well developed and well nourished, and had many purpuric spots on the legs, thighs, buttocks, abdomen and right forearm. There were many petechiae of varying size on the inner aspect of both arms. There were many bleeding points in the gums. Hemoglobin 62%, red blood cells 3,300,000, white blood cells 1,350; polymorphonuclears 25%, lymphocytes 75% and platelets 25,000. The bleeding time was thirty-three min-

1557. KUNTZEN, H.: *Ztschr. f. ärztl. Fortbild., Jena.*, 29:663, 1932.
1558. SMITH, ADELAIDE ROSS: J.A.M.A., 93:1970, 1929.

utes. On the basis of the history of exposure to benzene, and the marked leukopenia, a diagnosis of chronic benzene poisoning was made. He was given three transfusions, and was put on a diet of half a pound of liver daily. After a month of liver diet the reticulocytes reached 8.6%, their highest point. Liver therapy was continued for three months longer. A year later the patient was found to be normal, with the exception of a slight leukopenia, of 4,770, otherwise his blood picture was normal. He was entirely free from symptoms.

Tschernikoff, Gadaskin, and Kowschar[1559] observed a distinct dilatation of the pupils, and an increased flow of saliva, in dogs on which they made experiments. Nahum and Hoff[1560] state that benzol inhalation in the presence of small quantities of adrenalin will give rise to ventricular extrasystoles and ventricular tachycardia; it is only when large quantities of adrenalin are present in the blood that ventricular fibrillation ensues.

In both the clinical reports and in experiments, the danger of death from ventricular fibrillation occurs during the phase of induction or recovery from narcosis and periods of hyper-excitability and increased adrenalin liberation. Feil[1561] states that the severity of the disorders found in man depends upon the individual predisposition. The danger seems to be greater in children, in pregnant women, in obese individuals, and in subjects using alcohol. Whether the intoxication is acute or chronic, benzene acts chiefly on the central nervous system. This effect has been explained by the power which benzene has of dissolving lipoids.

Adler, Herzmark, and Selinger[1562] believe that workmen should be subjected to periodic examinations, and that those who give evidence of severe hyperthyroidism should not be admitted to this type of work, involving the use of benzol. Dr. Valentine, an industrial physician of Chicago, Illinois, in a personal communication related to me three cases from one

1559. Tschernikoff, A. M., Gadaskin, D., and Kowschar: *Naunyn-Schmeidebergs, Arch.*, 161:214, 1931.
1560. Nahum, L. H., and Hoff, H. E.: *J. Pharmacol. & Exper. Therap.*, 50:336, 1934.
1561. Feil, A.: *Presse méd.*, 40:1973, 1932.
1562. Adler, Herzmark, and Selinger, A.: *Arch. f. Gewerbepath. u. Gewerbehyg.*, 1:763, 1930.

factory, in one week, of severe hyperthyroidism in men cleaning out bottles which had contained benzol.

Albrecht[1563] reports a case of benzene intoxication in a man thirty-five years of age who had been employed for four years in a chemical factory, working with paints. During his illness a diagnosis of a brain tumor was given. The fundus of the eye showed the presence of a fresh hemorrhage, and he had a bilateral positive Babinski and Oppenheim, but after fourteen days the pyramidal symptoms disappeared and he made an uneventful recovery.

Flury and Wirth, by experiments on people and animals, found that the various solvents, especially the esters—methyl acetate, ethyl acetate, phthalic acid, diethyl ester, methyl glycol acetate, methyl alcohol, acetone, and ethylene glycol—under practical tests showed more or less severe irritation to the accessible mucous membranes of the eyes and respiratory tract, which may lead to increased inflammation. They state that subjects and animals become accustomed to the irritation of all solvents. Cases of hypersensitivity were not observed.[1564]

All of these experimental materials have a paralyzing effect on the central nervous system. The more volatile ones are similar in their action to narcotics, when inhaled. With the inhalation of narcotic concentrations a strong acid formation occurs in the blood, which leads to a peculiar deep narcosis, leading usually to the death of the animal. Also severe subsequent sickness and delayed cases of death are sometimes found. With the repeated inspiration of less than narcotic strength, deaths also occur among animals, especially with the methyl compounds. The repeated inhalation of the esters leads to definite blood changes, and the esters are evidently by no means as harmless as is often asserted.

The case to which I have previously alluded was that of a young man, twenty-nine years of age a machinist for a rubber cutting company. A fuse blew out which stopped the machine and fans, causing the benzol mixture to spill over the machines. He kept on cleaning these machines, and in about forty-five minutes began to feel very faint, dizzy and nauseated. Fresh air revived him, but he developed a severe

    1563. ALBRECHT: *Monatschr. f. Psychiat. u. Neurol.*, 82:108, 1932.
    1564. FLURY, F., and WIRTH, W.: *Arch. f. Gewerbepath. u. Gewer-behyg.*, 5:1-89, 1933.

headache and excruciating pains around the entire lower half of the body, buttocks, and abdomen. On reaching home he went to bed, and toward evening of the same day became worse. The next day the pain began to spread anteriorly and in all directions. The patient called a physician who prescribed a medicine, but this he vomited and even had hemoptysis. On the following day he vomited again, and the pain became worse. Then he developed a general malaise, weakness of the extremities, and fever. The patient was removed to a hospital. He gave a history of blood oozing from the gums for two weeks, pain in the upper third of thigh, pain in both extremities, headache, and high fever. His appetite was poor, and he felt nauseated, especially after meals. There was hemoptysis after retching, with a thoracic pain on the left side and a precordial pain. He had a nocturia four times a night, and a frequency every hour during the day. Nervous symptoms were headache, numbness, paresthesia, blurring of vision, tinnitus; stuporous for one day. Hyperesthenia of lower half of body from head of navel to toes. Cellulitis of right thigh. Patient on entering the hospital was acutely ill; there were small ecchymoses and brown patches, with marked pallor of face. Tenderness over gall-bladder region. Right upper thigh inflamed. Pain started in center of buttocks, radiating to groin, to middle thigh. Left lower sacral, third, was where tenderness started to lateral thigh and middle left buttocks. The reflexes were all normal. There was a large indurated area on the outer aspect of the right thigh. This was opened but no free pus was found. On June 9, 400 cc. of blood were given; on June 12, 400 cc.; and on June 18, 500 cc. The temperature varied from 100° to 104.8°. The blood count was: 950 white cells, 3,500,000 red cells, and hemoglobin 68%. This was not relieved by blood transfusions. The red count went down to 3,490,000, and hemoglobin 60% coagulation time was six minutes. Diagnosis in this case was made on a history of exposure to benzene, the extreme low white count, the low red count, and hemorrhages. Large doses of benzene may destroy the red cells, while small doses stimulate the production of red cells to 6,000,000. An overdose or too long exposure may cause hemorrhages in the skin and mucous membranes, anemia of a high grade, fever, and almost complete disappearance of leucocytes, as in the case above, with cellulitis of the right hip.

Smyth says: "Toluene being less volatile than benzene is also less toxic. Xylene is quite toxic, but less volatile than toluene, therefore less hazardous. Neither seems to be readily absorbed through the skin in toxic amounts." This seems unusual since benzene is toxic whether taken per mouth, inhaled, or absorbed through the skin.[1565]

Dieckoff describes a chronic case of poisoning from the swallowing of benzol in a thirty year old man who daily syphoned benzol in a mixing machine.[1566]

The nitro- and amino- groups and aromatics, produce about the same clinical picture. The latter in general are simple blood poisons, while the former in addition exert a direct action on the central nervous system. In light cases of poisoning from nitro- or amino- compounds, there is flushing of the face with a sense of fullness and throbbing pain in the head, burning sensation in the throat, and a feeling of tightness in the chest. More marked cases develop a violent throbbing headache, dizziness, roaring in the ears, and visual disturbances. With more severe poisoning the face becomes livid, the lips and tongue blue, the knees weak, and the gait staggering. The blue color of the face may persist for several days. In extreme cases cyanosis increases, muscular tremors develop, there are extreme weakness, cold skin, nausea, vomiting, abdominal cramps, quick shallow respiration, lowered blood pressure, and coma. The respirations become progressively slower and shallower; involuntary urination and defecation may occur, and convulsions, usually just before death. For this type of poisoning the skin is the most important portal of entry.

Treatment: Dassen recommends blood transfusions in the treatment of chronic benzol poisoning.[1567]

All patients with leukopenia should be removed from the source of employment. Those having symptoms such as bleeding from the nose and mouth should be immediately hospitalized and there treated by transfusions. The anemia is best treated by transfusions of 400 to 500 cc. of blood. Pentnucleo-

1565. SMYTH, H. F.: *J. Indust. Hyg.*, 13:87, 1931.

1566. DIECKOFF, J.: *Arch. f. Gewerbepath. u. Gewerbehyg.*, 3:549, 1932.

1567. DASSEN, R.: Abst. from *Semana med.*, 2:230, 1933, in *Chem. Abst.*, October 20, 1933, p. 5115.

tide has been recommended. In one case, however, in which I tried this drug it failed to have any effect, blood transfusions giving better results. Injection of liver extract and even eating half of a pound of liver a day has given good results. Splenectomy was also performed in one case.[1568] Arsenic and iron preparations can be used to advantage. Ninety to 120 grains of iron and ammonium citrate per day may be given until hemoglobin has reached the normal limits. In McClure's case after thirteen transfusions the red blood count rose to 5,280,000, and fourteen weeks later the count was still 4,270,000. X-ray of the long bones should be used for the stimulating effect upon the bone-marrow.

Hayhurst and Neiswander[1569] report a case which they treated by transfusions of whole blood and by bone marrow extract. Four years later the red blood count was still below 4,500,000. Physical examination by Dr. Russell M. Wilder, of the University of Chicago, gave the following report: "We find him in excellent condition; weight 70.1 kg; temperature 98.8°, pulse 68, blood pressure 114/60; urine: specific gravity 1.021 - 1.022, no albumin, or sugar, or sediment; Wassermann and Kahn negative; blood count: red cells 4,700,000 to 4,850,000; white blood cells, 4,700 to 4,850; hemoglobin 85 to 88%; polymorphonuclears 38-40, lymphocytes 7-10, small lymphocytes 13-47, mononuclears 6-8, eosinophils 1-2%; red cells appear normal although there is a slight anisocytosis."

Nahum and Hoff[1570] claim that benzol vapor produces an abnormal sensitivity of the heart to adrenalin, a common constituent of the blood, bringing about an irregularity in the heart beat which causes death. Excitement and physical activity predispose to the occurrence of sudden death by benzol. Excitement, moreover, causes a large amount of adrenalin to be poured into the system. This can be counteracted by an injection of acetyl-choline, which protected animals from death by ventricular fibrillation.

Grunberg[1571] enumerates the absolute contra-indications for benzol absorption: (1) tuberculosis of the lungs with unstable compensation; (2) well-marked functional neuroses; (3)

1568. McClure: *J.AM.A.*, September 9, 1916.
1569. Hayhurst, E. R., and Neiswander: *J.A.M.A.*, 96:269, 1931.
1570. Nahum, Louis H.: *Science News Letter*, April 28, 1934, p. 267.
1571. Grunberg, G.: *Gig., bezopass. i. pat. truda.*, 5-6:77, 1935.

diseases of the blood-forming organs; (4) eczema and dermatitis on exposed parts of the body; (5) kidney inflammation;
(6) anemia (not less than 65%).

Postmortem Appearances: The appearance of the body of
a person dying from benzol poisoning is that of an anemic individual, except where death occurs suddenly from asphyxiation by benzol. Bright red spots may be found upon the body.
The blood is found fluid and usually of a dark color. Hemorrhages may be found in the pleura, and the gastric and intestinal mucosa. Autopsy may also show bleeding from the nose,
gums, buccal membranes, and bowel.

Lenoir and Claude reported a case of myocardial infarcts
and hemorrhages under the endocardium seen at autopsy.[1572]

Postmortem examination usually discloses hemorrhage in
the brain and inner organs, with yellowish discoloration of the
bone-marrow, anemia, and fatty degeneration of the liver and
kidneys. One of the first autopsies to be reported was published by Sury-Bienz in 1888.[1573]

McCallum reported that the autopsy of Selling's first case
showed the following: Hemorrhages in skin, viscera, and
serous surfaces; pallor of the organs; blood pale and watery;
muscles a deep red color; some fatty degeneration of the heart
muscle, somewhat less in the liver; bone-marrow of femur
fairly consistent, of a dull ochre color, with abundance of
blood supply. Smears from the marrow suggested aplasia,
showing very few cells of any kind, the most numerous being
normal red cells slightly paler, extremely scanty leucocytes,
chiefly of lymphocytic or myeloblastic type, with reduced
chromatin.

Martland found hemorrhages in practically every organ
of the body—lungs, pancreas, gastric and intestinal mucous
membranes, etc. All of the abdominal organs showed unusual
congestion and there was bloody mucus in the air passages. On
section of the lung a distinct odor of benzene was given off
(this being a case of acute poisoning). There was an abnormal
quantity of phenol in the urine, but no benzene.[1574]

1572. Lenoir and Claude: *Bull. et mém. Soc. méd. d. hôp. de Paris,*
October 20, 1897.
1573. Sury-Bienz: *Vrtljschr f. gerichtl. Med.,* 49:138, 1888.
1574. Hamilton, Alice: Industrial Poisons in the United States,
462, 1929.

In Baker's case the autopsy showed secondary degenerative changes in the parenchymatous organs.[1575] The bone-marrow of the long bones was markedly altered as in aplastic anemia. Over the surface of each lung were numerous petechial hemorrhages in the pleura, with a small amount of blood-stained serum in each pleural cavity. Each lung was tremendously engorged and edematous throughout. The liver was markedly enlarged, weighing 2350 gm. The microscopical sections of the liver showed almost a complete, fatty metamorphosis of the liver cells. The capsule of the kidneys showed few petechial hemorrhages.

Serra[1576] quotes Dorner as having observed multiple sclerosis in a case of benzene poisoning which came to autopsy, and Stiefler observed in this connection an epileptic syndrome. In fatal cases Gaffe observed extensive hemorrhage of the lung which he considered characteristic of this type of poisoning.

Lederer[1577] reports the death of an individual in whom autopsy revealed complete maceration of the buccal mucosa; the tongue was covered with thick scales; the left lung was enlarged, whereas the right lung showed the presence of a brownish cloudy fluid; the spleen was considerably enlarged in all its dimensions, the capsule appearing under tension and smooth; the liver was also found to be enlarged, and both suprarenal bodies showed necrosis; the kidneys were much enlarged; the mucosa of the stomach was covered with dirty brownish-red substance; the bone-marrow of the femoral diaphysis showed a compact and mottled bone-marrow. The anatomical diagnosis was splenomegaly of Gaucher's type.

Mallory[1578] reported a case of an autopsy of a forty-four year old Canadian housewife who worked in a rubber factory for four years until one month before her present illness. The autopsy showed an aplastic anemia. The immediate cause of her death was sepsis. She developed a generalized septicemia with B. welchii, and in the short period intervening between death and her arrival at the morgue the body had blown up to an almost unrecognizable form.

1575. BAKER, FREDERICK H.: *Tr. Mass. Med.-Leg. Soc.*, 6:131, 1929.
1576. SERRA, CORNELIAS: *Morgagni*, 74:807, 1932.
1577. LEDERER, E.: *Arch. f. Gewerbepath. u. Gewerbehyg.*, 3:535, 1932.
1578. MALLORY, TRACY B.: *New England J. Med.*, 213:182, 1935.

Falconer[1579] reported a case of lymphatic leukemia following benzol poisoning in a white man, fifty-eight years of age,
employed by a can company. The blood studies showed the
following: red blood cells, 1,530,000; white cells, 8100 per ccm.
Differential: neutrophils, 62; lymphocytes, 32; monocytes, 6%.
Platelet count, 68,000. He recovered from the acute attack and
was given light work, but two years later was forced to give
up work entirely. On December 16, 1927, his white cell count
was 108,300. On February 1, 1928, he was re-admitted to a
hospital. His hemoglobin was 39%; white cell count, 108,000;
red cells, 1,520,000. On February 13 the white count had increased to 140,000; neutrophils 2%, and 98% lymphocytes:
34,000 platelets per ccm. Death occurred on February 16, 1928.
An autopsy verified the diagnosis of lymphatic leukemia.

Rohner, Baldridge, and Hausmann[1580] reported a case
of chronic benzene poisoning, with autopsy. The clinical picture was typical of chronic benzene poisoning. In the last few
days of life the man became delirious. Blood transfusions did
not seem to have any effect. Autopsy was similar to that mentioned previously.

Isolation and Tests: In a suspected case of benzene poisoning the tissues should be immediately removed to a refrigerator where they can be frozen and comminuted while in that
condition, using from 100 to 400 gm. and proceeding as directed
under Volatile Poisons (page 19). The distillate is collected
in about 25 cc. of carbon tetrachloride in an Erlenmeyer flask.
The distillate consists of a carbon tetrachloride layer and an
aqueous layer, placed in a Squibb's separatory funnel, well
shaken, and allowed to stand. After the two layers have made
a clear separation, the lower one (carbon tetrachloride) contains most of the benzene and is separated, placed in a clean
dry flask, and stoppered. The aqueous layer is extracted three
or four times with fresh portions of carbon tetrachloride, which
are combined into one. To this carbon tetrachloride solution
are added 10 cc. of a two-to-one mixture of fuming nitric sulphuric acid, and this is thoroughly shaken. The extraction
flask is best immersed in cold water, as there is heat evolved.
The benzene is converted into nitrobenzene and mononitroben-

1579. FALCONER, ERNEST H.: *Am. J. M. Sc.*, 186:353, 1933.
1580. ROHNER, BALBRIDGE, and HAUSMANN: *Arch. Path.*, 1:221, 1926.

zene. The carbon tetrachloride is evaporated on the water-bath, and the residue, consisting of nitrobenzene and the nitrating acids, is allowed to cool and is treated with 50 cc. of water. This is extracted several times with fresh portions of ether in a separatory funnel, which, upon evaporation of the ether, leaves nitrobenzene as a yellow residue with a characteristic odor, which on standing yields typical crystals. The nitrobenzene residue is weighed, and the amount of benzene present in the organ is calculated. The residue, after weighing, can be used for other tests. A small portion, about one-fifth, is taken up with 5 cc. of absolute alcohol and made alkaline with three drops of 30% sodium hydroxide. To this is added twice the volume of 1% fructose solution. An intense violet color results, which gradually fades. To another portion of the residue 10 cc. of water are added in a test-tube. The nitrobenzene is reduced by zinc-dust concentrated hydrochloric acid to aniline and phenyl di-aniline. A portion of the reduced material is made alkaline with alcoholic sodium hydroxide. One drop of chloroform is added, and the mixture heated. The characteristic odor of isonitrile is easily discerned.

To another portion of the mixed amines a few drops of 10% sodium nitrite are added, and then sodium carbonate until the first precipitate forms ($ZnCO_3$). Then add 3 cc. of 0.1% alkaline solution of beta-naphthol. An intense brown color results. Joachimoglu reports that this method is about 55% to 60% quantitative.[1581] Von Hans Jost discovered in printers an increased elimination of paired sulphuric acid, glycuronic acids, phenols, and hippuric acid.[1582]

Yant, Schrenk, Sayers, Horvath, and Reinhart[1583] came to the conclusion that there was a distinct and rapid increase in the percentage of inorganic sulphates in the total sulphates in the urine of dogs subjected to a variety of conditions of exposure to benzene.

Urine Sulphate Test as a Measure of Benzene Exposure:* A

1581. JOACHIMOGLU: *Biochem. Ztschr.*, 70:93, 1915.

1582. JOST: *Arch. f. Gewerbepath. u. Gewerbehyg.*, 3:491, 1932.

1583. YANT, W. P., SCHRENK, H. H., SAYERS, R. R., HORVATH, A. A., and REINHART, W. H.: *J. Indust. Hyg. & Tox.*, 18:68, 1936.

* YANT, W. P., SCHRENK, H. H., and PATTY, F. A.: *J. Indust. Hyg.*, 18:349, 1936; SCHRENK, H. H., YANT, W. P., and SAYERS, R. R.: *J.A.M.A.*, 107:849, 1936; YANT, W. P., SCHRENK, H. H., SAYERS, R. R., HORVATH, A. A., and REINHART, W. H.: *J. Indust. Hyg. & Tox.*, 18:69, 1936.

valuable test for evidence of benzene absorption is to determine the urine sulphate ratio, or the amount of inorganic sulphates in the urine divided by the amount of total sulphates. A distinct decrease in the inorganic sulphates is a definite indication of benzene exposure and for the removal of the individual from the place of work. If the sulphates return to normal rapidly after removal from his work it indicates there was an exposure to benzene or to a substance that causes similar sulphate changes. The following table (Yant et al.) gives the percentage of inorganic of the total sulphates:

TABLE LIV

PER CENT OF INORGANIC OF TOTAL SULPHATES IN THE URINE
OF CONTROLS AND PLANT EMPLOYEES

Inorganic sulphates percent of total sulphates	Percent of total persons examined	
	Controls (33)*	Plant Employees (60)*
85-100	81.8	16.7
81- 84	18.2	20.0
70- 80	0.0	23.3
60- 69	0.0	20.0
50- 59	0.0	8.3
40- 49	0.0	8.3
30- 39	0.0	1.7
†24- 29	0.0	1.7

* Number of persons in group.
† Lowest value found.

The urine specimen should be taken after the individual has been working three to four days and should not be collected on Monday if employee is off on Sunday.

Method of Analysis of Urine Specimens:*

Inorganic Sulphates: 25 cc. of urine, 100 cc. of water and 10 cc. of dilute-hydrochloric acid (one part concentrated HCl and four parts water by volume) are measured into a 200- to 250-cc. Erlenmeyer flask. If the urine is dilute 100 cc. of urine are taken and 4 cc. of concentrated HCl are added. Twenty-five cc. of water may also be added. To the urine a 5% barium chloride solution is added slowly, drop by drop. The urine solution should not be shaken, stirred, or otherwise disturbed while the barium chloride is being added. The solution is allowed to stand an hour or longer, according to convenience, then shaken up and filtered through a Gooch crucible. The pre-

* *J. Indust. Hyg. & Tox.*, January, 1936.

cipitate is washed with about 250 cc. of cold water, dried, ignited and weighed.

Specimen for above test should be placed on ice immediately after voiding unless test is made at once. Barium chloride should be added within twenty-four hours. (Folin's Method.) The sulphuric acid of the conjugated sulphates is set free by boiling with acid. This has been known for many years to occur with phenol poisoning and probably occurs with poisoning by other chemicals having the benzene ring.

Total Sulphates: 25 cc. of urine and 20 cc. of dilute hydrochloric acid (one to four), or 100 cc. of dilute urine* and 8 cc. of concentrated HCl, are boiled gently in an Erlenmeyer flask (200 to 250 cc.) for twenty to thirty minutes. The mouth of the flask should be covered with a small watch glass to retard loss of steam during the boiling. The flask is cooled in running water for two or three minutes and the contents diluted to about 150 cc. with cold water. To this cold solution 10 cc. of 5% barium chloride are added and the procedure continued as described under "inorganic sulphates."

No. 42 Whatman filter paper may be substituted for a Gooch crucible.

Garilov described the colorimetric process for the determination of benzene in the air.[1584] The air is passed through a mixture of sulphuric acid and fuming nitric acid (four to one), thus forming nitrobenzol. Dilute the mixture, make slightly alkaline, extract with ether, and reduce to aniline by treating with sulphuric acid and zinc dust, similar to the method described above for identification of benzene in organs. Neutralize with sodium carbonate, and add an excess of tartaric acid and calcium oxychloride solution until a permanent rose-violet color results. Compare with colors produced from known quantities of benzene. The results are accurate to about 3%, and the method may be used to determine benzene in gasoline.

Gadaskin[1585] developed a method for quantitative determination of benzene in blood, in which nitration acids are added directly to the blood and dinitrobenzene extracted and reduced with stannous chloride and hydrochloric acid. The solu-

---

* A dilute specimen may be recognized by its weak color or by specific gravity test of less than 1.005.

1584. GARILOV, A. A.: *Chem. Abst.*, 26:3547, 1932.

1585. GADASKIN, I. D.: *Biochem. Ztschr.*, 198:149, 1928.

tion is neutralized and m-phenylenediamine extracted with
ethei. To the aqueous solution of m-phenylenediamine, hydrochloride is added and the mixture oxidized with perhydrol to
form neutral violet. The aqueous solution of this compound
imparts a violet color to cotton, which varies in intensity with
the amount of benzene present in the blood. Gadaskin finds
this method for the qualitative determination of benzene in
blood sensitive enough to detect concentrations of benzene in
blood lower than the lethal concentration.

Yant, Schrenk, and Mautz[1586] removed benzene by bubbling nitrogen through the acidified mixture of water and the
specimen of material until it was finally in a fluid state. The
nitrogen sweeps the benzene vapors through the water condenser into the absorption division which contains the nitration acids. The dinitrobenzene formed is determined according
to the Smyth modification[1587] of the Elliot and Dalton method[1588] for determining small amounts of benzene in air. This
method is much shorter than that of Joachimoglu[1589] described
above. It also removes sources of error due to loss of benzene
through the water condenser. The nitrogen which removes the
benzene prevents the oxidation of benzol to phenols in the presence of biologic material. Dinitrobenzene is identified by a
method similar to that given for the fructose test using levulose. This test gives an intense violet color after two minutes,
but the color gradually fades. This test is specific for o- and m-
dinitrobenzene which are formed in the nitration of benzene.
The method was developed by Chavassieu and Morel.[1590]

The alpha-naphthol test also was applied to the dinitrobenzene residue, as given above. This is more sensitive than the
levulose test, but is not specific for m-dinitrobenzene.

Cook and Ficklen[1591] described a method for the determination of benzene in air in which the trap for collection of benzene

1586. Yant, W. P., Schrenk, H. H., and Mautz, P. H.: Rept. of Investigations, Dept of Interior, U. S. Bureau of Mines, No. 3282, August,
1935.
1587. Smyth, H. F.: J. Indust. Hyg., 11:338, 1929.
1588. Elliot, S., and Dalton, J.: Analyst, 44:132, 1919.
1589. Joachimoglu: Biochem. Ztschr., 70:93, 1915.
1590. Chavassieu and Morel: Compt. rend. Acad. d. sc., 143:966,
1906.
1591. Cook, Warren A., and Ficklen, J. B.: J. Indust. Hyg., 17:41,
1935.

is immersed in a solid carbon dioxide acetone coating contained in a Dewar flask. The benzene, together with a small portion of less water-miscible solvents, is frozen out in the trap, to which are added 5 cc. of 0.5% ferrous sulphate solution, followed by 2 cc. of 1% hydrogen peroxide solution. The trap is removed, stoppered, and shaken, and the contents poured out into a test-tube. If benzene is present in the amount of .005 cc. a characteristic brown color is produced two to five minutes after the reagents have been added, and if 0.01 to 0.05 cc. is present, in addition to the brown color a black precipitate is formed. Upon the addition of 1 cc. of double normal nitric acid the black, amorphous precipitate will dissolve; dilute with water and compare with standards. The reaction is complicated, and the method does not lend itself to precision results. However, it is sufficiently quantitative to estimate the amount of benzene in air within the limits required in an industrial hygiene investigation.

Fulweiler and Barnes,[1592] state that one part of benzene in 50,000,000 parts of alcohol may be detected with the ultraviolet spectroscope. This, however, is only a qualitative method.

PHENYLHYDRAZINE ($C_6H_5.NH.NH_2$)

PHENYLHYDRAZINE has a molecular weight of 108.08, a melting point of 20°C., and a boiling point of 244°C.

Subcutaneous injections in animals produce a profound anemia.* Phenylhydrazine causes hyperplasia of the spleen and a slight hyperplasia of the leukoblastic elements of the bone-marrow, has no primary effect on the erythroblastic elements, the reticulocytes or the blood platelets, and produces its effects essentially by hemolysis of the mature red cells.

Intravenous and subcutaneous doses are very toxic. Fatty degeneration of the liver has been noted in animals after large intravenous doses. Phenylhydrazine is given in the treatment of polycythemia vera only. Jaundice has been noted when a dosage of 2.5 gm. had been reached, with an accompanying anorexia, nausea and sometimes vomiting, also irritability of the bladder and itching of the skin. Dermatitis, excessive

---

1592. FULWEILER, W. H., and BARNES, J.: *J. Franklin Inst.*, July, 1922.
* For a review of the literature up to 1932, see Benzol Poisoning by CAREY P. McCORD, published by the Industrial Health Conservancy Laboratories, Cincinnati, Ohio.

hemolysis with a severe secondary anemia and a tendency to thrombosis have also been reported.

Phenylhydrazine is given in 0.2 gm. (three grains) daily by mouth for three or four days; then the dosage is gradually decreased as the hemoglobin falls below 100.*

TRICHLORETHYLENE (C_2HCl_3)

TRICHLORETHYLENE is a chemical derived from ethylene by the replacement of three hydrogen atoms with chlorine. It is a heavy, colorless liquid which rapidly volatilizes at ordinary temperature to a colorless, heavy gas with a pleasing, faintly ethereal or chloroform-like odor. The liquid has a density at 15.6°C. of 1.474, thus indicating that it is one and a half times as heavy as water. It boils at 85 to 86.2°C., and freezes at —126.4°F. (—88°C.). Its molecular weight is 131.4. Its vapors are 4.4 times as heavy as air at normal temperature. Entrance into the human body is usually by inhalation, although it may occur through the skin, which will become seriously burned, followed by general toxic symptoms. Trichlorethylene is related chemically to chloroform, and has a similar narcotic as well as anesthetic action. Probably there is no cumulative action from small amounts, or it would be noticed in those using it day after day for trifacial neuralgia. However, there are serious chronic sequelae following acute attacks of poisoning. These may consist of anesthesia in the region supplied by the trigeminal nerve, distributed over the greater part of the face and mouth although Eichert** says he found no anesthesia of the area innervated by the trigeminal nerve. Of more consequence is the atrophy of the optic nerve leading to loss of vision with loss of the corneal reflex of the eye. The most dangerous result from this chemical is that it leads to addiction. It is reported that men working with it will not inform the foreman of any illness for fear of losing their positions, thereby losing the opportunity of inhaling this drug and experiencing the pleasing effects which make them feel at peace with the world. When sprayed in the Bunsen flame, the vapors burn with a luminous flame in the heated zone. When sprayed on burning cotton the flame is extinguished when the cotton

---

* BASTEDO: Materia Medica Pharmacology and Therapeutics, 4th ed., W. B. Saunders and Co., 1937.
** EICHERT, H.: *J.A.M.A.*, 106:1652, 1936.

becomes dampened with trichlorethylene. When small portions of trichlorethylene are thrown upon a red-hot plate, flashes of flame are seen around the heated zone. The ignition temperature has been found to be 410°C.

Trichlorethylene is rapidly advancing in use as an industrial solvent. It is used for the removal of oils and fats from almost any substance. While it is a chemical agent known for many years, it was not until the World War that it was brought into widespread use.

Stuber reported 284 cases of trichlorethylene poisoning, 202 of which were acute and eighty-two chronic.[1593] Of the total, twenty-five were fatal, and in seventeen of these there was a loss of consciousness. In some there were symptoms of drunkenness, or dullness and confusion; in others there were general nervous symptoms with nausea and vomiting. One of the cases who died was held to be a case of phosgene poisoning.

In its more extensive use in dry cleaning, a greater number of cases of poisoning by this chemical can be anticipated.

Welwart found that toxic gases were formed when a fresh lot of trichlorethylene washing compound was made by charging the kettle with the required amount of solid potassium hydroxide which, on coming in contact with a few liters of liquid left in the kettle from the last operation, formed a concentrated hot potassium hydroxide solution.[1594] This decomposed the trichlorethylene into formate, carbon monoxide, ethylene, and traces of dichloracetylene.

Willcox claims to have seen a case of jaundice from trichlorethylene.[1595] Muller investigated its toxic action and failed to obtain any fatty degeneration with dichlorethylene in an unsaturated body while it was readily obtained with chloroform, carbon tetrachloride, and tetrachlorethane.[1596] Joachimoglu, in 1927, failed to demonstrate fatty degeneration in animals in seven to twenty-four days by inhalation, feeding, and ingestion.[1597] Lehmann, in 1911, found that a cat exposed to 0.07% trichlorethylene for six hours a day for ten to seventeen

1593. STUBER, K.: Arch. f. Gewerbepath. u. Gewerbehyg., 2:398, 1931.

1594. WELWART: Seifensieder Ztg., 56:26, 1929; Chem. Abst., 23: 3361, 1929.

1595. WILLCOX, W.: Lancet, 1:57, 1931.

1596. MULLER, J.: Arch. f. exper. Path. u. Pharmakol., 109:276, 1925.

1597. JOACHIMOGLU, G.: Berl. klin Wchnschr., 58:147, 1921.

days showed a loss of weight and subsequent death, but there was no degeneration of the internal organs. Carrieu, in 1927,[1598] and Nebuloni, in 1929,[1599] found congestion of the lungs, spleen, liver, and kidneys, with some inflammation of tracheal mucosa, in animals killed with the vapors of trichlorethylene. Castellino, in 1932, showed slight degeneration in rabbits.[1600]

Taylor[1600-A] found that the concentration of pure ethylene in air of 0.5% and 0.4% trichlorethylene vapor produced deep anesthesia in rats, while 0.2% gave only slight effects. Taylor exposed two dogs and a number of rats for six months, exposure lasting six hours a day, five days a week. The dogs were given 0.2% trichlorethylene. A concentration of 0.3% proved too high, and only two of the original six rats survived six months. All of the other animals survived. The histological examination of the livers and kidneys showed no signs of any degeneration. There was a slightly greater tendency of alveolar collapse in the lungs in the experimental rats as compared with the controls. There was no consolidation or edema. This collapse is generally observable in laboratory rats, and it appears that there is no evidence that the collapse observed was due to trichlorethylene. The absence of liver and kidney injury after long-continued exposure to trichlorethylene vapor is the most striking result of the experimental work. The report of Taylor is of extreme interest since liver damage has been reported in human cases, while in the animal experiments the organs were quite normal.

The Underwriters' Laboratories report on trichlorethylene[1600-B] gives the results of exposure of animals to vapor in concentrations of 0.6% to 1.0% by volume (2.0 to 3.4 pounds per 1000 cubic feet). Two minutes after the beginning of a five-minute exposure the guinea pigs breathed irregularly, and they coughed and rubbed their noses. Four minutes after the start of the test the animals showed considerable lack of concentration. The animals recovered within a day of the test and appeared to be normal during the remainder of the observation period. In the thirty-minute exposure the animals appeared

1598. CARRIEU, M. F.: *Rev. d'hyg.*, 49:348, 1927; *Presse méd.*, 76: 1199, 1926.
1599. NEBULONI, D. A.: *Med. d. lavoro*, 20:205, 1929.
1600. CASTELLINO, N.: *Folia med.*, 18:415, 1932.
1600-A. TAYLOR, H.: *J. Indust. Hyg. & Tox.*, 18:175, 1936.
1600-B. Miscellaneous Hazard No. 494, May 2, 1933.

semi-conscious within twenty minutes after the start of the test and were lying on the floor of the cage. Three guinea pigs removed from the room at the end of thirty minutes after the start of the test were semi-conscious and showed violent trembling, especially in the legs. All the animals appeared normal within thirty minutes after they were exposed to air but were very lethargic and weak. They recovered within a day after the test. Practically the same observations were noted with animals exposed for one hour.

In the two-hour test the animals were able to walk and eat within thirty minutes after they were exposed to air, but were very weak. They made a complete recovery within a day following the test. Where concentrations of 2.0% to 2.3% (6.7 to 7.7 pounds per 1,000 cubic feet) were used, they found that the guinea pigs were unconscious at the end of a two-hour period and showed occasional weak twitching movements. Two of the animals died within twenty minutes without regaining consciousness. The other animal appeared very lethargic and weak on the day following the test and showed some difficulty in breathing.

One of the animals which died following exposure to trichlorethylene vapor-air mixture for two hours was autopsied. The lungs were found to be hyperemic in general, and contained innumerable petechial hemorrhages throughout. The upper left lobe was particularly filled with such hemorrhages. There was some edema. The cut sections did not produce any pussy exudate. The liver was hyperemic, but otherwise normal. The heart was engorged with dark clotted blood, but otherwise normal. The spleen was pale and yellowish in color and unusually soft. The stomach and intestines contained semi-fluid contents. The intestinal contents were slightly colored with blood. Upon opening the abdominal cavity, a definite hyperemia and moderate edema of all the viscera was noted.

Recovery from trichlorethylene anesthesia is generally complete, but vertigo and dizziness occur sometimes. Striker, Goldblatt, Warm, and Jackson[1601] have investigated the use of this drug as an anesthetic and found no harmful consequence in any of the 304 cases investigated. Kramer[1602] reported no

1601. STRIKER, C., GOLDBLATT, S., WARM, I. S., and JACKSON, D. E.: Anesth. & Analg., 14:68, 1935.

1602. KRAMER, J.: Berl. klin Wchnschr., 58:149, 1921.

harmful after effects in any of the attempts to use it in cases of trigeminal neuralgia.

On the other hand, Stuber, included, in her reports of chronic trichlorethylene poisoning, damage to the liver, kidneys, optic and trigeminal nerve, ductless glands, sex organs, the skin, and the central nervous system.[1603] Plessner reported injury to the trigeminus, and subsequent apoplexy, due to the specific action of trichlorethylene.[1604] Gerbis, in 1928,[1605] and Kalinowsky, in 1927[1606] have shown that the action was in all probability due to some impurity.

Reese, of Johns Hopkins Hospital, in a personal communication to the author, gave a history of a man who had worked with trichlorethylene for fourteen months, five and six days a week, from 7:30 in the morning until 6:00, and sometimes until 10:00 to 12:00 at night. The patient worked in a small room (about 8 x 10 feet) with one door and window. The window was kept closed to prevent fumes from blowing into the shop. The door was always open. A drum-like machine was used in which the clothes were saturated in the trichlorethylene for ten to twelve minutes. The clothes were then removed from this drum by hand after the "tri" had been drained from a hopper below. Removal of the clothes took from three to four minutes, during which time the patient caught the fumes from the clothes full in the face. This was repeated fifty to sixty times a day. The hands were often covered with the substance for a short period at a time, and if there was any sweating, burning was rather marked. The skin seemed to dry excessively, and often cracked. Each day or two filters in the machine (saturated in "tri") had to be removed and cleansed by hand. In this room an exhaust fan was used which worked from the floor. This was kept in constant operation. According to the patient, this fan kept the room, in general, free from the fumes, but did not prevent him from receiving a good dose of the fumes while removing the clothes from the cleaning machine. The patient presented himself for examination with the complaint of loss of vision for a period of six weeks. Examination revealed that

1603. Quoted by DHERS, V.: *Med. du Trav.*, 5:127, 1933.
1604. PLESSNER, W.: *Berl. klin. Wchnschr.*, 53:25, 1916.
1605. GERBIS, H.: *Zentralbl. f. Gewerbehyg.*, 15:97, 1928.
1606. KALINOWSKY, L.: *Ztschr. f. d. ges. Neurol. u. Psychiat.*, 110: 245, 1927.

he had a toxic amblyopia, with central scotoma in each eye and vision reduced to 20/100 and 4/200. This blind spot included the area from the center of fixation to the normal blind spot as is seen in many toxic amblyopias. Since the first examination the condition has progressed. Nothing else was found in the general examination. Complete blood and spinal fluid studies were negative, and a neurological examination revealed no positive findings. There was a moderate blepharitis with crusting at the base of the cilia, and slight hyperemia of the conjunctivae. The young man became entirely incapacitated, and is now working in the Maryland School for the Blind.

Dhers states that precautionary measures should be established where people come in contact with trichlorethylene. He suggests the wearing of overalls and gloves to protect the skin which becomes dry and eczematous. He also suggests periodic medical examinations to detect signs of absorption.[1607]

Christianson describes a patient who, during the course of two months, had developed symptoms suggesting a disturbance of the upper respiratory tract. This condition developed after the patient had worked for half an hour vigorously cleaning a pair of shoes with trichlorethylene. Recovery was delayed for five months.[1608] A similar intoxication is reported by Koch in 1931, and, according to this author, confirms his assertion that trichlorethylene has properties directly injurious to the lungs. Roholm reports four cases of acute trichlorethylene poisoning in Copenhagen factories in December 1932.[1609]

Persson reports two cases of chronic poisoning by trichlorethylene in which there was a neuromyelitic complex which had not been described before in connection with this kind of poisoning.[1610] The patients were two men employed at the same factory in cleaning machine parts in a bath of trichlorethylene before plating them. The bath gave off vapor freely, and, owing to inadequate ventilation, the vapor was inhaled by the men. During their work they became giddy and had a feeling of being drunk all day; their gait became staggering. They also complained of headache, nausea, loss of appetite, and

1607. DHERS, V.: *Med. du Trav.*, July, 1933, p. 127.
1608. CHRISTIANSON, T.: Abst., *J.A.M.A.*, 101:2090, 1933.
1609. ROHOLM, K.: Abst., *J.A.M.A.*, 101:2090, 1933.
1610. PERSSON, H.: Abst., *Acta med., skandinav.*, 1934; also in *Bull. Hyg.*, 10:364, 1935.

tremoı. After cessation of work for six months they improvea sufficiently to resume work. However, at this time there was still some paresthesia in the feet with stiffness in the legs.

Eichert reported two cases of addiction, one in a man, aged fifty-two, who took by inhalation four ounces over a period of two days, and the other in a woman of the same age who took six ounces of trichlorethylene over a period of several days.[1611]

Kunz and Isenschmid described a case in which a worker used trichlorethylene to dislodge diamond powder from a steel cylinder.[1612] He evaporated daily about 100 to 300 cc., and found that the operation made him sleepy. After half a year his acuity of vision was greatly reduced, and at the end of the year he had to stop work. There was a pupillary difference and no reaction to light. Both pupils showed considerable change. Abnormal conditions were also seen in other parts of the body.

Starkenstein[1613] reports a case of epileptoid seizures with psychic disturbances, and Stuber[1614] collected eleven instances of nervous sequelae, headache, dizziness, anorexia, and disturbed heart action. Long continued exposure to trichlorethylene has been responsible for lesions in two of the cranial nerves, the optic and the trigeminus.

Baader reports a case of a man who worked with trichlorethylene for five years and then began to complain of great weariness, sometimes a feeling of drunkenness, with occasional vomiting.[1615] Gradually, he lost weight, sexual libido, and sharpness of vision. Baader found malnutrition and anemia, the hemoglobin being only 60%. Examination of the eyes revealed retrobulbar neuritis with pallor on the temporal side. This man proved to be a trichlorethylene addict. Another case of Baader's had optic atrophy with blindness, and he mentions a similar case seen by Zangger.

Disturbances of vision have been reported by Axenfeld,[1616]

1611. EICHERT: *J.A.M.A.*, 106:1653, 1936.
1612. KUNZ, E., and ISENSCHMID, R.: *Klin. Montasbl. f. Augenh.*, 94:577, 1935.
1613. Quoted by STUBER.
1614. STUBER, K.: *Arch. f. Gewerbepath. u. Gewerbehyg.*, 2:398, 1931.
1615. BAADER, E. W.: *Zentralbl. f. Gewerbehyg.*, N.S. 4:385, 1927.
1616. Quoted by STUBER.

by Plessner[1617] and by Teleky.[1618] In some there was loss of color sense without visible changes in the eye grounds. Therefore, the use of trichlorethylene should be thought of by ophthalmologists when disturbances of the optic nerve are seen in men working with solvents.

Plessner reported four very unusual cases of poisoning, in which the symptoms came on after a day or even half a day of exposure, and consisted of complete paralysis of the sensory fibers of the fifth nerve with no motor paralysis or involvement of the other nerves in that region.[1619]

Kalinowsky reported a case where there was complete loss of sensation in the face, mouth, and nose, with no motor paralysis, but with difficulty in speech and mastication, which seemed to be caused by loss of sensation.[1620] There was also a painless keratitis without photophobia. The second case reported by this author had like symptoms but not as severe, no loss of teeth and very slight keratitis. Here also sensory paralysis was permanent. There has been some doubt cast on Kalinowsky's cases, as chemical examination failed to show the presence of di-, tri-, or tetrachlorethylene.

As a solvent, trichlorethylene is among the most efficient known, and has very widespread uses in a large variety of industries. It will remove oils, fats, tar substances, waxes, gums, and resins very rapidly from metal, wool, silk, textiles, cottons, and leather without damage to them. It is used in the extraction of caffeine from coffee, and nicotine from tobacco. It serves in the removal of oil from olives, cocoa, maize, cottonseed, linseed, soy beans, and sugar mud, as well as in the extraction of grease from garbage, tankage, leather, and bones. As an insecticide, trichlorethylene destroys grape lice, and larvae of mosquitoes, as well as many other insects.

In arriving at a diagnosis of trichlorethylene poisoning, one must take into consideration the occupational history; also that damage to the optic nerve may be caused by many other conditions. For instance, it is reported that about 33.7% of such damage is due to locomotor ataxia, tabes—a common variety of syphilis; it is also seen in paresis. Therefore, care-

1617. PLESSNER: Berl. klin. Wchnschr, 33:25, 1916.
1618. Quoted by STUBER.
1619. PLESSNER: Berl. klin. Wchnschr., 33:25, 1916.
1620. KALINOWSKY, L.: Ztschr. f. d. ges. Neurol. u. Psychiat., 110: 245, 1927.

ful examination, including spinal fluid and blood examinations, should be made to determine the presence of this disease. The entire group of scleroses within the central nervous system presents frequent causative factors in the production of optic atrophy where there is destruction of various nerve areas with replacement by scar tissue. Chronic myelitis, inflammation of the spinal cord from any cause, sometimes is accompanied by destruction of the optic nerve. Fracture of the skull and heavy blows to the skull will lead to this condition. Focal infection from any source, and any other inflammatory process of this structure, will lead to damage very difficult to differentiate from that of trichlorethylene poisoning. Many intoxications caused by poisons other than trichlorethylene are followed by blindness due to the same type of nerve destruction. Certain of these may be used by the patient, either as medication or during his work. Many of the medicaments are sold in patent medicines. Filix mass, or male fern, used in the treatment of tapeworm, and quinine, serve as examples. Wood alcohol is found in some poisonous liquor. Atoxyl is used in the treatment of psoriasis, lichen planus, and many other skin diseases; this agent, containing 37% arsenic, will sometimes produce most serious optic atrophy. Nicotine, taken directly through accident or sometimes by excessive smoking, leads to serious loss of vision. Lead poisoning may be at fault, chronic malaria, diabetes, severe hemorrhages, and arteriosclerosis produce optic atrophy.

Fatal Dose: The relative toxicity of trichlorethylene as compared to chloroform is 1.7. McCord[1621] believes that 10,000 parts to 1,000,000 parts of air is definitely narcotic to man. In his study with rabbits, death occurred in two hours with concentrations of 20,000 parts of trichlorethylene to 1,000,000 parts of air; in two and a half hours with concentrations of 10,000 parts to 1,000,000; in fourteen to twenty-eight hours with concentrations of 5,000 parts per 1,000,000; in twenty-eight to forty-one hours with concentrations of 1,000 parts per 1,000,000; and in nineteen days there was one death with 500 parts per 1,000,000. New and Nonofficial Remedies gives the dose for use in the relief of facial neuralgia as fifteen drops by inhalation, repeated in a few minutes if necessary, with a limit of sixty drops in any twenty-four hours.

1621. McCord, Carey P.: *J.A.M.A.*, 99, 1932.

Inhalation of the vapor may be easily prevented by downward ventilation, since the vapor is about 4.4 times as heavy as air. Also a downward ventilation will reduce the amount inhaled practically to a minimum. Closed systems of dry cleaning and degreasing should be employed wherever practical.

Henderson and Haggard give the relative toxicity of a number of chlorinated hydrocarbons in comparison with carbon tetrachloride, as shown in the following table, taken from their book:[1622]

TABLE LV

RELATIVE LETHAL CONCENTRATIONS BY VOLUME IN
AIR, IF TOXICITY OF $CCl_4 = 1$

(Table arranged in ascending order of toxicity)

Methyl Chloride	CH_3Cl*	0.6
Tetrachlormethane (Carbon Tetrachloride)	CCl_4	1.0
Trichlormethane (Chloroform)	$CHCl_3$	2.2
Perchlorethylene	C_2Cl_4**	1.6
Trichlorethylene	C_2HCl_3**	1.7
Dichlorethylene	$C_2H_2Cl_2$	1.7
Pentachlorethane	C_2HCl_5**	6.2
Tetrachlorethane	$C_2H_2Cl_4$**	9.1

* WALLER, A. D.: *J.A.M.A.*, 53:9, 1919.

** HERRMANN, G.: Inaugural Dissertation; Wurzburg, C. Fuchs, 1911.

Tschentke gives the chemical examination of trichlorethylene for anesthesia.[1623]

Postmortem Appearances: An account of a postmortem by Vallee and Leclerq[1624] is vitiated by the fact that the victim suffered from a long standing liver disease. In a postmortem seen by Taylor the only effect was congestion of the viscera due to narcotic properties. Taylor has also done experimental work in trichlorethylene poisoning in rats, and histological examination of the livers, kidneys, lungs, tracheas, hearts, spleens, brains, and femurs of the rats showed no signs of any degeneration. These animals had been exposed to concentrations of 0.5% and 0.4% trichlorethylene vapor in the air. Strassmann reported a case of a boy who died after inhaling trichlorethylene vapor. Postmortem showed no characteristic findings, grossly.[1625]

1622. In their book "Noxious Gases," Monograph No. 35, 1927.
1623. TSCHENTKE, H. L.: *J. Indust. & Eng. Chem.*, 26:21, 1934.
1624. Quoted by TAYLOR, H.: *J. Indust Hyg. & Tox.*, 18:175, 1936.
1625. STRASSMANN, F.: *Aerztl. Sachverst.-Ztg., Berl.*, 37:51, 1931.

Tests: 1. Vitali's test gives a green flame when air contains trichlorethylene, similar to other chlorinated hydrocarbons.

2. The quantitative examination of the air can be conducted the same as given under Methyl Chloride (see page 438).

3. Obtain the boiling point if liquid is submitted. Trichlorethylene boils at 85 to 86.2°C. Its specific gravity is 1.474 at 15.6°C.

Treatment: Give inhalations of oxygen. For treatment of inhalation of decomposition products, such as hydrochloric

TABLE LVI

TOXICITY OF COMMON SOLVENTS

Solvent	Rapidly Fatal for Short Exposure P.P.M.	Maximum Amount That Can Be Inhaled for One Hour Without Serious Disturbances P.P.M.	Noxiousness Impossible to Breathe Several Minutes P.P.M.	Lethal Dose Cats Thirty Minutes P.P.M.	Lethal Dose Man Thirty Minutes P.P.M.
Carbon Disulphide			33000 (4)	33000 (4)	500–1000 (2)
Carbon Tetrachloride		4000–6300 (2)		63000 (2) (3)	48000–63000 (2)　(1)
Chloroform		5100–6200 (2)		25000 (2) (3)	
Pentachlorethane				44000 (2) (3)	
Gasoline	24300 (1)	4300–71 (2)	17000		
Dichlorethylene				9600 (2) (3)	
Perchlorethylene				31000 (2) (3)	
Tetrachlorethane				7300 (2) (3)	
Trichlorethylene				37000 (2) (3)	

1. U. S. Dept. of Interior, Bureau of Mines Technical Paper, 272, 1921.

2. HERRMANN, G.: Inaugural Dissertation; Wurzburg, C. Fuchs, 1911.

3. LEHMANN, K. B.: *Arch. f' hyg.*, 84:1, 1911.

4. Table taken from Publication of the National Safety Council Health Practices, Pamphlet No. 9; KOBERT: Kompendium der Toxikologie, 5th ed., Stuttgart, 45, 1912.

acid, chlorine, and phosgene, give intravenous injections of salyrgan and glucose.

CHLOROPRENE (2-CHLORO-BUTADIENE)

VON OETTINGEN, Hueper, Deichmann-Gruebler, and Wiley[1626] report that this substance is used extensively in chemical industries, it being the starting material for the synthetic rubber DuPrene. It is a colorless liquid of pungent odor, insoluble in water and pharmacologically inactive solvent. It polymerizes at moderately elevated temperatures with the formation of semi-solid particles. Experiments indicate that chloroprene is a toxic material which should be handled with the greatest precaution. The inhalation of vapors as low as 0.3 mg. per liter may cause toxic symptoms. With regard to the early detection of an incipient poisoning, the icteric index of the blood should be determined at intervals, and the urine should be tested for albumin, reducing substances, and bile pigments. Low blood pressure should be considered as an indication of possible incipient poisonings, as should also complaints of loss of appetite, indigestion, and catarrhal conditions of the respiratory tract.

Von Oettingen and Deichmann-Gruebler[1627] found that, in experiments with DuPrene in rubber sheeting, it was not liable to cause irritation of the skin or to liberate odorous or toxic gases at temperatures up to 75°C.

TETRAETHYL LEAD

TETRAETHYL was discovered by Löwig in 1852.[1628] By the term "tetraethyl" is meant the chemical substance, $Pb(C_2H_5)_4$, of a commercial grade of purity or higher. Tetraethyl lead is a colorless oily liquid, (specific gravity 1.659), with a sweetish odor. It has an appreciable vapor pressure at ordinary temperatures, one liter of air at usual temperatures containing 5 mg. of the material when saturated. It is miscible with fats and oils, insoluble in water, and soluble in alcohol and acetone.

Although it has been known for about three-quarters of a

1626. von Oettingen, W. F., Hueper, W. C., Deichmann-Gruebler, W., and Wiley, F. H.: *J. Indust. Hyg. & Tox.*, 18:240, 1936.

1627. von Oettingen, W. F., and Deichmann-Gruebler, W.: *J. Indust. Hyg. & Tox.*, 18:271, 1936.

1628. Löwig, C.: *J. prakt. Chem.*, 60:304, 1853.

century, no cases were reported in the literature until October, 1924, when Eldredge[1629] referred to a series reported to him by Thompson and Schoenleber. A total of 138 cases were included in their series, comprising forty-nine cases seen by Kehoe, in Dayton, Ohio, and seventy-one in Bayway, New Jersey, the remainder of the cases being in Deepwater, New Jersey. In July, 1925, Kehoe[1630] reported a series of non-fatal cases which were of a milder form.

* The effect of tetraethyl lead differs markedly from that of other compounds of lead because it is more rapidly absorbed and more soluble in fats, which properties lead to its concentration in the central nervous system and in the liver. Norris and Gettler[1631] reported the results of necropsy and the chemical examination of four cases. Reynolds[1632] reported a case of tetraethyl lead exposure of three weeks' duration. At the time of examination the patient presented a Parkinsonian syndrome, with mental lethargy which had developed gradually after the termination of the period of exposure. Kehoe reported the toxicity of tetraethyl to be a function of its lead content rather than a characteristic of the compound. Buck and Kumro[1633] found the minimum lethal dose for tetramethyl lead to be from 70 to 100 mg. per kilogram for rats when administered intraperitoneally, as compared with 10 mg. per kilogram for tetraethyl lead, and from 2 to 3 mg. per kilogram for tributyl and tripropyl lead chloride. The tetraethyl and tetramethyl lead were administered in solution in olive oil, while the trialkyl lead compounds were administered in a dilute alcoholic solution. The absorption was much slower in olive oil, thus making it difficult to have comparable results. The first three types of compounds behaved similarly in producing plumbism, and the trialkyl and tetra-alkyl salts were again similar but differed from the first three in their tendency to produce encephalopathy.

1629. ELDREDGE, W. A.: A Study of the Toxicity of Lead Tetra-Ethyl, Chemical War Service, Edgewood Arsenal, Med. Research Div., Report 29, October 5, 1924.

1630. KEHOE, R. A.: Tetraethyl Lead Poisoning: Clinical Analysis of a Series of Non-fatal Cases, J.A.M.A., 85:108, 1925.

1631. NORRIS, CHARLES, and GETTLER, A. O.: J.A.M.A., 85:818, September 12, 1925.

1632. REYNOLDS, P. E.: U. S. Vet. Bur. M. Bull., 5:147, February, 1928.

1633. BUCK, J. S., and KUMRO, D. M.: Toxicity of Lead Compounds, P. Pharmacol. & Exper. Therap., 38:161, 1930.

Poisoning in man may take place through skin absorption or through inhalation. Machle[1634] has given comparisons of the tetraethyl and trialkyl compounds as follows: "The process of absorption of tetraethyl lead is not usually accompanied with any symptoms except, perhaps, a degree of nausea due to the sweetish odor of the compound. Exposure to and absorption of trialkyl compounds of lead, on the other hand, are associated with a marked degree of irritation of serous and mucous membranes. In either event the onset of symptoms of intoxication is delayed somewhat, usually for from one to three hours in the case of tetraethyl lead, somewhat less in the case of triethyl lead salts. As is the case with many other general poisons, the interval between exposure and the onset of symptoms varies inversely with the dose; a person in whom well marked symptoms have developed within an hour after exposure may be assumed to have had a more significant exposure than another patient in whom no definite illness develops until four or even twelve hours have elasped. This delay in onset of symptoms is the result of at least two factors: (1) the decomposition of lead within the body with the liberation of water-soluble lead compounds, and (2) the delayed absorption from either the pulmonary epithelium or the skin. Delayed absorption from the enteric tract may also occur, but this is less likely to happen because of vomiting and purgation."

Symptoms: Severe, acute symptoms are preceded by a prodromal period varying from eighteen hours to eight days. In one case, reported by Machle, the symptoms first developed ten to twelve hours after exposure; moderate definite symptoms were manifested for eleven days, and then mania developed, thus constituting the longest interval between exposure and the onset of severe symptoms seen among these patients. "The stimulation of the central nervous system results in insomnia, which is uniformly present; sleep is difficult, broken and restless, and wild and terrifying dreams are constant. During the waking state, pallor and an anxious expression are usually seen; the patient is irritable and nervous and may give evidence of delusional interpretations or a depressive mood, or his state may stimulate an anxiety neurosis. Mental excitement may be marked, headache is usual and often severe, and

1634. MACHLE, W. F.: *J.A.M.A.*, 8:105, 1935.

vertigo is frequent." Anorexia, nausea and vomiting, or gastric disturbance, were the most constant symptoms attributable to the gastro-enteric tract, tending to be marked in the mornings, and customary in usual lead poisoning. Diarrhea occurred more often than constipation, although neither disturbance was regular or frequent. A metallic taste was complained of by many.

The systolic and the diastolic blood pressures are lowered, falling in some cases as low as 80 and 40. The average systolic pressure of Machle's series was 104. Symptoms similar to chronic lead poisoning were reported. Weakness, tremor, muscular pains, and ease of fatigue were regular and frequent symptoms. A subnormal temperature is a customary observation; the morning temperature is as low as 96°F. Complete recovery is from two to three weeks. Kehoe found, even in his moderately severe cases, that all symptoms had disappeared in six to ten weeks. Norris and Gettler[1635] reported visual and auditory disturbances, hallucinations, delirium, insomnia, and anemia.

Postmortem: Specific changes in the organs from tetraethyl lead poisoning are not seen. The autopsy reveals a generalized visceral congestion with slight parenchymatous degeneration, intense pulmonary congestion with edema and bronchial pneumonia, and peculiar yellowish discolorations of the skin and cortex of the brain. There were hemorrhagic foci in the bone marrow of the femur, and a slight degree of chronic leptomeningitis was noted with moderate cerebral congestion. The lungs resembled an appearance that is encountered in malignant influenza. The changes in the liver and kidneys, as in the heart, pancreas, adrenals and other organs, represent a more or less uniform type of response to a general noxious agent and cannot be considered a picture of tetraethyl lead poisoning.

Tests: Gettler isolated tetraethyl lead in the volatile distillate and estimated the lead, using the Fairhall method. In one case examined by Gettler, he found the amounts of lead shown in Table LVII.

The organs were digested and heated the same as in the Fairhall ashing method. The lead was precipitated by hydrogen sulphide, then converted to the sulphate and weighed as such.

1635. NORRIS, CHARLES, and GETTLER, A. O.: *J.A.M.A.*, 85:818, 1925.

TABLE LVII
LEAD FOUND IN ORGANS

Organ	Weight in Gm.	Weight Used in Gm.	Lead Found in Mg.	Total Mg. Found in Organ
Brain	1,250	250	4.78	23.90
Bone (vert.)	8,840	285	1.284	39.83
Blood	3,070	30	0.027	2.76
Lungs	1,540	250	1.09	6.71
Liver	1,400	250	8.54	47.82
Kidney	340	120	1.23	3.48

On May 20, 1925, a conference, called by the Surgeon General of the Public Health Service, met to consider the possible health hazards from the manufacture, distribution and the use of this compound as a substance to be added to gasoline.[1636] The committee reported that no menace to the public had been revealed, and that the risk to garage workers was far less than that present in some lead industries.

Treatment: If tetraethyl lead is splashed on the skin, it should be removed immediately by kerosene followed by tincture of green soap. The treatment, otherwise, is the same as for lead poisoning previously given: alkalinization by sodium bicarbonate, intravenous injections of calcium gluconate, the administration of bromides—instead of opium—and chloral for the delirium that is seen in these cases (see pages 154 et seq.).

NAPHTHALENE
(Molecular Weight 128.06)

NAPHTHALENE, $C_{10}H_8$, is a white crystalline mass, insoluble in alcohol, chloroform, ether, and oils. It melts at 80°C. (176° F.), and boils at 217.2° C. (422.96° F.). Poisoning has resulted from the inhalation of its vapors by individuals sleeping under bed-clothing that had been dusted with naphthalene as a moth powder.

The symptoms following the inhalation are headache, nausea, vomiting, profuse perspiration, neuritis optica, hematuria, and slight edema. Several cases of poisoning are reported in children who had eaten moth balls containing naphthalene.[1637] Poisoning has been reported from its application to open

1636. Public Health Bull. 163, Treasury Dept., U. S. Public Health Service, Washington, 1926.

1637. ZANGERLE: *Therap. Monatsh., Berl.,* 13:122, 1899; NASH: *Brit. M. J.,* 1:251, 1903.

wounds,[1638] and in persons to whom it had been administered as a vermifuge, or as an intestinal antiseptic in typhoid fever. When taken by mouth there is gastric irritation with vomiting and abdominal pain, a burning sensation in the urethra, pain in the bladder and kidney region, and occasionally strangury. The urine may be dark due to the presence of oxidation products of the drug, albumin and hemoglobin may be found in the urine. Acute nephritis and jaundice have been reported.

Poisonings have occurred from the chlorinated naphthalenes, as perchlor-naphthalene. It is produced as a substitute for resins, and rubber, and for the impregnation of textiles and insulating material. It is poisonous when inhaled, causing headache and a feeling of weakness, with uncertain gait. On the skin it causes folliculitis, similar to that seen in chlorine acne.

Of the hydrogenated naphthalenes, tetra- and deca- hydronaphthalene (tetraline, $C_{10}H_{12}$, and decaline, $C_{10}H_{18}$) are useful solvents for resins and fats. When used industrially, or in newly painted and polished rooms, they may produce headache, nausea, vomiting and irritation of the conjunctiva and of the mucous membranes of the nose and throat. Inhalation of tetralin leads to the excretion of an extraordinary grass-green urine, owing to the oxidation of the tetraline to tetralol.[1639]

No cases of general poisoning have been reported from anthracene, $C_{14}H_{10}$, or with phenanthrene. Anthraquinone, $C_{14}H_8O_2$, and alizarin, $C_{14}H_8O_4$, have caused acute cases of poisoning.

ACRIDINE
(Molecular Weight 179.08)

ACRIDINE, $C_{13}H_9N$, forms colorless crystalline needles. Its melting point is 107°C.; its boiling point 346°C. Its salts show a greenish-blue fluorescence. Injurious effects are occasionally seen when it is used industrially either in solid form or as a vapor. The symptoms consist of violent burning and itching, and sometimes inflammatory swelling of the skin and mucous membrane. Acridine is regarded as the effective irritating principle in tar, creosote, pitch, etc., which sensitize the skin to light.

Road tars, or the residues after coal tar distillation, find

1638. FRONMÜLLER: Memorabilien, 5:257, 1883.
1639. LESCHKE, E.: Clin. Tox., 236, 1934.

useful application as road construction materials. The chemical composition of road tar is very complex.[1640] Road tars retain small and variable amounts of many of the substances supposedly extruded under the influence of heat at lower temperatures. A coal tar from which all benzene has been distilled is a result of decomposition of other compounds, such as cyclohexanes, which on being heated break up into hydrogen and benzene. Road tars may contain a high content of benzene, and benzene poisoning may result from its handling. McCord states that there is no clinical picture of road tar poisoning. A case of road tar poisoning recently presented itself in which there were signs suggestive of the convulsions of phenol, at a later time the pulmonary edema of anthracene, and still later hemorrhages suggestive of benzene. McCord reports the case of a man thirty years of age, engaged in highway construction, who was poisoned by fumes emanating from the shut-off valve of a tank which had been opened earlier in the day. He became violently ill with convulsive seizures, and was taken to a hospital. On the seventh day he developed a severe hemorrhage. Six weeks later he presented a case of acute nephritis, with some blood in the urine during this period. Following this condition of multiple hemorrhage, nephritis, anemia, and wasting persisted until the man became neurasthenic and hysterical. He developed paralysis of the right leg and hemorrhagic lesions in the spinal cord.

Production of carcinoma in the various internal organs after application of tar has been reported as follows:

In rabbits, carcinoma of the breast[1641] in thirty-three months; of the stomach and intestines[1642] in two weeks; and of the rectum.[1643]

In rats, carcinoma of the bladder[1644] in one hundred and fifteen days; of the stomach[1645] in three hundred and forty-one days; and of the uterus[1646] in two hundred and forty-two days.

1640. McCord, Carey P.: J.A.M.A., 92:695, 1929.
1641. Yamagiwa, K., and Ichikawa, K.: J.A.M.A., 73:298, 1919.
1642. Ishibashi, M., and Ohtani, S.: Gann, Ergebn. d. Krebforsch. in Japan, Tokyo, 15:2, 1921.
1643. Leitch, A.: Compt. rend. Cong. du. Cancer, 39, 1923.
1644. Maisin, J., and Picard, E.: Compt. rend. Soc. de biol., 91:799, 1924.
1645. Menetrier, P.: Bull. de l'Ass. franc. p. l'étude du Cancer, Par., 13:563, 1924.
1646. Teutschlaender, M.: Ztschr. f. Krebsforsch., 23:161,1926.

In guinea pigs, carcinoma of the gall-bladder[1647] in from five and one-half to twelve months.

Woglom[1648] has given a very comprehensive review of the literature dealing with the production of tar carcinoma.[1649]

The author[1650] investigated the amount of tarry residue in thirty brands of cigarettes, and found the residue varied between 4.84% and 15.29%. The investigation was carried on with the idea of throwing some light on the increase of cancer of the tongue, larynx, pharynx, and lung, as the increase in cancer has been parallel to the increased consumption of tobacco. For instance, in 1905 the number of small cigarettes manufactured in America was 3,673,727,411; in 1930 it was 123,809,553,142, and in 1934 the total reached 125,699,859,298. Comparing these figures with the increase in cancer one is certainly led to believe that cigarette smoking is an important factor in causing cancer of the lung. In England during the period 1901-1910 the death rate was one per 100,000, increasing to 2.3 per 100,000 in 1927.

DIHYDROXYBENZENES

THE DIHYDROXYBENZENES, $C_6H_4(OH)_2$, pyrocatechol (pyrocatechin), resorcinol, and hydroquinol, have caused a few cases of poisoning in people sensitive to these drugs, or where they are used in excess.

Guaiacol (methyl-pyrocatechol) has caused severe poisoning and death.[1651] Most of the cases of poisoning have been caused (as previously mentioned with the dihydroxybenzenes) by prolonged use both internally and externally in the treatment of bronchitis and tuberculosis. The symptoms are irritation of the alimentary tract, loss of consciousness, fall of temperature, and collapse. Haenelt[1652] reported the death of a child from the application of 5% resorcinol in vaseline. The child died on the third day. Postmortem showed boggy lung, hemorrhages from the pleura and pericardium. The spleen was large, and all the organs were congested. The blood show-

1647. LEITCH, A.: *Brit. M. J.*, 2:451, 1924; KAZAMA, Y.: *Gann, Ergebn. d. Krebforsch. in Japan, Tokyo,* 16:14, 1922; *Japan M. World,* 4:277, 1924.

1648. WOGLOM, W. H.: *Arch. Path.*, 2:533 and 709, 1926.

1649. SIMONDS, J. P., and CURTIS, J. S.: *Arch. Path.*, 19:287, 1935.

1650. McNALLY, W. D.: *Am. J. Cancer*, 16:6, 1932.

1651. WYSS: *Deutsche med. Wchnschr.*, 20:296, 321, 1894.

1652. HAENELT, VON MARIE: *München. med. Wchnschr.*, 72:386, 1925.

ed methemoglobin and bilirubin 2.8%, hemoglobin 53%, and red cells 2,900,000.

CREOSOTE

CREOSOTE is a mixture of phenols obtained from wood tar. The U. S. P., XI, gives it as an almost colorless or yellowish, highly refractive, oily liquid, having a penetrating, smoky odor, and a burning caustic taste. It does not readily become brown on exposure to light. Creosote is inflammable, and burns with a luminous, smoky flame. About two drams (7.4 cc.) caused the death of an adult woman in thirty-six hours, while another patient recovered after drinking six drams, (22.2 cc.). The chief ingredients are guaiacol, pyrocatechin methyl ester $(C_6H_4(OCH_3)(OH)$, creosol $C_6H_3(CH_3)(OCH_3)(OH)$ methyl homopyrocatechin) and phloral (methyl creosol). For detecting carbolic acid in creosote Flückiger[1653] suggests mixing an aqueous solution of the sample with one-fourth its volume of ammonium hydroxide, wetting the inside of a porcelain dish with this solution, and carefully blowing bromine fumes onto the surface. A blue color appears if carbolic acid is present. If the sample contains only creosote, then the color is a dirty green or brown. An excess of bromine spoils the reaction. Cookson[1654] reports a case of a man sixty-eight years old who had worked for thirty-five years in a creosote factory, who developed a large fungating ulcer on the dorsum of the hand. Postmortem showed the organs healthy except for small epitheliomatous depositions in both lungs, both kidneys and the liver and two in the heart walls.

PYROGALLOL ($C_6H_6O_3$)
(Molecular Weight 126.05)

PYROGALLOL occurs as light, white or nearly white, odorless leaflets or fine needles. It is used in the form of an ointment in the treatment of disease, especially of psoriasis; it is also used in photography, in hair dyes, marking inks, etc. It is readily absorbed by the skin in the treatment of skin diseases, and in this manner has caused a few cases of poisoning.[1655] Pyrogallol melts between 130° and 133° C.

1653. FLÜCKIGER: Arch. d. Pharm., 113:30.
1654. COOKSON, H. A.: Brit. M. J., 1:368, 1924.
1655. NEISSER: Ztschr. f. klin. Med., Berl., 1:88, 1880; VOLLMAR: Ztschr. f. Med.-Beamte, Berl., 9:68, 1896.

The chief symptoms of poisoning by pyrogallol result from its effect upon the red blood-corpuscles; the latter become shrunken and lose their hemoglobin. The hemoglobin is converted into methemoglobin, and the blood assumes a reddish-brown color. Icterus may follow, and the decomposition products of the red corpuscles cause nephritis with the appearance of albumen, epithelial cells, and blood in the urine; or the nephritis may lead to uremia. These blood changes lead to headache, cyanosis, chills, vomiting, diarrhea, and strangury; the pulse becomes small, and the urine assumes a dark brown color due to the presence of oxidation products of the poison and of blood-pigment. In fatal cases the cyanosis becomes intense, tremors develop, and death occurs in a state of collapse.

The fatal dose is not known, but the application of 75 grains contained in 3.5 ounces of ointment is said to have been fatal. Recovery is reported from one dram of pyrogallic acid taken internally. Smith[1656] reported the death of a man who drank a quantity of alcohol containing about 250 grains of pyrogallol and died five days later from nephritis.

Treatment consists in removing the poison from the skin, and, if it has been taken by mouth, the washing out of the stomach. Methods to protect the kidneys should be instituted. Inhalations of oxygen have been used with some benefit.

Postmortem Appearances: If this substance has been applied to the skin, the point of application will be dark because of its great avidity for oxygen. The kidneys become enlarged and black; the pelvis of the kidneys, the ureters, and the bladder may contain a bloody liquid.

CRESOL

CRESOL is a mixture of three isomeric cresols obtained from coal tar. The preparation is stated to contain 35% orthocresol, 40% metacresol, and 25% paracresol. Of the three cresols the meta compound is less poisonous to mammals than phenol, the ortho is more poisonous than phenol, and the para still more so.[1657] Hale found tricresol to be about 0.9 as toxic as phenol.[1658]

1656. SMITH: *Pacific M. J.*, 34:456, 1891.
1657. WANDEL: *Arch. f. exper. Path. u. Pharmakol.*, 56:161, 1907.
1658. HALE: Bull. 88, Hyg. Lab., U. S. Pub. Health Service, 1913.

The symptoms are the same as those given under phenol (page 810).

Cresol is sold in the form of a suspension in water with soap. The liquor cresolic compositus of the U. S. P. is such a preparation; it is similar to the proprietary preparation "Lysol." Death has occurred from its use by suicides. However, for that purpose it has been replaced by the barbituric acid series. The Coroner's Office of Cook County in 1935 reported twenty-three deaths due to lysol. In 1936 there were 16 deaths due to lysol, 7 due to phenol. Of the 250 cases of poisoning reported in the Apotheker Zeitung for the years 1925-27, 10.8% were due to lysol.[1659]

Lysol is a clear, brown, oily fluid. It is composed of coal-tar cresols and soap solution. It is soluble in equal volumes of alcohol, ether, chloroform, and benzene. Lysol is excreted in the urine in the form of phenyl-glycuronic acid, sometimes in such amounts as to form glancing crystals. Lysol causes both local and general symptoms similar to those caused by carbolic acid, but the action on the intestine, kidney, and skin is even stronger. It boils between 198° and 203° C. (388.4° and 397.4° F.). At ordinary temperature the commercial cresol is a liquid containing all three cresols. It is insoluble in small quantities of 6% soda solution; with a large excess it forms crystalline scales, while carbolic acid is freely soluble in small or large quantities of alkaline solution. Bromin converts cresol into tribrom-cresol, but this is a liquid at ordinary temperatures, while tribrom-phenol is a solid. Ferric chloride gives a similar reaction as with phenol.

Fatal Period is the same as given under phenol.

Fatal Dose: Death occurred from the taking of one-half ounce of the poison, a physician being called a half hour after the ingestion. Recovery occurred in one case with prompt treatment following the ingestion of four ounces.

THYMOL

THYMOL, $C_{10}H_{14}O$, occurring in colorless crystals, often large, has a molecular weight of 150.11. It has an aromatic thyme-like odor and a pungent taste. One gm. of thymol is soluble in about 1,000 cc. of water, in about 1 cc. of alcohol, in 0.7 cc. of chloroform, in 1.5 cc. of ether, and in 1.7 cc. of olive

1659. LESCHKE: Clinical Toxicology, 261, 1934.

oil, at 25° C. It melts between 48° and 51° C. It is found in mouthwashes, toothpastes, and numerous patent medicines used for the treatment of colds. It is used extensively as an anthelmintic, especially in hookworm infections. In poisoning in man there are nausea, vomiting, depression, headache, confusion, and roaring in the ears, giddiness, and collapse. Severe symptoms have followed the taking of forty grains of thymol in ten-grain doses per hour, in a child four years of age.[1660] Sixty grains are said to have caused convulsions in a child of eight, and six gm. are said to have caused the death of an anemic individual.

Isolation: Thymol can be removed by distillation, the distillate being extracted with chloroform. The chloroform layer after evaporation leaves a residue of thymol. The thymol can be identified by its melting point. Thymol dissolved in glacial acetic acid and mixed with an equal volume of sulphuric acid, and slightly warmed, develops a violet-red color.

NAPHTHOL

TWO naphthols, the alpha- and beta- compounds may be made from naphthalene, as they bear the same relation to naphthalene that phenol does to benzene. The beta- compound has been used in medicine as an external application in various skin diseases, especially in scabies, and internally as an intestinal disinfectant and anthelmintic.

Beta-naphthol, $C_{10}H_8O$, has a molecular weight of 144.06. It occurs as pale, buff-colored, shining crystalline leaflets, or a white or yellowish-white, crystalline powder. It has a faint phenol-like odor, and is stable in air. One gram of betanaphthol is soluble in about 1,000 cc. of water, in 0.8 cc. of alcohol, in 17 cc. of chloroform, and in 1.3 cc. of ether, at 25° C. It sublimes readily when heated, and volatilizes with the vapors of alcohol and water. It melts between 120° and 122°C. (U. S. P., XI.)

Its physiological action is similar to that of phenol, but it is a more powerful antiseptic. It is readily absorbed through skin, and most cases of poisoning have resulted from its use in scabies; a-naphthol is said to be more poisonous.

The symptoms have been vomiting, unconsciousness, and irritation of the kidneys.

1660. ASHWORTH: *Australia M. J.*, 18:483, 1896.

Treatment is similar to that given for phenol poisoning.

Postmortem Appearance: Parenchymatous degeneration of the organs, and extensive changes in the skin have been reported.

Isolation and Tests: Beta-naphthol may be extracted from the stomach contents or from the vomited matter with alcohol. On evaporation of the alcohol the residue gives a blue color changing to green and then brown when warmed with potassium hydroxide and chloroform.

CARBOLIC ACID - PHENOL

POISONING by this chemical is not as frequent as formerly. In the registration area of the United States in 1909, 1,621 of the 3,376 cases of death due to poison were due to phenol. The reports of the Coroner's Office of Cook County, Illinois, for 1935 show only eight deaths due to carbolic acid and twenty-three due to cresol (lysol.) Phenol was a very popular poison until the druggist was prohibited by the State law from selling it in a greater strength than $33\frac{1}{3}\%$ phenol. During a period of thirteen years, from 1905 to 1919, I found that phenol caused 781 deaths of which 714 were suicides, forty-one accidental, and twenty-six undetermined. The number of men destroying their lives by this poison was twice that of the number of women during the same period. 545 men, 232 women and four children met death by this agency.[1661] Accidental poisonings have occurred from mistaking the solution of the phenol for other drugs or alcoholic drinks. In several instances the carbolic acid had been stored in whiskey flasks, the color resembling that of "Bourbon" and being responsible for the mistake. Criminal poisoning by this agency is rare because of the difficulty of its administration. Fatal cases have resulted from its application to the skin. This is shown by a case of Hamilton's[1662] in which a chemist stepped into a pool of phenol waste and did not remove his clothing. Two other cases of industrial phenol poisoning were reported by Patterson to Hamilton.[1662] The first was that of a workman who was unscrewing a cap on a phenol drum when some of the contents splashed out over him. The second

1661. McNally, W. D.: *Med. Rec.*, February 1, 1919.

1662. Hamilton, A.: *J.A.M.A.*, 68:1445, 1917. Hamilton, A.: Industrial Poisons, 491, 1929.

was that of a man whose clothes were saturated with a 10% phenol solution, and who died before medical aid arrived.

Pure phenol has the formula C_6H_6O, and a molecular weight of 94.05. According to the U. S. P., XI, it is colorless, interlaced or separate, needle-shaped crystals, or a white, or light pink, crystalline mass. It is obtained from coal tar or made synthetically. Carbolic acid has a characteristic, somewhat aromatic odor, and a burning taste. The crystals melt at from 40° to 43° C.; the boiling point is 181.5° C. It is soluble in about fifteen parts of water, but becomes liquid when ten parts of water are added to ninety parts of the crystals. It is very soluble in alcohol, glycerine, chloroform, ether, carbon disulphide, fixed or volatile oils, and in liquid petrolatum. Its vapor is inflammable.

Phenol is a general protoplasmic poison, hence it is a valuable antiseptic. It precipitates proteins, but the combination is loose, and the poison readily penetrates the tissues and causes necrosis. It exerts a numbing, or even an anesthetic, action upon the sensory nerves. Aside from its local action, phenol produces marked changes in the central nervous system. It is absorbed from the skin, and is inhaled in the form of vapor by the lungs. A part of the phenol absorbed is oxidized in the body to hydroquinol and pyrocatechol; a part is excreted in the urine unchanged, and a part in combination with sulphuric and glycuronic acids. These combinations are unstable and tend to undergo further oxidation, by which colored substances are formed which give to the urine a peculiar smoky appearance.

Symptoms: The drinking of carbolic acid leads to an erosion of the mucous membranes of the mouth, esophagus, and stomach, with severe burning. When applied to the skin, it causes a sense of tingling and numbness that may amount to almost complete anesthesia. In concentrated form, a white eschar is formed that falls off in a few days, leaving a bright brown stain. Gangrene has been reported when the evaporation of phenol has been prevented. I have seen scarring effects of a 3% phenol solution when used on the face. Numerous cases of phenol poisoning have caused eczema from its application to the skin in the form of lotions and ointments. The same condition has been reported from the use of sweat bands made of imitation leather, from the phenol that was included in the composition.

When taken internally, phenol causes a burning pain in the mouth, throat, and stomach. Vomiting usually results, but it is not as constant or persistent as with other corrosive poisons.

In concentrated form phenol acts as an energetic corrosive. Constitutional effects begin shortly after the poison is absorbed. In mild cases of poisoning the chief symptoms are headache, dizziness, and sometimes excitement with mild delirium; the countenance is pale, the respiration is irregular, and the pulse small. Even after recovery from the immediate effects of the poison, weakness persists for a long period of time. In severe cases of poisoning the patient becomes unconscious, the pulse is weak and rapid, and the respiration irregular. The skin is covered with a clammy sweat, is livid and blue. Death results from failure of respiration. Cases have been reported where there was an initial rise of temperature, followed by a fall. Convulsions rarely occur. Convulsions occur more frequently in cases of poisoning in children.[1663] The pupils are generally contracted and the cornea is insensitive. Occasionally consciousness may return and death occur later.

Fatal Dose: C. E., November 3, 1919, took an unknown amount of phenol, and died in less than three hours. Five hundred and thirteen gm. of stomach and content contained 10.686 gm. of phenol; 95 gm. of spleen contained 0.1150 gm. of phenol; 127 gm. of kidney contained 0.1298 gm. of phenol; 540 gm. of liver contained 0.6426 gm. of phenol; 496 gm. of bowel contained 0.2360 gm. of phenol. A woman died from twenty-two grains (1.4 gm.), while one dram (3.7 cc.) of the liquid phenol proved fatal in twenty-three hours to a girl seventeen years of age. The fatal dose as given by Falck is about one-half ounce (15 gm.). Much smaller quantities than this introduced into wounds or body cavities may cause death. In one case a uterine douche containing one dram (3.9 gm.) of phenol to a quart of water caused the death of a woman in one hour and forty minutes, the symptoms were a rise of temperature to 108.5°F., thirst, vomiting, and violent delirium. From fifteen to thirty grains may be regarded as a fatal dose under such circumstances.

Fatal Period: In a large percentage of cases death occurs within one or two hours, and is not often delayed beyond twelve hours. Death may occur from shock in a few minutes, or may

1663. ABRAHAMS: *Pediatrics*, 9:241, 1900.

result after several days from pneumonia by the aspiration of vomited matter into the lungs during unconsciousness.[1664]

Treatment: The stomach should be washed out with warm water containing calcium in an effort to make an insoluble compound. Sulphates and alcohol may be given in a strong solution, or sodium sulphate may be used in the wash water to delay the absorption. Alcohol is used as a solvent for removing the phenol rapidly from the skin and mucous membranes, and so prevents its escharotic action. I have seen two cases where whiskey was given after the taking of an unknown quantity of carbolic acid, the patients vomiting and recovering. In a third case, the same procedure was followed but death occurred. Macht gives an experimental study of lavage in acute carbolic acid poisoning.[1665]

Postmortem Appearances: Postmortem appearances vary with the strength of the phenol and the condition of the stomach at the time it was given. When taken by mouth the mucous membrane of the mouth, esophagus, and stomach may be white, corroded, and partly detached. If the case is of long duration, the patches are red. The urine is usually of a dark or dark-greenish color, unless death occurs very quickly. The odor of the poison may be noted upon opening the body. The blood is usually dark and fluid; the brain, the meninges, the lungs, the liver, and the spleen are often congested.

Isolation: Phenol will be found in the acid distillate. Distillation is continued until the distillate fails to respond to Millon's reagent. As carbolic acid is not soluble in petrolic ether to an appreciable extent, the distillate may be shaken with this solvent for the removal of various impurities, and the carbolic acid finally extracted with ether. As salicylic acid responds to many of the tests for carbolic acid, it should be excluded by making the distillate alkaline in the cold with sodium carbonate and extracting several times with ether. Under these conditions, carbolic acid is taken up by the ether, while sodium salicylate remains in the aqueous solution. The distillate should be subjected to quantitative determination, using the volumetric method of Koppeschaar,[1666] which is based on the formation

1664. SCHLEICHER: *Deutsche med. Wchnschr.,* 17:9, 1891; CAHN: *Therap. Monatsh., Berl.,* 25:431, 1911.

1665. MACHT, D. I.: *Bull. Johns Hopkins Hosp.,* 26:98, 1915.

1666. KOPPESCHAAR: *Ztschr. a. Chem.,* 15:233, 1876.

of tribromophenol, when bromine water is added in moderate excess to an aqueous solution of phenol:

$$C_6H_5OH + 3Br_2 = C_6H_2Br_3OH + 3HBr$$

Alkali bromide and bromate are now used instead of the bromine water, from which the bromine is liberated by hydrochloric acid, the reaction being as follows:

$$5NaBr + NaBrO_3 + 6HCl = 6NaCl + 3Br_2 + 3H_2O$$

The bromine thus set free, and not fixed by the phenol, is then determined by adding potassium iodide and titrating the liberated iodine with N/10 thiosulphate. The sodium bromide and bromate is prepared by adding bromine to 100 cc. of normal sodium hydroxide until the liquid becomes brown in color and smells distinctly of bromine, then heat the liquid till it becomes quite colorless. Cool and dilute to one liter.

> 1 cc. = 0.007992 gm. bromine.
> 1 cc. = 0.001568 gm. phenol.

Iodine x 15.68 ÷ 126.92 = 0.1235 = phenol.

Example:[1667] Five gm. carbolic powder are put into a 250-cc. flask, HCl added, and made up to the mark with water. The flask is shaken and the contents filtered. Fifty cc. of the filtrate (=1 gm. of sample) are measured into a stoppered bottle and 100 cc. of the bromide and bromate solution added, together with a little more HCl, and, after being well shaken, this is allowed to stand for fifteen minutes. KI solution is then added, the bottle is again shaken, and the iodine set free is titrated with N/10 thiosulphate. Suppose that 13.8 cc. of the latter are required, and that titration with iodine showed that 1 cc. of it = 0.0121 gm. iodine; also that 10 cc. of the bromide and bromate solution and KI required 10.5 cc. thiosulphate. Then 100 cc. of the bromide and bromate solution = 105 cc. N/10 thiosulphate, of which 105 —13.8=81.2 cc. represent the bromine absorbed, which has been determined in terms of iodine.

Hence 81.2 x .0121 x .1235 = .1214 gm. phenol, or 12.14%.

Tests: 1. Take 2 cc. of the acid distillate and add an equal quantity of Millon's reagent.[1668] Dissolve mercury in an equal weight of 63% nitric acid, warming gently to start the reaction, and dilute the product with twice its volume of water. After letting it stand overnight, decant the clear reagent. This will

1667. SUTTON, F.: Volumetric Analysis, 11th ed., 405, 1924.
1668. MILLON: *Compt. rend.*, 28:40, 1849.

detect one part in 2,000,000 parts of water, but the red color is also given by all monophenols and by proteins.

2. Phenol may be identified in very small amounts microscopically by the precipitation of tribromophenol, $C_6H_2Br_3OH$. Delicate one to 60,000. Out of a very dilute solution, crystals, 40 to 60 micra, or, upon long standing, a dense network of little rods of about 200 to 2000 micra, will be formed. Tribromophenol has a characteristic odor, and sublimes easily in beautiful needles. This is readily soluble in alkalis, and is again precipitated by the addition of an acid.

3. If a few drops of ferric chloride are added to 5 cc. of the acid distillate a blue-violet color will be formed in the presence of phenol. This color is retarded by the presence of a mineral acid, or ammonia, and fails entirely in the presence of alcohol.

4. When a fragment of para-diazobenzol-sulphonic acid is added to an alkaline solution of carbolic acid a yellow color is formed, which becomes very much lighter on the addition of acetic acid. When a crystal of sodium chloride is added to the mixture a light yellow precipitate which later forms light yellow platelets, 30 to 40 micra, appears.

5. To 5 cc. of the distillate add a drop of an alcohol solution of ethyl nitrate. Underlay with sulphuric acid by means of a pipet. A rose-colored ring will form at the surface of contact.[1669] Rodillon adds one drop of a 10% aqueous solution of $NaNO_2$ to 10 cc. of the suspected solution and overlays sulphuric acid with this mixture, when a double ring appears at the zone of contact, emerald green below and ruby red above. This reaction will show the presence of one part of carbolic acid in 2,000,000 parts of water.

6. If a solution of carbolic acid is warmed with one-fourth of its volume of ammonia and a few drops of calcium hypochlorite added, a blue color is produced, which disappears rapidly, but returns on the addition of more hypochlorite. To 25 cc. of the acid distillate add three drops of aniline and dilute from five to ten drops of the mixture with 10 cc. of water. Add as much sodium hypochlorite solution as will serve to change the blue color that is first formed into brown. After a few minutes add some of the original solution supposed to contain car-

1669. EIJKMAN: *Ztschr. f. anal. Chem.*, 22:576, 1883; see also RODILLON: *J. Chem.*, 7s., 23:136, 1921.

bolic acid, to which a few drops of ammonia have been added. In the presence of carbolic acid a permanent blue color will be obtained.

To differentiate between carbolic acid and the other phenols the suspected material can be extracted with chloroform. To a few cc. of the chloroform extract, a small piece of solid potassium hydroxide is added, and the whole slightly warmed. If carbolic acid is present, it turns red; naphthols, blue; thymol, dark red; pyrocatechin, yellowish-brown; resorcin, red; hydroquinon, yellowish-red to reddish-brown; pyrogallol and phloroglucin, reddish-yellow.

For the determination of phenol in cerebrospinal fluid Castex and Arnaudo[1670] recommend: To 10 cc. of the cerebrospinal fluid add 13 cc. of water, 1 cc. of 10% sodium tungstate, and 1 cc. of 2/3 N sulphuric acid, proceeding as with blood according to Theis and Benedict's method. A standard is made so that 10 cc.=0.0125 mg. phenol. The normal amount of phenols in the cerebrospinal fluid is between 0.20 and 0.36 mg. per 100 cc.

Dissolve one drop of phenol in 10 cc. concentrated hydrochloric acid in a glass mortar and add 0.5 gm. or more of a mixture of sodium nitrite (one part), and exsiccated sodium sulphate (two parts). Stir well and allow to stand for two to five minutes. Note the color, and then pour about 1 cc. of acid mixture into excess of 10% ammonia water and note the change in color. Carbolic acid gives a rich crimson color in two minutes. On pouring in more of the ammonia get a deep emerald green. If at crimson stage in the acid one to two drops of 38% formaldehyde be added and the mixture stirred, the color changes to a rich purple, and if it is now poured into a solution of ammonia a deep blue instead of a green is generally yielded. (Ortho cresol gives green, and formaldehyde changes it to blue, and ammonia to olive green. Meta cresol, para cresol, and cresol give no positive colors.) Beta naphthol and alpha naphthol in acid solution give crimson-purple and finally violet-purple after three to five minutes. These colors are destroyed by ammonia. Thymol, after stirring and being left for five minutes, gives a green color, changed to yellow with ammonia.

1670. CASTEX, M. R., and ARNAUDO, A. F.: *Prensa méd. argent.*, August 30, 1933.

One drop of phenol is dissolved in 5 to 10 cc. concentrated hydrochloric acid with a minute crystal of sodium nitrite; this is carefully and gradually heated nearly to boiling, cooled and diluted, and poured into an excess of 10% ammonia water. Carbolic acid, ortho and meta cresol give a deep blue color. With para cresol no such results were obtained. The official method of the A.O.A.C. may be used.* It depends upon the color developed by the use of Millon's reagent, comparing the color with a known phenol standard.

Para Cresol Test: An aqueous solution acidified with acetic acid together with a little sodium nitrite and a few drops of 1% to 2% copper sulphate solution, gives a rich wine red color, pink with water dilution. Guaiacol gives green color; orcinol, phloroglucinol, and the catechins give much less definite results—rather poor reds and purples, both before and after ammonia. Catechol gives a distinct but not intense bluish-green in the acid mixture, while pyrogallol gives a purplish color if heated with a nitrate in the acid solution, but not if a nitrite is used.

Behrens and Kley[1671] found that a saturated solution of phenol, if brought in contact with a cold saturated solution of paranitrosodimethylanilinenitrate, and with the addition of sodium acetate, yields a spider web-like aggregation of yellow transparent platelets (200 micra). More dilute solutions take a longer time but yield, on the other hand, better developed crystals (60 to 80 micra) of moderate polarization and linear extinction, and, in the margin of the test drop, fan-like branching crystals about 150 to 200 micra in size. Orthocresol gives a similar reaction with paranitrosodimethylaniline.

If phenol is evaporated in the presence of dilute nitric acid, trinitrophenol (picric acid) is formed, which with water gives a clear light yellow solution. If evaporated with ammonia there are formed yellow dendrites of ammonia picrate, which, then treated with water and thallonitrate, yield difficultly soluble crystals of thallopicrate which have a strong polarizing action and appear lemon-yellow in reflected light. (Differentiation from the cresols.)

Traces of phenol can be detected in the form of greenish-blue copper-like indophenol, by adding dimethylparapheny-

* Methods of Analysis, A.O.A.C., 4th ed., 73, 1935.
1671. BEHRENS and KLEY: Organische Mikrochemische Analyse, Zweite Auflage, 30:1922.

leidiamine and hydrogen peroxide to the solution, which previously has been made alkaline with sodium carbonate. The reaction takes about ten minutes and is not much accelerated by heating. It is a sensitive test, the only disadvantage being that the product obtained is of an amorphous nature which does not permit the differentiation from the other phenols.

Barac[1672] has described a spectrographic determination of phenol. To 20 cc. of urine add 0.5 to 2 cc. of aqueous phenol of known liter. To this add 5 cc. saturated Pb $(OAc)_2$ solution, and 3 cc. of 0.1 N NaOH, and filter. Combine an aliquot portion of the filtrate and an equal volume of saturated aqueous solution of Na_2HPO_4, and filter. Acidify the filtrate with concentrated hydrochloric acid and extract a known volume three times with ether. Bring the ether extract to volume, dry, and examine with the spectrograph.

SALICYLIC ACID

SALICYLIC ACID, $C_7H_6O_3$, has a molecular weight of 138.05. It occurs as colorless crystals, usually in fine needles, or a fluffy white, crystalline powder. It has a sweetish, afterwards an acrid, taste. It is stable in the air. One gram of salicylic acid is soluble in 460 cc. of water, in 2.7 cc. of alcohol, in 42 cc. of chloroform, in 3 cc. of ether, in 3 cc. of acetone, in 135 cc. of benzene, and in 52 cc. of oil of turpentine, at 25°C. (U.S.P.,XI).

The symptoms in a mild case of poisoning, such as is frequently seen in the treatment of acute rheumatism, are nausea and vomiting, a feeling of fullness in the head, with ringing in the ears, dimness of vision, profuse perspiration, confusion, and dullness. In large doses of the free acid there is an irritation of the throat and stomach, leading to vomiting and difficulty in swallowing; later there may be diarrhea. Flushing of the face, distressing dyspnea, weak pulse, subnormal temperature, and, in more severe cases, convulsions, coma, and perhaps death in a state of collapse occur. Delirium and hallucinations have been described. Mild nephritis is a frequent symptom. Eczema and other skin eruptions may appear, and dimness of vision and deafness may continue for days or weeks. An overdose causes nausea and vomiting, and long continued use of salicylic acid causes loss of appetite, diarrhea alternating with constipation, irritation of the kidneys, skin eruptions, and mental depression.

1672. BARAC, G.: *Compt. rend.*, 201:1433, 1935.

Fatal Dose: Death occurred in a patient suffering from acute rheumatism after taking over one ounce in four days.[1673] Death has been attributed to 4, 5, and 10 gm. I have given as high as 380 grains of sodium salicylate in a retention enema a number of times in acute arthritis, due to a Neisserian infection. Zumbroich[1674] reported the death of an infant from the application of a 10% ointment of salicylic acid to the head and neck.

Treatment: Wash out the stomach with sodium bicarbonate, 10 gm. to the pint. Milk, eggs, and vegetable oils may be given to allay the burning sensation.

Postmortem Appearances: A marked hyperemia of all the organs is usually present. Lesions of gastritis, enteritis, and acute parenchymatous nephritis have been found.

Isolation: Salicylic acid is found in the acid ether extract of the alkaloidal extraction. The ether is evaporated, leaving a residue of salicylic acid in a crystalline form.

Tests: 1. Salicylic acid sublimes after decomposition by rapid heating, a part of it is changed to carbon dioxide and phenol. It melts at 155° C. The crystals dissolve readily in sodium hydroxide and ammonium hydroxide, which, when acidified with acetic acid, slowly separate into short prisms, 30 to 40 micra in size.

2. To a small amount of the residue in a test-tube add 1 cc. of methyl alcohol, and a few drops of concentrated sulphuric acid. Cool, and heat again. In the presence of salicylic acid the odor of oil of wintergreen will be noticed.

3. When silver nitrate is brought in contact with a solution of sodium salicylate a white precipitate is formed which in a half-minute becomes crystalline. Out of a dilute solution small needles and leaf-like crystals are obtained. The precipitate of silver salicylate is very soluble in dilute ammonia.

4. The residue from the ether extract is dissolved in a little hot water. To the solution in the test-tube add four or five drops of 10% potassium nitrite solution, four or five drops of 50% acetic acid, and one drop of 10% cupric sulphate solution, and heat to boiling. After one or two minutes a blood red color will develop in the presence of salicylic acid.

Estimation: Make an aqueous solution of the residue with

1673. QUINCKE: *Berl. klin. Wchnschr.*, 19:710, 1882.
1674. ZUMBROICH: *Monatschr. f. Kinderh.*, 15:167, 1918.

the aid of 1 or 2 cc. of N/10 sodium hydroxide. For each determination measure out a volume corresponding to about 0.1 gm. of salicylic acid and dilute with water to about 100 cc. Next pipet a known volume of the bromide and bromate solution. Solution of sodium bromide and bromate made by dissolving 19.5 gm. of bromine in about 100 cc. of water containing 100 gm. of sodium hydroxide. The liquid thus obtained is boiled well and then diluted to two liters. The solution can be kept indefinitely. 0.138 gm. of salicylic acid corresponds to 0.480 gm. of free bromine, or as much as will be liberated by acid from about 50 cc. of the solution. N/10 sodium thiosulphate (24.822 gm. of the crystals per liter—1 cc.—equals 0.008 gm. bromine) is delivered into a stoppered bottle, add 5 cc. of strong hydrochloric acid, then the 100 cc. of the solution of the sample as above.

Another bottle containing an equal quantity of the bromine solution is similarly diluted and acidified, and left to stand side by side with the sample. Potassium iodide solution is then added to the contents of both bottles, and the liberated iodine titrated with N/10 thiosulphate. Starch solution may be added toward the end of the process, but it is important not to add it until the liquid is nearly decolorized by the thiosulphate.[1675]

ACETYLSALICYLIC ACID

ACETYLSALICYLIC ACID, $C_9H_8O_4$, has a molecular weight of 180.06. Its synonym is "aspirin". It occurs as colorless crystals, commonly tabular or needle-like, or a white crystalline powder. It is odorless, is stable in dry air, in moist air gradually hydrolyzing into salicylic and acetic acids. It melts not below 135° C. One gram of acetylsalicylic acid is soluble in about 300 cc. of water, in 5 cc. of alcohol, in 17 cc. of chloroform, and in from 10 to 15 cc. of ether, at 25° C. It is about one and one-half times as toxic for man as is sodium salicylate, and sometimes causes severe symptoms in medicinal doses. The reactions are similar to those of salicylic acid. It is used extensively by the laity, but, I have never seen a death from an overdosage.

The literature contains a large number of references to poisoning by aspirin in which there was edema of the face, a

1675. SUTTON: Volumetric Analysis, 11th ed., 406, 1924.

feeling of thickness of the tongue with inability to swallow, and an urticarial rash. Lewis[1676] reported a patient who had taken eighteen five-grain tablets, and a number of capsules of aspirin. He was taken to a hospital with symptoms of marked anemia, temperature 101.4°, pulse 120. During the day he vomited undigested milk, with no trace of blood. The following day the anemia was more profound, pulse 150 weak and irregular. An enema was administered, with little result. The vomiting continued at intervals. At 5:00 the next morning a large quantity of blood was passed by the bowel, and he rapidly became unconscious. No thought of an exploratory laparotomy could be entertained. He died a few hours later. Postmortem showed the ileum acutely congested, and the cecum and colon loaded with blood clots. On opening, the intestines were found to be uniformly inflamed. The mucous coat had apparently disappeared, leaving the submucous coat and blood vessels exposed and eroded. Bleeding from this large area had evidently been the cause of death. The other organs were in a normal condition.

In Hungary, more than 100 attempts at suicide have been made with aspirin. The mortality rate is about 0.5%.

A woman living in Detroit, Michigan, died in convulsions shortly after taking a dose of quinine and aspirin. No cause could be found for her death. [1677] Habituation has been reported by Macht, in which a man increased the dose from five grains to twenty-five to sixty grains per day, but even after two years had only a few toxic symptoms (constipation and slight digestive disturbances).[1678]

In the extraction of organs for the presence of aspirin, alcohol without the presence of an acid should be used. The alcohol is evaporated as usual under a vacuum and then extracted with ether. Aspirin will be found in the residue from the evaporation of the ether extract; with sulphuric acid or with sodium hydroxide, on boiling with water, it hydrolyzes to salicylic acid. The presence of these two substances with a melting point will serve to identify the presence of aspirin. Aspirin does not give a color with ferric chloride until it has been hydrolyzed, when it gives the reactions for salicylic acid.

1676. LEWIS, F. W.: *Lancet,* 4: 61, 1919.
1677. *Bull. Pharm.,* November, 1915, p. 456.
1678. MACHT: *Med. Rec.,* 94: 767, 1918.

TRINITROPHENOL — PICRIC ACID

TRINITROPHENOL, $C_6H_2(OH)(NO_2)_3$ 1:2:4:6, has a molecular weight of 229.05. It occurs as pale yellow prisms or scales, is odorless, and has an intensely bitter taste. Trinitrophenol explodes when heated rapidly, or when subjected to percussion. One gram of trinitrophenol is soluble in 78 cc. of water, 12 cc. of alcohol, 35 cc. of chloroform, 65 cc. of ether, and in 10 cc. of benzene, at 25° C. Trinitrophenol melts between 121° and 123° C. An aqueous solution is acid to litmus paper. (U.S.P. XI). It finds extensive use as a dressing for burns and in superficial wounds. It has caused several cases of dermatitis, and therefore it has been replaced by tannic acid. Cases of dermatitis and eczema have been reported in ammunition factories.

Symptoms: When the poison is taken internally, the symptoms begin with pain in the abdomen, vomiting, and diarrhea.[1679] The urine is at first dark yellow, but later becomes of a red-brown color; it contains no bile. There may be anuria and strangury. The vomited matter and the feces are stained yellow. The conjunctiva, and later the skin, assume a yellowish color, and the vision may become yellow. A part of the picric acid is excreted unchanged by the urine, but most is transformed by the liver into picramic acid. Eczema and itching are common results. Prostration, stupor, fever, and occasionally convulsions followed by collapse, have been observed. Toxic doses destroy the red corpuscles and produce gastroenteritis, hemorrhagic nephritis, and acute hepatitis.

Bapty[1680] reports the case of a nurse who had a 10% picric acid solution applied to the small vesicles of herpes zoster. The lesion became worse, there were red, raised areas on both forearms, the cheeks, and the neck, which spread over the whole body. The face was swollen, the eyes shut, and the urine was scanty and contained picric acid.

Fatal Dose: Fifteen to thirty grains have caused toxic symptoms, but recovery has followed the taking of ninety grains.[1681]

Treatment: Treatment consists in washing out the stom-

1679. ADLER: *Wien. med. Wchnschr.*, 30:819, 1880.
1680. BAPTY, W.: *Canad. M. A. J.*, 14:1207, 1924.
1681. HALLA: *Prag. med. Wchnschr.*, 7:490, 1882.

ach, thoroughly, with milk and whites of eggs, as they form soluble compounds with the poison. Give high colonic flushings. Intravenous injection of dextrose should be given, as this is believed to aid the reduction of the picric acid to the less poisonous picraminic acid.[1682]

Isolation: Picric acid will be found in the acid ether extract, after purification by the general method for alkaloids (page 30).

Tests: 1. Ammonia forms with yellow green crystals which strongly reflect light.

2. The addition of sodium hydroxide and a small amount of glucose to a solution of the picric acid will give a red color due to the formation of picraminic acid.

3. On warming an alkaline solution of a picrate with a concentrated solution of potassium cyanide, potassium isopurpurate is formed, which imparts a blood red color to the fluid.

4. Dye test: Place a strand of wool and one of cotton in a small amount of the solution which has been faintly acidified and warmed. The wool is stained but the cotton is not. The color may be removed from the wool by suspending it in dilute alkali.

5. Reduce the picric acid solution with a hydrochloric acid solution of stannous chloride; then add a little ferric chloride. A blue color is produced, owing to the production of amidophenol.

BENZALDEHYDE (C_6H_5CHO)

BENZALDEHYDE is a colorless liquid when pure, boiling at 180° C. (356° F.)., and having a characteristic odor. It gives all the ordinary aldehyde reactions. On oxidation it yields benzoic acid, and on reduction benzyl alcohol. It is found in the acid distillate, from which it is extracted with ether in a separatory funnel. The ether layer, upon spontaneously evaporating, leaves the benzaldehyde as an oily residue.

Detection: 1. Smell.

2. In a flask with a reflux condenser oxidize some of the benzaldehyde to benzoic acid by means of sulphuric acid and potassium dichromate. Distill with steam. Extract the distillate with ether, and test for the presence of benzoic acid.

1682. RYMSZA: Ein Beitrag. z. Toxikol. der Pikrinsaure, Dorpat, 1889.

3. One cc. of the distillate or a small amount of the suspected material is treated with concentrated sulphuric acid and phenol, and boiled. A deep red color is produced. Cool, add 10 cc. of water, and make alkaline with potassium hydroxide. This changes the color to blue-violet. If this is now acidified and extracted with ether, the color passes to the ether layer.

Estimation: Benzaldehyde is estimated by conversion to benzoic acid, which can then be weighed or titrated.

NITROBENZENE

NITROBENZENE, $C_6H_5NO_2$, is an oily liquid, of a pale yellow color, having a specific gravity of 1.186, and a boiling point of 205° C. (401° F). It is insoluble in water, and easily soluble in alcohol. The liquid burns readily with a luminous flame, and has a sweet taste, and an odor strongly resembling that of oil of bitter almonds. It is used extensively in the manufacture of anilin and of explosives, as a substitute for benzaldehyde (oil of bitter almonds) in perfumery and flavoring extracts, and as an ingredient of shoe dyes, floor polishes, inks, etc. It has caused many severe cases of illness, some with fatal results, when spilt upon clothes, or from wearing shoes dyed with liquids said to contain nitro-benzene.[1683] Poisoning has resulted from its application to the skin in the treatment of scabies, or as a delousing agent.[1684]

Symptoms: When taken internally there is a burning sensation, followed by numbness and tingling, but other symptoms may not appear for one to three hours. These are non-characteristic nervous symptoms, fatigue, nausea, headache, giddiness, skin irritation, and itching, sleeplessness, and palpitation of the heart. The gait is unsteady, the breath has the odor of bitter almonds, and coma may come on unexpectedly. Muscular twitchings, and involuntary evacuation of the feces and urine may occur. The temperature falls, and the respiration is frequently of the Cheyne-Stokes type. The blood damage is characterized by anemia, paleness, and cyanosis, especially noticeable by the blue color of the lips, which, in more severe cases spreads to the head, trunk, and limbs. The spectroscope usually shows the absorption bands of methemoglobin,

1683. STLFEL, R. E.: *J.A.M.A.*, 72:395, 1919; MINER: *J.A.M.A.*, 72:593, 1919; SANDERS: *J.A.M.A.*, 74:1518, 1920.
1684. WOLPE: *Deutsche med. Wchnschr.*, 46:100, 1920.

but often another absorption band, which has been called the nitrobenzene hemoglobin band, is present.[1685] The oxygen capacity of the blood in human cases of poisoning has been found greatly reduced, in one case being only 6.2 volumes per cent.[1686] The pupils may be contracted or dilated, and do not react to light; there may be nystagmus. The urine is dark, smells of nitrobenzene, and contains a reducing substance. The blood is chocolate colored, thick, and viscid. Death usually occurs from failure of respiration.

If the poison is absorbed through the skin or lungs the symptoms may appear rapidly, the patient may become dizzy, and faint, and collapse within a few minutes, and death may occur within an hour.[1687]

Chronic poisoning by nitrobenzene has been reported in industries, with languor, somnolence, breathlessness, blueness of the face, and sometimes failure of the sight as common symptoms. The urine is a dark maroon color; on warming it gives a characteristic odor of oil of bitter almonds.

Muehlberger found forty-seven cases of poisoning from shoe dyes reported in the literature.[1688] Of these twenty-five were from nitrobenzene, and twenty-one from aniline. Among the first cases reported are those of Landouzy, who cites ten instances in which aniline poisoning followed the use of black shoe dyes.[1689] Stone gives the clinical history and necropsy of a case due to the use of a black shoe dye. Stifel reported seventeen cases of nitrobenzene poisoning resulting from soldiers having their shoes dyed brown in order to match the color of their puttees.[1690] Muehlberger reported nine cases of shoe dye poisoning, six of which were known to have occurred from the use of shoe dyes containing aniline instead of nitrobenzene as a solvent.

Fatal Dose: Fifteen drops of nitrobenzene have proved fatal. Patients have recovered, under treatment,[1691] from 3.5

1685. FILEHNE: *Arch. f. exper. Path. u. Pharmakol.,* 9:329, 1878.

1686. LOEB, BOCK, and FITZ: *Am. J. M. Sc.,* 161:539, 1921.

1687. HAMILTON, A.: *J. Indust. Hyg.,* 1:200, 1919; THOMSEN: *München. med. Wchnschr.,* 68:399, 1921.

1688. MUEHLBERGER, C. W.: *J.A.M.A.,* 84:1987, 1925.

1689. LANDOUZY, L., and BROUARDEL, G.: *Bull. Acad. de méd., Par.,* 44:114, 1900. STONE, W. J.: *J.A.M.A.,* 43:977, 1904.

1690. STIFEL, R. E.: *J.A.M.A.,* 72:395, 1919.

1691. CISSEL: Abst., *Lancet,* 1:1521, 1894.

ounces (105 cc.). In one case coming under the author's observation, three ounces of nitrobenzene were taken by mistake for an alcoholic beverage, causing death in less than one hour. During the prohibition era in the United States a considerable number of cases of poisoning resulted from the drinking of alcohol containing nitrobenzene. Von Jaksch places the mortality at twenty per cent.[1692]

Fatal Period: Death may occur within three hours, as in the case of the author's, cited above, or within one hour after inhalation or absorption through the skin. Death may occur as late as forty-eight hours, and has been delayed for seventeen days.

Treatment: The stomach should be washed out with water containing epsom salts, which delays the absorption and solubility of the poison. Oils, milk, and alcohol should not be given, as they favor absorption. If the poison has been spilled upon the clothing, the skin should be immediately cleansed. Inhalations of oxygen and intravenous injection of glucose and sodium chloride should be given.

Postmortem Appearances: The face appears flushed and the lips livid. The organs have the odor of bitter almonds. Ecchymoses may be found in the esophagus, stomach, and duodenum. The icteric pigmentation of the skin may be so marked as to amount to a pronounced jaundice, but the increasing cyanosis, superimposed on this, often produces a dirty yellowish-gray color. The liver has the appearance of that of acute yellow atrophy. Edema of the lungs, and parenchymatous degeneration of all the organs, as well as small patches of necrosis in the liver were seen in a case reported by Schnopfhagen. Spectroscopic examination of the blood will show the presence of methemoglobin but no methematin.

Isolation: Nitrobenzene is found in the acid distillate, from which it is extracted with ether, the nitrobenzene being left as the residue after evaporation of the ether.

Tests: The nitrobenzene is reduced by zinc and hydrochloric acid to anilin: $C_6H_5O_2 + 6H + C_6H_5NH_2 + 2H_2O$. The aniline may be extracted with ether, and tests applied for its presence. Two drops of phenol, three drops of water, and a small piece of potassium hydroxide are carefully heated to boiling in

1692. VON JAKSCH: Die Vergiftungen, 325, 1912.

a small porcelain dish. Add 5 cc. of the volatile distillate and continue boiling. In the presence of nitrobenzene a carmine-red ring forms on the edge of the liquid, which changes to green on the addition of concentrated calcium hypochlorite solution.

DINITROBENZENE

METADINITROBENZENE (dinitrobenzol, $C_6H_4(NO_2)_2$) forms, when pure, colorless crystals melting at 90° C. (194° F.). It is used in the manufacture of explosives, and also as a dye intermediate; most cases of poisoning have occurred in connection with its manufacture or handling in the filling of shells. The poison may be absorbed through the lungs, or more frequently by the skin. Its physiological action and symptoms are similar to those of nitrobenzene.

Detection: Dinitrobenzene may be reduced by tinfoil and hydrochloric acid, to the three phenylene diamins (o, m, and p). Make the fluid alkaline with sodium hydroxide, and extract with ether. Take up the residue in a little water after evaporation of the ether. Acidify with dilute sulphuric acid, then add to this some of the dissolved residue. A yellow to red color is produced if it contains metaphenylenediamin.

TRINITROTOLUENE

TRINITROTOLUENE (T N T), $C_6H_2.CH_2.(NO_2)_3$, poisoning causes cyanosis of the cheeks and lips; the hands and hair become stained a yellowish brown. In more severe cases there is a high degree of exhaustion, fainting fits occur, and the blood and skin show the same changes, anemia, cyanosis, icterus, as in poisoning by mono- and di-nitrobenzene. There is the same damage as in acute yellow atrophy of the liver.

Trinitrotoluene is a fine crystalline yellow powder, melting at 82°C. (179.6°F.), sometimes used in the form of flakes or of fused yellowish-brown lumps. It is employed as a high explosive, chiefly in shells and grenades. During the World War it came into prominence as a toxic agent. The poisonings occurred not in the process of manufacture, but in the various manipulations involved in its handling, and in shell and grenade filling. The poison may be absorbed through the skin, the gastro-intestinal tract, or the lungs; the first channel seems to be the most important. Trinitrotoluene acts as an irritant at its point of entrance into the body, leading to dermatitis, gastric pain, etc. Among the toxic symptoms are pallor and cyanosis, dyspnea on exertion, dizziness, headache, fatigue, irritation. Blood abnormalities frequently occur, even in the minor grades of poisoning. Fragmented red cells were frequently found, giving evidence of a rapid increased destruction of red cells. Distinct increases of these cells indicates a considerable degree of poisoning. Among other red cell abnormalities noted were polychromatophilia; Howell-Jolly bodies; stippling; and increased numbers of reticulated cells, indicating increased activity on the part of the blood-forming organs. A leukocytosis and a relative lymphocytosis were common. There was a reduction in the hemoglobin percentage.

Postmortem Appearances: The liver shows extensive necrosis and atrophy, which cannot be distinguished from acute yellow atrophy. Microscopically a great part of the liver tissue is found to have undergone complete destruction associated with a proliferation of fibrous tissue. Death results from aplastic anemia, unassociated with jaundice. The symptoms included bleeding from the nose and gums, delirium, and coma, the hemoglobin may be 30%, and the red cells below a million, and, postmortem, aplastic bone-marrow.

Treatment: The workers should be protected by proper clothing, and should wear masks. The hands should be washed at the end of each working period with a 10% solution of sodium sulphide. Anemic and young individuals should be excluded from this type of employment; and blood examinations should be made frequently. In the treatment of jaundice, give calcium gluconate or glucose intravenously. The treatment of anemia is the same as that given under Benzol (page 776).

Detection: Trinitrotoluene is excreted in the urine as a chromogen conjugated with glycuronic acid. Extract the urine with ether. Discard this ether extract. Acidify the urine with one-half its bulk of 20% sulphuric acid, and extract twice with ether. Wash the combined ether extracts well with water, and then with dilute sodium carbonate solution to remove the acid. Dry this ether extract over anhydrous sodium sulphate. On treating this purified ether extract with alcoholic potash, a beautiful blue color is obtained.[1693]

1693. Med. Res. Council, No. 11:16, 1917, and No. 58:50, 1921; see also TUTIN: *Lancet,* 2:554, 1918.

ANILINE

ANILINE, $C_6H_5NH_2$, is a colorless, oily, inflammable liquid, of a peculiar odor and a burning aromatic taste, which may become brown on standing. Commercial aniline oil, which causes most cases of aniline poisoning, is a mixture of aniline, toluidine, nitrobenzene, and other benzene derivatives. It has basic properties and forms well defined salts. It boils at 184° C. (363° F.), and is sparingly soluble in water, but readily soluble in alcohol, chloroform, and ether. Most of the cases of poisoning are caused by the absorption through the skin, where workmen engaged in the use of this substance or its derivatives. Many cases are reported from rubber works where aniline is used in certain operations,[1694] also from the use of a wash for printers' ink which had aniline as one of its ingredients, and among dyers and painters. A number of cases of poisoning have occurred from the wearing of shoes dyed with aniline dyes contained in liquids, and from shoes which were cleaned with aniline.

The symptoms are the same as for nitrobenzene. The urine is dark, due to oxidation products of aniline. Convulsions may occur, and then coma, and sometimes death. The breath has an odor resembling that of coal tar. Anemia, skin eruptions, various nervous symptoms, and amblyopia have been observed among men employed for some time in aniline factories, and have been attributed to chronic poisoning by aniline. Complete recovery from aniline may not occur for a number of weeks.

Fatal Dose and Period: Twenty-five cc. of aniline oil caused the death of a young woman in twenty-four hours.[1695] Smith[1696] reported a case in which a woman died twelve hours after taking three ounces (90 cc.) of marking ink that consisted largely of aniline.

Treatment is the same as under Nitrobenzene (page 825).

Postmortem appearances are not characteristic. Methemoglobin is found in the blood, and the odor of aniline may be noted in the organs. There may be irritation of the gastric

1694. HAMILTON, A.: U. S. Bureau of Labor Statistics, Bull. 179, 1915; HARRINGTON: *Boston M. & S. J.*, 179:497, 1918.

1695. MÜLLER: *Deutsche med. Wchnschr.*, 13:27, 1887.

1696. SMITH: *Lancet*, 1:89, 1894.

mucosa and inflammation or degeneration of the cells of the liver, kidney, and heart. Sometimes edema of the lungs has been described.

Isolation: Aniline may be found in the alkaline distillate. If aniline is suspected, make alkaline with sodium hydroxide instead of magnesium oxide. The alkaline distillate can be extracted with ether and the following tests applied:

1. To 10 cc. of the distillate add three drops of chloroform and 2 cc. of an alcoholic potash solution. If very much aniline is present, a disagreeable odor will appear immediately. If only a very small amount is present, it will be necessary to warm the mixture before the odor will appear.

2. Bromine water added to the distillate will cause a flesh-colored precipitate of tribromaniline to appear.

3. To some of the residue from the ether extract add concentrated sulphuric acid, and a solution of potassium bichromate. A blue color is produced, which disappears in a few minutes. In the presence of water the color is either green or black.

COAL TAR DYES

FEW cases of poisoning occur from the handling of enormous quantities of aniline dyes. Where poisoning is reported, it is usually caused by chemicals other than the dye used in the process. Phenylenediamines are used for dyeing furs, and also for hair dyes, and cause symptoms in some people. The dye is mixed with hydrogen peroxide before use, and if completely oxidized its toxicity is lost. Since some persons wearing furs have a peculiar susceptibility to phenylenediamines, a severe dermatitis and even systemic poisoning may occur. The absorption of phenylenediamines causes salivation, nausea, vomiting, and diarrhea. Faintness with palpitation or paroxysmal tachycardia may occur, also symptoms of angioneurotic edema have been reported. Phenylenediamines and toluylenediamine can produce asthma-like attacks, especially in hypersensitive workers. These two substances are used in the fur-dyeing industry under the name of "ursol."

Triphenylmethane series of dyes have a local irritating action upon the skin.[1697] Injury to the hand has resulted from

1697. ERDHEIM: *Arch. f. klin. Chir.*, 106:91, 1914; *Arch. f. klin. Chir.*, 113:772, 1920; *Wien. klin. Wchnschr.*, 32:726, 1919; BALLIN and SALTZSTEIN: *J.A.M.A.*, 76:1333, 1921.

the breaking off, under the skin, of copying and indelible pencils containing methyl violet.

Bladder Tumors in Aniline Workers: The literature contains numerous references to the presence of malignant tumors in the bladder of aniline dye workers in the process of manufacturing. Hamilton[1698] has pointed out that in the production of amino compounds there is always the possibility of arsine being produced due to the action of the acid on the scrap iron, or zinc dust, used in the processes of the reduction. Hamilton suggests that the soot, pitch, and paraffin tumors—the chimney-sweepers' cancer and the epithelioma of briquet makers — (which have been long considered analogous to these "anilin" tumors) may be due to chronic arsenic poisoning. The development of the tumors is extremely slow, and takes, on the average, about seventeen years from the beginning of work in aniline. The first clinical signs consist of irritation of the mucous membrane of the bladder, with difficulty in passing urine, strangury, and hematuria.

ACETANILID (C₈H₉ON)
(Antifebrin: Molecular Weight 135.08)

ACETANILID is colorless, shiny crystals, usually scaly, or a white crystalline powder. It is odorless, and is stable in the air. One gram of acetanilid is soluble in 190 cc. of water, 3.4 cc. of alcohol, 3.7 cc. of chloroform, 17 cc. of ether, 4 cc. of acetone, 47 cc. of benzene, and in about 5 cc. of glycerine, at 25° C. Acetanilid melts between 113° and 115° C.

The most frequent source of poisoning has been from its indiscriminate use for headaches. Of 614 cases of poisoning reported by the physicians to the U. S. Department of Agriculture, 325 cases (53%) occurred when the drug was taken without a physician's prescription.

Symptoms: The toxic actions are manifest in acetanilid by marked and prolonged cyanosis, great weakness, prostration, and collapse; coldness of extremities, profuse sweating, with feeble shallow respiration, unconsciousness; occasionally marked restlessness, convulsions, and delirium; sometimes persistent vomiting and dyspnea; pupils dilated, sometimes con-

---

1698. KEBLER, MORGAN, and RUPP: Bull. 126, Bureau of Chemistry, 1909.

stricted. In mild cases of poisoning, cyanosis, especially marked under the finger nails, and on the extremities and lips, may be the first symptoms noted by the attending physician. The oxygen capacity of the blood is lowered, and methemoglobin can be detected by the spectroscope. Where life is prolonged for a few days a progressive destruction of the red corpuscles may be seen. There may be acute nephritis, suppression of urine, and acute jaundice.

Fatal Dose: Severe symptoms have followed the ingestion of doses of four to fifteen grains. A boy of seven died in two hours after a third dose of 4.5 grains of acetanilid and 0.38 grain of caffeine. Recovery has been reported from the ingestion of doses up to 120 grains.

Treatment: Wash out the stomach with charcoal, and treat symptomatically. Give camphor, or strychnine after marked depression. Intravenous injection of normal saline, or hypodermatoclysis, should be given. Where the acetanilid habit has been acquired, withdrawal of the drug may cause maniacal actions.

Isolation and Detection: Acetanilid will be found in the acid ether extract during the examination for alkaloids. Some of it may be found in the acid chloroform extract.

1. A small portion of the residue is warmed with alcoholic potash and a drop of chloroform. The offensive odor of isonitrile appears in the presence of acetanilid.

2. Add 1 cc. of a 2% potassium dichromate solution and 5 cc. sulphuric acid to some of the solvent residue and agitate. A red color develops, which soon changes to blue, blue-green, and finally fades.

3. Heat about 0.1 gm. of the suspected substance with 1 cc. hydrochloric acid and add a small quantity of a solution of calcium hypochlorite and phenol. A red color is produced, which changes to a fine blue on the addition of ammonia.

DINITROPHENOL $(C_6H_3(NO_2)_2OH)$

DINITROPHENOL (alpha-dinitrophenol (1-2-4) is a yellow crystalline powder, closely related to picric acid. Newspaper publicity, indicating that this was a useful drug for reducing weight, caused its indiscriminate sale by druggists. Soon the medical literature contained many warnings of its harmful effects.

The use of alpha-dinitrophenol was suggested by Tainter, Stockton and Cutting.[1699] They recommended its use in an initial dose of 100 mg. of the sodium salt orally, taken at meals, with an increase at weekly intervals until a dosage was established that would cause decrease of two to three pounds of weight weekly. In their early experience some of their patients had gastro-intestinal upsets of brief duration; some complained of feeling tired, and others thought their nervousness was increased. A few of the patients had attacks of dizziness, and a number had skin reactions that required stoppage of the drug. In 1935 these same authors[1700] studied 177 patients and found that almost invariably a therapeutically effective dose of dinitrophenol produced symptoms of increased heat production, and in a few individuals there was some dyspnea on exertion due to the increased need for oxygen. Some had a sensation of languor or muscular weakness. Beebe[1701] reports a woman, aged thirty-two, who showed high fever and rash after the injection of one 1.6-grain capsule daily for three days, and then two capsules daily for three days.

A case of granulopenia was reported by Hoffman, Butt and Hickey in 1934.[1702] In 1936 Imerman and Imerman[1703] reported two cases of granulopenia following oral administration of alpha-dinitrophenol. Five similar cases were reported by Bohn,[1704] Davidson and Shapiro,[1705] Dameshek and Gargill,[1706] and Silver.[1707] Peripheral neuritis has been reported by Madler.[1708] Cataracts have been reported by Boardman.[1709] Anemia, thrombocytopenia, and purpura have been also reported.

Poisoning from this substance was reported by munitions

1699. TAINTER, M. L., STOCKTON, A. B., CUTTING, W. C.: J.A.M.A., 101:1472, 1933.
1700. J.A.M.A., 105:332, 1935.
1701. BEEBE: Colorado Med., 32:30, 1935.
1702. HOFFMANN, A. M., BUTT, E. M., and HICKEY, N. G.: J.A.M.A., 102:1213, 1934.
1703. IMERMAN, S. W., and IMERMAN, C. P.: J.A.M.A., 106:1085, 1936.
1704. BOHN, S. S.: J.A.M.A., 103:249, 1934.
1705. DAVIDSON, E. N., and SHAPIRO, M.: J.A.M.A., 103:480, 1934.
1706. DAMESHEK, W., and GARGILL, S. L.: New England J. Med., 211:440, 1934.
1707. SILVER, S.: J.A.M.A., 103:1058, 1934.
1708. MADLER, J. E.: J.A.M.A., 105:12, 1935.
1709. BOARDMAN, W. W.: J.A.M.A., 105:108, 1935.

plants during the period of the World War.[1710] Dinitrophenol in small doses, such as is given for the reduction of weight, has repeatedly caused functional changes indicative of toxicity of the liver, heart, and muscles in a large percentage of patients in whom no special idiosyncrasy was observed. Six cases of severe neutropenia have occurred, two of them fatal.[1711]

Goldman and Haber* reported a case of acute complete granulopenia with death due to the ingestion of 21.80 mg. of dinitrophenol over a period of four months.

In cases observed by Massermann and Goldsmith[1712] it was found that the oxygen consumption rate of patients rose from a pre-treatment control mean of —69 ± 1.54 to 26.0 ± 2.95 under maximal dosage, the mean rise in metabolic rate being, therefore, 32.9 ± 3.31, and ranging from +8 to +52 in individual patients. Examination of these patients revealed that in eight instances no physiological change could definitely be attributed to the pharmacological action of the drug, while in four there was a decrease in spontaneous activity with deepening lethargy and torpor. The toxic effects were characterized by fall in blood pressure, tachycardia, acidosis, progressive stupor, and one death.

It has been noticed that the use of dinitrophenol has caused profuse sweating; the temperature may rise 3°. Fourteen grains of the drug have caused signs of high temperature with a pulse 20 to 390 beats over normal, and respiration 15 to 30 over normal. Larger doses raised the metabolic rate, temperature, respiratory rate, and pulse rate of animals until they died.

Lattimore[1713] reported a case of a twenty-nine year old woman who for several months took three to five tablets of dinitrophenol a day. She discontinued its use for about three months, and resumed taking five tablets a day, about one week before death. Autopsy revealed petechial hemorrhages over the arms and legs; the heart showed moderate myo-

1710. KOELSCH, F.: Centralbl. f. Gewerbehyg., 4:261, 1927; MAGNE, H., MAYER, A., and PLANTEFOL, L.: Ann. de physiol., 7:269, 1931; PERKINS, R. G.: U. S. Pub. Health Reports, 34:2335, 1919.

1711. MACBRYDE, C. M., and TAUSSIG, B. L.: J.A.M.A., 105:13, 1933.

* GOLDMAN, A., and HABER, M.: J.A.M.A., 107:2115, 1936.

1712. MASSERMANN, J. H., and GOLDSMITH, H.: J.A.M.A., 102:523, 1934.

1713. LATTIMORE, J. H.: J. Kansas M. Soc., 35:388, 1934.

carditis; lungs were negative; spleen twice the normal size and soft; its cut surface appeared to be semi-liquid; the liver was so soft that upon pressure the fingers would sink into it. Microscopic examination of the spleen and liver showed marked destruction and hemorrhage; in the kidneys there was marked destruction of the epithelial lining of the tubules, with hemorrhage into the glomeruli.

ACETOPHENETIDIN ($C_{10}H_{13}O_2N$)

ACETOPHENETIDIN (phenacetin) has a molecular weight of 179.11. It is a colorless, glistening, crystalline substance, usually scaly, or a fine white crystalline powder which is odorless, slightly bitter, and stable in the air. One gm. is soluble in 131 cc. of water, 15 cc. of alcohol, 14 cc. of chloroform, and in about 13 cc. of ether at 25° C. Its melting point is 128° to 129° C. (U.S.P., XI).

Acetophenetidin is less toxic than acetanilid, but the symptoms of poisoning are practically identical; they are weakness, dizziness, depression, collapse, cyanosis with a blue-black hue to the skin and mucous membranes, formation of methemoglobin, chocolate colored urine, and weak, rapid heart. Skin affections occur more frequently than with acetanilid. In the fatal cases some pre-existing disease was usually present which was aggravated by this drug. Six grains taken within two hours caused death in a woman aged seventy-six. Many cases have been reported of death from taking five to ten grains. Addiction to this drug does not occur as often as to acetanilid.

Tests: 1. If a mixture of acetanilid and acetophenetidin is warmed with so much water that about one-half of the quantity remains undissolved, then the solution will contain about eight times as much acetanilid as acetophenetidin. When the solution cools, there will be formed drops of acetanilid.

2. A mixture of acetanisidin and acetophenetidin can be treated in the same fashion, but it is not possible without addition of water to separate acetanilid from acetophenetidin.

3. In dilute hydrochloric acid, acetanisidin is just as easily soluble as acetanilid, whereas acetophenetidin is difficultly soluble in this acid.

4. If boiled with dilute sulphuric acid, acetanisidin is somewhat more resistant to decomposition than acetanilid. Acetic acid appears in the distillate, and the residue will con-

tain the difficultly soluble sulphate of para-anisidin which crystallizes in well-formed, short crystals. Acetophenetidin decomposes only after prolonged boiling, which is to be continued for at least ten minutes. The sulphate of para-acetophenetidin is so difficultly soluble that it can easily be separated from the sulphates of anilin and para-anisidin by means of water. It crystallizes in the form of long, colorless needles (300 micra) which become consolidated to delicate star-like formations.

5. With platinochloride and sodium iodide, para-acetophenetidin yields black crystals.

6. With sulphuric acid and potassium bichromate a yellowish-brown color will be obtained. With anilin a violet and blue color is obtained. Para-anisidin gives a similar reaction, so that it is easy to differentiate by this means between acetophenetidin and acet-para-anisidin.

ANTIPYRINE ($C_{11}H_{12}CN_2$)

ANTIPYRINE has a molecular weight of 188.11, and is composed of colorless crystals, or a white crystalline powder. It is odorless, and has a slightly bitter taste. One gm. of antipyrine is soluble in less than 1 cc. of water, 1.3 cc. of alcohol, 1 cc. of chloroform, and 43 cc. of ether, at 25° C. It melts between 111° and 113° C. Antripyrine has a physical action similar to that of acetanilid. It differs from that substance and acetophenetidin in not causing methemoglobin. It is excreted in the urine where it is detected by the ferric chloride reaction; part is in combination with sulphuric acid.

Symptoms: Skin rashes or eruptions often accompanied by edema and itching are the toxic effects due to the use of antipyrine. Larger doses may cause prostration and collapse, with pallor, cold perspiration, rapid and feeble pulse, and occasionally cyanosis. Nervous symptoms, such as restlessness or convulsions, disturbances of sensation or of hearing, rarely amblyopia, vertigo, delirium or coma also occur, as well as occasional albuminuria. Pollak[1714] reported a fatal case from the consumption of 17 gm. in two and a half days. Death followed within a short time the administration of twenty-two grains in a consumptive and fifteen grains in a patient suffering with angina pectoris. Alarming symptoms have followed the use of five, ten, and fifteen grains.

1714. POLLAK: *Wien. med. Wchnschr.,* 61:1555, 1911.

The treatment is the same as under Acetanilid (see page 831). Wash out the stomach; give inhalations of oxygen or artificial respiration. Treat symptomatically with strychnine, camphor, and digitalis as the condition warrants.

Tests: Antipyrine is found in the acid ether extract during the investigation for alkaloids. If antipyrine, acetophenetidin, and acetanilid are suspected, they should be extracted with acid chloroform in which they are more soluble.

1. The heating of acetanilid and acetophenetidin with sulphuric acid gives in the distillate acetic acid, while in the residue in the flask there will be formed the difficulty soluble sulphate of para-anisidin which crystallizes out as short prisms. Acetophenetidin requires a longer time for this change. A sulphate of paraphenacetin is formed, which changes over into the sulphate of anilin and para-anisidin. Long, colorless needles are formed.

2. With sulphuric acid and potassium dichromate a yellow-brown color appears (anilin gives a violet and blue color).

3. An aqueous solution of phenacetin with ferric chloride gives a red color, which is destroyed by mineral acids.

4. Add to a water solution of antipyrine a drop or two of a dilute solution of potassium nitrite, and acidify with sulphuric acid. The characteristic green color of nitrosoantipyrine is produced. The reaction serves for the detection of one part of antipyrine in 10,000 parts of water.

5. Treat a portion of the residue of the extract with dilute hydrochloric acid, and add a few drops of Mayer's reagent. If a precipitate is obtained, antipyrine is indicated.

6. To another portion of this same solution add a few drops of sodium bromate reagent. If a blue color appears, phenacetin is indicated.

AMINOPYRINE
(Aminopyrine—Amidopyrina; Molecular Weight 231.16)

DIMETHYLAMINOPHENYLDIMETHYLPYRAZOLON occurs as colorless, or white, small crystals, or a white crystalline powder. It is odorless, and is stable in the air. Aminopyrine melts between 107° and 109° C. One gm. of aminoprine is soluble in 18 cc. of water, in 1.5 cc. of alcohol, in 12 cc. of benzene, in 1 cc. of chloroform, and in 13 cc. of ether, at 25° C. Madison and Squire reported that the onset of primary granulocytopenia was directly preceded by the use of amidopyrine alone or in combination with a barbiturate.[1715] The disease appeared most frequently in persons readily accessible to the drug, such as physicians, nurses, and patients. Miller[1716] reported the histological changes in bone-marrow of dogs following amidopyrine. However, in their experiments, attempts to cause granulopenia have not always been successful. Amidopyrine orally administered may exert a toxic effect upon the bone-marrow with little evidence of the fact in the circulatory granular elements of the blood.

Darling, Parker, and Jackson[1717] conclude that the uniformity of the pathological changes in the bone-marrow suggests that agranulocytosis is probably a disease entity.

Dennis[1718] reported a series of experiments in rabbits which show great promise. He was impressed by the capability of certain pyogenic bacteria (streptococci, staphylococci, and pseudomonas aeruginosa) to produce in culture media a toxin, leucocidin, which destroyed white blood cells, especially granulocytes. Dennis quoted the work of Nakayama,[1719] Gay and Oram,[1720] Van de Velde,[1721] Reudiger,[1722] and Gheorghiewsky.[1723]

Kracke[1724] has suggested that the vast increase in the use of coal-tar benzol derivatives as therapeutic agents, in the past few years, may be responsible for the recent increase in the number of cases of agranulocytosis. Hoffman, Butt, Hickey, and Watkins[1725] have called attention to a relationship between these drugs and the disease. Seeman,[1726] however, noted that in thirteen of his thirty-six cases amidopyrine or its allies had

1715. MADISON, F. W., and SQUIRE, T. L.: *J.A.M.A.*, 102:755, 1934.

1716. MILLER, K.: *Science*, 80:320, 1934.

1717. DARLING, R. C., PARKER, F., JACKSON, H.: *Am. J. Path.*, 12:1, 1936.

1718. DENNIS, E. W.: *J. Exper. Med.*, 57:993, 1933.

1719. NAKAYAMA, Y.: *J. Infect. Dis.*, 27:86, 1920.

1720. GAY, F. P., and ORAM, FLORENCE: *Proc. Soc. Exper. Biol. & Med.*, 28:850, 1931.

1721. VAN DE VELDE, H.: *Cellule*, 10:403, 1894.

1722. REUDIGER, G. F.: *J.A.M.A.*, 44:98, 1905.

1723. GHEORGHIEWSKY, B. A.: *Ann. Inst. Pasteur*, 13:298, 1899.

1724. KRACKE, R.: *J. Lab. & Clin. Med.*, 17:993, 1932.

1725. HOFFMANN, A. M., BUTT, E. M., and HICKEY, N. G.: *J.A.M.A.*, 102:1212, 1934; WATKINS, C. H.: *Proc. Staff Meet., Mayo Clin.*, 8:713, 1933.

1726. SEEMAN, H.: *Ugesk. f. laeger.*, 96:237, 1934.

been taken, yet in fifteen there was definitely no history of such therapy. Jackson,[1727] in an analysis of twenty-seven cases in which complete and unequivocal data relative to medication were at hand, found that in only seven of them could the disease be properly regarded as directly traceable to the administration of these compounds. A special report of the Council on Pharmacy and Chemistry of the American Medical Association[1728] concludes that there is "no question that amidopyrine is very important in the production of granulocytopenia."

The diagnosis of agranulocytosis can be definitely made only when the white blood count is greatly reduced, usually below 1,000 cells per cubic millimeter, and when the granulocytes are either completely absent or found in very small numbers, and usually abnormal in character. Agranulocytosis occurs most commonly in mid-adult life. Jackson, in a series of 103 cases found the white blood count rarely to be as high as 25l)0 per cubic centimeter, and often 1000 or less. In this series of 103 cases, thirty had white counts less than 500, twenty-eight had white counts between 500 and 1000, thirty-eight had white counts between 1000 and 2000, and only seven had white counts between 2000 and 3000. Neutropenia of an extreme grade is the rule.

Treatment: Transfusions of blood have been helpful in a number of instances. Pentose nucleotide has been tried in other instances. Pentose nucleotide was introduced as "Nucleotide K 96," and is now marketed under the trade name of "Pentonucleotide." The dose recommended is one ampoule intramuscularly twice a day until the leucocyte count and granulocyte percentage have risen considerably.[1729] Fitz-Hugh,[1730] and Taussig[1731] treated four cases by x-ray with a mortality of 50%. Foran, Sheaff, and Trimmer reported remissions in five patients who received liver extract.[1732] The commercial preparation of the fraction "G" of Cohn was used in doses equiva-

1727. JACKSON, H., JR.:　Am. J. M. Sc., 188:482, 1934.

1728. J.A.M.A., 102:2183, 1934.

1729. JACKSON, H., JR., PARKER, F., JR., and TAYLOR, F. H. L.:　Am. J. M Sc., 184:297, 1932.

1730. FITZ-HUGH, T., JR., and COMROE, B.:　Am. J. M. Sc., 185:552, 1933.

1731. TAUSSIG, A. E., and SCHNOEBELEN, P. C.:　J.A.M.A., 97:1757, 1931.

1732. FORAN, F. L., SHEAFF, H. M., and TRIMMER, R. W.:　J.A.M.A., 100:1917, 1933.

lent to 100 gm. of fresh liver. This was injected intramuscularly, or diluted with 20 cc. of distilled water and injected intravenously every eight to twelve hours until improvement occurred. There is no remedy at the present time that will stop this condition in 60% of the cases.

CANTHARIDES

EVERY year two or three cases of poisoning by this substance occur in Cook County. Most of the cases seen by the author have been caused from its use as an aphrodisiac. In one case death occurred due to its use as an abortifacient. Severe poisoning and even death have resulted from its absorption through the skin to which it had been applied as a vesicant.

Cantharides (cantharis, U. S. P., XI, Spanish or Russian flies) consists of dried insects, cantharis vesicatoria (U. S. P., XI). Cantharides yields not less than 0.6% of cantharidin and not more than 10% of moisture. The powdered drug, or the tincture has usually been used, but a number of cases of poisoning have been reported from the use of the salts.

Symptoms: Applied to the skin, cantharides produces redness and pain, followed by vesicles which later collect to form blisters. When taken internally, similar conditions are formed on the mucous membrane as on the skin. There is an intense burning in the esophagus and stomach. There may be intense thirst with inability to swallow. Vomiting may occur, and the vomited material will contain blood and shreds of mucous membrane. Bloody diarrhea, with the most intense abdominal pain, occurs. There is weakness and a state of collapse, and death may occur in from sixteen to twenty-four hours after the poison is taken. There is irritation of the bladder with a constant desire to urinate, pain referred to the kidney with albuminuria, scanty urine, hematuria, and rapid pulse. The inflammation of the bladder and urethra produces pain, and frequently leads to priapism. In pregnant women abortion has resulted. Nephritis caused by this drug may lead to death. Chronic nephritis has been reported from its use. Powell[1733] and Wallace and Pellini[1734] show that cantharides produces a marked degree of acidosis, the renal injury not being an essential factor in this acidosis.

1733. POWELL: *Lancet*, 2:1296, 1907.
1734. WALLACE and PELLINI: *Arch. Int. Med.*, 28:711, 1921.

Twenty-five grains of the powdered drug have caused death; in another case recovery followed the ingestion of forty-two grains.

Fatal Period: In one case which the author saw, death occurred in eighteen hours. Life may be prolonged from one to fourteen days. In cases that are rapidly fatal the chief symptoms arise from the alimentary tract, the intense irritation of which leads to a shock-like condition. In the less acute cases death usually results from nephritis.

Treatment: The stomach should be washed out. Mucilaginous drinks and opiates should be given to allay the pain. Oil should not be used, as the cantharidin is readily soluble in it.

Postmortem Appearances: The postmortem appearances show a severe gastritis, enteritis, and nephritis. Cystitis and urethritis have also been observed. Vesicles may be found in the mouth and pharynx. An examination of the kidneys may show marked damage of the glomeruli and tubules, the picture being one of combined glomerulo-nephritis and nephrosis.

CANTHARIDIN ($C_{10}H_{12}O_4$)

CANTHARIDIN is the active principle of cantharides. It forms colorless, shining, neutral, rhombic leaflets, melting at 218°C., and subliming at higher temperature as white needles. Cantharidin is used principally in remedies for stimulation of the urinary and genital organs, and locally as a blistering agent. It is often combined with phosphorus, nux vomica, and zinc phosphide. It is soluble in acetone, chloroform, and ethyl acetate, but only very slightly soluble in cold water, and in petroleum ether. The fatal dose of cantharidin is not definitely known, but it is considered as about 30 mg. Cantharidin is readily absorbed from all surfaces, even the skin. When taken by mouth it produces burning in the mouth, great thirst with some inability to swallow, nausea, vomiting, and sometimes bloody diarrhea and tenesmus. The symptoms are comparable with those of Cantharides (see page 839).

Detection: The material is treated with water and 1 cc. of 10% sodium carbonate solution. Evaporate to dryness on the water-bath. The residue is taken up in 10 cc. of water and treated with 2 cc. of hydrochloric acid (one to four) and shaken out with chloroform. The chloroform extract is evaporated, the least traces of the solvent being blown out with an air current. The residue, after evaporation of the chloroform, may be applied to the flexor surface of the forearm to test out its vesicant action. Obtain the melting point, and note if the substance sublimes.

DIGITALIS

DIGITALIS (foxglove, digitalis folium P. I.) is the dried leaf of digitalis purpurea. The potency of digitalis shall be such that 0.1 gm. of it, when assayed as directed, shall possess an activity equivalent to not less than one U.S.P. digitalis unit. One U.S.P. unit is identical in potency with the International Digitalis Unit, as adopted in 1928 by the Permanent Commission on Biological Standardization of the Health Organization of the League of Nations. One International Digitalis Unit represents the activity of 0.1 gm. of the "International Standard Digitalis Powder" (U.S.P., XI).

The toxicity of digitalis is due to the presence of several glucosides; some of which occur also in the seeds. The most active of these is digitoxin, which occurs to the extent of 0.22% to 0.4% in leaves of average activity. It is insoluble in water. Other glucosides are digitalin, digitalein, and digitonin; the latter is almost inert physiologically.

A toxic dose of digitalis produces vomiting, cardiac irregularity, and sudden heart failure. A number of other drugs are used in medical practice that behave similarly to digitalis, such as squill, apocynum, and strophanthus.

The toxic phenomena may be grouped under: (1) digestive disturbances, usually characterized by nausea and vomiting; (2) cardiac irregularities, and (3) excessive doses causing fatalities. Digestive disturbances are not caused by the local irritation, and are best explained on the assumption that the emetic center is stimulated by reflexes set up by the cardiac actions. In addition to the nausea, great malaise, and often headache, which may be distressing, are noted. When these occur the drug should be discontinued. In the cardiac disturbances there is a drop in the pulse rate to below 50 with ventricular extrasystoles due to excessive vagus stimulation. An overdose of the drug may cause excessive vagus stimulation (sinus irregularity). Later a partial heart block may be seen if the conductivity of the heart was naturally low before the administration of the digitalis preparation.

Fatal Dose: A single massive dose of about 2.5 gm. may be fatal. Death has been caused by one ounce, 30 cc., of the tincture. Of the various constituents of digitalis, digitoxin is the most active. In the Koppe case[1735] one-thirtieth grain (0.002 gm.) of digitoxin caused most severe poisoning, and it is very probable that one-fifteenth grain (0.004 gm.) would ordinarily be fatal. Ampoules of a proprietary digitalis preparation caused several deaths, in 1915, in a Chicago hospital. The batch of material was immediately removed from the market and no further accidents occurred. Six to 7 cc. of digalen (presumably containing 1.8 to 2.1 mg. of "soluble digitoxin") caused extremely severe poisoning.

Digitoxin, $C_{34}H_{54}O_{11}$, crystallizes from a mixture of methyl alcohol and chloroform in slender anhydrous prisms melting at 243°C. (469°F.), or from dilute alcohol in hydrated crystals melting at 145°C. (293° to 302°F.). It is insoluble in hot or cold water, very slightly soluble in ether, and readily soluble in alcohol and chloroform.

Tests: 1. Concentrated sulphuric acid dissolves it with a greenish color, which is unchanged by the addition of bromine.

2. If a small portion of digitoxin is dissolved in 2 cc. of glacial acetic acid containing a trace of iron, and this solution floated upon 2 cc. of concentrated sulphuric acid containing a trace of iron, a brownish color appears at the zone of contact of the two solutions.

3. Lafon's Reaction: If a small portion of the glucoside is moistened with a drop or two of a mixture of equal parts of 95% alcohol and concentrated sulphuric acid, and a drop of very dilute solution of ferric chloride be mixed with this, an intense greenish-blue coloration is observed. Digitalin does not give this reaction.

4. Brissemont-Derrien's Reaction: Dissolve a portion of the glucoside in 2 cc. of the following solution (30 cc. of glacial acetic acid mixed with 20 cc. of 4% oxalic acid solution (reduced to glyoxalic acid by treatment with sodium amalgam until the reaction is neutral), and float the solution on 2 cc. of concentrated sulphuric acid. Digitoxin slowly develops a grayish-green color at the zone of contact, while digitalin strikes a cherry-red tone.

Digitalin, $C_{35}H_{56}O_{14}$, is a colorless, amorphous powder,

1735. KOPPE: *Arch. f. exper. Path. u. Pharmakol.*, 3:289, 1874.

melting at 217°C. (422.6°F.). It is very sparingly soluble in water, readily soluble in hot alcohol, and very sparingly soluble in ether and chloroform.

Tests: 1. Concentrated sulphuric acid colors pure digitalin orange-yellow. This solution soon becomes blood red, changing to cherry and then violet on the addition of a little bromine water.

2. Instead of the bromine water one may use Keller's reagent. Digitalin gives a cherry-red color at the zone of contact, the lower layer of the acetic acid solution being light yellow, changing to brownish.

Digitonin, $C_{54}H_{92}O_{28}$ or $C_{55}H_{94}O_{28}$, is classified with the saponins, and crystallizes in colorless needles, or in thick warty masses melting at 235°C. (455°F.). It dissolves in 600 parts of cold water and fifty parts of warm water to a turbid solution, but dissolves to a clear solution in fifty parts of 50% alcohol. Its solutions are levorotatory.

Tests 1. Concentrated sulphuric acid dissolves it with a red color, which is intensified by the addition of a drop of bromine water.

2. Concentrated hydrochloric acid dissolves digitonin, the solution becoming yellow and finally reddish-violet on heating or on long standing, with a slight greenish fluorescence. Digitalin dissolves in concentrated hydrochloric acid with a golden-yellow color, which changes to violet on standing.

Isolation and Detection: In the isolation of these glucosides from the gastro-intestinal content by the same process used for the isolation of alkaloids, digitoxin, and to a less extent digitalin and digitonin, will be obtained by extraction of the acid aqueous solution with chloroform.

Physiological Test: Whenever digitalis or its derivatives are suspected as a source of poisoning, physiological tests should be made on frogs or cats. The author uses frogs, as they are much easier to handle. Foster and VanDyke emphasize the temperature control in the frog assay method, and have effected this by means of a specially constructed water-bath.[1736] The heart is exposed, the beats counted, and then 1 or 2 mg. of suspected glucoside in solution in alcohol of not over 20% strength is injected into the lymph sac. If the material belongs to the digitalis series, the heart will become slower, will empty itself

1736. FOSTER and VANDYKE: *J. Am. Pharm. Ass.*, 22:381, 1933.

more completely at each systole, and will dilate less during diastole, until it finally stops in systole. Control tests should be run with known quantities of digitalis, using the same weight animal under the same experimental conditions.

Treatment: Wash out the stomach with a tannic acid solution. Give an emetic. Tincture of aconite can be given, but cautiously.

STROPHANTHUS

STROPHANTHUS (formerly in the U. S. P.) has caused severe and fatal poisoning. The symptoms are similar to those of digitalis poisoning, but the course is more rapid.

Strophanthinum (strophthanin) is a U.S.P. preparation. It is a glucoside obtained from strophanthus kombe Oliver. Strophanthinum, when assayed as directed, shall possess a potency equivalent to the activity of not less than 40% and not more than 60% of ouabain, when similarly assayed.

Death has occurred from the intravenous injection of strophanthinum. It may occur in a few hours, or it may occur in a few minutes, from doses less than 1 mg.

Strophanthin, $C_{40}H_{66}O_{19}3H_2O$, is a white or yellowish crystalline powder which melts at about 158°C. (316.4°F.). It contains varying proportions of water which it does not lose entirely without decomposition. If heated **in vacuo** to 80°C. (176°F.) it loses its water of crystallization, the anhydrous substance melting at 178° to 179°C. (352.4° to 354.2°F.). It is very soluble in water and in dilute alcohol, less soluble in dehydrated alcohol, and nearly insoluble in chloroform, ether or benzene.

Isolation: From the acid aqueous extract of the material under examination, a benzene extract is made to remove various impurities, and strophanthin is finally removed by shaking with amyl alcohol. Evaporation of the solvent leaves the residue containing the strophanthin.

Tests: 1. Treated with concentrated sulphuric acid, strophanthin turns emerald green, changing to brown. When warmed with the acid the green color changes to violet shades, and finally becomes black.

2. Add a trace of ferric chloride solution and a few mils (cc.) of sulphuric acid to an aqueous solution of the suspected residue. A reddish-brown precipitate is produced, which turns emerald green after one or two hours.

3. Sulphuric acid containing a little phenol gives a violet color, changing to green. Froehde's and Mandelin's reagents yield the same colors.

4. Strophanthin gives a red color when treated in turn with a solution of sodium nitroprusside and an alkali.

5. Tannic acid yields a precipitate with strophanthin, which dissolves in excess of the reagent.

OLEANDER

THE leaves and bark of the common ornamental shrub, Nerium oleander, contain two or more active principles belonging to the "digitalis series." The symptoms caused by eating the leaves have been vomiting, abdominal pain, vertigo, convulsive movements, insensibility, small, very slow pulse, and in some cases epileptiform convulsions followed by coma and death.

COTTON-ROOT BARK

COTTON-ROOT bark has been used to some extent as an emmenagogue, and has a reputation among the negroes in the south as being an abortifacient. A few cases of poisoning have been reported. The symptoms are rapid, weak pulse, dilated pupils, shallow respiration, great muscular relaxation, and sometimes abortion. Four ounces of fluid extract caused severe symptoms.

TANSY

TANSY, the leaves and tops of tanacetum vulgare, a common plant in the United States, contains a volatile oil in which thujon is present. Tansy formerly was used extensively by the laity as an abortifacient. A number of deaths have occurred from its use. When a large dose is taken internally, there is a sensation of warmth in the stomach; the pulse is weak and respirations become slow and irregular; there are muscular incoordination, convulsions, coma, and death. There is usually great irritation of the urinary tract, with albuminuria, strangury, hematuria, and painful erections.

One dram (3.7 cc.) of the oil has caused death in an hour and a quarter; 15 gm. caused death in less than two hours. A patient died twenty-six hours after taking an infusion of perhaps one-half ounce of the dry herb.

OIL OF PENNYROYAL

THE leaves and tops of hedeoma pulegioides are used as a carminative, using 5 to 10 gm., in one to two ounces, as an infusion. The oil (oleum hedeoma), in a dose of 0.2 cc. or three minims, has caused convulsions. The oil, in addition to its local effects, causes nephritis and fatty degeneration of the liver. The leaves and the oil are used by the laity as an emmenagogue, and have a reputation as an abortifacient. A few deaths have resulted, not only from the oil but the proprietary preparation containing the leaves as well as the oil. The chief symptoms are those of a gastro-intestinal irritant, collapse, unconsciousness, coma. Convulsions and dilated pupils may be seen. Macht reported a case of poisoning by pills in which there was a marked fatty degeneration of the liver.[1737]

NUTMEG

NUTMEG (myristica, U.S.P.) is often used as an emmenagogue, and as an abortifacient. The symptoms are mainly narcotic, but there may be excitement and motor stimulation with choreiform movements; a flushing of the face, staggering gait, drowsiness, stupor which may last from four to thirty hours; delirium, sometimes burning pain in the stomach; occasionally collapse with small thready pulse; dilated, sometimes contracted pupils. The symptoms usually appear within six hours, and recovery occurs in twenty-four hours. Hepatic necrosis has been demonstrated in cats.

Two nutmegs eaten by a boy of eight caused death in twenty-four hours.

APIOL

THERE have been a series of poisonings caused by apiol which has been used to produce menstruation or as an abortifacient. The causes of poisoning were not due to apiol itself but to a mixture of apiol and ortho-tricresyl phosphate which was accidentally made by a well known firm. The first cases of poisoning were observed in Holland in 1931. It was taken by women with menstrual disorders; they fell ill with severe polyneuritis and paralysis of the hands and feet.

1737. *J.A.M.A.*, 61:105, 1913.

OIL OF SAVIN

SAVIN is the tops of juniperus sabina, an evergreen growing in Europe, and said to occur also in the northern part of the United States. The active principle is contained in an oil which is closely related to oil of turpentine. I have seen a number of cases of death from its use as an abortifacient. The amount used by the individuals was not known. The symptoms are similar to those given under Tansy (see page 845). It is doubtful whether it has any specific action on the uterus. The abortion may be the indirect result of the hyperemia of the pelvic organs caused by the irritation of the intestines. Lewin has collected twenty cases in which abortion occurred, with nine deaths; also eleven cases of poisoning in which abortion did not occur, but in four of which death resulted.[1738]

Death may occur in twelve hours, or it may be delayed for four or five days. In a case described by Blyth, a woman died in about twenty-six hours from an unknown quantity of infusion of savin tops.[1739] Postmortem showed the pharynx was reddened and the gullet congested; the stomach was congested and contained savin tops. The odor of savin is usually noticed in the stomach and sometimes in other organs. The treatment is evacuation of the stomach and a general symptomatic regime.

OIL OF TURPENTINE

OIL OF TURPENTINE is obtained by distillation from the resin of pine trees, and contains principally the cyclic hydrocarbon, pinene. It is used chiefly as a solvent, but finds some use in medicine. When pure, oil of turpentine is composed of one or more terpenes, but, as usually seen, it contains oxidation products of these hydrocarbons. It is a colorless or light yellowish, highly inflammable oil, moderately soluble in alcohol and very slightly so in water. It has a hot, burning taste, and when applied to the skin causes irritation and redness. It has a characteristic odor.

The rectified oil of turpentine consists mainly of terebenthene. It is a mobile, colorless liquid with an odor of turpentine, and is highly refractive. Turpentine oil has a specific gravity of 0.864, and a boiling point of 156° to 160°C. (312.8° to 320°F.); it burns with a smoky flame. It is insoluble in water,

1738. LEWIN: Die Fruchtabtreibung durche Gifte, Berlin, 1905.
1739. BLYTH: Poisons, 4th ed., 475, 1906.

dilute acids, and dilute alkalis; it is soluble in absolute alcohol, ether, petroleum ether, chloroform, and benzene. It has been largely replaced by cheaper solvents, especially the petroleum distillates and the chlorinated hydrocarbons.

Poisoning has occurred from its use in medicine, also from accident, or occasionally from the use of the substance for the purpose of suicide, or, more frequently, for producing abortion. Its vapors are also poisonous, causing redness and swelling of the mucous membranes, with some exudation. In one individual, Mrs. W. C., the exposure to turpentine fumes for two weeks during very hot weather, I believe was responsible for the production of an exfoliative dermatitis from which the patient died. Turpentine vapors, and also the oil, taken internally, cause a nephritis, and repeated doses may cause a chronic nephritis. Repeated irritation of the respiratory tract may cause pneumonia. It is excreted by the lungs, and gives its characteristic odor to the expired air. It is also excreted in the urine, which acquires the odor of violets, showing reduced properties, since the turpentine is combined with glycuronic acid. When a large dose is taken internally, the symptoms are similar to those caused by oil of tansy. Painters exposed to the vapors in a closed space may have bronchitis, conjunctivitis, headache, dizziness, staggering, drowsiness, even unconsciousness, and often strangury and irritation of the kidneys with bloody urine.

The lethal dose is not known. A woman died in a few hours after taking about six ounces of the oil. An infant of fourteen weeks died in fifteen hours after swallowing half an ounce.

The treatment consists in the evacuation of the stomach, and the administration of demulcents and stimulants.

OIL OF CEDAR

THE literature since 1845 contains a record of only nineteen cases of cedar oil poisoning; thirteen were abortion cases, four of them ending fatally.[1740]

The symptoms are burning in the stomach, vomiting (sometimes bloody), violent convulsions, bloody froth at the mouth, irregular respiration, weak, slow and sometimes intermittent pulse, and cold, clammy skin.

1740. MCNALLY, W. D.: *Med. Rec.*, 1916.

Oil of cedar has a specific gravity of 0.928 and a refractive index of 1.471 at 7° C.

The symptoms appear soon after the poison is taken, often within a few minutes. Death occurred after ingestion of about one ounce within an hour;[1740] it has been delayed twenty-six hours.[1741] With treatment, recovery has followed the ingestion of one ounce. A few cases of accidental poisoning have been reported, one due to a pharmacist's error, and another when the oil was used in the treatment of gonorrhea. Wait[1742] reported four cases, in one of which a young man who had seduced a girl was convicted of her murder. In the second case a young woman, aged twenty-six, who took a "large spoonful" recovered with treatment. In a third case, a girl seventeen years of age took one ounce and recovered with treatment. In a fourth case a woman, aged thirty-two years, died within one hour after drinking an unknown amount. Branden[1743] reports a case in which a woman recovered after swallowing one dram. In Thompson and Archibald's case, in which an unknown amount was taken, the woman died.[1744] In Brown's case,[1745] the woman took one-half ounce of oil without aborting. The symptoms consisted of dizziness, frothing at the mouth, violent convulsions, unconsciousness, dyspnea, cold perspiration, and suppression of the urine for thirty-six hours. Other cases have been reported, but in no instance did a woman abort.

Postmortem Appearances: In the author's case, the gastric contents had a pronounced odor of oil of cedar. There was an edema of both lungs. The heart was normal in size, the myocardium, endocardium, and the valves appeared normal. There was an increase of the pericardial fluid. The peritoneum was smooth and glistening; the vessels of the omentum, mesentery and pelvis were deeply injected. The stomach was acutely dilated. The subserous vessels of the lesser and greater curvature were intensely engorged. Upon opening the stomach a strong odor of oil of cedar was noticed. The serosa of the small intestine appeared normal; there was a distinct hyperemia of the mucosa of the large intestine. The liver was slight-

1741. BOLLES: *Med. & Surg. Reports, Boston City Hosp.*, 2s., 2:270, 1877.

1742. WAIT, S. C.: *Boston M. & S. J.*, 40:469, 1849.

1743. St. Louis Clinique, 1908, p. 105.

1744. THOMPSON and ARCHIBALD: *Interstate M. J.*, 20:657, 1913.

1745. *Med. News,* 58:15, 1893.

ly enlarged, with intense congestion. The pancreas appeared normal. The spleen was of normal size. The kidneys were slightly enlarged, of a dark red color; the capsule stripped easily leaving a smooth surface. On section, both cortex and medulla appeared hyperemic. The urinary bladder was empty. The mucosa was hyperemic. The uterus was enlarged and contained a fetus of about six weeks gestation; the membranes were intact. The ovaries and tubes were markedly congested. The right ovary was enlarged, and upon section a corpus luteum of about 0.75 cm. in diameter was found.

Isolation: The well-diluted material is subjected to distillation with steam. The distillate is saturated with sodium chloride and shaken out in a separatory funnel with ether or odorless, low-boiling-point petroleum ether. The ether layer is separated and allowed to evaporate spontaneously.

Detection:

1. Odor.   2. Specific gravity.   3. Refractive index.

CAMPHOR ($C_{10}H_{16}O$)

CAMPHOR has a molecular weight of 152.12. It is a ketone obtained from cinnamomum camphora, and forms white, translucent crystaline masses that are almost insoluble in water but dissolve readily in alcohol, ether, benzene, oils, and chloroform. It has a penetrating, characteristic odor, a pungent, aromatic taste, and is readily pulverizable in the presence of a little alcohol, ether, or chloroform. One gm. of camphor is soluble in about 800 cc. of water, in 1 cc. of alcohol, in 0.5 cc. of chloroform, and in 1 cc. of ether at 25° C. It is freely soluble in carbon disulfide, in petroleum benzine, and in fixed and volatile oils. Its specific gravity is about 0.990 at 25° C. It melts between 174° and 177° C. Natural camphor has a specific rotation (alpha)$_D$, in a solution containing 10 gm. of camphor in 100 cc. of alcohol and using a 200-mm. tube, of between +41° and +42°. Under similar conditions the specific rotation (alpha)$_D$ of synthetic camphor is between +5° and —5°.

Most of the cases of accidental poisoning occur among children. Liniments containing camphor have been mistaken for castor oil with serious results. It is used extensively as a household remedy for colds, a practice that occasionally leads to mild cases of poisoning.

The first symptoms of camphor poisoning are usually a

burning sensation in the throat and stomach, vomiting, thirst, blurred vision, roaring in the ears, dizziness, headache, and rapid pulse. These symptoms are followed in from ten minutes to several hours by hallucinations, delirium, and convulsions; the latter may develop very suddenly. The pulse is irregular, and the breath and urine smell of camphor. Nausea, faintness, and loss of appetite may continue for several days.

Fatal Dose and Period: A child died after swallowing a quantity of camphor estimated as about fifteen grains (1 gm.). A child of sixteen months died in a few hours after taking 15 gm. of a 20% camphorated oil. In a case reported by Rubsamen, 170 cc. of 10% camphorated oil placed in the peritoneal cavity caused the usual symptoms, and death on the third day.[1746]

Treatment: Treatment consists of evacuation of the bowels and stomach with saline purgatives or calomel. Castor oil and alcohol should not be used, as they favor the absorption of the poison. Bromides and morphine may be used to relieve the convulsions.

The postmortem appearances are not characteristic, but the organs will have the odor of camphor.

Isolation: Camphor will be found in the acid distillate. The benzene extract is evaporated on a water-bath, the camphor remains as a residue. This can be purified by several recrystallizations from 50% alcohol. The melting point of camphor is 176° C. It has a characteristic odor and spontaneous volatility.

Test the solution under the polariscope.

The purified material, obtained by recrystallization, is dried and weighed as such.

MALE FERN

MALE FERN (Aspidium, U.S.P., the rhizome of Dryopteris Filix-mass or of D. Marginalis) yields an extract, official under the name of Oleoresina aspidii; a dark green, thick liquid usually depositing a granular, crystalline substance, which must be thoroughly mixed with the liquid portion before use. Its specific gravity is not less than 1.00 at 25°C.

The symptoms of poisoning are due to local irritation of the stomach and intestines and in part to the effects of stimu-

1746. RUBSAMEN: *Zentralbl. f. Gynäk., Leipz.,* **36**:1009, 1912.

lation and depression of the central nervous system. The chief symptoms are vomiting, purging, acute abdominal pain, muscular weakness, confusion and somnolence with twitching of the muscles or slight convulsive movements, headache, fever, dyspnea, collapse, coma, and death. One of the most serious symptoms is blindness, either temporary or permanent. In seventy-eight cases of poisoning collected by Sidler-Huguenin,[1747] eighteen of the patients became permanently blind in both eyes, while fifteen became blind in one eye. The lesion was atrophy of the optic nerve.

Fatal Dose and Period: Children have died from one or two drams. The fatal dose for adults has varied from five to six drams. Death has occurred from six to twenty hours after ingestion of the drug.

Treatment: Evacuate the stomach, being careful not to use fats or oils. Give mucilaginous drinks and stimulants after washing out the stomach.

Postmortem Appearances: Postmortem appearances are not characteristic . The stomach and bowels are congested and swollen and covered with small ecchymoses.

Isolation and Detection: The poisonous principle is extracted by ether. The residue contains an ethereal oil with filicic acid. The latter when saponified yields butyric acid and phloroglucin. A pine splinter moistened with hydrochloric acid is turned red by phloroglucin.

SANTONIN

SANTONIN, $C_{15}H_{18}O_3$, has a molecular weight of 246.14. It is made up of colorless crystals, usually tabular, or a white crystalline powder. Santonin is odorless, and nearly tasteless at first, but later developing a bitter taste. It is stable in the air, but rapidly becomes yellow on exposure to light. Santonin is almost insoluble in cold water, and only slightly soluble in boiling water. One gm. is soluble in 43 cc. of alcohol and in 1.7 cc. of chloroform at 25°C. It melts between 169° and 171°C. Solutions of santonin are levorotatory.

With 2 cc. of alcohol and potassium hydroxide the mixture develops a red color (U.S.P., XI).

Santonin is used almost exclusively as an anthelmintic to remove round worms from the intestine, and most cases of poi-

1747. SIDLER-HUGUENIN: *Cor.-Bl. f. schweiz. Aerzte,* 28:513, 1898.

soning have occurred from its medicinal use by the laity. The most outstanding symptom produced is xanthopsia, or "yellow sight" — objects that are brightly illuminated have a yellow tinge—and there are often other disturbances of color vision. This effect rarely continues for twenty-four hours, although, in one severe case of poisoning, complete blindness lasted for nearly a week. Occasionally there are disturbances of the senses of taste, smell, and hearing. The symptoms may begin in a few minutes, and consist of headache, dizziness, unsteady gait, dilated pupils, clonic convulsions, loss of consciousness, and also a fall of body temperature. Convulsions may continue for several days, or the patient may early pass into a condition of stupor. The urine is yellow and may be diminished in quantity.

Fatal Dose and Period: Nearly all cases of poisoning have occurred among children who have been given the drug as a remedy for round worms. Children from five to six years old have died in from thirty-five minutes to fifteen hours after taking six grains of santonin. Adults have recovered after eight to fifteen grains.

Treatment: Treatment consists of thorough evacuation of the stomach and bowels. Ether, chloroform, or chloral hydrate may be used to control the convulsions. In case of collapse the child may be placed in a warm bath with cold effusions.

There are no characteristic postmortem appearances.

Isolation: The tissue under examination is made into a thin paste with very dilute sodium hydroxide and digested at 30°C. (86°F.) with three times its volume of 96% alcohol for twenty-four hours. The liquid is filtered, the alcohol is distilled off, and the aqueous alkaline fluid is shaken out with benzene. As long as the liquid is alkaline, santonin will not be taken up by the benzene, and various impurities may thus be removed. The santonin can finally be removed with chloroform or benzene after the aqueous fluid has been acidified with hydrochloric acid.

Tests: 1. The material is placed on a watch glass and exposed to the sunlight for a day or two. On adding a drop of alcoholic solution of potassium hydroxide a characteristic red color is produced.

2. Santonin dissolved in concentrated sulphuric acid gives a yellow color. The crystals are surrounded by a violet ring as they join the solution if this solution is then diluted with an

equal volume of water and treated with ferric chloride a violet color is produced.[1748]

3. When fused with potassium hydroxide, santonin imparts a red color to the mass.

4. Alcoholic solution of santonin, plus two drops of alcoholic furfural solution and 2 cc. of sulphuric acid, warmed on a water-bath, gives a red color, which changes to violet and to blue.

VEGETABLE PURGATIVES

MOST of these cases of poisoning are accidental, although some have been due to the use of the drugs for criminal purposes—for committing murder or for securing abortion. After poisonous doses there is violent purgation accompanied by colic, tenderness in the abdomen; shock, collapse, and death may follow. Some of these drugs cause local irritation when applied to the skin. They may be divided into three classes according to their chemical properties: (1) purgative oils; (2) purgatives of the anthracene series; (3) the jalapin group.

PURGATIVE OILS
CROTON OIL

A FEW cases of poisoning have resulted from the administration of croton oil in candy or whiskey as a practical joke. Ellis[1749] reported a death due to its use for the latter. It is the most violent of all cathartics, one-half drop producing burning in the mouth and stomach, often vomiting, and after one-half to three hours several extensive fluid evacuations with much colic and tenesmus. It finds very little use in medical practice today. Twenty drops have been fatal, but recovery is said to have followed one-half ounce. The treatment consists of thorough evacuation of the stomach, opiates, and general symptomatic care. Applied externally, croton oil produces irritation proceeding to pustulation and even sloughing. Students in the author's laboratory class in Materia Medica have tasted the oil, reporting a burning sensation followed by marked edema and inflammation of the tongue.

At autopsy the mucous membrane of the alimentary tract is reddened and swollen, and hemorrhages may be found in the bowel.

1748. LINDO: *Chem. News*, 36:222, 1877.
1749. *Am. J. M. Sc.*, 65:436, 1874.

Croton oil is found in the acid petrolic ether extract in investigation for alkaloids. It will be mixed with fatty substances which are soluble in the petrolic ether. The residue may be tested for the presence of croton oil by rubbing a little on the inside of the arm and observing the hyperemia and vesication. Some of the residue may be given to laboratory animals.

There are no conclusive chemical tests for croton oil in amounts such as would be extracted from the gastro-intestinal tract.

ANTHRACENE PURGATIVES
ALOES

ALOES is the dried juice of the leaves of Aloe perryi Baker. Unground Socotrine aloe is a yellowish-brown to blackish-brown, opaque, smooth and glistening mass. The odor is characteristic. The active principles are pentosides, of which there are several varieties.

Aloin is a lemon yellow to dark yellow microcrystalline powder, or minute crystals. It is odorless, or has a slight odor of aloe. It darkens on exposure to light and air. Aloin is soluble in water, in alcohol, and in acetone; it is also soluble in ammonia water, and in solutions of alkali hydroxides, forming red solutions (or yellow solutions that become red) having a green fluorescence.

Poisoning with aloes has resulted from the use of too large medicinal doses, and from its use by the laity as an abortifacient. The chief symptoms of poisoning are colic, abdominal pains, purgation, and tenesmus; the stools usually contain blood. It is said to have a specific action upon the uterus.

The fatal dose is one-third to two-thirds ounce. The U.S.P. dose is four grains (0.25 gm.) for aloes, and one-fourth grain (0.015 gm.) for aloin.

JALAPIN AND ELATERIN PURGATIVES

THE most important members of this group are colocynth, elaterin, gamboge, jalap, podophyllum, and scammony. The drugs are often used in the form of resins or extracts; some of them are contained in most of the purgative pills. Death has resulted from excessive use of proprietary pills containing various drugs of this group. The action of all these substances is very similar; the symptoms following an overdose are vomiting, abdominal pain, violent purging, tenesmus, followed by great weakness, collapse, and death.

COLOCYNTH

COLOCYNTH (bitter apple), the fruit of citrullus colocynthis, contains several resinous bodies and an extremely bitter alkaloid. A number of deaths have followed large doses of colocynth; it has often been used as an abortifacient. Poisoning has occurred from inhalation of the powdered drug.

The symptoms are the usual ones of gastro-intestinal irritation. The fatal cases developed prostration, arrhythmic pulse, and collapse.

A few deaths have been reported from fifteen to thirty grains. Recovery followed seventy-five grains. A woman died in twenty-four hours after taking one and one-half teaspoonfuls of the powder. In another case death did not occur until forty hours after an unknown amount of the drugs had been taken.

Dragendorff and Johannson[1750] have isolated colocynth from the bodies of poisoned cats. The substance is colored first brown, then red, by Froehde's reagent, while Mandelin's reagent (0.5% solution of ammonium vanadate in sulphuric acid) produces a transient blood red color.

GAMBOGE

GAMBOGE is derived from garcinia hanburii. It has occasionally caused death when used as a purgative, and as an abortifacient. It caused a severe diarrhea in a patient, W. W., seen by the author. He had been using it in lithographing work. It was thought at first that the man had amebic dysentery. Repeated laboratory examinations failed to show the presence of the ameba. When he was removed from his employment and discontinued the use of gamboge the diarrhea stopped and the man regained forty-one pounds which he had lost.

Treatment is the same as for other purgatives.

Postmortem may show only intense congestion of the alimentary tract, with ecchymoses, and bloody serofibrinous exudates and adhesions; sometimes there is ulceration of the

1750. Ermittelung van Giften, Göttingen, 356, 1895.

entire gastro-intestinal canal. The peritoneum, liver, spleen, kidneys, and bladder have also been found congested.

ELATERIN

ELATERIN is a neutral principle obtained from a substance (elaterium) deposited by the juice of the fruit of the squirting cucumber (ecballium elaterium).

The fatal dose is placed at seven or eight grains, although an ill and feeble lady of seventy died seemingly from the purging caused by two-fifths of a grain.

After extraction, elaterin yields a carmine red color on treatment with concentrated sulphuric acid containing a trace of carbolic acid. Froehde's reagent gives a pink to yellow-green to deep green color.

PODOPHYLLUM

PODOPHYLLUM is the dried rhizome and roots of podophyllum peltatum, a common North American plant, also called "mandrake." It is usually dispensed in the form of resin or podophyllum, often called podophyllin, the active principle of which is podophyllotoxin.

The symptoms of poisoning consist of vomiting and purging, cold extremities, cold perspiration, and weak and thready pulse.

The fatal dose has been placed at five to ten grains.

Podophyllum and podophyllotoxin may be removed from the acid aqueous liquid, as in the examination of alkaloids, by shaking out with chloroform. Both substances are colored dark yellowish-green by Mandelin's reagent.

IVY AND SUMAC POISONING

POISONING usually results from direct contact with the plant, although this is not necessary; contact with articles of clothing, or with individuals, and perhaps animals, who have come into contact with the plant is sufficient. The poison is not volatile, but may be carried in the smoke from burning plants. Poisoning may come from a great variety of plants, including the vines and shrubs known as poison ivy (rhus radicans or toxicodendron), and poison oak (R. diversiloba, etc.), and the poison sumac shrub or tree (R. vernix); but the effects produced by all seem to be identical. The most common form of poisoning is a severe inflammation, and vesicular eruption of the skin. There is violent itching, redness, swelling, vesication, and, finally, desquamation. If the poison reaches the face, the swelling may be so great as almost entirely to obliterate the features; the patient may be unable to open his eyes for several days. The symptoms usually appear within twenty-four hours or may be delayed three or four days. It may occur on any part of the body.

Treatment: Wash the skin with hot water and soap, or with alcohol. This usually prevents further development of the poisoning. Tincture of rhus has been given internally— also intramuscularly for the immunization or "desensitization" or relief of individuals exposed to or suffering from ivy poisoning. A case is reported in which an infusion of the root was taken instead of sassafras tea; there was a rash resembling that of measles, with intolerable itching, suffusion of the eyes, and pain in the throat and stomach. The application of tincture of ferric chloride has been recommended. A few cases of poisoning, with at least one death, have resulted from the taking of rhus internally in order to secure immunity from the poison.

Detection: There are no chemical tests by which toxicodendron may be identified. Skin test may be applied from the infusion of the material suspected to have caused the poisoning. To an alcoholic infusion of the material is added an alcoholic solution of lead acetate, and the precipitated lead compound of toxicodendron is suspended in water and decomposed with ammonium sulphide. After filtering off the lead sulphide, the active principle is shaken out with ether. After evaporation of the ether, the residue will form characteristic eruptions when applied to the skin, and will detect one part in a million of the poison.

PICROTOXIN

PICROTOXIN is obtained from cocculus indicus, which is the dried fruit of Anamirta paniculata, a climbing shrub. The fruit is known as fish-berries, grains of paradise, and Levant nuts. The powdered berries have long been used as fish and bird poisons. Most cases of poisoning from picrotoxin have been accidental. The berries have been mistakn for wild cherries, for cubebs, or for pepper, with fatal results. Cocculus indicus contains about 1% of picrotoxin, which is a neutral body, acting, however, as a weak acid toward strong bases, and having the formula $C_{30}H_{34}O_{13}$. Picrotoxin is slightly soluble in cold water, more soluble in hot water, and readily soluble in alcohol, ether, and chloroform. It forms colorless crystals melting at from 192° to 200° C. (377.6° to 392° F.). It is odorless, but is intensely bitter. Five to 10 mg. may be given in the treatment of barbiturate poisoning.

Symptoms: If taken internally, there is a burning pain in the esophagus and stomach, followed shortly by salivation, nausea, vomiting, and diarrhea. There are weakness, confusion, dizziness, headache, drowsiness, cold, profuse perspiration, and unconsciousness; the face is pale, the pupils may be contracted or dilated; the respiration is at first rapid and labored, later it is slow. Convulsions usually begin early; in Sozinskey's case there was, every five minutes, a powerful general convulsion. Between convulsions there was complete relaxation. Each convulsion began with twitching of the muscles about the left corner of the mouth.

Fatal Dose and Period: No cases of death from pure picrotoxin have been reported. Death is said to have resulted from thirty-six grains of the powdered berries, which would equal about one-third grain of picrotoxin. Death has been reported in thirty minutes.

Treatment: The stomach should be washed out. Chloral hydrate may be given during the convulsions. Caution must be used in giving chloral hydrate in picrotoxin poisoning, for it kills in the same manner as picrotoxin, by paralysis of the respiratory center.

Postmortem Appearances: In animals killed by picrotoxin there may be hyperemia and edema of the lungs with hyperemia of the meninges, and occasionally redness of the mucous membrane of the stomach and esophagus.

Isolation: Picrotoxin is extracted from the aqueous solution as prepared under alkaloids with chloroform or amyl alcohol.

Tests: 1. A minute quantity of the suspected substance is evaporated to dryness with concentrated nitric acid, and the residue moistened with concentrated sulphuric acid. On the addition of an excess of potassium hydroxide the presence of 1/100,000 gm. of picrotoxin will be shown by the appearance of a brick-red color.

2. A drop of a 20% alcoholic solution of anisaldehyde

added to a solution of picrotoxin in sulphuric acid produces a blue-violet ring, becoming blue.*

3. Picrotoxin, boiled with vanillin-hydrochloric acid, gives a green color after a few minutes.

4. A mixture of picrotoxin and sucrose becomes red on treatment with concentrated sulphuric acid.

5. An aqueous solution of picrotoxin reduces Fehling's solution and ammoniacal silver oxide, but it gives no precipitate with neutral or basic lead acetate, Mayer's reagent, gold, platinic or mercuric chlorides, tannic acid, or most other general reagents for alkaloids.

6. A small particle of picrotoxin treated with two drops of an alcoholic solution of benzaldehyde (one to one) and then with a drop of concentrated sulphuric acid becomes red. If the liquid is agitated it obtains a reddish-violet color.

WATER HEMLOCK (CICUTA)

SEVERAL species of cicuta are very poisonous; the one most carefully studied is cicuta virosa, a common European plant which has long been known to be very toxic and which has been used for suicidal and also for homicidal purposes. In America, C. maculata (American water hemlock; wild hemlock; spotted hemlock; spotted parsley; snake-weed; beaver poison; musquash root; muskrat weed; cowbane; children's bane) is not identical with C. virosa, but is the most important. All parts of the plant are poisonous; the underground parts are especially dangerous. These have been mistaken, with fatal results, for horse-radish, parsnips, artichokes, sweet cicely, angelica, and other edible roots. Most of the cases have occurred in children. It has caused many deaths in cattle.

After the plant has been eaten, the symptoms begin within a few minutes, starting with dizziness, pain in the abdomen, salivation, violent and sometimes bloody vomiting, cold skin, profuse perspiration, slow, weak pulse, unconsciousness, and frequent violent epileptiform convulsions, as in picrotoxin poisoning. The pupils are usually widely dilated and do not react to light; the jaw may be firmly closed.

The fatal dose is not known. Death has occurred in one hour.

Treatment is the same as that for picrotoxin.

* MELZER, H.: *Ztschr. f. anal. Chem.*, 37:451, 1898.

There are no characteristic postmortem changes.

Detection for the presence of any remnants of the plant is best made by a microscopical examination of the vomited matter.

LAUREL

ANDROMEDOTOXIN has been found in kalmia latifolia ("broad-leaf laurel," "mountain laurel," "mountain ivy," etc.) and kalmia angustifolia ("narrow-leaf laurel" "lamb-kill," "dwarf laurel," etc.). Few cases of poisoning by laurel have been reported.

LOCAL ANESTHETICS

COCAINE HYDROCHLORIDE, long in use as the best and most reliable local anesthetic, has been largely supplanted by the newer drugs, because of the accidents causing illness or death of the patient. These accidents have decreased with increasing experience concerning the margin of safety with which cocaine can be used.

Considering the dangers attending its use, this highly toxic substance should be discarded. Research workers have found more than 100 local anesthetics to replace cocaine, but less than a dozen are found in common use. The reason for this failure to have more of the new anesthetics in daily use is that the substitutes could not replace cocaine in the various operations, as the extraction of teeth, operations upon the skin, and even in major operations.

A few of these anesthetics which have survived are as follows:

Alypin (New and Nonofficial Remedies, 43, 1932) is a brand of benzopropyl claimed to be the equal of cocaine, but it is not a mydriatic. It is used in ophthalmology in 2% to 4%; in rhinolaryngology, 5% to 10%. It is said not to produce disturbance of accommodation, and to be less toxic than cocaine. Death was reported in one case from the injection of 7.4 cc. of a 10% solution into the urethra and bladder; severe poisoning has been reported from small amounts. Epinephrine preparations may be added when a vasoconstrictor is desired.

Apothesine is a local anesthetic of the procaine rather than the cocaine type. It is effective for injection anesthesia, but not when applied to mucous membranes. Its absolute toxicity is less than that of cocaine, but twice that of procaine hydrochloride. It is used in 0.5% to 2% solutions, generally with epinephrine in sterile water.

Anesthesin (ethyl aminobenzoate, benzocaine), $C_6H_4NH_2$. $COO(C_2H_5)$ 1:4, U.S.P. XI., has a molecular weight of 165.09. It occurs as small, white or colorless crystals, or a white crystalline powder. It is odorless and is stable in the air. One gm. is soluble in about 2,500 cc. of water, 5 cc. of alcohol, 2 cc. of chloroform, 4 cc. of ether, and in from 30 to 50 cc. of expressed oil of almond or olive oil, at 25°C. It is soluble in dilute acids and melts between 88° and 90°C. The average dose is: metric, 0.3 gm.; apothecaries, 5 grs.

Butesin n-butyl-p-aminobenzoate, $C_6H_4NH_2COO$ (C_4H_9), is a white crystalline powder, odorless and tasteless, almost insoluble in water, and soluble in dilute acids, alcohol, chloroform, ether, benzene and fatty oils. It melts at 56° to 57°C. To a dilute hydrochloric acid solution of butesin (one to 100) add a few drops of sodium nitrite solution (one to ten), and then add 0.2 gm. betanaphthol in 10 cc. sodium hydroxide solution (10%). This gives a scarlet red precipitate. To a dilute hydrochloric acid solution of butesin, add a few drops of iodine solution, shake well, and let stand a few minutes. This will yield a dark-brown precipitate which changes to large, reddish-brown prisms.

Butesin Picrate—Dinormalbutyl-p-aminobenzoate-trinitrophenol, $(C_6H_4NH_2.COO.C_4H_9)_2.C_6H_2(NO_2)_3OH$, combines the anesthetic action of butesin with the antiseptic properties of trinitrophenol (picric acid). It is a yellow amorphous powder, odorless, and tasting slightly bitter. It is soluble in 2,000 parts of water, 100 parts of cottonseed oil; and is soluble in alcohol, chloroform, ether, and benzene, and melts between 109° and 110° C.

1. The aqueous solution is a greenish-yellow, which is intensified by alkali and decreased by acid.

2. To an acidulated solution of butesin picrate, add a few drops of sodium nitrite; then a slightly alkaline solution of betanaphthol added gives a salmon-colored precipitate which quickly darkens. When a 1% potassium cyanide solution is added, a purplish red color will appear.

Butyn is the normal sulphate of a base resembling the base of procaine hydrochloride. A committee of the Section on Ophthalmology of the American Medical Association[1751] reported the successful use of butyn in practically all operations on the eye and in some operations on the nose and throat. The committee concluded that butyn is more powerful than cocaine, a smaller quantity being required; that it acts more rapidly than cocaine; and that the action is more prolonged. So far as the experiences of the committee go butyn in the quantity required is less toxic than cocaine. The committee found butyn superior to cocaine in that it produces no drying of the tissues and no change in the size of the pupil, and that it has no ischemic effect. For ophthalmologic work, butyn is generally used in 2% solutions. A single application produced, within one minute, an anesthesia sufficient to permit the removal of superficially-placed foreign bodies. Butyn solutions may be sterilized by boiling. Butyn is soluble in less than its own weight of water at 20° C. It dissolves slowly in cold water, but rapidly in hot water. Alkali hydroxides and carbonates should not be added to butyn, as the free base is precipitated as a colorless oil.

Butyn, γ-dibutylaminopropyl-p-aminobenzoate-N-sulphate, $(NH_2.C_6H_4.COO(CH_2)_3.N(C_4H_9)_2)_2.H_2SO_4$, occurs as a colorless, odorless, solid, producing numbness when placed on the tongue. It melts at 98° to 100° C. It is soluble in equal parts of water, very soluble in alcohol and acetone, slightly soluble in chloroform, and insoluble in ether.

Tests: 1. Alkali hydroxides and carbonates precipitate butyn as a colorless oil. With soluble bicarbonate it is precipitated in crystalline form. When exactly neutralized with hydrochloric acid, the white hydrochloride crystallizes out of solution. Butyn hydrochloride melts at 151° C.

2. In a one to ten aqueous solution, potassium mercuric iodide yields a white precipitate; iodine solution a brown precipitate; gold chloride solution a brown precipitate; picric acid solution a yellow precipitate; and barium chloride solution gives a white precipitate which differentiates it from procaine hydrochloride.

3. To an aqueous solution (one to five) of butyn add two drops dilute of hydrochloric acid and two drops of sodium nitrite solution (10%), and then a solution of betanaphthol (0.2

1751. *J.A.M.A.*, 78:343, 1922.

in 10 cc. sodium hydroxide solution). This gives a scarlet red precipitate (phenacaine gives a white precipitate).

4. Dilute sulphuric acid plus potassium permanganate solution is colorless (distinction from cocaine).

Butyn is two and one half times as toxic as cocaine. When injected intravenously into cats it is about equal to cocaine.

Alypin — The hydrochloride of 2 - benzoxy - 2 dimethyl-aminomethyl - 1 - dimethylaminobutane, $CH_3.CH_2C(C_6H_5COO)$ $(CH_2N(CH_3)_2).CH_2N:(CH_3)_2.HCl$, occurs as a white, crystalline powder, odorless, with a bitter taste. It is very soluble in water, freely soluble in alcohol, and chloroform, and insoluble in ether. It is very stable. Its aqueous solutions may be sterilized by boiling, for not over five minutes.

Tests: 1. Aqueous solution (one to 100), plus potassium dichromate, gives an orange-yellow crystalline precipitate, soluble in hydrochloric acid.

2. Potassium permanganate gives a violet crystalline precipitate, turning brown on standing. It is precipitated by the general alkaloidal reagents.

Alypin is said to be equal to cocaine as an anesthetic, but is not mydriatic. It is claimed not to produce disturbances of accommodation and to be less toxic than cocaine, but this evidence is rather conflicting. Death was reported in one case from the injection of about 7.4 cc. of a 10% solution in the urethra and bladder. Severe poisoning has resulted from smaller amounts.*

Orthoform — Methyl m-amino-p-oxybenzoate, $C_6H_3.NH_2.$ $OH.CO.(CH_3)$, occurs as a fine, white crystalline powder that melts at 141° to 143° C. It is odorless and tasteless; almost insoluble in water, freely soluble in alcohol and ether. When crystallized from chloroform it sometimes forms white crystals, melting at 110° to 111° C.

Tests: 1. A hydrochloric acid solution of orthoform, upon the addition of sodium nitrite, is colored yellowish-red, and then there is a yellow precipitate, deepening to red on exposure to aid. The slight solubility of these preparations renders them unsuitable for injection, but their slow absorption tends toward safety. The anesthesia they produce is not as complete as that of the more soluble anesthetics, but their effect is more lasting. They are non-irritant and non-toxic.

* New and Nonofficial Remedies, A.M.A., **43**, 1932.

Metycaine—Benzoyl-y (2 methylpiperidino)-propanol hydrochloride, $C_6H_4COO(CH_2)_3NC_6H_{12}HCl$, occurs as a fine, white, crystalline, odorless powder. When applied to the tongue, it has a slightly bitter taste, followed by numbness. It is freely soluble in water, soluble in alcohol, and chloroform, insoluble in ether; permanent in the air; faintly acid to litmus paper; and optically inactive. It melts between 171° and 173° C.

Tests: 1. Alkali carbonates and hydroxides precipitate it as a white to a light yellowish oil.

2. Metycaine solution (one to ten) plus dilute sulphuric acid and potassium permanganate, is colorless (alypin gives a violet crystalline precipitate which soon disappears).

3. Gold chloride gives a yellow precipitate (distinction from apothesine which gives a lemon yellow).

4. Dilute hydrochloric acid, plus sodium nitrite solution (10%), plus betanaphthol solution (0.2 gm. in 10 cc. of 10% sodium hydroxide solution) gives a white, changing to yellow, and finally greenish yellow color.

Phenacaine (Holocaine)—Ethenyl-p-diethoxydiphenylamidine hydrochloride, $CH_3C: (NC_6H_4OC_2H_5) . (NH.C_6H_4OC_2H_5) . HCl + H_2O$, consists of small colorless crystals—odorless, bitter in taste, producing a numbness in the tongue. It is permanent in air; soluble in fifty parts of water, freely soluble in alcohol, and chloroform, insoluble in ether; and faintly alkaline to litmus. It melts at 189° C. On boiling in glass vessels, the aqueous solution becomes turbid, owing to the separation of a quantity of the base by the alkali in the glass.

Tests: 1. Chlorinated soda solution gives a flesh-colored precipitate. In a few minutes this changes to a violet-colored precipitate, and, if shaken with ether, the ether layer is colored Burgundy red.

Procaine Borate—1-amino-benzoyl-2-diethylaminoethanol-penta-m-borate, $C_6H_4NH_2COO.C_2H_4.N(C_2H_5)_2.5HBO_2$, occurs as a fine, white, odorless, crystalline powder. Its slightly bitter taste is followed by numbness. It is permanent in air; soluble in acetone, benzene chloroform, and ether; alkaline to litmus; and melts at 163° to 166° C. Procaine borate closely resembles procaine hydrochloride in its action and uses. Novocaine is a brand of procaine hydrochloride.

Procaine Nitrate — $C_6H_4.NH_2COO.C_2H_4.N(C_2H_5)_2.HNO_3$, consists of small colorless crystals, odorless and soluble in water and alcohol. Its melting point is between 100° and 102°C.

Willsteadt[1752] recommends the precipitation of novocaine with Reinecke salt (ammonium tetra rhodanatae-diamino-chromate), and with flavic acid. With both reagents we can obtain characteristic crystalline precipitates. With Reinecke's salts the precipitation is most sensitive, and a clouding is obtained even at a concentration of 0.1 mg. novocaine chlorohydrate per cc. Clouding appears immediately, and the precipitation is found after half a minute. With Reinecke's salt, with the members of the cocaine series, the following reagents were given:

With a 0.2 mg. procaine per cc. a heavy precipitate is obtained; with a concentration of 0.07 mg. per cc. of procaine an immediate clouding is obtained and later a precipitation; with 0.33 mg. per cc. of pantocaine, an immediate clouding results, and later a crystalline precipitate is formed; with 0.1 mg. per cc. of tutocaine, there is an immediate clouding and a delayed precipitate.

These precipitation reactions are of course, not specific, because, there are a series of compounds which can be precipitated by these reagents. Willsteadt, for the qualitative determination, found the compounds 1-amido 8 naphthol-4-sulfo acid the most sensitive reagent. As little as 1.3 gamma of novocaine chlorohydrate in 2 cc. of water can be detected by this method, but for colorimetric determination 1-amido-8-naphthol-3, 6-disulpho acid is of greater advantage. The concentration is 2.7 gamma in 2 cc. of water. The reaction is based on a diazo coupling. Other diazo compounds give the following results:

Diazotized amine	Color received with novocaine	Color of the blank
Aniline	yellow	colorless
p–nitraniline	yellow	yellow
Sulfanilic acid	colorless	colorless
Naphthionic acid	yellow, then red	yellow
1–naphthylamine–4, 8 disulpho acid	yellow, then red	yellow, remains permanent
1–amido–8–naphthol–3, 6 disulpho acid	reddish brown, later red	brownish-yellow, later brownish-red
Benzidine	yellow	colorless
o–Tolidine	yellow	yellow
Dianisidine	red	red

1752. WILLSTEADT, HARRY: *Biochem. Ztschr.*, 269:182, 1934.

In all these tests, three minutes after adding the reagent a little sodium acetate is added.

Betaeucaine Hydrochloridum — $C_5H_7N(CH_3)_3O(C_6H_5CO)$. HCl, occurs as white, odorless, crystalline powder, stable in air. It is soluble in thirty parts of water, thirty-five parts of alcohol, six parts chloroform; neutral to litmus paper; and melts at 268° C.

Tests: 1. Dissolve 0.1 gm. in 1 cc. of sulphuric acid. Keep at 100° C. for five minutes, and then mix cautiously with 2 cc. water. The aromatic odor of methyl benzoate becomes noticeable, and on cooling crystals of benzoic acid form.

2. Saturated aqueous solution with a solution of mercuric chloride gives a white, curdy precipitate.

3. Potassium chromate and dilute sulphuric acid gives a yellowish curdy precipitate.

4. Triturate about 0.05 gm. with about five times its weight of mercurous chloride and moisten with a few drops of water; no black color is produced. (Difference from cocaine hydrochloride.)

Assay: Dissolve about 0.5 gm. of eucaine hydrochloride, previously dried to constant weight at 100°C. and accurately weighed, in 100 cc. of neutral alcohol. Titrate this alcoholic solution with N/10 sodium hydroxide. Each cc. corresponds to 0.02837 gm. of eucaine hydrochloride.

Tutocaine (Butanim) — p - amino - benzoyldimethylaminomethyl - butanol - hydrochloride, $(CH_3)_2N.CH_2.CH(CH_3)CH$ $(CH_2)(O.CO.C_6H_4.NH_2)HCl$, is a light, ivory-colored crystalline powder. It is colorless, and its faintly bitter taste is followed by numbness. It is permanent in air; soluble in four parts of water, but difficultly soluble in alcohol; neutral to litmus; optically inactive and melts at 212° to 215° C.

Tests: 1. Alkali hydroxides and carbonates precipitate it as a light yellowish oil, which after some time solidifies and melts at not less than 81°C.

2. To an aqueous solution (one to five) add dilute hydrochloric acid and sodium nitrite solution (10%), and mix with a solution of betanaphthol in sodium hydroxide; this gives a scarlet red precipitate. (Phenacaine gives white precipitate.)

3. An aqueous solution (one to ten), with potassium mercuric iodide solution, gives a white precipitate.

4. With iodine solution there is a brown precipitate.

5. With gold chloride a brown precipitate is formed.

6. With picric acid, a yellow precipitate.

7. Nitric acid and silver nitrate give a white curdy precipitate.

8. Dilute hydrochloric acid and barium chloride cause no precipitation. (Distinction from butyn.)

9. With dilute sulphuric acid plus potassium permanganate solution, the color disappears immediately. (Distinction from cocaine.)

Tutocaine in 3% solution was found to be about four times as toxic as procaine hydrochloride by rapid intravenous injection into a cat. A fatality has been reported following the injection of 8 cc. of a 2% solution into the urethra.

Procaine Hydrochloridum, para-aminobenzoyl-diethylaminoethanol hydrochloride, $C_{13}H_{20}O_2N_2$.HCl, (molecular weight, 272.64) crystallizes from alcohol in fine colorless needles which melt at 156°C. (312.8°F.). One gm. is soluble in 0.6 cc. of water and in 30 cc. of alcohol at 25°C. It is slightly soluble in chloroform, and almost insoluble in ether. The aqueous solution is neutral and may be boiled without decomposition. From the water solution it is precipitated by gold chloride, iodine, mercuric potassium iodide, and picric acid.

Tests: Sodium hydroxide or sodium carbonate produces a colorless, oily precipitate, crystallizing on standing. Sodium bicarbonate causes no precipitate.

Procaine will be found in the alkaline ether extract and will respond to color reactions for the amino group.

Moser[1753] came to the conclusion that procaine injections, even if the substance be given in small doses, may be very dangerous.

Nupercaine — a-butyloxycinchoninic acid, — diethylethylenediamide hydrochloride — $C_9H_5N.OC_4H_9(2).CONH(CH_2)_2N-(C_2H_5)_2CHl$ (4)—is a local anesthetic. It is about five times as toxic as cocaine when it is injected intravenously into animals. Death has been reported after the subcutaneous injection of 135 cc. of a solution of 1 in 1,000. It occurs as a fine, white, crystalline, odorless powder; hygroscopic; very soluble in water. When there is one or more per cent of nupercaine present in an aqueous solution, the addition of potassium perchlorate causes nupercaine perchlorate to crystallize out. These crystals

1753. MOSER: *Zentralbl. f. Chir.*, 58:1703, 1931.

melt at 130° to 132° C. Silver nitrate causes a white percipitation in a nitric acid solution.

Ulilmann[1754] found nupercaine five times more toxic than cocaine in guinea pigs and rabbits. Lipschitz and Laubender[1755] found nupercaine, intravenously, two times as toxic as cocaine. Gessner and Naulieimer[1756] found nupercaine fifty times more toxic than procaine in guinea pigs, but seven to eight times more toxic in rats.

Case 1. Mandl[1757] reported the case of a man fifty years of age who was operated upon for an ulcer. One hundred and fifty cc. of a 0.1% nupercaine were introduced in the abdominal cavity after local procaine anesthesia. The operation took forty-five minutes, and in forty hours he was dead. The cause of death was given as shock of nupercaine.

Case 2. Jones[1758] reported a woman, fifty years of age, with an ovarian cyst. Spinal anesthesia, 15 cc. of one to 1500 nupercaine. Death occurred in three minutes.

Case 3. Steinbriick[1759] reported death during a diffuse peritonitis of a man sixty years of age, from a spinal anesthesia of 1.4 cc. of a 1% nupercaine.

Case 4. Keys and McSellan[1760] report five cases. A female, sixty-one years of age, was given 2 cc. of one to 200 solution of spinal anesthesia. She died in a few minutes after being put in Trendelenburg position.

Case 5. A man forty-four years of age had gangrenous cholelithiasis and was given 2 cc. of 1:200. He died during the operation following the injection.

Case 6. A young man with bronchitis died six hours after an abdominal operation, after being given spinal anesthesia.

Case 7. A patient died following the injection of 20 cc. of a 2% solution infiltrated for a tonsillectomy. Death occurred in a few minutes.

Case 8. This case was another fatality, the quantity given was not known.

1754. ULILMANN: Narkose u. Anaesth., 2:168, 1929.
1755. LIPSCHITZ and LAUBENDER: Klin. Wchnschr., 9:968, 1930.
1756. GESSNER and NAULIEIMER: Schmerz Narkose-Anaesth., 3:44, 1930.
1757. MANDL, F.: Zentralbl. f. Clin., 57:2966, 1930.
1758. JONES, W. H.: Lancet, 2:549, 1930.
1759. STEINBRIICK, H.: Zentralbl. f. Chir., 57:273, 1930.
1760. KEYS, E. S., and McSELLAN, A. M.: J.A.M.A., 96:2085, 1931.

Keys and McSellan recommend the safe dose for infiltration in 100 cc. to be one to 1000; for caudal 30 cc. to be one to 500; and for spinal fluid 2 cc. to be one to 200. Nupercaine is twenty times as toxic as procaine in man. Anesthesia is slightly delayed, more intense, and two to six times more lasting. Fawlkes reported dermatitis caused by using a nupercaine ointment.[1761]

Pantocaine is a local anesthetic, which advantageously replaces cocaine. It melts between 147 and 148° C. Its molecular weight is 298. It has alkaloidal characteristics. Crystals of pantocaine picrate are formed with picric acid. With nitric acid beautiful yellow colorations are obtained. After evaporation, alcoholic potash gives a purple red color, which becomes red on slight heating, and also an odor is produced which is suggestive of carbylamine. It has a chlorine content of 17.75, and nitrogen 9.25. Melissinos and Netto[1762] found that the lethal dose for the guinea pig is not more than 43 mg. per kilo weight of animal. The fatal dose, as given by the manufacturers, is 30 mg. per kilogram of animal. As compared with cocaine, it has been found that the minimum lethal dose for the guinea pig is 50 mg. per kilo body weight, against 30 mg. found for pantocaine. Therefore pantocaine is much more toxic than cocaine. Baumecker[1763] reports a case of a man seventy-three years old who was admitted early in the morning to a clinic, complaining of urinary retention and stating that he did not void for the last eighteen hours. Catheterization was tried, and when some blood appeared the manipulation was discontinued. After three hours of futile attempt the urethra was anesthetized with a 1% solution of pantocaine in the attempt to resume catheterization. After two minutes the patient suddenly lost consciousness, turned pale, and expired. Postmortem examination revealed a severe stricture of the posterior urethra, and at that place the lumen of the urethra was also completely obliterated. Very little of the pantocaine had reached the bladder. The cause of death was explained as follows: The catheter had probably entered the blind canal destroying the tissue and the small blood vessels. The pantocaine solution had followed the same way as the catheter, and dissolved the thrombi, occluding these

1761. FAWLKES, R. W.: *J.A.M.A.*, 100:1171, 1933.
1762. MELISSINOS and NETTO: *Ann. de méd. lég.*, 13:386, 1933.
1763. BAUMECKER, H.: *Zentralbl. f. Chir.*, 59:1431, 1932.

vessels, and had reached the blood stream. Therefore the process should correspond to a pantocaine injection given intravenously.

Fanburg[1764] reported a case in which, after several months of occasional application of nupercaine ointment to eczema of dorsum feet to relieve itching, there developed erythematous vesication, with swelling and pruritis of feet, legs, thighs, arms, and neck. This patient was sensitive to nupercaine. Darnel[1765] reported two deaths due to an anesthesia with spinocaine. Both deaths occurred in women who underwent a cholecystectomy.

Seeger[1766] reports a case of death after a tonsillectomy. The patient was twenty-six years old, and was referred to a otolaryngological clinic for the operation. He had previously been given 0.01 gm. of morphine and 0.001 gm. of atropine subcutaneously, and the pharynx was swabbed with a 10% solution of cocaine with the addition of one-third of its volume of a one-per-thousand adrenaline solution. The patient was removed to the operating table, and the peritonsillar tissue on both sides was infiltrated with 12 to 15 cc. of 0.5% novocaine solution which contained 3 mg. adrenaline per 100 cc. The patient felt oppressed and had palpitation, and after four minutes became suddenly pale and lost consciousness, the respiration and pulse suddenly stopped, and death occurred after a few gasping breaths. Camphor, lobeline, and adrenaline given intracardially gave no results. The postmortem examination revealed the following: Hypoplasia of the aorta and adrenal medulla, lipomatosis of the heart, small punctate hemorrhages in the pleura and epicardium; the lungs were in part hyperemic; there was struma nodosa parenchymatosa, anemia of the brain, and no evidence of embolism.

Another case was that of a patient forty-six years old who had been given 0.001 gm. of atropine; the pharyngeal and laryngeal mucosa were painted with a 10% cocaine solution plus one-third of its volume of one to 1000 adrenaline, followed by a subcutaneous infiltration of the surgical field with 50 cc. of a 1% novocaine solution, with 3 mg. of adrenaline per 100 cc. Immediately following the injection the patient complained of

1764. FANBURG, S. J.: J.A.M.A., 101:30, 1933.
1765. DARNEL, R.: Zentralbl. f. Chir., 58:1123, 1931.
1766. SEEGER, T.: Arch. f. Ohren-, Nasen-u. Kehlkopfh., 49:132, 1932.

violent pain in the region of the neck. The pulse was rapid and small, and after two minutes the patient suddenly became pale and no pulse could be obtained and the respiration stopped. Postmortem examination revealed the following: The pericardial sac contained about 100 cc. of a clear serous fluid, the heart chambers were dilated and filled with uncoagulated blood. The myocardium was heavily infiltrated with fat tissue, which in places reached the endocardium. The lungs were large, heavy, and from the cut surface there oozed a foamy brown red fluid. The tissue contained much air. The pathological and anatomical diagnosis was an acute dilatation of a hypertrophic and lipomatous heart, with an acute edema of the lungs which were already indurated and emphysematous.

Snapp[1767] reports the death of a twenty-six year old physician who was given 20 cc. of a 0.5% novocaine solution to which four drops of a one to 1000 solution of adrenaline were added, injected in the usual manner into the peritonsillar tissue. Immediately after the injection, nausea and pallor followed. He vomited, and had violent spasms, marked cyanosis, mydriasis, and sudden death. All attempts at resuscitation failed.

Mayoux[1768] reports a case of a woman twenty years of age who was to undergo a tonsillectomy. She was given an identical treatment as outlined above. There was collapse in five minutes, pallor, tremor, of the upper extremities, and stopping of the respiration and pulse, followed by death.

Mayer, Skillein, and Sonnenschein[1769] made a report of a questionnaire, which was sent to 150 laryngologists of the United States. In 1920, on the basis of the answers, they published reports on eighteen fatal cases resulting from the administration of local anesthesia, four of which were due to novocaine, and all four occurred in connection with tonsillectomies as follows: Sudden death occurred after the peritonsillar injection of 3.7 cc. of a 0.75% novocaine solution (plus 0.13 adrenaline, one to 1000).

Mayer, in 1928, reports four more deaths due to novocaine and anesthesia.[1770]

1767. SNAPP, C. F.: *Ann. Otol., Rhinol. & Laryngol.*, 37:974, 1928.
1768. MAYOUX, R.: *Ann. d. mal. de l'orielle, du larynx*, 47:577, 1928.
1769. MAYER, E., SKILLEIN, R. H., and SONNENSCHEIN, R.: *Laryngoscope*, 30:443, 1920; *J.A.M.A.*, 77:1336, 1921.
1770. MAYER, EMIL: *J.A.M.A.*, 90:1290, 1928.

Other cases have been reported by Bledgrad,[1771] Becker,[1772] Simpson,[1773] Mendoza[1774] Brutt,[1775] Wiemann,[1776] Becker,[1777] Kappis,[1778] Hartung, [1779] Waldapfel,[1780] Hering,[1781] and Schoemaker.[1782]

Riechen[1783] reported two cases of death in two young men, twenty and twenty-eight years of age, respectively. Each patient received 65 cc. of procaine by injection. Decker[1784] observed in a patient the occurrence of a total amaurosis, without any apparent changes in the fundus. The blindness usually recedes after a few days, and after a transitory period, in which there is a central scotoma, the patient recovers completely. Many cases of intoxication with novocaine are seen because of the individual hypersensitivity, and this cannot always be ascertained before the injection. Gebele[1785] reports a patient dying on the twelfth day from the after-effects of the injection of 120 cc. of 0.5% novocaine-suprarenine solution. Klotz[1786] reported 151 fatal cases of local anesthesia. One-half of these cases were due to cocaine, and one-quarter were due to novocaine.

Fatal poisonings by vagus stimulation with paralysis of the heart action and respiration with collapse have been observed by Wiemann, Eideus,[1787] and Hering.[1788]

1771. BLEDGRAD, N.: *Acta oto-laryng.*, 4:305, 1922; *Acta oto-laryng.*, 6:426, 1924.

1772. BECKER, H. M.: *Zentralbl. Laryng.*, 159, 1920.

1773. SIMPSON: *Zentralbl. Laryng.*, 159, 1920.

1774. MENDOZA: Cited by CANUYT: *Ann. d. mal. de l'orielle, du larynx*, 48:433, 1929.

1775. BRUTT, H.: *Deutsche med. Wchnschr.*, 21:577, 1918.

1776. WIEMANN, O.: *Zentralbl. f. Chir.*, 698, 1919.

1777. BECKER, J.: *Zentralbl. f. Chir.*, 50:1695, 1923.

1778. KAPPIS, M.: *Zentralbl. f. Chir.*, 517, 1920.

1779. HARTUNG, H.: *Zentralbl. f. Chir.*, 186, 1922.

1780. WALDAPFEL, R.: *Deutsche Ztschr. f. Chir., Leipz.*, 219:179, 1929.

1781. HERING, F.: *Zentralbl. f. Chir.*, 827, 1920.

1782. SCHOEMAKER, J.: *Tijdschr. v. inland. Geneesk.*, 63:1999, 1919.

1783. RIECHEN, F.: *Ztschr. f. Untersuch. d. Lebensmitt.*, 63:557, 1932.

1784. DECKER: *Deutsche med Wchnschr.*, 8:22, 1922.

1785. GEBELE: *Deutsche Ztschr. f. Clin.*, 233:618, 1931.

1786. KLOTZ, ANDRE: Less accidents mortels de l'anesthene locale—Paris Louve et Cie., 1929.

1787. EIDEUS: *Arch. f. klin. Chir., Berl.*, 122:1922.

1788. SCHAPS., *Deutsche Ztschr. f. Chir.*, 158, 1920. BUITT: *Deutsche med. Wchnschr.*, 44:577, 1918.

EPINEPHRINE
(Molecular Weight 183.11)

E PINEPHRINE, $C_9H_{13}O_3N$, (also called adrenaline and su-
prarenine) is the active principle of the medulla of the
suprarenal gland. It can be prepared synthetically. It behaves
as a feeble base, and might be classed with the alkaloids. Its
solutions are very unstable unless a preservative is added. It is
a white or light brownish, microcrystalline, odorless powder,
gradually darkening on exposure to the air.

Epinephrine is very slightly soluble in water and in alcohol. It is insoluble in ether, in chloroform, in acetone, or in
fixed or volatile oils. Epinephrine combines with acids, forming salts which are readily soluble in water, and from these solutions the base may be precipitated by ammonia water or alkali carbonates. An acid solution of epinephrine is not visibly
affected by solutions of trinitrophenol, tannic acid, phosphomolybdic acid, mercuric potassium iodide, or platinic chloride.
A slight acid, aqueous solution of epinephrine (one in 1000)
gives, with the ferric chloride test solution, an emerald green
color, turning to cherry red and finally to brown on standing.
Other oxidizing agents produce pink, red, and violet colors,
which change to brown. Fixed alkali hydroxides cause the solution to darken on standing, but do not precipitate the epinephrine. It is slightly alkaline to litmus paper. The average
hypodermic dose is 0.005 gm. (1/120 grain).

Epinephrine is used locally for arresting hemorrhages, and
increasing the anesthetic effects of cocaine; hypodermically in
bronchial asthma; intravenously for tiding over acute circulatory collapse. Epinephrine leaves the blood stream rapidly and
is then destroyed, especially in the liver, so that the effects of
an intravenous injection are of very short duration. It is poorly absorbed from mucous membranes, and its absorption from
subcutaneous injections is delayed by its vasoconstrictor effect,
so that the response is relatively slight, except as regards especially sensitive conditions, such as asthma, or in hypersensitive
individuals. Epinephrine may resuscitate hearts that have apparently stopped, although the chance of revival diminishes
rapidly, and permanent success is scarcely possible if the circulation has stopped for longer than ten minutes. If the collapse is merely threatened, the epinephrine (0.02 to 0.10 mg.)
may be injected into the jugular vein or carotid artery, and re-

peated at intervals. If the pulse cannot be felt, epinephrine should be administered by intracardiac injection, 0.5 to 1 mg. (0.5 to 1 cc. of one to 1000) is injected slowly, directly into the heart (right ventricle) with a long fine needle.

The toxic effects of epinephrine may be seen in acute cardiac dilatation, pulmonary edema, ventricular fibrillation, terminating in death. These usually follow intravenous injections and are especially liable to occur if the heart is already weakened or over-excitable, in cardiac disease, or as the result of chloroform or other cardiac poisons. Where there is a cardiac insufficiency the hypodermic injection of 1 mg. generally produces distinct dilatation and extrasystoles.[1789]

In animals, excessive doses of epinephrine produce vomiting, excitement, debility, bloody diarrhea, hematuria, ascending central paralysis, great fall of temperature, occasionally convulsions, complete prostration, and death by respiratory or cardiac paralysis. Rabbits show multiple pulmonary hemorrhages, probably associated with edema.[1790]

Fatal Dose: The fatal dose is about 500 times the therapeutic dose; 0.1 to 0.6 mg. per kilogram intravenously, or 2.5 to 10 mg. per kilogram hypodermically may cause death. Schmidt claims that atropine decreases the toxicity of epinephrine. The toxic effects are usually the result of the peripheral actions. Dentists seldom use epinephrine with a local anesthetic, as they have found many susceptible patients. After injection of the anesthetic there occur tremors, palpitation, precordial distress, increased rate of respiration, and even fainting in the chair, which not only alarms the patient, but also the dentist. After the local application, tremors, anxiety and nervousness, palpitation, precordial distress, increased rate of pulse and respiration, rise of blood pressure and temperature, and sometimes hyperglycemia have been reported. The hypersusceptibility occurs especially in patients of nervous temperament; most markedly in those with toxic goiter, also in patients with a hypertension.

Tests: Epinephrine in strong solutions gives a precipitate with the general alkaloidal reagents. A simultaneous reduction

1789. Loeper, M., DuBois, and Wagner: Compt. rend. Soc. de biol., 81:85, 1918. Roth, D.: Deutsche med. Wchnschr., 905, 1914.

1790. Schmidt, Leo: Exper. Med., 9:285, 1919; Chem. Abst., 14:979, 1919.

occurs with phosphomolybdic and phosphotungstic acids.

1. With a solution of one to 1000, a drop of sodium hydroxide gives a yellow color, gradually becoming brown.

2. With a very dilute ferric chloride solution an emerald green color is obtained, which changes to a blood red upon the addition of ammonia.

3. Reduction takes place with Nessler's reagent, gold chloride solution, ammoniacal silver.

Frankel Allers Test: To a solution of adrenalin add iodic acid or potassium iodide; with phosphomolybdic acid a rose-red to eosin-red color is obtained. This will be changed to a reddish-brown by the addition of ammonia. This test is delicate one to 300,000.

Kobayashi[1791] describes a new colorimetric method for the quantitative determination of adrenaline in the blood. The Folin, Cannon and Dennis colorimetric method produces a blue color with sodium tungstate; the color is also given by uric acid. Adrenaline gave a violet color with phosphotungstic acid $(H_7P(W_2O_7)_6)$, which is proportional to the adrenaline content of the blood. Solutions should contain at least 0.2 mg. per cent of adrenaline. In tests on various substances, only vitamin C and hydroquinone gave similar colors. Blood obtained from the ear veins of normal rabbits contained 29.2 to 126.2, or an average of 73.5_r per liter; carotid blood 228 to 447, or an average or 323_r per liter. After adrenalectomy no adrenaline could be detected in the circulating blood.

EPHEDRINE
(Molecular Weight 165.13)

EPHEDRINE, $C_{10}H_{15}ON$, is an alkaloid derived from ephedra equistina Bunge, ephedra sinica Stapf and other species of ephedra. The U. S. P., XI, gives it as an unctuous, almost colorless solid, or white to colorless crystals or granules. Ephedrine is soluble in water, alcohol, chloroform, ether, and in liquid petrolatum, the latter becoming turbid if the ephedrine is not dry. It melts between 34° and 40°C., the variability in the melt-point is due to the differences in the moisture content. Solutions of ephedrine are strongly alkaline to moistened litmus

1791. KOBAYASHI, S.: *Jap. J. M. Sc. Tr., IV., Pharmacol.,* 8 No. 3; *Proc. Japan Pharmacol. Soc.,* 9:152, 1935; see also *Chem. Abst.,* 30: No. 10, 3455, 1936.

paper. The U. S. P., XI, recognizes ephedrine hydrochloridum $C_{10}H_{15}ON.HCl$, having a molecular weight of 201.60, and ephedrine sulfas, $(C_{10}H_{15}ON)_2.H_2SO_4$, having a molecular weight of 428.33. The effects on the circulation, intestines, bronchi, iris, etc., agree in nearly every detail with those of epinephrine. The chief differences are that the rise of blood pressure is more lasting, and that the cardiac stimulation makes it more effective than epinephrine in the lighter grades of hemorrhages, and in histamine, peptone, anaphylactic, and traumatic shock.[1792] Dermatitis medicamentosa due to ephedrine was reported by Bullen.[1792] In 1929 Scheer[1792] reported a case of erythematous rash with many small vesicles on skin and face and hands, with edema of face, occurring from the use of ephedrine in oil as a nasal spray. Ayres and Anderson reported erythematous eruptions followed by desquamation in two cases.[1792]

Tests: Ephedrine gives a melting point of 40°C., with chloral hydrate a compound melting between 214°C. and 216°C. Gold chloride gives yellow needles with a melting point between 128° and 131°C. The gold salt, when heated with water, gives an odor of benzaldehyde, at the same time methylamine is split off, the odor of which is apparent after the addition of caustic soda. An olive green color is obtained when an alcoholic solution of ephedrine is heated with carbon disulphide and copper sulphate, due to the formation of thiocarbonic acid derivatives.

1792. SOLLMANN: A Manual of Pharmacology, 3rd ed., 446, 1927. BULLEN, S.: J. Allergy, 3:485, 1932. SCHEER: Arch. Dermat. & Syph., 20:641, 1929. AYRES and ANDERSON: J.A.M.A., 97:437, 1932.

FOOD POISONING AND FOOD-BORNE
INFECTIONS

WITH a history of food poisoning, the physician should tabulate all the food eaten by those infected. Having this information, one food will be found to have been the source of the trouble. In an examination of three mass food poisonings, the offending substance was found to be in a hollandaise sauce used on broccoli. Poisoning may be due to injurious chemicals. Such was the case of the mass poisoning in 1914, when arsenic was introduced in soup by a cook named Jules Crones, at the Mundelein Banquet, held at the Chicago Athletic Club. Poisoning may be due to bacterial decomposition of the food itself, or to some unusual condition of the individual partaking of the food. Under the latter would be included the cases of food sensitization or idiosyncrasy best considered in texts on allergy.

Food poisoning, due directly to some constituent of the food may depend upon the presence of: (1) Metallic or organic poison, introduced by accident, negligence, or design, into food originally normal; (2) organic poison naturally present in the animal or plant tissues of which the food is composed; (3) pathogenic bacteria in the food, or (4) poisonous substances produced in the food by microbic activity.[1793]

1. Metallic or Organic Poisons:

Arsenic is the chief metallic poison added to foods. It was the poison of choice of Jules Crones, previously alluded to. In one instance enough arsenic trioxide was added to a large can of herring to kill 100 people. Poison may be added to candy or selected dishes of food in such a manner that one person will be poisoned. An illustration is that of a man desiring to kill his wife, who injected strychnine into a piece of chocolate candy and placed it fifth in the first row. His wife obtained the fifth and fatal piece of candy.

An extensive beer poisoning outbreak in 1900 was due to the arsenic in the sulphuric acid which was used to prepare the glucose, in which outbreak thousands of beer-drinkers were affected, a number fatally.

Lead poisoning has been traced to water in new lead pipes,

1793. JORDAN, E. O.: Legal Medicine and Toxicology, PETERSON, HAINES and WEBSTER, 2:803, 1923.

and to lead contamination of foods and drink in contact with this metal. Poisonings from eating tin, zinc, and copper in foods are very rare.

2. Poisons Present in Normal Animal or Plant Tissue:

An example of this would be the eating of poisonous mushrooms. Fatal cases of oxalic acid poisoning due to eating rhubarb leaves have been reported. I have seen a number of cases of poisoning due to the use of butter and to the drinking of milk from cows that had eaten white snake root. (See under snake root poisoning, page 605.)

3. Pathogenic Bacteria and Other Organisms:

The presence of pathogenic micro-organisms in the food seems to be the factor most commonly responsible for the large explosive outbreaks of characteristic food poisoning. The outbreaks usually classed under the head of food poisoning are due more frequently to infection with bacilli closely related to, but not identical with, the typhoid bacillus.

Food-borne infection results from the ingestion of food contaminated with the micro-organisms causing infectious diseases such as typhoid and paratyphoid fevers, diphtheria, scarlet fever, streptococcic sore throat, Asiatic cholera, poliomyelitis, and other acute infections which produce definite symptoms. The articles of diet which are said to produce food poisoning are meats, fish, oysters, canned foods, cheese, ice cream, and mushrooms and other poisonous plants mistaken for edible varieties. Meat that has caused intoxication may be from animals that were infected, or it may be contaminated by flies and dust after the animal has been slaughtered. Numerous cases of poisoning have been reported where sausage, ham, and other meats were eaten raw. Poisonings have been less frequent since the public has been educated to refrigerate all types of food products. The paratyphoid is regarded as one of the chief causes of meat infections. If meat is kept for several days the bacteria in it propagate rapidly, and it becomes highly poisonous.[1794] Meat may carry the organisms and toxins of a number of specific diseases, tuberculosis, typhoid fever, and botulism. It may also harbor and transmit trichina (trichinella spiralis), taenia saginate (beef tapeworm), taenia echinococcus, and other animal parasites that are pathogenic to man. Canned

1794. HARRIS, SEALE: Tice's Practice of Medicine, 8:89, 1935.

meats and canned fish that are opened and allowed to stand a day or two without refrigeration, or without heating before serving, may be a source of poisoning.

The symptoms associated with the commoner forms of meat poisoning are those usually associated with gastro-intestinal disturbances. There may be nausea, profuse vomiting, and diarrhea, accompanied by fever, headache, and other manifestations. The period intervening between the partaking of the food and the appearance of the symptoms is very short, usually five to six hours. The symptoms occur in two hours, and may be delayed for thirty hours.

Sausage and uncooked ham seem to be the greatest offenders. Gärtner[1795] isolated a bacillus from the meat, intestines, and spleen of a cow that was killed because it had enteritis. The owner sold the meat and it was responsible for fifty-eight cases of poisoning. The bacillus enteritidis has been found in a number of meat poisonings, causing outbreaks attributed to the bacillus enteritidis.[1795] These outbreaks involved about 2,000 cases, with twenty deaths. "Most investigators in Germany, where the majority of food poisoning outbreaks have occurred, or have at least been bacteriologically studied, are of the opinion that bacillus suipestifer (the same in their opinion as B. paratyphosus B) is much more widely distributed than B. enteritidis and that it occurs, especially in certain regions, as in the southern part of the German Empire, affecting quite commonly the intestinal tract of healthy human beings. These paratyphoid carriers, it is supposed, may contaminate food through handling or preparation just as typhoid carriers are known to do."

In a number of food poisoning outbreaks, bacilli belonging to the proteus group of Hauser[1796] have been found in the infested food and the bodies of affected persons, and these bacilli have been held responsible.

4. Poisonous Products of Bacteria and Other Organisms:

The best known example of poisoning by means of bacterial products is botulism. The name botulism, first applied to sausage poisoning in general, has come to have a more specific meaning, and is now properly used for the form of

1795. GARTNER: *Breslau ärtzl. Ztschr.*, 10:249, 1888. MAYER: *Deutsche Vrljschr. f. Offentl. Ges.*, 45:44, 1913.
1796. HAUSER: Ueber Faulnissbakterien, Leipzig, 1885.

intoxication due to the products of a specific micro-organism, bacillus botulinus (clostridium botulinum). Van Ermengen[1797] discovered bacillus botulinus in 1885 in ham, which had caused a number of cases of illness.

The author saw probably the first two fatal cases of botulinus poisoning which occurred in Chicago. In 1915, two women ate home canned pimentos, with symptoms appearing within eight hours. Two cases of poisoning by botulism due to imported canned onions with one death occurred in Chicago on January 23, 1929. The chief complaints were sore throat, and the patient had difficulty in swallowing; felt dizzy, and continued to see double as he had the day previously. The conjunctiva was infected. Eyelids showed slight ptosis; pupils were widely dilated but equal, and responded very slightly to light. Pulse was 100. Temperature was not taken. Patient seemed entirely rational and gave a clear account of his own and his brother's illness. He stated that he felt all right except for his eyes. This patient was given polyvalent botulinus antitoxin and recovered. Washings from the can of onions showed the presence of B. botulinus type B.[1798]

The public uses the words "ptomaine poisoning" to cover any illness resulting from the ingestion of food. This has been discarded by the physicians, who know that in many instances the poisoning is due to bacterial infection of man by food. Illustration of this came with the isolation of the bacillus enteritidis from a fatal case of meat poisoning, and the isolation of the bacillus botulinus, the growth of which, and the elaboration of an extracellular toxin in the food, caused a few deaths and many cases of illness. Many cases of botulinus came from the packing of ripe olives. More precautions and care in the packing of the olives in the last ten years have practically eliminated olives as a source of botulism.

Many cases of food poisoning result from the eating of cream pastry, such as cream puffs, and cream-filled cakes and pies. In 1929, 111 cases were investigated by the Health Department of the City of Chicago. The Health Department then made a ruling, early in 1930, forbidding the selling of such pastry during the months of July, August, and September. This had the absolute effect of preventing illness from this cause.

1797. VAN ERMENGEN: *Ztschr. f. Hyg.*, 26:1, 1897.
1798. KOEHLER, G.: *Illinois M. J.*, April, 1930.

Samples of cream puffs and all their ingredients were tested for poison and found to be negative. The feces and urine of the workers in the bakery were found negative. Bacteriologic examination showed the presence of an organism in the custard that corresponded closely to Escherich's paragruenthali. This is related to the B. coli group. Jordan[1799] claims that the staphylococcus was responsible for this type of infection. Geiger, Crowley, and Gray[1799] reported an outbreak of food poisoning due to nut ice-cream. The cultures showed staphylococcus aureus, which may have been the cause of the outbreak. Barber[1799] reported several cases of milk poisoning due to a strain of staphylococcus albus occurring in the udder of an apparently healthy cow. Fresh milk containing the staphylococcus did not apparently produce illness, but on standing the milk became poisonous. Experiments showed that various strains of staphylococci of diverse origin and different cultural characters are capable of generating in broth a substance, which, when taken by mouth, produces gastro-intestinal disturbances. This substance is destroyed by boiling, and is either destroyed or greatly weakened by being heated at from 60° to 65° for thirty minutes.

A theory was advanced that a mixture of other foods was a contributory factor in causing illness, rather than the consuming of the cream puffs. To discredit this theory a large bakery placed at my disposal five dozen cream puffs daily for three weeks, which I gave to students in my class. These cream puffs were sometimes twenty-four hours old, yet not one case of illness resulted though two to three puffs were eaten daily during this period, with other types of food. An examination of the cream puffs that had been kept in a bakery twenty-four hours showed that the bacterial count had risen from 500 to 130,000 to 2,300,000. In one instance the count went up to 24,000,000 per gm. of sample. In a mass poisoning, where 1,589 guests were served at a convention banquet, an outbreak of food poisoning occurred which was apparently due to affected crab meat. An examination of the crab meat by Geiger, Greer, and White[1800] showed an organism which

1799. JORDAN, E. O.: *J.A.M.A.*, 94:1648, 1930. GEIGER, J. C., CROWLEY, A. B., and GRAY, J. P.: *J.A.M.A.*, 105:1980, 1935. BARBER, M. A.: *Philippine J. Sc.*, 9:515, 1914.

1800. GEIGER, J. C., GREER, F. E., and WHITE, J. L.: *Am. J. Pub. Health*, May, 1928, p. 602.

resembled culturally very closely the salmonella suipestifer.

Seligmann[1801] reported that, since 1931, duck egg poisoning has become more frequent in Germany. A series of almost forty-eight mass poisonings were collected by Fromme. A very impressive mass poisoning was observed in September, 1934, in a Berlin hospital. Only those served a certain mayonnaise, none of them patients, seventy-seven in all, were affected. The chief symptom was a diarrhea, at first painless, later associated with diffuse colic, which persisted even after the diarrhea had stopped. The stools were brownish, mixed with mucus, and a little blood was present in a few cases. The temperature varied between 102.2° and 103.1°. In 20% of the cases it dropped slightly on the second day. The stools or the urine, sometimes both, contained an organism of the paratyphoid group, identified serologically and by the non-formation of a wall of mucus, as belonging to the Breslau strains, although it was not very pathogenic to mice, and showed negative rhamnose and tartrate reactions. Breslau and Gärtner bacilli were the exciting organisms found in most of the cases from the duck egg infection.

Stone[1802] reported a case of botulinus from the ingestion of ripe fruit. According to Rosenau,[1802] a total of ninety-one outbreaks of botulism have been reported in the United States and Canada since 1899, involving 345 persons, with a death rate of 61.7%. Autopsy in one of Stone's cases revealed, as the most important observations, acute parenchymatous changes, involving the brain, heart muscle, liver, spleen, and kidney, with marked acute fatty degeneration of the heart muscle and liver. Many of the outbreaks of botulism are due to the so-called "cold-pack" process of home canning.[1803]

Caprio[1803] reported an outbreak of botulism in a family of five, in which three deaths were caused after eating a jar of home preserved peppers.

In the Grafton, North Dakota, outbreak of food poisoning, Dr. Cary, in a personal communication (February, 1931) stated that it was due to type A of bacillus botulinus. The autopsy

1801. SELIGMANN, E.: Schweiz. med. Wchnschr., 65:550, 1935.

1802. STONE, W. J.: J.A.M.A., 92:2019, 1929. ROSENAU, M. J.: in Cecil's Textbook of Medicine, W. B. Saunders Company, Philadelphia, 533, 1927.

1803. J.A.M.A., 92:1868, 1929. CAPRIO, F. S.: J.A.M.A., 106:687, 1936.

of one of the individuals showed a congestion of the basal ganglion, chromatolysis of ganglionic cells, and disappearance of Nissl granules. There was an engorgement of liver sinusoids, liver cells were bile-tinged in areas, the bile duct was not distended. The spleen showed congestion, distribution of brownish pigments in pulp. Blood in the larger vessels was bile-tinged. The stomach contained multiple areas of congestion; hemorrhages were not observed. There was congestion of the kidney, with multiple hemorrhages into the tubules, granular deposits of brownish pigments in periphery of tubules, blood in the larger vessels showed similar changes and tinging. The congestion of the brain, meninges, liver, kidney, and stomach reported in this case have been reported in a number of other cases dying from botulism.[1804] Kosher and associates reported their observation in detail on baccillus botulinus infection in canned spinach.[1804]

Symptoms: The symptoms of botulism differ from those of paratyphoid meat poisoning. An intense toxic action upon the nervous system is especially characteristic. The onset is slower, the first symptoms beginning about twelve to twenty-four hours after the meal. Constipation is common. Nausea, gastric pain, and diarrhea are frequently absent, but may occur. There are invariably visual disturbances, such as dilation of the pupils and double vision, with difficulty in swallowing and speaking. The central nervous system, in general, is profoundly affected, exhaustion is great, and recovery is greatly prolonged. The pulse is sometimes small and rapid, occasionally slow. Consciousness is not impaired. The temperature is usually subnormal, but may be high. There is a progressive loss of muscular action, death usually resulting from respiratory failure. The bacilli are quickly destroyed by boiling. In the case of the pimentos, 0.2 cc. of the juice from the can was sufficient to cause death of a full grown rabbit, whereas 5 cc. when brought to the boiling point for five minutes was given to a dog without effects.

Two types of bacillus botulinus have been found in the United States. The spores are 0.6 to 0.9 micron by 2 to 6 micra in size. They are alike culturally, but are entirely dis-

1804. Editor, *J.A.M.A.*, 77:483, 1921; SEMERAK, C. B.: *J. Infect. Dis.*, 2:29, 1921; EDMUNDS, C. W.: 81:542, 1923. *J.A.M.A.*, 77:1250, 1921; see also EDMUNDS, C. W., and KEIPER, G. F.: *J.A.M.A.*, 87:494, 1924; DICKSON, E. C.: *J.A.M.A.*, 80:185, 1923.

tinct in their immunologic relations. Specific antitoxins can be produced for the two types of B. botulinus (designated as Type A and Type B) by the same methods as those used for the production of diphtheria antitoxin. In animal experiments the antitoxin exerts considerable therapeutic effect, in human botulism outbreaks but little success has so far been obtained by the administration of botulism antitoxin. This may be due partly to the fact that antitoxin prepared from the B strain has no effect in neutralizing the A toxin, and conversely, partly to the failure of using the antitoxin before the disease has progressed too far.

Treatment: In the treatment it is important to empty the stomach as soon as the symptoms of poisoning appear. A drastic cathartic should be given, such as croton oil, to clear out the bowels. The treatment is symptomatic. The specific antitoxin A and B should be given in every case where a diagnosis of botulism poisoning is made.[1805]

Ergot poisoning is caused by the poisonous substance, or ergot, produced in rye and other grains due to the growth of a parasitic fungus, Claviceps purpurea. In times of famine, when spoiled grain was used, many deaths were caused from this source.

Certain types of food are allowed to become ripe and more or less decomposed before being eaten. This is seen among those who prefer game that has been hanging for some time, or beef that has been aged to such an extent that it is covered with mold. Savage[1806] states that "a study of the evidence along these accessory lines of inquiry singularly fails to bring forward any evidence associating the consumption of food in a state of incipient putrefaction with illness in those who consume it."

In 1870 an Italian named Selmi studied basic substances removed from a cadaver which he called "ptomaines." Similar substances are found in living tissues, giving all the alkaloidal reactions, and also called ptomaines. Gantier calls this group of substances leukomaines. Normal tissue may produce substances (creatine, creatinine, tyrosine, leucine, glycine) which give the general reactions of alkaloids. In

1805. BURKE, VICTOR, ELDER, J. DOHRMAN, and PISCHEL: *Arch. Int. Med.,* 27:265, 1921.

1806. SAVAGE, W. C.: *J. Hyg.,* 20:69, 1921.

1865 Panun[1807] isolated from putrefying meat a substance, soluble in water but insoluble in absolute alcohol and heat, which in its effects resembled curare and snake venom. Bergmann and Schmiedelberg isolated from putrefying yeast a crystalline substance which was very poisonous and which they called sepsin.

In the alkaline ether extracts of human organs there will be found substances giving tests for amines, and it is only after purification of these extracts that one is able to differentiate them from the vegetable alkaloids. Guareschi[1808] subdivides these substances into ten different headings: (1) aliphatic and aromatic amines; (2) diamines; (3) hydramines; (4) guanidines; (5) amino acids; (6) pyridine and oxipyridine bases; (7) ptomaines produced by bacteria in various diseases, called pato-amines; (8) ptomaines of unknown structure; (9) ptomaines or poisons of putrefied alimentary products; (10) putrefactive. They contain the elements carbon, hydrogen, nitrogen, and some of them contain oxygen.

Amines: The amines are bases originating from ammonia and built on the same type. The poisonous ones are monamines, diamines, and the quaternary ammonia bases. They usually occur in the form of oily liquids which are colorless and volatile. Others are amorphous, and are either monoacid or biacid bases. Some of these ptomaines are strong bases, forming crystalline salts and absorbing carbon dioxide from the air. They usually have a strong penetrating odor, which persists for a long time when in contact with skin or clothing. Their salts are unstable, particularly in the presence of a strong mineral acid, and the base changes rapidly in contact with air. They also possess reducing properties. They reduce iodic acid, gold chloride, silver bromide, potassium bichromate in sulphuric acid, and potassium ferricyanide. The toxicity varies greatly. Some of the amines which have been extracted from human viscera are not toxic to guinea pigs or fish, in amounts of a few mg. Methylamine, ethlyamine, propylamine, dimethylamine, trimethylamine, triethylamine, phenylethylamine, betaine, amidovalinanic acid, cystine. nemidine, midine and pyschyamine, and neuridine are not

1807. PANUN: *Virchows Arch. f. Path. Anat.*, 27:28, 29, 1865.
1808. GUARESCHI: Introducione allo Studio Degli Alcaloidi, 422, 1892.

toxic. Putrescine and cadaverine are not very toxic. Butiamine, isoamylamine, exylamine, ethylidenediamine, choline, muscarine, neurine, methylguanidine, glycocyamidine, hydrolutidine, hydrocholidine, piarvoline, tetamine, escombrine, aselline, sucolatoxine, morrhuic acid, hydrocoridine, midatoxine, mitilotoxine, gadinine, tifotoxine, coridine, moribuine, lusotoxin, and thyrotoxin are toxic.

Bettink and Van Dissel's reagent* is prepared as follows: Two grams of crystallized ferric chloride are dissolved in 2 cc. of 1% hydrochloric acid, the mixture is diluted to 100 cc., and 0.5 gm. of chromic anhydride are added. The substance to be tested is dissolved in a drop of 1% hydrochloric acid and introduced into the mixture, and potassium ferricyanide is added, and Prussian-blue is immediately obtained.

Diamines: Diamines are formed in putrefactive processes, generally in the presence of an abundance of nitrogen. Ethylidenediamine was found by Brieger in putrid haddock, in the filtrate from the mercury chloride precipitate: guanidine, neuridine, a base isomeric with ethylenediamine ($C_2H_3N_2$), muscarine, and triethylamine. Neuridine, $C_5H_{14}N_2$, is a diamine, and is apparently the most common basic product of putrefaction. It has been obtained from the putrefaction of gelatin, horseflesh, fish, and from the yolk of eggs. It is usually accompanied by choline, from which it can be separated by converting the bases into hydrochlorides, choline hydrochloride being soluble in absolute alcohol, neuridine scarcely so. Neuridine is not poisonous.

Cadaverine is formed in putrid animal matter, and in cultures of the genus spirillum. It may be formed synthetically by dissolving trimethylcyanide in absolute alcohol, and then reducing with sodium. Cadaverine forms well-defined crystalline salts as well as compounds with metals. Cadaverine hydrochloride crystallizes in needles which are deliquescent, or from an alcoholic solution in plates. The crystals are insoluble in absolute alcohol, but readily soluble in 96% alcohol. Putrescine hydrochloride is difficultly soluble in 96% alcohol. The aurochloride contains 61.5% gold, melting at 188° C. It crystallizes partly in cubes and partly in

*BETTINK and VAN DISSEL: *Niew. Tijdsch. v. Pharm. Nederl.*, 1884, y. tambien. Berichte d. Deutsche Chem. Gesellsch, 379, 1884.*

needles, and is easily soluble in water. Other salts are the picrate and oxalate.

Putrescine, $C_4H_{12}N_2$, tetramethylenediamine, is a clear liquid, free base, with a semen-like odor, boiling at about 135° C. It is a common base in putrefying animal substances, and also occurs in the urine in cases of cystinuria. Putrescine forms crystalline salts, putrescine hydrochloride, the platinochloride, the aurochloride, the picrate, and dibenzoylputrescine. Putrescine is not poisonous. It can be identified by the melting points of its salts.

Paraphenylenediamine occurs in the form of tubular crystals, melting point 140° C, boiling point 267° C. Metaphenylenediamine is a crystalline substance, melting point 63°, boiling point 276° C. Both these diamines are poisonous. Metaphenylenediamine produces in the dog the symptoms of an aggravated influenza with continual sneezing and hoarse cough, in large doses ending in coma and death. Paraphenylenediamine produces exophthalmia, the tissues of the eyes undergoing complete alteration.[1809]

Tyrotoxicon (diazobenzol), $C_6H_5N_2(OH)$, is found in milk and egg products allowed to undergo putrefaction.

Leukomaines are produced in muscle and in the glands. These leukomaines, also called physiological alkaloids, are formed continuously in the living cell, and are eliminated in general by the excretory organs (kidneys and sweat glands). Leukomaines have been divided into five different headings: (1) xanthinic and uric acid leukomaines; (2) mono- and diaminoleukomaines; (3) creatinine leukomaines; (4) amino-acids; (5) miscellaneous leukomaines.

The first group comprises substances such as xanthine, adenine, guanine, hypo-xanthine, methyl-xanthine, pseudoxanthine, para-xanthine, and carnine. The second group includes the diamine leukomaines such as leurine, cadaverine, neuridine and gerontine.

The third group includes substances such as creatine, creatinine, cruso-creatinine, xantho-creatinine and amphicreatine.

The amino-acids, the fourth group, are the following: hippuric acid, leucine, alanine, histidine, and tyrosine.

The miscellaneous group includes spermine, plasmanine, protamine, and undetermined leukomaines.

1809. BLYTH, A. W.: Poisons, Their Effects and Detection, 519, 1906.

Methods of Extraction: Various methods have been devised for the separation of the amines. A special method can be found for practically each that are desires to separate. The methods of Gautier and Breiger may be followed. The one of Breiger, although being long, gives better results. The material is finely comminuted, boiled with 0.5% hydrochloric acid for three to five minutes, the insoluble portion filtered off, and the filtrate evaporated the same as described under alkaloids (see page 31). The residue is evaporated to the consistency of a syrup, is treated with 96% alcohol, filtered, and the filtrate treated with lead acetate and the precipitate filered off.

The filtrate is again evaporated to a syrupy consistency, and treated with 96% alcohol. This is again filtered, the alcohol is evaporated, water is added, and the lead is removed by hydrogen sulphide. The filtrate is then again evaporated to the consistency of syrup, and treated with alcohol and bichloride of mercury. By the different solubility of certain amines in water, some separation of the mercury salts takes place when water is added.

The mercury filtrate is freed from mercury and evaporated, the excess of hydrochloric acid being carefully neutralized by means of soda. It is again treated with alcohol, so as to separate the inorganic substances as much as possible. The alcohol extract is evaporated, dissolved in water, neutralized with soda, acidulated with nitric acid, and precipitated with phosphomolybdic acid. The phosphomolybdic acid precipitate is decomposed with neutral lead acetate, which process may be facilitated by heating on the water-bath. Remove the lead by hydrogen sulphide, and evaporate as before to a syrupy consistency. Alcohol is added, by which process many basic toxins are eliminated as hydrochlorates, or they can be converted into double salts for the purpose of separation. Attempts should be made to make other salts, such as gold and platinum, the melting points of these salts giving an idea of the amine present in its purity. This being a cumbersome and tedious method, the work should be done in a room entirely separated from that where toxicological examinations are made, for the lead used in the biological material causes the desks and the surroundings to become contaminated with lead.

MUSHROOM POISONING

AS LONG as people will gather mushrooms in the fields and woods, just so long will we have mushroom poisoning. Occasionally poisoning occurs from the ingestion of mushrooms which though non-poisonous when fresh, have undergone some decomposition, causing illness. Cases of poisoning occur from eating the white, or deadly amanita (amanita phalloides); sometimes also from the fly agaric (amanita muscaria), the false morel (helvella), and, less often, other poisonous fungi.

AMANITA PHALLOIDES

FORD[1810] has found seventy to eighty species of mushrooms that are poisonous to man. The amanita has been described under many names. In England and America the term "toadstool" is usually applied to mushrooms of any type. Roch[1811] reported 381 cases, with 188 deaths, a mortality of 49%. Ford,[1811] who has had wide experience with poisonous mushrooms, reported 204 cases, with 153 deaths, which were traced to species clearly identified as amanita phalloides, a mortality of 75%. This type of mushroom is more abundant at certain seasons of the year, as late summer, in August or September. It has an excellent taste, so that no warning is given to its victims at the time of eating.

The amanita phalloides, the so-called white amanita, or deadly amanita, grows to a height of about four to six inches, the stalk being one-half to three-quarters of an inch in diameter, and the upper expanded top or pileus having a diameter of three to four inches. "The stalk is set in an expanded cup or volva often called the 'poison cup,' which is set in the ground sometimes at a considerable depth and attached by fine threads of mycelium to the roots below. On the lower part of the stalk there may be small, rather feathery, flakes which are easily brushed off and which are remnants of the universal volva in which the growing plant was originally enclosed. The upper part of the stalk has attached to it a filmy, delicate ring or annulus about one-half to one inch from

1810. FORD, W. W.: *J. Pharmacol. & Exper. Therap.*, 29:305, 1926.
1811. ROCH, M.: Les empoisonnements par les champignons, Geneva, 1913. FORD, W. W.: *Bull. Johns Hopkins Hosp.*, 18: No. 193:123, 1907.

the junction of the pileus and the stalk. This is often adherent to the lower part of the pileus. The pileus is usually smooth on top, and is provided on its under surface with a series of gills sometimes until covered by the annulus or veil. Attached to the gills are the spores, pure white in color. The entire plant is of a peculiar dead white, except for the upper portion of the pileus, which may be chalky white, smoke colored, delicately yellow or slightly greenish. Many botanists separate the species into different varieties according to the color of the pileus. As the plants mature they take on a somewhat obscure dirty brownish-white color, and as they begin to decay they are often grayish-brown. The form which often appears in the early Spring is small and pure white in color. This is usually called amanita verna or the 'destroying angel' of Bulliard. It is indistinguishable from amanita bisporigera of Atkinson. The 'deadly amanita' is very common in woods and along the borders of the roads, especially during the latter part of August and September. It usually grows singly. When dried it has quite a characteristic odor."

Symptoms: The tymptoms of amanita phalloides poisoning begin after six to fifteen hours, with extreme abdominal pain, vomiting, and diarrhea. Vomitus and feces may contain undigested food, blood, and mucus. Anuria is seen occasionally. The patient becomes weak. Jaundice, cyanosis, and coldness of the skin, especially the extremities, develop within two or three days. Drowsiness, followed by coma, and death in from four to five days is the usual course, although recovery from mushroom poisoning has been known when small quantities were eaten and when the stomach was promptly evacuated. Eye symptoms, such as trismus are rare, and the pupils are usually normal in size, reacting to light and accommodation. When the meal has been chiefly mushrooms severe intoxication may cause death within forty-eight hours. Children are more susceptible to intoxication, and the mortality is much greater than with adults. Patients may recover during the course of a week, but are not normal for about a month. Schultz laid stress upon the nervous ocular symptoms, such as trismus.

Postmortem Appearances: Postmortem examination shows a considerable gastro-enteritis, with swelling of the follicles and lymph glands, as well as degeneration of the liver, with fatty infiltration to an extent usually associated only with phosphorus poisoning. Maschka noticed a fatty degeneration of the internal organs. In addition there is fatty degeneration of the kidneys, heart, and muscles. In the brain there are degenerative changes of the ganglion cells and the neuroglia. Sahli[1812] found the gross lesions including the subpleural and intrapulmonary hemorrhages, and noted in addition a general atrophy of the panniculus adiposus. Schürer,[1813] in an autopsy on a child of five years, who died thirty-five hours after ingestion of a fungi thought to be amanita phalloides, noted an inflammation of the ileum and colon; swelling of the mesenteric glands; fatty degeneration of the heart and skeletal muscles; fatty degeneration of the liver, particularly in the periphery of the acini; fatty degeneration of the kidney, and advanced degenerative changes in the cells of the central nervous system. Miller[1814] described the pathologic anatomy of four cases which he believed to be "phalloides" poisoning. He calls attention to the minute and massive hemorrhages in the intestines and to the absence of jaundice. On microscopic examination he found frequent degeneration and fatty infiltration of the endothelial cells of the blood-vessels, degeneration and fatty infiltration of the epithelial cells of the adrenals, with an increase of lipoid material and advanced fatty degeneration of the cells of the kidney, which were totally replaced by fat. The other changes were similar to those reported by other investigators.

Active Principle of Amanita Phalloides: The active principle of amanita phalloides was named amanita hemolysin. The non-hemolytic substance present in the extracts after heating, the amanita toxin, it being regarded as the poison after ingestion of the fungi, is responsible for death in man. Kobert found a substance which was a powerful hemolytic, or hemotoxic, dissolving the corpuscles of a variety of animals in dilutions as high as one in 125,000 of the dried material. Kobert called this substance phallin. On the basis of Ford's[1815] experiments, he concluded that the blood destroying substance in amanita phalloides cannot be the active

1812. SAHLI: See STUDER, SAHLI, and SCHARER: Nitth. der Naturfors. Gesellsch., 81, 1885.
1813. SCHÜRER, J.: Deutsche med. Wchnschr., 38:548, 1912.
1814. MILLER: Berl. klin. Wchnschr., 4:1164, 1918.
1815. FORD, W. W.: J. Infect. Dis., 3:192, 1906; J. Exper. Med., 8: 437, 1906; J. Infect. Dis., 5:116, 1908.

principle, and plays at most only a subsidiary role when the fungi are eaten raw. Subsequently Abel and Ford[1816] demonstrated that, on the treatment of aqueous extracts of the fungus with methyl alcohol, a voluminous precipitate appears which contains the amanita hemolysin, while the amanita toxin remains in solution. The methyl alcohol precipitate taken up in water contains a very small amount of coagulable protein, which may be removed by the addition of freshly prepared metaphosphoric acid and by uranyl acetate. After removal the solutions contain inorganic salts and a pigmentary substance, the greater bulk of the solution being a glucoside which reduces Fehling's solution and ammoniacal silver nitrate, after hydrolysis with mineral acids gives an abundant precipitate with neutral or basic lead acetate and tannic acid, and does not ferment with brewer's yeast. Furthermore, these solutions give several tests for pentoses, including a purplish-violet color on heating gently with a-naphthol and sulphuric acid, and a cherry-red color after similar treatment with phloroglucinol and hydrochloric acid with a drop of ferric chloride solution. In addition, the solutions always contain nitrogen, as evidenced by positive Laissaigne tests. On the basis of these and other reactions, Abel and Ford concluded that the amanita hemolysin is not a toxalbumin, but a nitrogenous glucoside easily decomposed by acids and yielding a pentose and a volatile base or bases, such as ammonia and methylamine. The reactions of the isolated glucoside were practically the same as those of the original solution after freeing from protein and various impurities. "The hemolytic strength of the solution remained intact and in certain preparations showed an activity in a dilution of one to 300,000, thus making it the most powerful blood-laking substance known. It was not, however, regarded by them as the active principle. This is contained in alcoholic solutions of the fungus and may be precipitated from these solutions by phosphotungstic acid. It has been shown by Schlesinger and Ford[1817] that after several reprecipitations by phosphotungstic acid and the removal of impurities by such reagents as silver nitrate and basic lead acetate the amanita toxin can be isolated in con-

1816. *Arch. f. exper. Path. u. Pharmacol.,* Schmiedeberg Festschrift, 1908; *J. Biol. Chem.,* 2:273, 1907.
1817. SCHLESINGER and FORD: *J. Biol. Chem.,* 3:279, 1907.

siderable purity. It was found to be highly resistant to boiling in aqueous and alcoholic solutions, to be slowly affected by acids at room temperature but rapidly destroyed by boiling acids. It did not reduce Fehling's solution either before or after prolonged treatment with 5 to 10% hydrochloric acid. The amanita toxin did not react with any of the alkaloidal precipitants nor did it give any of the alkaloidal color reactions. It did not give the Biuret test or Millon's reaction. Because of these reactions the amanita toxin was regarded by Schlesinger and Ford as neither a glucoside, an alkaloid, nor a protein in the generally accepted sense. Since, however, it contained nitrogen and sulphur, the latter as conjugate sulphuric acid, and on fusion with potassium hydrate gave off the odor of amines and indol and gave the characteristic pyrrol-red test, it was concluded by Schlesinger and Ford that the toxin is probably either an indol derivative or an aromatic phenol so combined with an amine group that it readily forms an indol or pyrrol ring."

On injection into animals the amanita toxin produces an acute intoxication in which the lesions closely resemble those seen in man in fatal cases, including the hemorrhages and the wide spread necrosis and fatty degeneration of the cells of the internal organs, especially the liver and the kidneys. With the evidence at hand there can be little doubt but that this body is the active principle. The amanita hemolysin is also poisonous to small animals on subcutaneous inoculation, producing wide spread destruction of the red blood corpuscles with hemoglobinuria, and microscopically an increased pigmentation, especially in the spleen and liver. Since these lesions are not observed in man the amanita hemolysin probably has no effect when the cooked fungi are ingested.

AMANITA MUSCARIA LINNAEUS

FARLOW[1818] gives the following description of amanita muscaria: "The fly agaric (amanita muscaria), so called because decoctions of it are used for killing flies, is in most places, at least in the northern and eastern parts of the country, a common species, often a good deal more abundant than the common mushroom. It is found during the summer along road-

1818. FARLOW: Bull. 15, U. S. Dept. of Agriculture, Div. of Veg. Phys. and Path., 1898.

sides, on the borders of fields, and especially in groves of con-
iferous trees. It prefers a poor soil, of gravelly or sandy character, and occurs only exceptionally in the grassy pastures
preferred by the common mushroom. It grows singly and not
in groups, and attains a large size, being one of the most striking toadstools. It differs from the common mushroom in having gills which are always white, never pink nor purple, and in
having a hollow stem which is bulbous at the base and clothed
with irregular, fringy scales on the lower part. The pileus
varies in color from a brilliant yellow to orange and a deep red,
the yellow and orange being more frequent than the red. The
surface is polished (and sometimes sticky) having scattered
over it a larger or smaller number of prominent, angular warty
scales, which can be easily scraped off. The gills and stalk are
white, and there is a large membranous collar, which hangs
down from the upper part of the stem." The close resemblance
of amanita muscaria to certain edible amanitas, in particular
to amanita caesaria, one of the most highly prized edible mushrooms has led to many cases of poisoning. This is particularly
true among the foreign-born inhabitants of America, who mistake the poisonous amanita muscaria of this country for the
edible amanita caesaria of Europe. The amanita caesaria of
Europe is apt to have a yellowish color and the amanita muscaria a reddish brown, while the amanita muscaria in America
is usually yellow and the amanita caesaria reddish brown.

Symptoms: The symptoms of poisoning by amanita muscaria may follow immediately after it is eaten, or may be delayed from one to six hours. The patients begin to show an
excessive salivation, perspiration, and lacrimation, accompanying a violent retching and vomiting, with a profuse diarrhea and
watery stools. The pulse is slow and irregular, the respiration
accelerated, and the patient dyspneic, the bronchi being filled
with mucus. The pupils are usually dilated. Mental symptoms
appear rapidly, giddiness with confusion of ideas, and rarely
hallucinations. The patient becomes excited, shrieking,
dancing, jumping, and may even have fits of raving madness.
Occasionally gastro-intestinal disturbances will be the outstanding feature, at other times the mental and nervous symptoms may predominate. The patients may fall into a deep
sleep, lasting several hours, from which they awaken exceedingly weakened, with definite signs of a change for the best. In

some cases of poisoning the pupils are contracted and fail to react to light and accommodation.

Mecke[1819] reported several intoxications with red fissim fungus. In two cases he reported that the patients had eaten fried mushrooms. One-half hour later the symptoms appeared They had violent abdominal pain, nausea, alternating sensations of heat and cold, perspiration, headache and congestion of the head. There was an increased salivation, blurring of vision, and diarrhea. A quantitative examination of the mushroom revealed a muscarine content of 0.36%.

Treatment: Wash out the stomach, as given under amanita phalloides.

Muscarine is found in very small quantities in amanita muscaria. It is, however, extremely active and persists for a long time in the dried plant. "It acts directly upon the sympathetic or autonomic nervous symptom, producing an increased secretion from the various glands of the body by its stimulation of the terminal filaments of the secretory nerves and a paralysis of the heart and respiration by a corresponding stimulation of the inhibitory nerve endings of the vagus nerve. Atropine, by its depressing action upon the same nerves which muscarine stimulates, is a perfect physiologic antidote for muscarine and also for synthetic muscarine, which may be prepared by the oxidation of cholin. The presence of muscarine in suspected materials may be easily demonstrated on the frog's heart. Applications of small quantities to the cardiac muscle produce an immediate stopping of the heart is diastole. This is quickly overcome by the application of a dilute solution of atropine. It is said that peasants used decoctions of it to induce drunkenness.[1820]

Postmortem Appearances: Postmortem findings are not characteristic in amanita muscaria poisoning. The degenerative changes in the internal organs as noted with the amanita phalloides are absent. There is never a fatty degeneration of the liver, kidneys, or heart.

A large number of other amanitas are deadly poisons, their properties being identical with those of amanita phalloides. The identification of these various species requires the work of

1819. MECKE, W.: *Arch. f. exper. Path. u. Pharmakol.*, 175:23, 1934.
1820. FORD, W. W.: Legal Medicine and Toxicology, PETERSON, HAINES and WEBSTER, 817, 1923.

chemists and botanists. The most important of these, according to Ford, are amanita porphyria, amanita strobiliformis, amanita radicata, amanita chlorincama, amanita mappa, amanita morrissii, amanita citrina, and amanita crenulata.

HELVELLA, OR GYROMYTRA ESCULENTA

THE morchella esculenta are non-poisonous. The false morels (helvella esculenta) contain the poisonous helvellic acid, and in some cases, if not all, a second poison whose nature is not yet known. Helvellic acid is a powerful hemolytic agent, whereas the second, unknown poison, has an injurious effect on the capillaries and the central nervous system.

The symptoms of poisoning usually occur within the first few hours after ingestion consisting of nausea, vomiting, gastric pains and diarrhea. Neither the vomiting nor the diarrhea is as violent as in poisoning by the amanita. There is stupor, dilatation of the pupils, enlargement of liver and spleen, and tubular damage to the kidneys, with albuminuria. In some cases death follows from acute yellow atrophy of the liver. In the absence of liver atrophy, the prognosis is favorable. Rost believes that all varieties of helvella are poisonous. Since helvellic acid and other poisonous substances are soluble in hot water, they are not destroyed by boiling.[1821]

Treatment is the same as for the other fungi, giving injections of glucose to protect the liver.

1821. See also OLMER, D.: *Gaz. d. hôp.*, 100:1218, 1927; ROCH and GAUTIER, P: *Rev. méd. de la Suisse Rom.*, 27:799, 1927; MUTO, K.: *J. Jap. Soc. Cet. Sc.*, 6:24, 1927; 49:255, 1928; GUTZEIT, R.: *Deutsche med. Wchnschr.*, 55:1342, 1929.

DEATH FROM POWDERED GLASS

THE use of powdered glass as an agency for the destruction of life is very rarely seen. In the examination of many thousands of alleged cases of poisoning, I have had only two where glass had been used. Although glass and other mechanical irritants are frequently spoken of as poisons, they are not such in the true acceptation of the word. Their effects are not produced after absorption, but are purely mechanical and local. They do not, consequently, come strictly under the head of poisons, but are included in the statutes under the expression "other noxious things." Pounded glass is frequently as dangerous as an efficient poison. There can be no doubt that the ingestion of particles of glass of a certain size may lead to an injury of the mucous membrane of the stomach and intestines such as to cause death. In the Clugston case, previously referred to (page 229), Clugston was given one-fourth ounce of powdered glass on July 4, in a dish of oatmeal. He had some discomfort—pain in the stomach and diarrhea, but recovered in a few days. One month later his wife pounded up more glass and gave him a second dose. This time the amount of the dose was slightly increased, the exact amount not being known. It is known, however, that it was close to one-half ounce. Clugston again became ill, but again recovered and returned to work. His wife then resorted to arsenic from which he finally died. At the autopsy a piece of glass was found in the appendix, one-fourth to one-half centimeter in its greatest diameter.

In Russia death due to the criminal administration of glass is frequent.[1822] It was a favorite means of destroying certain of the lower animals, such as dogs, rats, and mice, until it was found that arsenic and barium were more efficient. Powdered glass is not very efficient as a poison or we should see more cases due to its use. From results of experiments and from experience of professional glass-eaters there is an indication that it is far less dangerous than is commonly supposed. Simmons and Glahm[1823] fed ground glass to a number of dogs for varying periods of time. The dogs were then killed and postmortem examinations made. As a result of their experiments they give the following conclusions: "The ingestion of ground or powdered glass has no toxic effect and produces no lesion, eith-

1822. *Virchows Jahresb.*, 1:505, 1893.
1823. SIMMONS and GLAHM: *J.A.M.A.*, 71:2127, 1918.

er gross or microscopic, on the gastro-intestinal tract of dogs."

Mode of Action: Sharp-cornered articles may act in several ways. The piece may cause perforation of the wall of the stomach or bowel, with the usual consequence of such perforation. Owing to the defensive actions on the part of the intestine, perforation by such articles is relatively rare. The action of a large number of pieces may set up a widespread irritation and inflammation, arising from the subsequent local infection, causing an acute or subacute gastro-enteritis, and this is probably the chief cause of suffering and death produced by these articles. It seems likely that in the case of professional glass-eaters the repeated wounding of the mucous membrane may lead to some sort of immunity which prevents an infection that might easily occur in other persons.

Symptoms: The symptoms produced by swallowing broken glass are generally due to irritation of the mucous membrane of the stomach and intestines, and are consequently similar to those of gastro-enteritis produced by other agencies. This was noted in the case of Clugston, where the gastro-enteritis was his first complaint. Generally there is a sharp pain in the stomach and later in the intestines, and sometimes nausea and vomiting, the vomited material being streaked with blood. The bowels are generally constipated, but sometimes there is diarrhea, the passage of stools being attended by pain, and the material passed usually mixed with blood. In case of perforation of the stomach or intestines collapse usually supervenes and the patient soon dies.

Fatal Dose and Fatal Period: It is impossible to state what the fatal dose of ground glass is. It has already been pointed out that large quantities of the substance may be taken without any seemingly harmful results. In the Clugston case the dose was close to one-half ounce, in the second attempt. The result depends largely upon the condition of the stomach as to the presence or absence of much food, upon the size and sharpness of the fragments of glass, and also upon individual susceptibility. In a case reported by Hebb[1824] a large teaspoonful of pounded glass caused the death of a child of eleven months. The patient may die from perforation of the stomach or bowels or from acute gastro-enteritis, or he may lin-

1824. HEBB: *Midland Med. & Surg. Rep.*, 1:47, 1829.

ger with subacute or chronic trouble for many days or weeks, and finally die from the remote effects of the irritant. In a fatal case reported by Reichardt,[1825] death occurred six days after ingestion of the powdered glass.

Treatment: If the case is seen early, the stomach should be evacuated. The patient should be given pieces of orange with long fibres of cotton. The cotton and the fibers of orange wind around the particles of glass and prevent them from injuring the mucous membrane of the stomach and bowel. It is the best treatment that the author has found and has resorted to many times for children who have swallowed bobby-pins and safety pins. The child should be given several oranges with cotton. The bobby-pins and safety pins upon being passed forty-eight to seventy-two hours later, are completely enveloped in the cotton fiber. If the bowels do not move, an injection of a mucilaginous or oily material should be given.

Pain should be treated by the use of opiates and hot applications, and collapse guarded against by the external use of warmth and the internal administration of cardiac and general stimulants, such as small doses of alcohol, ether, ammonium carbonate, and strychnine. If the symptoms point to perforation of the stomach or bowels, a surgical operation should be resorted to promptly.

Postmortem Appearances: Postmortem appearances are such as are commonly observed in cases of gastro-enteritis and are found almost entirely in the gastro-intestinal tract. There is a redness of the mucous membrane, which is covered with tenacious mucus and frequently streaked with blood. Perforations in the stomach and intestines should be carefully looked for, and if found the abdominal cavity should be searched for particles of glass which may have escaped into it. In the Clugston case there was found a piece of glass in the appendix. In Reichardt's case,[1825] already referred to, erosions were found in the pharynx, stomach, duodenum, and upper part of small intestines; and in the case of a boy of twelve years, described by Bronowski,[1826] many ulcers were found on the mucous membrane of the stomach and intestine, and in both the powdered glass was discovered in form resembling sand.

Chemical Examination: The contents of the stomach and

1825. REICHARDT: *Arch. d. Pharm.*, 2s., 91:9, 1882.
1826. BRONOWSKI: *Virchows Jahresb.*, 1:505, 1893.

intestines and vomited matter and feces may be washed in a
stool-sieve and any particles left on the sieve examined as
described here.   After the digestion of the stomach or
bowels by the Fresenius and von Babo method, the solution is
filtered, and the glass will be found upon the filter paper. However, if other substances of a mechanical nature are suspected,
they should be looked for before the destruction of the organic
matter. The particles of glass separated by either washing or
digestion may be identified by the following properties: (a)
They are transparent or translucent; if the glass, however, has
an exceedingly irregular surface, this property may be largely
lacking.   (b) The surface is more or less irregular, with sharp,
uneven angles, by which it may be distinguished from the regularly crystalline bodies.   (c) They are fusible when heated on
a platinum foil; sand or other forms of silica do not fuse. The
globules adhere to the foil and may show sufficient transpar-
ency for lines to be seen through them, and even for the reading of letters. (d) They are ductile. (e) When glass is heated
in a platinum dish with hydrofluoric acid it dissolves and the
silica disappears, leaving a residue consisting of the fluorides
of the metals from which the glass was made. Quartz or silica,
for which glass might be mistaken, would disappear wholly
under this test. The examination of this residue for metals may
show the original composition of the glass. In the examination
greatest care must be taken so that the material is not contaminated by pieces of glass accidentally derived from vessels or
other apparatus. The discovery of a few pieces of glass in the
stomach may sometimes be due to the accidental swallowing
of pieces of glass from glass vessels which contained food.

In an alleged case of criminal poisoning by glass, tried a
few years ago in New Jersey, Dr. John Marshall demonstrated
that the fragments of glass found in the organs of the deceased,
upon chemical examination, could have been introduced by the
screwing down of the cover of the Mason fruit jar in which the
organs were sent to the chemist. Splintering of small pieces
of glass in the use of fruit jars is by no means uncommon. Small
pieces of glass are occasionally found in food from accidental
contamination. Simmons and Glahm report that of 120 specimens of food submitted to them for examination, particles of
glass were found in seventeen; in thirteen of these it was evident that the glass was accidentally present.

BLOOD

THE importance of having articles submitted for the presence of blood in cases of homicide justified itself so many times in the experiences of the author, while chemist to the Coroner of Cook County, that he believes it should be a routine for coroners and police officials to collect and submit all substances that contain suspicious stains to the chemist for examination.[1827]

Although clothing may not contain blood stains, it may contain dust, sawdust, or fibers, which would connect the individual with the alleged crime.

Everything that appears in the least degree suspicious should be taken, such as articles of clothing or bedding, pieces of wall paper, curtains, stains found on woodwork or floor, or substances containing suspicious stains found in the neighborhood of the deceased, on the person of the accused or suspected, and any implements or weapons that may possibly have any connection with the case. Before removing the stains for analysis, the expert should make notes giving their relative position and direction with respect to the body. If the articles submitted by the authorities are wet, they should be allowed to dry, spread out, and then examined carefully for the presence of stains. If the body has been removed from the house, stains may be found on the linoleum in the kitchen, on the stairs leading to the basement, on the stairs going out of the basement, or on the adjacent woodwork. Woodwork and all articles submitted should be separately marked by the authorities and by the expert to whom the same has been submitted. Photographs should always be taken of the stains. After all suspected substances are in the possession of the expert, they should be kept under lock and key. They should be submitted preferably in person, as sometimes there is a point for argument by the defense (which causes embarrassment both to the prosecutor and expert) in the tracing of such evidence from the time the substance was removed from the source of crime until it reached the laboratory. If it is impossible on account of distance to submit the articles in person, they may then be sent by express,

1827. Material in this section is taken largely from the author's chapter on the medicolegal examination of blood and blood stains in the 2nd ed. of "Legal Medicine and Toxicology," by PETERSON, HAINES and WEBSTER, 1923.

the seals and wrappers and twine serving for identification at the time of the trial.

The expert must make a minute examination of the substances that are submitted. This examination should be made not only by the unaided eye, but also by means of magnifying glasses, both by daylight and by artificial light, since it often happens that small blood-stains can be detected much more readily by artificial light than by daylight. They should also be examined by ultraviolet light. Every spot that appears suspicious should be described and located, and its nature later determined by chemical tests or microscopic examination. Each article received should be carefully described, together with a detailed statement of the results of the preliminary examination in each case. The most important kinds of stains submitted for medicolegal examination are: (1) Blood-stains. (2) Stains containing blood, such as menstrual, lochial, and nasal, after epistaxis. (3) Seminal stains, as in cases of alleged rape, adultery, or sodomy. (4) Stains containing mucus or pus, such as nasal, leukorrheal, and gonorrheal.

BLOOD-STAINS

THE expert is more frequently required to examine stains for blood than for anything else, and he is requested to determine, in the first place, whether the stain is a blood-stain or whether it contains blood or not; secondly, if it is a blood-stain, whether the blood is from a mammal, a bird, a fish, or a reptile; and thirdly, if the blood is mammalian, is it that of any given species of mammal. It is often alleged by the accused in cases of homicide that the blood-stains in question were made by the blood of a fish, bird, reptile, or other animal. In such cases the work may be narrowed down to determining whether the blood in the stain is consistent with that of the animal mentioned, or consistent with its being human blood. When no data are given, the expert must present the result of his investigation, and state whether or not these results are consistent with the stain being that of human blood.

There are also other questions that the expert may be required to decide, as, for example, in cases where there is no doubt but that the blood in the stain is human, as in the case of blood-stains or pools of blood found in the immediate neighborhood of the victim of a homicide, the approximate length of time which had elapsed since the escape of the blood and the finding of the body must be determined. Again, an opinion is often requested concerning the direction from which the blood must have come in order to have produced a given stain. To throw light on these questions, it is necessary that one understands some of the physical and chemical properties of blood.

Blood contains a pale, straw-colored fluid having a specific gravity of about 1.028. In this fluid are suspended the red and white blood corpuscles, and the blood platelets, the latter, up to the present time, having no medicolegal importance. After the escape of the blood from the vessels coagulation occurs, leaving the blood serum as a clear, limpid fluid exuding from the clot. This consists of a solution in water of various protein substances, and of several inorganic salts, the principal of which is sodium chloride. The constituents of blood serum have a primary importance in the medicolegal examination of blood in connection with the serum, precipitin, or biologic test.

Of the solid constituents of blood, the red blood cells are the only ones that at the present time have a practical medicolegal value. They contain hemoglobin, which imparts the red color to the blood. The difference in the color of the arterial and venous blood is due to the varying proportion of oxygen held in combination with the hemoglobin. The number of the red cells in the blood varies in different animals and in different individuals. The number varies somewhat in different persons in health, and in some diseases the number differs greatly from the normal. Authorities agree that the average number of the red blood cells in the blood of healthy adult human beings is from 4,500,000 to 5,000,000 per cubic millimeter. Wormley has calculated, estimating the number as 5,000,000 per cubic millimeter, that one grain of human blood contains 825,000,000 red cells, and therefore, that the weight of a single red cell is approximately 1/800,000,000 grain. The blood of the rabbit contains about 3,500,000 red cells per cubic millimeter, and that of the goat about 18,000,000 per cubic millimeter.

The white cells exist in healthy human blood to the extent of approximately 7,000 per cubic millimeter. Although their proportion to the red blood-cells in health is about one to 700, in some diseases their relative proportion may be much in excess of this, and in rare instances may be increased even to the proportion of one white to two or three red cells. As yet, however, they have no practical value in the usual medicolegal examination of blood-stains. It has been suggested to apply the Zondek hormone test to blood spots to show whether the blood is from a pregnant woman or not, and to show the difference of male and female.[1828]

The coagulation of blood is of importance in certain medicolegal cases. It is well known that when blood is drawn into a dish and allowed to stand, it separates into two portions, a solid mass, the clot or coagulum, red in color and containing all the solid elements of the blood, and a nearly colorless liquid portion, the blood-serum. The time required for the complete coagulation of the blood varies in different animals, and under unlike circumstances the time required may differ in blood from the same animal. For instance, the blood of the fowl begins to coagulate in one and a half minutes; that of the rabbit, sheep, and pig in from a half to one and a half minutes; that of the horse and ox in from five to thirteen minutes; that of the dog in from one to three minutes; that of man in from three to four minutes—and the coagulation is complete in human blood as a rule in from nine to ten minutes. In the case of bird blood, coagulation is rapid and the coagulum large, while in cold, blooded animals the coagulation is slow and the coagulum small.

The following circumstances increase the rapidity of the coagulation: Increase in temperature; exposure of a large surface of blood to the air, as, for instance, when it is collected in a shallow dish; contact with numerous points of some foreign bodies, as when stirred or beaten with a number of wires, or, as in the case of many stains submitted to medicolegal examination, when a small drop falls on a rough surface. The following conditions may delay, or even prevent, coagulation: Exposure to cold, as for instance, if cooled rapidly to the freezing point coagulation will not take place for an hour or so; contact with oily or greasy substances; admixture with syrupy liquids; and heating the blood quickly to a temperature of 56°C. (132.8°F.)— which entirely prevents coagulation.

Blood is a viscid fluid, this viscidity often rendering it possible to determine in certain blood-stains the direction from

1828. GORONCY, ASCHEIM: *Deutsche med. Wchnschr.*, 58:662, 1932.

which it came. When a minute drop of blood meets an object after having been propelled from an artery, it forms an oval or pear-shaped stain if the surface upon which it impinges be more or less oblique, and the bulk of the blood is driven to the farther end of the stain. The same results may follow the force of a blow caused by some blunt instrument, such as a club, striking in a pool of blood. If, however, the surface upon which the blood impinges be vertical and of such a nature that it does not immediately absorb the blood, then the bulk of the blood which has been driven to the farther part of the stain, will, if the blood came from below upward, gravitate back to the lower

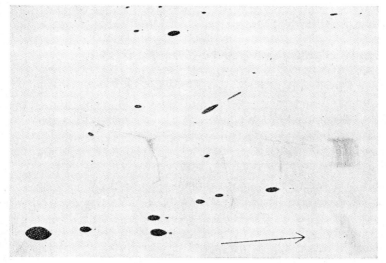

FIG. 21
The Direction of Blood Impingement

portion. If the surface happens to be rough, like that of a shaggy overcoat cloth, the coagulation takes place so rapidly that this gravitation does not occur, so that, if a drop of blood be propelled from near the surface of the ground upward against the surface of a rough overcoat, that surface being vertical, it will be found on examination after the stain has become dry that the bulk of the blood is in the upper portion of the stain, which is generally the smaller end. The importance of being able to determine the direction from whence the blood came in order to form the stains found in certain cases is self-evident and needs no further discussion.

Drying of Blood: The time required for blood to dry is also important. For example, in a case of double murder the appearance of the blood beneath the two bodies showed that a considerable length of time had elapsed between the deaths of the two individuals. A drop of blood dries much more slowly than a drop of water of the same size. The character of the surface on which the blood falls also has considerable bearing on the time required for complete drying. If the surface be an absorbent one, so that the blood may permeate the substance itself, as in the case of a piece of unstarched cotton or linen cloth, the drying takes place quite rapidly. But if the surface be a non-absorbent one, as that of a piece of glass or a board having a smooth surface, and also in the case of some kinds of dense woven fabrics, the time required for the drying of a drop of blood is much greater than that of a drop of water of equal size. A large drop of blood requires proportionally a longer time to dry than a small drop. For instance, a drop of blood allowed to fall from the end of a finger on a piece of glass, the drop measuring three-eighths inch in diameter, required one hour and five minutes for complete drying under favorable conditions—namely, in a room with an open fire and a temperature of 71° F. (21.6° C.). A drop of similar size on a piece of soft pine board in a room in which the temperature was only 65° F. (18.3° C.), and with the atmosphere not so dry as in the previous instance, did not undergo any perceptible change for half an hour, and in one hour it had only begun to shrink and have a glazed appearance on the edge. This glazed appearance gradually extended toward the center of the drop, and the drying became complete in exactly two hours. Therefore, from one to two hours is required for a single drop of blood to dry.

These facts show how necessary it is to observe carefully every blood-stain in the medicolegal cases submitted for investigation. The number, exact location, shape, color, and whether or not the individual stains have a different density in different parts, must be noted. From the facts obtained by simple inspection, which should be made as quickly as possible after the receipt of the substances to be examined, important information may possibly be gained with reference to the age of the stain, the direction from which the blood emanated, and perhaps some idea of the force with which it was propelled.

Color of Blood-Stains: Rust stains are often confused with blood-stains and submitted by authorities to the expert. In a number of instances I have saved accused men from being held for murder, when I established the fact that the stains were not made by blood. For example, in the Jennie Constance case, two men, L. P., and J. B., were held as suspects. Pipe and clothing containing suspicious stains were submitted to me. I found these stains to be rust. Later David Shanks, a colored man, confessed and paid the penalty for the crime.

If a blood-stain be recent, the time elapsed since the stain was made can sometimes be determined within narrow limits by observing carefully its color. A freshly made blood-stain, after it has become dry, under ordinary circumstances has a bright scarlet color. Upon exposure to ordinary daylight this color gradually changes to a dull brown during a period of about ten days, after which time the color does not change materially; therefore if a given stain has been exposed only to light and air under ordinary conditions for less than ten days, some opinion can be formed as to the approximate age of the stain. It must be borne in mind, however, that there are conditions which hasten this change of color, as: continuous exposure to direct sunlight; the application of a high degree of heat, such as might be obtained by a hot iron or the heating of the substance containing the stain on a stove or in an oven; or treating the stain with certain preservatives, like alcohol, naphtha, or formalin, which will very rapidly change the color to a dull brown.

Solubility of Blood-Stains: Schwarzacher[1829] gives a curve showing the solubility of the stain in water, exposed to various lengths of time.

In the case of a recently shed blood on clothing or weapons, an extract can be made with salt solution or distilled water. When the stain has been exposed to heat or chemicals, the extraction takes a longer time and it may be necessary to use some other solvent. Katayama[1830] found that blood-stains, whether dried in porcelain dishes and though exposed to a temperature of 80° C. (176° F.) for an indefinite

1829. SCHWARZACHER: *Deutsche Ztschr. f. d. ges. gerichtl. Med.*, 15:119, 1930.

1830. KATAYAMA: *Vrtljschr. f. gerichtl. Med., Berl.*, 49:269, 1888.

length of time, or to 100° C. (212° F.) for an hour, were still soluble in distilled water within twenty-four hours: if heated to 140° C. (284° F.) for one hour the stains were soluble only in caustic potash of a specific gravity of 1.017 diluted with three volumes of water just before use, or in glacial acetic acid. If the stain was exposed to 135° to 143° C. (275° to 289.4° F.) it lost its power of reacting to the guaiac or Van Deen test; and if exposed to over 145° C. (293° F.) it lost its power to form Teichmann's crystals. Sutherland[1831] obtained very little extraction with a potassium cyanide solution in the case of stains heated to 140° C. (284° F.) for two hours, but he obtained crystals of hematin chloride in extracts made with glacial acetic and concentrated sulphuric acid. Ferrai found that blood exposed to a temperature of 130° C. (266° F.) for an hour, 140° C. (284° F.) for twenty minutes, or 160° C. (320° F.) for five minutes, yields an extract with which the serum reaction cannot be obtained. If the stain has been exposed to formaldehyde the solubility is greatly altered, rendering Pfaff's scale unreliable. This scale is based on the solubility of the blood in a solution of arsenous acid, one to 120. Fresh blood dissolves at once; blood two to three days old, within fifteen minutes; three to eight days old, within thirty minutes; two to four weeks old, within one to two hours; four to six weeks old, within three to four hours; and blood a year or more old dissolves in from four to eight hours.

To extract a stain, scrape off a fragment if the stain be on a hard surface as of wood or metal, the particles being allowed to fall on a piece of white paper. If the stain be on cloth, a portion of the stained part and a portion of the unstained part, very essential in colored fabrics for control, should be removed and cut into small pieces. Then small particles of the stain or parts of the cloth are placed in a small test-tube of about 2 cc., adding about 1 cc. of salt solution, and stirring with a clean glass rod. This will give sufficient solution for the chemical and spectroscopic test. For the precipitin test the extract must be filtered or centrifuged to obtain an absolutely clear solution.

Many substances resembling blood-stains are found on articles submitted by officials. Iron rust and stains of red paint

1831. SUTHERLAND: Blood-stains, 6, 1907.

containing iron seldom present a glazed appearance, but may be confusing on clothing until a chemical examination reveals the presence of iron. The rust or paint stains are not soluble in the usual solvents, but are soluble in warm hydrochloric acid.

The addition of a drop of potassium ferrocyanide yields the Prussian-blue reaction in the presence of iron. This test should be made with unstained parts, especially with garments, as salts of iron are frequently employed as mordants. The addition of ammonia to the stain extract changes the reddish hue of vegetable coloring matter to a greenish-crimson or bluish-black, while blood pigment remains unaltered. Red or reddish-brown stains due to anilin dyes become yellow on the addition of nitric acid, while blood pigment does not undergo such change in color.

Methods of Identifying Blood-Stains: The methods employed in the identification of blood-stains are: (1) Chemical; (2) optical; (3) microscopical examination; (4) the precipitin, biologic, or serum test; and (5) the isoagglutinin test.

The chemical and optical methods are used for the purpose of detecting hemoglobin or its decomposition products. They serve also to detect the protein contained in the stain, but do not enable us to distinguish between proteins of different species.

The detection of hemoglobin, however, shows us with certainty the presence of blood, but since hemoglobin is contained in the blood of many animals, its detection throws no light upon the nature of the animal from which the blood in any given stain came. To determine this latter question resort is had to the microscopic examination of the blood cells in the stains and especially to the precipitin test. By means of these methods of investigation it is usually possible to determine whether the blood is of human or animal origin. As pointed out on page 960, hemoglobin may have antigenic properties, and it is possible that use may be made thereof in the identification of blood.

Hemoglobin and Its Decomposition Products: Hemoglobin is the red coloring-matter of the blood, being found in the blood of all vertebrates with the exception of two, amphioxus and leptocephalus, and in many of the invertebrates. It carries the oxygen to the tissues, with which it forms two compounds, oxyhemoglobin and methemoglobin. In oxyhemoglobin the oxygen is loosely combined with the pigment and separates from it readily, while in methemoglobin the combination is much more stable. Solutions of oxyhemoglobin have the bright cherry-red color seen in arterial blood, while the darker color of venous blood is that of a solution of hemoglobin largely deprived of its oxygen. The color of a solution of methemoglobin is brown. Solutions of these three substances when examined with the spectroscope show different absorption bands, which will be discussed shortly.

Hemoglobin contains iron; it also forms distinct compounds with nitric oxide (NO_2), and carbon monoxide, the solutions of which give characteristic absorption spectra. The carbon monoxide hemoglobin has medicolegal importance in cases of poisoning by illuminating gas and fumes from burning charcoal; poisoning by illuminating gas is common, owing to the large percentage of carbon monoxide in illuminating gas. It is this compound that imparts the bright cherry-red color to the blood and tissues in cases of poisoning by this gas.

Hemoglobin is quite easily decomposed by various agencies. If a solution of it be heated to boiling, the color changes to brown, due to the decomposition of the hemoglobin into a brown pigment (hematin), and a protein (globin). This pigment hematin is quite important medicolegally, as it is formed from hemoglobin by many agencies to which blood-stains may be exposed, and also because it is formed during some of the principal chemical tests for blood.

Hematin contains all the iron of the hemoglobin from which it was derived. It is insoluble in water, alcohol, and ether, but is soluble in alkaline hydroxides and in alcohol containing sulphuric acid. Solutions of hematin give characteristic absorption spectra. If a solution of hematin be treated with ammonium sulphide or some other reducing agent, a pigment called hemochromogen is formed; this pigment was formerly designated reduced hematin.

Another decomposition product of importance in medicolegal examination of some blood-stains is hematoporphyrin, or iron-free hematin. This pigment is produced from hemoglobin or hematin by the action of agencies which remove the iron from these compounds; some of these agencies are conditions to which blood-stains may be subjected accidentally or intentionally, as has been shown by Liman, Kratter and Hammerl.[1832] When this decomposition has taken place in a blood stain, the application of the ordinary tests will not reveal the presence of blood pigment, and it is necessary to resort to special methods for the recognition of the hemochromogen or the hematoporphyrin by means of the spectroscope.

If blood-stained articles are treated with naphtha or benzene, or certain deodorizers or disinfectants, the blood pigment will be so decomposed that it cannot be detected by the ordinary chemical tests. At the same time the red blood cells will be fixed to such an extent that they resist subsequent treatment with water.

Chemical Tests for Blood: The principal chemical tests for blood are the following:

1. Teichmann's, or the hemin, test.
2. Sodium tungstate test.
3. Guaiacum test.
4. Benzidin test.
5. Phenolphthalin test.
6. Protein tests.

Teichmann's Test: This is by far the most important test for blood pigment, and is extremely delicate. It is made in the following manner:

If the blood-stain is dried, a small fragment should be removed with the point of a knife and transferred to a glass slide. If the stain be a diffused one, or if the blood while still fresh has soaked into the fabric, as in the case of a stain on cotton or linen cloth, then it suffices to scrape a small portion of the stain with the knife point, collecting the dust thus removed on a glass slide. The fragment of dried blood, or the dust, is then treated on a slide with a small drop of water in which has been dissolved a minute fragment of sodium chloride. This drop is evaporated to dryness by gentle heat, the dried residue covered with a cover-glass, a drop of glacial acetic acid allowed to run under the cover-glass, and the slide again gently heated until bubbles of gas are seen to form in the liquid under the cover glass. This shows that the glacial acetic acid has been heated to the boiling point. If now, the slide is allowed to cool, the microscope will reveal the characteristic crystals of chloride of

1832. LIMAN, KRATTER and HAMMERL: *Vrtljschr f. gerichtl. Med.*, *Berl.*, 4:41, 62. 1892.

hematin in case the stain examined contained blood. These crystals of chloride of hematin are called "hemin" crystals, which have a characteristic form.

The normal hemin crystals have a yellow to chocolate brown color, and separate in the form of small rhombic plates. They naturally vary a little in size according to the rapidity of their formation. Sometimes two or more arrange themselves in the form of a cross or a rosette. Sometimes, particularly if the fragment of dried blood on the slide was of considerable size, the form of the crystals in some parts of the preparation may be somewhat modified, some assuming a pointed, oval shape, and in some the outlines may be a little irregular; in all cases, however, a sufficient number of the normal perfect crystals will be seen to render their identification positive.

The test depends on the principles, first, that hematin is formed from the decomposition of the hemoglobin by heat, and, secondly, that the hematin in solution in boiling glacial acetic acid unites with the chlorine of the salt to form chloride of hematin, which is soluble in boiling glacial acetic acid, crystallizing from this solvent on cooling.

Precautions: Care should be taken in heating the slide so as not to raise the temperature sufficiently to decompose the hematin in the first dry residue obtained. If the temperature is raised to about 142° C. (287.6° F.), no hemin crystals will be formed.

Further, on heating the slide after the addition of glacial acetic acid, the temperature should not be raised sufficiently to produce active boiling of the acid, since active ebullition may carry all the pigment beyond the edge of the cover glass, which might prevent the detection of the hemin crystals.

The hemin test will not detect blood pigment in bloodstains that have been heated to a high temperature, that have been subjected to the prolonged action of naphtha, solution of aluminum chloride, or bromochloralum, or that have been exposed for a long time to direct sunlight.

Wachholz[1833] found that all concentrated mineral and organic acids may be used for the test, and recommends that a one to 10,000 solution of concentrated sulphuric, lactic, or glacial acetic acid in 90 to 95% alcohol be used, as they boil readily and the crystals are not destroyed by excessive heat. Two drops of

1833. WACHHOLZ: *Vrtljschr. f. gerichtl. Med., Berl.*, 21:227, 1901.

a 34% hydro-bromic acid in 5 cc. of formic acid give colored crystals which stand out more prominently than when sodium chloride and glacial acetic acid are used.

The Sodium Tungstate Test: This test is of great value in the case of diffused blood-stains caused by the action of water on the original stain, as in unsuccessful attempts to wash a blood-stain from cloth, and in cases in which the blood exists in solution in water or some other aqueous fluid, such as urine. By means of this test all the blood pigment is precipitated from its aqueous solution, and thus concentrated to a small volume in the form of a precipitate that can be tested by the hemin test or subjected to spectroscopic examination.

In the case of a diffused blood-stain in which the blood pigment has been largely diluted with water and spread over a large surface of cloth or other fabric, the application of the hemin test in the ordinary way will generally fail to detect the blood pigment. It is, therefore, necessary first to remove all the blood from a considerable piece of the cloth, concentrate to a small volume, and identify it by one or more of the other tests. This is best done in the following manner: A piece of the cloth of sufficient size—the amount required depending on the extent to which the blood has been diluted, this being determined generally by simple inspection — is removed and placed in an evaporating dish or wine glass containing distilled water in which has been dissolved a crystal or two of potassium iodide. In this the fabric is soaked with frequent stirring and pressing by means of a glass rod, so as to facilitate the thorough washing out of the pigment from the cloth. The fluid is poured off into a flask or test-tube, according to the amount used, and the process repeated once or twice with fresh portions of water and potassium iodide, and finally the fluid is entirely pressed out from the cloth. These united washings are then filtered so as to remove all solid particles, strongly acidulated with acetic acid, and treated with a few cc. of a saturated solution of sodium tungstate also strongly acidulated with acetic acid. In case the fluid is deeply colored with blood pigment, 5 to 10 cc. of the tungstate solution may be necessary. If there is much blood pigment present in the fluid, the addition of the sodium tungstate solution will produce a distinct, light-colored precipitate, which will be quite bulky, but which, on boiling the fluid in the flask or test-tube, will become aggregated in the form of dense, chocolate-colored flocculi. These can be collected on a filter paper, washed with water, dried, and tested by the hemin test; or, spectroscopically, by dissolving a part in very dilute sodium or ammonium hydroxide, when the spectrum of hematin in alkaline solution may be seen.

If there be not a sufficient amount of blood pigment to impart any perceptible color to the extract obtained by washing, the addition of the sodium tungstate solution will cause perhaps only a very slight turbidity. In this case the mixture is actively boiled and set aside for a day or two to settle completely. The tungstate precipitate of the blood pigment will be found in the light sediment at the bottom. The supernatant clear fluid should then be decanted from the sediment, and the latter transferred to a watch glass, in which it is washed by collecting it in the center of the watch glass by gently rotating the latter, and the supernatant fluid removed by introducing carefully strips of blotting or filter paper. In this way, by careful manipulation, the precipitate is finally collected in only a drop or two of water, which is transferred to a glass slide, evaporated by gentle heat, and the hemin test applied.

A number of oxidation reactions have been applied to blood stains, guaiacum, benzidin, phenolphthalin, and fluorescein, giving the best results.

The Guaiacum Test: This test depends on the principle that if a solution of blood pigment be treated with a few drops of very dilute tincture of guaiacum and then with a drop or two of a solution of hydrogen peroxide a blue color is immediately produced. This test is also called Van Deen's test. Van Deen, however, used ozonized oil of turpentine instead of the hydrogen peroxide solution, but the latter is preferable, since it is purer and can always be obtained.

A minute fragment of the stain, or a few fibers of the stained fabric, is placed in a small porcelain evaporating dish or crucible, treated with a drop of water in order to dissolve a portion of the pigment, and then with a few drops of the guaiacum alone; a drop or two of the solution of hydrogen peroxide is then added, and, if there is the slightest trace of blood pigment present, a blue color will be produced immediately.

This test is an extremely delicate one, and will, according to Wormley, react with blood pigment in a solution of only one part in 5,000. It will also react with old stains as well as with fresh ones; if the stain be very old, however, it is necessary to soak it for a longer time in water. A piece of moistened filter paper pressed for a moment on a blood-stain will generally remove enough of the coloring matter to give this reaction; in this case the tincture of guaiacum and the hydrogen peroxide are applied directly to the paper. This is a valuable and practical preliminary test. A suspected spot is covered with a piece of moistened filter paper and the latter pressed on the spot for a moment, the paper removed, and the spot on the paper tested. If no blue color be produced on the paper, it is positive that the stain is not a blood-stain; if, however, a blue color is produced, it is an indication that the stain may contain blood, the presence of which must be confirmed by other tests or methods of examination. The tincture of guaiacum used in this test must be freshly prepared, and must be made from perfectly clear pieces of the resin, which should be obtained from the center of a freshly broken clear lump.

Schaer[1834] has modified the test as follows: A fragment of the blood-stain, especially if it is an old stain, is moistened with very dilute acetic acid for a few minutes and then treated with a solution containing 1% of guaiacum and from 70 to 75% of chloral hydrate. Then, if no blue color appears, there is added a drop or two of the following solution of hydrogen peroxide: 15 cc. of a 3 to 5% solution of hydrogen peroxide free from acid, with 25 cc. alcohol, 5 cc. chloroform, and 1.5 cc. glacial acetic acid. The blue color will appear immediately if blood pigment is present.

There are many substances other than blood pigment that will produce a blue color with the guaiacum test. The following have been shown by different observers to be capable of producing this same reaction: Potato skin, casein glue, many compounds of iron, particularly the chloride, acetate, and citrate, and to a slight degree, ferric hydroxide, which is always present in iron-rust; according to Huenefeld,[1835] ferric sulphate, iron alum, cupric sulphate and nitrate, the double chloride of gold and sodium, manganese dioxide, potassium permanganate; and, according to Wesener, indigo, so that the test is not reliable in the case of stains on cloth that has been dyed with indigo.

1834. SCHAER: *J. Pharm.*, 361, 1899.
1835. HUENEFELD: Die Blutproben vor Gericht.

Practically, therefore, the negative result obtained by this test is of greater value than the positive result, since it shows that the stain in question does not contain blood pigment in such a form as to be soluble in the ordinary solvents.

Phenolphthalin Test: Phenolphthalin is a more delicate and useful reagent than guaiacum. With phenolphthalin Delearde and Benoit[1836] were able to detect blood in a dilution of one part in 1,000,000, and Kastle[1837] recognized blood at a dilution of one part in 80,000,000.

In order to prepare this reagent, phenolphthalein is dissolved in a considerable excess of 30%, sodium hydroxide solution and boiled with an excess of zinc dust until a few drops of the strongly alkaline liquid no longer give the color of phenolphthalein after neutralization with hydrochloric acid and the addition of sufficient alkali to give a slightly alkaline reaction. The solution is then decanted from the excess of zinc dust, and the phenolphthalin is precipitated by acidifying with hydrochloric acid. The substance is then collected on a filter and purified by several crystallizations from water and alcohol in the following manner: The phenolphthalin is dissolved in the smallest quantity of boiling alcohol in which it will dissolve, filtered if necessary, and cold water gradually added with constant stirring until the compound is precipitated out as a white crystalline precipitate. From three to five crystallizations are carried out in precisely this manner, and in this way phenolphthalin is finally obtained in the form of a white crystalline compound entirely free from all traces of phenolphthalein.

One of the great advantages of phenolphthalin in work of this kind is that we know we are dealing with a perfectly definite compound the purity of which can be determined simply and easily whenever desired, and which, on oxidation passes into another equally definite compound, the smallest amount of which can be readily detected by means of an alkali, and which may be determined very accurately by colorimetric methods.

Alkaline Phenolphthalin: This reagent is prepared by dissolving 0.032 gm. of phenolphthalin in 21 cc. of N/10 sodium hy-

1836. DELEARDE and BENOIT: *Compt. rend. Soc. de biol.*, 64:990, 1908.
1837. KASTLE: Bull. 51, Hyg. Lab., 1909.

droxide and adding sufficient water to make the volume of the solution up to 100 cc. This reagent may also be prepared by bringing together 1 cc. of N/10 sodium hydroxide with some-what more phenolphthalin than will dissolve in this quantity of alkali, diluting with 10 to 20 cc. of water, filtering, and adding to the filtrate 20 cc. of N/10 sodium hydroxide and sufficient water to make up to 100 cc. Since phenolphthalin itself is prac-tically insoluble in water, and since 1 cc. of N/10 sodium hy-droxide neutralizes exactly 0.032 gm. of the compound, we ob-tain a solution by the latter mode of procedure of the same con-centration as that prepared by the first method, no weighing being required.[1837]

When first prepared, the alkaline solution of phenolphtha-lin is perfectly colorless. On long standing, however, it gradu-ally acquires a faint color, due to the oxidation of traces of the compound by atmospheric air. Then to 1 cc. of the alkaline phenolphthalin reagent add 0.5 cc. of the extract and one drop of 3% hydrogen peroxide. In five minutes a deep purplish red or pink color will be obtained in the presence of blood. The control test is made by mixing 0.5 cc. of distilled water, 1 cc. of the reagent, and a drop of peroxide; if the reagent has been properly prepared only a trace of pink will be found. Kastle reports that animal tissues in many cases retard the oxidation of phenolphthalin under the influence of blood. If a positive test is obtained, care should be taken in this as in the other oxi-dation tests, to exclude oxidases or peroxidases by boiling, and the salts of heavy metals and other oxidizing agents by chemi-cal methods.

Benzidin Test: This is also a very delicate test for blood. To a saturated solution of benzidin in alcohol or glacial acetic acid freshly prepared, or to a small amount of benzidin about the size of a grain of rice, placed on a white tile with a few drops of glacial acetic acid, add an equal volume of 3% hydrogen per-oxide and 0.5 cc. of the solution under examination. Make a control test, substituting water for the unknown solution. A greenish-blue color is obtained in the presence of blood. The benzidin reaction serves to detect blood when present in a dilu-tion of one part in 300,000.

The fluorescence of hemoglobin derivatives, especially hematoporphyrin, is recommended as a sensitive test for blood pigment.

Fuld finds rhodamine B very sensitive as a reagent: Take 0.2 gm. of the dye in 50 cc. of alcohol, add 5 gm. zinc dust and 4 cc. of 10% NaOH, add to the boiling alcohol; on the addition of 3% hydrogen peroxide this gives a red color with blood in a dilution of one part in 10,000,000.

The Protein Test: This test is of comparatively little value, since there are so many substances other than blood that contain protein. It depends on the fact that if a solution of protein, such as must be contained in a solution of blood or a blood-stain, be heated to near the boiling point of water (after faint acidulation if alkaline or neutral), the protein is coagulated. If the solution contains at the same time blood pigment, this latter will be carried down with the coagulated protein, and will impart to it a more or less brownish tint. Practically, in the testing of blood stains, this reaction is obtained during the first part of the hemin test. On evaporation of a drop of the solution of a blood-stain on a glass slide, when the temperature reaches approximately 75° or 80° C. (167° or 176° F.), the drop may be seen to become turbid. This is due to the coagulation of the protein, there usually being in an ordinary blood-stain a sufficient quantity of protein in solution. This reaction alone does not serve to distinguish between a stain containing blood and one containing any other albuminous fluid.

Spectroscopic Test for Blood: The spectroscopic test for blood pigment depends on the fact that when a solution of hemoglobin, its compounds, or decomposition products, is placed in front of the slit of a spectroscope, certain rays of light will be absorbed, thus producing dark bands called absorption bands in certain portions of the solar spectrum. The position of these bands varies with solutions of the different blood pigments, since these different pigments absorb different rays of light. The discovery of the absorption bands of oxyhemoglobin by Hoppe-Seyler in 1862 gave an impetus to this method of examination, resulting later in the discovery of the peculiar bands formed by solutions of the other compounds of hemoglobin and its colored decomposition products.

When a sufficient amount of blood can be obtained for examination, whether in the fresh state or in the form of a dried stain as in the case of the drying of a small pool of blood, a sufficient quantity of solution of blood pigment may easily be made to permit of its examination with the ordinary large laboratory

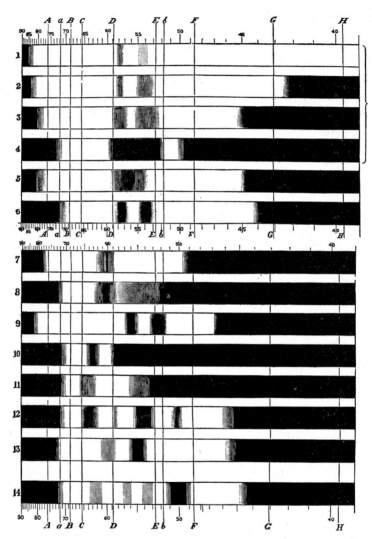

Spectra: 1, 2, 3, 4, oxyhemoglobin of various degrees of concentration; 5, hemoglobin; 6, CO-hemoglobin; 7, 8, hematin in alkaline solution, dilute and concentrated; 9, hemochromogen (Stokes' reduced hematin); 10, methemoglobin; 11, acid hematin (blood treated with acetic acid); 12, acid hematin in alcoholic solution; 13, acid hematoporphyrin; 14, alkaline hematoporphyrin.

FIG. 22
Appearance of Bands Produced by
Solutions of Oxyhemoglobin, and by
Hemoglobin, Hematin, etc.

spectroscopes. The position of the absorption bands may be located by means of the scale with which the better instruments are provided. It frequently happens, however, that the amount of material at hand in medicolegal cases is not sufficient to yield the required quantity of solution. In such cases resort must be had to one of the smaller spectroscopes, and in some cases to the so-called microspectroscope, which is, more properly speaking, a spectroscopic eyepiece applied to the tube of a microscope. Of the smaller spectroscopes, the most convenient is the Vogel's direct vision pocket-spectroscope, which can be mounted on a block. It is provided with a prism and reflector so arranged that two spectra may be obtained—one of the light that passes through the solution of the suspected stain, and the other either the ordinary solar spectrum or a spectrum caused by light passing through a solution of some known blood pigment for the purpose of comparison. This direct vision spectroscope requires but an extremely small amount of solution, which may be contained in small half-dram phials set into holes bored in the block at the proper points. These points are so chosen that the light passing through the center of the fluid will pass directly into the slit of the spectroscope, or will be reflected into it by the mirror and prism. In looking through the instrument thus arranged the two spectra will be seen, one just above the other.

In most instances the blood-stains are so small that the spectroscopic eyepiece must be used in a microscope. The instrument usually used is the spectroscopic eyepiece of Sorby or Abbe. For the description of these instruments the reader is referred to works on optical apparatus, or to a catalog of the manufacturers of microscopes and microscopic accessories.

Oxyhemoglobin: The characteristic spectrum of oxyhemoglobin can be seen only in very dilute solution. If a solution containing about 0.75% be examined in a layer 1 cm. (0.4 inch) thick, most of the rays of light will be absorbed between the lines D and b, thus forming a single large absorption band. On diluting the solution still further, this large absorption band resolves itself into two bands that are very distinct; one, the darker and more distinct but narrower of the two, is called a, and lies very near the line D, while the wider but less distinct band, called b, lies near the line E. The first four spectra in Fig. 22 show the appearance of the bands produced by solutions of oxyhemoglobin in different degrees of concentration. These four spectra are taken from Preyer's plates[1838] with the addition of the wave-length scale by Gamgee.

Hemoglobin: As mentioned, the oxygen contained in oxyhemoglobin is loosely combined, so that it can be removed from the oxyhemoglobin easily by either mechanical means or chemical agents. It may be exhausted by a vacuum-pump or removed by the action of reducing agents, such as a dilute solution of ammonium sulphide, or a solution of ferrous sulphate to which a small quantity of citric or tartaric acid has been added, and then just enough ammonia to render it faintly alkaline, (Stokes' reagent). From this treatment there results a solution of hemoglobin that has a darker color than that of oxyhemoglobin. If this solution be examined with a spectroscope, a single absorption band, called Y, is seen occupying the space between the positions formerly occupied by the oxyhemoglobin bands, a and b. It is generally less sharply defined than the oxyhemoglobin bands.

Methemoglobin: This, as mentioned, is also a compound of hemoglobin and oxygen, but a much more stable one, the oxygen consequently being removed from it with much greater difficulty. It is sometimes formed from hemoglobin in the living body, as in the case of hemoglobinuria and of potassium chlorate poisoning. Putrefaction also changes some of the hemoglobin into methemoglobin. An old blood-stain that has been exposed to direct sunlight contains some methemoglobin.

A solution of methemoglobin examined with the spectroscope shows a dark absorption band in the red between C and D, lying a little nearer to C than to D (see spectrum 10; also No. 4, on the Plate). If properly diluted, two faint bands may be seen between D and E, in a position similar to the oxyhemoglobin bands; and still a fourth band has been described in the blue, between B and H.

Carbon Monoxide Hemoglobin: This stable compound is formed by the action of carbon monoxide (CO) on hemoglobin or oxyhemoglobin. It is of medicolegal importance in cases of poisoning by carbon monoxide, which results from the inhalation of illuminating gas containing it, such as water-gas, or from the inhalation of the fumes from burning charcoal. Solu-

1838. PREYER: Die Blut-Krystalle, Jena, 1871.

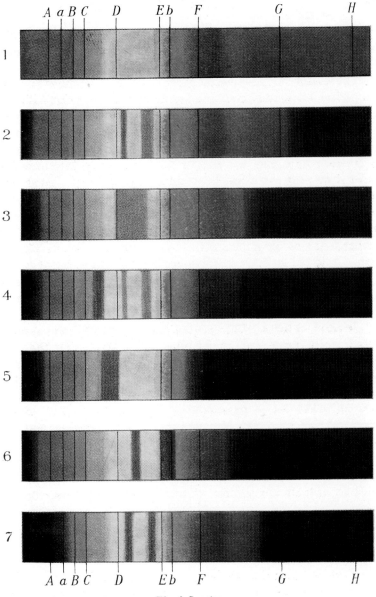

Blood Spectra

1. Solar spectrum.
2. Oxyhemoglobin.
3. Hemoglobin.
4. Methemoglobin in dilute solution.
5. Hematin in alkaline solution.
6. Hemochromogen, or reduced hematin.
7. Carbon-monoxide hemoglobin.
    (From Peterson and Haines, Legal Medicine and
            Toxicology, 1904)

tions of this compound have a bright cherry-red color, which is seen in the blood and tissues of those poisoned with carbon monoxide. This peculiar color can be preserved in such cases by adding to the blood an equal volume of a concentrated solution of borax. Solutions of carbon-monoxide hemoglobin give a spectrum similar to that of oxyhemoglobin, except that the two bands lie a little nearer to the violet end of the spectrum. It can be distinguished from the oxyhemoglobin spectrum, however, by the fact that it remains unchanged on heating the specimen under examination with ammonium sulphide.

Hematin: The recognition of this pigment is of importance in those cases in which the stain has been subjected to the action of agencies that cause decomposition of the hemoglobin. In order to extract the hematin from a blood-stain so as to prepare it for spectroscopic examination it is necessary to treat the stain, or a portion of it, with a dilute alkali (sodium or ammonium hydroxide), with glacial acetic acid, or with alcoholic solution of sulphuric acid, since hematin is insoluble in water, alcohol, and ether.

The acid and the alkaline solutions of hematin give different spectra. The spectrum of hematin in alkaline solution has a dark band between C and D, lying near D, and if sufficiently concentrated, overlapping D, while the violet end of the spectrum will be almost absorbed. (See spectra 7 and 8, and the Plate.) The spectrum of hematin in acid solution has an absorption band between C and D, very close to the line C (see spectrum 11). In an alcoholic sulphuric acid solution properly diluted the spectrum may have four bands, one between C and D, nearer C; a very faint band, not always visible, just to the right of D; a broad band between D and E, nearer E; and the fourth band between b and F, a little nearer b (spectrum 12).

Hemochromogen, or Reduced Hematin: This is produced by treating an alkaline solution of hematin with a reducing agent, such as ammonium sulphide or Stokes' reagent. Its solutions give a well defined absorption band midway between D and E and a fainter band between B and E. (See spectrum 9, and the Plate.) On exposure to the air an alkaline solution of hemochromogen absorbs oxygen and is reconverted into hematin.

Hematoporphyrin: This is formed by dissolving blood pigment in concentrated sulphuric acid or by heating it with concentrated hydrochloric acid. The solution in concentrated sulphuric acid gives a spectrum having two bands, one faint and to the left of D, and the other more distinct, between D and E (see spectrum 13). In dilute alkaline solution its spectrum has four bands, one faint and midway between C and D, the second and third rather faint, and having a position similar to the A and B oxyhemoglobin bands; and the fourth, a broad dark band reaching from b nearly to F (spectrum 14).

Method of Examination: The method of treating a blood-stain for spectroscopic examination varies according to the quantity of material at disposal and according to the age of the blood-stain i.e., whether the hemoglobin is present in the stain unchanged or has been decomposed by agencies mentioned above. If plenty of material be available and the blood pigment be mostly undecomposed, a portion of the stain can be treated with a little water or dilute salt solution, and examined directly with the direct vision spectroscope, and the oxyhemoglobin bands recognized; the solution should then be treated with a little reducing agent and the single band of hemoglobin obtained. If the blood pigment has become partially decomposed in the stain, the spectrum of methemoglobin may be seen either alone or combined with the oxyhemoglobin spectrum. If so greatly decomposed that it no longer yields any color to water, it should be treated with a little dilute sodium hydroxide; the resulting solution will give the spectrum of hematin in alkaline solution if the stain contained blood. Ammonium sulphide added to this solution gives the spectrum of hemochromogen. By using glacial acetic acid instead of dilute sodium hydroxide on a stain that is insoluble in water, the spectrum of hematin in acid solution may be seen. If the stain has been heated to a high temperature, so that hematoporphyrin has been formed, a fragment of the stain must be treated with concentrated sulphuric acid, which will dissolve it, giving a purplish red solution showing the spectrum of hematoporphyrin in acid solution.

If the amount of material be minute, so that it is necessary to use a microspectroscope, the best method of examination to be employed is that recommended by Richardson:

"Procure a glass slide with a circular excavation in the center, called by dealers a concave center, and moisten it around the edges of the cavity with a small drop of diluted glycerine. Thoroughly clean a thin glass cover slip about one-eighth inch larger than the excavation; lay it on white paper, and upon it place the tiniest visible fragment of a freshly dried blood clot. This fragment will weigh from 1/50000 to 1/25000 grain. Then, with a cataract needle, deposit on the center of the cover, near your blood spot, a drop of glycerine about the size of a small period, and with a dry needle gently brush the blood to the brink of your microscopic pond, so that it may be just moistened by the fluid. Finally, invert your slide upon the thin glass cover in such a manner that the glycerined edges of the cavity in the former may adhere to the margins of the latter, and, turning the slide face upward, transfer it to the stage of the microscope. By this method it is obvious that we obtain an extremely minute quantity of strong solution of hemoglobin whose point of greatest density, generally in the center of the clot, is readily found under a one-fourth-inch objective, and tested by the adjustment of the spectroscope eye-piece. After a little practice it will be found quite possible to modify the bands by the addition of sulphuret of sodium solution, as advised by Preyer.

"In cases of this kind, where the greatest possible economy, or even parsimony, of the material is needful, I would advise the following mode of procedure for proving and corroborating your proof of the existence of blood, so that its presence in a stain may be affirmed with absolute certainty:

"From a suspected blood spot upon metal, wood, paper, muslin, or cloth, scrape with a fine, sharp knife two, three or more minute particles of the reddish substance, causing them to fall near the middle of a large, thin glass cover slip. Apply in close proximity to them a very small drop of 0.75% salt solution, bring the particles of supposed blood clot to its edge, and proceed as I have already directed.

"After thus examining the spectrum of the substance you may generally, by rotating the stage, cause the colored fluid to partly drain away from the solid portion, wherein, under favorable circumstances, should the specimen be blood, the granular white blood globules become plainly visible, as do also cell walls of the red discs. Among the latter, if your mental and physical vision be keen enough, you can, by the aid of a 1/25 immersion lens and an eye-piece micrometer, measure a series of corpuscles accurately enough to discriminate human blood from that of an ox, pig, horse, or sheep."

Since there are a few substances, solutions of which give a spectrum somewhat resembling that of oxyhemoglobin, such as solutions of alkanet root in alum and those of cochineal, the spectroscopic examination should not be restricted to the recognition of the spectrum of oxyhemoglobin alone. The stain should be treated with the different reagents, so as to obtain several of the blood spectra. The solution of oxyhemoglobin, should, after the oxyhemoglobin bands have been recognized, always be converted into hemoglobin and again examined, since the vegetable solutions mentioned above are not changed by the action of reducing agents.

The methods of examination heretofore described enable us to determine simply the presence of the coloring matter of blood, which throws no light whatever upon the kind of blood, since the red coloring matter—hemoglobin—is contained in the blood of all vertebrates except the **amphioxus** and **leptocephalus,** [1839] and in that of many of the invertebrates.

In order to obtain any information as to the nature of the animal from which the blood in question originated, resort must be had to the microscopic investigation, for the purpose of determining if possible the form and size of the red blood cells and to the precipitin or biologic test.

Microscopic Examination of Blood: The red blood cells vary in different animals. In birds, reptiles, and fish the corpuscle is oval in shape and has a distinct nucleus, while in most mammals it is a circular, biconcave disc without a nucleus; in the camel and llama tribe, however, the red cells are oval in shape, but have no nucleus. The distinction between any kind of blood having nucleated red cells and one having nonnucleated red cells offers no difficulty whatever, even in the case of dried stains, since the nuclei are very stable and not readily destroyed, and can be very easily recognized by their high density. The microscopic distinction between the different kinds of mammalian blood presents much greater difficulty, since, with the exception of the camel tribe, the only difference is in the size of the red blood cells. This difference in size lies within such narrow limits that in some cases the positive distinction, by the microscope, between the blood of certain different animals is absolutely impossible, particularly after

1839. LANKESTER: *Proc. Roy. Soc.*, 21:71, 1872.

the blood has been dried. In other cases, however, the difference in size is so marked that there is no difficulty in distinguishing between them if the red cells have not been decomposed. This distinction is made by measuring the diameter of a large number of red cells and thus determining the average size. This requires the use of the highest powers of the microscope and the most delicate and accurate scales for measuring.

In the microscopic examination of blood stains the expert is not required to state with certainty from what animal the blood originated in any given case. He is only required to make a complete scientific investigation of the stains in question, to state the facts as he finds them, and with what those facts are consistent. He must state whether or not a stain contains blood, and, if blood be present and he has been able to obtain the red blood cells for microscopic investigation, whether or not these red blood cells are nucleated or non-nucleated; if non-nucleated, what is the average size of the red blood cells found. Only perfect red blood cells must be measured. In some cases it is alleged by the accused that the blood stains were caused by slaughtering or dressing a bird or a fish, or some animal, as a pig, ox, or sheep. In such cases it is obviously necessary for the expert to state only whether or not the red blood cells he found in the stain were or were not consistent with the explanation advanced. If the red cells he found were non-nucleated circular discs, the blood forming that stain could not have emanated from a bird, fish or reptile. If he finds that the average diameter of the red blood cells is greater than 1/3500 inch, the blood in that stain could not have emanated from any animal whose red blood cells are smaller than 1/4000 inch, and, therefore, could not have come from a pig, ox, horse, sheep, or goat.

As to the structure of the red blood cells authorities differ. Many of the older physiologists considered the blood cells as having a distinct cell-wall containing a fluid colored with a red pigment, while others thought they consisted of a stroma or network that is colorless, elastic, and made up of a protein substance the interstices of which contain the coloring-matter. This latter theory appears to be supported by the weight of evidence.

When the red blood cells of mammalian blood are treated with water, or with any fluid the density of which is less than that of the blood serum, they undergo a distinct change in form, owing to the absorption of water and the loss of their own contents by osmosis. They first lose their biconcavity, then become biconvex, and finally spheric. While this change is taking place the distance between the two edges diminishes, so that finally the diameter of the cell, which has become spheric is only about two-thirds of the original diameter when the cell had its normal biconcave shape. At the same time its density has disappeared, so that it is much more difficult to see, the outline of the cell being a mere line. Finally, if this influence continues, the cells become entirely destroyed.

A similar change in the form and size of many of the red blood cells takes place when the blood dries slowly, so that, in preparing a blood stain for microscopic examination, that portion of the stain should be selected that has dried most quickly, since there it would be expected to find a larger proportion of cells that have preserved their normal shape and size than in the center of the clot, where the drying has taken place more slowly.

When blood is treated with saline solutions of greater density than blood serum, the red cells become shrunken or shriveled and the edges irregular, or what is termed "crenated," but they do not lose their density and color. The red blood cells are generally destroyed by acids and alkalis. Thus, while there are many agencies that may cause a diminution in the size of the red blood cells, as yet none is known outside the living body that will cause an increase in their size or diameter. The influence of disease upon the size and form of the red blood cells will be referred to later .

The size of the red blood cells differs considerably in various animals, and to a certain extent within narrow limits in the same animal. As a rule, in animals having nucleated cells they are much larger than in those having non-nucleated cells, as, for instance, in one of the Louisiana reptiles (Amphiuma), the red cell is about 1/350 inch in its long diameter, large enough to be seen by the unaided eye. Of the mammals, as will be seen by the table, the elephant has the largest red blood cells, the average size being 1/2745 inch. In medicolegal cases generally the question arises only as to the distinction between the blood of man and that of the domestic animals in the case of mammalian blood stains. In these the red blood cells vary in their average diameter from about 1/6000 to 1/3000 inch. As will be seen from the table, the authorities differ but slightly with reference to the average diameter of the human red blood cell. All agree that it is between 1/3300 and 1/3200 inch. Gulliver and Formad place the average at 1/3200 inch; Wormley at 1/3250 inch; the French Committee appointed by the Medicolegal Society of France in 1873, at 1/3257 inch; Masson gives the same diameter, and Carl Schmidt places it at 1/3300 inch. Formad states, as the result of a large series of measurements, that 90% of the red blood cells will measure between 1/3300 and 1/3100 inch, only 10%, therefore, falling outside of these limits, which he considers the normal. The smallest red blood cell is 1/3800 and the largest 1/2900 inch. Hayem,[1840] states that in every 100 red blood cells about twelve will be larger than the average and about twelve smaller than the average.

The dog, pig, horse, ox, cow, cat, sheep, and goat are the only domestic mammals whose blood is liable to be of importance in medicolegal cases with reference to its distinction from human blood. Of these, the blood of the dog approaches most nearly in size to human blood.

The average diameter of the red blood cell in dog's blood is about 1/3550 inch, while that of all the other animals mentioned is less than 1/4000 inch; the red cells of the ox, pig, horse, and cat vary from 1/4400 to 1/4200 inch; the red blood cell of the sheep is about 1/5000, and that of the goat still smaller, less than 1/6000 inch. The size of the goat's blood cell is, therefore, approximately one-half that of the human.

Table LVIII on page 930 gives the average measurements as reported by various hematologists. The older authorities, Gulliver and Carl Schmidt, obtained their results with low magnifying powers of the microscope, which agree astonishingly with the results obtained by others using higher powers and much better instruments. The figures given are in vulgar fractions of an inch, which is the scale almost universally used in this country, and which it is necessary to use in court, since the average juryman knows nothing about the metric scale. Where the original measurements were given in thousands of a millimeter*

1840. HAYEM: Du Sang, Paris, 1889.

* A thousandth of a millimeter is equal to 0.00003937 inch. It is often called a micromillimeter, or micron, and is represented by the Greek letter μ. These terms are frequenty used in connection with the measurement of microscopic objects.

AVERAGE SIZE OF THE RED BLOOD-CELLS

MAMMALS	Gulliver	Wormley	Formad	REPTILES		Gulliver	Wormley
Ibex.................		1-6445		Tortoise	Long diam.	1-1252	1-1250
Goat.................	1-6366	1-6189	1-6100	(land)	Short "	1-2216	1-2200
Sloth................	1-2865			Turtle	Long "	1-1231	
Platypus (duck-billed)..	1-3000			(green)	Short "	1-1882	
Capybara............	1-3190	1-3164		Boa Con-	Long "	1-1440	1-1245
Seal.................	1-3281			strictor	Short "	1-2400	1-2538
Woodchuck..........	1-3484			Viper.....	Long "	1-1274	
Musk-deer...........	1-12325				Short "	1-1800	
Beaver..............	1-3325			Lizard....	Long "	1-1555	
Porcupine...........	1-3369				Short "	1-2743	
Llama Long diameter	1-3361	1-3201					
Short "	1-6229	1-6408		**BATRACHIANS**			
Camel Long "	1-3123	1-3331		Frog......	Long diam.	1-1108	1-1089
Short "	1-5876	1-5280			Short "	1-1821	1-1801
				Toad.....	Long "	1-1043	
BIRDS					Short "	1-2000	
Chicken Long diameter	1-2102	1-2080		Triton....	Long "	1-848	
Short "	1-3436	1-3483			Short "	1-1280	
Turkey.. Long "	1-2045	1-1894		Proteus...	Long "	1-400	
Short "	1-3598	1-3444			Short "	1-727	
Duck.... Long "	1-1937	1-1955		Amphiuma	Long "	1-363	1-358
Short "	1-3424	1-3504		tridactylum	Short "	1-615	1-622
Pigeon... Long "	1-1973	1-1892					
Short "	1-3643	1-3804		**FISHES**			
Goose... Long "	1-1836			Trout.....	Long diam..	1-1524	
Short "	1-3839				Short "	1-2460	
Quail.... Long "	1-2347			Perch.....	Long "	1-2099	
Short "	1-3470				Short "	1-2824	
Dove.... Long "	1-2005			Pike......	Long "	1-2000	
Short "	1-3369				Short "	1-3555	
Sparrow. Long "	1-2140			Eel.......	Long "	1-1745	
Short "	1-3500				Short "	1-2842	
Owl..... Long "	1-1763			Lamprey (Circular).....		1-2134	
Short "	1-4076			Lamprey (diam. of nucleus)....		1-6400	

MAMMALS	Gulliver	Wormley	Formad	Richardson	C. Schmidt, 1848	French Medicolegal Society, 1873	Masson, 1885	Dragendorff	Woodward
Man.......	1-3200	1-3250	1-3200	1-3224	1-3330	1-3257	1-3256	1-3300	1-3092
Monkey....	1-3412	1-3382	......	1-3395					
Opossum...	1-3557	1-3145							
Guinea-pig..	1-3538	1-3223	1-3400	......	......	......	1-3300	......	1-3213
Kangaroo...	1-3440	1-3410							
Musk-rat...	1-3550	1-3282							
Dog.......	1-3532	1-3561	1-3580	1-3542	1-3630	1-3479	1-3577	1-3628	1-3246
Rabbit....	1-3607	1-3653	1-3662	......	1-3968	1-3681	1-3628	1-3968	
Rat.......	1-3754	1-3652	......	......	1-3968				
Mouse.....	1-3814	1-3743			1-4166				
Pig........	1-4230	1-4268	1-4250	1-4230	1-4098	1-4233	1-4098	1-4098	
Ox........	1-4267	1-4219	1-4200	1-4267	1-4385	1-4535	1-4233	1-4385	
Horse......	1-4600	1-4243	1-4310	......	1-4456	1-4535			
Cat........	1-4404	1-4372	......	......	1-4535	1-3907	1-4456	1-4535	
Elk........	1-3938	1-4384							
Buffalo.....	1-4586	1-4351							
Wolf (prairie)	1-3600	1-3422	1-3450						
Bear (black)	1-3693	1-3656							
Hyena.....	1-3735	1-3644							
Squirrel (red)	1-4000	1-4140							
Raccoon....	1-3950	1-4084							
Elephant...	1-2745	1-2738							
Leopard....	1-4319	1-4390							
Hippo'mus..	1-3429	1-3560							
Rhinoceros.	1-3765	1-3649							
Whale.....	1-3099	......	......	1-3090					
Tapir......	1-4000	1-4175							
Lion.......	1-4322	1-4143							
Ocelot.....	1-4220	1-3885							
Mule......		1-3760							
Ass........	1-4000	1-3620							
Ground-squirrel...		1-4200							
Bat........	1-4175	1-3966							
Sheep......	1-5300	1-4912	1-5000	1-5300	1-5649	1-5080	......	1-5649	

they have been reduced to vulgar fractions of an inch.[1841]

Method of Examination: In determining the size of the normal red blood cells of man and different animals two methods have been adopted: One consists in preparing a thin layer of fresh blood and measuring the red cells while still suspended in the serum, and the other in preparing a very thin layer of dried blood and measuring those cells that have retained their normal form.

In making a layer of fresh blood sufficiently thin for this purpose care must be taken that the slides and cover-glasses are perfectly clean and free from grease or dust. A very small drop of blood is then placed on the slide by touching the slide to the drop as it issues from a wound made by pricking the lobe of the ear or the tip of the finger with a sharp needle or lancet. The drop on the slide should be immediately covered with a perfectly clean cover-glass, when the blood will spread out under the cover-glass, if the drop has not been too large, in so thin a layer that most of the red blood cells will be seen lying on their flat surface and not arranged in rouleaux, as would be the case if the size of the drop were too large or the glasses not perfectly clean. If on examination under a low power field the specimen is found to be a satisfactory one, the edge of the cover-glass should be surrounded with a thin layer of oil or cement of some kind, so as to prevent evaporation. It may then be examined and the diameter of those red cells which have not been distorted, measured.

Most observers have found, however, that it is more convenient to use the dried preparation than the fresh. The red blood cells are very slightly flattened by the mechanical process adopted in making a very thin layer, but this flattening is of no practical importance, since the diameter of the red cells is so slightly increased that the increase is not perceptible, even with the highest powers. A larger number of the blood cells are distorted in making a thin dried layer than in making the fresh preparation, and only the perfectly round cells in mammalian blood should be selected for measurement.

Very thin layers of dried blood may be made by placing a small drop of fresh blood on the edge of a ground-glass slide,

1841. The first two columns of the table are taken from the appendix to the 2nd of WORMLEY's Micro-Chemistry of Poisons, 733 et seq.

and drawing that edge quickly over the surface of another slide, or over the surface of a clean cover-glass. When the layer is sufficiently thin, it will dry almost immediately. This thin layer, if prepared on a slide, may be covered with a cover-glass which can be fixed on the slide with paraffin, and the red blood cells, which are of normal shape, may be measured directly. If the preparation has been made on a cover-glass, the cover-glass may be inverted on a glass slide, fixed in the same way, and the normal red cells measured; or the red blood cells on the slide or cover may be fixed and rendered insoluble by heating to 120° C. (248° F.). The specimen may then be mounted in Canada balsam and the red cells measured at some convenient time. Or if desired, the thin layer, after being heated, may be stained with fuchsin or eosin, washed with water, dried, and mounted in balsam. The staining of the red cells makes the edges a little more sharply defined and renders the measuring a little less tiresome.

By the method used in preparing thin layers of blood for clinical examination, a better preparation will be obtained, and one containing a smaller proportion of distorted red cells. This method consists in placing a very small drop of the blood, drawn, with the same precautions on an absolutely clean cover-glass, covering with another cover-glass, and as soon as the blood has spread out drawing the two cover-glasses apart quickly, taking care to keep them in the same plane while drawing them apart. Very satisfactory thin layers of dried blood may thus be obtained. These thin layers may be treated as mentioned in the preceding paragraph, and the normal red blood cells measured. The white blood cells are also perfectly preserved in this way.

The method of treating a dried blood-stain for the purpose of bringing out the red blood cells to their normal shape and of freeing them from extraneous matter so that their edges may be brought plainly into view is very different. A minute fragment of the dried blood-stain is removed with the point of a knife or a pair of sharp-pointed scissors, transferred to a glass slide, and moistened with some liquid menstruum that will serve to soften and gradually disintegrate the clot but will not destroy the blood cells. Various menstrua have been proposed, some preferring alkaline fluids, others acid ones, and still others neutral solutions.

Virchow's liquid consists of a 30 or 33% solution of caustic potash. Roussin recommended a mixture of three parts of glycerol, one part of sulphuric acid, and water to a specific gravity of 1.028. Ranvier's liquid is made by dissolving 2 gm. of potassium iodide in 100 gm. of water, and saturating this solution with iodine. Vibert used a solution of one-half part of corrosive sublimate, two parts of common salt, and 100 parts of water. Paccini's fluid is made by dissolving in a mixture of 300 parts of water and 100 of glycerol, two parts of common salt and one part of corrosive sublimate. Wormley recommended simply a small quantity of distilled water, adding approximately the amount originally present in the dried specimen under examination. If the stain is a very old one, so as to require long soaking in the menstruum, he recommends a dilute solution of glycerol, one having a specific gravity of 1.030, and in cases of very old stains, which disintegrate with difficulty, he advises the addition of a little caustic potash to the glycerine or the water. Satisfactory results are obtained from a solution of potassium acetate of a specific gravity of 1.030. The addition of a little formalin to this solution improves it by preventing the formation of any fungus growth. Finally 0.9% sodium chloride solution may be used. The cells may be stained in various ways (fuchsin, eosin) to render them more distinct.

Care must be taken, in selecting portions of a dried stain for microscopic examination and measurement, to take the dried fragments from some portions of the stain that has dried quickly. If the specimen be taken from the center of a mass of dried blood which has required several hours to dry, the red cells will have taken up a sufficient amount of water to render them spherical, and, therefore, unfit for measurement. The particle of stain thus selected should be moistened with whatever menstruum the observer prefers, covered with a thin cover-glass, and sealed with cement to prevent the evaporation of the fluid. If the blood has dried in a very thin layer on some non-absorbent surface, the thin film may be scraped from the surface with a sharp knife upon a glass slide, and the cells fixed by heating to 120° C. (248° F.), or by moistening them with a mixture of equal parts of absolute alcohol and ether before treatment with the fluid. The slide should be examined from time to time with a low power, and as soon as cells of the normal form are seen, they may be measured with the high powers. It will be found that the dried blood in some stains disintegrates much more slowly than in others, and, other conditions being equal, the older the stain, the longer the time required. A stain a few days old disintegrates rapidly, so that measurements should be made as soon as the preparation is completed. Distorted and swollen red cells must not be measured.

More satisfactory results are obtained where the blood has fallen on a non-absorbent surface. When possible the examiner should select a dried crust as thin as possible. If the blood has fallen on a piece of linen or cotton cloth in small quantity, so that it has penetrated the fiber of the cloth immediately, as a general rule only unsatisfactory results can be obtained, because the cells adhere tightly to the individual fibers, which, while moist, are somewhat swollen and contract on drying. By this contraction the adherent blood cells frequently become so distorted as to become unfit for measurement. In such cases a satisfactory result can usually be obtained only when, for some reason or other, complete absorption of the fresh blood has been prevented, as, for instance, if the cloth happened to be more or less starched or if the drop of the fresh blood was a little too large to be completely absorbed at once. Nucleated blood cells can, however, readily be seen under these circumstances. The difficulty of discrimination occurs only in the case of mammalian blood stains.

Blood corpuscles may be transferred from a stain by placing a solution of celloidin on the suspected spot and allowing it to dry; the resulting pellicle may be removed and examined under a cover-glass under which acetone saturated with eosin is introduced to stain the corpuscles (Dominicis). The best results are obtained with stains on metals, weapons, and stones, and other non-absorbent surfaces. The margins of the blood spots, or thin layers, are best suited. Transfer of blood-stains from textile and absorbent materials is more difficult, and a thicker pellicle of celloidin is necessary.

Blood-stains which have been subjected after drying to long continued action of moisture are generally unsuitable for microscopic measurement, since the red cells absorb a sufficient amount of water to render them abnormal. If the stain has been formed on a non-absorbent surface and has been kept dry, a sufficient number of the red cells will preserve their normal form, so as to be suitable for microscopic measurement, for an indefinite number of years. Blood-stains on iron can be satisfactorily examined only if the iron has been kept completely dry, so that rusting of the iron has not taken place. If, however, the iron has rusted at the point where stained, not only the blood cells may be totally destroyed, but the blood pigment may also be decomposed.

Blood-stains are frequently submitted to the expert in which an attempt has been made to wash off the blood with water. Thorough washing will, of course, remove all traces of blood from cloth, but it frequently happens that a hasty attempt to remove the blood-stain, particularly from cloth having a rough surface, will leave a sufficient number of particles of unchanged blood to render satisfactory examination and measurement possible. If a blood-stain on cotton or linen cloth is treated with water the blood pigment is taken up by the water and carried along with it, so that after drying, the whole portion of the cloth that has been wet will show a yellowish stain, but the color will be deeper and browner at the edge than in the center. This is called a diffused or a washed stain, the edges of which, after drying, may be of a deeper brown color, while an inch or two from the edge the color is of a much lighter tint. Sea-water removes the blood from a dried stain much more slowly than fresh water.

In the examination of blood-stains great care should be taken to note every peculiarity of each individual stain. As has been mentioned, the form of the stain, together with the distribution of the blood in it, may show from which direction the blood making the stain started. Note should be made as to whether the stain is a spatter or a smudge, or whether it has the appearance of having been wiped or washed. Careful examination should also be made to determine the presence in the stain of any foreign substances, such as hairs, epithelial cells, spermatozoa, pieces of tissue, muscular fibers, or adipose tissue, bits of bone, etc. It may happen that the presence of such substances will throw light on the nature of the blood making the stain. For instance, any hair found in a blood stain may resemble that of the victim and be unlike that of the accused, or in case the tissues have been much bruised by a blunt instrument, or perhaps bones fractured and crushed, it is not uncommon to find small particles of tissue, or even a minute fragment of bone, mixed with the blood. Sometimes these foreign substances may be detected by gross inspection; at other times the fragments may be so minute that their presence can be detected only by a microscopic examination.

The following table, taken from Wormley's article, gives the results obtained by him in the examination of dried blood-stains made by different kinds of mammalian blood, the nature of the blood in some instances being unknown to him at the time of examination:

TABLE LIX
WORMLEY'S MEASUREMENTS. EXAMINATION OF OLD BLOOD-STAINS

Animal	Age of Stain	Remarks	Average Inch	Fresh Blood Inch
(1) Human ...	2 months	Stain; unknown	1-3358	1-3250
(2) Human ...	2½ months	Stain	1-3236	1-3250
(3) Human ...	3 months	Stain	1-3384	1-3250
(4) Human	19 months	Clot	1-3290	1-3250
(5) Elephant	13 months	Clot	1-2849	1-2738
(6) Dog	4 months	Trace of stain; unknown	1-3626	1-3561
(7) Rabbit ...	18 months	Clot	1-3683	1-3653
(8) Ox	16 months	Stain	1-4544	1-4219
(9) Ox	32 months	Stain; unknown	1-4495	1-4219
(10) Ox	4½ years	Clot	1-4535	1-4219
(11) Buffalo	18 months	Clot	1-4312	1-4351
(12) Goat	17 months	Stain	1-5897	1-6189
(13) Ibex	18 months	Clot	1-6578	1-6445

Influence of Disease on the Red Blood Cells: It is well known that in certain diseases the red blood cells may be altered, both in size and form, and also in the relative proportion of the red and the white blood cells. Some diseases will diminish their size, as high fever, diphtheria, and septicemia. In pernicious anemia we find many red cells much smaller than normal, even to one-half the normal diameter, called microcytes. Many of the red cells are also distorted (poikilocytes), and some of the red cells in this disease are nucleated. In other forms of anemia we may also find some of the modifications in the form and the size of the red blood cells. In leukemia the number of the red cells in the fresh blood is very greatly reduced, the red cells vary in size and form, and many are nucleated.

There seems to be no record in medicolegal literature of blood stains from persons suffering from any of these diseases having been submitted to legal investigation. The only error that would be caused by such conditions would be the greater probability of considering the blood to be that of an animal rather than of human origin.

Other Stains Containing Blood:

Diagnosis of these can be made by finding other foreign substances mixed with the blood cells, such as epithelial cells of various kinds, pus, dried mucus, spermatozoa, etc.

Menstrual Stains: The possibility of determining whether or not a blood stain was caused by menstrual blood depends largely on the amount of hemorrhage. This, as is well known, differs with various women, and also in the same woman at various times. If the flow be scanty, as at the very beginning or end of the menstrual period, the menstrual blood will have mixed with it a large number of epithelial cells from the vagina. If, however, the flow is abundant, a stain may be made by menstrual blood, particularly a small stain, which does not contain any demonstrable vaginal cells.

The vaginal cells are large polygonal, squamous, epithelial cells, somewhat similar to those from the mucous membrane of the mouth, but having on the average a somewhat larger nucleus. Sometimes we see a vaginal cell with two nuclei. These cells may be exfoliated singly or in small patches containing several layers of cells. If the vagina be inflamed, as in leukorrhea or gonorrhea, these cells will be exfoliated from the membrane in much larger number, and mixed with pus-corpuscles. Possibly a cylindrical or ciliated cell from the lining membrane of the uterus may be seen mixed with the blood.

If, therefore, we find mixed with the red blood cells a number of vaginal epithelial cells we may state that the stain in question is consistent with its having been made by menstrual blood. If, however, we do not find any vaginal cells mixed with the blood, we would not be warranted in concluding that the stain was not made by menstrual blood.

The location of the stains, as on bedding or under-clothing, may possibly be of service in deciding the question as to the menstrual origin of the blood stain in question. In uncleanly women these stains are said to be found more frequently on the back part of an undergarment than on the front.

Nasal Blood Stains: The detection of nasal blood stains depends upon precisely the same principle as that of menstrual stains, namely, the finding of various cylindrical and ciliated cells from the mucous membrane of the nose mixed with blood. If there is but little hemorrhage and the stain be made by forcibly blowing the nose, the blood will be mixed with more or less mucus and cells, and, when such a stain becomes dry, it presents a different appearance from an ordinary blood stain; it is paler and more bulky and, after being moistened, if there is much dried mucus present, it will swell up and have a more or less elastic consistency.

If the hemorrhage from the nose has been profuse, a large portion of the blood may not have mixed with it any of the mucous secretion or any of the cells, so that stains may be made from blood coming from the nose which do not differ in any way from a pure blood-stain. In such cases the location of the stain in question may show whether or not it could have been made by blood coming from the nose. For instance, in a case in which the accused alleged that the blood on his clothing was due to nose bleed, a horizontal spatter of blood was found between the folds of a turn-down collar, in such a position that it could not have come from the nose while the collar was around the neck.

As in the case of menstrual stains, therefore, we can only state that a stain in which are found coagulated mucus and cells mixed with the blood is consistent with its having originated from the nose. If we do not find such an admixture, we cannot say that the stain was not caused by nose bleed unless it is so located that it would be impossible for the blood coming from the nose to have been placed in that position.

THE PRECIPITIN TEST FOR BLOOD

SPEAKING generally, the only course now known in tracing protein substances back to their source, that is, to the species from which they came, is by means of their immune reactions; and in the case of blood and other animal products, practically the only method for purposes of biologic differentiation is the precipitin test. Complement fixation may be used also, but it is more sensitive—almost too sensitive—and more complicated, and in this country this test is not in current use for the identification of blood spots for medicolegal purposes. Because the determination of the ultimate source of blood spots and stains often is vital to the administration of justice, the precipitin test is of special forensic value and interest. The test has been used in this country for the identification of blood for forensic purposes since it was introduced, although probably not so widely as it might have been; but it does not appear that any standard method of procedure even with respect to certain essential points as yet has become established, and there are scarcely any adequate detailed descriptions of the test.[1842] The succeeding statements are taken with minor changes from an article by Hektoen.[1843]

The precipitin test rests on the fact that when a suitable animal is injected with foreign protein, its serum, when mixed with a solution of the foreign protein, will form a precipitate. This reaction is due to the accumulation in the blood of the injected animal of newly produced substances, which are called precipitins. By foreign protein is meant protein from some other source than the species to which the animal injected belongs. Thus serum for the identification of blood is obtained by injecting rabbits (the animal nearly always used for this purpose) with the blood or serum of an animal of a different species, the exact species in each case depending on the kind of blood one intends to test for with the resulting precipitin serum is limited to proteins of the same kind as those that were injected; indeed, the precipitin test owes its practical value to this fact.

The Production of Precipitin Serum: At present we know of only two animals that are good and suitable precipi-

---

1842. The literature up to about 1908 on precipitins and their medicolegal use is indexed fully in Vol. 13 of the 2nd Series of the Index Catalogue of the Library of the Surgeon-General's office, U. S. Army, Washington, D. C. Reference is made also to NUTTALL: "Blood Immunity and Blood Relationship," 1904; GRAHAM-SMITH and SANGER: "The Biological or Precipitin Test for Blood Considered Mainly from Its Medicolegal Aspect," *J. Hyg.*, 3:258, 1903; SUTHERLAND: "Blood Stains: Their Detection, and the Determination of Their Source," 1907; BORDET: "Studies in Immunity," collected and translated by F. P. GAY, 1909; UHLENHUTH and STEFFENHAGEN: "Die biologische Eiweiss-Differenzierung Mittels der Präzipitation unter besonderer Berücksichtigung der Technik," Kolle and Wassermann Handbuch, 3:256, 1913; HUNT and MILLS: "Some Experience Bearing on the Medicolegal Value of the Precipitin Test for Human Blood," *Boston M. & S. J.*, 176:48, 1917; STOKES and STONER: "The Use of the Precipitin Test for the Detection of Human Blood in Criminal Trials," *Boston M. & S. J.*, 177:65, 1917.

1843. HEKTOEN, LUDVIG: The Precipitin Test for Blood, *J.A.M.A.*, 70:1273, 1918.

tin producers for practical purposes, the rabbit and the domestic fowl. Hitherto the rabbit has been used almost altogether, Sutherland,[1844] in India, being the only one to use the fowl on a large scale. Of the two the fowl seems to be the more ready and reliable producer, but fowl serum must be handled with special care because of the tendency under certain conditions to give non-specific reactions. So long as rabbits are plentiful, it would seem best, at least in this country, not to change to the fowl except for special purposes, as when it is necessary to test directly for rabbit blood. In any case, young, healthy, previously unused animals should be selected; they should be kept under hygienic conditions and given enough good food. It is always advisable to inject several rabbits at the same time, especially when antihuman precipitin is to be produced, because in some rabbits the response to the injection may be rather insignificant.

Either whole blood, defibrinated or citrated, or serum may be injected; the results appear to be about the same. As we deal with whole blood in the identification of blood spots, there may be an advantage in using antiserum produced by whole blood;[1845] this may be counterbalanced, however, by the fact that serum is somewhat richer in proteins. Blood should not be injected intravenously because of the danger of sudden death. To produce antihuman precipitins, albuminous urine and various transudates have been injected also; but the best results are secured from blood or serum, and in these days when patients are bled so frequently from the veins for diagnostic tests, there is no difficulty in obtaining the required human blood or serum, which need not be absolutely fresh provided it is free from bacteria. The injection of rabbits with washed human corpuscles, now so often practised in order to produce an amboceptor for the Wassermann test, frequently gives as a by-product in sufficient

1844. SUTHERLAND, W. D.: "Note on 2,643 Medicolegal Cases, in which 6,566 Articles, Suspected to be Blood-Stained, were Examined," *Indian J. M. Research, Calcutta*, 3:205, 1915.

1845. That hemoglobin is antigenic, seems certain. At any rate, strong precipitin serum may be obtained by injecting rabbits with aqueous extracts of carefully washed red corpuscles, this antiserum acting specifically on such extracts and possibly on similar extracts from related species, but not at all or only slightly on the corresponding serums. HEKTOEN, LUDVIG, and SCHULHOF, Kamil on Specific Erythroprecipitins, *J. Infect. Dis.*, 31:32, 1922.

concentration for practical use specific precipitins for the proteins in human blood.

In the immunization of rabbits, good results may be obtained with various methods that differ more or less in minor details. The tendency is to inject smaller quantities of blood or serum than formerly. Several rabbits should be injected at the same time because, as stated, there is great individual variation in the power to produce precipitins, especially anti-human. A good way is to inject from 1 to 2 cc. of serum intravenously, repeat in six days or so, and then after six or eight days to inject 4 to 5 cc. intraperitoneally. Or from 5 to 6 cc. of blood or serum may be injected intraperitoneally four or five times at intervals of six days or so. In either case the serum should be tested about the seventh day after the last injection, because at this time the precipitin content reaches its high point; and it remains at this point only a few days the tests must be made promptly so that if the serum is found to be potent, goodly quantities may be collected while the precipitin still runs high. It has been found that the danger of death from anaphylactic reactions when the last injections are given may be avoided by first giving a small so-called desensitizing injection, 1 or 0.5 cc. intravenously or intraperitoneally.

The intravenous injections of increasing quantities of human serum, say 1, 2, 3, 4, and 5 cc., at three-day intervals may yield strong precipitin serum also. In this case it is best to begin testing the serum of the injected rabbits as early as the fourth day after the last injection.

A rapid method of immunization consists in giving intraperitoneal injections of increasing quantities—5, 10, 15 cc.—on three successive days. The same total quantity of antigen injected at one time may also give good results. As a rule, the precipitin in either case reaches its acme about the ninth to the twelfth day or thereabouts. If serum is used, the injections may be made intravenously. This so-called rapid method yields more reliable results with beef, sheep, horse, swine, cat, and chicken blood or serum than with human, and it is probably that in the last case the desired result will be obtained oftener by repeated injections at longer intervals.[1846]

1846. HEKTOEN, LUDVIG: On the Production of Precipitins. *J. Infect. Dis.*, 14:403, 1914.

In the case of the fowl a single intraperitoneal injection of 20 cc. of blood or serum usually in ten or twelve days yields a precipitin serum of sufficient strength for practical purposes.[1847]

It is not necessary to describe the details of injections, bleeding, and collection of serum. At every step scrupulous effort must be made to prevent contamination; contaminated serum is useless because it may give misleading reactions. Sterile serum may be kept for months in the cold sealed in ampoules in quantities without much loss of potency. It is best to store serum in small bottles or tubes, each of 1 or 2 cc., so that there need be no danger of contaminating a large quantity each time a little is to be use. A small amount of chloroform is added as a preservative.

Occasionally rabbit serum is opalescent; such serum is useless because when put in test mixtures one cannot tell for certain whether precipitates are formed or not. In order to avoid opalescence of the serum, it is recommended to allow the animal to fast for eighteen hours or so before it is bled. In the case of fowl, only roosters should be used, as the serum of hens often cannot be used because of the fat content.

Tests of Precipitin Serum: To identify blood or other protein substances it is necessary to use precipitin serum of some degree of potency and of a strictly limited range of action.

Test for Strength: Various methods have been used to determine the strength of a precipitin serum, but we shall mention only the simple method of finding the highest dilution in salt solution of the antigen—the serum or blood of the species used in the injection—with which the precipitin serum forms a precipitate within a few minutes at ordinary room temperature.

Small, perfectly clean and perfectly clear glass tubes are best, the lumen being about 0.5 cm. in diameter. In each of a series of such tubes in a small rack is placed a small quantity of antigen dilution, the first tube receiving the lowest dilution, the next higher, etc. (for example, one to 500, one to 1,000, one to 1,500, one to 2,000, etc.); there is now introduced by means of a capillary pipet about 0.1 cc. of antiserum at the

1847. HEKTOEN, LUDVIG: The Production of Precipitins by the Fowl, *J. Infect. Dis.*, 22:561, 1918.

bottom of each tube, special care being taken to get a precise line of contact between the two fluids. The antiserum can be run in slowly at the side of the tube; being heavier than the diluted antigen it will go to the bottom of the tube, but the line of contact will not be quite so sharp as when it is introduced at the bottom with a pipet. The tubes, which are kept at room temperature, are now watched for the formation of a grayish-white percipitate at the plane of contact between the fluids.

If a precipitate forms almost at once in the antigen dilution of one to 1,000, the antiserum is strong enough to be used in blood tests for forensic purposes. An antiserum that forms a precipitate almost at once in thousandfold dilution of the antigen usually gives reactions in much higher dilutions— one to 20,000 or higher after a longer time, say twenty minutes. The strength or titer of antiserum may be designated by the dilution of antigen with which it forms a definite precipitate within a given time, at room temperature. For instance, if an antihuman serum gives a precipitate within twenty minutes in a dilution of human serum or blood of one to 20,000, its strength or titer may be said to be one to 20,000 at twenty minutes.

The precipitin reaction is observed best by holding the tubes near a black, flat object (book cover, ruler) held directly in the path of the light; the precipitate, at first composed of fine particles, and sharply defined, may become more flocculent and sink to the bottom.

To make tests with dilutions of the whole blood, the corpuscles are laked by means of water; the normal salt content is restored by adding the required amount of 1.8% salt solution (double strength of physiologic sodium chloride solution), and further dilutions are made with salt solution of the usual strength. When fowl antiserum is used, the salt content of all dilutions should be 1.8%, as then there is less danger of non-specific reactions. When fowl antiserum is taken out of the ice box it should be left at the room temperature for an hour or two before it is used.

In place of the contact or ring method, some observers simply mix the antiserum with the antigen; a positive reaction now appears in the form of a diffuse cloudiness of the whole mixture. This is not as precise and sensitive as the contact method, and is not recommended for practical blood tests.

Tests for Specificity: Because of the relationship of species, almost every strong precipitin serum may form precipitates with proteins, at least in low dilutions, of species related to that species, the blood proteins of which were used for the production of serum. Indeed, any strong antimammalian serum may react in low dilutions—one to ten or so—of mammalian serums or blood generally. This is the mammalian reaction of Nuttall.[1848] In the case of kindred species, the precipitin affinities often are more marked; for instance, an antigoat serum may react in high dilutions of sheep and beef as well as of goat serum or blood. Further examples of closely related groups are the horse, ass, and mule; the dog,

TABLE LX

SPECIFICITY OF PRECIPITIN IN SERUM OF RABBIT INJECTED WITH
HUMAN BLOOD

Blood	Highest dilution giving precipitate with antihuman serum after twenty minutes at room temperature
Fish	1:10
Chicken	1:10
Rabbit	0
Guinea-pig	1:10
Rat	1:10
Cat	1:10
Dog	1:10
Swine	1:10
Sheep	1:10
Beef	1:10
Horse	1:10
Goat	1:10
Monkey (Macacus rhesus)	1:100
Human	1:5000

wolf, and fox; the domestic fowl, turkey, goose, duck and pigeon; the hare and the rabbit, each with more or less pronounced common precipitin reactions. Man and monkey, from the highest down, constitute another group with special precipitin inter-reactions between the members. How it is possible by the precipitin test to identify the blood of the individual species is discussed later. As each antiserum may vary in the number and strength of its group and of its precipitins, and as it must be known to be free from non-specific reactions before it is used, it is necessary, besides fixing its potency, to determine the exact range of its action. The test for specificity is carried

1848. NUTTALL: Blood Immunity and Blood Relationship, 1904.

out in the same manner in general as the test for potency; that is to say, tubes are prepared in the same manner with dilutions of as many other serums or bloods beside that used in the

TABLE LXI

PRECIPITIN TESTS FOR BLOOD

MATERIAL	KIND OF BLOOD PRESENT	REMARKS
Blood on hat, coat, vest, shirts, and trousers.	Human	The accused claimed the spots were caused partly by fish, partly by calf blood.
Blood on blade and inside handle of knife.	Human	
Blood on miner's shirt.	Human	In this case, efforts had been made to wash away the blood, but deep in the texture of the shirt the threads were still incrusted with blood.
Blood on shoes and shoe-strings.	Human	
Blood on brick, window-shade, coat.	Human	
Blood on handle of pickax.	Human	
Blood on hammer and handkerchief.	Human	
Crust of blood on ax.	Human	Ax found in ruins of house burned down after triple murder.
Blood on dollar bill.	Human	
Blood on coat and trousers.	Human	
Blood on bedclothes.	Human	
Blood on old newspaper.	Rabbit	Antirabbit chicken serum used.
Blood on paper money, shirt, trousers, shoes, gun barrel.	Human	
Smears of blood on the neck of a bottle.	Human	
Blood on shirt.	Human	
Blood on shavings.	Human	
Blood on hair, wall-paper, and floor.	Human	
Blood on shoe-string.	Human	
Blood on trousers.	Not human	
Blood on paper.	Human	
Blood on shoes.	Rabbit	Antirabbit chicken serum used.
Blood on pocket.	Beef–Human	Accused worked at beef killing in stockyards.
Blood on wall of barn.	Beef–Human	The spots were said to have been left by a calf as it ran about after dehorning.
Blood on automobile door handle.	Human	Handle broke off in boy's back.

production of the serum as seem necessary to afford a thorough test, certainly not less than two, the antiserum added as before, and the results noted. At the same time the antiserum is tested with salt solution only to determine whether any precipitate then forms.

A usable antiserum must be perfectly clear; it must have a certain minimum specific precipitin strength, and it must not give any misleading non-specific reactions. To illustrate: If an antihuman serum is perfectly clear; if it forms a precipitate practically at once in a one to 1,000 or higher dilution of human blood or serum; and if with that of any other species, then in very low dilutions only, say from one in ten to one in 100, and much more slowly, save possibly in the case of the monkey (group reaction); and if it does not form any precipitate with salt solution, then it may be used in tests for human blood for forensic purposes.

Preparation of Material for Precipitin Test: Materials submitted for blood tests usually are stains and spots on any of the great variety of objects on which blood may fall or be smeared. Among the articles submitted by the police to the Coroner's Office of Cook County, Chicago, for examination of suspected spots and stains, may be mentioned knives, firearms, axes, wrenches, hatpins, automobile fenders, spades, forks, shoes and gloves; all kinds of wearing apparel, towels, rake, paper, board, baseball bats, flooring, grass, paper money, stone, mortar, cement, earth, etc. The first question to decide is whether the suspicious spots and stains consist of blood, and for this purpose we have the chemical, microscopic, and spectroscopic methods which have been described. It is necessary to determine whether spots and stains are made by blood, not only because blood may be simulated by paint, fruit juices, and in other ways, but also because spots and stains made by protein materials other than blood may react in the same way as blood to the precipitin test. For instance, antihuman serum alone will not distinguish spots by human blood from spots by other human protein-containing material such as albuminous urine, purulent sputum, exudates, and transudates. All the antihuman serum can tell us is that the spots are made by human proteins, and whether they are made by blood must be determined by the general tests for blood.

All glassware and other articles used in the precipitin test must be absolutely clean and sterile. It is best in all final tests to use tubes that are practically new, because tubes that have been boiled and sterilized many times may be no longer clear. A good supply of fresh, sterile pipets should be on hand.

Salt solution (0.9%) is the best general solvent for extracting proteins from material to be tested. If practicable, crusted material may be scraped off, ground up carefully, and mixed with a small quantity of salt solution; or it may be necessary to place small pieces of cloth, paper, or other substances, straw, cork, rubber, wood, leather, lime, mortar, etc., including some or all of a suspected spot, directly into the solution. Whenever possible, extracts should be made also of unspotted parts of the substratum for purposes of control tests. In case of lime-containing material a cloudiness may result that will clear on passing CO_2 into the extract.

How long to continue the extraction depends on the quantity and solubility of the protein in question; if it is to be kept up for more than one or two hours, it is better to put the mixture in the refrigerator and to add a little chloroform to restrain the growth of bacteria. The passage of protein into solution is indicated if bubbles made by blowing through the fluid with a pipet tend to persist (foam test); also if cloudiness develops on application of the nitric acid heat test. As only a dilute solution—one to 1,000—is needed for the precipitin test, extracts of blood usually must be diluted with salt solution. When the nitric acid heat test causes only a faint opalescence in a blood dilution, its strength is regarded as about one to 100. Comparative foam tests, with known blood dilutions being used as the standard, also help to fix the strength of an extract. A one to 1,000 dilution of blood is practically colorless by transmitted light. The extracts should be clear as water; turbid extracts must be cleared by filtration or centrifugation. The reaction must be neither strongly acid nor alkaline to litmus; for neutralization, 0.1% sodium hydroxide or hydrochloric acid solution should be used; dilutions of blood at one to 1,000 rarely need the reaction corrected, but extracts of wood, bark, and leather may contain acids that cause cloudiness in rabbit serum.

Stains that do not extract well with salt solution may give better results if treated with a 1% solution of potassium cyanide; the alkalinity should be corrected with tartaric acid.[1849]

1849. SUTHERLAND, Ref. 1844.

In case of cloth with suspicious stains that yield no information on being scraped or soaked, it is a good plan to cut out small pieces from the stains and tease them apart. The single threads running in the depth of the stained part may be found incrusted with blood, i.e., covered with small crusts which contain red blood corpuscles or in which the blood is demonstrable in other ways. Even when the cloth has been washed recently, incrustations may be found in the depth, especially, of course, if the cloth is of a heavy variety.

The Actual Test and Controls: The precipitin test requires a number of careful controls to guard against error; the antiserum must be tested with salt solution, with the blood against which it is known to act, and with other bloods in order to be certain that it gives a specific reaction only. Samples of various kinds of blood should be kept on hand for control tests. For this purpose blood may be dried in drops on filter paper or linen, each drop being made by a definite quantity (0.1 or 0.05 cc.); or the blood may be kept in the cold, diluted as described, say one to 100 in salt solution. As the reactive power of blood kept in solution is said to weaken gradually, too long intervals

---

TABLE LXII
SCHEME FOR PRECIPITIN TEST

Tubes	
1	Extract of blood on shirt + antiserum.
2	Extract of blood on shirt + normal serum (estimated dilution of blood in Tubes 1 and 2, 1:1000.)
3	Extract of bloodless part of shirt + antiserum.
4	Salt solution + antiserum.
5	Human blood or serum 1:1000 + antiserum.
6	Blood or serum other than human 1:1000 + antiserum.
7, 8, etc.	Same as Tube 6, but with different bloods.

---

must be avoided before new solutions are prepared. To avoid still other chances of error, the extract of the unknown blood must be tested with normal rabbit serum or, if fowl antiserum is used, with normal fowl serum, and the extract of blood-free parts of the substratum on which the unknown blood was situated is to be tested with antiserum. These precautions must be observed in connection with every forensic precipitin test—nothing is taken for granted. Assuming now that spots on a shirt that have been shown to consist of blood are to be tested for human blood, the precipitin test may be conducted in accord with the scheme presented in Table LXII it being understood that the quantity of extract or control solution in each tube is 0.5 cc. and of antihuman rabbit serum or normal rabbit serum, 0.1 cc. These quantities may be reduced if desired in order to save material; indeed, the test may be made in capillary tubes if necessary.

If a typical precipitate develops within a minute or two in Tubes 1 and 5 while no precipitate forms in any of the other tubes after standing for twenty minutes, all at the room temperature, then the conclusion is warranted that the blood on the shirt is human blood. Some observers would add: provided monkey blood can be excluded.

Having obtained a positive reaction with the extract under the aforesaid conditions, it would be well to determine next the highest approximate dilution of the extract that reacts with the antiserum after twenty minutes at room temperature, thus still further verifying the specificity of the reaction.

Usually the only questions asked are whether certain spots and stains are due to blood, and if so, to human blood; but sometimes it becomes necessary to determine if possible the exact species of blood that is not human. The scheme for human is applicable in general with, of course, such changes as to antiserums and controls as are indicated in the given case from the facts at hand. If the blood corpuscles are preserved, it may be possible to determine from the absence or presence of nuclei whether or not one is dealing with mammalian blood. Often tests with various antiserums may be made before a positive reaction occurs, and it must not be forgotten that absence of reaction may be due not only to failure to hit on the right antiserum, but also to changes in the unknown blood whereby it has lost its power to react.

The question whether more than just one kind of blood is present in the material to be examined may be raised. It has been found that in mixtures each kind of blood present can be identified by the precipitin test; in such cases, antiserums of as high potency as possible should be used, as it may be difficult otherwise to detect proteins present in small amounts.

The claim may be made that a blood-stain which reacts with antihuman serum is not made by human blood, but by the blood of an animal, e. g., dog—falling on clothing or other articles stained before or afterward with albuminous human urine or some other product containing human protein. In such cases the corpuscles in the stain should be studied with special care to determine, if possible, whether they are consistent in size, shape, and structure with the claims advanced, and then additional precipitin tests should be made as indicated, and react, with anticanine serum if it is claimed that dog blood is present. In cases such as now assumed erythroprecipitin (antihemoglobin?) serums (see Refs. page 940) may prove to be of decisive value if it becomes established that they can act specifically on derivatives from the red corpuscles of different species.

Factors that May Interfere with the Reaction: The power of blood to react with precipitin may be reduced or completely destroyed by alcohol, by formaldehyde, cresol, corrosive sublimate, and other germicides, by acids and alkalies and other chemicals, by peptic digestion, by decomposition, and by heat. Badly decomposed blood may react, but it is difficult to obtain clear extracts. Fluid blood is said to lose power to react on being heated at from 60° to 90° C. (140° to 194° F.), but dried blood may resist heating at 150° C. (302° F.). Rust also is said to change blood so that it reacts less readily. Blood-stains on shoes blackened over may be detected after neutralization of the solution. In such cases the shoe strings should be examined carefully; in two instances the accused washed off blood from the shoes but not from the strings. Blood in spots from fifteen to sixty years old has been identified successfully, but certain statements that materials from thousand-year old mummies may give the precipitin reaction have been contradicted.

Dried blood resists harmful influences much better than fluid, and if blood found in the fluid state is to be kept for later tests it is better to dry the samples on filter paper than to keep them in fluid form in which they may decompose. Under no circumstances should blood or bloody material for the precipitin test be put in alcohol, because alcohol causes changes that interfere with the test.

Other Uses of the Precipitin Test: The precipitin test may be of value also in the identification of bone and other tissue, the origin of which is in doubt, as perhaps only fragments and scraps are at hand. When dissolved, the proteins in and of the tissues give the same general response to the precipitin test as the proteins of the blood of the species concerned. The only exception to this rule is furnished by the crystalline lens, which is unique, as it reacts only to serum produced by injections of lens substance, and that without regard to species. Bone should be reduced to powder, washed thoroughly with ether or benzin to remove the fat, dried, and then extracted with salt solution. Tissue of other nature may be treated according to the same principles. Such extracts are tested in the same general way as blood extracts.

Putting white of egg in urine to simulate albuminuria, and spattering non-human blood on clothing and bedding to feign spitting of blood, have been detected by the precipitin test. The test has been used extensively in certain European countries to detect adulterations of meat products, particularly sausages, and other foods, as flour and honey; it has been found of value, too, in the administration of game laws.[1850]

Special Method for the Differentiation of Blood of Closely Related Animals. Examples of related animals with more or less common precipitin reactions have been given. In thousandfold dilution a blood may react so much more promptly with its own antiserum than even lower dilutions of related blood that commonly no difficulty arises, provided the limits as to the dilution and time are followed exactly as prescribed and the necessary controls included in the test. Nuttall's experiments, to which we have referred, were made according to a totally different plan, the blood dilution being several times lower than one to 1,000, and the mixtures allowed to stand for several hours. To repeat: A reaction between an antihuman serum and a thousandfold blood dilution is diagnostic of human blood, provided it becomes evident within a few moments and that within twenty minutes at room temperature no reaction occurs between the same antiserum and like dilutions of the bloods selected for the control tests. Sutherland[1851] made a special study of blood stains of many varieties of monkeys, his tests being made with the dilutions and time limit just set forth, and in no instance, not even in the case of the orang utan, did he get a positive result with antihuman serum; consequently, special methods do not seem necessary to distinguish human from monkey blood. These observations should be repeated so that, if possible, final

---

1850. GAY: *J. Med. Research,* 19:219, 1908; CLARKE: *Univ. California Publ., Path.,* 2:131, 1914.

standards may be fixed. In this country the question whether ape or monkey blood may be present is not likely to arise, because the circumstances, as a rule, preclude that such blood can be present.

That differentiation may be difficult is illustrated by the ruminant group. Antibeef serum, for instance, may react in high dilution of beef, sheep, goat, and perhaps also other ruminant blood. Indeed, any antiruminant serum may react with any ruminant blood in considerable dilution. although not with equal promptness in all cases. Several expedients have been recommended in this and similar cases:

1. Specific Absorption. (Weichardt.) This is based on the principle that by mixing, let us say, antibeef serum with goat serum and then removing the resulting precipitate, the special antigoat precipitin will be removed.

2. Cross Immunization. (Uhlenhuth.) This consists in obtaining precipitin serum from one animal for the proteins of a related animal. Injecting certain Old World monkeys with human serum, Uhlenhuth obtained antihuman precipitins, but this result seems to be quite exceptional, as neither Sutherland[1851] nor Berkeley[1852] was able to confirm it. Uhlenhuth was able to demonstrate hare blood on a cane by means of antihare precipitins developed in the rabbit, antihare fowl serum reacting equally well with hare and rabbit blood; he also found that the fowl produces antipigeon precipitin and the pigeon antifowl, but cross immunization failed in the case of the horse-ass and goat-sheep.

3. Dilution of the Antiserum and of the Suspected Blood. Dilution of an antiserum may so weaken certain confusing group precipitins as to cause their practical elimination and still leave the main precipitins strong enough to give a specifically diagnostic reaction under the conditions prescribed for forensic practice. For diluent, Sutherland and Mitra[1853] recom-

1851. SUTHERLAND: "The Applicability to Medicolegal Practice in India of the Biochemical Test for the Origin of Blood Stains," Scientific Memoirs by Officers of the Medical and Sanitary Depts. of the Government of India, 39, 1910.

1852. BERKELEY: "The Impossibility of Differentiation between Monkey Blood and Human Blood by means of Antisera derived from Monkeys," Univ. California Publ., Path., 2:105, 1913.

1853. SUTHERLAND and MITRA: "Misleading Reactions Obtained with Precipitating Antisera, and How to Avoid Them," Indian M. J., 1:707, 1914.

mend normal serum of the same kind as the antiserum.

It is, of course, in the low blood dilutions that antiserums of high potency give the most marked group reactions. As the dilutions of the bloods of a group are increased, the reaction narrows down more and more, and in high dilutions there may be no question as to its specificity. Hence, determination of the highest dilution in which a suspected blood reacts with a given antiserum, if properly controlled, may solve the problem.

4. Special Study of Rapidity and Measure of Reaction. Hamburger[1854] recommends that in the case of a stain that reacts with antiruminant serum, for instance, separate parts of the extract be tested with antigoat, antisheep, and antibovine serum in the usual way, and the results carefully noted. The antiserum that gives the most rapid and profuse precipitate supplies the clue.

Systematic detailed studies should be made on the blood of closely related animals in order to determine more fully to what extent differentiation can be made by these and possibly other methods.

Suggestions to the contrary[1855] notwithstanding, it is not possible to distinguish between different human races, and far less between individuals, by means of the precipitin test.

MEDICOLEGAL APPLICATION OF HUMAN BLOOD ISO-AGGLUTINATION

THE expert is frequently asked in the examination by the defense attorney if he knows to what group the blood belongs. Therefore it is necessary to apply blood grouping tests. The expert may also be called into court regarding

1854. HAMBURGER: Gerechtlijk onderzoek van bloed en anders lichaamsvochten," Tijdschr. v. strafrecht, 17:82, 1904. Zur Differenzierung des Blutes 'Eiweiss biologische verwandter Tierspecies: eine Erweiterung der ulichen serodiagnostischen Methode, Deutsche med. Wchnschr., 31:212, 1905. Here it may be noted that WELCH and CHAPMAN have pointed out that the weight of the precipitate under certain conditions serves to distinguish between related proteins. WELSH and CHAPMAN: On the Differentiation of Proteins of Closely Related Species by Precipitin Reaction, J. Hyg., 10:177, 1910.

1855. MALLET: The Serum Precipitation Test for the Identification of Blood Stains, Virginia Med. Semimonth., 285, 1903-04; Tr. Med. Soc. Virginia, 49, 1903-04. BRUCK: Die biologische Differenzierung von Affenarten und der menschlichen Rassen durch spezifische Blutreaktion, Berl. klin. Wchnschr., 44:798, 1907.

this same blood grouping as an aid in determining parentage. The inheritance of the iso-agglutinative group-specific substances in human blood appears to follow Mendelian laws.[1856]

With regard to the stain on clothing, it has the value of connecting the blood of the diseased with the blood-stains found on the accused. However, it is possible that the blood may have had an entirely different origin; the circumstances in the case must be carefully considered. The expert must let the jury weigh this evidence. The sera of some individuals will glutinate the cells of others. All human blood may be divided into four groups.

Serums of group A and B (2 and 3) can be procured from a hospital laboratory; the diluting medium of 0.9% sodium chloride and 1% sodium citrate in distilled water in small test-tubes and glass slides should be provided. Add three drops of fresh blood from the finger tip to 2 cc. of citrate solution in a small test-tube. Invert the tube several times to mix the cells. Mark one end of a glass slide A, and the other end B. With a glass pipet place a large drop of group A (two serum) at the end A. In the opposite end put a drop of group B (3 serum). Into the serum add a drop of the salt emulsion taken from the patient. Rotate gently. If the glutination is marked it may be seen with the naked eye in fifteen minutes as a fine brick dust. Examine each end of the slide under a low power objective. When sera A and B agglutinate the cells, the blood belongs to the group AB of the Landsteiner (group 1 Moss). If the serum of B alone produces agglutination, the cells belong to the group A (Group 2 Moss), but if the cells are agglutinated only by A they belong to group B (Group 3 Moss). If neither serum agglutinates the cells, they belong to group O (Group 4 Moss), provided groups A and B test sera are potent.

Stains found on clothing, instruments, walls, floors, or wherever the blood may be spattered, can be compared with the blood group of the suspected criminal or of the deceased. Wash the cells with normal saline and if they appear distinct

1856. OTTENBERG: Medical Application of Human Blood Grouping, J.A.M.A., 77:682, 1921; 78:983, 1922. Hereditary Blood Qualities, J. Immunol., 6:363, 1921; Medicolegal Application of the Blood Group, J.A.M.A., 78:89, and 79:180, 1922.

under the microscope try the effect of group A and then group B serum upon them. It may be necessary to allow the test to stand for one hour using a concave slide to prevent evaporation. When the cells are disintegrated so that their agglutination cannot be detected, immerse the particles of blood-stain in a minimum of saline, centrifuge, and try the agglutionation effect of the clear fluid on cells known to be in A and B groups. If the cells of A and B groups are agglutinated the unknown blood is group B. If the cells of B are agglutinated, the unknown blood is group A. If the cells of neither group are agglutinated, the unknown blood is group AB. The same technique is followed in the selection of a donor. Some confusion has arisen from the fact that there are three different groups. Landsteiner in 1900 discovered the human blood groups and showed that they depend upon the existence of two corpuscular substances known as A and B and the two corresponding hemagglutinins anti-A and anti-B. The constitution of the four human blood groups with respect to these substances is shown in the following:

	I Universal Donor	II	III	IV Universal Recipient
Serum	Anti-A Anti-B	Anti-B	Anti-A	No Agglutinins
Cells	0	A	B	AB
Frequency in U.S.A.	45%	42%	10%	3%

The Committee of Hygiene of the League of Nations states that the groups be designated with respect to agglutinable elements A and B as follows: International, Jansky and Moss. Blood transfusion is a safe procedure if the donor belongs to the same blood group as the patient. The extremely rare accidents that have happened in spite of this precaution have not proved to be due to any incompatibility of the transfused blood that could be detected with any known test. The courts recognize blood grouping characteristics existing between the child, mother and father. Dunger and Hertzfelt[1857] from the comparison of the blood groups of the child, mother, and supposed father state that an accused man has one

1857. DUNGER and HERTZFELT: *Ztschr. f. Immunitätsforch. u. exper. Therap.*, 6:284, 1910. See BERNSTEIN: *Klin. Wchnschr.*, 3:4195, 1924.

chance in six of proving that he could not have been the father of the child.[1858]

Because of the regularity of the blood group scheme it was obvious from the outset that the underlying blood properties are constitutional, and following the rediscovery of Mendel's laws by de Vries, Correus and Tschermals, these individual blood properties were shown to be hereditary, and subject to the Mendelian rules. The falsely accused man and the true father may belong to the same group. The average chance of excluding paternity is about one to seven.[1859] For the population of Germany these figures are somewhat high, about one to six.

Groups of Parents	Groups of Children	Exclusive
O x A	O	A,B A B
O x A	O, A	
O x B	O, B	A, A B
A x B	O, AB, AB, O, B	A,A B
O x A B	A B	O, A B
A x A B	A, B., A B	O, A B
B x A B	B, B, A B	O
A B x A B	A, B, A B	O

After having established by chemical test that the stain contains blood and the extracts of the stain respond to the precipitin reaction for human blood, one may use the two methods, the examination for iso-agglutination and that for agglutinogens.

The test for agglutins consists in adding a trace of the whole blood or a fragment of the stain or an extract of it to suspensions of bloods of group A and B. If possible the tests should include the blood of the victim and the accused person. Precautions must be taken in order to avoid error due chiefly to the presence of agglutinating substances other than iso-agglutinins or to pseudo-agglutination. For this reason control tests with blood of group O are essential. Iso-agglutinins are still active in dried blood after many months or even a longer interval, but they may deteriorate sooner, and consequently no conclusions can be drawn from negative results. Several authors have reported that the properties

1858. HOOKER and BOYD: *J. Crim. Law.*, 25: 187, 1934.
    1859. HOOKER, S. B., and BOYD, A. C.: *J. Immunol.*, 16: 451, 1929. WIERNE, A. S.: *J. Immunol.*, 24: 483, 1933.

of A and B are detectable by suitable technique not only in blood and organs but also in secretions, such as saliva, seminal fluid, mucus, and sweat.

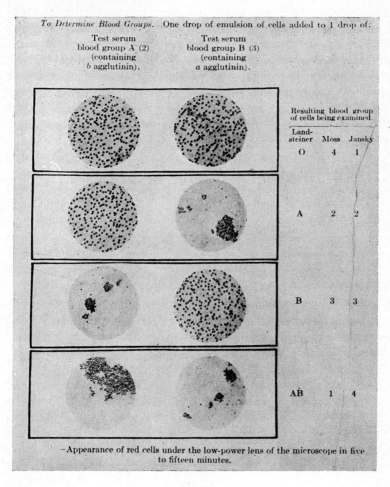

To Determine Blood Groups. One drop of emulsion of cells added to 1 drop of:

FIG. 23
Blood Groups
(Laboratory Medicine, Nicholson, 1934)

If the cells can be obtained, an extract of the stain is made with normal saline. A drop of a cell emulsion made as described above from known group II and one from group III donors is added to the slide. If no agglutination occurs, the stain is from the blood of a person belonging to group I.

If cells from group III are agglutinated but not in group II, then the individual is in group II. The reverse is true if agglutination takes place in group II but not in group III, then the individual is in group III. If the extract agglutinates both groups then the serum in the stain came from group IV. The group of the stain having been identified, and if by comparison with the blood of the accused it falls into the same group as that of the accused, the test does not aid very much. However, if the blood group of the stain on the clothing or the weapons of the accused tallies with that of the deceased, important evidence is added to that already obtained by the prosecutor. (Fig. 23, page 957.)

This test may be of aid in cases of disputed paternity. Early in life group peculiars appear, the specific agglutinating ability of the red cells beginning at birth and the agglutinating power of the serum arising during the first year and remaining unchanged throughout the life of the individual.

Landsteiner[1860] has added three additional agglutinogen characteristics. M. N., and MN which in tests of non-paternity increase a falsely accused man's possibilities of exoneration to one chance in three or four. Blood grouping is valuable in connection with other characteristics. In a recent case, H. vs. H., in the Circuit Court, a comparison of the head, eyes, and face of the child with that of the father, hardly made it necessary for a blood grouping test. The mother and son were in group B, the father in group B. The father then could be in O, A, B, A B. The New York legislature amends the law relating to the support and education of children born out of wedlock and proceeds to establish paternity, by providing "the court, on motion of the defendant, shall order the making of one or more blood-grouping tests by a duly licensed physician and the results thereof may be received in evidence."[1861] The prosecution is not given the right to demand a specimen of blood from the defendant. Too much should not be expected from the serologist in the examinations of stains on clothing, rags or weapons exposed to the weather or fire, as the cells and serum may be altered.

"When immune serums obtained by injecting rabbits with human blood were exhausted with certain bloods of a given

1860. LANDSTEINER: *J.A.M.A.,* 103:1041, 1934.
1861. Laws of New York, 1935, c.198.

group, it was found that some of the serums still agglutinated other bloods of the same group but not the blood used for the absorption. In this way individual blood properties were demonstrated[1862] entirely independent of the blood groups, two of which, designated as M and N, were found to be applicable to the investigation of cases of disputed paternity. The properties of M and N define three types of human blood, namely the types M, N, MN, depending on which of the agglutinogens are present. The frequency of these types in the white population examined is approximately 30% M, 20% N, and 50% MN."

Martinet* reports that after repeated transfusions where the M and N factors have been crossed between the donor and the patient, sensitization to the M and N factors sometimes appears. In man, anti-M and anti-N hemolysins are apparently formed without the formation of the agglutinins as in the rabbit.

1862. LANDSTEINER, KARL, and DEVINE, PHILIP: J. Exper. Med., 47:757, 1928; 48:731, 1928.

* MARTINET, RENE: Arch. Int. Med., 11:573, 1936.

MEDICOLEGAL EXAMINATIONS
OF SEMINAL STAINS

IN CASES of alleged rape or sodomy the recognition of seminal stains on clothing or other substances may be of great medicolegal importance. The articles usually submitted for examination are underclothing, wearing apparel, pieces of bed clothing; in some cases scrapings from the skin or mucous membrane of the alleged victim, such as dried masses from the neighborhood of the genitals or adherent to the hair, or scrapings of mucus from the vagina. The stains may be simple or complex. They may consist of pure dried seminal fluid, or of seminal fluid mixed with other fluids or secretions. The appearance of a dried seminal stain varies according to circumstances, particularly according to the nature of the surface on which the stain is made. If, on a non-absorbent surface, such as a piece of wood or iron, or on heavy woolen cloth or velvet, it dries, forming a grayish scale on the surface, a portion can easily be removed with the point of a knife-blade or a needle for microscopic examination. If cotton or linen has been starched, so as to render it comparatively non-absorbent, a seminal stain will have the same scaly appearance. If the cotton or linen is soft, the dried seminal stain will give it a feeling of having been starched. The usual color of the stain is grayish, or it may have a yellowish tint, and in old men the stain may have a reddish tint. When the stain is viewed by direct sunlight or under an electric light a faint irregular outline may be determined.

The Florence Test: Seminal stains are detected with absolute certainty only by the recognition of the characteristic morphologic elements, the spermatozoa, by microscopic examination. The seminal fluid consists of an admixture of the secretion of several glands, being a solution of various organic and inorganic substances especially rich in phosphates, and the characteristic spermatozoa and numerous cells coming from the mucous membranes lining the different portions of the genital tract. Seminal fluid contains nucleoproteins, albumin, and a proteose-like substance. A crystalline substance called spermin was first isolated from seminal fluid by Schreiner in 1878. It is said to have the formula C_2H_5N, and gives all the general reactions of an alkaloid. It is soluble in water and absolute alcohol, but very slightly soluble in ether; its solutions have an alkaline reaction. Spermin is not characteristic to the seminal fluid of man, but has been found in that of some animals, also in sputum, blood, and some of the animal tissues. The views as to the nature of this base are not unanimous. Florence[1863] claims to have discovered an alkaloidal body that he finds only in the seminal fluid of man, which gives a characteristic crystalline precipitate with a concentrated solution of iodine in potassium iodide. Florence has not been able to obtain these crystals with the seminal fluid of any other animal, nor from any other fluid or tissue. This substance Florence calls virispermin. This test is one of extreme delicacy, a single fibril of cloth upon which is a dried seminal stain sufficing to yield numerous crystals when the test is properly made. The reagent consists of: potassium iodide 1.65 gm., iodine 2.54 gm., and distilled water 30.00 gm. These proportions correspond to the formula KI_3. (?)* The iodine dissolves quickly in the solution of potassium iodide, and it is only necessary to mix the materials together in a glass-stoppered bottle and allow it to stand for a short time, when the reagent will be ready for use.

The test is made in the following manner: A minute fragment of the stained fabric is carefully removed with fine-pointed forceps and sharp-pointed scissors, transferred to a glass slide, treated with a small drop of distilled water, and allowed to soak for a minute or two, and a minute drop of the iodine reagent is added to it in such a way that the two drops of fluid come in contact at their edge, and immediately are covered with a cover-glass. If the suspected stain contained any dried seminal fluid, the examination with the microscope will show a very large number of brown crystals that resemble in appearance the hemin crystals obtained with Teichmann's test for blood.

If the stain be on a non-absorbent piece of wood, it is sufficient to remove a minute fragment of the scale with the point of a knife, transfer it to a glass slide, and treat it in the same manner.

This test, while it is not all that Florence claimed for it, is extremely valuable as a preliminary test. It has the same val-

1863. FLORENCE: Du Sperme et des Taches de Sperme en Medecine Legale, 1897.

* (Potassium has valence of one; Iodine one, five and seven).

ue as a preliminary test for seminal stains that the guaiacum test has as a preliminary test for blood stains. If the characteristic crystals are obtained in any given stain, it shows that the stain may be a seminal stain, and an examination must be made for the detection of the spermatozoa, which must be found also in order to be able to state with certainty that the stain in question is of seminal origin. If, however, no crystals are obtained with this test with any given stain, it shows with certainty that the stain does not contain any dried seminal

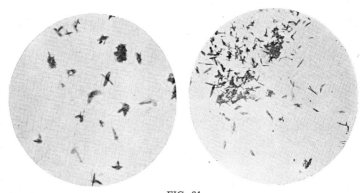

FIG. 24

Crystals obtained from a single thread, one-eighth inch long, cut from the stained portions of a child's chothing in a case of attempted rape

fluid. In treating an ordinary seminal stain in this way, as a general rule, a brown precipitate can be seen to form at the instant the two drops come in contact upon the glass slide, and this brown precipitate, on microscopic examination, is seen to consist of the characteristic crystals. The seminal stains are determined only by the recognition of the characteristic morphological elements by microscopical examination. If the seminal fluid forming a stain is mixed with other secretions, the appearance of the dried stain would, of course, be modified accordingly.

The Barberio Test: With an aqueous solution of picric acid added to a newly voided, putrefied or macerated semen, Barberio obtained yellow microcrystal-like needles, of rhomboidal shape, three or four times as long as wide. Occasionally forms like two cones with bases together appeared. The crystals can be preserved on the slide after removing the excess picric acid with distilled water, absorbing the water with filter paper, and mounting in balsam. The reaction may be obtained with stains as old as six years, and probably after a longer time. If the stain has been submitted to a temperature higher than 150° C. (302° F.), a poor reaction is obtained; at 200° C. (392° F.) crystals cannot be obtained. Lecha-Marzo,[1864] who gives an extended review of the whole subject, tested fresh and putrefied brain, liver, kidneys, lungs, spleen, nasal and vaginal discharges, blood, pus, perspiration, white and yolk of eggs, and some vegetable juices with Barberio's method and obtained negative results. With saliva, rounded crystals were obtained, but they were easily distinguished from those of semen.

While many methods have been proposed for obtaining crystalline precipitates, none seems to be absolutely specific for semen. Thus crystals are produced on the addition of the Florence reagent to solutions of the decomposition products of lecithin, which is one of the constituents of many animal tissues. Lecithin decomposes during putrefaction or drying, so that the Florence reaction may be obtained with extracts of tissues that contain lecithin if they have decomposed and are old. This does not, however, detract from the value of the test as a preliminary one, as it still remains the most valuable of any chemical test recommended so far for seminal stains. For the positive recognition of a seminal stain, however, it is necessary to obtain perfect spermatozoa.

Detection of Spermatozoa: The spermatozoa, as is well known, are tadpole-shaped bodies having an ovoid head and a tail nine or ten times longer than the head. The length of the head of human spermatozoa is very constant and about 1/3600 inch, being therefore, as long as the diameter of the human red blood cell. If seen on its side, the head of a spermatozoon appears more or less pear-shaped. In the examination of stained spermatozoa it will be seen that the anterior third of the head is less dense than the posterior two-thirds, and is stained less deeply.

The spermatozoa are stable and not readily destroyed, so that they may be detected in stains many years old if the stain has not been subjected to too much washing or exposure. These bodies, after they become dry, are so very brittle, that

1864. LECHA-MARZO: *Progesso Clin.*, 6:267, 1918.

the tail is easily separated from the head, and for this reason it is so difficult to obtain many perfect spermatozoa in the examination of old dried seminal stains.

For the positive recognition of spermatozoa it is necessary to find perfect bodies with head and tail complete, since there are other bodies, such as certain spores, sometimes found in old stains, which much resemble the heads alone, and there are numerous substances, such as bacteria or bits of the fibrils of cloth, which frequently resemble the tails alone. Therefore great care should be exercised in the handling of any substances suspected to contain seminal stains which are to be submitted for medicolegal examination. They should not be subjected to unnecessary handling or rubbing, and should be submitted in as fresh a condition as possible.

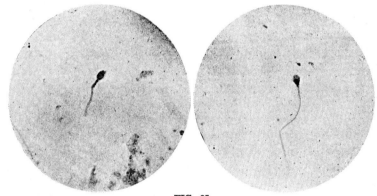

FIG. 25
Human Spermatozoa

If the stain is a scaly one, as by the drying of the fluid on a non-absorbent surface, the detection of the spermatozoa is comparatively easy. A fragment of the stain, removed with the point of a knife, should be transferred to a glass slide, treated with a drop of distilled water, and allowed to soak for several hours under conditions that will prevent the rapid evaporation of the water. The scales should then be gently separated with fine needles, treated with a drop of the staining solution, covered with a cover-glass, and examined directly with the microscope. Sometimes a better preparation can be made by first soaking the particles of stain with water on a cover-glass for several hours; then pick to pieces, and allow to dry. When dry, pass the cover-glass three or four times through a flame, or heat it in an air-bath to 115° C. (239° F.) for fifteen to twenty minutes, so as to fix the spermatozoa on the glass, in the same manner that blood cells are fixed previous to staining. Then treat the dry residue on the cover-glass with staining solution, wash off the superfluous stain, and dry. This preparation can be mounted dry, sealing the cover-glass with paraffine, or it can be mounted in Canada balsam, or in any other desirable menstruum.

If the stain is on unstarched cotton or linen cloth, the detection of the spermatozoa is much more difficult. The spermatozoa are apt to cling to the fibrils so tenaciously that it is difficult to separate them without breaking the head from the tail. Care should be taken to select for the examination a thread of the cloth near the center of the stain. The cloth should first be examined with the lens in order to see, if possible, if one side contains more dried stain than the other. For instance, stains have been found that yielded an abundance of spermatozoa on one side of the cloth, while none could be found on the other, although the Florence reaction could be obtained on both sides. Also the liquid portion of the seminal fluid may be spread for quite a distance on a piece of linen or cloth, while the solid bodies, the spermatozoa and cells may be limited to the center portion of the stain; in this case the Florence reaction will be obtained from the edge of the stain as well as from the center, but the spermatozoa can be isolated only from the central portion of the stain.

The best method to prepare such a stain for microscopic examination is to carefully cut from near the center of the stain, with a pair of fine-pointed scissors, a few individual threads of cloth from one-sixteenth to one-eighth inch long, and treat each piece of thread on a glass slide or cover-glass with a small drop of water, allowing it to soak at least two hours, the evaporation of the water being prevented. Some think that the soaking should continue from twelve to twenty-four hours. Numerous preparations should be made, since it frequently happens, even in well-marked seminal stains, that careful search will fail to detect unbroken spermatozoa in one or more of the preparations. After sufficiently prolonged digestion the small fragment of thread should be very carefully separated into its individual fibrils by manipulating with sharp-pointed needles. It can then be stained and examined.

To prevent the breaking of spermatozoa on cloth Wondson[1865] recommends that the cloth be fixed in Müller's fluid for twenty-four hours at 37° C. (98.6° F.), washed in several changes of water, blotted, and laid flat on a slide, drying the slide slowly and staining with 1% watery solution of eosin, washing, and drying. Hankin[1866] suspends the stained cloth for a moment in boiling water, cools, places it in a 2% potassium cyanide solution for two minutes, washes in distilled water, and teases out the threads on a slide before mixing and staining.

Baecchi[1867] proposed a staining method for cloth as follows: Place the piece of cloth, say 1 cm. square, in 1% acid fuchsin or methylene-blue; wash in 1% hydrochloric acid; dry in air or dehydrate in absolute alcohol; clear in xylol; mount in Canada balsam. If the spots are not fresh place for one-half hour to twenty-four hours in 20 to 30% ammonium hydroxide solution and then in distilled water.

Moist material, such as mucus obtained from the uterus or vagina, may be placed upon a glass slide, stained, and examined at once for the detection of spermatozoa. According to Florence, the spermatozoa of none of the domestic animals has the pear-shaped profile of human spermatozoa. The following table by Boston[1868] gives the measurements of various spermatozoa in micra:

TABLE LXIII
MEASUREMENTS OF VARIOUS SPERMATOZOA

| | Total Length | Heads | | Tail Length |
		Length	Width	
Man	51–58	4–6	3–4	41–53
Dog	67–74	4–8	3–4	59–67
Rabbit	51–66	6–9	3–4	45–60
Horse	64–67	6–8	6	54–60
Bull	87–93	9	6	77–83
Sheep	83	9	3	74
Cat	58–74	7	3–4	53–66

Ellerman[1869] stains an isolated thread with erythrosin, places it in ammonia water for one minute, washes in water,

1865. WONDSON: *Brit. M. J.,* 2:501, 1908.
1866. HANKIN: *Brit. M. J.,* 2:126, 1906.
1867. BAECCHI: *Vrtljschr. f. gerichtl. Med.,* 43:1, 1912.
1868. BOSTON: *J. Applied Microscopy,* 4:1360, 1901.
1869. ELLERMAN: *Vrtljschr. f. gerichtl. Med.,* 42:116, 1911.

then stains in iron hematoxylin for two minutes, dries, and mounts in balsam. The spermatozoa are black; the fibers not stained.

The Biologic Test: Farnum[1870] has proposed a biologic test for human semen that is based on the same principles as the serum test for blood. He prepared rabbits by injecting into the peritoneal cavity from 5 to 10 cc. of either semen or testicular emulsion at intervals of from two to six days, the rabbits receiving from five to eight injections. The test was made in a similar manner to the serum test for blood. He found that the serum obtained from the blood of rabbits prepared with human semen gave a distinct reaction with both recent and old emulsions of human semen in salt solution, and also with human seminal stains which have been dried and kept for thirty-four days, these stains being extracted with salt solution and filtered. More recent observations by Hektoen[1871] tend to confirm Farnum's results, as they indicate that there is a specific antigenic substance peculiar to human semen. Whether this precipitin reaction or other immune reactions, such as the anaphylactic test suggested by Lecha-Marzo, are practicable for the detection of semen in medicolegal work, remains to be demonstrated. At present the precipitin test holds out promise enough to merit thorough trial.

Having determined that the stain was made by seminal fluid, apply the same technique as for the grouping of blood, which will determine the group from which it came. Blood from the accused can then be typed and give valuable evidence for or against the accused.

1870. FARNUM, C. G.: *J.A.M.A.*, 37:1721, 1901.
1871. HEKTOEN, LUDVIG: *J.A.M.A.*, 78:704, 1922.

HAIR AND OTHER FIBERS

THE expert is occasionally required to examine hair or fibers found at the scene of a crime; on weapons, clothes, and from the wall paper, and flooring, and many other places that might have some bearing upon the investigation of the crime. If hair from the accused has been found in the hand of the deceased, valuable evidence may be obtained. The hair may have been altered by bleaching with hydrogen peroxide, or if it was gray it may have been darkened with sulphur, lead, mercury, silver, aniline dyes, phenylene-diamines, pyrogallol, and plant extracts. Where decomposition of a dead body has advanced or where the victim has been decapitated, valuable information for identification purposes may be obtained from the axillary and pubic hairs. Occasionally hair in these places is also dyed. When only a few hairs are submitted for identification of their source, the task is often very difficult. The distinctive features of hairs that are recognized by even low powers 200 to 300 diameters are: (1) The shingled or terraced ("imbricated") surface; (2) the distinction between cortex and medulla; (3) the pigment granules in the cortex; (4) the cells composing the medulla; and (5) the transition in structure from shaft to root, and the peculiar sheath of the latter. All of these features are not found in a single specimen, but, fortunately, positive identification can be made through the detection of several of them.

At first it must be established whether the hairs are of animal or vegetable origin. A rough test, if sufficient material is available, is to burn a few of the fibers in air; vegetable fibers burn readily without disagreeable odor and leave a sharply burnt end; animal hairs burn with difficulty, emit an odor of burnt feathers, and show a fused or rounded and curved end. Take a small quantity of the fiber or other material submitted and put it in a test-tube with 1 cc. of water and two drops of alcoholic solution of alphanaphthol and 1 cc. of sulphuric acid. If the fibers are vegetable they will dissolve and the liquid will become a deep violet color, whereas if they are of animal origin no violet color will be seen in the fluid. A strong mineral acid added to the material and heated causes disintegration of a hair into its component cells. Thymol and sulphuric acid color linen and cotton fibers violet, but give no color with wool, hair, or silk. Microscopically the appearance of woody fibers can readily be recognized, and usually a decision can be made between cotton, linen, silk, and animal hairs, unless they have been chemically treated.

The hairs can be mounted in paraffine in sections made in the same manner, which gives additional information.

The animal hairs that require consideration are those which, living or dead, enter into the human environment— the domesticated quadrupeds, the parasitic rodents, the animals whose skins are converted into clothing and some types of wearing apparel. The hairs of these represent different types, and can be distinguished positively from human hair. (See Fig. 26.)

A question often presented to the microscopist in a legal inquiry is whether hairs admittedly human can be identified as the product of a given individual; whether they must have grown on the body of a certain person, and could not have been furnished by any other. While similarity in color and size with those of a given individual may be marked, there is nothing peculiarly characteristic in the hairs of one person to distinguish them from the hairs of many others of similar complexion. Occasionally the detection of abnormalities in hair or disease from a suspected source would naturally furnish a probability, but not a certainty, of a common origin. This is one of the most difficult problems that confronts the microscopist.

The expert is frequently asked from what part of the body these hairs are derived. The long, soft hairs from the scalp and beard are distinguished both by their length and by their gradual tapering from root to point. The short, thick, stiff hairs from the eyelashes and the eyebrows, while averaging almost the same thickness as scalp hairs at the root, taper rapidly toward the point, the short, slender flexible hairs, from the general surface of the body, the so-called lanugo or down, have, on the average, a much smaller diameter than other hairs, even than the equally short but thick hairs from the eyelashes. These downy hairs, moreover, frequently exhibit no pigment granules in the cortex, and the medullary canal is apt to be relatively small and is frequently absent.

Scalp hairs average 1/350 inch in the male, 1/450 in the female. The variations in different persons, may, however,

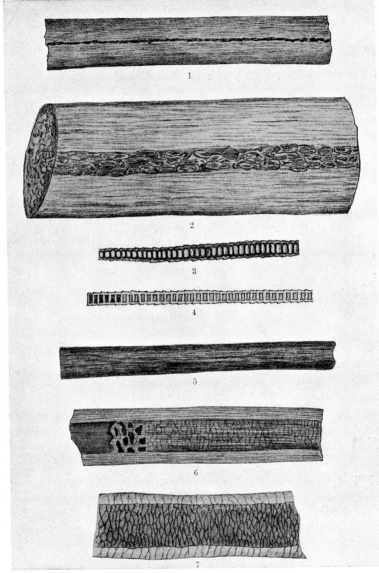

1, Hair of ox (x200). 2, Pig's bristle (x200). 3, Cat's hair (x200). 4, Mouse's hair (x200). 5, Horse's hair (x200). 6, Donkey's hair (x200). 7, Goat's hair (x200).

FIG. 26
Animal Hairs
[From Text-book of Legal Medicine and Toxicology Peterson and Haines Vol. II, 1904, W. B. Saunder & Co.]

be extreme—from 1/1000 to 1/200 inch. Hairs from the beard and mustache are usually the thickest of the body, ranging from 1/250 to 1/150 inch; they usually exhibit the greatest diameter on the chin and upper lip, shading off in diameter as they approach the scalp above and below. Hairs from the eyebrows, lids, axillae, and pubic region, present about the same diameter at their roots as do those of the scalp. Here again great variations are found in different individuals. The downy hairs and hair from the hairy parts of the body average from 1/2000 to 1/1000 inch in diameter near the root. The downy hairs of the fetus and of the newborn infant contain no pigment and no medullary canal. The hairs of children before puberty frequently have no medullary canal; they are relatively slender when compared with hairs of the same length and locality from adults.

Animal hairs, including human hair, consist of a root embedded in the hair follicle, and a shaft. Examination under the microscope reveals that most hairs have three well-defined layers. (1) An outer layer of transverse cells known as the cuticle. These cells are imbricated, the lower ends of the cells being covered by the upper ends of the next layer. (2) A middle layer or cortex consisting of longitudinal fibers. (3) An inner layer of various shaped cells forming the core or medulla.

The medulla is seldom, if ever, present through the entire length of the hair.[1872] When present it sometimes contains numerous air bubbles which, together with the paucity of pigment, produce the lighter shades of hair peculiar to certain individuals. The root of the hair, except for the fact that it is immediately invested with a hair follicle, does not in any way differ in structure from the hair shaft. The hair follicle in transverse section varies in different races from circular to elliptical form. In the Chinese race the diameter of the follicle and the hair is 100 x 77 to 85, in the European 100 x 62 to 72, and in the Negro 100 x 40 to 60. The more elliptical the form of the follicle the greater the curl of the hair. Hairs are being continuously shed and regenerated, the average life of a hair of the scalp being stated as 1,600 days.[1873]

Cotton fibers consist of long tubular cells which when seen under the microscope appear as flat ribbon-like bands twisted

1872. JORDAN, H. E.: Textbook of Histology, 281, 1923.
1873. STOHR.

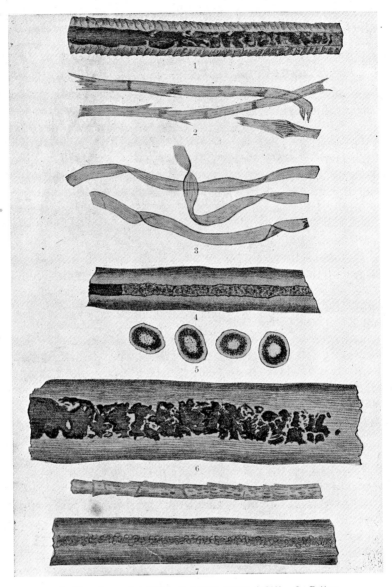

1, Sheep's wool (x200). 2, Linen fibers (x200). 3, Cotton fibers (x200). 4, Hair from human head (x200). 5, Transverse sections of hairs from human head (x200). 6, Hair from human beard (x200). 7, Hairs from back of hand (x200).

FIG. 27
Wool, Fibers, and Human Hairs
[Peterson and Haines, 1904]

like a corkscrew. Linen fibers show cross lines or folds about which the fiber is often swollen. Silk consists of long clear threads devoid of all cellular structure. The fibers of wool are easily distinguished under the microscope on account of the ease with which the epidermal scales can be observed and the wavy appearance of the fibers. (See Fig. 27.) The scales are translucent, and the cortical layer shows through them.

The hair of the common goat is formed almost entirely of true hairs. They occur as broad scales, the ends of which are wavy, but not serrated. The fiber layer or cortex is very narrow. The hair of the cow consists partly of soft wool hairs, without medulla, and partly of stiffer hairs with medulla. The epidermal scales are finely dentate, cylindrical, and very closely arranged. The cortical layer is thin and striate. The medulla is very broad, and is composed of a single row of distinct cells with fissures between them filled with air. Hairs from the body of the horse have a large medulla which occupies about two-thirds of the total diameter, and which consists of one or two rows of narrow leaf-shaped cells. The hairs of the cat have a thin irregular epidermal layer which envelops the fibers and gives a toothed appearance to the outline. The cortex is well developed. The medulla occupies half to three-fifths of the diameter of the hair and contains a single row of narrow regular cells with well-defined walls. Rabbit hairs are of importance, since they find commercial use in the imitation of many furs. The epidermal scales on these hairs are thick, and their forward edges terminate in a sharp point. The cortical layer is not apparent. The medulla consists of a single row of regular cells at the base; this rapidly increases as we pass up the fiber until there may be six to eight rows of cells. Rat hair is similar in structure to that of the cat; the medulla is well developed, and consists usually of well-defined pigmented cells with an apparent space between each cell. In parts of the hair two to three rows of smaller cells may be seen. Toward the extremity the hair appears to be jointed, each cell fitting into the one underneath.

The hair of exhumed bodies contains its original color. The hair of mummies 2,000 to 3,000 years old frequently contains its original black color. The importance of examination of the hair in chronic arsenical poisoning has already been referred to.

MEDICOLEGAL ASPECTS OF X-RAYS
AND OTHER FORMS OF RADIANT ENERGY*

DURING the last decades the x-ray has been used with growing frequency as a partial basis for the settlement of claims following injury, and, to a less extent, following disease. The practitioner is considered negligent who fails to give his patient the benefit of x-ray service before and after manipulation of fractured bones. The industrial boards and the courts are called upon to appraise a continuous series of inferences derived from x-ray studies and certified by "experts" whose qualifications seem acceptable. The expert is seldom a "Friend of the Court" but is employed by either the plaintiff or the defendant to explain his x-ray interpretations before a lay jury who have had no special training or experience in evaluating the findings without the aid of such expert testimony, except in a minor number of rather obvious fracture cases where "he who runs may read." The arbitrator or jury must then listen to the interpretations by experts employed by the opposing side and determine for the court and for the public between any variations in testimony given. This system of introducing evidence is probably parallel to that used in subjects outside the x-ray field but may often times result in a miscarriage of justice for the various reasons to be discussed.

A question of malpractice is occasionally brought up against a doctor in cases where an excessive amount of x-rays or other radiant energy has been applied either in the course of diagnosis or treatment. Burns by x-rays, radium, ultra-violet or infra-red rays, and by short wave length radio rays, are not common and may result in temporary or permanent damage. When in the course of treatment of malignancies or other intractable disease where only high doses of radiant energy are of benefit it becomes necessary to apply x-rays or radium to the point where some permanent tissue damage is probable or certain, the patient should be informed of this fact before witnesses or in writing before the high dosage is administered. This eliminates the surprise element and gets the patient's concurrence in a procedure instituted solely for his benefit although carrying an element of danger. Shocks and burns caused by electric currents are in a somewhat different category, since damaging amounts are not purposely given.

* By HOLLIS E. POTTER, M.D., Chicago.

Roentgenographic evidence is most commonly invoked in law during the adjustment of claims involving injury or disease in the bony parts of the body. Detecting the presence and extent of fracture or displacement in bones of the extremities is or should be a relatively simple procedure. Injuries to the head and to the trunk of the body involve factors both technical and inferential which require a higher type of skill and experience. Problems connected with the spine and skull demand many years of rather special experience and study to qualify a medical graduate in correctly evaluating the many structural changes meaningful or meaningless to a discussion of the case.

Radiographic demonstration of foreign bodies oftimes has a legal aspect. In gunshot wounds one may recognize the presence and something of the character and location of projectiles. Foreign bodies in the eye may be identified and localized with considerable accuracy. In dentistry sometimes small metallic objects such as brooches and partial plates may be inspired or swallowed. Claims of swallowed bits of crockery, broken glass, and other materials in restaurant food are not infrequent. The x-ray has its limitations in showing small fragments of semi-opaque materials, whereas tiny masses of heavy metals are quite demonstrable. Swallowed or inspired pins among office workers and dress makers is a fairly common problem.

Particularly in the late years much attention has been focused on pulmonary disease in certain industries. Pneumonoconiosis, and especially that division known as silicosis, produces a nodular, a linear, and conglomerate fibrosis demonstrable by x-rays, and because of its frequent association with tuberculosis that whole question is brought up. The x-ray properly plays a prominent role in evaluating, these cases, but the interpretation of normal chest films together with the identification of nodular, linear, and amorphous scars from previous disease, and the differentiation from a number of significant diseases caused by wholly different stimuli, is quite necessary. One's ability to identify and differentiate silicosis from an x-ray standpoint obviously depends on his familiarity with the x-ray characters of all pulmonary lesions as to their number, size, and distribution, as well as their density, their marginal definition, and their internal pattern.

It would be beyond the scope of this chapter to enumerate

the many other situations after injury or disease in which the x-ray findings as commonly used in civil practice might assume a legal aspect. Its many applications to the discovery or verification of disease in the gastro-intestinal system, the vascular system, the urinary system, etc., might at any time become legally significant.

Fluoroscopy, independent of radiography, should seldom have medicolegal importance. In order to amplify the identification of films certain States have specified that supplementary observations made with the screen, and the finding of lesions the same as is exhibited by films, greatly amplifies the value of the testimony. Makers of such laws did not perhaps realize that in the majority of cases minor bone changes in the heavy parts of the body can be detected with no degree of accuracy, if at all, by the fluoroscopic screen. It, therefore, does not detract from the validity of the radiographic proof of a lesion if it is overlooked by the screen. Fluoroscopy has a definite value in a limited number of situations. Thus, the relationship of fragments in extremity fractures may be well appreciated, whereas a simple fissure fracture without displacement may not even be recognized. Fluoroscopy of the chest and of the constantly moving viscera of the gastro-intestinal tract gives vital information regarding function, and aids in planning the radiographic attack.

1. **Difference of opinion** as to the interpretation of x-ray films is sometimes legitimate, because at certain stages of development lesions caused by somewhat different stimuli may have certain x-ray characters in common. The life history of a changing lesion is best studied on a series of films made at various stages of its growth. Then the study assumes more definite character, and points of differentiation generally appear.

Much more common are the differences in opinion which arise from one of the following causes:

A. Imperfect technique: While routine technique has improved with the years it is an amazing fact that even today poor technical results are more common than the opposite. The modern x-ray machine is an instrument of precision, but in its operation a number of human factors enter which modify the results to an extent quite beyond the scope of a technique chart. The operator should have beforehand a reasonable suspicion of the character and location of a lesion, and not rest until he has exhausted the possibilities of his method in showing it. He may be excused when patient willfully or consciously fails to cooperate. If the medical and lay public realized that often the diagnostic value of x-rays lay in the last 10% of technical excellence the matters of propinquity and convenience would bear less weight in planning for an x-ray study.

B. Variations in the so-called "normal": Just as there are differences in the anatomic structures of the nose and other facial features due to age, physical type, nutrition, etc., one sees differences in the architecture of the osseous system and organs of the body of various individuals properly considered healthy.

C. Actual anomalies or gross variations from the average normal are rather more common than formerly thought. A study of a thousand unselected spines will reveal 6 to 8% of anomalies at the lumbosacral region, besides a much larger number of minor variations in type or proportion. Anomalies are more common in certain parts of the body, but may occasionally be found anywhere. After a large anatomic and x-ray experience one comes instinctively to classify them into groups according to type and degree, since they show great tendency to repeat about the same features and to exhibit characteristics peculiar to themselves. Only a familiarity with these characters prepares one to differentiate them from injuries and from acquired disease.

D. Overlapping shadow structures are sometimes misinterpreted when viewing a single film made through a complex of structures lying at different depth levels. Relatively few parts of the body studied by x-rays are overlaid and underlaid by structures of an entirely homogenous nature so that their shadow presents no pattern of its own in addition to the individual part studied. In case of disagreement from such overlap, clarification is obtained by using more than one film made at somewhat different angles.

It cannot be called a favorite device of radiologists to hide or distort shadow outlines or densities by the use of other than the standard angles of projection, but in careless or single exposures overlaps may have to be explained to the novice. The custom of discarding all but one film for use in adjustment of claims is to be condemned.

E. Because of pre-existing injuries a misinterpretation may be made in which the old changes are wrongfully ascribed to a recent accident. In any refracture it may be difficult to separate in an exact manner the changes due to the old and the new. Most valuable in this connection is a set of films made at various stages after the first injury.

Bony callus grows differently at different ages and in different bones of the body. Linear skull fractures may heal to the point of disappearance in six months, or in other cases be plainly visible two years after injury. Minor fractures of the skull, spine, and pelvis are not infrequently overlooked in general practice, treated as contusions and sprains, and first come to diagnosis in a second injury where the question of liability required careful x-ray study. A radiologist who does a mass of non-legal work on the urinary and gastro-intestinal tract well realizes how often these long forgotten injuries come to light in the lumbar region.

In case a fracture has undergone normal union and the injured part regained normal function a second fracture in the general region will usually show some differentiating signs which enable one to recognize approximately what took place at the time of the first and at the time of the second injury. Refracture of partly healed bones gives more difficulty.

F. Pre-existing arthritis, epiphysitis, osteochondritis, and Schmorl's disease produce changes at joint margin and in nearby bony structures which must be recognized as such before being ascribed to injury. A discussion of the relation between osteo-arthritis and injury deserves an entire chapter. Arthrosis is a word which better expresses the fact that certain spurs and bridges are present at articular margins. These are so commonly unaccompanied by pain that the word arthritis should be reserved for those joints which are involved in a clinical sense. Unfortunately we cannot by x-rays give any valuable estimate as to the clinical activity of osteo-arthrosis unless the spurs and other bony changes show new or incomplete ossification which increases to maturity during the early months after an injury. Inflammation of the ligaments and regional soft tissues present in an active arthritis is invisible to x-rays.

Pathologic fractures in which the bone gave way easily because of pre-existing tumor, cyst, tuberculosis, etc., can be identified on films critical enough to show bone structure. The pathology uncovered may mean vastly more to the patient than the injury. It will modify considerably the medicolegal aspect.

The question of aggravation is often brought up whenever the x-rays show the changes of pre-existing disease, however inert it seemed to be before the accident. There is seldom anything shown by x-rays which tends to prove or disprove aggravation in any given case. Occasionally, however, serial films give the most positive proof of aggravation.

2. Limitations of the radiograph in determining the extent of injury: While x-rays daily contribute worlds of information in the tangible form so acceptable to the adjustment of legal claims, it seems appropriate to insist at this point that x-ray findings should be used only for what they are worth in determining the extent of injury, the loss of function, or the degree of lasting disability. A considerable fracture-dislocation of the spine may occur without serious injury to the cord, whereas another looking about the same to x-rays may have sustained a complete cord section. The real seriousness of the case may be outside the province of x-rays. Great legal stress is often laid on a simple linear fracture in the vault of the skull because the x-ray shows it beyond the shadow of a doubt. Basal fractures, subarachnoid hemorrhage, etc., may be far more serious but escape x-ray visualization entirely.

For the sake of justice it is somewhat unfortunate that x-ray demonstrations appeal to the sense of sight and on this account gain greater credence than evidence appealing only to the ears or other sense organs. It is well known among attorneys that a "good x-ray case" will go farther in court than many another cases of greater disability and no x-ray findings. It is unfortunate for a claimant if he has had a fearfully painful sprain of the back in which x-rays show no fracture, no anomaly, and no pre-existing bone changes from disease.

3. Medicolegal x-ray testimony: The only legitimate object in medicolegal testimony is to explain to the court what in truth the x-ray has shown of significance to the case in hand. This should be done in the simplest possible form, because those who listen and decide have had limited experience or perhaps no experience in judging upon the validity of the statements made. Originally it was perhaps assumed that anything shown by x-ray films can be seen and therefore appreciated by anyone with good eyes. The history of the growth of x-rays in

diagnosis has been, however, that so many complexities have
arisen (outside of technique) that mistakes can only be reduced to a minimum by the development of a whole new special group of workers in medicine. In non-legal procedure,
men in this special field often enter into prolonged consultation
with the general practitioner or other specialist before finally
evaluating the significance of x-ray findings in one of their
cases. In legal practice the personal demonstration and explanation of x-ray findings has been found just as necessary
for much the same reasons.

The witness desiring to give an honest straightforward ex-
position of the case finds that he is obliged to conform to the
practice of submitting to an inquisition conducted by two opposing attorneys, one of whom is anxious to make you over-
state the truth while the other wishes to discount your every
utterance. You are, therefore, placed in a position where you
are forced by question and answer to assert and defend each
point to be brought out. Your own attorney may obstruct you
in this by not asking you the right questions. If he is wise he
will give you your head at some point early in the interview,
so that you may set up your points and the reasons therefor,
lest any be neglected. If you are wise you will seize an early
opportunity to present a definite number of points to support
your inference and aid in any way possible to have these points
treated logically and systematically. If you are prepared to
state it as your opinion that x-rays show a fracture of the first
lumbar vertebra for four reasons, you will probably not be diverted till all four have been duly considered. These must be
defended against attack by the opposing side.

It will seem to you that in a court where you have been
sworn to speak all and nothing but the truth and you have done
so to your great satisfaction, your cross-examiner assumes
nothing of the kind. He will set traps and pitfalls into which
you will innocently fall unless wary in your answers and wise
to the ways of lawyers. If he asks you if the x-ray appearances
of a fractured hip are not similar in some respects to those seen
in tuberculosis and you agreeably reply that they are similar in
certain . . . he stops you and tells the jury you said they were
similar and assumably identical. Your answer must be that
they are not similar except in those minor respects (which you
were about to relate when he cut you off and made a poor wit-

ness of you). You must know that "normal" means the average of that seen in a large number of healthy individuals, rather than simply "perfect," for only One is admitted to have been perfect. Just as he is subtly offensive, you are forced by the system in vogue to assume a defensive mental attitude. Always this is possible and consistent with your direct testimony if your case is valid. If your case is not valid you have no business on the stand. According to his code if he is not able to discount the testimony you have given with reference to a subject in your special field he will try to discount you and will do so unless you are alert.

4. **The x-ray medicolegal racket:** Because of its mysterious painless penetration and its strange appeal through the sense of sight, x-rays have been seized upon by unscrupulous lawyers and doctors as the central basis of proof for manufacturing evidence of injury or disease where none existed. In the same manner x-ray films showing overlaps, anomalies, arthrosis, or other pre-existing disease have been willfully introduced as evidence of a traumatic lesion. Minor bone changes due to trauma have been willfully exaggerated, in the presence of these relatively innocent and unrelated conditions.

It is an open secret that x-ray films of the chest showing active and healed tuberculosis, chronic bronchitis, bronchiectasis, fibrosis associated with asthma, etc., have been the foundation of a wholesale claim for damage in recent years. The x-ray plays a most important role in determining the presence and extent of silicosis long before it is disabling, and through its aid many worthy workmen have been awarded just compensation.

Certain mistakes in diagnosis are excusable, but when it becomes quite apparent that doctors and lawyers are united to willfully deceive a court of justice there can be no excuse. More often than not the patient and his lawyer were first deceived when the attending physician innocently gave them an incorrect opinion as to the extent of injury based upon the faulty interpretation of an incompetent radiologist. In such cases the blame is laid upon the x-ray when in fact it should be laid upon the persons who failed to recognize the truths set forth. The x-ray is becoming discredited for these mistakes of ignorance made in its name. No wonder an improper claim is entered, and no wonder a review or trial of the case gives the impression that it has been purposely built up around an improper x-ray inference.

When used properly, and in the light of our present day knowledge x-rays, are a most valuable adjunct in determining the extent of injury. They present most convincing evidence in a large majority of bone injuries, and most important information in certain diseases of soft tissues. In the best civil practice the overlapping shadow structures, the anomalies, the pre-existing injuries and disease, are recognized as such and are given their true evaluation. It is rather too much to expect that the average judge, attorney, or juryman can do the same, but legal methods of presenting evidence and judging therefrom were devised long before x-rays were discovered.

Historically, there is no perfect agreement as to who first introduced the radiograph into court as evidence. In a personal communication, Judge Ben B. Lindsay, of Denver, claimed that he was the first. Very early in the history of x-rays he tried a case of fractured neck of femur and offered in evidence radiographs made by Dr. George B. Stover, of that city. The court refused their admission, but later admitted the x-ray evidence when Dr. Stover brought an x-ray apparatus into the court room and went through the various steps of making further radiographs before all assembled.

SPECTROGRAPHIC ANALYSIS

SPECTROGRAPHIC examination of small amounts of human tissues have demonstrated the presence of many substances. Many chemical elements difficult to determine by the usual means are identified readily by this method.

Sheldon and Ramage[1874] washed small pieces of organs in distilled water to free from blood, placed them in a steam-bath, and dried to constant weight. Where fat was present, this was removed by drying on ashless filter paper. The dried material was then ground to a powder and a small amount of this powder used for obtaining the spectrum. The amount of powder used was 0.05 gm. This was rolled in a small piece of ashless filter paper and then burnt in an oxy-coal-gas flame before the slit of a quartz spectrograph, a quartz lens being used to focus the image of the flame on the slit. Plates five inches by four

1874. SHELDON, J. H., and RAMAGE, H.: *Biochem. J.*, 25:1608, 1931.

inches, suitably placed in the holder, cover the region from the red to beyond 2,800. Standard solutions were prepared, having different percentage composition. The brilliance of the lines obtained upon burning the papers charged with the standard solutions varies with the amount of solution used, and, since it is possible to obtain the photographs of 16 spectra on the one photographic plate, four of these were devoted to the standard solutions. The intensity of the lines of an element in a specimen compared with that in the different strengths of the standard solution is a method which can be put to a quantitative as well as qualitative use.

Using this technique, the authors were able to detect up to 0.05 gm. of a specimen; caesium, barium, cadmium, gallium, indium, thallium, bismuth, chromium, cobalt nickel, ruthenium, rhodium, palladium, and iridium. Other elements that have been described in the plant and animal tissues are not included in this list, the more important of which are tin, zinc, aluminum, and titanium. These can be detected when an arc spectrum is employed. They are in the ultraviolet region of the spectrum beyond wave length 3,108. The methods, while extremely delicate and of interest to the biochemist, are not being used by the toxicologist.

Gerlach and Ruthardt[1875] reported the quantitative determination of copper in tissue by means of spectro-analysis with the report of a case of questionable copper sulphate intoxication. The same scientists[1876] used a quantitative spectrographic analysis of determination in tissues for manganese. Scott and Williams reported a new development in histospectrography.[1877]

1875. GERLACH, W., and RUTHARDT, K.: Beitrage Zur Pathologischen Anatomie, 92:347, 1933.

1876. GERLACH, W., and RUTHARDT, K.: *Virchows Arch. f. Path. Anat.,* 292:52, 1934.

1877. SCOTT, G. H., and WILLIAMS, P. S.: *Proc. Soc. Exper. Biol. and Med.,* 32:505, 1934.

SILICOSIS AND ASBESTOSIS

SILICOSIS may be appropriately termed a "depression disease," because in America prior to 1930 little was heard of silicosis, while now hundreds of alleged cases have come to the attention of the medical and legal fraternities. Hippocrates, in his "Epidemics"[1878] was the first to mention the symptoms which we recognize today as signs of silicosis. George Bower[1879] mentioned asthma due to inhalation of dust in the blood and lungs. Lohneiss,[1880] referring to miners, described the effects on them: "The dust and stone fall upon the lungs, the men have lung disease, breathe with difficulty, and at last take consumption." Very little was written on the subject until 1717, when Ramazzini wrote a book on "Diseases of Tradesmen,"[1881] incorporating his views from a personal investigation of mines and industry. The description he has portrayed of silicosis has changed but little up to the present time.

The literature was sporadic in nature. Every thirty or forty years someone would write about disease of the lungs. The first report with microscopic demonstration of silica was made by Peacock.[1882] Greenhow was the first to find the crystalline and small angular bodies, and to identify positively the presence of silicon dioxide by means of hydrofluoric acid.

The first time the term "silicosis" was used appears to have been by Rovida,[1883] in 1871. After 1930 the literature contained numerous references to the etiology, symptomatology, pathology, chemistry of dust, and quantitative determinations of silica in postmortem material. Following the Conference at Johannesburg, South Africa, in August, 1930, the literature was greatly augmented by contributions from every country.

The Committee on Pneumonokoniosis of the Industrial Hygiene Section of the American Public Health Association[1884] defined silicosis as "a disease due to breathing air containing

1878. HIPPOCRATES: 4-Epid., M. 13, Trans. by FARR, 120, 1780.
1879. COLLIS, EDGAR L.: Milroy Lectures: Industrial Pneumonoconiosis, Georgii Agricolae, 1557; translated by HERBERT HOOVER.
1880. LOHNEISS, G. E.: Bericht von Bergwercken, 56, 1690.
1881. RAMAZZINI: De morbus arta ficium diatribe, 1717.
1882. PEACOCK: Brit. & Foreign M. Rev., 11:263, 1860.
1883. ROVIDA: Un caso di silicosis del polmini con analisi chemica, 1871.
1884. Am. Pub. Health Ass'n. Year Book, 1932-1933.

silica (SiO_2), characterized anatomically by generalized fibrotic changes and the development of miliary nodulation in both lungs, and clinically by shortness of breath, decreased chest expansion, lessened capacity for work, absence of fever, increased susceptibility to tuberculosis, (some or all of which symptoms may be present), and by characteristic x-ray findings."

In case of death, diagnosis must rest upon two findings: The characteristic fibrotic changes seen in section of the lung on microscopic examination, and by chemical examination showing an excess of silicon dioxide, 1.13 mg. or more per gm. of dried tissue. The normal lungs contain 1.13 mg. of silicon dioxide per gm. of dried tissue.[1885] As silica is a normal constituent of all the food we eat and the water we drink, it is natural that we should find it in all tissues of the body. It is a normal constituent of connective tissue, skin, blood, bone, urine, feces, and saliva of men. The silica in the lung in case of silicosis is derived chiefly by inhalation. Men engaged as grinders, stone cutters, or in occupations where the dust contains silica, are prone to develop silicosis in a concentration of 10 million parts per cubic foot of air, if the dust is 35% silica. The most harmful dusts are those of 3 micra or under. Cement and coal dust favorably modify silicosis.

The author advanced the theory that the fibrosis in the lungs in silicosis is caused by the chemical action of fluorides in the blood upon the silicon dioxide. The presence of fluorides with silica causes silicosis to appear at an earlier date in experimental animals than in animals dusted with pure silica.

To make a diagnosis it is absolutely necessary to have a history of the occupation and exposure of each workman in the silica-containing dust; to have a complete physical examination, and to have x-ray pictures. Detection in the sputum of particles of dust known to be associated with the pneumonokoniosis may assist in diagnosing the occupational sign of the attack. However, knowing the occupation of the man, one would expect to find in his sputum the particular type of dust he had been inhaling. Policard and Magnin[1886] conclude "that the microscopic and chemical examination of the sputum is no aid in the diagnosis of silicosis." They only confirm etiological data much more easily obtained in some other way.

1885. McNALLY, W. D.: *J.A.M.A.*, 101:584, 1933.
1886. *Presse méd.*, 38:875, 1930.

The inhalation of silica causes an inflammation with the development of fibrous tissue in small, well defined nodules. These nodules are more dense than the lung tissue, and are seen in the x-ray pictures.

Three stages of silicosis are recognized. The most usual symptoms are slight shortness of breath on exertion, non-productive cough, and recurrent colds. There may be less ability to expand the chest than usual, and the elasticity of the chest may be impaired. Usually the normal breath sounds may be somewhat harsh, roughened, and shortened. The cough is usually the first symptoms. At first it is both paroxysmal and non-productive and later is accompanied by scanty expectoration. Later on, the outstanding symptom is dyspnea. The second stage is often manifested by continuation of the shortness of breath on exertion and frequently pains in the chest; as the fibrosis increases and reduces the lung ventilation the symptoms become more marked. A patient may not lose weight, and may appear robust, but shortness of breath, may interfere with his working efficiency. The chest expansion is notably decreased, and chest movements apparently are smaller. In the third stage there is pain in the side, which is probably due to early pleuritis. There is an absence of fever; night sweats are common. The patient, as a rule, is pale; his chest is flattened anteriorly; the expansion of the chest is more limited than in the other two stages; there are local areas of dullness, and the inspiratory breath sounds are shortened, roughened, or more harsh. In the third stage, hemoptysis, loss of strength, and gastro-intestinal symptoms are pronounced. The symptoms increase in severity as the disease progresses. Tuberculosis may intervene at any time. It may be twenty years before the patient is incapacitated. In some instances, however, death has occurred within one and a half years from the time of exposure to silicon dioxide.

Both silicosis and tuberculosis may be present at the same time, and the term "tuberculosilicosis" has been applied to this condition. When there are no cavities, one of the outstanding clinical findings would be a reduced vital capacity, i.e., the volume of air that can be expelled from the lungs after a full inspiration would show a reduction from the normal.

When the individual dies and material is removed at the autopsy, the pathological and chemical examination is the final word as to whether or not the case is one of silicosis. The history, the x-ray and clinical findings are subordinate to these findings. In *Industrial Medicine,* February, 1935,[1887] the author suggested that no lump sum settlement should be made in silicosis cases, but that monthly payments be made with the proviso that at the time of death an autopsy be performed and the lungs examined for chemical and microscopical evidence of disease caused by inhaling dust. The following tables, LXIV and LXV, give an analysis of normal lungs and lungs from persons having had various degrees of silicosis. Table LXV is of interest as it gives the occupation of the individual, and reports of investigators from various parts of the world.

TABLE LXIV
ANALYSES OF LUNGS

Case	Age	Ash %	per Gram Mg. of SiO₂ of Dried Tissue
579	6 Mos. Fetus	1.05	.11
580	2 Days Old	5.32	.50
590	3 Yrs. Old	5.21	.21
806	5 Days Old	3.20	.12
596	Full Term	5.36	.077
311[1]	81 Years	6.71	1.86
312[1]	63 Years	5.61	.92
441[1]	40 Years	6.17	1.21
15[2]	51 Years	9.85	.72[3]
17[2]	43 Years	5.53	1.90
18[2]	28 Years	3.50	.80
6[4]	23 Years	4.77	1.10
16[4]	72 Years	4.40	1.10
1[5]	Normal		1.40 (Colorimetric)
2[5]	Fetus		.09

1. McNALLY, W. D.: *J.A.M.A.,* 101:584, 1933.
2. GIESE, WILLY: Beitrage Zur Pathologischen Anatomie und Zur Allgemeinen Pathologie, 1932-33.
3. Hydrochloric Acid insoluble which is nearly all silica.
4. CUMMINS, S. L., SLADDEN, A. F.: *J. Path. & Bact.,* 33:11, 1930.
5. KING, E. J., STANTIAL, H., and DOLAN, M.: *Biochem. J.,* 27: 1004-1005.

The prognosis in silicosis is unfavorable. The silica once lodged in the lung remains there forever, and the lung tissue is never restored to normal. Susceptibility to pneumonia and tuberculosis is increased in all stages of silicosis, especially in the last.

When an autopsy is performed, upon opening the thoracic

1887. "Silicosis—An Old Disease Revived."

cavity there are usually dense adhesions, and it is with difficulty that the thoracic organs can be removed. The adhesions are usually adherent on the lateral, mediastinal and posterior surfaces, with more extensive adhesions from the latter surface. The lungs are not collapsed, but stand out as if a cast had been

TABLE LXV
ANALYSES OF LUNGS, VARIOUS OCCUPATIONS

Case	Author	% SiO₂ in Dried Lung	Remarks
1	Giese[1]	2.24	Stone cutter
3	"	7.98	Miner
5	"	3.50	Foundryman
8	Hackman[2]	2.35	Miner
14	"	3.12	Stone cutter
30	"	5.53	Miner, stone c.
1	McCrea[3]	1.39	African gold m.
4	"	4.47	African gold m.
6	"	2.81	African gold m.
503	McNally[4]	1.40	Mill stone sharp.
300	"	2.60	Granite cutter
446	"	1.09	Zinc miner
1	Pancoast and Pendergrass[5]	1.81	Sand blaster
4	" " "	2.45	Sand blaster
40	Sladden[6]	1.72	Coal miner
41	"	1.78	Potter
42	"	1.80	Coal miner
1	Smith and Wikoff[7]	2.16	Driller
4	" " "	2.69	Driller
6	" " "	1.98	Laborer
3	King, Stantial and Dolan[8]	3.64	
4	" " " "	1.70	
5	" " " "	.81	

1. GIESE, WILLY: Beitrage Zur Pathologischen Anatomie und Zur Allgemeinen Pathologie, 1932-33. (Figures are for Hydrochloric Acid insoluble.)

2. HACKMAN, C.: Beitrage Zur Pathologischen Anatomie und Zur Allmeinen Pathologie, 90, 1932-33.

3. McCREA, JOHN: The Ash of Silicotic Lungs, South African Inst. for Med. Research, Pub. 3, p. 122, 1933.

4. McNALLY, W. D.: *J.A.M.A.,* 101:584, 1933.

5. PANCOAST and PENDERGRASS: *Am. J. Roentgenol.,* 26:556, 1931.

6. SLADDEN, A. F.: *Lancet,* 225:123, 1933.

7. SMITH and WIKOFF: *Am. J. Pub. Health,* 23:12, 1252, 1933.

8. KING, STANTIAL and DOLAN: *Biochem. J.,* 27:1004-1005.

made. The lungs are not much increased in size, but show an increase in weight. On section, the lung of a typical case of silicosis will show a dull slate gray, the surface uniformly studded with discrete firm black nodules. The air spaces are emphysematous. The large bronchi are thickened by fibrosis.

The peribronchial lymph glands along the bifurcations of the large bronchi are enlarged and black in color, and, upon section, cut with difficulty and give a gritty feeling. The cut sections are gray, with areas of black scattered throughout. The lung cuts with difficulty and may show irregular spherical masses of dense fibrous tissue scattered over the surface.

The pathology of silicosis is well summarized in the statement on the Medical Aspects of Silicosis made at the International Conference on Silicosis in Johannesburg, South Africa,

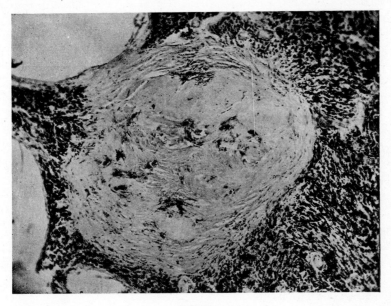

FIG. 28
A Silicotic Nodule

August 13 to 27, 1930. It was agreed that the microscopic pathological changes that may be produced by the prolonged inhalation of silica dust are:

1. The development of a condition designated in South Africa as a dry bronchiolitis characterized by an accumulation of dust-filled phagocytes in or in relation to the terminal bronchioles, with possibly some desquamation of their epithelium.

2. The accumulation of dust-containing phagocytes about and in the intrapulmonary lymphoid tissue and their transportation through the lymphatics into the tracheobronchial lymph

nodes. (The conditions described above under (1) and (2) do not constitute the disease silicosis.)

3. The gradual development of fibrous tissue within such accumulations of phagocytes and the formation of characteristic nodules of hyaline fibrous tissue.

4. Degenerative changes in these foci.

5. The hyaline nodules increase in size by extension at their periphery. Coalescence of adjacent nodules takes place and brings about involvement of further areas of the lungs. (The conditions described under (3), (4) and (5) constitute the disease silicosis.) (See Fig. 28.)

The pleura are nearly always thickened, and contain deposits of dust. The interlobular septa are thickened and contain dust. The primary lesion of silicosis is located in the tracheo-bronchial lymph nodes, and a chemical analysis of a large number of lymph nodes shows increased amounts of silicon dioxide as the disease advances in the lung. The nodule is characteristic and pathognomonic for silicosis, consisting of a discrete mass of hyaline connective tissue surrounded by layers of fibrous tissue. In some nodules the hyaline material will contain dust, in other sections there will be no dust. (See method of micro-incineration under Methods of Collecting Dust, page 994.)

The dust count should not exceed 10,000,000 particles per cubic foot when collected by the Greenburg Impinger method, and counted with about 110 diameters magnification. This is equivalent to 300 particles per cubic centimeter (referring to silica dust exposure). This is the standard used in South Africa, Ontario, Wisconsin, and Oklahoma.

In South Africa the degree with which an individual is affected with silicosis has been divided into various stages:[1888] "First, rather more fibrosis than usual; second, more fibrosis than usual; third, ante-primary; fourth, primary; fifth, secondary." In the United States, the stages are called first, second, and third. "The first stage means that definite physical damage to the lungs has been found, and that such damage has resulted from exposure to dust. The second stage means that definite and specific physical signs of silicosis are or have been present, and that capacity for work has been impaired by the disease, though not seriously. The third stage means that specific physi-

1888. RUSSELL, A. E.: J. Lancet, 22:605, 1933.

cal signs of silicosis are or have been present, and that capacity
for work has been seriously and permanently impaired by the
diseases."[1889] (For the complete literature on the various phases
of pneumonokoniosis, refer to The Pneumonokoniosis Series by
Davis, Salmonsen and Earlywine.)[1890]

Sweany[1891] states that tuberculosis with silicosis renders a
roentgenographic examination difficult or impossible in the
majority of patients affected with silicosis, because of atypical
characteristics or the location of the lesions.

Denny, Robson and Irwin* found in animal experiments
that rabbits dusted with quartz, to which less than 1% of
metallic aluminum dust had been added, showed practically no
fibrosis at the end of treatment.

McCord, Kasper and Fredrick** state that ethyl silicate is
used as a vehicle and solvent in paints and lacquers, as a stone
preservative, in heat resistant coatings, as a cement bonding
agent for refractories and other materials, and as a strengthening or hardening agent in sand molds, brick textile products and
the like. Small quantities of ethyl silicate are used in dentistry
for sealing of dental surfaces.

Tetraethyl-ortho-silicate, $Si(OC_2H_5)_4$, is a limpid water-
white liquid, boiling at 165.5°C. Its density is 0.933 20/20 and
its vapor pressure is relatively low. Air saturated with ethyl
silicate vapor at room temperatures (25°C.) will contain approximately 17 mg. per liter of the vapor.

Regardless of the method of administration, but with regard to dosage and time element, the administration of ethyl
silicate invariably leads to a characteristic response to which
most other manifestations apparently are related. This basic
injury is at the location of marked hemorrhage into the air
sacs, with some rupturing of alveolar tissues. This change may
appear well within ten minutes following intraperitoneal in-

1889. SAYERS, R. R., et al.: U. S. Bureau of Mines Tech. Paper, 545.
1890. BOOK I: The Pneumonokonioses (Silicosis)— Bibliography
and Laws; BOOK II: The Pneumonokonioses (Silicosis)—Literature and
Laws of 1934; BOOK III: The Pneumonokonioses (Silicosis)—Literature
and Laws, Chicago Medical Press, Chicago.
1891. SWEANY, H. C.: Pathologic Interpretations of Roentgenologic
Shadows in Pneumoconiosis, J.A.M.A., 106:1965, 1936.
  * Canad. M. A. J., 37, 1937.
  ** McCORD, CAREY P., KASPER, JOSEPH A., and FREDRICK, WILLIAM
G.: The Toxicity of Organic Silicon Compounds 1. Tetraethyl-Ortho-
Silicate. Manuscript from the Detroit Department of Health, 1937.

troduction of minute quantities of ethyl silicate and without occurrence of the demonstrable local injury within the abdominal cavity. To a limited extent, the capillaries of the heart and heart muscle are likewise injured by ethyl silicate. If death be not immediate, hemolysis may take place leading to hematuria and anomalies in blood counts. Also, in those animals surviving for a few days, an acute nephritis regularly may be demonstrated.

From their animal experiments the authors found that ethyl silicate possesses highly injurious properties.

The minimal lethal dose, when introduced intravenously into rabbits, is approximately 0.2 ml. per kilo of body weight; death usually takes place within one hour. The minimal lethal dose for rats, when administered intraperitoneally, is approximately 0.06 ml. per 100 gm. of body weight; with rare exception, death takes place within four days.

DETERMINATION OF SILICON DIOXIDE

THE whole lung is cut into small pieces and dried. After drying it is ground to sixty-mesh. Some fibrous material may have to be cut with scissors and ground in a mortar. Ten to twenty gm. of this well mixed powder are weighed into a platinum dish and the moisture determined, so as to be able to calculate all the silicon dioxide and other minerals to the dry basis. The sample is then ashed in the electric muffle, using about 5 gm. of the sample at a time, as the material may foam over if a larger sample is used. After the organic matter is all destroyed, a gray to reddish colored ash is obtained. Cool, weigh, and report as ash. If ashed over a flame the destruction of organic matter may be hastened by the addition of ammonium nitrate, or pure hydrogen peroxide. (The loss in weight is due to water of crystallization, carbon dioxide, and the destruction of the organic matter in the tissues.) The ash at this stage may be examined by petrographic or chemical methods, or a combination of the two, but the examination is best made on the original lungs, as ashing causes a change in the appearance of the mineral present. The ash is now digested with dilute hydrochloric acid, evaporated to dryness, and this process repeated three times. The residue is heated on the electric plate with strong hydrochloric acid for one hour. Warm water is added and the residue washed, dried upon an ashless filter paper, and ignited in a platinum crucible. It is then cooled, and weighed as "hydrochloric acid insoluble." A slight loss of silica may occur at this stage of the analysis, owing to the presence of fluorides, which the author found to be present in all tissues in the body. The ash still contains some iron and aluminum. The residue is treated with cold hydrofluosilicic acid for twenty-four to forty-eight hours, which separates silicates, leaving the free silica. The residue is washed with warm water upon a small ashless filter paper, dried, and ignited in a platinum crucible. The residue is weighed as silicon dioxide. As a further check the residue in the platinum crucible is treated with hydrofluoric acid, warmed slowly under a hood, ignited, cooled in a desiccator, and weighed, the loss in weight being calculated as silicon dioxide.

Lematte and Kohane[1892] have advised the use of perchloric acid and 1% boric acid to prevent the loss of silica due to fluorides. Where it is desired to obtain the total silica, both free and combined, the ash as obtained above is fused with about four parts of a mixture of potassium and sodium carbonates, digested upon the hot plate with warm water, filtered, and evaporated to dryness with an excess of hydrochloric acid. The dry residue is treated three times in the same manner with hydrochloric acid, pulverizing the white residue each time. The final residue is taken up with dilute hydrochloric acid, and washed with warm water upon a small ashless filter paper until tests for chlorides are negative. The paper is dried, ignited, cooled, weighed, and calculated as silicon dioxide, which can be checked by adding hydrofluoric acid as above. The filtrate after treating with hydrochloric acid can be examined for the presence of other minerals. The filtrate in the fusion method cannot be used for the quantitive analysis of sodium or potassium, as these have been added.

For the colorimetric determination of silica[1893] as the silicomolydate, reference should be made to the papers published by King.

A micro-method has been devised where histological sections mounted on a slide can be ignited in the muffle and ex-

1892. LEMATTE; KOHANE: *Compt. rend. Acad. d. sc.*, 196:575, 1933.
1893. KING, E. J.: *J. Biol. Chem.*, 80:25, 1928; see also *Chem. Abst.*, *J. Am. Chem. Soc.*, 50:2395, 1928. SCHWARTZ, M. C.: *Indust. & Eng. Chem., Anal. Ed.*, 6: No. 5, 364, 1934.

amined for the presence of silica. Examining these under the
polarized light will show the presence of free silica.

METHODS OF COLLECTING DUST

VARIOUS methods have been used in collecting samples.
We formerly used the sugar-tube method, supplanting it
by the Palmer water spray apparatus. The Bureau of Mines
at the Pittsburgh Station[1894] made comparative tests of the

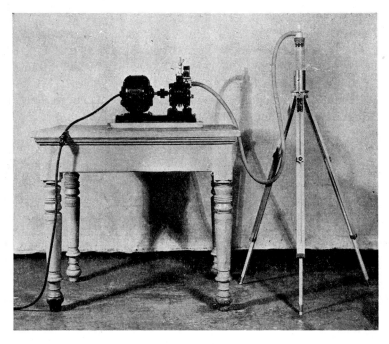

FIG. 29
The Impinger

various methods in use and a new instrument, the Impinger,
was evolved (Fig. 29). "In this instrument, the air to be sam-
pled is drawn through a glass tube and impinged at a high
velocity into a graduated tube containing water. The dust is
momentarily arrested, wetted by the collecting fluid, and in
this manner trapped. The apparatus possesses an efficiency of
94% to 97.5% when sampling finely divided silica dust suspension at the rate of one cubic foot per minute." A portion of the

1894. U. S. Pub. Health Reports, 47:654, March 18, 1932.

collecting fluid is removed to a Sedgwick Rafter Counting Cell for microscopic count to determine the number of particles present. An eyepiece micrometer known as a "Whipple Disk" is placed in the eyepiece of the microscope in making the counts. The great objection to this form of apparatus is the weight, as one person cannot carry both parts of the apparatus and tripod. Collecting the dust in this manner gives the chemist an opportunity to weigh the amount of dust collected to determine the amount of organic matter, inorganic matter, how much dust is is in the form of silicates, and how much is free silica or other minerals, all of which can be determined quantitatively. The nature of the organic matter in the air can also be determined chemically and microscopically.

Irwin[1895] states that the micro-incineration method is an aid in the diagnosis of silicosis. Micro-incineration should be regularly included in the microscopic examination of any lung where siliceous fibrosis is suspected, not with any dogmatic predictions in mind but rather as a means towards a more certain diagnosis and a better understanding of the pathogenesis of siliceous fibrosis.[1896]

ASBESTOSIS

ASBESTOSIS is a pneumonokonioses caused by the inhalation of asbestos dust. Although the exact differences between silicosis and asbestosis are not well defined, anatomic and radiologic observations have shown that the appearance of asbestos fibrosis seems to be sufficiently distinctive to avoid confusion, asbestos causing a softer, more delicate, and more diffuse type of fibrotic changes. A full medical and industrial history is emphasized as an aid to differential diagnosis.

Asbestos exists in two chief forms, amphibole, and serpentine. The minerals of amphibole and serpentine are known commercially as asbestos, and are used extensively in the manufacture of incombustible boards, paper, cloth, covering for oil and steam pipes, yarn and rope, and for packing valves.

1895. Irwin, D. A.: *Canad. M. A. J.*, 31:140, 1934.
1896. Dust References: Sartorius, F., and Jotten, K. W.: *Zentralbl. f. Gewerbehyg.*, 21:65, 1934; Tillson, B. F.: *Eng. & Mining J.*, 135:306, 1934; Meiter, E. G.: *Nat. Safety News*, 29:34, 1934; Meller, H. B.: *J. Franklin Inst.*, 217:709, 1934; McNally, W. D., and Sander, O. A.: *J. Am. Insurance*, 11:21, 1934; McNally, W. D., and Sweeney, H., *Nat. Underwriters*, 31:38, 40, 1934.

Most of the asbestos comes from Canada, and is the serpentine N Chrystole. The Canadian asbestos is a hydrated magnesium silicate containing no free silica, but about 44% of combined silica, 43% magnesium, nearly 13% of water, and traces of iron and nickel. The silica is combined chiefly with calcium, magnesium, sodium, iron, aluminum, and potassium. At the present time it is estimated that there are nearly 12,000 individuals employed in the chief asbestos plants in the United States, of whom 10,000 might be exposed to asbestos dust.[1897] Gardner and Cummings,[1898] and Gloyne,[1899] state that the nodular formation found so distinctive of silicosis is not found in asbestosis. While silicosis is predominantly parenchymatous, asbestosis is mainly interstitial. The clinical picture of asbestosis is milder than that of silicosis.[1900] The individual with marked asbestosis will greatly resemble the individual with silicosis. There is the same dyspnea on exertion, the same dry cough, and the more or less indefinite physical signs elicited by the stethoscope. The asbestosis patient is apt to be pasty looking, while the silicotic patient is apt to be very robust in appearance. Lanza states that x-ray appearances are not as clear cut or distinctive as in silicosis and do not lend themselves to ready grouping into progressive stages. "There are less evident pathologic changes in these films and the shadows are finer, more granular and softer than in silicosis. The asbestos film gives the impression of ground glass, and there is no nodulation with the consequent tendency of the nodules to coalesce and give dense opaque somewhat different shadows, occupying the lower third of the lung, except in far advanced cases, when the shadows may occupy the major portion of the lung."

As under silicosis, one must obtain a very careful occupational history. "Associated with exposure to asbestos dust is the occurrence in the sputum and pulmonary tissues of a peculiar formation known as asbestos bodies. These asbestos bodies have been described by a number of observers, and are due apparently to the action of the tissues on the asbestos fiber. It is commonly agreed they are not diagnostic and indicate

1897. LANZA, A. J.: *J.A.M.A.*, 106:368, 1936.
1898. GARDNER, L. U., and CUMMINGS, D. E.: *J. Indust. Hyg.*, 13:65, 1931.
1899. GLOYNE, S. R.: *Tubercle*, 14:445, 1933.
1900. LANZA, A. J., MCCONNELL, W. J., and FEHNEL, J. W.: U. S. Pub. Health Report, 50:1, 1935.

merely that the individual has been exposed to asbestos dust.[1901]

Many of the workers in asbestos have a terminal death of tuberculosis. Such was the case of L. P., aged forty, who died on January 13, 1935, and who had a history of working for fourteen years in an asbestos factory. The postmortem showed that the lung on the right and left sides was bound down by dense adhesions. The left lung contained many small tuberculous cavities. One large cavity was found in the upper lobe. On section the lung showed, in addition to the small cavities, areas of anthracosis, and the peribronchial lymph nodes were moderately enlarged. The tricuspid valves were negative. The aortic valves were slightly calcified. The mitral valve would not admit the small finger, and there were areas of calcification. The myocardium was pale, but firm. Grossly there was no pathology in any of the other organs. Microscopical examination showed a chronic fibrous and caseous tuberculosis of lung and peribronchial lymph node. There were many giant cells, also areas of caseous pneumonia, and fibrous tissue with brownish-black granular pigment, fibrous myocarditis, chronic interstitial changes in the kidney, chronic tuberculosis of the spleen. Anatomic diagnosis showed asbestosis, anthracosis, and silicosis. On chemical examination, the right lung contained 3.72 mg. of silicon dioxide per gm. of dried tissue, and the left lung contained 3.98 mg. per gm. of dried tissue.[1902]

1901. MEREWEATHER, WOOD, W. B., and GLOYNE, S. R.: *Lancet, 2*: 1383, 1934.

1902. Asbestosis References: AMENDOLA, O.: *Morgagni,* 76:16, 1934, *Indust. Bull.,* 13:95, 1934; *Safety Eng.,* 68:74, 1934; BEGER, P. J.: *Deutsche med. Wchnschr.,* 60: 231, 1934; BEGER, P. J.: *Med. Klin.,* 30: 1222, 1258, 1934; ELLMAN, P.: *Brit. J. Radiol.,* 7:281, 1934; MEREWEATHER, E. R. A.: *Tubercle,* 15:69, 1933; 109, 1933; 152, 1934; STEWART, M. J.: *J. Tech. Methods,* 13:70, 1934; WOOD, W. B., and GLOYNE, S. R.: *Lancet,* 2:1383, 1934.

RADIUM

RADIUM in the human body is found, for the most part, evenly distributed throughout the skeleton. Small traces have been found in the viscera, and one case is recorded in which the lungs contained a relatively large amount. All information available indicated that radium in the body of a person who is radioactive is deposited mainly in the bones of the skeleton, and that the amount which occurs in the different bones is approximately proportional to the weight of the bones.

Radium poisoning occurs when a few micrograms of radium, or other alpha-ray emitting radioactive substances, become fixed in the system. Its action lies principally in destroying the blood-producing centers and in weakening the bones. Modes of entrance include those of ingestion by breathing of radioactive substances by watch dial painters, chemists and miners, drinking of radium water nostrums, and intravenous or other forms of injections of radium by physicians. From 60 to 90% of radium taken into the system is eliminated principally in the feces (90%) and in the urine (10%). Some radium is lost in the expired air, none in perspiration. Necrosis of the jaw, osteogenic sarcoma, and regenerative anemia are among the most common symptoms of radium poisoning. Martland[1903] has described several cases of typical aplastic anemia of the regenerative type, while lymphatic leukemia was described by von Jagic.[1904]

Examination of the blood of those using radium-active dial paint shows a polynuclear leucopenia. Alpha rays are much more destructive to human bones than either beta or gamma. Most cases of poisoning by radium which occur in women who work with luminous paint, come from their moistening and pointing the brushes with their lips and tongues. St. George, Gettler, and Muller[1905] were able to detect radioactivity in the body of a dial-painter exhumed five years after death.

An osteitis affecting the bones of the jaws, followed by suppuration, has been reported from the effects of radium. Osteitis of the femur, humerus, and of the cranial bone, has been reported by several investigators.*

1903. MARTLAND, H. S.: *Arch. Path. & Lab. Med.*, 2:465, 1926.
1904. VON JAGIC: *Berl. klin. Wchnschr.*, 48:1220, 1911.
1905. ST. GEORGE, A. V., GETTLER, A. O., and MULLER, R. H.: *Arch. Path.*, 7:397, 1929.
* TELEKY, L: *Wien. Klin. Wchnschr.*, 19, 1937.

If, upon examination of workers in radioactive substances, a polynuclear leucopenia is found, they should be removed immediately from the source of employment, and given iron and liver preparations, and blood transfusion to aid in the formation of new blood.

Female workers using a radioactive luminous paint containing 0.7 to 3.0 mg. of radium per 100 gm. developed symptoms of the disease, one to several years after the beginning of employment. The symptoms were those of general weakness, progressive anemia, and necrosis of the jaw. In fifteen cases death resulted from a secondary infection, leading to general sepsis. The radioactive substances are deposited in the phagocytes of the liver, spleen, and marrow. The expired air when examined with an electroscope shows the presence of radioactive bodies.

Dominici, Petit, and Jaboin[1906] injected into the jugular vein of horses 1 mg. of radium sulphate (insoluble). They found that this salt is eliminated rapidly in the beginning, but the elimination gradually slows down and part of the salt remains fixed in the organism. The radioactivity persists for over six months. The authors state that the radium which remains in circulation gives off an emanation which diffuses into the blood and is transported to the entire organism. It is thus logical that this prolonged diffusion is capable of acting in the entire structure of the tissues so as to modify their physiological function.

Castle, Drinker, and Drinker[1907] described a novel condition affecting five workers who were applying a luminous paint containing radium which caused necrosis of the jaw.

Weil and Lacassagne[1908] observed two men, both of strong constitution who had worked for two or three years with a radioactive substance of the thorium group. Both died with a blood dyscrasia. One patient presented the picture of an aplastic pernicious anemia, the other of a myeloid leukemia.[1909]

1906. DOMINICI, H., PETIT, G., and JABOIN, A.:   *Compt. rend. Acad. d. sc.,* 150:726, 1910.

1907. CASTLE, W. B., DRINKER, KATHERINE R., and DRINKER, CECIL K.:   *J. Indust. Hyg.,* 7:371, 1925.

1908. WEIL, EMILE, and LACASSAGNE, ANTONI: *Bull. Acad. de. méd., Paris,* 93:237, 1925.

1909. References to special phases of radium poison:

LEAKE, J. P.: "Radium Poisoning," *J.A.M.A.,* 98:1077, 1932. And: "Some Unrecognized Dangers in the Use and Handling of Radioactive Substances," *J.A.M.A.,* 85:1769, 1925.

GRANZOW, J.: "Action of Radium on Vital Organs (Heart, Spleen, Liver), on Structure and Function of Female Genitals, and on Offspring," *Arch. f. Gynäk.*, 151:612, 680, 1932.

THOMAS, H. E., and BRUMER, F. H.: "Chronic Poisoning in Rats," *Am. J. Roentgenol.*, 29:641, 662, 1933.

IMBERT, L., and IMBERT, R.: "Generalized Lesions: Experiments on Rats," *Bull. Acad. de méd., Paris.*, 109:229, 236, 1933.

DROSCHL, H.: "Repeated Occurrence of Cancer in Physicians Working with Radium Case," *Ztschr. f. Krebsforsch., Jena.*, 38:274, 1933.

LERICKE, J. R., and FONTAINE, R.: "Ulcerous Radiodermatitis of Sixteen Years Duration Cured by Perlaterial Sympathectomy and Skin Grafts: Case," *Lyon chir.*, 30:107, 1933.

IVES, J. E., KNOWLES, F. L., and BRITTEN, R. R.: "Health Aspects of Radium Dial Painting: Measurements of Radioactivity in Workers," *J. Indust. Hyg.*, 15:433, 1933.

SCHWARTZ, L., MAKEPEACE, F. C., and DEAN, H. T.: "Health Aspects of Radium Dial Painting," *J. Indust. Hyg.*, 15:447, 1933.

CASTANO, C. A., and RICCI, G:. "Clinical Study of Complications of Roentgen and Radium Therapy," *Prensa méd. argent.*, 20:2341, 1933.

VOLTZ, F.: "Intestinal Hemorrhage Following Roentgen and Radium Therapy for Dysmenorrhea: Medicolegal Aspects," *Deutsche Ztschr. f. d. ges. gerichtl. Med.*, 22:221-234, 1933.

FOVEAU DE COURMELLES: "Radiodermatitis," *Rev. de path. comparée*, 33:1395, 1933.

NOVAK, F. V.: "Intoxication by Radium and Radioactive Substances," *Casop. lék. cesk.*, 72:1225, 1933.

STOKLAS, J.: "Radioactivity of Atmosphere as Factor in Development of Mountain Sickness in Joachimstal and Schneeberg," *Deutsche med Wchnschr.*, 59:1199, 1933.

THOMAS, J. M.: "Burns," *Brit. M. J.*, 2:55, 1933.

BLOOMFIELD, J. J., and KNOWLES, R. L.: "Health Aspects of Radium Dial Painting: Occupational Environment," *J. Indust. Hyg.*, 15:368, 1933.

KNOWLES, R. L., BRITTEN, R. H., SCHWARTZ, L., and THOMPSON, R. L.: "Health Aspects of Radium Dial Painting," *J. Indust. Hyg.*, 15:362, 1933.

BILTRIS, R.: "Malignant Tumors in Guinea Pigs after Introduction of Radium," *Bull. Assoc. franç. p l'etude du cancer*, 22:438, 1933.

EVANS. R. D.: "Poisoning: Review of Present Knowledge," *Am. J. Pub. Health*, 23:1017, 1933.

KOELSCH, F.: "Industrial Health Injuries Caused by Radium Energy," *Jahresk. f. ärztl. Fortbild.*, 24:1, 1933.

RATTI, A.: "Lesions Due to Radiation: Clinical Study," *Atti d. Cong. ital. di radiol. med.*, Part 1, 6:1, 1933.

FOVEAU DE COURMELLES: "Radioclasis: Harmful Effects of Radiation," *J. de méd. de Paris*, 53:597, 1933.

OSGOOD, E. E.: "Action of Benzol, Roentgen Rays, and Radium on Blood and Blood-forming Organs," *Ann. Int. Med.*, 6:771, 1932.

AUBERTIN, C.: "Blood Diseases of Radiologists Due to Radium and Roentgen Radiation," *Monde méd., Paris*, 42:555, 1932.

VOLTZ, F.: "Cause and Prevention of Injuries: Memo. to Committee on Hygiene of League of Nations," *Radiol. Rundschau.*, 1:20, 1932.

DAVIS, J. S.: "Burns from Radium," *Tr. South. S. A.*, 44:227, 1931.

NIELSEN, J.: "Chronic Occupational Poisoning: Discussion Based on Case of Leukemia in Radium Worker," *Acta radiol.*, 13:385, 1932.

DHERS, V.: "Professional Dangers," *Rev. d'actinol.*, 8:171, 1932.

BITES AND STINGS

POISONOUS snakes belong to two groups: The colubrine (Colubridae), and the viperine (Viperidae). In dangerous snakes the poison fangs are placed anteriorly, attached to the maxilla, which in the poisonous Colubridae is long and lies horizontally while in the Viperidae it is short and lies vertically. The viperine snakes are characterized by a triangular head and tubular poison fangs, and are the most important of the poisonous snakes in America. The rattlesnake (Crotalus), the copperhead (Ancistrodon contortrix), and the water moccasin (A. piscivorus), are found in all parts of the United States. There are many harmless snakes which resemble the poisonous. The poisonous snakes have black bands bordered by two yellow ones, while the harmless snakes have a yellow band bordered by two black ones. The poisonous coral snakes have transverse rings of black, vermillion, and yellow. When striking the snake must open its jaws widely and bend back the neck, as the fangs are directed backward. The fangs are then brought forward and erected by the sphenopterygoid muscles. The poison fangs are grooved or perforated and connected with the poison glands which resemble the salivary glands and may be nearly an inch in length. When the fangs enter tissue the jaws close and the pressure exerted causes the venom to pour out of the poison glands. The symptoms following the bite vary according to the species of the snake. There is considerable local pain at the point of the bite, the part becoming red and swollen. An extravasation of blood is produced with great rapidity near the point of entrance of the bite. This action is probably due to endotheliolysin, which destroys the endothelial lining of blood vessels. Thirst is intense, and the surface of the body is covered with cold perspiration. There may be nausea, vomiting, and cardiac depression. The poison of the cobra acts much faster than the venom of the vipers. The symptoms produced are similar to those of a glossopharyngeal paralysis. Both venoms cause at first, a feeling of stimulation, then depression. The pulse becomes weaker, the respiration slower, the heart beats for about a minute after failure of respiration.

Treatment: Apply a tight ligature above the site of the bite. Make a deep incision around the fang punctures, apply suction with the mouth and irrigate with a strong solution of potassium permanganate. In the absence of the permanganate solution, empty the powder from a .32 caliber shell and burn the punctured skin with the lighted nitrocellulose or gun powder. This is usually ineffective in the case of the cobra bite because of the time elapsing before treatment is started. It is also ineffective with any other bite after absorption has taken place. Alcohol cannot be considered of value; it may, however, be given as a stimulant. Inject 100 to 200 cc. of antivenin into the area bitten. With the concentrated sera much less may be given. A rattlesnake injects about 225 mg. of venom, the moccasin about 150 mg. and the copperhead about 45 mg. One ampoule of antivenin neutralizes 20 or more mg. of the venom of any American pit viper (rattlesnake, moccasin or copperhead). Each ampoule contains 10 cc. If a physician is not present, the antivenin can be injected into the loose cellular tissue and the patient then taken to the nearest physician. Antitoxins have been prepared against both viperine and colubrine venoms and these are specific; thus a colubrine antivenin will not be of value against a viperine bite. Blood transfusion should be given to correct the anemia. The fatal period is from a few minutes to twelve hours. If more than twenty hours have elapsed, death will occur from exhaustion or infection.

Spider Bites: Ginsburg[1910] reports that since 1935, fifty-four cases of black widow spider (Latrodectus mactans, black, with one or more red spots on the dorsal abdomen) poisoning have been treated in the General Hospital of Fresno County, California, making a total of ninety-six cases treated with no fatalities. Acute symptoms set in within one-half to two hours. There is increasing pain and muscular spasm, leading to a picture simulating an acute abdominal condition, with rigidity, fever, leukocytosis, and even nausea and vomiting. The presence of muscle spasms in the extremities, the increased blood pressure and spinal fluid pressure, the absence of true tenderness in the painfully contracted muscles, and the profuse perspiration aid in the differential diagnosis. Such exceptional manifestations as shock or circulatory collapse, local or generalized skin eruptions, edema or necrosis, and residual nerve lesions, although occasionally reported, are not commonly encountered and should not be stressed in the description of the usual case.[1911]

1910. GINSBURG, H. M.: *California & West. Med.,* 46:361, 1937.
1911. BOGEN, E., LOOMIS, R. N.: *Calif. & West. Med.,* 45:31, 1936.

The treatment should be confined to a simple antiseptic application. Relief of pain may be secured by the use of hydrotherapy, by spinal puncture, by the intravenous injection of 20 cc. of a 10% solution of magnesium sulphate, and the intravenous injection of 10 cc. of a 10% solution of calcium gluconate. The above authors believe that calcium gluconate is much more effective than the use of opiates as recommended by Kobert.[1912]

Mechanical measures for the destruction of the spider are most generally advised. The broom, fly swatter, or a folded newspaper may be used to kill it. The spider should be destroyed by burning or other means, as the sac may contain hundreds of spiderlings. Bogen and Loomis recommend the use of naphthalene, the commercial moth-ball material, for the fumigation of small boxes and chests; for large completely sealable chambers fumigation with sulphur dioxide from sulphur candles. The poison of the spider contains toxalbumin. There are no special tests identifying this poison.

Scorpion bites may have a very serious effect in children. The bite of the Butus quinquestriatus is practically 50% fatal.

The venom of bees is ejected through the sting which is at the end of the abdomen. The venom contains formic acid and neurotoxin. The sting should be removed from the bite with a scalpel or forceps and the wound bathed with alcohol or ammonia. If the bite is on the nose or near the eye, caution should be used in bathing with these agents. Hot boric acid compresses can be applied to reduce the swelling. Hansen[1913] reported a case of death in an adult, from a single sting on the leg.

Certain fish of the genus Muraena have well developed teeth close to a poison sac which excretes a venom introducing it into the wound made by the bite. The sting-rays (Trygonidae) have a barbed spine which is connected with a poison apparatus. The Trachinus draco and the Scorpaena scropha are poisonous fish which have a grooved spine passing through each of its gill covers which is connected with a poison gland.[1914] Following an injection of the venom from these fish

1912. KOBERT, R.: Kompendium der Toxikologie, 194, 1912.

1913. HANSEN: Ungesk. f. laeger, September 20, 1921.

1914. STITT: Practical Bacteriology, Blood Work Parasitology, 535, 1923.

"a sensation of suffocation follows and the victim may become delirious. At times collapse and death result."

Certain eels (Muraena) have "ichthyotoxin" in their blood which acts in a manner similar to snake poison. When the eel serum is injected under the skin of a dog, edema and extravasation of blood appear. With large amounts of the poison the tissue becomes gangrenous or an ulcer may form.

The Physalia, or man-of-war, is found in the water and along some of our southern beaches, especially Florida. Its purple crested bladder may distend to four inches in diameter and its long locomotive tentacles stretch out thirty feet long. The stings of man-of-war are painful, but leave with hot applications of boric acid.

WAX

HALOWAX is a trade name for a compound composed of chlorinated naphthalene combined with chlorinated substitution products, waxes, bitumens and synthetic resins. These products are used among manufacturers of electrical insulation and in the radio industry for condensers.

Kronenberg,[1915] in a personal communication, states that the Illinois Department of Health, Division of Industrial Hygiene, has contacted a plant in this kind of manufacture where nineteen females were sufferers of a dermatitis. In two other plants contacted, three additional cases were reported. This group of cases arose in an environment in which the chlorinated napthalene products were used in a molten state to impregnate condensers and for "flashing" the condensers. The principal complaint was the skin eruption, chiefly located about the forehead, face, back and buttocks. Two of the cases showed similar lesions of both thighs. The skin lesion was characteristic of an acne-like eruption. There were also demonstrable large blackheads and small cysts of the skin. Three of the cases complained of constipation and gastric discomfort. They described it as "feeling gassy and heartburn." The icterus index on one of the cases was 5.0, and on another 5.6. No evidence of jaundice was recorded.

The solid chlorinated naphthalene products, when held in a molten state, produce vapors and it is these vapors that must be controlled.

The present opinion is that inhalation plays the chief role in causing intoxication.

Experiments at the present stage, October 2, 1937, indicate a sharp increase in toxicity when the chlorination of naphthalene exceeds 53% chlorine. The penta and hexa chloronapththalenes (62.6% chlorine) have been shown to produce a persistent degree of liver damage over a period of time. A temporary safe limit of concentration in the air of one milligram per cubic meter has been suggested.

Better ventilation, and an adequate personal protection of the worker which includes shower and bathing facilities and daily garment change, have been urged by Kronenberg.

1915. KRONENBERG, M. H., Chief of Division and Industrial Medical Supervisor, Department of Health, Division of Industrial Hygiene.

INDEX